INSTRUCTOR RESOURCES FOR NURSING EXCELLENCE

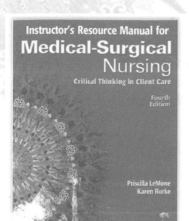

Instructor's Resource Manual for
Medical-Surgical
Nursing
Critical Thinking in Client Care

Fourth Edition

Priscilla LeMone
Karen Burke

Instructor's Resource Manual
ISBN: 0-13-198572-8
This manual helps faculty plan and manage the medical-surgical nursing course. It includes a brand new "Strategies for Success" module which discusses Learning Theories, Planning for Instruction, How to Use Effective Pedagogies, Assessing Learning, and more!
Presented in an easy-to-use tabular format, the manual includes
- detailed lecture notes organized by learning objectives
- Suggestions for Classroom Activities
- Suggestions for Clinical Activities
- Test Item File with comprehensive rationales

Instructor's Resource DVD-ROM
ISBN: 0-13-198569-8
This DVD-ROM includes all the textbook resources that instructors need to teach medical-surgical nursing courses.

- Comprehensive **PowerPoint** presentations that integrate lecture slides, images, animations or videos, and other resources into a single file
- **Classroom Response System** questions set in PowerPoint slides (Ask your Prentice Hall representative for more information about hardware to enhance your presentation)
- Complete **Image Gallery** in PowerPoint
- **TestGen** Test Item Files with questions in all NCLEX-RN® formats, including questions mapped to the chapter learning objectives and the clinical competencies
- Link to the **Prentice Hall Instructor's Resource Center** for additional resources
  Alternate CD-ROM versions are available to faculty who cannot use the DVD-ROM version.
  ISBN: 0-13-235058-0

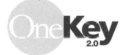

Online Course Management Systems

For Students	For Instructors
Exam Review Questions	Test Item Files
Case Studies	PowerPoint Presentations
Media Gallery Resources	Discussion Board
MediaLinks	Class Announcements
Email Communication	

For a Preview, go to:

http://cms.prenhall.com/webct/ index.html

http//cms.prenhall.com/ blackboard/index.html

Student Assessment…Real Nursing Skills…Remediation…The path to student success and nursing excellence!

An easy-to-use adaptive online tool that allows instructors and students to measure performance and adapt course content without investing additional time or resources! Nursing instructors today need to

PRENTICE HALL
mynursinglab™
Nursing Excellence for the Next Generation.

measure student competence and understanding of nursing concepts as they progress through the curriculum. *MyNursingLab* saves instructors time by providing quality feedback and ongoing individualized assessments for students, and an easy to use method to organize and adapt course materials including assignable homework. *MyNursingLab* is a user-friendly site giving students the opportunity to test themselves on key concepts and skills. Students can track their own progress through the course and use their customized study plan activities to remediate and help them achieve success in the classroom, in clinicals, and ultimately on the NCLEX-RN®.
To take a tour and see the power of *MyNursingLab*, go to **www.prenhall.com/nursing**.

Ask your Prentice Hall Representative about package options for your curriculum.

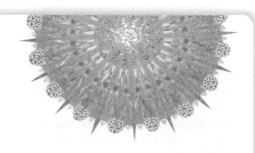

NURSING EXCELLENCE STARTS HERE

Dear Future Nurse,

We wrote this fourth edition of *Medical-Surgical Nursing: Critical Thinking in Client Care* to provide you with the knowledge and the skills you need to care for adult clients and to help you achieve nursing excellence when you enter practice.

As you have discovered in school, nursing students are expected to build upon a foundation of knowledge from basic sciences, social sciences, nursing fundamentals, and nursing experience. In this course, you will develop the skills to synthesize and analyze critically your knowledge to build your clinical competence and achieve that nursing excellence.

With this in mind, we developed a simple-to-complex presentation of material that helps build your skills as you learn about medical-surgical nursing: skills for the classroom, skills for clinical, skills for success on the NCLEX-RN® exam, and skills for your future as a professional nurse.

Here's how your textbook will help you achieve nursing excellence:

1. **Build upon your foundational knowledge** by reading your textbook and using its resources to help you learn the material and prepare for class.
2. **Hone your clinical skills** using the helpful information provided in textbook boxes and applications on the Prentice Hall Nursing MediaLink DVD-ROM and Companion Website.
3. **Prepare for NCLEX-RN® success** with the questions at the end of each book chapter, on the student DVD-ROM, and the Companion Website at **www.prenhall.com/lemone**.
4. **Build Clinical Competence** using our new end-of-unit review that helps you synthesize and apply the concepts you learned from all the chapters in a body system unit.

As you begin your medical-surgical nursing course, we wish you the best of luck, and we encourage you to contact us at **NursingExcellence@prenhall.com** to let us know what you think of our book and its resources.

We appreciate you using our book!

Sincerely,

Priscilla LeMone

Karen Burke

HOW YOUR BOOK IS ORGANIZED

PART I   **MEDICAL-SURGICAL NURSING PRACTICE**

Unit 1   Dimensions of Medical-Surgical Nursing   3
- 1   Medical-Surgical Nursing   4
- 2   Health and Illness in the Adult Client   18
- 3   Community-Based and Home Care of the Adult Client   35

Unit 2   Alterations in Patterns of Health   52
- 4   Nursing Care of Clients Having Surgery   53
- 5   Nursing Care of Clients Experiencing Loss, Grief, and Death   84
- 6   Nursing Care of Clients with Problems of Substance Abuse   101
- 7   Nursing Care of Clients Experiencing Disasters   125

Unit 3   Pathophysiology and Patterns of Health   146
- 8   Genetic Implications of Adult Health Nursing   147
- 9   Nursing Care of Clients Experiencing Pain   169
- 10   Nursing Care of Clients with Altered Fluid, Electrolyte, and Acid-Base Balance   194
- 11   Nursing Care of Clients Experiencing Trauma and Shock   254
- 12   Nursing Care of Clients with Infections   286
- 13   Nursing Care of Clients with Altered Immunity   328
- 14   Nursing Care of Clients with Cancer   368

PART II   **NUTRITIONAL-METABOLIC PATTERNS**

Unit 4   Responses to Altered Integumentary Structure and Function   421
- 15   Assessing Clients with Integumentary Disorders   422
- 16   Nursing Care of Clients with Integumentary Disorders   439
- 17   Nursing Care of Clients with Burns   486

Unit 5   Responses to Altered Endocrine Function   516
- 18   Assessing Clients with Endocrine Disorders   517
- 19   Nursing Care of Clients with Endocrine Disorders   533
- 20   Nursing Care of Clients with Diabetes Mellitus   562

Unit 6   Responses to Altered Nutrition   603
- 21   Assessing Clients with Nutritional and Gastrointestinal Disorders   604
- 22   Nursing Care of Clients with Nutritional Disorders   629
- 23   Nursing Care of Clients with Upper Gastrointestinal Disorders   655
- 24   Nursing Care of Clients with Gallbladder, Liver, and Pancreatic Disorders   696

PART III   **ELIMINATION PATTERNS**

Unit 7   Responses to Altered Bowel Elimination   740
- 25   Assessing Clients with Bowel Elimination Disorders   741
- 26   Nursing Care of Clients with Bowel Disorders   753

Unit 8   Responses to Altered Urinary Elimination   827
- 27   Assessing Clients with Urinary Elimination Disorders   828
- 28   Nursing Care of Clients with Urinary Tract Disorders   845
- 29   Nursing Care of Clients with Kidney Disorders   882

PART IV   **ACTIVITY-EXERCISE PATTERNS**

Unit 9   Responses to Altered Cardiac Function   934
- 30   Assessing Clients with Cardiac Disorders   935
- 31   Nursing Care of Clients with Coronary Heart Disease   957
- 32   Nursing Care of Clients with Cardiac Disorders   1021

Unit 10   Responses to Altered Peripheral Tissue Perfusion   1074
- 33   Assessing Clients with Hematologic, Peripheral Vascular, and Lymphatic Disorders   1075
- 34   Nursing Care of Clients with Hematologic Disorders   1101
- 35   Nursing Care of Clients with Peripheral Vascular Disorders   1153

Unit 11   Responses to Altered Respiratory Function   1208
- 36   Assessing Clients with Respiratory Disorders   1209
- 37   Nursing Care of Clients with Upper Respiratory Disorders   1228
- 38   Nursing Care of Clients with Ventilation Disorders   1265
- 39   Nursing Care of Clients with Gas Exchange Disorders   1320

Unit 12   Responses to Altered Musculoskeletal Function   1378
- 40   Assessing Clients with Musculoskeletal Disorders   1379
- 41   Nursing Care of Clients with Musculoskeletal Trauma   1398
- 42   Nursing Care of Clients with Musculoskeletal Disorders   1432

PART V   **COGNITIVE-PERCEPTUAL PATTERNS**

Unit 13   Responses to Altered Neurologic Function   1502
- 43   Assessing Clients with Neurologic Disorders   1503
- 44   Nursing Care of Clients with Intracranial Disorders   1527
- 45   Nursing Care of Clients with Cerebrovascular and Spinal Cord Disorders   1578
- 46   Nursing Care of Clients with Neurologic Disorders   1616

Unit 14   Responses to Altered Visual and Auditory Function   1668
- 47   Assessing Clients with Eye and Ear Disorders   1669
- 48   Nursing Care of Clients with Eye and Ear Disorders   1691

PART VI   **SEXUALITY-REPRODUCTIVE PATTERNS**

Unit 15   Responses to Altered Reproductive Function   1742
- 49   Assessing Clients with Reproductive System and Breast Disorders   1743
- 50   Nursing Care of Men with Reproductive System and Breast Disorders   1767
- 51   Nursing Care of Women with Reproductive System and Breast Disorders   1793
- 52   Nursing Care of Clients with Sexually Transmitted Infections   1836

BUILD YOUR CLINICAL COMPETENCE TO ACHIEVE NURSING EXCELLENCE

1. BUILD UPON YOUR FOUNDATIONAL KNOWLEDGE

Building upon your experience from anatomy, physiology, and fundamentals courses, each body system unit begins with an assessment chapter. Reviewing this chapter gives you the foundation for the nursing care chapters that follow.

ANATOMY AND PHYSIOLOGY REVIEW ▶

The Anatomy and Physiology Review for each body system reviews structures and functions essential for understanding the assessment, pathophysiology, and nursing care that come later.

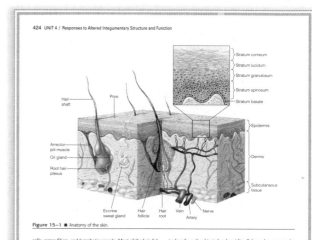

424 UNIT 4 / Responses to Altered Integumentary Structure and Function

Stratum corneum
Stratum lucidum
Stratum granulosum
Stratum spinosum
Stratum basale
Hair shaft
Pore
Epidermis
Arrector pili muscle
Oil gland
Root hair plexus
Dermis
Subcutaneous tissue
Eccrine sweat gland
Hair follicle
Hair root
Vein
Nerve
Artery

Figure 15–1 ■ Anatomy of the skin.

cells, nerve fibers, and lymphatic vessels. Most of the hair follicles, sebaceous glands, and sweat glands are located in the dermis. The dermis consists of a papillary and a reticular layer. The papillary layer contains ridges that indent the overlying epidermis. It also contains capillaries and receptors for pain and touch. The deeper, reticular layer contains blood vessels, sweat and sebaceous glands, deep pressure receptors, and dense bundles of collagen fibers. The regions between these bundles form lines of cleavage in the skin. Surgical incisions parallel to these lines of cleavage heal more easily and with less scarring than incisions or traumatic wounds across cleavage lines.

Superficial Fascia
A layer of subcutaneous tissue called the superficial fascia lies under the dermis. It consists primarily of adipose (fat) tissue and helps the skin adhere to underlying structures.

Glands of the Skin
The skin contains sebaceous (oil) glands, sudoriferous (sweat) glands, and ceruminous glands. Each of these glands has a different function.

Sebaceous glands are found all over the body except on the palms and soles. These glands secrete an oily substance called **sebum**, which usually is ducted into a hair follicle. Sebum softens and lubricates the skin and hair and also decreases wa-

ter loss from the skin in low humidity. Sebum also protects the body from infection by killing bacteria. The secretion of sebum is stimulated by hormones, especially androgens. If a sebaceous gland becomes blocked, a pimple or whitehead appears on the surface of the skin; as the material oxidizes and dries, it forms a blackhead. Acne vulgaris is an inflammation of the sebaceous glands.

There are two types of sweat glands: eccrine and apocrine. Eccrine sweat glands are more numerous on the forehead, palms, and soles. The gland itself is located in the dermis; the duct to the skin rises through the epidermis to open in a pore at the surface. Sweat, the secretion of the eccrine glands, is composed mostly of water but also contains sodium, antibodies, small amounts of metabolic wastes, lactic acid, and vitamin C. The production of sweat is regulated by the sympathetic nervous system and serves to maintain normal body temperature. Sweating also occurs in response to emotions.

Most apocrine sweat glands are located in the axillary, anal, and genital areas. The secretions from apocrine glands are similar to those of sweat glands, but they also contain fatty acids and proteins. Apocrine glands are a remnant of sexual scent glands. Ceruminous glands are modified apocrine sweat glands. Located in the skin of the external ear canal, they secrete yellow-brown waxy cerumen. This substance provides a sticky trap for foreign materials.

GENETIC CONSIDERATIONS
Neurologic Disorders

- In all types of spinocerebellar ataxia, there is degeneration of the spinal cord and cerebellum, resulting in loss of muscular coordination and spasticity.
- One recently confirmed risk factor for Parkinson disease is a positive family history of the disease. This neurodegenerative disease affects more than half a million people, manifested by tremor, muscular stiffness, and difficulty with balance and walking.
- Although multiple sclerosis (MS) is not directly inherited, genetic factors may influence a predisposition to MS within families as well as the severity and course of the disease.
- Narcolepsy, a sleep disorder, does have a familial connection.
- Huntington disease is an inherited degenerative disorder that leads to dementia. It currently affects approximately 30,000 Americans, with an additional 150,000 at risk for inheriting the disease from their parents.
- Fredreich's ataxia is a rare inherited disease that causes a progressive loss of voluntary muscle coordination and enlargement of the heart.
- Essential tremor, as a primary disorder, affects as many as 3 to 4 million people. In more than half of cases, essential tremor is inherited as an autosomal dominant trait, meaning that children of an individual with the disease have a 50% chance of also developing the disorder.
- Epilepsy is one of the most common neurological diseases, characterized by abnormal cell firing in the brain that causes recurring seizures. Recent evidence suggests that there may be a genetic predisposition in up to 70% of cases.
- Charcot-Marie-Tooth syndrome is the most common inherited peripheral neuropathy in the world, characterized by a slowly progressive degeneration of the muscles of the foot, lower leg, hand, and forearm.
- Alzheimer's disease (AD) is a leading cause of death in adults, increasing in incidence with age and more common in women. AD tends to run in families, with mutations in 4 genes believed to be responsible for the disease.
- Amyotrophic lateral sclerosis (ALS) is a neurologic disease that causes progressive degeneration of motor neurons in the brain and spinal cord, resulting in paralysis and death. Chromosome abnormalities have been linked to familial ALS.
- Although Tay-Sachs disease is most often considered a disease of children, there is a chronic adult form that causes neuron dysfunction and psychosis.

◀ GENETIC CONSIDERATIONS

This box lists specific genetic issues for each body system that help you incorporate relevant questions when you take a client health history.

◀ DIAGNOSTIC TESTS

This table summarizes key diagnostic tests used for disorders of each body system and the related nursing care.

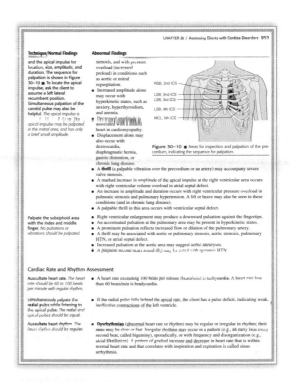

▲ ASSESSMENTS WITH ABNORMAL FINDINGS

Organized in a new, two-column format, the assessment section provides easy-to-follow steps that include normal findings, as well as abnormal findings that might be present.

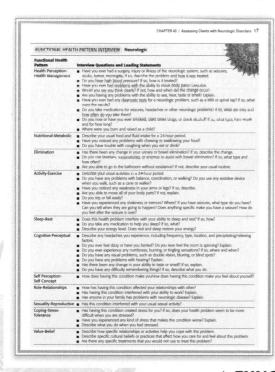

▲ FUNCTIONAL HEALTH PATTERN INTERVIEW

This table provides you with sample assessment questions related to functional health patterns so you can plan your interviews during a client health history and physical assessment.

2. HONE YOUR CLINICAL SKILLS

Use the special application boxes to help prepare for clinical experiences.

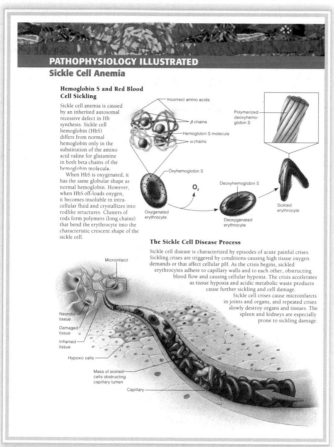

PATHOPHYSIOLOGY ILLUSTRATED

Sickle Cell Anemia

Hemoglobin S and Red Blood Cell Sickling

Sickle cell anemia is caused by an inherited autosomal recessive defect in Hb synthesis. Sickle cell hemoglobin (HbS) differs from normal hemoglobin only in the substitution of the amino acid valine for glutamine in both beta chains of the hemoglobin molecule.

When HbS is oxygenated, it has the same globular shape as normal hemoglobin. However, when HbS off-loads oxygen, it becomes insoluble in intracellular fluid and crystallizes into rodlike structures. Clusters of rods form polymers (long chains) that bend the erythrocyte into the characteristic crescent shape of the sickle cell.

Incorrect amino acids
β chains
Polymerized deoxyhemoglobin S
Hemoglobin S molecule
α chains
Oxyhemoglobin S
O_2
Deoxyhemoglobin S
Oxygenated erythrocyte
Deoxygenated erythrocyte
Sickled erythrocyte

The Sickle Cell Disease Process

Sickle cell disease is characterized by episodes of acute painful crises. Sickling crises are triggered by conditions causing high tissue oxygen demands or that affect cellular pH. As the crisis begins, sickled erythrocytes adhere to capillary walls and to each other, obstructing blood flow and causing cellular hypoxia. The crisis accelerates as tissue hypoxia and acidic metabolic waste products cause further sickling and cell damage.

Sickle cell crises cause microinfarcts in joints and organs, and repeated crises slowly destroy organs and tissues. The spleen and kidneys are especially prone to sickling damage.

Microinfarct
Necrotic tissue
Damaged tissue
Inflamed tissue
Hypoxic cells
Mass of sickled cells obstructing capillary lumen
Capillary

▲ NURSING CARE OF THE OLDER ADULT

This box prepares you with essential guidelines to provide nursing care for older adults you will see in clinical settings.

▲ PATHOPHYSIOLOGY ILLUSTRATED

The 3-D art brings the concepts to life—visual illustrations of disease processes help you better understand pathophysiology and its impact on the body.

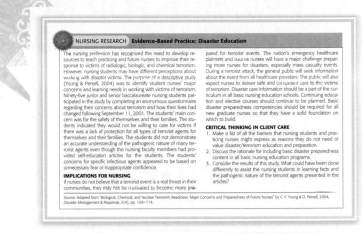

▲ NURSING RESEARCH BOXES

These evidence-based practice boxes focus on research into specific topics and relate it to current nursing care. Critical thinking questions show you how research can be applied to nursing care.

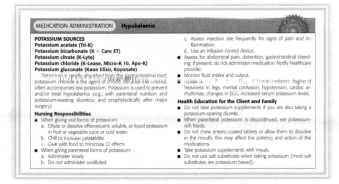

▲ MEDICATION ADMINISTRATION BOXES

This box prepares you to administer the most common drugs you will encounter in treating disorders within the chapter, as well as related nursing responsibilities and client-family teaching.

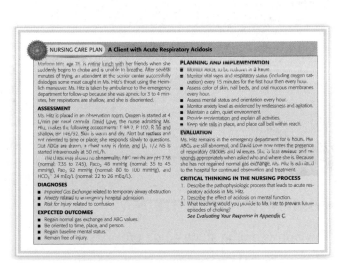

▲ NURSING CARE PLANS

Learn how to construct nursing care plans by studying the case study model presented in your book, including assessment, diagnoses, expected outcomes, planning and implementation, and evaluation. Critical thinking questions give you more opportunity to apply what you learn.

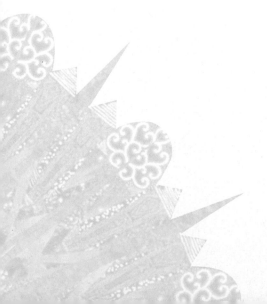

3. PREPARE FOR NCLEX-RN® SUCCESS

Take advantage of multiple opportunities to prepare yourself for the NCLEX-RN®. We offer unique sets of test questions at the end-of-chapter, on the student Prentice Hall Nursing MediaLink DVD-ROM, on your textbook Companion Website, and in the Study Guide.

TEST YOURSELF NCLEX-RN® REVIEW ▶

At the end of each chapter, test your application and analysis of the chapter concepts within NCLEX®-style review questions. Answers and comprehensive rationales appear in Appendix C.

TEST YOURSELF NCLEX-RN® REVIEW

1 The key difference between emergencies and disasters is that:
1. emergencies are controlled.
2. disasters result from man made errors.
3. emergencies can typically be handled by available emergency services.
4. disasters typically involve the local emergency services and no other agencies.

2 Which of the following is NOT true regarding nurses' responsibilities in disaster preparedness?
1. Nurses have a responsibility to the public to be knowledgeable about disaster preparedness and response.
2. Nurses must have a personal and family plan as a part of their disaster preparedness and response plan.
3. Nurses will be the leaders in the incident command structure set up at the site of the disaster.
4. Nurses who are prepared for disasters will be better able to help themselves, their families, and their communities in a

5 Which of th
equipment
1. PPE pro
2. Eye, fac
PPE pro
3. PPE sh
and/or
4. Healthc
strict ha

6 Which of th
1. Decont
downw
2. Decont
the dis
3. Decont
hospita
4. Decont

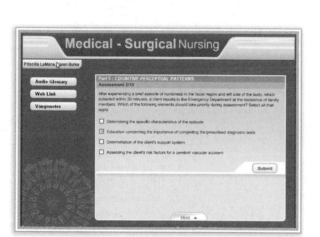

◀ PRENTICE HALL NURSING MEDIALINK DVD-ROM

Packaged with your textbook, the Student DVD-ROM provides you with additional practice NCLEX®-style tests and feedback with rationales for right and wrong answers. Each question is coded to the step in the Nursing Process, Cognitive Level, and the Category of Client Need according to the NCLEX-RN® Test Plan.

A CD-ROM version of this student resource can be purchased online at www.MyPearsonStore.com using ISBN: 0-13-235057-2

COMPANION WEBSITE ▶

This bonus online study guide provides even more NCLEX-RN® review questions with instant feedback, and rationales for all answers help you learn the material and prepare you for course exams.

www.prenhall.com/lemone

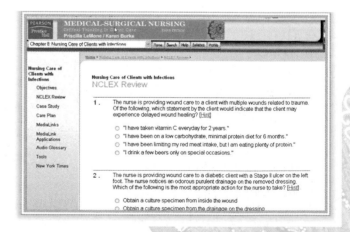

STUDENT STUDY GUIDE

ISBN: 0-13-198570-1

Using your Study Guide, you can test yourself with NCLEX-RN® review questions in each chapter.

4. BUILD YOUR CLINICAL COMPETENCE

Finally, to achieve nursing excellence, you need to synthesize and apply the concepts you learned from all the chapters in a body system unit. At the end of each unit in your textbook, Building Clinical Competence gives you the opportunity to pull the unit material together by practicing skills needed to care for multiple patients simultaneously. This activity has three parts:

FUNCTIONAL HEALTH PATTERN ACTIVITY ▶

Through this activity you will learn more about how disorders discussed in the unit affect clients' functional health status. The Functional Health Pattern is further defined, priority nursing diagnosis are identified, and critical thinking questions allow you to apply your learning.

CLINICAL SCENARIO ▶

Each clinical scenario presents you with multiple clients. The critical thinking questions ask you to set priorities while managing multiple clients, preparing you for NCLEX® questions that test prioritization and safe nursing care. To be successful, you need to apply not only knowledge from across the unit but also principles related to setting priorities and maintaining patient safety.

CASE STUDY WITH CONCEPT MAP ▶

Read the Case Study and review the Concept Map that diagrams the priority diagnosis. Go to the student DVD-ROM and use the concept mapping software to practice organizing and representing a priority nursing diagnosis in a concept map that you build on your own.

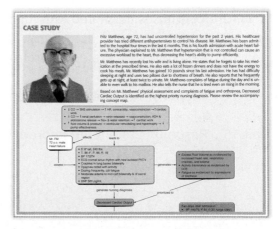

On the Next Page, *you will find a list of all the* **Building Clinical Competence** *activities and where to find them in your textbook.*

BUILDING CLINICAL COMPETENCE

Use the Building Clinical Competence features to review for unit exams in your course.

Unit 1	Dimensions of Medical-Surgical Nursing	Pages 49-51
Unit 2	Alterations in Patterns of Health	Pages 143-145
Unit 3	Pathophysiology and Patterns of Health	Pages 416-418
Unit 4	Responses to Altered Integumentary Structure and Function	Pages 513-515
Unit 5	Responses to Altered Endocrine Function	Pages 600-602
Unit 6	Responses to Altered Nutrition	Pages 735-737
Unit 7	Responses to Altered Bowel Elimination	Pages 824-826
Unit 8	Responses to Altered Urinary Elimination	Pages 929-931
Unit 9	Responses to Altered Cardiac Function	Pages 1071-1073
Unit 10	Responses to Altered Peripheral Tissue Perfusion	Pages 1205-1207
Unit 11	Responses to Altered Respiratory Function	Pages 1375-1377
Unit 12	Responses to Altered Musculoskeletal Function	Pages 1497-1499
Unit 13	Responses to Altered Neurologic Function	Pages 1665-1667
Unit 14	Responses to Altered Visual and Auditory Function	Pages 1737-1739
Unit 15	Responses to Altered Reproductive Function	Pages 1854-1856

BUILD YOUR CLINICAL COMPETENCE TO ACHIEVE NURSING EXCELLENCE

Medical-Surgical
Nursing
Critical Thinking
in Client Care

VOLUME TWO
FOURTH EDITION

Priscilla LeMone, RN, DSN, FAAN
Associate Professor Emeritus
Sinclair School of Nursing
University of Missouri Columbia
Columbia, Missouri

Karen Burke, RN, MS
Education Consultant
Oregon State Board of Nursing
Portland, Oregon

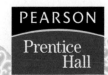

PEARSON

Prentice
Hall

Upper Saddle River, New Jersey 07458

Publisher: Julie Levin Alexander
Publisher's Assistant: Regina Bruno
Editor-in-Chief: Maura Connor
Acquisitions Editor: Pamela Fuller
Editorial Assistant: Melisa Baez
Development Editor: Kim Wyatt
Managing Editor, Development: Marilyn Meserve
Managing Production Editor: Patrick Walsh
Production Liaison: Cathy O'Connell
Production Editor: Lynn Steines, Carlisle Publishers Services
Manufacturing Manager: Ilene Sanford
Design Director and Cover Designer: Mary Siener
Photographer: Patrick Watson
Director of Marketing: Karen Allman
Senior Marketing Manager: Francisco Del Castillo
Marketing Coordinator: Michael Sirinides
Associate Editor: Michael Giacobbe
Media Development Editor: John J. Jordan
New Media Project Manager: Tina Rudowski
Composition: Carlisle Publishing Services, Inc.
Printer/Binder: RR Donnelley Willard
Cover Printer: Phoenix Color
Cover photo: Kaleidoscope: Caribbean Blues, Paula Nadelstern, artist; Karen Bell, photographer

Notice: Care has been taken to confirm the accuracy of information presented in this book. The authors, editors, and the publisher, however, cannot accept any responsibility for errors or omissions or for consequences from application of the information in this book and make no warranty, express or implied, with respect to its contents. The authors and publisher have exerted every effort to ensure that drug selections and dosages set forth in this text are in accord with current recommendations and practice at time of publication. However, in view of ongoing research, changes in government regulations, and the constant flow of information relating to drug therapy and drug reactions, the reader is urged to check the package inserts of all drugs for any change in indications of dosage and for added warnings and precautions. This is particularly important when the recommended agent is a new and/or infrequently employed drug.

Pearson Education Ltd.
Pearson Education Singapore, Pte. Ltd.
Pearson Education Canada, Ltd.
Pearson Education—Japan
Pearson Education Australia PTY, Limited

Pearson Education North Asia Ltd.
Pearson Educación de Mexico, S.A. de C.V.
Pearson Education Malaysia, Pte. Ltd.
Pearson Education, Upper Saddle River, New Jersey

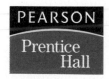

10 9 8 7 6 5 4 3

ISBN-13: 978-0-13-171310-9
ISBN-10: 0-13-171310-8

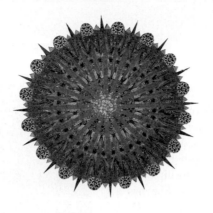

Dedication

I dedicate this book to Oz, who fills my days with sunshine.

Priscilla LeMone

I dedicate this book to Louise, mentor and friend; the woman who sets the standard for always striving to make a difference for the future of nursing.

Karen Burke

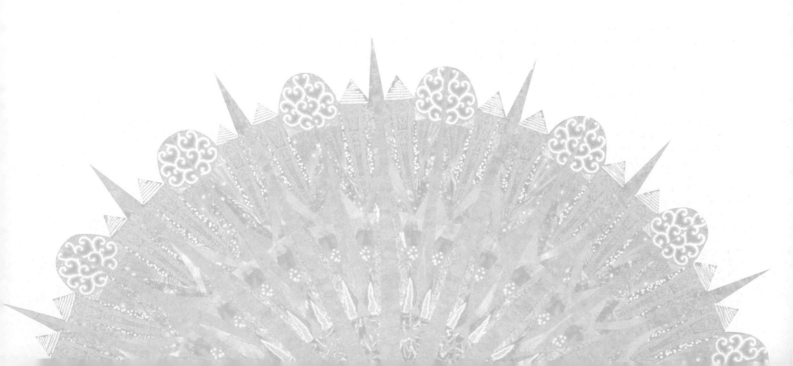

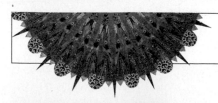

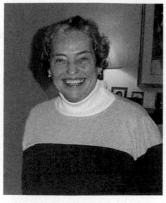

PRISCILLA LEMONE, RN, DSN, FAAN

Priscilla LeMone spent most of her career as a nurse educator, teaching medical-surgical nursing and pathophysiology at all levels from diploma to doctoral students. She has a diploma in nursing from Deaconess College of Nursing (St. Louis, Missouri), baccalaureate and master's degrees from Southeast Missouri State University, and a doctorate in nursing from the University of Alabama–Birmingham. She is retired as an Associate Professor Emeritus, Sinclair School of Nursing, University of Missouri–Columbia, but continues to keep up to date in nursing as an author of nursing textbooks.

Dr. LeMone had numerous awards for scholarship and teaching during her more than 30 years as a nurse educator. She is most honored for receiving the Kemper Fellowship for Teaching Excellence from the University of Missouri–Columbia, the Unique Contribution Award from the North American Nursing Diagnosis Association, and for being selected as a Fellow in the American Academy of Nursing.

She believes that her education gave her solid and everlasting roots in nursing. Her work with students has given her the wings that allow her love of nursing and teaching to continue through the years.

Recently married after 8 years of widowhood, Dr. LeMone lives in Ohio. When she has time, she enjoys traveling, gardening, and reading fiction.

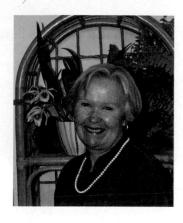

KAREN M. BURKE, RN, MS

Karen Burke has practiced nursing in direct care and as a nurse educator and administrator. She is currently the Education Consultant for the Oregon State Board of Nursing. In this role, she serves as a consultant to new and existing nursing education programs in the state.

Ms. Burke entered nursing with a diploma from Emanuel Hospital School of Nursing in Portland, Oregon, later completing baccalaureate studies at Oregon Health & Science University (OHSU), and a master's degree at the University of Portland. She retired as the Director of Health Occupations at Clatsop Community College in Astoria, Oregon. Ms. Burke currently is a member of the steering committee for the Oregon Consortium for Nursing Education, and is actively involved in the Education Committee of the Oregon Nursing Leadership Council. She is coauthor of another text, *Medical-Surgical Nursing Care* (2nd edition) with Priscilla LeMone, Elaine Mohn-Brown, and Linda Eby.

Ms. Burke strongly values the nursing profession and the importance of providing a strong education in the art and science of nursing for all students preparing to enter the profession. Her diverse experience has prepared her to relate to nursing students at all levels and in diverse programs.

Ms. Burke divides her time between a house in the country with her husband Steve and spoiled cat, and a small condo in the city. She and Steve love to garden, travel, and spend time with their extended family. Ms. Burke enjoys a passion for quilting, accumulating and gradually completing multiple UFOs (unfinished objects).

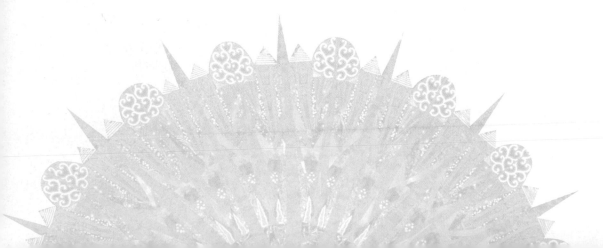

CONTRIBUTORS

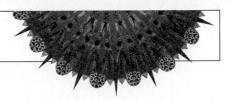

We extend a deep, sincere thanks to our contributors, who gave their time, effort, and expertise so willingly to the development and writing of chapters and resources that help foster our goal of achieving nursing excellence through building your clinical competence.

TEXTBOOK CONTRIBUTORS

Jane Bostick, PhD, RN
Assistant Professor of Clinical Nursing
University of Missouri–Columbia
Columbia, Missouri
Chapter 6: Nursing Care of Clients with Problems of Substance Abuse

Nancy R. Bowers, MSN, RN, CNS
Associate Professor
University of Cincinnati–Raymond Walters College
Cincinnati, Ohio
Chapter 8: Genetic Implications of Adult Health Nursing

Cheryl DeGraw, MSN, RN, CRNP, CNE
Nursing Instructor
Florence–Darlington Technical College
Florence, South Carolina
End-of-Unit features

Marianne Fasano, MEd, MSN, BSN
Assistant Director of Nursing
Pasco–Hernando Community College
New Port Richey, Florida
Unit Concept Maps

Mei R. Fu, PhD, RN, MS, MA, APRN-BC, BS, BA
Assistant Professor, Course Coordinator
New York University
New York, New York
Chapter 14: Nursing Care of Clients with Cancer

Joanne C. Langan, PhD, RN
Chair, Division of Mental Health, Family, Community, and Systems Nursing
Assistant Professor
Saint Louis University, School of Nursing
St. Louis, Missouri
Chapter 7: Nursing Care of Clients Experiencing Disasters

Elaine Mohn-Brown, EdD, RN
Nursing Professor
Chemeketa Community College
Salem, Oregon
Chapter 17: Nursing Care of Clients with Burns

Helen Sandkuhl, MSN, CEN, TNS, FAEN
Director of Nursing, Emergency Services
Saint Louis University Hospital
St. Louis, Missouri
Chapter 11: Nursing Care of Clients Experiencing Trauma and Shock

Marjorie Whitman, MSN, RN, AOCNS
Nurse Clinician
University of Missouri Hospital
Columbia, Missouri
Chapter 4: Nursing Care of Clients Having Surgery
Chapter 9: Nursing Care of Clients Experiencing Pain
Chapter 12: Nursing Care of Clients with Infections
Chapter 13: Nursing Care of Clients with Altered Immunity
Chapter 19: Nursing Care of Clients with Endocrine Disorders
Chapter 20: Nursing Care of Clients with Diabetes Mellitus

STUDENT AND INSTRUCTIONAL RESOURCE CONTRIBUTORS

Katrina Allen, MSN, RN, CCRN
Nursing Instructor
Faulkner State Community College
Bay Minette, Alabama
Companion Website

Christina Baumer, PhD, RN, CNOR, CHES
Division Chair, Continuing Education
Program Director, Surgical Technology
Lancaster General College of Nursing and Health Sciences
Lancaster, Pennsylvania
Study Guide

Sharon F. Beasley, MSN, RN
Nursing Instructor
Technical College of the Lowcountry
Beaufort, South Carolina
Companion Website
Student DVD-ROM

Michelle Buchman, RN, BSN, BC
Educational Support Services LLC
St. John's Marian Center
Chesterfield, Missouri
Study Guide

Donna L. Bumpus, MSN
Assistant Professor
Lamar University
Beaumont, Texas
Instructor's Resource Manual

Joy Burnard, MSN, RN, CDE
Adjunct Faculty
Point Loma Nazarene University
Bakersfield, California
Companion Website

Barbara M. Carranti, MS, RN, CNS
Instructor, Department of Nursing
Le Moyne College
Syracuse, New York
Companion Website

Kim Cooper, MSN, RN
Nursing Department Chair, Assistant Professor
Ivy Tech Community College of Indiana
Terre Haute, Indiana
Student DVD-ROM

Nina R. Cuttler, MSN, APRN, BC
Nursing Instructor
Central Carolina Technical College
Sumter, South Carolina
Student DVD-ROM

Vera Dauffenbach, EdD, MSN, RN
Associate Professor, Director of the Graduate Program
Bellin College of Nursing
Green Bay, Wisconsin
Companion Website

Katherine H. Dimmock, EdD, MSN, RN, JD
Nursing Dean and Professor
Columbia College of Nursing
Milwaukee, Wisconsin
Companion Website
Student DVD-ROM

Susan A. Erlewine, MSN, RN, CHPN
Assistant Professor
Hocking College School of Nursing
Nelsonville, Ohio
Companion Website

Pamela Fowler, MSN, BSN
Assistant Professor of Nursing
Rogers State University
Claremore, Oklahoma
Instructor's Resource Manual

Polly C. Haigler, PhD, RN, BC
Clinical Associate Professor
University of South Carolina
Columbia, South Carolina
Student DVD-ROM

Michelle Helderman, MSN, RN
Nursing Instructor
Ivy Tech Community College
Terre Haute, Indiana
Companion Website

Amy Herrington, MSN, RN, CEN
Critical Care Staff Development Specialist
University of Kentucky Healthcare
Lexington, Kentucky
Companion Website

Ann Isaacs, MS, APRN, BC
Professor of Nursing
Luzerne County Community College
Nanticoke, Pennsylvania
Companion Website
Student DVD-ROM

Tricia Jenkins, RN, MBA, PhD
Assistant Professor
Florida Atlantic University
Boca Raton, Florida
Instructor's Resource CD-ROM

Cathleen E. Kunkler, MSN, RN, ONC
Instructor, Nurse Education
Corning Community College
Corning, New York
Companion Website

Dawna Martich, MSN, RN
Clinical Trainer
American Healthways
Pittsburgh, Pennsylvania
Instructor's Resource CD-ROM

Mary Ann Siciliano McLaughlin, MSN, RN
Nurse Educator
Hospital of the University of Pennsylvania
Philadelphia, Pennsylvania
Companion Website

Linda Oakley-Clancy, MSN, RN
Assistant Professor
Manatee Community College
Bradenton, Florida
Companion Website

Mary Jean Ricci, MSN, RN
Assistant Professor
Holy Family University
Philadelphia, Pennsylvania
Companion Website

Tami J. Rogers, DVM, MSN, BSN
Professor of Nursing
Valencia Community College
Orlando, Florida
Companion Website
Student DVD-ROM

Christine M. Thomas, MSN, DNSc, RN
Assistant Professor
West Chester University
West Chester, Pennsylvania
Companion Website
Student DVD-ROM

Shellye Vardaman, MSN, RN, BC
Assistant Professor
Troy University
Troy, Alabama
Instructor's Resource CD-ROM

Loretta Wack, MSN, RN
Associate Professor
Blue Ridge Community College
Weyers Cave, Virginia
Companion Website

Julie Will, MSN, RN
Associate Professor
Ivy Tech Community College
Terre Haute, Indiana
Companion Website

Kathleen Wilson, MSN, RN
Nursing Professor
Houston Community College
Houston, Texas
Companion Website
Student DVD-ROM

Charlotte Wisnewski, PhD, RN, BC, CDE
Assistant Professor
University of Texas Medical Branch
Galveston, Texas
Student DVD-ROM

Nancy H. Wright, RN, BS, CNOR
Professor of Nursing
Virginia College
Birmingham, Alabama
Instructor's Resource Manual

Annette Zampelli, MSN, CRNP
Nursing Professor
Pennsylvania State Hershey Medical
Center and School of Nursing
Hershey, Pennsylvania
Companion Website
Instructor's Resource Manual

Dawn Zwick, MSN, RN, CNP
Lecturer, Graduate Program
Kent State University
Kent, Ohio

THANK YOU

Our heartfelt thanks go out to our colleagues from schools of nursing across the country who have given their time generously during the past two years to help us create this exciting new edition of our book. These individuals helped us plan and shape this textbook and resources by reviewing chapters, art, designs, and more. **Medical-Surgical Nursing: Critical Thinking in Client Care,** fourth edition, has reaped the benefit of your collective experience as nurses and teachers, and we have made many improvements due to your efforts, insights, suggestions, objections, encouragement, and inspiration. Among those who gave us their encouragement and comments are the following:

ACADEMIC REVIEWERS

Theresa Adelman, MSN, RN, CEN, TNS,
Methodist College of Nursing

Sheila Alexander, PhD, RN,
University of Pittsburgh

Catherine A. Andrews, PhD, RN,
Edgewood College

Vivian F. Austin, RN, MSN,
Macon State College

Michael Beach, MSN, APRN,
University of Pittsburgh

Deborah Becker, MSN, CRNP, BC,
University of Pennsylvania

Margaret Bellak, MN,
Indiana University of Pennsylvania

Carol Bence, MS, RN,
Indiana Wesleyan University

Alice Blazeck, RN, DNSC,
University of Pittsburgh

Donna Bowles, EdD, MSN, RN,
Indiana University Southeast

Judith E. Breitenbach, MS, RN,
Towson University

Debra J. Brown, PhD, RN, FNP, ANP, BC,
University of North Carolina–Chapel Hill

Michelle Buchman, RN, BSN, BC,
St. John's Marian Center

Donna L. Bumpus, MSN, RN,
Lamar University

Susan E. Caulkins, MSN, APRN, BC,
Central Carolina Technical College

Cynthia L. Dakin, PhD, RN,
Northeastern University

Barbara Ann D'Anna, DSL, MSN, RN, CNOR,
Anne Arundel Community College

Maggie Davis, MSN, RN,
Central Florida Community College

Rosalinda DeLuna, RN, CCRN,
Indiana University Northwest

Linda Denison, APRN, BC,
University of Wisconsin

Wanda Dooley, MSN, APRN, BC, FNP,
Northern Virginia Community College

Phyllis Dubendorf, MSN, RN, CRNP,
University of Pennsylvania

Elizabeth Farren Corbin, PhD, FNP, RN,
Baylor University

Marianne Fasano, Med, MSN, RN, CRNI, CWOCN, PCCN,
Pasco–Hernando Community College

Patricia Fowler, MSN, RNC, CNS,
University of Texas–El Paso

Kathleen W. Free, MSN, RNC, ARNP,
Indiana University Southeast

Arlinda Garner, MS, RN,
College of the Mainland

Janet Goeldner, MSN, RN, AOCN,
University of Cincinnati–Raymond Walters College

Sung Hi Gwak, MSN, CCRN, RN, BC,
Borough of Manhattan Community College

Becky Haglund, MN, RN,
Santa Ana College

Polly Haigler, PhD, RN, BC,
University of South Carolina

Barbara A. Hannah, EdD, MS, CPAN, BS,
University of Oklahoma

Anne Helm, MSN, RN,
Owens Community College

Carolyn Insley, MS, MN, RN, BSN,
Fort Hays State University

Vanessa Johnson, PhD, MS, BSN,
University of Oklahoma

Catherine B. Kaesburg, MSN, RN, CNS,
Illinois State University

Sarah Keeling, MN, RN, BSN,
Georgia Perimeter College

Bonnie Kirkpatrick, MS, RN, CNS,
Ohio State University

Andrea Knesek, MSN, BC,
Macomb Community College

Cheryl Lantz, MS, RN, BSN,
Dickinson State University

Rhonda Lawes, RN, MS,
University of Oklahoma

Catherine Lazo-Miller, MS, RN,
Indiana University Northwest

Jennifer Leisegang, MSN, RN, ARNP,
Whatcom Community College

Christine Linert, MSN, RN, OCN,
Collin County Community College

Kit Mallow, MSN, RN,
Gogebic Community College

Hyacinth Martin, MSED, MA, RN,
Borough of Manhattan Community College

Jill M. Mayo, MSN, RN,
Mississippi College

Ellen McAvoy, MA, RN,
Hillsborough Community College

Arlene McGrory, DNSc, RN,
University of Massachusetts–Lowell

Gail Meagher, MSN, RN,
Odessa College

Ann Merrill, MS, MA, BSN,
University of Oklahoma

Brenda Michel, EdD, MS, RN,
Lincoln Land Community College

Sue Ellen Miller, MSN, RN, CNE,
Forsyth Technical Community College

Jo Mizzi, MBA, RN,
Highline Community College; Bellevue Community College; Overlake Hospital and Medical Center

Elise Muller-Lindgren, RN, MN, CHPN,
Highline Community College

Judy Ogans, MS, RN,
University of Oklahoma

Gina Oliver, PhD, RN,
University of Missouri–Columbia

Wendi Palermo, MSN, RN,
McNeese State University

Karen Peel, MN, CCRN,
University of South Carolina

Rebecca A. Phillips, PhD, RN,
University of Oklahoma

Bill Powell, PhD, RN, FNP,
University of North Carolina–Chapel Hill

Tara McMillan Queen, RN, AA, BSN, MN, ANP-C, GNP,
Mercy School of Nursing

Colleen Quinn, MSN, RN,
Broward Community College

Anita K. Reed, MSN, RN,
St. Elizabeth School of Nursing

Tami J. Rogers, BSN, MSN, DVM,
Valencia Community College

Pamela Johnson Rowsey, PhD, RN,
University of North Carolina–Chapel Hill

Megan Sary, MSN, RN,
Merritt College

Jeannie Short, MSN, RN,
Indiana Wesleyan University

Annette S. Stacy, MSN, RN, AOCN,
Arkansas State University

Judith Stauder, MSN, RN,
Stark State College of Technology

Cecilia Tolson, MSN, CNOR, RN,
Owens Community College

Shirley E. Van Zandt, MSN, MPH, CRNP,
Johns Hopkins University

Benita Walton-Moss, DNS, APRN, BC,
Johns Hopkins University

Antoinette Willsea, MSN, RN,
Piedmont College

Kathleen M. Woodruff, MS, CRNP,
Johns Hopkins University

Annette Zampelli, MSN, CRNP,
Penn State Hershey Medical Center

CLINICAL REVIEWERS

Randall Beaton, PhD, EMT,
University of Washington

Pamela Bilyeu, RN, BSN, CNOR, CURN, ONC,
Saint Vincent Healthcare

William P. Carrick, MSN, BSN,
McLean Hospital; Cab Health and Recovery

Cynthia Christensen, MSN, CVN, ARNP-BC,
Ben Collins D.O.

Cathy Cormier, MN, RN,
Southeastern Louisiana State University

Caroline Kuhlman, MSN, APRN-BC, ACON,
Massachusetts General Hospital

Debra J. Lenhart, MSN, RN,
Oklahoma University

Connie Miller, MSN, FNP-C, CDE, BC-ADM,
Cheyenne Crossroads Clinic

Bonnie Pedraza, MSN, RN, CCRN,
University of Wisconsin–Milwaukee

Joanne Farley Serembus, EdD, RN, CCRN,
Roxborough Memorial Hospital

Colleen Marie Totero, MSN, RN, ANCC, APNP, CCRN,
University of Wisconsin

Denise York, MEd, MS, CNS, RNC,
Columbus State Community College

STUDENT REVIEWERS

Julie Bauder,
Johns Hopkins University School of Nursing

Lorna Benoit,
Essex Community College

Lori Bunalski,
The College of New Jersey

Marla Greco,
Pennsylvania State University

Jessica Kramer,
The College of New Jersey

Kristina Smith,
University of Maryland

Emily Watson,
The College of New Jersey

Melissa Whitty,
The College of New Jersey

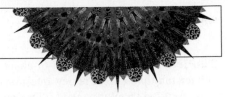

This is a wonderful time to become a nurse! We have all heard about the nursing shortage, especially as it relates to the aging of the population. In fact, the need for new nurses is projected to be at or greater than one million by 2010. While this problem will have to be faced as a society as a whole, it means that your knowledge and skills will be in great demand to meet healthcare needs well into the future. We wrote this book to help you build those skills.

Nursing students are expected to build on knowledge of basic sciences, social sciences, and the fundamentals of nursing to synthesize and critically analyze new skills necessary to ensure clinical competence. We revised and updated the fourth edition of *Medical-Surgical Nursing: Critical Thinking in Client Care* to provide you with the knowledge and skills you need to care for adult clients to promote health, facilitate recovery from illness and injury, and provide support when coping with disability or loss.

Throughout the text, we make every effort to communicate that both nurses and adult clients may be male or female; and that clients require holistic, individualized care regardless of their age or racial, cultural, or socioeconomic background.

OUR GOAL—HELPING YOU ACHIEVE CLINICAL COMPETENCE BY BUILDING ON YOUR SKILLS

Our focus in writing this book is to provide you with knowledge that provides a base for clinical judgment and that can be applied to provide safe, individualized, and competent clinical nursing care. Our easily understood, straightforward style will help you integrate concepts in pathophysiology, pharmacology, and interdisciplinary healthcare interventions into prioritized nursing care. We developed multiple learning strategies to help you succeed—audio, illustrations, teaching tips, and video and animation media. We include boxes, tables, special features and illustrations, as well as synthesis and critical thinking exercises, so you can build your skills for class, for clinical, for NCLEX®, and for practice.

We believe that students learn best within a nursing model of care with consistent organization and understandable text. Starting with the first edition, we have held fast to our vision that this textbook:

- Maintains a strong focus on nursing care as the essential element in learning and doing nursing, regardless of the age of the client or the setting for care.
- Provides a proper balance of physiology, pathophysiology, pharmacology, and interdisciplinary care on which to base safe, competent, and individualized nursing care.
- Emphasizes the nurse's role as an essential member of the interdisciplinary healthcare team.
- Uses functional health patterns and the nursing process as the structure for providing nursing care in today's world by prioritizing nursing diagnoses and interventions specific to altered responses to illness.

- Fosters critical thinking and decision-making skills as the basis for nursing excellence in clinical practice.
- Continues to believe that the person receiving care has not only a personal experience with health and illness, but is also an active participant in maintaining and/or regaining health. Within this philosophy, we regard that person as a client, rather than a patient, in this textbook. The client may be an individual, a family, or a community.

ORGANIZATION

The book is organized into 52 chapters in six major parts, organized by functional health patterns. Each part opens with a concept map illustrating the relationship of each functional health pattern to possible nursing diagnoses. The parts are then divided into units based on alterations in human structure and function. Each unit with a focus on altered health states opens with an assessment chapter. On the accompanying DVD-ROM, students find a comprehensive review of anatomy and physiology complete with animations, three-dimensional structures, and exercises. This draws upon the student's prerequisite knowledge, and serves to reinforce basic principles of anatomy and physiology as applied to physical assessment.

Following the assessment chapter in each unit, the nursing care chapters provide information about major conditions and diseases. Each of these nursing care chapters follows a consistent format, including three key components:

PATHOPHYSIOLOGY The discussion of each *major* illness or condition begins with incidence and prevalence with an overview of pathophysiology, followed by manifestations and complications. *Focus on Cultural Diversity* boxes demonstrate how race, age, and gender affect differences in incidence, prevalence, and mortality. *Pathophysiology Illustrated* art brings physiologic processes to life.

INTERDISCIPLINARY CARE Interdisciplinary care considers treatment of the illness or condition by the healthcare team. The section includes information about specific tests necessary for diagnosis, medications, surgery and treatments, fluid management, dietary management, and complementary and alternative therapies.

NURSING CARE Because illness prevention is critical in health care today, this section begins with health promotion information. We discuss nursing care within a context of priority nursing diagnoses and interventions, with rationales provided for each intervention. Boxes that present information essential to client care are *Nursing Care, Meeting Individualized Needs, Practice Alerts, Medication Administration, Nursing Research,* and *NANDA, NIC, and NOC Linkages*. Last, for each major disorder or condition, we provide a narrative *Nursing Care Plan* that begins with a brief case study, followed by the steps of the nursing process. Critical thinking questions specific to the care plan conclude with a section called *Evaluate Your Response* that provides additional guidance for critical thinking. Suggested guidelines are found in Appendix C.

CHAPTER REVIEW This end-of-chapter section concludes with ten multiple-choice review questions to reinforce comprehension of the chapter content. (The correct answers with rationales are found in Appendix C.) The *EXPLORE MediaLink* feature encourages students to use the DVD-ROM and the Companion Website to apply what they have learned from the textbook through critical thinking and interactive exercises.

What's New in the Fourth Edition

We carefully reviewed the third edition of this book to ensure current content and the necessary knowledge to educate the next generation of nurses. New features of the fourth edition include:

- We divided the chapter objectives into Learning Outcomes and Clinical Competencies. Learning Outcomes show you the knowledge you'll gain, while Clinical Competencies demonstrate how you will apply that knowledge.
- We changed the heading "Collaborative Care" to "Interdisciplinary Care" to better illustrate the role of each member of the healthcare team in providing safe, research-based, client-centered care.
- We added a list of key terms to the beginning of each chapter, and these terms are then printed in bold type and defined at the first occurrence within text. You can learn the correct pronunciation of all terms on the Audio Glossary, found on the textbook's Companion Website.
- We added new chapters and content to make the book absolutely current and clinically relevant.
  - Chapter 7: Nursing Care of Clients Experiencing Disasters
  - Chapter 8: Genetic Implications of Adult Health Nursing
  - Chapter 38: Nursing Care of Clients with Ventilation Disorders
  - Chapter 39: Nursing Care of Clients with Gas Exchange Disorders
- We redesigned the assessment chapters that begin each body system unit to provide students with a more structured, easy-to-use overview for assessment of that body system. The new format includes:
  - A list of needed equipment at the beginning of each chapter.
  - Increased review of normal anatomy and physiology of the system being assessed.
- The assessment section of the chapter is divided as follows:
  - *Diagnostic Tests* This section includes diagnostic test tables and a narrative summary. The tables include the name of the test, the purpose and description of the test, and related nursing care.
  - *Genetic Considerations* This section reminds you of the relevant genetic-based information to gather during the health history.
  - *Health Assessment Interview* This interview not only summarizes and prioritizes the questions to ask, but also provides an interview guide based on functional health patterns.
  - The *Physical Assessment* section is in a new, easy-to-read two-column format that demonstrates how to perform the assessment, with normal and abnormal findings.
- We added a box titled *Fast Facts* to highlight and summarize important data about the prevalence and incidence of selected disorders and other featured content.
- An end-of-unit review for each of the 15 units, called *Building Clinical Competence,* synthesizes what you've learned in the unit and applies the knowledge to specific cases. The feature includes:
  - A functional health pattern expansion that includes further discussion and critical thinking questions;
  - A clinical scenario involving a priority issue reflection piece that synthesizes underlying concepts and includes a variety of questions that allow students to apply different skills; and
  - A case study with concept map that further synthesizes material using the nursing process.

SPECIAL FEATURES

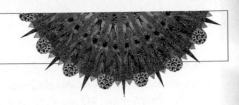

ASSESSMENT OF THE CLIENT

Bowel Assessments 748
Cardiac Assessments 952
Ear and Hearing Assessments 1687
Endocrine Assessments 529
Eye and Vision Assessments 1676
Female Reproductive System Assessments 1761
Hematologic, Peripheral Vascular, and Lymphatic Assessments 1092
Integumentary Assessment 431
Male Reproductive System Assessments 1749
Musculoskeletal Assessments 1391
Neurologic Assessments 1519
Nutritional and Gastrointestinal Assessments 620
Reflex Assessments with Abnormal Findings 1523
Respiratory Assessments 1092
Special Neurologic Assessments with Abnormal Findings 1524
Urinary Assessments 842

BUILDING CLINICAL COMPETENCE

Alterations in Patterns of Health 143
Dimensions of Medical-Surgical Nursing 49
Pathophysiology and Patterns of Health 416
Responses to Altered Bowel Elimination 824
Responses to Altered Cardiac Function 1071
Responses to Altered Endocrine Function 600
Responses to Altered Integumentary Structure and Function 513
Responses to Altered Musculoskeletal Function 1497
Responses to Altered Neurologic Function 1665
Responses to Altered Nutrition 735
Responses to Altered Peripheral Tissue Perfusion 1205
Responses to Altered Reproductive Function 1854
Responses to Altered Respiratory Function 1375
Responses to Altered Urinary Elimination 929
Responses to Altered Visual and Auditory Function 1737

DIAGNOSTIC TESTS

Cardiac Disorders 944
Ear Disorders 1684
Endocrine System 523
Eye Disorders 1674
Female Reproductive System 1756
Gastrointestinal Disorders 615
Hematologic, Peripheral Vascular, and Lymphatic Disorders 1087
Integumentary System 428
Intestinal Disorders 744
Male Reproductive System 1746
Musculoskeletal System 1387
Neurologic System 1514
Respiratory System 1217
Urinary System Disorders 835

FOCUS ON CULTURAL DIVERSITY

BiDil for Treating Heart Failure in African Americans 1035
Cirrhosis 711
Cultural Aspects of Terminal Illness Care 89
Gallstones 697
Heart Disease 958
HIV/AIDS 349
Hypertension in African Americans 1157
Incidence and Mortality for Breast Cancer in Women 1822
Incidence and Prevalence of IBD 782
Inherited Hemolytic Anemias 1106
Lactase Deficiency 798
Obesity 631
Risk and Incidence of Cancer 370
Risk and Incidence of Diabetes Mellitus 564
Risk and Incidence of Prostate Cancer 1783
Risk Factors for Stroke 1580
Risk for Testicular Cancer 1774
Sickle Cell Anemia 1107
Substance Use and Ethnicity 105
Tuberculosis 1281

FUNCTIONAL HEALTH PATTERNS INTERVIEW

Endocrine System 528
Hematologic, Peripheral Vascular, and Lymphatic Systems 1090
Integumentary System 429
Intestinal Tract 747
Musculoskeletal System 1390
Neurologic System 1517
Nutritional Status and Gastrointestinal System 618
Respiratory System 1221
The Cardiac System 951
The Ear 1685
The Eye 1675
The Female Reproductive System 1759
The Male Reproductive System 1748
Urinary System 840

GENETIC CONSIDERATIONS

Adult Polycystic Kidney Disease 884
Alcoholic Fathers and Their Sons 104
Cardiac Disorders 950
Chronic Obstructive Pulmonary Disease 1331
Clients with Marfan Syndrome 1057
Cystic Fibrosis 1340
Ear Disorders 1684
Endocrine System 527
Eye Disorders 1674
Female Reproductive System Disorders 1755
Focus on Hemophilia 1143

Focus on Lymphoma 1129
Hematologic, Peripheral Vascular, and Lymphatic Disorders 1089
Integumentary System 427
Intestinal Tract 746
Male Reproductive System Disorders 1747
Musculoskeletal Disorders 1389
Neurologic Disorders 1513
Nutritional and Gastrointestinal System 614
Primary Lymphedema 1199
Respiratory Disorders 1220
Thoracic Aortic Aneurysms 1172
Urinary System 839

MEDICATION ADMINISTRATION

Acne Medications 459
Acute Renal Failure 905
Addison's Disease 555
Alzheimer's Disease 1621
Antianginal Medications 973
Antibiotic Therapy 319
Anticoagulant Therapy 1189
Antidiarrheal Preparations 756
Antidysrhythmic Drugs 1006
Antifungal Agents 450
Antihypertensive Drugs 1161
Antiplatelet Drugs 976
Antiprotozoal Agents 780
Antiretroviral Nucleoside Analogs 357
Antispasmodics in Spinal Cord Injury 1600
Antituberculosis Drugs 1288
Antiviral Agents 322
Asthma 1327
Blood Transfusion 264
Calcium Salts 230
Cholesterol-Lowering Drugs 967
Chronic Pancreatitis 728
Cirrhosis 717
Colloid Solutions 279
Decongestants and Antihistamines 1230
Diuretics for Fluid Volume Excess 210
Drugs to Treat Anemia 1112
Drugs to Treat Obesity 634
Drugs Used to Prevent and Treat Nausea and Vomiting 673
Drugs Used to Treat GERD, Gastritis, and Peptic Ulcer Disease 665
Drugs Used to Treat Stomatitis 658
Genital Warts 1842
Glaucoma 1710
Gout 1446
Headaches 1545
Heart Failure 1033
Hyperkalemia 225
Hyperthyroidism 538
Hypokalemia 221

Hypothyroidism 544
Immunosuppressive Agents 345
Immunosuppressive Agents for SLE 1474
Increased Intracranial Pressure 1539
Inflammatory Bowel Disease 787
Insulin 573
Intravenous Insulin 586
Laxatives and Cathartics 759
Magnesium Sulfate 235
Multiple Sclerosis 1631
Myasthenia Gravis 1649
Narcotic Analgesics 182
Neurogenic Bladder 871
Neuromuscular Blockers 1356
Nonsteroidal Anti-Inflammatory Drugs 179
Oral Hypoglycemic Agents 578
Osteoporosis 1437
Paget's Disease 1442
Parkinson's Disease 1637
Seizures 1550
Shock 278
Tamoxifen 1825
Therapeutic Baths 441
The Woman with Dysmenorrhea 1802
Topical Burn Medications 501
Urinary Anti-Infectives and Analgesics 850
Vitamin and Mineral Supplements 645

NANDA, NIC, AND NOC

Acute Brain Injury 1562
Acute Myocardial Infarction 994
Acute Renal Failure 913
Altered Bowel Motility 757
Alzheimer's Disease 1625
Amputation 1426
Anemia 1115
Appendicitis or Peritonitis 769
ARDS 1371
Brain Tumor 1575
Breast Cancer 1831
Cancer 411
Cervical Cancer 1815
Chronic Pain 190
Cirrhosis 723
CNS Infection 1568
Colorectal Cancer 809
Compound Fracture 1420
COPD 1340
Cushing's Syndrome 553
DVT 1193
Endometriosis 1812
Experiencing Death Anxiety 97
Experiencing Trauma 268

Eye Infection or Inflammation 1696
Fluid Volume Deficit 209
Gastric Cancer 693
GERD 667
Glaucoma 1713
Having Surgery for Prostate Cancer 1789
Hearing Deficit 1733
Heart Failure 1039
Hemophilia 1146
Herpes Zoster 455
HIV Infection 365
Hypertension 1166
Infection 325
Inflammatory Bowel Disease 795
Influenza 1205
Inner Ear Disorder 1728
Laryngeal Cancer 1262
Leukemia 1128
Lung Cancer 1317
Major Burn 511
Malignant Lymphoma 1136
Malignant Melanoma 471
Malnutrition 650
Multiple Sclerosis 1634
Nasal Trauma 1248
Obesity 640
Osteoarthritis 1457
Osteoporosis 1440
Pancreatitis 731
Parkinson's Disease 1642
Peptic Ulcer Disease 688
Peripheral Vascular Disease 1180
Pneumonia 1276
Potassium Imbalance 223
Pulmonary Embolism 1352
Respiratory Acidosis 250
Respiratory Failure 1365
Rheumatoid Arthritis 1469
SCI 1606
Seizures 1553
Shock 283
Stomatitis 659
Stroke 1592
Substance Abuse Problem 120
The Postoperative Client 80
Tuberculosis 1293
Type 1 DM 596
Urinary Incontinence 879
Viral Hepatitis 710

NURSING CARE OF THE OLDER ADULT

Cardiac Dysrhythmias 996
Chronic Venous Stasis 1196

End-of-Life Checklist 95
Fluid Volume Deficit 203
Heart Failure 1023
Hypertension 1157
Infections 315
Minimizing the Risk for UTI and UI 873
Older Adults with Cancer 371
Peripheral Vascular Disease 1178
Pneumonia 1268
Pressure Ulcer Prevention 474
Renal Failure 914
Tuberculosis 1282
Variations in Assessment Findings—Hypothyroidism 545
Variations in Assessment Findings—Shock 280

NURSING CARE PLAN

A Client Experiencing Loss and Grief 98
A Client Experiencing Withdrawal from Alcohol 119
A Client Having Surgery 81
A Client with a Below-the-Knee Amputation 1425
A Client with a Bladder Tumor 867
A Client with a Brain Tumor 1573
A Client with Acute Appendicitis 768
A Client with Acute Glomerulonephritis 892
A Client with Acute Myelocytic Leukemia 1125
A Client with Acute Myocardial Infarction 991
A Client with Acute Pancreatitis 729
A Client with Acute Renal Failure 912
A Client with Acute Respiratory Acidosis 249
A Client with Acquired Immunity 303
A Client with AD 1622
A Client with Addison's Disease 556
A Client with a Hip Fracture 1418
A Client with Alcoholic Cirrhosis 721
A Client with a Major Burn 507
A Client with a Migraine Headache 1547
A Client with an SCI 1603
A Client with ARDS 1370
A Client with a Seizure Disorder 1552
A Client with a Stroke 1588
A Client with a Subdural Hematoma 1561
A Client with Bacterial Meningitis 1567
A Client with Cancer 403
A Client with Cholelithiasis 702
A Client with Chronic Pain 191
A Client with Colorectal Cancer 807
A Client with COPD 1338
A Client with Coronary Artery Bypass Surgery 983
A Client with Cushing's Syndrome 551
A Client with Cystitis 853
A Client with Deep Venous Thrombosis 1191
A Client with End-Stage Renal Disease 924
A Client with Fluid Volume Excess 212

The Client with Acne   457

Pathophysiology **457**

   INTERDISCIPLINARY CARE   458

   NURSING CARE   459

The Client with Pemphigus Vulgaris   460

   INTERDISCIPLINARY CARE   460

   NURSING CARE   460

The Client with Lichen Planus   460

The Client with Toxic Epidermal Necrolysis   460

Pathophysiology **460**

   INTERDISCIPLINARY CARE   461

The Client with Actinic Keratosis   461

The Client with Nonmelanoma Skin Cancer   461

Incidence **461**, Risk Factors **461**, Pathophysiology **462**

   INTERDISCIPLINARY CARE   463

   NURSING CARE   464

The Client with Malignant Melanoma   465

Incidence **465**, Risk Factors **466**, Pathophysiology **466**

   INTERDISCIPLINARY CARE   467

   NURSING CARE   468

The Client with a Pressure Ulcer   472

Incidence **472**

   INTERDISCIPLINARY CARE   472

   NURSING CARE   473

The Client with Frostbite   476

The Client Undergoing Cutaneous and Plastic Surgery   477

Cutaneous Surgery and Procedures **477**, Plastic Surgery **478**

   NURSING CARE   479

The Client with a Disorder of the Hair   481

Pathophysiology **481**

   INTERDISCIPLINARY CARE   482

   NURSING CARE   482

The Client with a Disorder of the Nails   483

Pathophysiology **483**

   INTERDISCIPLINARY CARE   483

   NURSING CARE   483

CHAPTER 17 Nursing Care of Clients with Burns   **486**

Types of Burn Injury   487

Thermal Burns **487**, Chemical Burns **487**, Electrical Burns **488**, Radiation Burns **488**

Factors Affecting Burn Classification   488

Depth of the Burn **489**, Extent of the Burn **490**

Burn Wound Healing   493

The Client with a Minor Burn   493

Pathophysiology **493**

   INTERDISCIPLINARY CARE   493

   NURSING CARE   493

The Client with a Major Burn   494

Pathophysiology **494**

   INTERDISCIPLINARY CARE   497

   NURSING CARE   505

Unit 5 Responses to Altered Endocrine Function   516

CHAPTER 18 Assessing Clients with Endocrine Disorders   **517**

Pituitary Gland **518**, Thyroid Gland **520**, Parathyroid Glands **520**, Adrenal Glands **520**, Pancreas **521**, Gonads **521**

An Overview of Hormones   521

Assessing Endocrine Function   522

Diagnostic Tests **522**, Genetic Considerations **527**, Health Assessment Interview **527**, Physical Assessment **527**

CHAPTER 19 Nursing Care of Clients with Endocrine Disorders   **533**

The Client with Hyperthyroidism   534

Pathophysiology and Manifestations **534**

   INTERDISCIPLINARY CARE   537

   NURSING CARE   538

The Client with Hypothyroidism   541

Pathophysiology and Manifestations **541**

   INTERDISCIPLINARY CARE   543

   NURSING CARE   543

The Client with Cancer of the Thyroid   546

The Client with Hyperparathyroidism   547

Pathophysiology and Manifestations **547**

   INTERDISCIPLINARY CARE   547

   NURSING CARE   547

The Client with Hypoparathyroidism   548

Pathophysiology and Manifestations **548**

   INTERDISCIPLINARY CARE   548

   NURSING CARE   548

The Client with Hypercortisolism (Cushing's Syndrome)   548

Pathophysiology **549**, Manifestations **549**

   INTERDISCIPLINARY CARE   549

   NURSING CARE   550

The Client with Chronic Adrenocortical Insufficiency (Addison's Disease)   553

Pathophysiology **553**, Manifestations **553**, Addisonian Crisis **553**

   INTERDISCIPLINARY CARE   554

   NURSING CARE   554

The Client with Pheochromocytoma   557

The Client with Disorders of the Anterior Pituitary Gland   557

Pathophysiology and Manifestations **557**

   INTERDISCIPLINARY CARE   558

   NURSING CARE   558

The Client with Disorders of the Posterior Pituitary Gland   558

Pathophysiology and Manifestations **558**

   INTERDISCIPLINARY CARE   559

   NURSING CARE   559

CHAPTER 20 Nursing Care of Clients with Diabetes Mellitus **562**

Incidence and Prevalence 563

Overview of Endocrine Pancreatic Hormones and Glucose Homeostasis 564

Hormones **564**, Blood Glucose Homeostasis **564**

Pathophysiology of Diabetes 564

Type 1 Diabetes **565**, Type 2 Diabetes **566**, Diabetes in the Older Adult **567**

INTERDISCIPLINARY CARE 568

Complications of Diabetes 582

Acute Complications: Alterations in Blood Glucose Levels **582**, Chronic Complications **587**

NURSING CARE 590

Unit 6 Responses to Altered Nutrition 603

CHAPTER 21 Assessing Clients with Nutritional and Gastrointestinal Disorders **604**

Nutrients 605

Carbohydrates **606**, Proteins **606**, Fats (Lipids) **607**, Vitamins **608**, Minerals **608**, The Mouth **610**, The Pharynx **610**, The Esophagus **610**, The Stomach **611**, The Small Intestine **612**, The Accessory Digestive Organs **612**

Metabolism 613

Assessing Nutritional Status and Gastrointestinal Function 613

Diagnostic Tests **614**, Genetic Considerations **614**, Health Assessment Interview **614**, Physical Assessment **619**

CHAPTER 22 Nursing Care of Clients with Nutritional Disorders **629**

The Client with Obesity 630

Incidence and Prevalence **630**, Risk Factors **631**, Overview of Normal Physiology **631**, Pathophysiology **631**

INTERDISCIPLINARY CARE 632

NURSING CARE 638

The Client with Malnutrition 641

Incidence and Prevalence **641**, Pathophysiology **641**

INTERDISCIPLINARY CARE 642

NURSING CARE 648

The Client with an Eating Disorder 650

Anorexia Nervosa **650**, Bulimia Nervosa **650**, Binge-Eating Disorder **651**

INTERDISCIPLINARY CARE 651

NURSING CARE 652

CHAPTER 23 Nursing Care of Clients with Upper Gastrointestinal Disorders **655**

The Client with Stomatitis 656

Pathophysiology and Manifestations **656**

INTERDISCIPLINARY CARE 657

NURSING CARE 658

The Client with Oral Cancer 660

Pathophysiology and Manifestations **660**

INTERDISCIPLINARY CARE 660

NURSING CARE 661

The Client with Gastroesophageal Reflux Disease 663

Pathophysiology **663**, Manifestations **663**

INTERDISCIPLINARY CARE 664

NURSING CARE 666

The Client with Hiatal Hernia 667

The Client with Impaired Esophageal Motility 668

The Client with Esophageal Cancer 669

Manifestations **669**

INTERDISCIPLINARY CARE 669

NURSING CARE 670

The Client with Nausea and Vomiting 671

Pathophysiology **671**

INTERDISCIPLINARY CARE 672

NURSING CARE 672

The Client with Gastrointestinal Bleeding 674

Pathophysiology **674**

INTERDISCIPLINARY CARE 674

NURSING CARE 675

The Client with Gastritis 677

Pathophysiology **677**

INTERDISCIPLINARY CARE 678

NURSING CARE 679

The Client with Peptic Ulcer Disease 680

Risk Factors **680**, Pathophysiology **680**, Manifestations **681**, Complications **681**, Zollinger-Ellison Syndrome **684**

INTERDISCIPLINARY CARE 684

NURSING CARE 685

The Client with Cancer of the Stomach 688

Risk Factors **688**, Pathophysiology **688**, Manifestations **689**

INTERDISCIPLINARY CARE 689

Complications **689**

NURSING CARE 691

CHAPTER 24 Nursing Care of Clients with Gallbladder, Liver, and Pancreatic Disorders **696**

The Client with Gallstones 697

Physiology Review **697**, Pathophysiology and Manifestations **697**

INTERDISCIPLINARY CARE 698

NURSING CARE 701

The Client with Cancer of the Gallbladder 703

The Client with Hepatitis 705

Pathophysiology and Manifestations **705**

INTERDISCIPLINARY CARE 707

NURSING CARE 709

The Client with Cirrhosis 710

Pathophysiology **710**, Manifestations and Complications **711**

INTERDISCIPLINARY CARE 716

NURSING CARE 720

The Client with Cancer of the Liver 723
Pathophysiology **724**, Manifestations **724**
INTERDISCIPLINARY CARE 724
NURSING CARE 724
The Client with Liver Trauma 724
Pathophysiology and Manifestations **725**
INTERDISCIPLINARY CARE 725
NURSING CARE 725
The Client with Liver Abscess 725
Pathophysiology and Manifestations **725**
INTERDISCIPLINARY CARE 725
NURSING CARE 725
The Client with Pancreatitis 726
Physiology Review **726**, Pathophysiology **726**
INTERDISCIPLINARY CARE 727
NURSING CARE 729
The Client with Pancreatic Cancer 731
Pathophysiology and Manifestations **731**
INTERDISCIPLINARY CARE 732

PART **ELIMINATION PATTERNS** **738**

III Unit 7 Responses to Altered Bowel
Elimination 740

CHAPTER 25 **Assessing Clients with Bowel Elimination
Disorders** **741**
The Small Intestine **742**, The Large Intestine **742**
Assessing Bowel Function 743
Diagnostic Tests **743**, Genetic Considerations **745**, Health Assessment
Interview **745**, Physical Assessment **746**

CHAPTER 26 **Nursing Care of Clients with Bowel
Disorders** **753**
The Client with Diarrhea 754
Pathophysiology **754**, Manifestations **754**, Complications **754**
INTERDISCIPLINARY CARE 755
NURSING CARE 755
The Client with Constipation 758
Pathophysiology **758**, Manifestations **758**
INTERDISCIPLINARY CARE 758
NURSING CARE 761
The Client with Irritable Bowel Syndrome 762
Pathophysiology **762**, Manifestations **762**
INTERDISCIPLINARY CARE 762
NURSING CARE 763
The Client with Fecal Incontinence 763
Pathophysiology **764**
INTERDISCIPLINARY CARE 764
NURSING CARE 765
The Client with Appendicitis 766
Pathophysiology **766**, Manifestations **766**, Complications **767**

INTERDISCIPLINARY CARE 767
NURSING CARE 767
The Client with Peritonitis 769
Pathophysiology **769**, Manifestations **769**, Complications **770**
INTERDISCIPLINARY CARE 770
NURSING CARE 771
The Client with Gastroenteritis 773
Pathophysiology **773**, Manifestations **773**, Complications **774**
INTERDISCIPLINARY CARE 776
NURSING CARE 777
The Client with a Protozoal Bowel Infection 777
Pathophysiology and Manifestations **778**
INTERDISCIPLINARY CARE 779
NURSING CARE 779
The Client with a Helminthic Disorder 779
Pathophysiology **779**
INTERDISCIPLINARY CARE 779
NURSING CARE 780
The Client with Inflammatory Bowel Disease 782
Ulcerative Colitis **784**, Crohn's Disease **785**
INTERDISCIPLINARY CARE 786
NURSING CARE 792
The Client with Sprue 796
Pathophysiology **796**
INTERDISCIPLINARY CARE 797
NURSING CARE 797
The Client with Lactase Deficiency 798
Manifestations **798**
INTERDISCIPLINARY CARE 798
NURSING CARE 799
The Client with Short Bowel Syndrome 799
INTERDISCIPLINARY CARE 799
NURSING CARE 799
The Client with Polyps 800
Pathophysiology **800**, Manifestations **801**
INTERDISCIPLINARY CARE 801
NURSING CARE 801
The Client with Colorectal Cancer 801
Pathophysiology **802**, Manifestations **802**, Complications **802**
INTERDISCIPLINARY CARE 802
NURSING CARE 805
The Client with a Hernia 809
Pathophysiology **809**, Manifestations **810**, Complications **810**
INTERDISCIPLINARY CARE 810
NURSING CARE 810
The Client with Intestinal Obstruction 811
Pathophysiology **811**
INTERDISCIPLINARY CARE 812
NURSING CARE 813

The Client with Diverticular Disease   814
  Pathophysiology **815**
    INTERDISCIPLINARY CARE   816
    NURSING CARE   817
The Client with Hemorrhoids   818
  Pathophysiology and Manifestations **818**
    INTERDISCIPLINARY CARE   819
    NURSING CARE   819
The Client with an Anorectal Lesion   820
  Anal Fissure **820**, Anorectal Abscess **820**, Anorectal Fistula **820**,
  Pilonidal Disease **821**
    NURSING CARE   821

Unit 8 Responses to Altered Urinary Elimination   827

CHAPTER 27 Assessing Clients with Urinary
Elimination Disorders   **828**
  The Kidneys **829**, The Ureters **834**, The Urinary Bladder **834**, The
  Urethra **835**
Assessing Urinary System Function   835
  Diagnostic Tests **835**, Genetic Considerations **838**, Health Assessment
  Interview **838**, Physical Assessment **839**

CHAPTER 28 Nursing Care of Clients with Urinary
Tract Disorders   **845**
The Client with a Urinary Tract Infection   846
  Physiology Review **847**, Pathophysiology and
  Manifestations **847**
    INTERDISCIPLINARY CARE   849
    NURSING CARE   851
The Client with Urinary Calculi   855
  Incidence and Risk Factors **855**, Physiology Review **855**,
  Pathophysiology **855**, Manifestations **856**, Complications **857**
    INTERDISCIPLINARY CARE   857
    NURSING CARE   859
The Client with a Urinary Tract Tumor   862
  Incidence and Risk Factors **862**, Pathophysiology **862**,
  Manifestations **863**
    INTERDISCIPLINARY CARE   863
    NURSING CARE   865
The Client with Urinary Retention   869
  Physiology Review **869**, Pathophysiology **869**,
  Manifestations **869**
    INTERDISCIPLINARY CARE   869
    NURSING CARE   869
The Client with Neurogenic Bladder   870
  Pathophysiology **870**
    INTERDISCIPLINARY CARE   870
    NURSING CARE   872
The Client with Urinary Incontinence   872
  Incidence and Prevalence **872**, Pathophysiology **872**
    INTERDISCIPLINARY CARE   873
    NURSING CARE   876

CHAPTER 29 Nursing Care of Clients with Kidney
Disorders   **882**
Age-Related Changes in Kidney Function   883
The Client with a Congenital Kidney Malformation   883
The Client with Polycystic Kidney Disease   884
  Pathophysiology **884**, Manifestations **885**
    INTERDISCIPLINARY CARE   885
    NURSING CARE   885
The Client with a Glomerular Disorder   885
  Physiology Review **885**, Pathophysiology **886**
    INTERDISCIPLINARY CARE   889
    NURSING CARE   891
The Client with a Vascular Kidney Disorder   894
  Hypertension **894**, Renal Artery Occlusion **894**, Renal Vein Occlusion
  895, Renal Artery Stenosis **895**
The Client with Kidney Trauma   895
  Pathophysiology and Manifestations **895**
    INTERDISCIPLINARY CARE   895
    NURSING CARE   896
The Client with a Renal Tumor   896
  Pathophysiology and Manifestations **896**
    INTERDISCIPLINARY CARE   896
    NURSING CARE   897
The Client with Acute Renal Failure   899
  Incidence and Risk Factors **899**, Physiology Review **900**,
  Pathophysiology **900**, Course and Manifestations **902**
    INTERDISCIPLINARY CARE   902
    NURSING CARE   910
The Client with Chronic Renal Failure   913
  Pathophysiology **914**, Manifestations and Complications **915**
    INTERDISCIPLINARY CARE   918
    NURSING CARE   923

PART IV **ACTIVITY AND EXERCISE PATTERNS**   **932**

Unit 9 Responses to Altered Cardiac
Function   934

CHAPTER 30 Assessing Clients with Cardiac Disorders   **935**
  The Pericardium **936**, Layers of the Heart Wall **937**, Chambers and
  Valves of the Heart **937**, Systemic, Pulmonary, and Coronary
  Circulation **938**, The Cardiac Cycle and Cardiac Output **939**, The
  Conduction System of the Heart **941**, The Action Potential **941**
Assessing Cardiac Function   943
  Diagnostic Tests **943**, Genetic Considerations **943**, The Health
  Assessment Interview **943**, Physical Assessment **950**

CHAPTER 31 Nursing Care of Clients with Coronary
Heart Disease   **957**
The Client with Coronary Heart Disease   958
  Incidence and Prevalence **958**, Physiology Review **959**,
  Pathophysiology **959**, Risk Factors **962**
    INTERDISCIPLINARY CARE   965
    NURSING CARE   968

The Client with Angina Pectoris 969

Pathophysiology **969**, Course and Manifestations **970**

INTERDISCIPLINARY CARE 970

NURSING CARE 972

The Client with Acute Coronary Syndrome 974

Pathophysiology **974**, Manifestations **975**

INTERDISCIPLINARY CARE 975

NURSING CARE 979

The Client with Acute Myocardial Infarction 979

Pathophysiology **982**, Manifestations **984**, Complications **985**

INTERDISCIPLINARY CARE 986

NURSING CARE 991

The Client with a Cardiac Dysrhythmia 994

Physiology Review **995**, Pathophysiology **996**

INTERDISCIPLINARY CARE 1004

NURSING CARE 1013

The Client with Sudden Cardiac Death 1015

Pathophysiology **1016**, Manifestations **1016**

INTERDISCIPLINARY CARE 1016

NURSING CARE 1018

CHAPTER 32 Nursing Care of Clients with Cardiac Disorders **1021**

The Client with Heart Failure 1022

Incidence, Prevalence, and Risk Factors **1022**, Physiology Review **1023**, Pathophysiology **1024**, Classifications and Manifestations of Heart Failure **1025**, Complications **1027**

INTERDISCIPLINARY CARE 1027

NURSING CARE 1036

The Client with Pulmonary Edema 1039

Pathophysiology **1040**, Manifestations **1040**

INTERDISCIPLINARY CARE 1040

NURSING CARE 1041

The Client with Rheumatic Fever and Rheumatic Heart Disease 1042

Incidence, Prevalence, and Risk Factors **1042**, Pathophysiology **1042**, Manifestations **1043**

INTERDISCIPLINARY CARE 1043

NURSING CARE 1044

The Client with Infective Endocarditis 1045

Incidence and Risk Factors **1045**, Pathophysiology **1045**, Manifestations **1045**, Complications **1046**

INTERDISCIPLINARY CARE 1046

NURSING CARE 1047

The Client with Myocarditis 1048

Incidence and Risk Factors **1049**, Pathophysiology **1049**, Manifestations **1049**

INTERDISCIPLINARY CARE 1049

NURSING CARE 1049

The Client with Pericarditis 1049

Pathophysiology **1050**, Manifestations **1050**, Complications **1050**

INTERDISCIPLINARY CARE 1051

NURSING CARE 1052

The Client with Valvular Heart Disease 1053

Physiology Review **1054**, Pathophysiology **1054**

INTERDISCIPLINARY CARE 1059

NURSING CARE 1061

The Client with Cardiomyopathy 1063

Pathophysiology **1063**

INTERDISCIPLINARY CARE 1066

NURSING CARE 1067

Unit 10 Responses to Altered Peripheral Tissue Perfusion 1074

CHAPTER 33 Assessing Clients with Hematologic, Peripheral Vascular, and Lymphatic Disorders **1075**

Red Blood Cells **1076**, Red Blood Cell Production and Regulation **1076**, Red Blood Cell Destruction **1078**, White Blood Cells **1079**, Platelets **1079**, Hemostasis **1079**, Structure of Blood Vessels **1082**, Physiology of Arterial Circulation **1082**, Factors Influencing Arterial Blood Pressure **1085**

Assessing Hematologic, Peripheral Vascular, and Lymphatic Function 1086

Diagnostic Tests **1087**, Genetic Considerations **1088**, Health Assessment Interview **1088**, Physical Assessment **1091**

CHAPTER 34 Nursing Care of Clients with Hematologic Disorders **1101**

The Client with Anemia 1102

Physiology Review **1102**, Pathophysiology and Manifestations **1102**

INTERDISCIPLINARY CARE 1110

NURSING CARE 1112

The Client with Myelodysplastic Syndrome 1115

Pathophysiology **1115**, Manifestations **1115**

INTERDISCIPLINARY CARE 1115

NURSING CARE 1116

The Client with Polycythemia 1117

Pathophysiology **1117**

INTERDISCIPLINARY CARE 1117

NURSING CARE 1118

The Client with Leukemia 1118

Physiology Review **1118**, Pathophysiology **1119**, Manifestations **1119**, Classifications **1119**

INTERDISCIPLINARY CARE 1122

NURSING CARE 1125

The Client with Malignant Lymphoma 1129

Incidence and Risk Factors **1129**, Pathophysiology **1129**, Course **1131**

INTERDISCIPLINARY CARE 1131

NURSING CARE 1133

The Client with Multiple Myeloma 1136

Incidence and Risk Factors **1136**, Pathophysiology **1136**, Manifestations **1136**

INTERDISCIPLINARY CARE 1137

NURSING CARE 1137

The Client with Neutropenia 1138

Pathophysiology and Manifestations **1138**

INTERDISCIPLINARY CARE 1139

NURSING CARE 1139

The Client with Infectious Mononucleosis 1139

Pathophysiology and Manifestations **1139**

INTERDISCIPLINARY CARE 1139

The Client with Thrombocytopenia 1139

Pathophysiology **1140**

INTERDISCIPLINARY CARE 1141

NURSING CARE 1141

The Client with Hemophilia 1142

Physiology Review **1142**, Pathophysiology **1142**, Manifestations **1143**

INTERDISCIPLINARY CARE 1144

NURSING CARE 1144

The Client with Disseminated Intravascular Coagulation 1146

Pathophysiology **1146**, Manifestations **1147**

INTERDISCIPLINARY CARE 1148

NURSING CARE 1148

CHAPTER 35 Nursing Care of Clients with Peripheral Vascular Disorders 1153

Physiology Review **1154**

The Client with Primary Hypertension 1155

Incidence and Risk Factors **1156**, Pathophysiology **1157**, Manifestations **1158**, Complications **1158**

INTERDISCIPLINARY CARE 1158

NURSING CARE 1163

The Client with Secondary Hypertension 1167

The Client with Hypertensive Crisis 1168

The Client with an Aneurysm 1170

Pathophysiology and Manifestations **1170**

INTERDISCIPLINARY CARE 1173

NURSING CARE 1173

The Client with Peripheral Vascular Disease 1176

Incidence and Risk Factors **1176**, Pathophysiology **1176**, Manifestations and Complications **1176**

INTERDISCIPLINARY CARE 1177

NURSING CARE 1178

The Client with Thromboangiitis Obliterans 1180

Incidence and Risk Factors **1180**, Pathophysiology and Course **1180**, Manifestations and Complications **1180**

INTERDISCIPLINARY CARE 1182

NURSING CARE 1182

The Client with Raynaud's Disease 1182

Pathophysiology and Manifestations **1182**

INTERDISCIPLINARY CARE 1182

NURSING CARE 1183

The Client with Acute Arterial Occlusion 1184

Pathophysiology **1184**, Manifestations **1184**

INTERDISCIPLINARY CARE 1184

NURSING CARE 1185

The Client with Venous Thrombosis 1186

Pathophysiology **1186**

INTERDISCIPLINARY CARE 1188

NURSING CARE 1190

The Client with Chronic Venous Insufficiency 1194

Pathophysiology **1194**, Manifestations **1194**

INTERDISCIPLINARY CARE 1194

NURSING CARE 1195

The Client with Varicose Veins 1195

Incidence and Risk Factors **1195**, Pathophysiology **1196**

INTERDISCIPLINARY CARE 1197

NURSING CARE 1197

The Client with Lymphadenopathy 1199

The Client with Lymphedema 1199

Pathophysiology and Manifestations **1200**

INTERDISCIPLINARY CARE 1200

NURSING CARE 1200

Unit 11 Responses to Altered Respiratory Function 1208

CHAPTER 36 Assessing Clients with Respiratory Disorders 1209

The Upper Respiratory System **1210**, The Lower Respiratory System **1211**

Factors Affecting Ventilation and Respiration 1213

Respiratory Volume and Capacity **1214**, Air Pressures **1214**, Oxygen, Carbon Dioxide, and Hydrogen Ion Concentrations **1215**, Airway Resistance, Lung Compliance, and Elasticity **1216**, Alveolar Surface Tension **1216**

Blood Gases 1216

Oxygen Transport and Unloading **1216**, Carbon Dioxide Transport **1216**

Assessing Respiratory Function 1217

Diagnostic Tests **1217**, Genetic Considerations **1219**, Health Assessment Interview **1220**, Physical Assessment **1222**

CHAPTER 37 Nursing Care of Clients with Upper Respiratory Disorders 1228

The Client with Viral Upper Respiratory Infection 1229

Pathophysiology **1229**, Manifestations and Complications **1229**

INTERDISCIPLINARY CARE 1230

NURSING CARE 1231

The Client with Respiratory Syncytial Virus 1231

The Client with Influenza 1231

Pathophysiology **1232**, Manifestations **1233**, Complications **1233**

INTERDISCIPLINARY CARE 1233

NURSING CARE 1234

The Client with Sinusitis 1235

Physiology Review **1235**, Pathophysiology **1235**, Manifestations and Complications **1236**

INTERDISCIPLINARY CARE 1236

NURSING CARE 1237

The Client with Pharyngitis or Tonsillitis 1238

Pathophysiology and Manifestations **1238**, Complications **1239**

INTERDISCIPLINARY CARE 1239

NURSING CARE 1239

The Client with a Laryngeal Infection 1240

Epiglottitis **1240**, Laryngitis **1241**

The Client with Diphtheria 1241

Pathophysiology and Manifestations **1241**

INTERDISCIPLINARY CARE 1241

NURSING CARE 1241

The Client with Pertussis 1242

Pathophysiology **1242**, Manifestations **1242**

INTERDISCIPLINARY CARE 1242

NURSING CARE 1243

The Client with Epistaxis 1243

Pathophysiology and Manifestations **1243**

INTERDISCIPLINARY CARE 1243

NURSING CARE 1244

The Client with Nasal Trauma or Surgery 1246

Pathophysiology and Manifestations **1246**, Complications **1246**

INTERDISCIPLINARY CARE 1246

NURSING CARE 1247

The Client with Laryngeal Obstruction or Trauma 1249

Pathophysiology and Manifestations **1249**

INTERDISCIPLINARY CARE 1249

NURSING CARE 1250

The Client with Obstructive Sleep Apnea 1250

Risk Factors **1250**, Pathophysiology **1250**, Manifestations **1250**, Complications **1250**

INTERDISCIPLINARY CARE 1251

NURSING CARE 1251

The Client with Nasal Polyps 1252

Pathophysiology and Manifestations **1252**

INTERDISCIPLINARY CARE 1252

NURSING CARE 1252

The Client with a Laryngeal Tumor 1252

Risk Factors **1253**, Pathophysiology and Manifestations **1253**

INTERDISCIPLINARY CARE 1254

NURSING CARE 1258

CHAPTER 38 Nursing Care of Clients with Ventilation Disorders **1265**

The Client with Acute Bronchitis 1266

Pathophysiology and Manifestations **1266**

INTERDISCIPLINARY CARE 1266

NURSING CARE 1267

The Client with Pneumonia 1267

Physiology Review **1267**, Pathophysiology **1267**

INTERDISCIPLINARY CARE 1270

NURSING CARE 1274

The Client with Severe Acute Respiratory Syndrome 1276

Pathophysiology **1276**, Manifestations and Complications **1278**

INTERDISCIPLINARY CARE 1278

NURSING CARE 1278

The Client with Lung Abscess 1280

INTERDISCIPLINARY CARE 1280

NURSING CARE 1280

The Client with Tuberculosis 1280

Incidence and Prevalence **1280**, Pathophysiology **1281**

INTERDISCIPLINARY CARE 1283

NURSING CARE 1289

The Client with Inhalation Anthrax 1293

The Client with a Fungal Infection 1294

Pathophysiology **1294**

INTERDISCIPLINARY CARE 1294

NURSING CARE 1295

The Client with Pleuritis 1295

The Client with a Pleural Effusion 1295

Pathophysiology and Manifestations **1295**

INTERDISCIPLINARY CARE 1296

NURSING CARE 1296

The Client with Pneumothorax 1297

Pathophysiology **1297**

INTERDISCIPLINARY CARE 1299

NURSING CARE 1300

The Client with Hemothorax 1302

The Client with a Thoracic Injury 1302

Pathophysiology and Manifestations **1302**

INTERDISCIPLINARY CARE 1303

NURSING CARE 1304

The Client with Inhalation Injury 1305

Pathophysiology and Manifestations **1305**

INTERDISCIPLINARY CARE 1306

NURSING CARE 1307

The Client with Lung Cancer 1308

Incidence and Risk Factors **1308**, Pathophysiology **1308**, Manifestations **1309**, Complications and Course **1311**

INTERDISCIPLINARY CARE 1311

NURSING CARE 1313

CHAPTER 39 Nursing Care of Clients with Gas Exchange Disorders 1320

The Client with Asthma 1321

Incidence and Risk Factors 1321, Physiology Review 1322, Pathophysiology 1322, Manifestations and Complications 1323

INTERDISCIPLINARY CARE 1324

NURSING CARE 1326

The Client with Chronic Obstructive Pulmonary Disease 1330

Incidence and Risk Factors 1330, Pathophysiology 1331, Manifestations 1332

INTERDISCIPLINARY CARE 1333

NURSING CARE 1336

The Client with Cystic Fibrosis 1340

Incidence and Prevalence 1340, Pathophysiology 1341, Manifestations 1342

INTERDISCIPLINARY CARE 1342

NURSING CARE 1342

The Client with Atelectasis 1343

The Client with Bronchiectasis 1344

The Client with an Occupational Lung Disease 1344

Physiology Review 1344, Pathophysiology and Manifestations 1345

INTERDISCIPLINARY CARE 1346

NURSING CARE 1346

The Client with Sarcoidosis 1346

The Client with Pulmonary Embolism 1347

Incidence and Risk Factors 1347, Physiology Review 1347, Pathophysiology 1347, Manifestations 1348

INTERDISCIPLINARY CARE 1348

NURSING CARE 1349

The Client with Pulmonary Hypertension 1352

Pathophysiology 1352, Manifestations 1352, Complications 1352

INTERDISCIPLINARY CARE 1353

NURSING CARE 1353

The Client with Acute Respiratory Failure 1353

Pathophysiology 1354, Manifestations and Course 1354

INTERDISCIPLINARY CARE 1355

NURSING CARE 1361

The Client with Acute Respiratory Distress Syndrome 1365

Manifestations 1366

INTERDISCIPLINARY CARE 1366

NURSING CARE 1367

Unit 12 Responses to Altered Musculoskeletal Function 1378

CHAPTER 40 Assessing Clients with Musculoskeletal Disorders 1379

The Skeleton 1380, Muscles 1381, Joints, Ligaments, and Tendons 1383

Assessing Musculoskeletal Function 1386

Diagnostic Tests 1386, Genetic Considerations 1388, Health Assessment Interview 1388, Physical Assessment 1389

CHAPTER 41 Nursing Care of Clients with Musculoskeletal Trauma 1398

The Client with a Contusion, Strain, or Sprain 1399

Pathophysiology and Manifestations 1399

INTERDISCIPLINARY CARE 1399

NURSING CARE 1400

The Client with a Joint Dislocation 1400

Pathophysiology 1401, Manifestations 1401

INTERDISCIPLINARY CARE 1401

NURSING CARE 1401

The Client with a Fracture 1401

Pathophysiology 1401, Fracture Healing 1402, Manifestations 1402, Complications 1403

INTERDISCIPLINARY CARE 1407

Fractures of Specific Bones or Bony Areas 1412

NURSING CARE 1416

The Client with an Amputation 1421

Causes of Amputation 1421, Levels of Amputation 1421, Types of Amputation 1421, Amputation Site Healing 1422, Complications 1422

INTERDISCIPLINARY CARE 1423

NURSING CARE 1424

The Client with a Repetitive Use Injury 1427

Pathophysiology 1427

INTERDISCIPLINARY CARE 1428

NURSING CARE 1428

CHAPTER 42 Nursing Care of Clients with Musculoskeletal Disorders 1432

The Client with Osteoporosis 1433

Risk Factors 1433, Pathophysiology 1434, Manifestations 1435, Complications 1435

INTERDISCIPLINARY CARE 1435

NURSING CARE 1437

The Client with Paget's Disease 1441

Pathophysiology 1441, Manifestations 1441, Complications 1441

INTERDISCIPLINARY CARE 1441

NURSING CARE 1443

The Client with Gout 1443

Pathophysiology 1444, Manifestations 1444, Complications 1444

INTERDISCIPLINARY CARE 1445

NURSING CARE 1447

The Client with Osteomalacia 1447

Pathophysiology 1448, Manifestations 1448

INTERDISCIPLINARY CARE 1448

NURSING CARE 1449

The Client with Osteoarthritis 1449

Risk Factors 1450, Pathophysiology 1450, Manifestations 1450, Complications 1450

INTERDISCIPLINARY CARE 1451

NURSING CARE 1455

The Client with Muscular Dystrophy 1458
Pathophysiology 1458, Manifestations 1458
INTERDISCIPLINARY CARE 1458
NURSING CARE 1458

The Client with Rheumatoid Arthritis 1459
Pathophysiology 1459, Joint Manifestations 1460, Extra-Articular
Manifestations 1461, Increased Risk of Coronary Heart Disease 1461
INTERDISCIPLINARY CARE 1461
NURSING CARE 1466

The Client with Ankylosing Spondylitis 1469
Pathophysiology 1470, Manifestations 1470
INTERDISCIPLINARY CARE 1470
NURSING CARE 1470

The Client with Reactive Arthritis 1470
Manifestations 1470
INTERDISCIPLINARY CARE 1470
NURSING CARE 1470

The Client with Systemic Lupus Erythematosus 1471
Pathophysiology 1471, Manifestations 1471
INTERDISCIPLINARY CARE 1473
NURSING CARE 1474

The Client with Polymyositis 1476
Manifestations 1476
INTERDISCIPLINARY CARE 1476
NURSING CARE 1476

The Client with Lyme Disease 1476
Pathophysiology 1476, Manifestations 1477, Complications 1477
INTERDISCIPLINARY CARE 1477
NURSING CARE 1477

The Client with Osteomyelitis 1477
Pathophysiology 1477, Manifestations 1478
INTERDISCIPLINARY CARE 1478
NURSING CARE 1480

The Client with Septic Arthritis 1481
Pathophysiology 1481, Manifestations 1481
INTERDISCIPLINARY CARE 1481
NURSING CARE 1481

The Client with Bone Tumors 1481
Pathophysiology 1482, Manifestations 1482
INTERDISCIPLINARY CARE 1482
NURSING CARE 1483

The Client with Systemic Sclerosis (Scleroderma) 1484
Pathophysiology 1485, Manifestations 1485
INTERDISCIPLINARY CARE 1485
NURSING CARE 1486

The Client with Sjögren's Syndrome 1486
Pathophysiology 1486
INTERDISCIPLINARY CARE 1486
NURSING CARE 1486

The Client with Fibromyalgia 1486
Pathophysiology 1487, Manifestations 1487
INTERDISCIPLINARY CARE 1487
NURSING CARE 1487

The Client with Spinal Deformities 1487
Pathophysiology 1488
INTERDISCIPLINARY CARE 1489
NURSING CARE 1489

The Client with Low Back Pain 1490
Pathophysiology 1490, Manifestations 1490
INTERDISCIPLINARY CARE 1491
NURSING CARE 1491

The Client with Common Foot Disorders 1492
Pathophysiology 1492
INTERDISCIPLINARY CARE 1493
NURSING CARE 1493

PART V COGNITIVE AND PERCEPTUAL PATTERNS 1500

Unit 13 Responses to Altered Neurologic
Function 1502

CHAPTER 43 Assessing Clients with Neurologic
Disorders 1503
Nerve Cells, Action Potentials, and Neurotransmitters 1504, The
Central Nervous System 1505, The Peripheral Nervous System 1509,
The Autonomic Nervous System 1511
Assessing Neurologic Function 1512
Diagnostic Tests 1512, Genetic Considerations 1513, Health
Assessment Interview 1513, Physical Assessment 1516

CHAPTER 44 Nursing Care of Clients with Intracranial
Disorders 1527
The Client with Altered Level of Consciousness 1529
Pathophysiology 1529, Prognosis 1532
INTERDISCIPLINARY CARE 1532
NURSING CARE 1533

The Client with Increased Intracranial Pressure 1535
Pathophysiology 1535, Manifestations 1536, Cerebral Edema 1537,
Hydrocephalus 1537, Brain Herniation 1537
INTERDISCIPLINARY CARE 1538
NURSING CARE 1541

The Client with a Headache 1542
Pathophysiology 1542
INTERDISCIPLINARY CARE 1543
NURSING CARE 1544

The Client with Epilepsy 1547
Incidence and Prevalence 1547, Pathophysiology 1548,
Manifestations 1548
INTERDISCIPLINARY CARE 1549
NURSING CARE 1551

The Client with a Skull Fracture 1554

Pathophysiology **1555**
INTERDISCIPLINARY CARE   1555
NURSING CARE   1555
The Client with a Focal or Diffuse Traumatic Brain Injury   1556
Pathophysiology **1556**
INTERDISCIPLINARY CARE   1559
NURSING CARE   1560
The Client with a Central Nervous System Infection   1563
Pathophysiology **1564**
INTERDISCIPLINARY CARE   1566
NURSING CARE   1566
The Client with a Brain Tumor   1569
Incidence and Prevalence **1569**, Pathophysiology **1569**,
Manifestations **1569**
INTERDISCIPLINARY CARE   1570
NURSING CARE   1572

**CHAPTER 45 Nursing Care of Clients with Cerebrovascular
           and Spinal Cord Disorders   1578**
The Client with a Stroke   1579
Incidence and Prevalence **1579**, Risk Factors **1579**,
Pathophysiology **1580**, Manifestations **1582**, Complications **1582**
INTERDISCIPLINARY CARE   1584
NURSING CARE   1586
The Client with an Intracranial Aneurysm   1592
Incidence and Prevalence **1592**, Pathophysiology **1592**,
Manifestations **1592**, Complications **1593**
INTERDISCIPLINARY CARE   1593
NURSING CARE   1594
The Client with an Arteriovenous Malformation   1595
Pathophysiology **1595**
INTERDISCIPLINARY CARE   1595
NURSING CARE   1595
The Client with a Spinal Cord Injury   1595
Incidence and Prevalence **1595**, Risk Factors **1595**, Pathophysiology
1596, Manifestations **1597**, Complications **1598**
INTERDISCIPLINARY CARE   1599
NURSING CARE   1601
The Client with a Herniated Intervertebral Disk   1607
Incidence and Prevalence **1607**, Pathophysiology **1607**, Lumbar Disk
Manifestations **1608**, Cervical Disk Manifestations **1608**
INTERDISCIPLINARY CARE   1608
NURSING CARE   1610
The Client with a Spinal Cord Tumor   1612
Classification **1612**, Pathophysiology **1612**, Manifestations **1612**
INTERDISCIPLINARY CARE   1613
NURSING CARE   1613

**CHAPTER 46 Nursing Care of Clients with Neurologic
           Disorders   1616**
Dementia   1617
The Client with Alzheimer's Disease   1617

Incidence and Prevalence **1618**, Risk Factors and Warning Signs **1618**,
Pathophysiology **1618**, Manifestations **1619**
INTERDISCIPLINARY CARE   1620
NURSING CARE   1621
The Client with Multiple Sclerosis   1626
Incidence and Prevalence **1626**, Pathophysiology **1626**,
Manifestations **1626**
INTERDISCIPLINARY CARE   1627
NURSING CARE   1632
The Client with Parkinson's Disease   1635
Incidence and Prevalence **1635**, Pathophysiology **1635**,
Manifestations **1635**, Complications **1637**
INTERDISCIPLINARY CARE   1637
The Client with Huntington's Disease   1642
Pathophysiology **1642**, Manifestations **1642**
INTERDISCIPLINARY CARE   1643
NURSING CARE   1643
The Client with Amyotrophic Lateral Sclerosis   1645
Pathophysiology **1645**, Manifestations **1645**
INTERDISCIPLINARY CARE   1645
NURSING CARE   1646
The Client with Myasthenia Gravis   1647
Pathophysiology **1647**, Manifestations **1648**, Complications **1648**
INTERDISCIPLINARY CARE   1649
NURSING CARE   1651
The Client with Guillain-Barré Syndrome   1653
Pathophysiology **1653**, Manifestations **1653**
INTERDISCIPLINARY CARE   1653
NURSING CARE   1654
The Client with Trigeminal Neuralgia   1655
Pathophysiology **1655**, Manifestations **1656**
INTERDISCIPLINARY CARE   1656
NURSING CARE   1656
The Client with Bell's Palsy   1657
Pathophysiology **1657**, Manifestations **1657**
INTERDISCIPLINARY CARE   1658
NURSING CARE   1658
The Client with Creutzfeldt-Jakob Disease   1658
Pathophysiology **1659**, Manifestations **1659**
INTERDISCIPLINARY CARE   1659
NURSING CARE   1659
The Client with Postpoliomyelitis Syndrome   1659
Pathophysiology **1659**, Manifestations **1659**
INTERDISCIPLINARY CARE   1659
NURSING CARE   1660
The Client with Rabies   1660
Pathophysiology **1660**, Manifestations **1660**
INTERDISCIPLINARY CARE   1660
NURSING CARE   1660

The Client with Tetanus — 1661

Pathophysiology **1661**, Manifestations **1661**

INTERDISCIPLINARY CARE — 1661

NURSING CARE — 1661

The Client with Botulism — 1661

Pathophysiology **1662**, Manifestations **1662**

INTERDISCIPLINARY CARE — 1662

NURSING CARE — 1662

Unit 14 Responses to Altered Visual and Auditory Function — 1668

CHAPTER 47 Assessing Clients with Eye and Ear Disorders — 1669

Extraocular Structures **1670**, Intraocular Structures **1671**, The Visual Pathway **1672**, Refraction **1673**

Assessing the Eyes — 1673

Diagnostic Tests **1673**, Genetic Considerations **1674**, Health Assessment Interview **1674**, Physical Assessment of the Eyes and Vision **1674**

The External Ear **1680**, The Middle Ear **1682**, The Inner Ear **1683**, Sound Conduction **1683**, Equilibrium **1683**

Assessing the Ears — 1683

Diagnostic Tests **1683**, Genetic Considerations **1684**, Health Assessment Interview **1684**, Physical Assessment of the Ears and Hearing **1686**

CHAPTER 48 Nursing Care of Clients with Eye and Ear Disorders — 1691

The Client with Conjunctivitis — 1692

Pathophysiology and Manifestations **1692**

INTERDISCIPLINARY CARE — 1694

NURSING CARE — 1695

The Client with a Corneal Disorder — 1695

Physiology Review **1696**, Pathophysiology and Manifestations **1696**

INTERDISCIPLINARY CARE — 1697

NURSING CARE — 1698

The Client with a Disorder Affecting the Eyelids — 1700

Pathophysiology and Manifestations **1700**

INTERDISCIPLINARY CARE — 1701

NURSING CARE — 1701

The Client with Eye Trauma — 1701

Pathophysiology and Manifestations **1701**

INTERDISCIPLINARY CARE — 1702

NURSING CARE — 1703

The Client with Uveitis — 1703

The Client with Cataracts — 1704

Incidence and Risk Factors **1704**, Pathophysiology **1704**, Manifestations **1704**

INTERDISCIPLINARY CARE — 1704

NURSING CARE — 1705

The Client with Glaucoma — 1706

Incidence and Risk Factors **1706**, Pathophysiology **1706**

INTERDISCIPLINARY CARE — 1708

NURSING CARE — 1711

The Client with Age-Related Macular Degeneration — 1713

Pathophysiology **1714**, Manifestations **1714**

INTERDISCIPLINARY CARE — 1714

NURSING CARE — 1714

The Client with Diabetic Retinopathy — 1714

Pathophysiology and Manifestations **1715**

INTERDISCIPLINARY CARE — 1715

NURSING CARE — 1716

The Client with a Retinal Detachment — 1716

Pathophysiology and Manifestations **1716**

INTERDISCIPLINARY CARE — 1716

NURSING CARE — 1717

The Client with Retinitis Pigmentosa — 1717

The Client with HIV Infection — 1718

The Client with an Enucleation — 1718

The Client with Otitis Externa — 1718

Pathophysiology and Manifestations **1719**

INTERDISCIPLINARY CARE — 1719

NURSING CARE — 1720

The Client with Impacted Cerumen or a Foreign Body — 1721

Pathophysiology and Manifestations **1721**

INTERDISCIPLINARY CARE — 1721

NURSING CARE — 1721

The Client with Otitis Media — 1721

Pathophysiology **1721**

INTERDISCIPLINARY CARE — 1722

NURSING CARE — 1723

The Client with Acute Mastoiditis — 1723

Pathophysiology and Complications **1723**, Manifestations **1724**

INTERDISCIPLINARY CARE — 1724

NURSING CARE — 1724

The Client with Chronic Otitis Media — 1724

The Client with Otosclerosis — 1725

The Client with an Inner Ear Disorder — 1726

Pathophysiology and Manifestations **1726**

INTERDISCIPLINARY CARE — 1727

NURSING CARE — 1727

The Client with an Acoustic Neuroma — 1729

The Client with Hearing Loss — 1729

Pathophysiology and Manifestations **1729**

INTERDISCIPLINARY CARE — 1730

NURSING CARE — 1732

PART VI SEXUALITY AND REPRODUCTIVE PATTERNS — 1740

Unit 15 Responses to Altered Reproductive Function — 1742

CHAPTER 49 Assessing Clients with Reproductive System and Breast Disorders **1743**

The Breasts **1744**, The Penis **1744**, The Scrotum **1744**, The Testes **1744**, The Ducts and Semen **1745**, The Prostate Gland **1745**, Spermatogenesis **1745**, Male Sex Hormones **1745**

Assessing the Male Reproductive System **1746**

Diagnostic Tests **1746**, Genetic Considerations **1747**, Health Assessment Interview **1747**, Physical Assessment **1747**

The Breasts **1751**, The External Genitalia **1751**, The Internal Organs **1752**, Female Sex Hormones **1753**, Oogenesis and the Ovarian Cycle **1754**, The Menstrual Cycle **1754**

Assessing the Female Reproductive System **1755**

Diagnostic Tests **1755**, Genetic Considerations **1755**, Health Assessment Interview **1758**, Physical Assessment **1760**

CHAPTER 50 Nursing Care of Men with Reproductive System and Breast Disorders **1767**

The Man with Erectile Dysfunction **1768**

Pathophysiology **1769**

INTERDISCIPLINARY CARE **1769**

NURSING CARE **1770**

The Man with Ejaculatory Dysfunction **1771**

The Man with Phimosis or Priapism **1771**

Pathophysiology **1771**

INTERDISCIPLINARY CARE **1771**

NURSING CARE **1772**

The Man with Cancer of the Penis **1772**

Pathophysiology **1772**

INTERDISCIPLINARY CARE **1772**

NURSING CARE **1772**

The Man with a Benign Scrotal Mass **1772**

Pathophysiology **1772**

NURSING CARE **1773**

The Man with Epididymitis **1773**

INTERDISCIPLINARY CARE **1773**

NURSING CARE **1773**

The Man with Orchitis **1774**

INTERDISCIPLINARY CARE **1774**

The Man with Testicular Torsion **1774**

The Man with Testicular Cancer **1774**

Risk Factors **1774**, Pathophysiology **1774**, Manifestations **1774**

INTERDISCIPLINARY CARE **1775**

NURSING CARE **1775**

The Man with Prostatitis **1776**

Pathophysiology and Manifestations **1776**

INTERDISCIPLINARY CARE **1777**

NURSING CARE **1777**

The Man with Benign Prostatic Hyperplasia **1777**

Risk Factors **1777**, Pathophysiology **1777**, Manifestations **1778**, Complications **1778**

INTERDISCIPLINARY CARE **1778**

NURSING CARE **1781**

The Man with Prostate Cancer **1782**

Risk Factors **1783**, Pathophysiology **1783**, Manifestations **1783**, Complications **1784**

INTERDISCIPLINARY CARE **1784**

NURSING CARE **1786**

The Man with Gynecomastia **1789**

The Man with Breast Cancer **1790**

CHAPTER 51 Nursing Care of Women with Reproductive System and Breast Disorders **1793**

Disorders of Female Sexual Function **1794**

Pathophysiology **1795**

NURSING CARE **1795**

The Perimenopausal Woman **1795**

The Physiology of Menopause **1795**, Manifestations **1796**

INTERDISCIPLINARY CARE **1796**

NURSING CARE **1796**

The Woman with Premenstrual Syndrome **1798**

Pathophysiology **1798**, Manifestations **1798**

INTERDISCIPLINARY CARE **1798**

NURSING CARE **1800**

The Woman with Dysmenorrhea **1800**

Pathophysiology **1800**, Manifestations **1800**

INTERDISCIPLINARY CARE **1800**

NURSING CARE **1802**

The Woman with Dysfunctional Uterine Bleeding **1802**

Pathophysiology **1802**

INTERDISCIPLINARY CARE **1803**

NURSING CARE **1804**

The Woman with a Uterine Displacement **1805**

Pathophysiology **1805**, Manifestations **1805**

INTERDISCIPLINARY CARE **1806**

NURSING CARE **1807**

The Woman with a Vaginal Fistula **1807**

The Woman with Cysts or Polyps **1808**

Pathophysiology **1808**, Manifestations and Complications **1808**

INTERDISCIPLINARY CARE **1808**

NURSING CARE **1809**

The Woman with Leiomyoma **1809**

Pathophysiology **1809**, Manifestations **1809**

INTERDISCIPLINARY CARE **1810**

NURSING CARE **1810**

The Woman with Endometriosis **1810**

Pathophysiology **1810**, Manifestations **1810**

INTERDISCIPLINARY CARE **1810**

NURSING CARE **1811**

The Woman with Cervical Cancer **1812**

Risk Factors **1812**, Pathophysiology **1812**, Manifestations **1813**

INTERDISCIPLINARY CARE **1813**

NURSING CARE **1814**

The Woman with Endometrial Cancer 1816

Risk Factors **1816**, Pathophysiology **1816**, Manifestations **1816**

INTERDISCIPLINARY CARE 1816

NURSING CARE 1817

The Woman with Ovarian Cancer 1817

Risk Factors **1817**, Pathophysiology **1818**, Manifestations **1818**, Complications **1818**

INTERDISCIPLINARY CARE 1818

NURSING CARE 1819

The Woman with Cancer of the Vulva 1819

Pathophysiology **1819**, Manifestations **1819**

INTERDISCIPLINARY CARE 1819

NURSING CARE 1820

The Woman with a Benign Breast Disorder 1820

Pathophysiology and Manifestations **1820**

INTERDISCIPLINARY CARE 1822

NURSING CARE 1822

The Woman with Breast Cancer 1822

Risk Factors **1822**, Pathophysiology **1823**, Manifestations **1823**

INTERDISCIPLINARY CARE 1824

NURSING CARE 1827

CHAPTER 52 Nursing Care of Clients with Sexually Transmitted Infections **1836**

Incidence and Prevalence **1837**, Characteristics **1837**, Prevention and Control **1838**

The Client with Genital Herpes 1838

Pathophysiology **1839**, Manifestations **1839**

INTERDISCIPLINARY CARE 1839

NURSING CARE 1840

The Client with Genital Warts 1840

Pathophysiology **1840**, Manifestations **1841**

INTERDISCIPLINARY CARE 1841

NURSING CARE 1841

The Client with a Vaginal Infection 1842

Pathophysiology and Manifestations **1842**

INTERDISCIPLINARY CARE 1843

NURSING CARE 1844

The Client with Chlamydia 1844

Pathophysiology **1844**, Manifestations **1844**, Complications **1845**

INTERDISCIPLINARY CARE 1845

NURSING CARE 1845

The Client with Gonorrhea 1845

Pathophysiology **1845**, Manifestations **1845**, Complications **1846**

INTERDISCIPLINARY CARE 1846

NURSING CARE 1846

The Client with Syphilis 1846

Pathophysiology **1847**, Manifestations **1847**

INTERDISCIPLINARY CARE 1848

NURSING CARE 1849

The Client with Pelvic Inflammatory Disease 1850

Pathophysiology **1851**, Manifestations **1851**, Complications **1851**

INTERDISCIPLINARY CARE 1851

NURSING CARE 1851

Appendix A Standard Precautions A–1

Appendix B 2007–2008 NANDA-Approved Nursing Diagnoses A–2

Appendix C Test Yourself and Evaluate Your Response Answers A–3

Glossary G–1

Index I–1

UNIT 9

Responses to Altered Cardiac Function

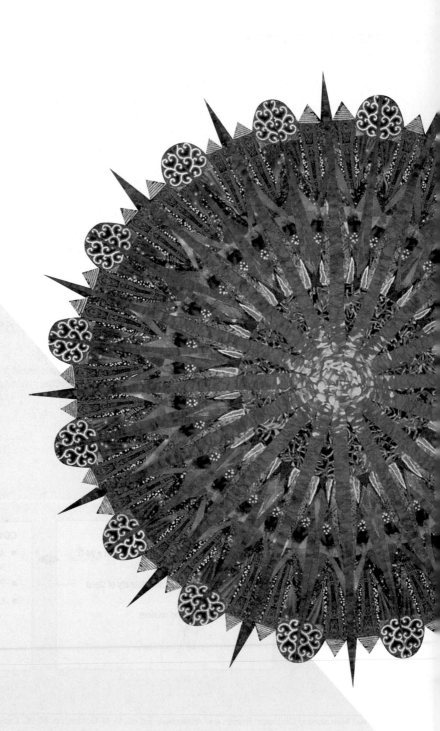

CHAPTER 30
Assessing Clients with Cardiac Disorders

CHAPTER 31
Nursing Care of Clients with Coronary Heart Disease

CHAPTER 32
Nursing Care of Clients with Cardiac Disorders

CHAPTER 30 Assessing Clients with Cardiac Disorders

LEARNING OUTCOMES

- Describe the anatomy, physiology, and functions of the heart.
- Trace the circulation of blood through the heart and coronary vessels.
- Identify normal heart sounds and relate them to the corresponding events in the cardiac cycle.
- Explain cardiac output and the influence of various factors in its regulation.
- Describe normal variations in assessment findings for the older adult.
- Identify manifestations of impaired cardiac structure and functions.

CLINICAL COMPETENCIES

- Assess an ECG strip and identify normal and abnormal cardiac rhythm.
- Conduct and document a health history for clients having or at risk for having alterations in the structure and functions of the heart.
- Conduct and document a physical assessment of cardiac status.
- Monitor the results of diagnostic tests and report abnormal findings.

EQUIPMENT NEEDED

- Stethoscope with a diaphragm and a bell
- Good light source
- Watch with a second hand
- Centimeter ruler

MEDIALINK

Resources for this chapter can be found on the Prentice Hall Nursing MediaLink DVD accompanying this textbook, and on the Companion Website at http://www.prenhall.com/lemone

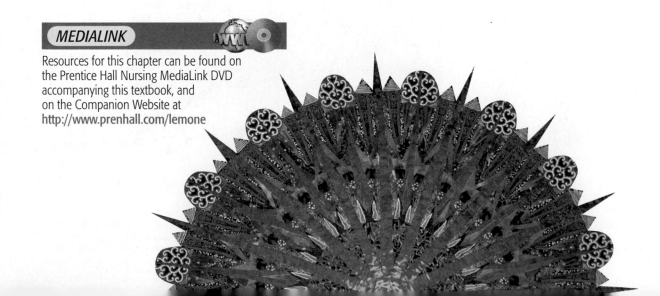

The heart, a muscular pump, beats an average of 70 times per minute, or once every 0.86 second, every minute of a person's life. This continuous pumping moves blood through the body, nourishing tissue cells and removing wastes. Deficits in the structure or function of the heart affect all body tissues.

Changes in cardiac rate, rhythm, or output may limit almost all human functions, including self-care, mobility, and the ability to maintain fluid volume status, respirations, tissue perfusion, and comfort. Cardiac changes may also affect self-concept, sexuality, and role performance.

ANATOMY, PHYSIOLOGY, AND FUNCTIONS OF THE HEART

The heart is a hollow, cone-shaped organ approximately the size of an adult's fist, weighing less than 1 lb. It is located in the mediastinum of the thoracic cavity, between the vertebral column and the sternum, and is flanked laterally by the lungs. Two-thirds of the heart mass lies to the left of the sternum; the upper base lies beneath the second rib, and the pointed apex is approximate with the fifth intercostal space, midpoint to the clavicle (Figure 30–1 ■).

The Pericardium

The heart is covered by the pericardium, a double layer of fibroserous membrane (Figure 30–2 ■). The pericardium encases the heart and anchors it to surrounding structures, forming the pericardial sac. The snug fit of the pericardium prevents the heart from overfilling with blood. The outermost layer is the parietal pericardium, and the visceral pericardium

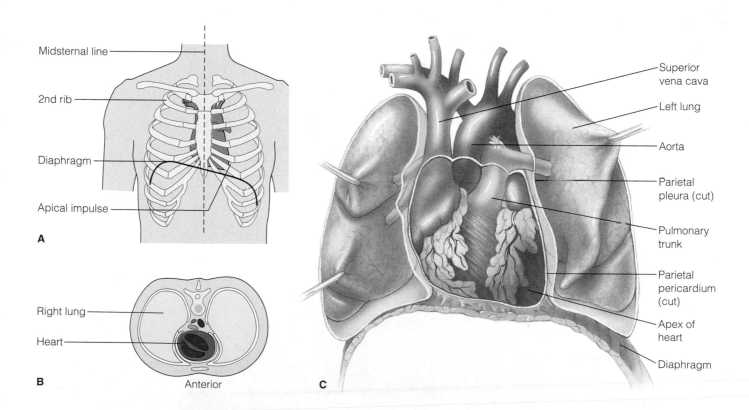

Figure 30–1 ■ Location of the heart in the mediastinum of the thorax. *A,* Relationship of the heart to the sternum, ribs, and diaphragm. *B,* Cross-sectional view showing relative position of the heart in the thorax. *C,* Relationship of the heart and great vessels to the lungs.

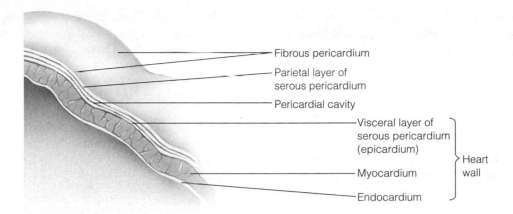

Figure 30–2 ■ Coverings and layers of the heart.

(or epicardium) adheres to the heart surface. The small space between the visceral and parietal layers of the pericardium is called the pericardial cavity. A serous lubricating fluid produced in this space cushions the heart as it beats.

Layers of the Heart Wall

The heart wall consists of three layers of tissue: the epicardium, the myocardium, and the endocardium (see Figure 30–2). The epicardium covers the entire heart and great vessels, and then folds over to form the parietal layer that lines the pericardium and adheres to the heart surface. The myocardium, which is the middle layer of the heart wall, consists of specialized cardiac muscle cells (myofibrils) that provide the bulk of contractile heart muscle. The endocardium, which is the innermost layer, is a thin membrane composed of three layers; the innermost layer is made up of smooth endothelial cells that line the inside of the heart's chambers and great vessels.

Chambers and Valves of the Heart

The heart has four hollow chambers, two upper atria and two lower ventricles. They are separated longitudinally by the interventricular septum (Figure 30–3 ■).

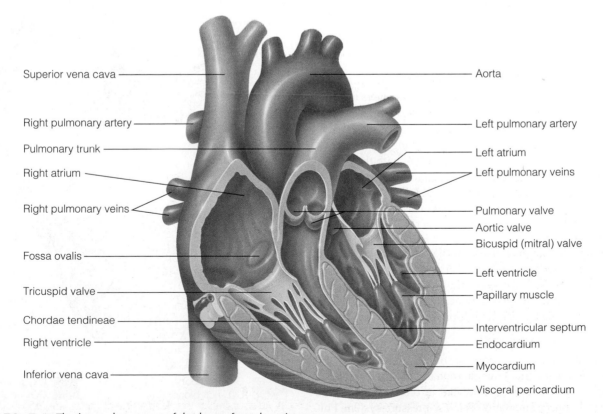

Figure 30–3 ■ The internal anatomy of the heart, frontal section.

The right atrium receives deoxygenated blood from the veins of the body: The superior vena cava returns blood from the body area above the diaphragm, the inferior vena cava returns blood from the body below the diaphragm, and the coronary sinus drains blood from the heart. The left atrium receives freshly oxygenated blood from the lungs through the pulmonary veins.

The right ventricle receives deoxygenated blood from the right atrium and pumps it through the pulmonary artery to the pulmonary capillary bed for oxygenation. The newly oxygenated blood then travels through the pulmonary veins to the left atrium. Blood enters the left atrium and crosses the mitral (bicuspid) valve into the left ventricle. Blood is then pumped out of the aorta to the arterial circulation.

Each of the heart's chambers is separated by a valve that allows unidirectional blood flow to the next chamber or great vessel (see Figure 30–3). The atria are separated from the ventricles by the two atrioventricular (AV) valves; the tricuspid valve is on the right side, and the bicuspid (or mitral) valve is on the left. The flaps of each of these valves are anchored to the papillary muscles of the ventricles by the chordae tendineae. These structures control the movement of the AV valves to prevent backflow of blood. The ventricles are connected to their great vessels by the semilunar valves. On the right, the pulmonary (pulmonic) valve joins the right ventricle with the pulmonary artery. On the left, the aortic valve joins the left ventricle to the aorta.

Closure of the AV valves at the onset of contraction (systole) produces the first heart sound, or S_1 (characterized by the syllable "lub"); closure of the semilunar valves at the onset of relaxation (diastole) produces the second heart sound, or S_2 (characterized by the syllable "dub").

Systemic, Pulmonary, and Coronary Circulation

Because each side of the heart both receives and ejects blood, the heart is often described as a double pump. Blood enters the right atrium and moves to the pulmonary bed at almost the exact same time that blood is entering the left atrium. The circulatory system has two parts: the pulmonary circulation (moving blood through the capillary bed surrounding the lungs to link with the gas exchange system of the lungs), and the systemic circulation, which supplies blood to all other body tissues. In addition, the heart muscle itself is supplied with blood via the coronary circulation.

Systemic Circulation

The systemic circulation consists of the left side of the heart, the aorta and its branches, the capillaries that supply the brain and peripheral tissues, the systemic venous system, and the vena cava. The systemic system, which must move blood to peripheral areas of the body, is a high-pressure system.

Pulmonary Circulation

The pulmonary circulation consists of the right side of the heart, the pulmonary artery, the pulmonary capillaries, and the pulmonary vein. Because it is located in the thorax near the heart, the pulmonary circulation is a low-pressure system. Pulmonary circulation begins with the right side of the heart. De-

oxygenated blood from the venous system enters the right atrium through two large veins, the superior and inferior venae cavae, and is transported to the lungs via the pulmonary artery and its branches (Figure 30–4 ■). After oxygen and carbon dioxide are exchanged in the pulmonary capillaries, oxygen-rich blood returns to the left atrium through several pulmonary veins. Blood is then pumped out of the left ventricle through the aorta and its major branches to supply all body tissues. This second circuit of blood flow is called the systemic circulation.

Coronary Circulation

The heart muscle itself is supplied by its own network of vessels through the coronary circulation. The left and right coronary arteries originate at the base of the aorta and branch out to encircle the myocardium (Figure 30–5A ■), supplying blood, oxygen, and

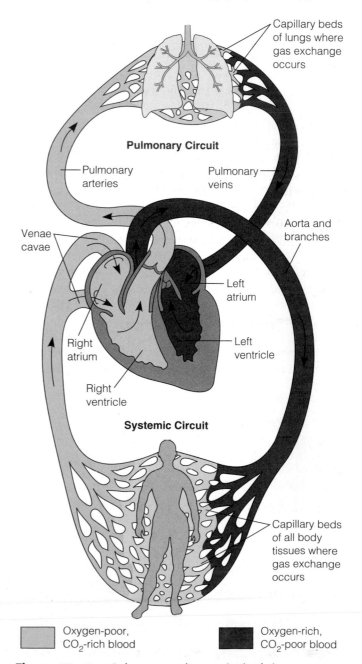

Capillary beds of lungs where gas exchange occurs

Pulmonary Circuit

Pulmonary arteries

Pulmonary veins

Aorta and branches

Venae cavae

Left atrium

Right atrium

Left ventricle

Right ventricle

Systemic Circuit

Capillary beds of all body tissues where gas exchange occurs

Oxygen-poor, CO_2-rich blood

Oxygen-rich, CO_2-poor blood

Figure 30–4 ■ Pulmonary and systemic circulation.

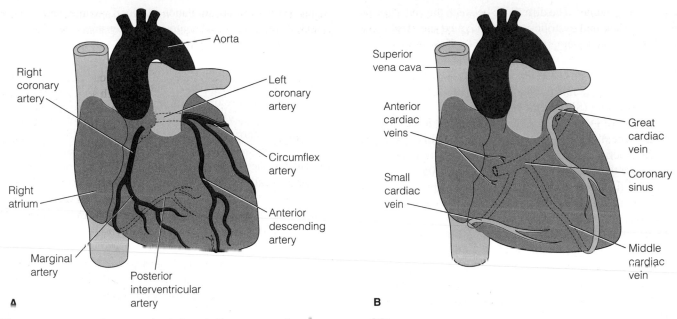

Figure 30–5 ■ Coronary circulation. *A*, Coronary arteries; *B*, coronary veins.

nutrients to the myocardium. The left main coronary artery divides to form the anterior descending and circumflex arteries. The anterior descending artery supplies the anterior interventricular septum and the left ventricle. The circumflex branch supplies the left lateral wall of the left ventricle. The right coronary artery supplies the right ventricle and forms the posterior descending artery. The posterior descending artery supplies the posterior portion of the heart. While ventricular contraction delivers blood through the pulmonary circulation and the systemic circulation, it is during ventricular relaxation that the coronary arteries fill with oxygen-rich blood. After the blood perfuses the heart muscle, the cardiac veins drain the blood into the coronary sinus, which empties into the right atrium of the heart (Figure 30–5B).

Blood flow through the coronary arteries is regulated by several factors. Aortic pressure is the primary factor. Other factors include the heart rate (most flow occurs during diastole, when the muscle is relaxed), metabolic activity of the heart, and blood vessel tone (constriction).

The Cardiac Cycle and Cardiac Output

The contraction and relaxation of the heart constitutes one heartbeat and is called the cardiac cycle (Figure 30–6 ■). Ventricular filling is followed by ventricular systole, a phase during which the ventricles contract and eject blood into the pulmonary and systemic circuits. Systole is followed by a relaxation phase known as diastole, during which the ventricles refill, the atria contract, and the myocardium is perfused. Normally, the complete cardiac cycle occurs about 70 to 80 times per minute, measured as the heart rate (HR).

During diastole, the volume in the ventricles is increased to about 120 mL (the end-diastolic volume), and at the end of systole, about 50 mL of blood remains in the ventricles (the

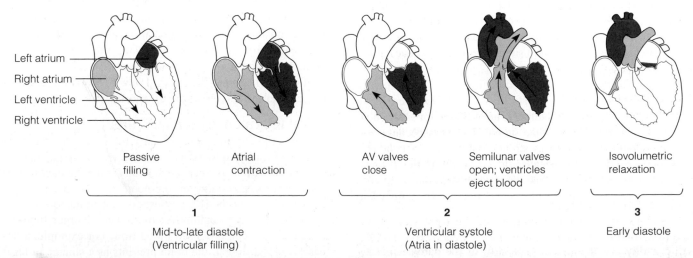

Figure 30–6 ■ The cardiac cycle has three events: (1) ventricular filling in mid-to-late diastole, (2) ventricular systole, and (3) isovolumetric relaxation in early diastole.

end-systolic volume). The difference between the end-diastolic volume and the end-systolic volume is called the **stroke volume (SV)**. Stroke volume ranges from 60 to 100 mL/beat and averages about 70 mL/beat in an adult. The **cardiac output (CO)** is the amount of blood pumped by the ventricles into the pulmonary and systemic circulations in 1 minute. Multiplying the stroke volume (SV) by the heart rate (HR) determines the cardiac output: SV × HR = CO. The **ejection fraction** is the stroke volume divided by the end-diastolic volume and represents the fraction or percent of the diastolic volume that is ejected from the heart during systole (Porth, 2005). For example, an end-diastolic volume of 120 mL divided by a stroke volume of 80 mL equals an ejection fraction of 66%. The normal ejection fraction ranges from 50% to 70%.

The average adult cardiac output ranges from 4 to 8 L/min. Cardiac output is an indicator of how well the heart is functioning as a pump. If the heart cannot pump effectively, cardiac output and tissue perfusion are decreased. Body tissues that do not receive enough blood and oxygen (carried in the blood on hemoglobin) become **ischemic** (deprived of oxygen). If the tissues do not receive enough blood flow to maintain the functions of the cells, the cells die (cellular death results in necrosis or infarction).

Activity level, metabolic rate, physiologic and psychologic stress responses, age, and body size all influence cardiac output. In addition, cardiac output is determined by the interaction of four major factors: heart rate, preload, afterload, and contractility. Changes in each of these variables influence cardiac output intrinsically, and each also can be manipulated to affect cardiac output. The heart's ability to respond to the body's changing need for cardiac output is called **cardiac reserve**.

Heart Rate

Heart rate is affected by both direct and indirect autonomic nervous system stimulation. Direct stimulation is accomplished through the innervation of the heart muscle by sympathetic and parasympathetic nerves. The sympathetic nervous system increases the heart rate, whereas the parasympathetic vagal tone slows the heart rate. Reflex regulation of the heart rate in response to systemic blood pressure also occurs through activation of sensory receptors known as baroreceptors or pressure receptors located in the carotid sinus, aortic arch, venae cavae, and pulmonary veins.

If heart rate increases, cardiac output increases (up to a point) even if there is no change in stroke volume. However, rapid heart rates decrease the amount of time available for ventricular filling during diastole. Cardiac output then falls because decreased filling time decreases stroke volume. Coronary artery perfusion also decreases because the coronary arteries fill primarily during diastole. Cardiac output decreases during bradycardia if stroke volume stays the same, because the number of cardiac cycles is decreased.

Contractility

Contractility is the inherent capability of the cardiac muscle fibers to shorten. Poor contractility of the heart muscle reduces the forward flow of blood from the heart, increases the ventricu-

lar pressures from accumulation of blood volume, and reduces cardiac output. Increased contractility may stress the heart.

Preload

Preload is the amount of cardiac muscle fiber tension, or stretch, that exists at the end of diastole, just before contraction of the ventricles. Preload is influenced by venous return and the compliance of the ventricles. It is related to the total volume of blood in the ventricles: The greater the volume, the greater the stretch of the cardiac muscle fibers, and the greater the force with which the fibers contract to accomplish emptying. This principle is called Starling's law of the heart.

This mechanism has a physiologic limit. Just as continuous overstretching of a rubber band causes the band to relax and lose its ability to recoil, overstretching of the cardiac muscle fibers eventually results in ineffective contraction. Disorders such as renal disease and congestive heart failure result in sodium and water retention and increased preload. Vasoconstriction also increases venous return and preload.

Too little circulating blood volume results in a decreased venous return and therefore a decreased preload. A decreased preload reduces stroke volume and thus cardiac output. Decreased preload may result from hemorrhage or maldistribution of blood volume, as occurs in third spacing (see Chapter 10 ∞).

Afterload

Afterload is the force the ventricles must overcome to eject their blood volume. It is the pressure in the arterial system ahead of the ventricles. The right ventricle must generate enough tension to open the pulmonary valve and eject its volume into the low-pressure pulmonary arteries. Right ventricle afterload is measured as pulmonary vascular resistance (PVR). The left ventricle, in contrast, ejects its load by overcoming the pressure behind the aortic valve. Afterload of the left ventricle is measured as systemic vascular resistance (SVR). Arterial pressures are much higher than pulmonary pressures; thus, the left ventricle has to work much harder than the right ventricle.

Alterations in vascular tone affect afterload and ventricular work. As the pulmonary or arterial blood pressure increases (e.g., through vasoconstriction), PVR and/or SVR increases, and the work of the ventricles increases. As workload increases, consumption of myocardial oxygen also increases. A compromised heart cannot effectively meet this increased oxygen demand, and a vicious cycle ensues. By contrast, a very low afterload decreases the forward flow of blood into the systemic circulation and the coronary arteries.

Clinical Indicators of Cardiac Output

For many critically ill clients, invasive hemodynamic monitoring catheters are used to measure cardiac output in quantifiable numbers. However, advanced technology is not the only way to identify and assess compromised blood flow. Because cardiac output perfuses the body's tissues, clinical indicators of low cardiac output may be manifested by changes in organ function that result from compromised blood flow. For example, a decrease in blood flow to the brain presents as a change in level of consciousness. Other manifestations of decreased cardiac output are discussed in Chapters 10 and 31 ∞.

Cardiac index (CI) is the cardiac output adjusted for the client's body size, also called the client's body surface area (BSA). Because it takes into account the client's BSA, the cardiac index provides more meaningful data about the heart's ability to perfuse the tissues and therefore is a more accurate indicator of the effectiveness of the circulation.

BSA is stated in square meters (m^2), and cardiac index is calculated as CO divided by BSA. Cardiac measurements are considered adequate when they fall within the range of 2.5 to 4.2 L/min/m^2. For example, two clients are determined to have a cardiac output of 4 L/min. This parameter is within normal limits. However, one client is 5 feet, 2 inches (157 cm) tall and weighs 120 lb (54.5 kg), with a BSA of 1.54 m^2. This client's cardiac index is 4 ÷ 1.54, or 2.6 L/min/m^2. The second client is 6 feet, 2 inches (188 cm) tall and weighs 280 lb (81.7 kg), with a BSA of 2.52 m^2. This client's cardiac index is 4 ÷ 2.52, or 1.6 L/min/m^2. The cardiac index results show that the same cardiac output of 4 L/min is adequate for the first client but grossly inadequate for the second client.

The Conduction System of the Heart

The cardiac cycle is perpetuated by a complex electrical circuit commonly known as the intrinsic conduction system of the heart. Cardiac muscle cells possess an inherent characteristic of self-excitation, which enables them to initiate and transmit impulses independent of a stimulus. However, specialized areas of myocardial cells typically exert a controlling influence in this electrical pathway.

One of these specialized areas is the sinoatrial (SA) node, located at the junction of the superior vena cava and right atrium (Figure 30–7 ■). The SA node acts as the normal "pacemaker"

of the heart, usually generating an impulse 60 to 100 times per minute. This impulse travels across the atria via internodal pathways to the atrioventricular (AV) node, in the floor of the interatrial septum. The very small junctional fibers of the AV node slow the impulse, slightly delaying its transmission to the ventricles. It then passes through the bundle of His at the atrioventricular junction and continues down the interventricular septum through the right and left bundle branches and out to the Purkinje fibers in the ventricular muscle walls.

This path of electrical transmission produces a series of changes in ion concentration across the membrane of each cardiac muscle cell. The electrical stimulus increases the permeability of the cell membrane, creating an action potential (electrical potential). The result is an exchange of sodium, potassium, and calcium ions across the cell membrane, which changes the intracellular electrical charge to a positive state. This process of depolarization results in myocardial contraction. As the ion exchange reverses and the cell returns to its resting state of electronegativity, the cell is repolarized, and cardiac muscle relaxes. The cellular action potential serves as the basis for electrocardiography (ECG), a diagnostic test of cardiac function.

The Action Potential

Movement of ions across cell membranes causes the electrical impulse that stimulates muscle contraction. This electrical activity, called the *action potential*, produces the waveforms represented on ECG strips.

In the resting state, positive and negative ions align on either side of the cell membrane, producing a relatively negative charge within the cell and a positive extracellular charge (Figure 30–8 ■). The cell is said to be polarized. The negative resting membrane

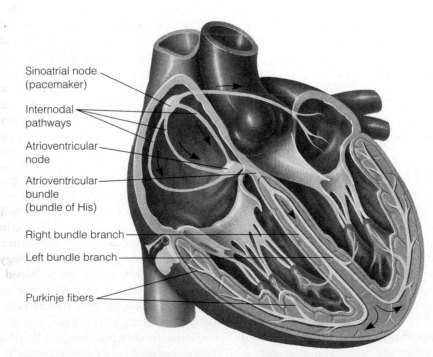

Sinoatrial node
(pacemaker)

Internodal
pathways

Atrioventricular
node

Atrioventricular
bundle
(bundle of His)

Right bundle branch

Left bundle branch

Purkinje fibers

Figure 30–7 ■ The intrinsic conduction system of the heart.

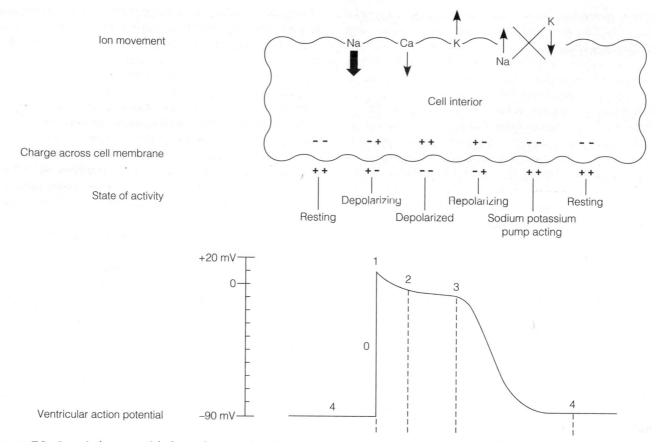

Figure 30–8 ■ Action potential of a cardiac muscle cell. In the resting state (phase 4), the cell membrane is polarized; the cell's interior has a negative charge compared to that of extracellular fluid. On depolarization (phase 0), sodium ions diffuse rapidly across the cell membrane into the cell, and calcium channels open. In the fully depolarized state (phase 1), the cell's interior has a net positive charge compared to its exterior. During the plateau period (phase 2), calcium moves into the cell and potassium diffusion slows, prolonging the action potential. In phase 3, calcium channels close, the sodium-potassium pump removes sodium from the cell, and the cell membrane again becomes polarized with a net negative charge.

potential is maintained at about −90 millivolts (mV) by the sodium-potassium pump in the cell membrane.

Depolarization

Two types of ion channels function to produce the electrical changes that occur during the depolarization phase: the fast sodium channels and the slow calcium channels. A fast action potential occurs in atrial and ventricular muscle cells and the Purkinje conduction system and uses the fast sodium channels. The slow type occurs in the SA and AV nodes, which use the slow calcium channels. The action potential for contraction of the heart is initiated in the SA node. When a resting cell is stimulated by an electrical charge from a neighboring cell or by a spontaneous event, its cell membrane permeability changes. Sodium ions enter the cell, and the membrane becomes less permeable to potassium ions. Addition of positively charged ions to intracellular fluid changes the membrane potential from negative to slightly positive at +20 to +30 mV. This change in the electrical charge across the cell membrane is called depolarization.

As the cell becomes more positive, it reaches a point called the threshold potential. When the threshold potential is

reached, an action potential is generated. The response to the action potential in the myocardial muscle cells causes a chemical reaction of calcium within the cell. This, in turn, causes actin and myosin filaments to slide together, producing cardiac muscle contraction. The action potential spreads to surrounding cells, causing a coordinated muscle contraction. As soon as the myocardium is completely depolarized, repolarization begins.

Repolarization

Repolarization returns the cell to its resting, polarized state. During rapid repolarization, fast sodium channels close abruptly, and the cell begins to regain its negative charge. During the plateau phase, muscle contraction is prolonged as slow calcium-sodium channels remain open. When these channels close, the sodium-potassium pump restores ion concentration to normal resting levels. The cell membrane is then polarized, ready for the cycle to start again. Each heartbeat represents one cardiac cycle, with one depolarization and repolarization cycle and one complete cardiac muscle contraction and relaxation (systole and diastole).

Normally, only pacemaker cells demonstrate automaticity. Pacemaker cells have a resting potential that is much less negative (-70 to -50 mV) than other cardiac muscle cells. Their threshold potential also is lower than that of other myocardial cells. These differences result from constant leakage of sodium and potassium ions into the cell.

Myocardial cells have a unique protective property, the refractory period, during which they resist stimulation. This property protects cardiac muscle from spasm and tetany. During the absolute refractory period, depolarization will not occur no matter how strongly the cell is stimulated. It is followed by the relative refractory period, during which a greater than normal stimulus is required to generate another action potential. During the supernormal period that follows, a mild stimulus will cause depolarization. Many cardiac dysrhythmias are triggered during the relative refractory and supernormal periods.

ASSESSING CARDIAC FUNCTION

Cardiac function is assessed by findings from diagnostic tests, a health assessment interview to collect subjective data, and a physical assessment to collect objective data. Sample documentation of an assessment of cardiac function is included in the box below.

Diagnostic Tests

The results of diagnostic tests of cardiac function are used to support the diagnosis of a specific disease, to provide information to identify or modify the appropriate medications or therapy used to treat the disease, and to help nurses monitor the client's responses to treatment and nursing care interventions. Diagnostic tests to assess the structures and functions of the heart are described on pages 944–946 and summarized in the following bulleted list. More information is included in the discussion of specific disorders in Chapters 31 and 32 ∞.

- The primary test used to identify the risk of coronary artery disease (CAD) or to monitor treatment for alterations in lipid levels is a measurement of lipid components of cholesterol, triglycerides, and lipolipids in the blood.
- Noninvasive tests of cardiac structure and function include a chest x-ray and stress/exercise tests. The treadmill test is the most basic exercise test, with diagnostic ability to measure cardiac perfusion enhanced by administering IV ra-

dioisotopes during the test. A treadmill exercise test is often combined with other tests to evaluate cardiac function under stress. The exercise thallium or technetium test is probably the most useful noninvasive test to monitor and diagnose CAD.

- Abnormal areas of the heart may be identified and evaluated by an MRI to locate areas of myocardial infarction, a CT scan to quantify calcium deposits in coronary arteries, or a PET test to evaluate myocardial perfusion and myocardial metabolic function.
- Echocardiograms are conducted in conjunction with Dopplers and color flow imaging to produce audio and graphic data about the motion, wall thickness, and chamber size of the heart and of the blood flow and velocity.
- A transesophageal echocardiogram (TEE) allows visualization of structures adjacent to the esophagus to visualize cardiac and extracardiac structures, including mitral valve and aortic valve pathology, left atrium intracardiac thrombosis, acute dissection of the aorta, endocarditis, and ventricular function during and after surgery.
- A cardiac catheterization with either coronary angiography or coronary arteriography may be performed to identify CAD or cardiac valvular disease, to determine pulmonary artery or heart chamber pressures, to obtain a myocardial biopsy, to evaluate artificial valves, or to do angioplasty or stent of an area of CAD.
- Pericardiocentesis is a procedure done to remove fluid from the pericardial sac for diagnostic or therapeutic purposes. It may also be an emergency procedure to treat cardiac tamponade.

Regardless of the type of diagnostic test, the nurse is responsible for explaining the procedure and any special preparation needed, for assessing for medication use that may affect the outcome of the tests, for supporting the client during the examination as necessary, for documenting the procedures as appropriate, and for monitoring the results of the tests.

Genetic Considerations

When conducting a health assessment interview and physical assessment, it is important for the nurse to consider genetic influences on health of the adult. During the health assessment interview, ask about family members with health problems affecting cardiac function, or of a family history of high cholesterol levels or early onset coronary artery disease. During the physical assessment, assess for any manifestations that might indicate a genetic disorder (see the box on page 950). If data are found to indicate genetic risk factors or alterations, ask about genetic testing and refer for appropriate genetic counseling and evaluation. Chapter 8 ∞ provides further information about genetics in medical-surgical nursing.

The Health Assessment Interview

A health assessment interview to determine problems with cardiac structure and function may be conducted during a health screening, may focus on a chief complaint (such as

---

SAMPLE DOCUMENTATION
Assessment of Cardiac Function

56-year-old male admitted to cardiac critical care unit from ED to rule out myocardial infarction. States he has pain in the middle of his chest that is "like a heavy pressure"; 6 on a 10-point scale. Skin cool, slightly moist. BP 190/94 right arm and 186/92 left arm (both reclining). Apical pulse 92, regular and strong. No pulse deficit. Respirations 28. Apical impulse non-palpable, no visible heaves or thrusts. S_1 and S_2 auscultated without murmurs or clicks. S_4 noted.

DIAGNOSTIC TESTS of Cardiac Disorders

NAME OF TEST Lipids

PURPOSE AND DESCRIPTION Blood lipids are cholesterol, triglycerides, and phospholipids. They circulate bound to proteins, and so are known as lipoproteins. Lipids are measured to evaluate risk for CAD and to monitor effectiveness of anti-cholesterol medications.

Normal values:
Cholesterol: 140–200 mg/dL
Triglycerides: 40–190 mg/dL

HDL: Men=37–70 mg/dL
Women=40–88 mg/dL
LDL: <130 mg/dL
(*Note:* Normal values may vary by laboratory.)

RELATED NURSING CARE Cholesterol levels alone may be measured at any time of the day, regardless of food or fluid intake. When measuring triglycerides and lipoproteins (HDL and LDL), fasting for 12 hours (except for water) with no alcohol intake for 24 hours prior to the test is recommended.

NAME OF TEST Electrocardiogram (ECG)

PURPOSE AND DESCRIPTION See Boxes 30–1 and 30–2.

RELATED NURSING CARE No special preparation is needed.

NAME OF TEST Chest x-ray

PURPOSE AND DESCRIPTION An x-ray of the thorax can illustrate the contours, placement, and chambers of the heart. It may be done to identify heart displacement or hypertrophy, or fluid in the pericardial sac.

RELATED NURSING CARE No special preparation is needed.

NAME OF TEST Stress/exercise tests
- Treadmill test

PURPOSE AND DESCRIPTION Stress testing is based on the theory that CAD results in depression of the ST segment with exercise. Depression of the ST segment and depression or inversion of the T wave indicates myocardial ischemia. When the client is walking on a treadmill machine, the work rate of the heart is changed every 3 minutes for 15 minutes by increasing the speed and degree of incline by 3% each time. Clients exercise until they are fatigued, develop symptoms, or reach their maximum predicted heart rate.

RELATED NURSING CARE *For all stress/exercise tests:* Ask the client to wear comfortable shoes, and to avoid food, fluids, and smoking for 2 to 3 hours before the test, assess for events that contraindicate the tests: recent myocardial infarction; severe, unstable angina; controlled dysrhythmias; congestive heart failure; or recent pulmonary embolism.

NAME OF TEST Thallium/technetium stress test (myocardial imaging perfusion test, cardiac blood pool imaging)

PURPOSE AND DESCRIPTION *Thallium stress test:* Thallium-201, a radioisotope that accumulates in myocardial cells, is used during the stress test to evaluate myocardial perfusion. Second scans are done 2 to 3 hours later when the heart is at rest; this is to differentiate between an ischemic area and an infarcted or scarred area of myocardium.

Exercise technetium perfusion test: Technetium 99m-laced compounds are administered and a scan is done to evaluate cardiac perfusion, wall motion, and ejection fraction. This is probably the most useful noninvasive test to diagnose and monitor CAD.

RELATED NURSING CARE Assess medications; those that affect the blood pressure or heart rate should be discontinued for 24 to 36 hours prior to the test (unless the test is being done to monitor the effectiveness of the medications).

NAME OF TEST Nuclear persantine [dipyridamole] stress test

PURPOSE AND DESCRIPTION This test is used when the client is not physically able to walk on the treadmill. Persantine, given IV, dilates the coronary arteries and increases myocardial blood flow. Coronary arteries that are narrowed from CAD cannot dilate to increase myocardial perfusion.

RELATED NURSING CARE Client is NPO after midnight except for water. Food, fluids, and drugs that contain caffeine should be avoided for 24 hours prior to the test, as should decaffeinated fluids. Some drugs, such as theophylline preparations, are discontinued for 36 hours prior to the test.

NAME OF TEST Nuclear dobutamine stress test

PURPOSE AND DESCRIPTION Dobutamine is an adrenergic drug that increases myocardial contractility, heart rate, and systolic blood pressure, which increases coronary oxygen consumption and thus increases coronary blood flow.

RELATED NURSING CARE Client is NPO after midnight except for water. Discontinue beta-blockers, calcium channel blockers, and ACE inhibitors for 36 hours prior to the test. Do not administer nitrates for 6 hours prior to the test.

NAME OF TEST Magnetic resonance imaging (MRI)

PURPOSE AND DESCRIPTION An MRI may be used to identify and locate areas of myocardial infarction.

RELATED NURSING CARE Assess for any metallic implants (such as pacemaker, body piercing, or artificial joint), which would contraindicate the test.

DIAGNOSTIC TESTS of Cardiac Disorders (continued)

NAME OF TEST Computed tomography (CT) scan

PURPOSE AND DESCRIPTION A CT scan may be conducted to quantify calcium deposits in coronary arteries.

RELATED NURSING CARE Assess for allergy to iodine or seafood if contrast medium is to be administered.

NAME OF TEST Cardiolite scan

PURPOSE AND DESCRIPTION Used to evaluate blood flow in different parts of the heart. Cardiolite (technetium 99m sestamibi) is injected IV. In a dipyridamole cardiolite scan, dipyridamole (Persantine) is injected to increase blood flow to coronary arteries. These scans may be done in conjunction with a treadmill test.

RELATED NURSING CARE See information in this table for treadmill test. Instruct the client to avoid intake of caffeine for 12 hours before having a test with dipyridamole cardiolite.

NAME OF TEST Positron emission tomography (PET)

PURPOSE AND DESCRIPTION Two scans are performed following injection of radionuclides, and the resulting images compared for myocardial perfusion and myocardial metabolic function. A stress test (treadmill) may be a part of the test. If the myocardium is ischemic or damaged, the images will be different. Normally, the images will be the same.

RELATED NURSING CARE Assess client's blood glucose: For accurate metabolic activity images, the blood glucose level must be between 60 and 140 mg/dL. If exercise is included in the test, the client will need to be NPO and avoid smoking and caffeine for 24 hours prior to the test.

NAME OF TEST Blood pool imaging

PURPOSE AND DESCRIPTION Following intravenous injection of technetium 99m pertechnetate, sequential evaluation of the heart can be performed for several hours. Useful for evaluation of cardiac status following myocardial infarction and congestive heart failure and effectiveness of cardiac medications. Can be done at the client's bedside.

RELATED NURSING CARE No special preparation is needed.

NAME OF TEST Echocardiogram

- M-mode
- Two-dimensional (2-D)
- Cardiac Doppler
- Color Doppler
- Stress echocardiogram

PURPOSE AND DESCRIPTION Echocardiograms use a transducer to record waves that are bounced off the heart, and to record the direction and flow of blood through the heart in audio and graphic data. An *M(motion)-mode echocardiogram* records the motion, wall thickness, and chamber size of the heart. A *2-D echocardiogram* provides a cross-sectional view of the heart. *Color flow imaging* combines 2-D echocardiography and Doppler technology to evaluate the speed and direction of blood flow through the heart, which can identify pathology such as leaky valves. *Stress echocardiography* combines a treadmill test with ultrasound images to evaluate segmental function and wall motion. If the client is not physically able to exercise, IV dobutamine may be administered and ultrasound images taken.

RELATED NURSING CARE No special preparation is needed; see related nursing care for the client having a treadmill test for a stress echocardiogram.

NAME OF TEST Transesophageal echocardiography (TEE)

PURPOSE AND DESCRIPTION Allows visualization of adjacent cardiac and extracardiac structures to identify or monitor mitral and aortic valve pathology, left atrium intracardiac thrombus, acute dissection of the aorta, endocarditis, perioperative left ventricular function, and intracardiac repairs during surgery. A transducer (probe) attached to an endoscope is inserted into the esophagus, and images are taken. Concurrent IV contrast medium, Doppler ultrasound, and color flow imaging may be used.

NAME OF TEST Cardiac catheterization (coronary angiography, coronary arteriography)

PURPOSE AND DESCRIPTION A cardiac catheterization may be performed to identify CAD or cardiac valvular disease, to determine pulmonary artery or heart chamber pressures, to obtain a myocardial biopsy, to evaluate artificial valves, or to perform angioplasty or stent an area of CAD. The test is performed by inserting a long catheter into a vein or artery (depending on whether the right side or the left side of the heart is being examined) in the arm or leg. Using fluoroscopy, the catheter is then threaded to the heart chambers or coronary arteries or both. Contrast dye is injected and heart structures are visualized and heart activity is filmed. The test is done for diagnosis and before heart surgery.

Right cardiac catheterization: The catheter is inserted into the femoral vein or antecubital vein and then threaded through the inferior vena cava into the right atrium to the pulmonary artery. Pressures are measured at each site and blood samples can be obtained for the right side of the heart. The functions of the tricuspid and pulmonary valves can be observed.

Left cardiac catheterization: The catheter is inserted into the brachial or femoral artery and advanced retrograde through the aorta to the coronary arteries and/or left ventricle. The patency of the coronary arteries and/or functions of the aortic and mitral valves and left ventricle can be observed.

NURSING CARE: CARDIAC CATHETERIZATION

Before the Procedure

- Explain the procedure to the client.
- No food or fluids are allowed for 6 to 8 hours before the test.

(continued)

DIAGNOSTIC TESTS of Cardiac Disorders (continued)

- Assess for allergies to seafood, iodine, or iodine contrast dyes (if previous tests have been done). If an allergic response to the dye is possible, antihistamines (such as Benadryl) or steroids may be administered the evening before and the morning of the test.
- Assess for use of aspirin or NSAIDs (risk of bleeding), Viagra (risk of heart problems), or history of kidney disease (dye used may be toxic to the kidneys).
- Discontinue oral anticoagulant medications. Heparin may be ordered to prevent thrombi.
- An IV of 5% D_5W is started at a keep-vein-open rate (to be available if emergency drugs have to be administered).
- Establish baseline of peripheral pulses.
- Take and record baseline vital signs.

Procedure

- Client is positioned on a padded table that tilts. A local anesthetic is used at the site of catheter insertion. ECG leads are applied and vital signs are monitored during the procedure.

The client lies supine and is asked to cough and deep breathe frequently. The procedure takes 1/2 to 3 hours.
- Tell the client that a hot, flushing sensation may be felt for a minute or two when the dye is injected.

After the Procedure

- Monitor vital signs every 15 minutes for the first hour and then every 30 minutes until stable. Assess cardiac rhythm and rate for alterations. Assess peripheral pulses distal to the insertion site.
- Assess client for complaints of chest heaviness, shortness of breath, and abdominal or groin pain.
- Monitor catheter insertion site for bleeding or hematoma.
- Administer pain medications as prescribed.
- Instruct client to remain on bed rest for 6 to 12 hours (or as ordered). If a collagen-like plug was inserted after removal of the catheter, only a 2- to 3-hour bed rest is necessary.
- Encourage oral fluids unless contraindicated (i.e., if the client has congestive heart failure).

NAME OF TEST Pericardiocentesis

PURPOSE AND DESCRIPTION This procedure is performed to remove fluid from the pericardial sac for diagnostic or therapeutic purposes. It may also be done as an emergency procedure for the client with cardiac tamponade (which may result in death). A large-gauge (16 to 18) needle is inserted to the left of the xiphoid process into the pericardial sac and excess fluid is withdrawn (see Figure 30–9 ■). The needle is attached to an ECG lead to help determine if the needle is touching the epicardial surface, thus preventing piercing of the myocardium.

NURSING CARE: PERICARDIOCENTESIS

Before the Procedure

- Gather all supplies:
  a. Pericardiocentesis tray
  b. ECG machine and electrode patches
  c. Emergency cart with defibrillator
  d. Dressing
  e. Culture bottles (if indicated)
- Reinforce teaching and answer questions about the procedure or associated care. Provide emotional support.
- Ensure that informed consent has been obtained.
- Provide for privacy.
- Obtain and document baseline vital signs.
- Connect the client to a cardiac monitor; obtain a baseline rhythm strip for comparison during and after the procedure.
- Connect the precordial ECG lead of the hub of the aspiration needle using an alligator clamp.

During the Procedure

- Follow standard precautions.
- Position seated at a 45- to 60-degree angle. Place a dry towel under the rib cage to catch blood or fluid leakage.
- Observe the ST segment for elevation and the ECG monitor for signs of myocardial irritability (PVCs) during the procedure. These indicate that the needle is touching the myocardium and should be withdrawn slightly.

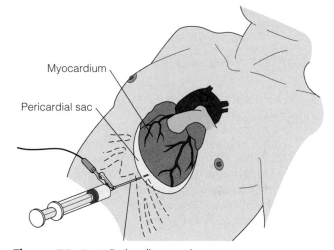

Myocardium

Pericardial sac

Figure 30–9 ■ Pericardiocentesis.

- Notify the physician of changes in cardiac rhythm, blood pressure, heart rate, level of consciousness, and urine output. These may indicate cardiac complications.
- Monitor central venous pressure (CVP) and blood pressure closely. As the effusion is relieved, CVP will decrease, and BP will increase.

After the Procedure

- Document the procedure and the client's response to and tolerance of the procedure.
- Continue to monitor vital signs and cardiac rhythm every 15 min during the first hour, every 30 min during the next hour, every hour for the next 24 hours.
- Record the amount of fluid removed as output on the intake and output record.
- If indicated, send a sample of aspirated fluid for culture and sensitivity and laboratory analysis.
- Assess heart and breath sounds.

BOX 30–1 Electrocardiogram

The electrocardiogram (ECG) is a graphic record of the heart's activity. Electrodes applied to the body surface are used to obtain a graphic representation of cardiac electrical activity. These electrodes detect the magnitude and direction of electrical currents produced in the heart. They attach to the electrocardiograph by an insulated wire called a lead. The electrocardiograph converts the electrical impulses it receives into a series of waveforms that represent cardiac depolarization and repolarization. Placement of electrodes on different parts of the body allows different views of this electrical activity, much like turning the head while holding a camera provides different views of the scenery. ECG waveforms and patterns are examined to detect dysrhythmias as well as myocardial damage, the effects of drugs, and electrolyte imbalances.

ECG waveforms reflect the direction of electrical flow in relation to a positive electrode. Current flowing toward the positive electrode produces an upward (positive) waveform; current flowing away from the positive electrode produces a downward (negative) waveform. Current flowing perpendicular to the positive pole produces a biphasic (both positive and negative) waveform. Absence of electrical activity is represented by a straight line called the isoelectric line.

ECG waveforms are recorded by a heated stylus on heat-sensitive paper. The paper is marked at standard intervals that represent time and voltage or amplitude (see Figure 1). Each small box is 1 mm^2. The recording speed of the standard ECG is 25 mm/second, so each small box represents 0.04 second. Five small boxes horizontally and vertically make one large box, equivalent to 0.20 second. Five large boxes represent 1 full second. Measured vertically, each small box represents 0.1 mV.

Both bipolar and unipolar leads are used in recording the ECG. A bipolar lead uses two electrodes of opposite polarity (negative and positive). In a *unipolar* lead, one positive electrode and a negative reference point at the center of the heart are used. The electrical potential between the two monitoring points is graphically recorded as the ECG waveform.

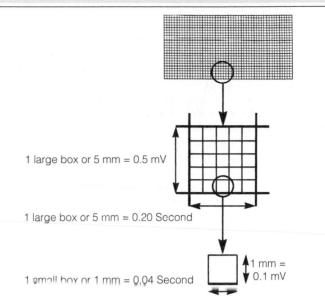

1 large box or 5 mm = 0.5 mV

1 large box or 5 mm = 0.20 Second

1 small box or 1 mm = 0.04 Second

1 mm = 0.1 mV

1) Time and voltage measurements on ECG paper at a recording speed of 25 mm/second.

The heart can be viewed from both the frontal plane and the horizontal plane (see Figure 2). Each plane provides a unique perspective of the heart muscle. The frontal plane is an imaginary cut through the body that views the heart from top to bottom (superior–inferior) and side to side (right–left). This perspective of the heart is analogous to a paper doll cutout. It provides information about the inferior and lateral walls of the heart. The horizontal plane is a cross-sectional view of the heart from front to back (anterior–posterior) and side to side (right–left). Information regarding the anterior, septal, and lateral walls of the heart, as well as the posterior wall, are obtained from this view.

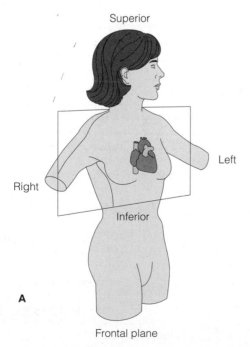

Superior

Left

Right

Inferior

A

Frontal plane

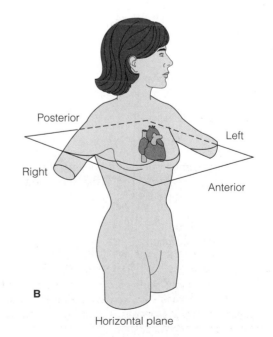

Posterior

Left

Right

Anterior

B

Horizontal plane

2) Planes of the heart. *A*, Frontal plane, *B*, horizontal plane.

(continued)

BOX 30–1 **Electrocardiogram** (continued)

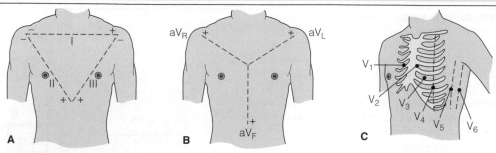

3) Leads of the 12-lead ECG. *A,* Bipolar limb leads I, II, III; *B,* Unipolar limb leads aV$_R$, aV$_L$, aV$_F$; *C,* Unipolar precordial leads V$_1$ to V$_6$.

A standard 12-lead ECG provides a simultaneous recording of six limb leads and six precordial leads (see Figure 3). The limb leads provide information about the heart in the frontal plane and include three bipolar leads (I, II, III) and three unipolar leads (aV$_R$, aV$_L$, and aV$_F$). The bipolar limb leads measure electrical activity between a negative lead on one extremity and a positive lead on another. The unipolar limb leads (called augmented leads) measure the electrical activity between a single positive electrode on a limb (right arm [R], left arm [L], or left leg [F for foot]), and the center of the heart.

The precordial leads, also known as chest leads or V leads, view the heart in the horizontal plane. They include six unipolar leads (V$_1$, V$_2$, V$_3$, V$_4$, V$_5$, and V$_6$), which measure electrical activity between the center of the heart and a positive electrode on the chest wall.

The cardiac cycle is depicted as a series of waveforms, the P, Q, R, S, and T waves (see Figure 4).

■ The *P wave* represents atrial depolarization and contraction. The impulse is from the sinus node. The P wave precedes the QRS complex and is normally smooth, round, and upright. P waves may be absent when the SA node is not acting as the pacemaker. Atrial repolarization occurs during ventricular depolarization and usually is not seen on the ECG.

■ The *PR interval* represents the time required for the sinus impulse to travel to the AV node and into the Purkinje fibers. This interval is measured from beginning of P wave to beginning of QRS complex. If no Q wave is seen, the beginning of the R wave is used. The PR interval is normally 0.12 to 0.20 second (up to 0.24 second is considered normal in clients over age 65). PR intervals greater than 0.20 second indicate a delay in conduction from the SA node to the ventricles.

■ The *QRS complex* represents ventricular depolarization and contraction. The QRS complex includes three separate waves: The Q wave is the first negative deflection, the R wave is the positive or upright deflection, and the S wave is the first negative deflection after the R wave. Not all QRS complexes have all three waves; nonetheless, the complex is called a QRS complex. The normal duration of a QRS complex is from 0.06 to 0.10 second. QRS complexes greater than 0.10 second indicate delays in transmitting the impulse through the ventricular conduction system.

■ The *ST segment* signifies the beginning of ventricular repolarization. The ST segment, the period from the end of the QRS complex to the beginning of the T wave, should be isoelectric. An abnormal ST segment is displaced (elevated or depressed) from the isoelectric line.

■ The *T wave* represents ventricular repolarization. It normally has a smooth, rounded shape that is usually less than 10 mm tall. It usually points in the same direction as the QRS complex. Abnormalities of the T wave may indicate myocardial ischemia or injury, or electrolyte imbalances.

■ The *QT interval* is measured from the beginning of the QRS complex to the end of the T wave. It represents the total time of ventricular depolarization and repolarization. Its duration varies with gender, age, and heart rate; usually, it is 0.32 to 0.44 second long. Prolonged QT intervals indicate a prolonged relative refractory period and a greater risk of dysrhythmias. Shortened QT intervals may result from medications or electrolyte imbalances.

■ The *U wave* is not normally seen. It is thought to signify repolarization of the terminal Purkinje fibers. If present, the U wave follows the same direction as the T wave. It is most commonly seen in hypokalemia.

Sinoatrial node

Atrioventricular node

QRS complex

R

Ventricular depolarization

Atrial depolarization

Ventricular repolarization

P

T

Q

S

ST Segment

PR Interval

Time(s)   0   0.2   0.4   0.6   0.8

QT Interval

4) Normal ECG waveform and intervals.

BOX 30–2 Interpreting an ECG

Interpreting an ECG strip to determine the cardiac rhythm is a skill that takes practice to learn and master. Many methods are used to analyze ECGs. It is important to use a consistent method for ECG analysis. Identifying and interpreting complex dysrhythmias requires advanced skills and knowledge obtained through further training. One method follows:

- *Step 1: Determine rate.* Assess heart rate. Use P waves to determine the atrial rate and R waves for the ventricular rate. Several approaches can determine the heart rate.
  - Count the number of complexes in a 6-second rhythm strip (the top margin of ECG paper is marked at 3-second intervals), and multiply by 10. This provides an estimate of the rate and is particularly valuable if rhythms are irregular.
  - Count the number of large boxes between two consecutive complexes, and divide 300 (the number of large boxes in 1 minute) by this number. For example, there are 6 large boxes between two R waves; 300 divided by 6 equals a ventricular rate of 50 bpm. Memorize the following sequence for rapid rate determination: 300, 150, 100, 75, 60, 50, 43. One large box between complexes equals a rate of 300; two, a rate of 150; three, a rate of 100; and so on.
  - Count the number of small boxes between two consecutive complexes, and divide 1500 (the number of small boxes in 1 minute) by this number. For example, there are 19 small boxes between two R waves; 1500 divided by 19 equals a ventricular rate of 79 bpm. This is the most precise measurement of heart rate
- *Step 2: Determine regularity.* Regularity is the consistency with which the P waves or QRS complexes occur. In a regular rhythm, all waves occur at a consistent rate. Rhythm regularity is determined by measuring the interval between consecutive waves. Place one point of an ECG caliper (a measuring device) on the peak of the P wave (for atrial rhythm) or the R wave (for ventricular rhythm). Adjust the other point to the peak of the next wave, P to P or R to R (see the figure in this box). Keeping the calipers set at this distance, evaluate intervals between consecutive waves. The rhythm is *regular* if all caliper points fall on succeeding wave peaks. Alternately, use a strip of blank paper on top of the ECG strip, marking the peaks of two or three consecutive waves. Then move the paper along the strip to consecutive waves. Wave peaks that vary by more than one to three small boxes (depending on the rate) are *irregular*. Irregular rhythms may be *irregularly irregular* (if the intervals have no pattern) or *regularly irregular* (if a consistent pattern to the irregularity can be identified).

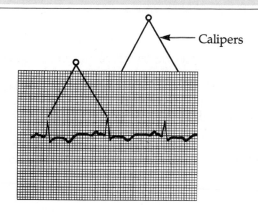

Calipers

- *Step 3: Assess P wave.* The presence or absence of P waves helps determine origin of the rhythm. All the P waves should be alike in size and shape (*morphology*). If P waves are not seen or they differ in shape, the rhythm may not originate in the sinus node.
- *Step 4: Assess P to QRS relationship.* Determine the relationship between P waves and QRS complexes. There should be one and only one P wave for every QRS complex, because the normal stimulus for ventricular contraction originates in the sinus node.
- *Step 5: Determine interval durations.* To evaluate impulse transmission through the cardiac conduction system, measure the PR interval, QRS duration, and QT interval. To measure, count the number of small boxes from the beginning of the interval to the end, and multiply by 0.04 second. Then determine whether the interval duration is within its normal limits. For example, the PR interval is 3.5 small boxes wide, or 0.14 second. This is within the normal limits of 0.12 to 0.20 second. This interval should be consistent, not varying from beat to beat. A PR interval greater than 0.20 second or one that varies from beat to beat is abnormal.

  The QRS complex duration is normally between 0.06 and 0.10 second. A QRS complex greater than 0.12 second indicates delayed ventricular conduction.

  The QT interval is normally 0.32 to 0.44 second. It varies inversely with the heart rate: The faster the heart rate, the shorter the QT interval. As a general rule, the QT interval should be no more than half the previous R–R interval. A prolonged QT interval indicates a prolonged relative refractory period of the heart.
- *Step 6: Identify abnormalities.* Note the presence and frequency of *ectopic* (extra) beats, deviation of the ST segment above or below the baseline, and abnormalities in waveform shape and duration.

chest pain), or may be part of a total health assessment. If the client has a problem with cardiac function, analyze its onset, characteristics, course, severity, precipitating and relieving factors, and any associated symptoms, noting the timing and circumstances. For example, ask the client:

- What is the location of the chest pain you experienced? Did it move up to your jaw or into your left arm?
- Describe the type of activity that brings on your chest pain.
- Have you noticed any changes in your energy level?

- Have you felt light-headed during the times your heart is racing?

The interview begins by exploring the client's chief complaint (e.g., chest pain, palpitations, or shortness of breath). Describe the client's chest pain in terms of location, quality or character, timing, setting or precipitating factors, severity, aggravating and relieving factors, and associated symptoms (Table 30–1).

Explore the client's history for heart disorders such as angina, heart attack, congestive heart failure (CHF), hypertension

GENETIC CONSIDERATIONS
Cardiac Disorders

- Familial hypercholesterolemia is a single gene disorder that results in atherosclerosis and CAD, which may occur at an earlier age than in the general population (i.e., before age 55 in men and age 65 in women). However, increased cholesterol levels may also be inherited and are a risk factor for CAD in both men and women.
- Marfan's syndrome is an autosomal-dominant inherited disorder that affects the skeleton, the eyes, and the cardiovascular system. The cardiovascular effects are a dilatation of the proximal aorta and aortic dissection associated with degeneration of the elastic fibers in the tunica media of the aorta. There may also be thoracic aortic aneurysms.
- Supraventricular aortic stenosis (SVAS) is a genetic vascular disorder resulting in an hourglass-shaped stenosis of the ascending aorta. It may also affect other major arteries, including the pulmonary, carotid, cerebral, renal, and coronary arteries.
- Hypertropic cardiomyopathy, a disease of sarcomere proteins, has a genetic transmission.
- Williams syndrome is a rare genetic disorder characterized by characteristic "elfin-like" features and heart and blood vessel problems (as well as other physical problems).
- Long QT syndrome (LQTS) is an inherited genetic disorder that results from structural abnormalities of the potassium channels in the heart, leading to dysrhythmias. This can result in unconsciousness, and may cause sudden cardiac death in teenagers and young adults when exposed to stressors ranging from exercise to loud sounds.

TABLE 30–1 Assessing Chest Pain

CHARACTERISTIC	EXAMPLES
Location	Substernal, precordial, jaw, back Localized or diffuse Radiation to neck, jaw, shoulder, arm
Character/quality	Pressure; tightness; crushing, burning, or aching quality; heaviness; dullness; "heartburn" or indigestion
Timing: onset, duration, and frequency	Onset: Sudden or gradual? Duration: How many minutes does the pain last? Frequency: Is the pain continuous or periodic?
Setting/precipitating factors	Awake, at rest, sleep interrupted? With activity? With eating, exertion, exercise, elimination, emotional upset?
Intensity/severity	Can range from 0 (no pain) to 10 (worst pain ever felt)
Aggravating factors	Activity, breathing, temperature
Relieving factors	Medication (nitroglycerin, antacid), rest; there may be no relieving factors
Associated symptoms	Fatigue, shortness of breath, palpitations, nausea and vomiting, sweating, anxiety, light-headedness or dizziness

(HTN), and valvular disease. Ask the client about previous heart surgery or illnesses, such as rheumatic fever, scarlet fever, or recurrent streptococcal throat infections. Also ask about the presence and treatment of other chronic illnesses such as diabetes mellitus, bleeding disorders, or endocrine disorders. Review the client's family history for CAD, HTN, stroke, hyperlipidemia, diabetes, congenital heart disease, or sudden death.

Ask the client about past or present occurrence of various cardiac symptoms, such as chest pain, shortness of breath, difficulty breathing, cough, palpitations, fatigue, light-headedness or dizziness, fainting, heart **murmur**, blood clots, or swelling. Because cardiac function affects all other body systems, a full history may need to explore other related systems, such as respiratory function and/or peripheral vascular function.

Review the client's personal habits and nutritional history, including body weight; eating patterns; dietary intake of fats, salt, fluids; dietary restrictions; hypersensitivities or intolerances to food or medication; and the use of caffeine and alcohol. If the client uses tobacco products, ask about type (cigarettes, pipe, cigars, snuff), duration, amount, and efforts to quit. If the client uses street drugs, ask about type, method of intake (e.g., inhaled or injected), duration of use, and efforts to quit. Include questions about the client's activity level and tolerance, recreational activities, and relaxation habits. Assess the client's sleep patterns for interruptions in sleep due to dyspnea, cough, discomfort, urination, or stress. Ask how many pillows the client uses when sleeping. Also consider psychosocial factors that may affect the client's stress level: What is the client's marital status, family composition, and role within the family? Have there been any changes? What is the client's occupation, level of education, and socioeconomic level? Are resources for support available? What is the client's emotional disposition and personality type? How does the client perceive his or her state of health or illness, and how able is the client to comply with treatment?

Interview questions categorized by functional health patterns are listed in the table on the next page.

Physical Assessment

Physical assessment of cardiac function may be performed either as part of a total assessment or alone for clients with suspected or known problems with cardiac function. Assess the heart through inspection, palpation, and auscultation over the precordium (the area of the chest wall overlying the heart). Normal age-related findings for the older adult are summarized in Table 30–2. Before beginning the assessment, collect all required equipment and explain the techniques to the client to decrease anxiety. A quiet environment is essential to hear and assess heart sounds accurately.

The client may sit or lie in the supine position. Movements over the precordium may be more easily seen with tangential

FUNCTIONAL HEALTH PATTERN INTERVIEW   The Cardiac System

Functional Health Pattern	Interview Questions and Leading Statements
Health Perception-Health Management	■ Have you ever had any problems with your heart, such as angina (pain), heart attack, or disease of the valves? If so, describe. What was used to treat these problems? ■ Have you been diagnosed with high blood pressure? If so, how is it treated? ■ Do you have a history of rheumatic fever, scarlet fever, or strep throat infections? If so, describe them and their treatment. ■ Have you had your cholesterol checked recently? What is it? If you have high cholesterol, how is it treated? ■ Have you ever had tests to check the function of your heart? Describe them if so. ■ Do you take any medications to make your heart function more effectively, such as aspirin, those to control your heart rate, anticoagulants, or diuretics? How often do you take them? ■ Do you have a pacemaker? At what age and for what problem? How do you check the batteries? ■ Do you smoke, chew tobacco, or use snuff? If so, how often and how much? ■ Do you drink alcohol? If so, what type, how much, and for how long? ■ Are you able to manage your activities of daily living and work independently? Explain.
Nutritional-Metabolic	■ Describe your food and liquid intake in a 24-hour period. How often do you eat fried foods, fast foods, or meat? ■ How much salt do you use on food? ■ Do you eat high-fiber foods? If so, what are they and how often? ■ Have you had a recent weight gain or loss? Explain. ■ Have you noticed any change in color of your skin; for example, pale or dusky or flushed? If so, do you know what causes this? ■ Have you had any swelling in your feet or legs? Where and how much? What do you do to relieve it? ■ Do you feel tired during the day? What do you do when you are tired?
Elimination	■ Has a heart problem interfered with your usual bowel and bladder elimination? Explain.
Activity-Exercise	■ Describe your usual activity in a 24-hour period. ■ Has there been any change in your ability, energy, or strength to perform your usual activities (such as bathing, cleaning house, yard work, shopping)? If so, explain. ■ Do you ever have to stop and rest while doing daily activities? Explain. ■ Do you notice shortness of breath with certain activities? If so, what are they? How long does this last? What do you do to breathe better? ■ Describe any cough you have had. Was it dry or wet? Do you cough up mucus? If so, what color is it? How long have you had the cough? ■ Have you experienced any numbness or tingling, dizziness or light-headedness, or palpitations? Describe if so. ■ Have you ever used oxygen?
Sleep-Rest	■ How long do you sleep each night? Do you feel rested after you sleep? ■ Does your heart problem interfere with your ability to sleep and rest? Explain. ■ How many pillows do you use at night? ■ Where do you sleep at night (e.g., in a recliner to breathe more easily)? ■ Do you ever feel short of breath while you are resting or sleeping? Does this wake you up if so? Explain.
Cognitive-Perceptual	■ Describe any chest pain you have experienced. When did it occur? Where was it located? On a scale of 0 to 10, with 10 being the worst pain you have ever had, rate the pain and describe it (for example, burning, crushing, stabbing, squeezing, heavy, tight). ■ What were you doing when the pain began, for example, were you working or resting? Did it begin suddenly or gradually? How long did it last? ■ Did you have any other symptoms with the pain, such as nausea or vomiting, sweating, racing heart, pale skin, palpitations? ■ What made the pain worse? What did you do to try to relieve the pain? Did that work?
Self-Perception-Self-Concept	■ How does having this condition make you feel about yourself?
Role-Relationships	■ How does this condition affect your relationships with others? ■ Has having this condition interfered with your ability to work? Explain.

(continued)

FUNCTIONAL HEALTH PATTERN INTERVIEW   The Cardiac System (continued)

Functional Health Pattern	Interview Questions and Leading Statements
Sexuality-Reproductive	■ Has this condition interfered with your usual sexual activity? ■ Have you ever had chest pain during sexual activity? What do you do for it? ■ Do you use a slower pace or different positions that are less stressful for you during sexual activities? Does this help?
Coping-Stress-Tolerance	■ Has having this condition created stress for you? ■ Have you experienced any kind of stress that makes this condition worse? Explain. ■ Describe what you do when you feel stressed.
Value-Belief	■ Describe how specific relationships or activities help you cope with this problem. ■ Describe specific cultural beliefs or practices that affect how you care for and feel about this problem. ■ Are there any specific treatments that you would not use to treat this problem?

lighting (in which the light is directed at a right angle to the area being observed, producing shadows). Assess the following types of movements:

■ The **apical impulse** is a normal, visible pulsation (**thrust**) in the area of the midclavicular line in the left fifth intercostal space. It can be seen on inspection in about half of the adult population. (The apical impulse was previously called the point of maximal impulse [PMI] but this is no longer used because a maximal impulse may occur in other areas of the precordium as a result of abnormal conditions.)

■ **Retraction** is a pulling in of the tissue of the precordium; a slight retraction just medial to the midclavicular line at the area of the apical impulse is normal and is more likely to be visible in thin clients.

■ **Pulsations** (other than the normal apical pulsations), which may be called **heaves** or **lifts**, are considered abnormal. They may occur as the result of an enlarged ventricle.

TABLE 30–2 Age-Related Cardiac Changes

AGE-RELATED CHANGE	SIGNIFICANCE
Myocardium: ↓ efficiency and contractibility. Sinus node: ↑ in thickness of shell surrounding the node, and a ↓ in the number of pacemaker cells	■ Decreased cardiac output when under physiologic stress with resulting tachycardia that lasts longer. The person may require rest time between physical activities.
Left ventricle: Slight hypertrophy, prolonged isometric contraction phase and relaxation time; ↑ time for diastolic filling and systolic emptying cycle.	■ Stroke volume may increase to compensate for tachycardia, leading to increased blood pressure.
Valves and blood vessels: Aorta is elongated and dilated, valves are thicker and more rigid, and resistance to peripheral blood flow increases by 1% per year.	■ Blood pressure increases to compensate for increased peripheral resistance and decreased cardiac output.

CARDIAC ASSESSMENTS

Technique/Normal Findings	Abnormal Findings

Apical Impulse Assessment

First using the palmar surface and then repeating with finger pads, palpate the precordium for symmetry of movement	■ An enlarged or displaced heart is associated with an apical impulse lateral to the midclavicular line (MCL) or below the fifth left intercostal space (ICS). ■ Increased size, amplitude, and duration of the apical impulse are associated with left ventricular volume overload (increased afterload) in conditions such as HTN and aortic

Technique/Normal Findings	Abnormal Findings

and the apical impulse for location, size, amplitude, and duration. The sequence for palpation is shown in Figure 30–10 ■. To locate the apical impulse, ask the client to assume a left lateral recumbent position. Simultaneous palpation of the carotid pulse may also be helpful. *The apical impulse is not palpable in all clients. The apical impulse may be palpated in the mitral area, and has only a brief small amplitude.*

stenosis, and with pressure overload (increased preload) in conditions such as aortic or mitral regurgitation.

- Increased amplitude alone may occur with hyperkinetic states, such as anxiety, hyperthyroidism, and anemia.
- Decreased amplitude is associated with a dilated heart in cardiomyopathy.
- Displacement alone may also occur with dextrocardia, diaphragmatic hernia, gastric distention, or chronic lung disease.

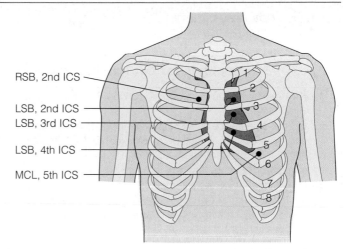

RSB, 2nd ICS
LSB, 2nd ICS
LSB, 3rd ICS
LSB, 4th ICS
MCL, 5th ICS

Figure 30–10 ■ Areas for inspection and palpation of the precordium, indicating the sequence for palpation.

- A **thrill** (a palpable vibration over the precordium or an artery) may accompany severe valve stenosis.
- A marked increase in amplitude of the apical impulse at the right ventricular area occurs with right ventricular volume overload in atrial septal defect.
- An increase in amplitude and duration occurs with right ventricular pressure overload in pulmonic stenosis and pulmonary hypertension. A lift or heave may also be seen in these conditions (and in chronic lung disease).
- A palpable thrill in this area occurs with ventricular septal defect.

Palpate the subxiphoid area with the index and middle finger. *No pulsations or vibrations should be palpated.*

- Right ventricular enlargement may produce a downward pulsation against the fingertips.
- An accentuated pulsation at the pulmonary area may be present in hyperkinetic states.
- A prominent pulsation reflects increased flow or dilation of the pulmonary artery.
- A thrill may be associated with aortic or pulmonary stenosis, aortic stenosis, pulmonary HTN, or atrial septal defect.
- Increased pulsation at the aortic area may suggest aortic aneurysm.
- A palpable second heart sound (S_2) may be noted with systemic HTN.

Cardiac Rate and Rhythm Assessment

Auscultate heart rate. *The heart rate should be 60 to 100 beats per minute with regular rhythm.*

- A heart rate exceeding 100 beats per minute (beats/min) is tachycardia. A heart rate less than 60 beats/min is bradycardia.

Simultaneously palpate the radial pulse while listening to the apical pulse. *The radial and apical pulses should be equal.*

- If the radial pulse falls behind the apical rate, the client has a pulse deficit, indicating weak, ineffective contractions of the left ventricle.

Auscultate heart rhythm. *The heart rhythm should be regular.*

- **Dysrhythmias** (abnormal heart rate or rhythm) may be regular or irregular in rhythm; their rates may be slow or fast. Irregular rhythms may occur in a pattern (e.g., an early beat every second beat, called bigeminy), sporadically, or with frequency and disorganization (e.g., atrial fibrillation). A pattern of gradual increase and decrease in heart rate that is within normal heart rate and that correlates with inspiration and expiration is called sinus arrhythmia.

MEDIALINK

Dysrhythmia Animation

Technique/Normal Findings	Abnormal Findings

Heart Sounds Assessment

See guidelines for cardiac auscultation in Box 30–3.

BOX 30–3 Guidelines for Cardiac Auscultation

1. Locate the major auscultatory areas on the precordium (see Figure 30–11).
2. Choose a sequence of listening. Either begin from the apex and move upward along the sternal border to the base, or begin at the base and move downward to the apex. One suggested sequence is shown in Figure 30–11.
3. Listen first with the client in the sitting or supine position. Then ask the client to lie on the left side, and focus on the apex. Lastly, ask the client to sit up and lean forward. These position changes bring the heart closer to the chest wall and enhance

auscultation. Carry out the following steps when the client assumes each of these positions:

a. First, auscultate each area with the diaphragm of the stethoscope to listen for high-pitched sounds: S_1, S_2, murmurs, pericardial friction rubs.
b. Next, auscultate each area with the bell of the stethoscope to listen for lower pitched sounds: S_3, S_4, murmurs.
c. Listen for the effect of respirations on each sound; while the client is sitting up and leaning forward, ask the client to exhale and hold the breath while you listen to heart sounds.

Identify S_1 (first heart sound) and note its intensity. At each auscultatory area, listen for several cardiac cycles. See Figure 30–11 ■ for auscultation areas. *S_1 is loudest at the apex of the heart.*

- An accentuated S_1 occurs with tachycardia, states in which cardiac output is high (fever, anxiety, exercise, anemia, hyperthyroidism), complete heart block, and mitral stenosis.
- A diminished S_1 occurs with first-degree heart block, mitral regurgitation, CHF, CAD, and pulmonary or systemic HTN. The intensity is also decreased with obesity, emphysema, and pericardial effusion. Varying intensity of S_1 occurs with complete heart block and grossly irregular rhythms.

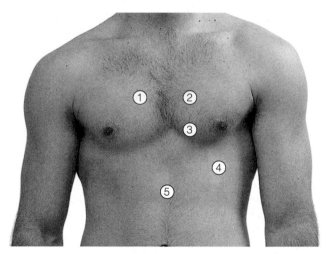

Figure 30–11 ■ Areas for auscultation of the heart.

Listen for splitting of S_1. *Splitting of S_1 may occur during inspiration.*

- Abnormal splitting of S_1 may be heard with right bundle branch block and premature ventricular contractions.

Identify S_2 (second heart sound) and note its intensity. *S_2 immediately follows S_1 and is loudest at the base of the heart.*

An accentuated S_2 may be heard with HTN, exercise, excitement, and conditions of pulmonary HTN such as CHF and cor pulmonale.
- A diminished S_2 occurs with aortic stenosis, a fall in systolic blood pressure (shock), and increased anteroposterior chest diameter.

Listen for splitting of S_2. *No splitting of S_2 should be heard.*

- Wide splitting of S_2 is associated with delayed emptying of the right ventricle, resulting in delayed pulmonary valve closure (e.g., mitral regurgitation, pulmonary stenosis, and right bundle branch block).
- Fixed splitting occurs when right ventricular output is greater than left ventricular output and pulmonary valve closure is delayed (e.g., with atrial septal defect and right ventricular failure).
- Paradoxical splitting occurs when closure of the aortic valve is delayed (e.g., left bundle branch block).

Identify extra heart sounds in systole. *Extra heart sounds are not present.*

- Ejection sounds (or clicks) result from the opening of deformed semilunar valves (e.g., aortic and pulmonary stenosis).
- A midsystolic click is heard with mitral valve prolapse (MVP).

Technique/Normal Findings	Abnormal Findings
Identify the presence of extra heart sounds in diastole. *Extra heart sounds are not present in diastole.*	■ An opening snap results from the opening sound of a stenotic mitral valve. ■ A pathologic S_3 (a third heart sound that immediately follows S_2, called a ventricular gallop) results from myocardial failure and ventricular volume overload (e.g., CHF, mitral or tricuspid regurgitation). ■ An S_4 (a fourth heart sound that immediately precedes S_1, called an atrial gallop) results from increased resistance to ventricular filling after atrial contraction (e.g., HTN, CAD, aortic stenosis, and cardiomyopathy). ■ A combined S_3 and S_4 is called a summation gallop and occurs with severe CHF.
Identify extra heart sounds in both systole and diastole. *No extra heart sounds should be heard during systole and diastole.*	■ A pericardial friction rub results from inflammation of the pericardial sac, as with pericarditis.

Murmur Assessment

Identify any murmurs. Note location, timing, presence during systole or diastole, and intensity. Use the following scale to grade murmurs: I = Barely heard II = Quietly heard III = Clearly heard IV = Loud V = Very loud VI = Loudest; may be heard with stethoscope off the chest. A thrill may accompany murmurs of grade IV to grade VI. Note pitch (low, medium, high), and quality (harsh, blowing, or musical). Note pattern/shape, crescendo, decrescendo, and radiation/transmission (to axilla, neck). *No murmurs should be heard.*	■ Midsystolic murmurs are heard with semilunar valve disease (e.g., aortic and pulmonary stenosis) and with hypertrophic cardiomyopathy. ■ Pansystolic (holosystolic) murmurs are heard with AV valve disease (e.g., mitral and tricuspid regurgitation, ventricular septal defect). ■ A late systolic murmur is heard with MVP. ■ Early diastolic murmurs occur with regurgitant flow across incompetent semilunar valves (e.g., aortic regurgitation). ■ Middiastolic and presystolic murmurs, such as with mitral stenosis, occur with turbulent flow across the AV valves. ■ Continuous murmurs throughout systole and all or part of diastole occur with patent ductus arteriosus.

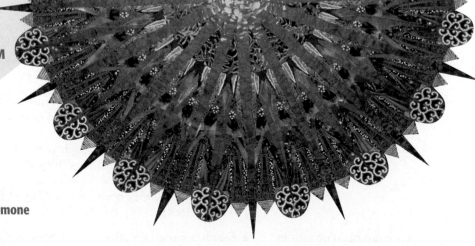

EXPLORE MediaLink

Prentice Hall Nursing MediaLink DVD-ROM
Audio Glossary
NCLEX-RN® Review

Animation/Videos
Cardiac A&P
Dysrhythmias
Heart Sounds
Hemodynamics
Oxygen Transport

COMPANION WEBSITE www.prenhall.com/lemone
Audio Glossary
NCLEX-RN® Review
Care Plan Activity: Cardiac Catheterization
Case Study: Chest Pain
MediaLink Application: Heart Sounds
Links to Resources

TEST YOURSELF NCLEX-RN® REVIEW

1 Which circulatory process supplies the heart with blood?
1. the systemic circulation
2. the pulmonary circulation
3. the coronary circulation
4. the hepatic circulation

2 The amount of blood pumped by the ventricles in 1 minute is known as:
1. heart rate.
2. ventricular contraction.
3. stroke volume.
4. cardiac output.

3 During what part of the cardiac cycle is the myocardium perfused?
1. prior to atrial filling
2. prior to ventricular relaxation
3. during diastole
4. during pulmonary perfusion

4 A client who is hemorrhaging has decreased preload. What physiologic event will follow?
1. increased afterload
2. increased ejection fraction
3. decreased cardiac output
4. decreased action potential

5 What physiologic process is responsible for the electrical impulse that stimulates myocardial contraction?
1. action potential
2. cardiac reserve
3. cardiac potential
4. ventricular contraction

6 The intensity of chest pain may be assessed by asking which question?
1. "Did the pain move into your left arm?"
2. "Was your pain relieved by resting or worse when you were busy?"
3. "On a scale of 0 (no pain) to 10 (worst pain), what number was your pain?"
4. "Was the pain a pressure, a burning, or a tightness?"

7 Which of the following is the most basic exercise stress test?
1. treadmill test
2. lipid profile
3. echocardiogram
4. cardiac catheterization

8 At what anatomic location would you assess the apical impulse?
1. left midclavicular, fifth intercostal space
2. left substernal, sixth intercostal space
3. right midaxillary, second intercostal space
4. right nipple line, any intercostal space

9 Your client's pulse rate is 50. You would document this as:
1. tachycardia.
2. bradycardia.
3. hypertension.
4. hypotension.

10 When auscultating heart sounds, where would S_1 be heard most loudly?
1. over the clavicles
2. at the apex of the heart
3. at the carotid pulse
4. at the base of the heart

See Test Yourself answers in Appendix C.

BIBLIOGRAPHY

Amella, E. (2004). Presentation of illness in older adults: If you think you know what you're looking for, think again. *American Journal of Nursing, 104*(10), 40–52.

Bench, S. (2004). Clinical skills: Assessing and treating shock. A nursing perspective. *British Journal of Nursing, 13*(12), 715–721.

Bickley, L., & Szilagyi, P. (2007). *Bates' guide to physical examination and history taking* (9th ed.). Philadelphia: Lippincott.

Burger, C. (2004). Emergency: Hypokalemia. Averting crisis with early recognition and intervention. *American Journal of Nursing, 104*(11), 61–65.

Coviello, J. (2004). Cardiac assessment 101: A new look at the guidelines for cardiac homecare patients. *Home Healthcare Nurse, 22*(2), 116–123.

Dulak, S. (2004). Hands-on help assessing heart sounds. *RN, 67*(8), 24ac1–4.

Eliopoulos, E. (2005). *Gerontological nursing* (6th ed.). Philadelphia: Lippincott Williams & Wilkins.

Harvey, S. (2004). Coronary heart disease. The nursing assessment and management of patients with angina. *British Journal of Nursing, 13*(10), 598–601.

Hayes, D. (2004). Bradycardia: Slow heart rate. Think fast! *Critical Care Choices, 4*(10), 12, 15.

Jarvis, C. (2004). *Physical examination & health assessment.* St. Louis, MO: Mosby.

Kee, J. (2005). *Prentice Hall handbook of laboratory & diagnostic tests with nursing implications.* Upper Saddle River, NJ: Prentice Hall.

Lindsey, J. (2005). Heart sounds: Do you hear what I see? *Journal of Emergency Medical Services, 30*(4), 104, 106.

MedlinePlus Medical Encyclopedia. (2004). *Cardiac catheterization.* Retrieved from http://www.nlm.nih.gov/medlineplus/ency/article/003419.htm.

Milewixz, D., & Seidman, C. (2000). Genetics of cardiovascular disease. *Circulation, 102* (Supplement 4), IV–103.

Murdaugh, J. (2003). Fatigue—a general diagnostic approach. *Australian Family Physician, 32*(11), 873–876, 935–936.

National Institutes of Health. (2003). *Genes and disease: The heart and blood vessels.* Retrieved from http://www.ncbi.nlm.nih.gov/books/bv.fcgi?rid=gnd.section.239

Porth, C. (2005). *Pathophysiology: Concepts of altered health states* (7th ed.). Philadelphia: Lippincott.

Tanabe, P., Steinmann, R., Kippenhan, M., Stehman, C., & Beach, C. (2004). Undiagnosed hypertension in the ED setting—an unrecognized opportunity by emergency nurses. *Journal of Emergency Nursing, 30*(3), 225–229, 292–297.

Weber, J., & Kelley, J. (2006). *Health assessment in nursing* (3rd ed.). Philadelphia: Lippincott.

CHAPTER 31 Nursing Care of Clients with Coronary Heart Disease

LEARNING OUTCOMES

- Discuss the coronary circulation and electrical properties of the heart.

- Compare and contrast the pathophysiology and manifestations of coronary heart disease and common cardiac dysrhythmias.

- Describe interdisciplinary and nursing care for clients with coronary heart disease and/or cardiac dysrhythmias.

- Relate the outcomes of diagnostic tests and procedures to the pathophysiology of cardiac disorders and implications for client responses to the disorder.

- Discuss nursing implications for medications and treatments used to prevent and treat coronary heart disease and dysrhythmias.

- Describe nursing care for the client undergoing diagnostic testing, an interventional procedure, or surgery for coronary heart disease or a dysrhythmia

CLINICAL COMPETENCIES

- Assess functional health status of clients with coronary heart disease and/or a dysrhythmia, including the impact of the disorder on the client's ability to perform activities of daily living and usual tasks.

- Use knowledge of the normal anatomy and physiology of the heart in caring for clients with coronary heart disease.

- Monitor clients with coronary heart disease or dysrhythmias for expected and unexpected manifestations, reporting and recording findings as indicated.

- Use assessed data to select nursing diagnoses, determine priorities of care, and develop and implement individualized nursing interventions for clients with coronary heart disease and dysrhythmias.

- Administer medications and treatments for clients with coronary heart disease and dysrhythmias safely and knowledgeably.

- Integrate interdisciplinary care into nursing care planning and implementation for clients with coronary heart disease and dysrhythmias.

- Provide appropriate teaching for prevention, health promotion, and self-care related to coronary heart disease and dysrhythmias.

- Evaluate the effectiveness of nursing interventions, revising or modifying the plan of care as needed to promote, maintain, or restore functional health for clients with coronary heart disease or dysrhythmias.

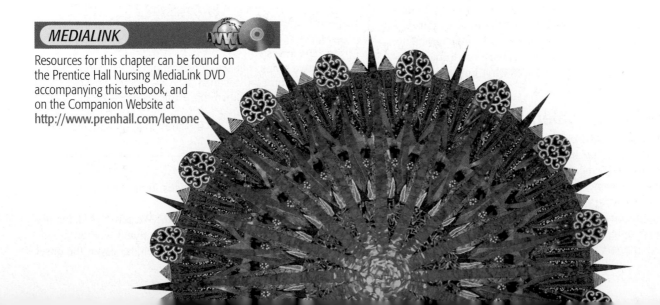

MEDIALINK

Resources for this chapter can be found on the Prentice Hall Nursing MediaLink DVD accompanying this textbook, and on the Companion Website at
http://www.prenhall.com/lemone

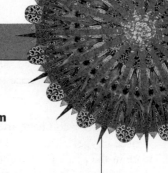

acute coronary syndrome (ACS), *974*
acute myocardial infarction (AMI), *982*
angina pectoris, *969*
atherosclerosis, *959*
atrial kick, *996*

cardiac arrest, *1002*
cardiac rehabilitation, *990*
cardiovascular disease (CVD), *958*
collateral channels, *959*
coronary heart disease, *958*
dysrhythmia, *985*
ectopic beats, *996*

heart block, *996*
ischemia, *969*
normal sinus rhythm (NSR), *1000*
pacemaker, *1008*
paroxysmal, *1000*
sudden cardiac death, *1015*

Impaired blood flow to the myocardium, changes in the conduction of electrical impulses through the heart, and structural changes in the heart itself affect the heart's ability to fulfill its major purpose: to pump enough blood to meet the body's demand for oxygen and nutrients. Impaired cardiac function, no matter what the underlying cause, affects the client's ability to participate in exercise and activities and to fulfill life roles. Disruptions in cardiac function affect other organ systems as well, potentially leading to organ system failure and death.

Cardiovascular disease (CVD) is a generic term for disorders of the heart and blood vessels. CVD is the leading cause of death and disability in the United States. Over 64 million people have some type of cardiovascular disease. The economic costs of CVD, both direct and indirect, to the nation are estimated at $368 billion annually (National Heart, Lung, and Blood Institute [NHLBI], 2004).

On an encouraging note, however, the incidence of new CVD cases per year is decreasing. Public education aimed at reducing fat intake, increasing exercise, and lowering cholesterol levels

have made people more aware of risk factors associated with CVD. The mortality rate from heart disease peaked in 1963 and has shown a slow but steady decline since that time.

This chapter focuses on disorders of myocardial blood flow (coronary heart disease) and cardiac rhythm. Disorders of cardiac structure and function are discussed in Chapter 32 ∞. Review the normal anatomy and physiology and nursing assessment of the heart in Chapter 30 ∞ before proceeding with this chapter.

DISORDERS OF MYOCARDIAL PERFUSION

THE CLIENT WITH CORONARY HEART DISEASE

Coronary heart disease (CHD), or *coronary artery disease (CAD)*, affects 13.2 million people in the United States and causes more than 500,000 deaths annually (NHLBI, 2004). CHD is caused by impaired blood flow to the myocardium. Accumulation of atherosclerotic plaque in the coronary arteries is the usual cause. Coronary heart disease may be asymptomatic, or may lead to angina pectoris, acute coronary syndrome, myocardial infarction (MI or heart attack), dysrhythmias, heart failure, and even sudden death.

Incidence and Prevalence

Many risk factors for CHD can be controlled through lifestyle modification. In fact, with increased public awareness of risk factors related to CHD, mortality rates are declining by about 3.3% per year. Nevertheless, CHD remains a major public health problem. Heart disease is the leading cause of death for all U.S. ethnic groups except Asian females (NHLBI, 2004). See the accompanying box. Nurses are in a prime position to encourage and support positive lifestyle changes by teaching

FOCUS ON CULTURAL DIVERSITY
Heart Disease

- Native Americans (American Indians and Alaska Natives) have the highest prevalence of coronary heart disease, followed by whites, African Americans, Mexican Americans and native Hawaiians, and Asian Americans.
- People with less than a high school diploma have the highest rate of CHD; people with a bachelor's degree or higher have the lowest.
- Economic status is a factor; the rate of CHD in people with a family income of less than $35,000 per year have a significantly higher rate than those with incomes greater than $75,000 per year.
- Regionally, the rate of CHD is highest in the South and lowest in the West.

and promoting healthy living practices. Individual choices can and do affect health.

The highest incidence of CHD is in the Western world, mainly in white males age 45 and older. Both men and women are affected by coronary heart disease; in women, however, the onset is about 10 years later because of the heart-protective effects of estrogen. After menopause, women's risk is equal to that of men.

Physiology Review

The two main coronary arteries, the left and the right, supply blood, oxygen, and nutrients to the myocardium. They originate in the root of the aorta, just outside the aortic valve. The *left main coronary artery* divides to form the anterior descending and circumflex arteries. The *anterior descending* artery supplies the anterior interventricular septum and the left ventricle, including the apex of the heart. The *circumflex* branch supplies the lateral wall of the left ventricle. The *right coronary artery* supplies the right ventricle and forms the posterior descending artery. The *posterior descending* artery supplies the posterior portion of the heart (see Figure 30–5).

Blood flow through the coronary arteries is regulated by several factors. Aortic pressure is the primary factor. Other factors include the heart rate (most flow occurs during diastole, when the muscle is relaxed), metabolic activity of the heart, blood vessel tone (constriction), and collateral circulation. Although there are no connections between the large coronary arteries, small arteries are joined by **collateral channels**. If large vessels are gradually occluded, these channels enlarge, providing alternative routes for blood flow (Porth, 2005).

Pathophysiology

Coronary atherosclerosis is the most common cause of reduced coronary blood flow.

Atherosclerosis

Atherosclerosis is a progressive disease characterized by *atheroma* (plaque) formation, which affects the intimal and medial layers of large and midsize arteries. See *Pathophysiology Illustrated: Coronary Heart Disease* on pages 960–961.

Atherosclerosis is initiated by unknown precipitating factors that cause lipoproteins and fibrous tissue to accumulate in the arterial wall. Although the precise mechanisms are unknown, abnormal lipid metabolism and injury to or inflammation of endothelial cells lining the artery appear to be key to its development.

In the bloodstream, lipids are transported attached to proteins called apoproteins. High levels of certain *lipoproteins,* a type of apoprotein, increase the risk of atherosclerosis. *Low-density lipoproteins*, which are high in cholesterol, carry cholesterol to peripheral tissues where some of it is released to be taken up and incorporated into cells for use in producing energy. *Very-low-density lipoproteins*, large molecules primarily composed of triglycerides and cholesterol, carry triglycerides to muscle and fat cells. When the triglycerides are released into these tissues, the remainder of the molecule is a low-density lipoprotein. *High-density lipoproteins*, in contrast, attract cholesterol, returning it from peripheral tissues to the liver.

Hyperlipidemia itself may damage arterial endothelium. Other potential mechanisms of vessel injury include excessive pressures within the arterial system (hypertension), toxins found in cigarette smoke, infections, and inflammation (Copstead & Banasik, 2005). Endothelial damage promotes platelet adhesion and aggregation, and attracts leukocytes to the area.

At the site of injury, *atherogenic* (atherosclerosis-promoting) lipoproteins collect in the intimal lining of the artery. These lipoproteins appear to actually bind with the extracellular portion of the vessel endothelium. Macrophages migrate to the injured site as part of the inflammatory process. Contact with platelets, cholesterol, and other blood components stimulates smooth muscle cells and connective tissue within the vessel wall to proliferate abnormally. Although blood flow is not affected at this stage, this early lesion appears as a yellowish fatty streak on the inner lining of the artery. Fibrous plaque develops as smooth muscle cells enlarge, collagen fibers proliferate, and blood lipids accumulate. The lesion protrudes into the arterial lumen and is fixed to the inner wall of the intima. It may invade the muscular media layer of the vessel as well. The developing plaque not only gradually occludes the vessel lumen but also impairs the vessel's ability to dilate in response to increased oxygen demands. Fibrous plaque lesions often develop at arterial bifurcations or curves or in areas of narrowing. As the plaque expands, it can produce severe stenosis or total occlusion of the artery.

The final stage of the process is the development of *atheromas,* complex lesions consisting of lipids, fibrous tissue, collagen, calcium, cellular debris, and capillaries. These calcified lesions can ulcerate or rupture, stimulating thrombosis. The vessel lumen may be rapidly occluded by the thrombus, or it may embolize to occlude a distal vessel.

Plaque formation may be *eccentric,* located in a specific, asymmetric region of the vessel wall, or *concentric,* involving the entire vessel circumference. Manifestations of the process usually do not appear until about 75% of the arterial lumen has been occluded.

Atherosclerosis tends to develop where arteries *bifurcate* or branch. Certain vessels have a higher likelihood of being affected, including the coronary arteries (the left anterior descending artery in particular), the renal arteries, the bifurcation of the carotid arteries, and branching sections of peripheral arteries. In addition to obstructing or occluding blood flow, atherosclerosis weakens arterial walls, and is a major cause of aneurysm in vessels such as the aorta and iliac arteries.

Myocardial Ischemia

Myocardial cells become ischemic when the oxygen supply is inadequate to meet metabolic demands. The critical factors in meeting metabolic demands of cardiac cells are coronary perfusion and myocardial workload. Coronary perfusion can be affected by several different mechanisms:

- One or more vessels may be partially occluded by large, stable areas of plaque.
- Platelets can aggregate in narrowed vessels, forming a thrombus.
- Normal or already narrowed vessels may spasm.
- A drop in blood pressure may lead to inadequate flow through coronary vessels.
- Normal autoregulatory mechanisms that increase flow to working muscles may fail (Copstead & Banasik, 2005).

Coronary Heart Disease

Coronary heart disease usually is due to *atherosclerosis*, occlusion of the coronary arteries by fibrous, fatty plaque. Coronary heart disease is manifested by *angina pectoris, acute coronary syndrome,* and/or *myocardial infarction.* Risk factors for coronary heart disease include age (over 50 years), heredity, smoking, obesity, high serum cholesterol levels, hypertension, and diabetes mellitus. Other factors, such as diet and lack of exercise, also contribute to the risk of CHD.

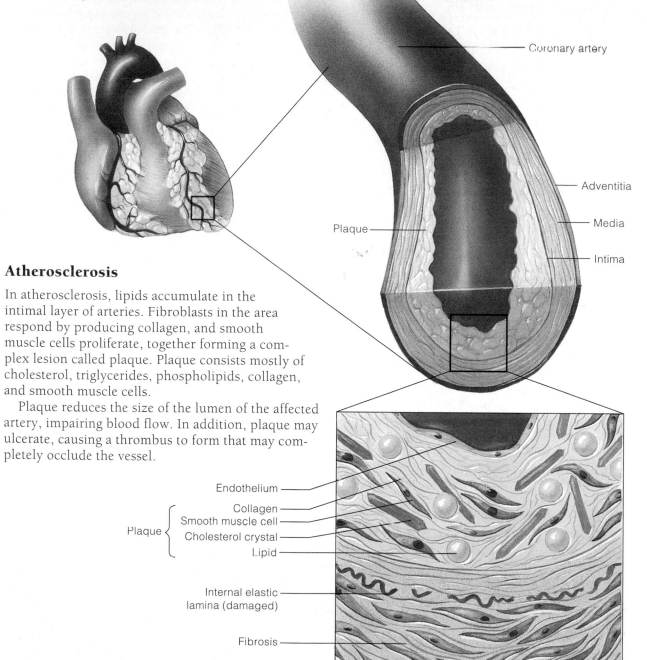

Coronary artery

Adventitia

Media

Intima

Plaque

Atherosclerosis

In atherosclerosis, lipids accumulate in the intimal layer of arteries. Fibroblasts in the area respond by producing collagen, and smooth muscle cells proliferate, together forming a complex lesion called plaque. Plaque consists mostly of cholesterol, triglycerides, phospholipids, collagen, and smooth muscle cells.

Plaque reduces the size of the lumen of the affected artery, impairing blood flow. In addition, plaque may ulcerate, causing a thrombus to form that may completely occlude the vessel.

Endothelium

Collagen

Smooth muscle cell

Cholesterol crystal

Lipid

Plaque

Internal elastic lamina (damaged)

Fibrosis

Angina Pectoris

Angina is characterized by episodes of chest pain, usually precipitated by exercise and relieved by rest. When myocardial oxygen needs are greater than partially occluded vessels can supply, myocardial cells become ischemic and shift to anaerobic metabolism. Anaerobic metabolism produces lactic acid that stimulates nerve endings in the muscle, causing pain. The pain subsides when the oxygen supply again meets myocardial demand.

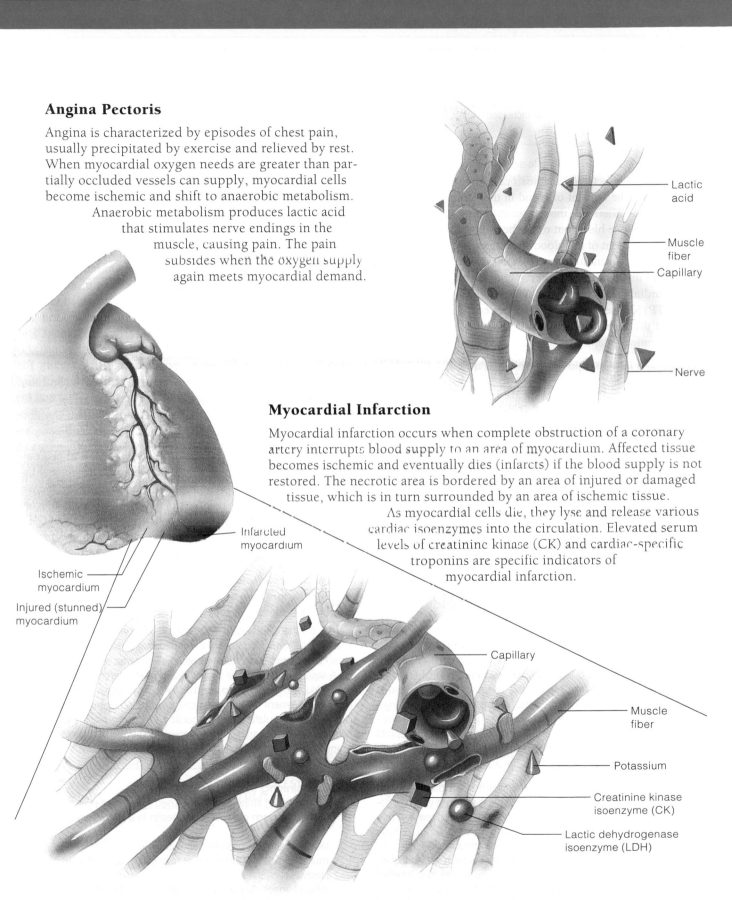

Lactic acid

Muscle fiber

Capillary

Nerve

Myocardial Infarction

Myocardial infarction occurs when complete obstruction of a coronary artery interrupts blood supply to an area of myocardium. Affected tissue becomes ischemic and eventually dies (infarcts) if the blood supply is not restored. The necrotic area is bordered by an area of injured or damaged tissue, which is in turn surrounded by an area of ischemic tissue. As myocardial cells die, they lyse and release various cardiac isoenzymes into the circulation. Elevated serum levels of creatinine kinase (CK) and cardiac-specific troponins are specific indicators of myocardial infarction.

Infarcted myocardium

Ischemic myocardium

Injured (stunned) myocardium

Capillary

Muscle fiber

Potassium

Creatinine kinase isoenzyme (CK)

Lactic dehydrogenase isoenzyme (LDH)

(VLDL) molecules. Elevated triglycerides also contribute to the risk for CHD.

CIGARETTE SMOKING *Cigarette smoking* is an independent risk factor for CHD, responsible for more deaths from CHD than from lung cancer or pulmonary disease (Woods et al., 2004). The effects of smoking on the cardiovascular system are dose dependent (NCEP, 2002). The male cigarette smoker has two to three times the risk of developing heart disease of the nonsmoker; the female who smokes has up to four times the risk. For both men and women who stop smoking, the risk of mortality from CHD is reduced by half. Second-hand (or environmental) tobacco smoke also increases the risk of death from CHD, by as much as 30% (Woods et al., 2004). Tobacco smoke promotes CHD in several ways. Carbon monoxide damages vascular endothelium, promoting cholesterol deposition. Nicotine stimulates catecholamine release, increasing blood pressure, heart rate, and myocardial oxygen use. Nicotine also constricts arteries, limiting tissue perfusion (blood flow and oxygen delivery). Further, nicotine reduces HDL levels and increases platelet aggregation, increasing the risk of thrombus formation.

FAST FACTS

■ Cigarette smoking is the leading independent risk factor for coronary heart disease and a primary target of risk factor management.

OBESITY *Obesity* (excess adipose tissue), generally defined as a body mass index (BMI) of 30 kg/m^2 or greater, and fat distribution affect the risk for CHD. Obese people have higher rates of hypertension, diabetes, and hyperlipidemia. In the Framingham study, obese men over age 50 had twice the incidence of CHD and acute myocardial infarction (MI) of those who were within 10% of their ideal weight. Central obesity, or intra-abdominal fat, is associated with an increased risk for CHD. The best indicator of central obesity is the waist circumference. A waist-to-hip ratio of greater than 0.8 (women) or 0.9 (men) increases the risk for CHD.

PHYSICAL INACTIVITY *Physical inactivity* is associated with a higher risk of CHD. Research data indicate that people who maintain a regular program of physical activity are less prone to developing CHD than sedentary people. Cardiovascular benefits of exercise include increased availability of oxygen to the heart muscle, decreased oxygen demand and cardiac workload, and increased myocardial function and electrical stability. Other positive effects of regular physical activity include decreased blood pressure, blood lipids, insulin levels, platelet aggregation, and weight.

DIET *Diet* is a risk factor for CHD, independent of fat and cholesterol intake. Diets high in fruits, vegetables, whole grains, and unsaturated fatty acids appear to have a protective effect. The underlying factors are not clear, but probably relate to nutrients such as antioxidants, folic acid, other B vitamins, omega-3 fatty acids, and other unidentified micronutrients (NCEP, 2002).

EMERGING RISK FACTORS Recent research demonstrates a link between elevated serum *homocysteine levels* and CHD.

Until menopause, women have lower homocysteine levels than men, which may partially explain their lower risk for CHD. Homocysteine levels are negatively correlated with serum folate and dietary folate intake; that is, increasing folate intake lowers homocysteine levels.

Based on evidence that aspirin and antiplatelet therapies reduce the risk for MI, *clot-promoting factors* are identified as CHD risk factors. *Inflammation* also has recently been identified as a risk factor. Inflammatory processes may increase the development of atherosclerotic plaque, and are implicated in plaque rupture (NCEP, 2002). Inflammation also promotes clot formation at the site of ruptured plaque. Although identified as risk factors, it is not generally recommended that clients routinely be tested for these factors.

METABOLIC SYNDROME The *metabolic syndrome,* a group of metabolic risk factors occurring in an individual, is a strong risk factor for CHD (Box 31–2). The metabolic syndrome has emerged as a risk factor for premature CHD that is equal to cigarette smoking. Three underlying causes of metabolic syndrome have been identified: overweight/obesity, physical inactivity, and genetic factors. It is closely associated with *insulin resistance,* impaired tissue responses to insulin. Genetic factors play a role in insulin resistance, as do the acquired factors of abdominal obesity and physical inactivity (NCEP, 2002).

RISK FACTORS UNIQUE TO WOMEN Risk factors unique to women include *premature menopause, oral contraceptive use,* and *hormone replacement therapy (HRT).* At menopause, serum HDL levels drop and LDL levels rise, increasing the risk of CHD. Early menopause (natural or surgically induced) increases the risk of CHD and MI. Women who have bilateral oophorectomy before age 35 without hormone replacement are eight times more likely to have an MI than women experiencing natural menopause. Estrogen replacement therapy reduces the risk of CHD and MI in these women. Oral contraceptives, by contrast, increase the risk for myocardial infarction, particularly in women who also smoke. This increased risk is due to the tendency of oral contraceptives to promote clotting, and their effects on blood pressure, serum lipids, and glucose tolerance (Woods et al., 2004). The Women's Health Initiative randomized trial of HRT showed an increased risk for CHD in previously healthy women taking a commonly prescribed combination of estrogen and progestin (Writing Group, 2002). This well-controlled research study (see the box on the next page) was terminated early when it showed a small but significant increased risk for CHD, stroke, pulmonary embolism, and invasive breast cancer in women taking HRT.

BOX 31–2 Characteristics of the Metabolic Syndrome

■ Abdominal obesity
■ Abnormal blood lipids (low HDL, high triglycerides)
■ Hypertension
■ Elevated fasting blood glucose
■ Clotting tendency
■ Inflammatory factors

NURSING RESEARCH   Evidence-Based Practice: Postmenopausal Women

The Women's Health Initiative (WHI) is studying the risks and benefits of strategies to reduce the incidence of heart disease, breast and colorectal cancer, and fractures in postmenopausal women (Writing Group, 2002). A group of 161,809 postmenopausal women between ages 50 and 79 were originally enrolled in WHI trials. Of these women, a subgroup of 16,608 women with intact uteri became part of a randomized trial to assess the risks and benefits of HRT, using the most frequently prescribed combined hormone (estrogen and progestin [Prempro]) replacement in the United States.

After a mean of 5.2 years of follow-up, this study was stopped due to convincing evidence that the risk for invasive breast cancer exceeded the benefits of HRT. The study also demonstrated increased risks for coronary heart disease, stroke, deep vein thrombosis, and pulmonary embolism, although overall mortality was not affected. HRT reduced the risk for colorectal cancer and hip fracture in this study group. The risk for CHD appears to be independent of other CHD risk factors such as age, ethnicity, hypertension, diabetes, smoking, obesity, and other identified risk factors.

IMPLICATIONS FOR NURSING

Nurses often are in the position of advising women about menopause, its manifestations, and hormone replacement ther-

apy. While HRT does reduce unpleasant menopausal effects such as night sweats and hot flashes, and it reduces the risk of osteoporosis and subsequent fractures, it carries associated risks. Advise each client about the risks and benefits of HRT, clearly presenting the evidence. Suggest alternative strategies to reduce menopausal symptoms, such as complementary medicines (see Chapter 51 ∞). Encourage measures such as weight-bearing exercise, calcium supplements, and a diet high in fiber and antioxidants to reduce the risks for osteoporosis, fracture, and colorectal cancer. Ultimately, each client will make her own decision about postmenopausal HRT.

CRITICAL THINKING IN CLIENT CARE

1. What factors might you suggest that a client consider when deciding whether to use HRT for menopausal manifestations and risks?
2. In this study, the increased risk for CHD was not related to the duration of time taking HRT, whereas the increased risk for stroke and invasive breast cancer emerged more than 1 year after randomization (stroke in the second through fifth year of the study, breast cancer within several years following randomization). Will this data affect your advice to menopausal women inquiring about HRT? If so, how?

FAST FACTS

- Risk factors for coronary heart disease are those factors that promote atherosclerosis and plaque development.
- Angina pectoris, acute coronary syndromes, and myocardial infarction are the manifestations of myocardial ischemia and coronary heart disease due to atherosclerosis.
- Atherosclerosis also is the primary underlying cause of stroke and peripheral vascular disease; therefore, the risk factors for atherosclerosis also are the risk factors for coronary heart disease, including angina, acute coronary syndromes, and myocardial infarction.

INTERDISCIPLINARY CARE

Care of clients with coronary heart disease focuses on aggressive risk factor management to slow the atherosclerotic process and maintain myocardial perfusion. Until manifestations of chronic or acute ischemia are experienced, the diagnosis often is presumptive, based on history and the presence of risk factors.

Diagnosis

Laboratory testing is used to assess for risk factors such as an abnormal blood lipid profile (elevated triglyceride and LDL levels and decreased HDL levels).

- *Total serum cholesterol* is elevated in hyperlipidemia. A *lipid profile* includes triglyceride, HDL, and LDL levels as well, and enables calculation of the ratio of HDL to total cholesterol. The ratio should be at least 1:5, with 1:3 being the ideal ratio. Elevated lipid levels are associated with an increased risk of atherosclerosis (see Table 31–3). In clients with a

strong family history of premature CHD or familial hypercholesterolemia, *lipoprotein (a)* also may be measured. Elevated levels of Lp(a) may independently increase the risk of CHD. Other subsets of blood lipids may also be measured in selected clients. See Chapter 30 ∞ for nursing care related to lipid profile studies.

Diagnostic tests to identify subclinical (asymptomatic) CHD may be indicated when multiple risk factors are present.

- *C-reactive protein* is a serum protein associated with inflammatory processes. Recent evidence suggests that elevated blood levels of this protein may be predictive of CHD.
- The *ankle-brachial blood pressure index (ABI)* is an inexpensive, noninvasive test for peripheral vascular disease that may be predictive of CHD. The systolic blood pressure in the brachial, posterior tibial, and dorsalis pedis arteries is measured by Doppler. An ABI of <0.9 in either leg indicates the presence of peripheral arterial disease and a significant risk for CHD.
- *Exercise ECG testing* may be performed. ECGs are used to assess the response to increased cardiac workload induced by exercise. The test is considered "positive" for CHD if myocardial ischemia is detected on the ECG (depression of the ST segment by greater than 3 mm; see Figure 31–1), the client develops chest pain, or the test is stopped due to excess fatigue, dysrhythmias, or other symptoms before the predicted maximal heart rate is achieved.
- *Electron beam computed tomography (EBCT)* creates a three-dimensional image of the heart and coronary arteries that can reveal plaque and other abnormalities. This noninvasive test requires no special preparation, and can identify clients at risk for developing myocardial ischemia.

■ *Myocardial perfusion imaging* (see the section on angina that follows) may be used to evaluate myocardial blood flow and perfusion, both at rest and during stress testing (exercise or mental stress). These diagnostic tests are further explained in Chapter 30 ∞ and the section on angina. Perfusion imaging studies are costly, and therefore not recommended for routine CHD risk assessment.

Risk Factor Management

Conservative management of CHD focuses on risk factor modification, including smoking, diet, exercise, and management of contributing conditions.

SMOKING Smoking cessation reduces the risk for CHD within months after quitting and improves cardiovascular status. People who quit reduce their risk by 50%, regardless of how long they smoked before quitting. For women, the risk becomes equivalent to a nonsmoker within 3 to 5 years of smoking cessation (Woods et al., 2004). In addition, stopping smoking improves HDL levels, lowers LDL levels, and reduces blood viscosity. All smokers are advised to quit. Health promotion activities focus on preventing children, teenagers, and adults from starting to smoke.

DIET Dietary recommendations by the National Cholesterol Education Program (2002) include reduced saturated fat and cholesterol intake, and strategies to lower LDL levels (Table 31–4). Most fats are a mixture of saturated and unsaturated fatty acids. The highest proportions of saturated fat are found in whole-milk products, red meats, and coconut oil. Nonfat dairy products, fish, and poultry as primary protein sources are recommended. Solidified vegetable fats (e.g., margarine, shortening) contain *trans* fatty acids, which behave more like saturated fats. Soft margarines and vegetable oil spreads contain low levels of *trans* fatty acids, and should be used instead of butter, stick margarine, and shortening. Monounsaturated fats, found in olive, canola, and peanut oils, actually lower LDL and cholesterol levels. Certain

TABLE 31–4 Dietary Recommendations to Reduce Total Cholesterol, LDL Levels, and CHD Risk

NUTRIENT	RECOMMENDATION
Calories	Adjusted to attain/maintain desirable body weight
Total fat	25%–35% of total calories
■ Saturated fats	■ <7% of total calories
■ Polyunsaturated fat	■ Up to 10% of total calories
■ Monounsaturated fat	■ Up to 20% of total calories
■ Cholesterol	■ <200 mg/day
Carbohydrate (primarily complex carbohydrates, such as whole grains, fruits, and vegetables)	50%–60% of total calories
Dietary fiber	20–30 g/day
Protein	About 15% of total calories

Source: Compiled from *Adult Treatment Panel III Final Report* by the National Cholesterol Education Program, 2002.

cold-water fish, such as tuna, salmon, and mackerel, contain high levels of omega-3 fatty acids, which help raise HDL levels, and decrease serum triglycerides, total serum cholesterol, and blood pressure.

In addition, increased intake of soluble fiber (found in oats, psyllium, pectin-rich fruit, and beans) and insoluble fiber (found in whole grains, vegetables, and fruit) is recommended. Folic acid and vitamins B_6 and B_{12} affect homocysteine metabolism, reducing serum levels. Leafy green vegetables (e.g., spinach and broccoli) and legumes (e.g., black-eyed peas, dried beans, and lentils) are rich sources of folate. Meat, fish, and poultry are rich in vitamins B_6 and B_{12}. Vitamin B_6 also is found in soy products; B_{12} is in fortified cereals. Increased intake of antioxidant nutrients (vitamin E, in particular) and foods rich in antioxidants (fruits and vegetables) appears to increase HDL levels and have a protective effect on CHD.

In middle-aged and older adults, moderate alcohol intake may reduce the risk for CHD (NCEP, 2002). Consumption of no more than two drinks per day for men or one drink per day for women is recommended. A drink is 5 ounces of wine, 12 ounces of beer, or 1.5 ounces of whiskey. People who do not drink alcohol, however, should not be encouraged to start consuming it as a heart-protective measure.

People who are overweight or obese are encouraged to lose weight through a combination of reduced calorie intake (maintaining a nutritionally sound diet) and increased exercise. High-protein, high-fat weight loss programs are not recommended for weight reduction.

EXERCISE Regular physical exercise reduces the risk for CHD in several ways. It lowers VLDL, LDL, and triglyceride levels, and raises HDL levels. Regular exercise reduces the blood pressure and insulin resistance. Unless contraindicated, all clients are encouraged to participate in at least 30 minutes of moderate intensity physical activity 5 to 6 days each week. To achieve weight loss and prevent weight gain, 60 to 90 minutes of moderate intensity exercise daily is recommended (U.S. Department of Health and Human Services, 2005).

HYPERTENSION Although hypertension often cannot be prevented or cured, it can be controlled. Hypertension control (maintaining a blood pressure lower than 140/90 mmHg) is vital to reduce its atherosclerosis-promoting effects and to reduce the workload of the heart. Management strategies include reducing sodium intake, increasing calcium intake, regular exercise, stress management, and medications. Hypertension management is discussed in Chapter 35 ∞.

DIABETES Diabetes increases the risk of CHD by accelerating the atherosclerotic process. Weight loss (if appropriate), reduced fat intake, and exercise are particularly important for the diabetic client. Because hyperglycemia apparently also contributes to atherosclerosis, consistent blood glucose management is vital. See Chapter 20 ∞ for a detailed discussion about diabetes and blood glucose management.

Medications

Drug therapy to lower total serum cholesterol and LDL levels and to raise HDL levels now is an integral part of CHD management. It is used in conjunction with diet and other lifestyle changes, and is based on the client's overall risk for CHD.

Drugs used to treat hyperlipidemia act specifically by lowering LDL levels. The goal of treatment is to achieve an LDL level of <130 mg/dL (NCEP, 2002). Medications to treat hyperlipidemia are not inexpensive; the cost–benefit ratio needs to be considered, because long-term treatment may be required. The four major classes of cholesterol-lowering drugs are statins, bile acid sequestrants, nicotinic acid, and fibrates. The nursing implications and client teaching for these drug classes are outlined in the Medication Administration box below.

MEDICATION ADMINISTRATION   Cholesterol-Lowering Drugs

STATINS
Lovastatin (Mevacor)
Pravastatin (Pravachol)
Simvastatin (Zocor)
Fluvastatin (Lescol)
Atorvastatin (Lipitor)

Statins inhibit the enzyme HMG-CoA reductase in the liver, lowering LDL synthesis and serum levels. The statins are first-line treatment for elevated LDL, used in conjunction with diet and lifestyle changes. Although their side effects are minimal, they may cause increased serum liver enzyme levels and myopathy.

Nursing Responsibilities
- Monitor serum cholesterol and liver enzyme levels before and during therapy. Report elevated liver enzyme levels.
- Assess for muscle pain and tenderness. Monitor CPK level if present.
- If taking digoxin concurrently, monitor for and report digoxin toxicity.

Health Education for the Client and Family
- Promptly report muscle pain, tenderness, or weakness; skin rash or hives, or changes in skin color; abdominal pain, nausea, or vomiting.
- Do not use these drugs if you are pregnant or plan to become pregnant.
- Inform your doctor if you are taking any other medications concurrently.

BILE ACID SEQUESTRANTS
Cholestyramine (Questran)
Colestipol (Colestid)
Colesevelam (Welchol)

Bile acid sequestrants lower LDL levels by binding bile acids in the intestine, reducing its reabsorption and cholesterol production in the liver. They are used in combination therapy regimens and for women who are considering pregnancy. Their primary disadvantages are inconvenience of administration due to bulk and gastrointestinal side effects such as constipation.

Nursing Responsibilities
- Mix cholestyramine and colestipol powders with 4 to 6 oz of water or juice; administer once or twice a day as ordered with meals.
- Store in a tightly closed container.

Health Education for the Client and Family
- Promptly report constipation, severe gastric distress with nausea and vomiting, unexplained weight loss, black or bloody stools, or sudden back pain to your doctor.
- Drinking ample amounts of fluid while taking these drugs reduces problems of constipation and bloating.
- Do not omit doses as this may affect the absorption of other drugs you are taking.

NICOTINIC ACID
Niacin (Nicobid, Nicolar, Niaspan, others)

Nicotinic acid in both prescription and nonprescription forms lowers total and LDL cholesterol and triglyceride levels. The crystalline form and Niaspan, a prescription extended release tablet, also raise HDL levels. Because the doses required to achieve significant cholesterol-lowering effects are associated with multiple side effects, nicotinic acid generally is used in combination therapy, particularly with the statin drugs.

Nursing Responsibilities
- Give oral preparations with meals and accompanied by a cold beverage to minimize GI effects.
- Administer with caution to clients with active liver disease, peptic ulcer disease, gout, or type 2 diabetes.
- Monitor blood glucose, uric acid levels, and liver function tests during treatment.

Health Education for the Client and Family
- Flushing of face, neck, and ears may occur within 2 hours following dose; these effects generally subside as treatment continues. Alcohol use during nicotinic acid therapy may worsen this effect.
- Report weakness or dizziness with changes in posture (lying to sitting; sitting to standing) to your doctor. Change positions slowly to reduce the risk of injury.

FIBRIC ACID DERIVATIVES
Gemfibrozil (Lopid)
Fenofibrate (Tricor)
Clofibrate (Atromid-S)

The fibrates are used to lower serum triglyceride levels; they have only a slight to modest effect on LDL. They affect lipid regulation by blocking triglyceride synthesis. They are used to treat very high triglyceride levels, and may be used in combination with statins.

Nursing Responsibilities
- Monitor serum LDL and VLDL levels, electrolytes, glucose, liver enzymes, renal function tests, and CBC during therapy. Report abnormal values.
- Up to 2 months of treatment may be required to achieve a therapeutic effect; rebound, with decreasing benefit, may occur in the second or third month of treatment.

Health Education for the Client and Family
- Take with meals if the drug causes gastric distress.
- Promptly report flulike symptoms (fatigue, muscle aching, soreness, or weakness) to your doctor.
- Do not use this drug if you are pregnant or plan to become pregnant. Use reliable birth control measures while taking this drug.
- Contact your doctor before stopping this drug and before taking any over-the-counter preparations.

The statins, including lovastatin (Mevacor), pravastatin (Pravachol), simvastatin (Zocor), and others, are first-line drugs for treating hyperlipidemia. They effectively lower LDL levels and may also increase HDL levels. The statins can cause myopathy; all clients are instructed to report muscle pain and weakness or brown urine. Liver function tests are monitored during therapy, because these drugs may increase liver enzyme levels.

The other cholesterol-lowering drugs, such as the bile acid sequestrants, nicotinic acid, and fibrates, are primarily used when combination therapy is required to effectively lower serum cholesterol levels. They also may be used for selected clients, such as younger adults, women who wish to become pregnant, or to specifically lower triglyceride levels.

Clients at high risk for MI are often started on prophylactic low-dose aspirin therapy. The dose ranges from 80 to 325 mg/day (Tierney et al., 2005). In women, the benefit of low-dose aspirin in reducing the risk for CHD is not clear prior to age 65 (NHLBI, 2005). Aspirin is contraindicated for clients who have a history of aspirin sensitivity, bleeding disorders, or active peptic ulcer disease. Angiotensin-converting enzyme (ACE) inhibitors or angiotensin receptor blockers also may be prescribed for high-risk clients, including diabetics with other CHD risk factors.

Complementary Therapies

Diet and exercise programs that emphasize physical conditioning and a low-fat diet rich in antioxidants have been shown to be effective in managing CHD (Box 31–3). Supplements of vitamins C, E, B_6, B_{12}, and folic acid may be beneficial. Other potentially helpful complementary therapies include herbals such as ginkgo biloba, garlic, curcumin, and green tea; and consumption of red wine, foods containing bioflavonoids, and nuts. Emphasize the need for clients to talk to their physician prior to taking any herbal preparations, as interactions with prescribed drugs are common. Behavioral therapies of benefit for clients with CHD include relaxation and stress management, guided imagery, treatment of depression, anger/hostility management, and meditation, tai chi, and yoga.

BOX 31–3 Complementary Therapies: Diet for CHD

Two diet programs have been shown to have a beneficial effect on CHD. The *Pritikin diet* is basically vegetarian, high in complex carbohydrates and fiber, low in cholesterol, and extremely low in fat (<10% of daily calories). Egg whites and limited amounts of nonfat dairy or soy products are allowed. The Pritikin program requires 45 minutes of walking daily and recommends multivitamin supplements, including vitamins C and E and folate.

The *Ornish diet* also is vegetarian, although egg whites and a cup of nonfat milk or yogurt per day are allowed. No oil or fat is permitted, even for cooking. Two ounces of alcohol a day are permitted. The Ornish program also calls for stress reduction, emotional social support systems, daily stretching, and walking for 1 hour three times a week.

NURSING CARE

Nurses are instrumental in educating adults about their risk for coronary heart disease, promoting participation in screening programs to identify that risk, and teaching all clients measures to reduce their risk for CHD.

Health Promotion

Present information about healthy lifestyle habits to community and religious groups, school children (grades K through 12), and through the print media. In promoting healthy lifestyle habits, nurses can positively affect the incidence, morbidity, and mortality from CHD.

Strongly encourage all clients to avoid smoking in the first place, and to stop all forms of tobacco use. Discuss the adverse effects of smoking and the benefits of quitting. Provide information about dietary recommendations to maintain a healthy weight and optimal cholesterol levels. Discuss the benefits and importance of regular exercise. Finally, encourage clients with cardiovascular risk factors to undergo regular screening for hypertension, diabetes, and abnormal blood lipids.

Assessment

Nursing assessment for CHD focuses on identifying risk factors.
- *Health history:* Current manifestations such as chest pain or heaviness, shortness of breath, weakness; current diet, exercise patterns, and medications; smoking history and pattern of alcohol intake; history of heart disease, hypertension, or diabetes; family history of CHD or other cardiac problems.
- *Physical examination:* Current weight and its appropriateness for height; body mass index; waist-to-hip ratio; blood pressure; strength and equality of peripheral pulses.

Nursing Diagnoses and Interventions
Imbalanced Nutrition:
More than Body Requirements

This nursing diagnosis may be appropriate for clients who are obese, have a waist-to-hip ratio greater than 0.8 (female) or 0.9 (male), or whose diet history or serum cholesterol levels indicate a need to reduce fat and cholesterol intake. See Chapters 21 ∞ and 22 for more information about assessing obesity.
- Encourage assessment of food intake and eating patterns to help identify areas that can be improved. *Clients often are unaware of their fat and cholesterol intake, particularly when many meals are eaten away from home. Careful assessment increases awareness and allows the client to make conscious changes.*
- Discuss American Heart Association and therapeutic lifestyle change (TLC) dietary recommendations, emphasizing the role of diet in heart disease. Provide guidance regarding specific food choices with healthy alternatives. *Specific diet information and suggestions help the client make better food choices.*
- Refer to a clinical dietitian for diet planning and further teaching. Suggest cookbooks that offer low-fat recipes to encourage healthier eating, and provide American Heart Association and American Cancer Society recipe pamphlets and information

on low-fat eating. *These resources provide tools for the client to use as eating patterns change.*

- Encourage gradual but progressive dietary changes. *Drastic changes in eating patterns may cause frustration and discourage the client from maintaining a healthy diet over the long term.*
- Discourage use of high-fat, low-carbohydrate, or other fad diets for weight loss. *These diets may adversely affect serum cholesterol and triglyceride levels, and often are too drastic to maintain over the long term.*
- Encourage reasonable goals for weight loss (e.g., 1.0 to 1.5 lb per week and a 10% weight loss over 6 months). Provide information about weight loss programs and support groups such as Weight Watchers and Take Off Pounds Sensibly (TOPS) *Gradual but steady weight loss is more likely to be sustained. Recognized programs that emphasize healthy eating provide support and incentive for making lifetime dietary changes.*

Ineffective Health Maintenance

Clients with risk factors for CHD may be unable to identify or independently manage their risk factors.

- Discuss risk factors for CHD, stressing that changing or managing those factors that can be modified reduces the client's overall risk for the disease. *Clients with significant nonmodifiable risk factors may be discouraged, reducing their ability to eliminate or control modifiable risk factors.*
- Discuss the immediate benefits of smoking cessation. Provide resource materials from the American Heart Association, the American Lung Association, and the American Cancer Society. Refer to a structured smoking cessation program to increase the likelihood of success in quitting. *Long-time smokers may assume that the damage from smoking has already been done, and quitting would not be "worth the price."*
- Help the client identify specific sources of psychosocial and physical support for smoking cessation, dietary, and lifestyle changes. *Support persons, groups, and aids such as nicotine patches help the client achieve success and provide encouragement during difficult times (such as withdrawal symptoms).*
- Discuss the benefits of regular exercise for cardiovascular health and weight loss. Help identify favorite forms of exercise or physical activity. Encourage planning for 30 minutes of continuous aerobic activity (i.e., walking, running, bicycling, swimming) four to five times a week. Encourage identification of an "exercise buddy" to help maintain motivation. *Engaging in preferred activities with a partner maintains motivation and increases the likelihood of maintaining an exercise program. Encourage continuation of the plan, even when days are missed. Exercise is cumulative, so increasing the duration of exercise on subsequent days can "make up" for a lost day.*
- Provide information and teaching about prescribed medications such as cholesterol-lowering drugs. Discuss the relationship between hypertension, diabetes, and CHD. *Teaching is important to promote understanding of and compliance with the prescribed drug regimen.*

Community-Based Care

Encourage participation in some form of cardiac rehabilitation program. Formal programs provide comprehensive assessment of, interventions for, and teaching of clients with cardiac disease. Monitored exercise and information about risk factors help clients identify ways to lower their risk for CHD.

Because clients themselves are primarily responsible for maintaining the lifestyle changes necessary to reduce the risk of CHD, provide teaching and support as outlined in the previous section. Assist the client to make healthy choices and reinforce positive changes. Emphasize the importance of regular follow-up appointments to monitor progress.

THE CLIENT WITH ANGINA PECTORIS

Angina pectoris, or *angina*, is chest pain resulting from reduced coronary blood flow, which causes a temporary imbalance between myocardial blood supply and demand. The imbalance may be due to coronary heart disease, atherosclerosis, or vessel constriction that impairs myocardial blood supply. Hypermetabolic conditions such as exercise, thyrotoxicosis, stimulant abuse (e.g., cocaine), hyperthyroidism, and emotional stress can increase myocardial oxygen demand, precipitating angina. Anemia, heart failure, ventricular hypertrophy, or pulmonary diseases may affect blood and oxygen supplies as well, causing angina.

Pathophysiology

The imbalance between myocardial blood supply and demand causes temporary and reversible myocardial ischemia. **Ischemia**, deficient blood flow to tissue, may be caused by partial obstruction of a coronary artery, coronary artery spasm, or a thrombus. Obstruction of a coronary artery deprives cells in the region of the heart normally supplied by that vessel of oxygen and nutrients needed for metabolic processes. Cellular processes are compromised as ATP stores are depleted. Reduced oxygen causes cells to switch from aerobic metabolism to anaerobic metabolism. Anaerobic metabolism causes lactic acid to build up in the cells. It also affects cell membrane permeability, releasing substances such as histamine, kinins, and specific enzymes that stimulate terminal nerve fibers in the cardiac muscle and send pain impulses to the central nervous system. The pain radiates to the upper body because the heart shares the same dermatome as this region. Return of adequate circulation provides the nutrients needed by cells, and clears the waste products. More than 30 minutes of ischemia irreversibly damages myocardial cells (necrosis).

Three types of angina have been identified:

- *Stable angina* is the most common and predictable form of angina. It occurs with a predictable amount of activity or stress, and is a common manifestation of CHD. Stable angina usually occurs when the work of the heart is increased by physical exertion, exposure to cold, or by stress. Stable angina is relieved by rest and nitrates.
- *Prinzmetal's (variant) angina* is atypical angina that occurs unpredictably (unrelated to activity), and often at night. It is

caused by coronary artery spasm with or without an atherosclerotic lesion. The exact mechanism of coronary artery spasm is unknown. It may result from hyperactive sympathetic nervous system responses, altered calcium flow in smooth muscle, or reduced prostaglandins that promote vasodilation.

- *Unstable angina* occurs with increasing frequency, severity, and duration. Pain is unpredictable and occurs with decreasing levels of activity or stress and may occur at rest. Clients with unstable angina are at risk for myocardial infarction. Unstable angina is discussed further in the section on acute coronary syndromes that follows.

Silent myocardial ischemia, or asymptomatic ischemia, is thought to be common in people with CHD. Silent ischemia may occur with either activity or with mental stress. Mental stress increases the heart rate and blood pressure, increasing myocardial oxygen demand (McCance & Huether, 2006). Like symptomatic angina, silent myocardial ischemia is associated with an increased chance of myocardial infarction and death (Kasper et al., 2005).

FAST FACTS

- Stable angina occurs with a predictable amount of activity or stress.
- Unstable angina occurs with increasing frequency and severity; it may occur at times unrelated to activity or stress.
- Prinzmetal's angina is the only type of angina not necessarily related to coronary heart disease and atherosclerosis, developing due to coronary artery spasm.

Course and Manifestations

The cardinal manifestation of angina is chest pain. The pain typically is precipitated by an identifiable event, such as physical activity, strong emotion, stress, eating a heavy meal, or exposure to cold. The classic sequence of angina is activity–pain, rest–relief. The client may describe the pain as a tight, squeezing, heavy pressure, or constricting sensation. It characteristically begins beneath the sternum and may radiate to the jaw, neck, shoulder, or arm. Less characteristically, the pain may be felt in the jaw, epigastric region, or back. Anginal pain usually occurs in a *crescendo–decrescendo* pattern (increasing to a peak, then gradually decreasing) and typically lasts 2 to 5 minutes. It generally is relieved by rest. Additional manifestations of angina include dyspnea, pallor, tachycardia, and great anxiety and fear.

Women frequently present with atypical symptoms of angina, including indigestion or nausea, vomiting, and upper back pain. The manifestations of angina are summarized in the accompanying box.

The severity of angina can be graded by the degree to which it limits the client's activities. Class I angina does not occur with ordinary physical activities. It is prompted by strenuous, rapid, or prolonged physical exertion. Class II angina may develop with rapid or prolonged walking or stair climbing, whereas Class III angina significantly limits ordinary physical activities. The client with Class IV angina may have angina at rest, as well as with any physical activity (Kasper et al., 2005).

MANIFESTATIONS of Angina

- Chest pain: Substernal or precordial (across the chest wall); may radiate to neck, arms, shoulders, or jaw
- Quality: Tight, squeezing, constricting, or heavy sensation; may also be described as burning, aching, choking, dull, or constant
- Associated manifestations: Dyspnea, pallor, tachycardia, anxiety, and fear
- Atypical manifestations: Indigestion, nausea, vomiting, upper back pain
- Precipitating factors: Exercise or activity, strong emotion, stress, cold, heavy meal
- Relieving factors: Rest, position change; nitroglycerin

INTERDISCIPLINARY CARE

The management of stable angina focuses on maintaining coronary blood flow and cardiac function. Stable angina often can be managed by medical therapy. Measures to restore coronary blood flow are discussed in the section on acute coronary syndrome. As for CHD, risk factor management is a vital component of care for the client with angina (see the preceding section of this chapter).

Diagnosis

The diagnosis of angina is based on past medical history and family history, a comprehensive description of the chest pain, and physical assessment findings. Laboratory tests may confirm the presence of risk factors, such as an abnormal blood lipid profile and elevated blood glucose. Diagnostic tests provide information about overall cardiac function.

Common diagnostic tests to assess for coronary heart disease and angina include electrocardiography, stress testing, nuclear medicine studies, echocardiography (ultrasound), and coronary angiography.

ELECTROCARDIOGRAPHY A resting ECG may be normal, may show nonspecific changes in the ST segment and T wave, or may show evidence of previous myocardial infarction. Characteristic ECG changes are seen during anginal episodes. During periods of ischemia, the ST segment is depressed or downsloping, and the T wave may flatten or invert (Figure 31–1 ■). These changes reverse when ischemia is relieved. For more details about the ECG, its waveforms, and its uses, see Box 30–1 in Chapter 30 ∞.

STRESS ELECTROCARDIOGRAPHY Stress electrocardiography (exercise stress test) uses ECGs to monitor the cardiac response to an increased workload during progressive exercise. See the Diagnostic Tests box in the previous chapter for more information about exercise stress tests.

RADIONUCLIDE TESTING Radionuclide testing is a safe, noninvasive technique to evaluate myocardial perfusion and left ventricular function. The amount of radioisotope injected is very small; no special radiation precautions are required during or after the scan. Thallium-201 or a technetium-based radiocompound is injected intravenously, and the heart is scanned with a radiation detector. Ischemic or infarcted cells of the

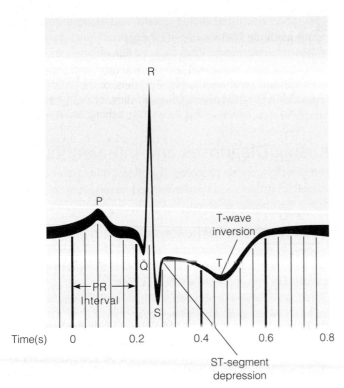

Figure 31–1 ■ ECG changes during an episode of angina. Note characteristic T-wave inversion and ST-segment depression of myocardial ischemia.

myocardium do not take up the substance normally, appearing as a "cold spot" on the scan. If the ischemia is transient, these spots gradually fill in, indicating the reversibility of the process. With severe ischemia or a myocardial infarction, these areas may remain devoid of radioactivity.

Left ventricular function can also be evaluated. Whereas the ejection fraction, or portion of blood ejected from the left ventricle during systole, normally increases during exercise, it may actually decrease in coronary heart disease and stress-induced ischemia.

Radionuclide testing may be combined with pharmacologic stress testing for clients who are physically unable to exercise or to detect subclinical myocardial ischemia. A vasodilator is injected to induce the same ischemic changes that occur with exercise in the diseased heart. Coronary arteries unaffected by atherosclerosis dilate in response to the drugs, increasing blood flow to already well-perfused tissue. This reduces flow to ischemic muscle, called *myocardial steal syndrome.*

ECHOCARDIOGRAPHY *Echocardiography* is a noninvasive test that uses ultrasound to evaluate cardiac structure and function. It may be done at rest, during supine exercise, or immediately following upright exercise to evaluate movement of the myocardial wall and assess for possible ischemia or infarction. *Transesophageal echocardiography (TEE)* uses ultrasound to identify abnormal blood flow patterns as well as cardiac structures. In TEE, the probe is on the tip of an endoscope inserted into the esophagus, positioning it close to the posterior heart (especially the left atrium and the aorta). It avoids interference by breasts, ribs, or lungs. See the Diagnostic Tests box

in Chapter 30 ∞ for more information about and the nursing care for clients undergoing these tests.

CORONARY ANGIOGRAPHY *Coronary angiography* is the gold standard for evaluating the coronary arteries. Guided by fluoroscopy, a catheter introduced into the femoral or brachial artery is threaded into the coronary artery. Dye is injected into each coronary opening, allowing visualization of the main coronary branches and any abnormalities, such as stenosis or obstruction. Narrowing of the vessel lumen by more than 50% is considered significant; most lesions that cause symptoms involve more than 70% narrowing. Vessel obstructions are noted on a coronary artery "map" that provides a guide for tracking disease progression and for elective treatment with angioplasty or cardiac surgery. During angiogram, the drug ergonovine maleate may be injected to induce coronary artery spasm and diagnose Prinzmetal's angina. See the Diagnostic Tests box in Chapter 30 for nursing care of clients undergoing coronary angiography.

Medications

Drugs may be used for both acute and long-term relief of angina. The goal of drug treatment is to reduce oxygen demand and increase oxygen supply to the myocardium. Three main classes of drugs are used to treat angina: nitrates, beta blockers, and calcium channel blockers.

NITRATES Nitrates, including nitroglycerin and longer-acting nitrate preparations, are used to treat acute anginal attacks and prevent angina.

Sublingual nitroglycerin is the drug of choice to treat acute angina. It acts within 1 to 2 minutes, decreasing myocardial work and oxygen demand through venous and arterial dilation, which in turn reduce preload and afterload. It may also improve myocardial oxygen supply by dilating collateral blood vessels and reducing stenosis. Rapid-acting nitroglycerin is also available as a buccal spray in a metered system. For some clients, this may be easier to handle than small nitroglycerin tablets.

> **PRACTICE ALERT**
> ■ Sublingual nitroglycerin tablets and nitroglycerin spray are the only medications appropriate to treat an acute anginal attack.

Longer-acting nitroglycerin preparations (oral tablets, ointment, or transdermal patches) are used to prevent attacks of angina, not to treat an acute attack. The primary problem with long-term nitrate use is the development of *tolerance,* a decreasing effect from the same dose of medication. Tolerance can be limited by a dosing schedule that allows a nitrate-free period of at least 8 to 10 hours daily. This is usually scheduled at night, when angina is less likely to occur.

Headache is a common side effect of nitrates, and may limit their usefulness. Nausea, dizziness, and hypotension are also common effects of therapy.

BETA BLOCKERS Beta blockers, including propranolol, metoprolol, nadolol, and atenolol, are considered first-line drugs to treat stable angina. They block the cardiac-stimulating effects of norepinephrine and epinephrine, preventing anginal attacks by reducing heart rate, myocardial contractility, and blood pressure, thus reducing myocardial oxygen demand. Beta blockers may be used alone or with other medications to prevent angina.

Beta blockers are contraindicated for clients with asthma or severe COPD (see Chapter 39 ∞) because they may cause severe bronchospasm. They are not used in clients with significant bradycardia, or AV conduction blocks, and are used cautiously in heart failure. Beta blockers are not used to treat Prinzmetal's angina because they may make it worse.

CALCIUM CHANNEL BLOCKERS Calcium channel blockers reduce myocardial oxygen demand and increase myocardial blood and oxygen supply. These drugs, which include verapamil, diltiazem, and nifedipine, lower blood pressure, reduce myocardial contractility, and, in some cases, lower the heart rate, decreasing myocardial oxygen demand. They are also potent coronary vasodilators, effectively increasing oxygen supply. Like beta blockers, calcium channel blockers act too slowly to effectively treat an acute attack of angina; they are used for long-term prophylaxis. Because they may actually increase ischemia and mortality in clients with heart failure or left ventricular dysfunction, these drugs are not usually prescribed in the initial treatment of angina. They are used cautiously in clients with dysrhythmias, heart failure, or hypotension.

The nursing implications of antianginal medications are summarized in the Medication Administration box on the next page.

ASPIRIN The client with angina, particularly unstable angina, is at risk for myocardial infarction because of significant narrowing of the coronary arteries. Low-dose aspirin (80 to 325 mg/day) is often prescribed to reduce the risk of platelet aggregation and thrombus formation.

NURSING CARE

The focus of nursing care for clients with angina is similar to the interdisciplinary care focus: to reduce myocardial oxygen demand and improve the oxygen supply. Angina usually is treated in community settings; the primary nursing focus is education.

Health Promotion

In addition to health promotion measures identified for CHD, emphasize the importance of active CHD risk factor management to slow progression of the disease. Encourage clients to stop smoking. Discuss the use of cholesterol-lowering drug therapy with clients who have hypercholesterolemia. Encourage regular aerobic exercise and a diet based on American Heart Association or National Cholesterol Education Program guidelines.

Assessment

Focused assessment data for the client with angina includes the following:

- *Health history:* Chest pain, including type, intensity, duration, frequency, aggravating factors, and relief measures; associated symptoms; history of other cardiovascular disorders, peripheral vascular disease, or stroke; current medications

and treatment; usual diet, exercise, and alcohol intake patterns; smoking history; use of other recreational drugs.

- *Physical assessment:* Vital signs and heart sounds; strength and equality of peripheral pulses; skin color and temperature (central and peripheral); physical appearance during pain episode (e.g., shortness of breath, apparent anxiety, color, diaphoresis).

Nursing Diagnoses and Interventions

High-priority nursing problems for clients with angina include ineffective cardiac tissue perfusion and management of the prescribed therapeutic regimen.

Ineffective Tissue Perfusion: Cardiac

The pain of angina results from impaired blood flow and oxygen supply to the myocardium. Nursing interventions can both prevent ischemia and shorten the duration of pain.

- Keep prescribed nitroglycerin tablets at the client's side so one can be taken at the onset of pain. *Anginal pain indicates myocardial ischemia. Nitroglycerin reduces cardiac work and may improve myocardial blood flow, relieving ischemia and pain.*
- Start oxygen at 4 to 6 L/min per nasal cannula or as prescribed. *Supplemental oxygen reduces myocardial hypoxia.*
- Space activities to allow rest between them. *Activity increases cardiac work and may precipitate angina. Spacing of activities allows the heart to recover.*
- Teach about prescribed medications to maintain myocardial perfusion and reduce cardiac work. Emphasize that long-acting nitrates, beta blockers, and calcium channel blockers are used to *prevent* anginal attacks, not to *treat* an acute attack. *It is important for the client to understand the purpose and use of prescribed drugs to maintain optimal myocardial perfusion.*
- Instruct to take sublingual nitroglycerin before engaging in activities that precipitate angina (e.g., climbing stairs, sexual intercourse). *This prophylactic dose of nitroglycerin helps maintain cardiac perfusion when increased work is anticipated, preventing ischemia and chest pain.*
- Encourage to implement and maintain a progressive exercise program under the supervision of the primary care provider or a cardiac rehabilitation professional. *Exercise slows the atherosclerotic process and helps develop collateral circulation to the heart muscle.*
- Refer to a smoking cessation program as indicated. *Nicotine causes vasoconstriction and increases the heart rate, decreasing myocardial perfusion and increasing cardiac workload.*

Risk for Ineffective Therapeutic Regimen Management

Denial may be strong in the client with angina pectoris. Because many people think of the heart as the locus of life itself, problems such as angina remind people of their mortality, an uncomfortable fact. Denial may lead to "forgetting" to take prescribed medications or to attempting activities that will precipitate angina. Some clients, by contrast, may become "cardiac cripples," afraid

MEDICATION ADMINISTRATION   Antianginal Medications

ORGANIC NITRATES
Nitroglycerin (Nitropaste, Nitro-Dur, Nitro-Bid, Nitrol, Transderm-Nitro, Nitrogard, Nitrodisc, Tridil)
Isosorbide dinitrate (Isordil)
Isosorbide mononitrate (ISMO)
Amyl nitrite

Nitrates dilate both arterial and venous vessels, depending on the dose. Coronary artery vasodilation increases blood flow and myocardial oxygen supply. Venous dilation allows peripheral blood pooling, reducing venous return, preload, and cardiac work. Arterial dilation reduces vascular resistance and afterload, also reducing cardiac work. Sublingual nitroglycerin (NTG) tablets are used to treat and prevent acute anginal attacks (when taken prophylactically before activity). Nitrates are administered sublingually, by buccal spray, or intravenously for immediate effect; or orally or topically for sustained effect.

Nursing Responsibilities
- Dilute intravenous nitroglycerin before infusing; use only glass bottles for the mixture. Nitroglycerin adheres to PVC bags and tubing, affecting the amount of drug that is delivered. Use non-PVC infusion tubing.
- Wear gloves when applying nitroglycerin paste or ointment to prevent absorbing the drug through the skin. Measure dose carefully and spread evenly in a 2- by 3-inch area.
- Remove nitroglycerin patches or ointment at night to help prevent tolerance.

Health Education for the Client and Family
- Use only the sublingual, buccal, and spray forms of nitrates to treat acute angina.
- If the first nitrate dose does not relieve angina within 5 minutes, take a second dose. After 5 more minutes, you may take a third dose if needed. If the pain is unrelieved or lasts for 20 minutes or longer, seek medical assistance immediately.
- Carry a supply of nitroglycerin tablets with you. Dissolve sublingual nitroglycerin tablets under the tongue or between the upper lip and gum. Do not eat, drink, or smoke until the tablet is completely dissolved.
- Keep sublingual tablets in their original amber glass bottle to protect them from heat, light, and moisture. Replace your supply every 6 months.
- You may experience a burning or tingling sensation under the tongue and develop a transient headache when you take the drug. These are expected; the headache will diminish over time.
- Use caution when standing from a sitting position; nitroglycerin may make you light-headed.
- Rotate ointment or transdermal patch application sites. Apply to a hairless area; spread ointment evenly without rubbing or massaging. Remove the patch or residual ointment at bedtime daily. Apply a fresh dose in the morning.
- If you are using a long-acting nitrate, keep a supply of immediate-acting nitrates to treat acute angina.

BETA BLOCKERS
Atenolol (Tenormin)
Metoprolol (Lopressor)
Propranolol (Inderal)
Nadolol (Corgard)

Beta blockers decrease cardiac workload by blocking beta receptors on the heart muscle, decreasing heart rate, contractility, myocardial oxygen consumption, and blood pressure. Beta blockers also reduce *reflex tachycardia* (an increased heart rate in response to stimuli such as increased SNS activity or vasodilation), which may develop with other antianginal drugs. Beta blockers are frequently prescribed as antianginal and antihypertensive agents.

Nursing Responsibilities
- Document heart rate and blood pressure before administering the medication. Withhold drug if the heart rate is below 50 bpm or the blood pressure is below prescribed limits. Notify the physician.
- Assess for and report possible contraindications to therapy, including heart failure, bradycardia, AV block, asthma, or COPD.
- Concurrent use of beta blockers and calcium channel blockers increases the risk for heart failure; notify the physician if these drugs are prescribed together.
- Do not abruptly discontinue these drugs after long-term therapy, as this can increase heart rate, contractility, and blood pressure, and cause fatal dysrhythmia, myocardial infarction, or stroke.

Health Education for the Client and Family
- Beta blockers help prevent angina but will not relieve an acute attack. Keep a supply of fast-acting nitrates on hand for acute anginal attacks.
- Do not suddenly stop taking this medication. Discuss discontinuing this medication with your doctor.
- Take your pulse daily. Do not take the drug, and contact your doctor, if your heart rate is below 50 bpm. Check your blood pressure frequently.
- Report a slow or irregular pulse, swelling or weight gain, or difficulty breathing to your doctor.

CALCIUM CHANNEL BLOCKERS
Nifedipine (Adalat, Procardia)
Diltiazem (Cardizem)
Verapamil (Isoptin, Calan)
Bepridil (Vascor)
Felodipine (Plendil)
Isradipine (DynaCirc)
Nicardipine (Cardene)
Nimodipine (Nimotop)

Calcium channel blockers are used to control angina, hypertension, and dysrhythmias. By blocking the entry of calcium into cells, these drugs reduce contractility, slow the heart rate and conduction, and cause vasodilation. Calcium channel blockers increase myocardial oxygen supply by dilating the coronary arteries; they decrease the workload of the heart by lowering vascular resistance and oxygen demand. Calcium channel blockers are often prescribed for clients with coronary artery spasm (Prinzmetal's angina).

Nursing Responsibilities
- Do not mix verapamil in any solution containing sodium bicarbonate. Administer IV push verapamil over 2 to 3 minutes.
- Document blood pressure and heart rate before administering the drug. Withhold the drug if the heart rate is below 50 bpm. Notify the physician.

(continued)

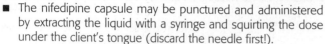

MEDICATION ADMINISTRATION   **Antianginal Medications (continued)**

- The nifedipine capsule may be punctured and administered by extracting the liquid with a syringe and squirting the dose under the client's tongue (discard the needle first!).
- Use caution when giving a calcium channel blocker with other cardiac depressants, such as beta blockers. Concomitant administration with nitrates may cause excessive vasodilation.
- Manifestations of toxicity include nausea, generalized weakness, signs of decreased cardiac output, hypotension, bradycardia, and AV block. Report these findings immediately. Maintain intravenous access, and slowly administer intravenous calcium

chloride. Do not infuse large volumes of fluid to treat hypotension as heart failure may result.

Health Education for the Client and Family
- Take your pulse before taking the drug. Do not take the drug and notify physician if your heart rate drops below 50 bpm.
- Keep a fresh supply of immediate-acting nitrate available to treat acute anginal attacks. Calcium channel blockers will not work fast enough to relieve an acute attack.

---

to engage in activities because of anticipated chest pain. Their inactivity may actually hasten the atherosclerotic process and inhibit collateral circulation development, worsening angina.

- Assess knowledge and understanding of angina. *Assessment allows tailoring of teaching and interventions to the needs of the client.*
- Teach about angina and atherosclerosis as needed, building on current knowledge base. *This can help the client understand that angina is a manageable disease and that pain can usually be controlled and the disease progress slowed.*
- Provide written and verbal instructions about prescribed medications and their use. *Written instructions reinforce teaching and are available to the client for future reference.*
- Stress the importance of taking chest pains seriously while maintaining a positive attitude. *Although it is vital to recognize the significance of chest pain and deal with it appropriately, it is also important to maintain a positive outlook.*
- Refer to a cardiac rehabilitation program or other organized activities and support groups for clients with coronary heart disease. *Programs such as these help the client develop risk factor management strategies, maintain a program of supervised activity, and gain coping skills.*

Community-Based Care

Many clients with stable angina manage their pain effectively, continuing to live active and productive lives. To promote effective management of this disorder, include the following topics in teaching for home care:

- Coronary heart disease and the processes that cause chest pain, including the relationship between the pain and reduced blood flow to the heart muscle
- Use and effects (desired and adverse) of prescribed medications; importance of not discontinuing medications abruptly
- Nitroglycerin use for acute angina: always carry several tablets (not the entire supply); prophylactic use before activities that often cause chest pain; take tablet at first indication of pain rather than waiting to see if the pain develops; seek immediate medical assistance if three nitroglycerin tablets over 15 to 20 minutes do not relieve the pain
- The importance of calling 911 or going to the emergency department immediately for unrelieved chest pain

- Appropriate storage of nitroglycerin: This unstable compound needs to be stored in a cool, dry, dark place; no more than a 6-month supply should be kept on hand.

For the client who has undergone cardiac surgery, also include the following:
- Respiratory care, activity, and pain management
- The importance of actively participating in rehabilitation
- Manifestations of infection or other potential complications and their management.

THE CLIENT WITH ACUTE CORONARY SYNDROME

Acute coronary syndrome (ACS) is a condition of unstable cardiac ischemia. ACS includes unstable angina and acute myocardial ischemia with or without significant injury of myocardial tissue. Although the term ACS may, in some cases, be applied to acute myocardial infarction (myocardial tissue death), myocardial infarction is discussed separately in the next section of this chapter. An estimated 1.4 million Americans are admitted to the hospital annually with ACS (Kasper et al., 2005).

FAST FACTS
- Acute coronary syndrome (severe cardiac ischemia), a common cause of hospital admission, includes unstable angina and acute myocardial infarction.
- Unstable angina is characterized by injury to myocardial cells; with prompt restoration of blood flow, muscle tissue recovers.
- Myocardial infarction is characterized by necrosis and death of myocardial cells; scar tissue forms and functional muscle is lost.
- ACS is the most common identified cause of sudden cardiac death (American Heart Association [AHA], 2005a).

Pathophysiology

ACS is a dynamic state in which coronary blood flow is acutely reduced, but not fully occluded. Myocardial cells are injured by the acute ischemia that results. Most people affected by ACS have significant stenosis of one or more coronary arteries.

ACS is precipitated by one or more of the following processes: (1) rupture or erosion of atherosclerotic plaque with formation of a blood clot that does not fully occlude the vessel; (2) coronary artery spasm (e.g., Prinzmetal's angina); (3) progressive vessel obstruction by atherosclerotic plaque or restenosis following a percutaneous revascularization (PCR) procedure; (4) inflammation of a coronary artery; or (5) increased myocardial oxygen demand and/or decreased supply (e.g., acute blood loss or anemia) (Braunwald et al., 2002). Of these, ruptured or eroded plaque is the predominant pathophysiology underlying ACS (AHA, 2005a). Plaque rupture often is triggered by hemodynamic factors such as increased heart rate, blood flow, and blood pressure in response to a surge of sympathetic nervous system (SNS) activity. Increased SNS activity also is thought to contribute to the higher incidence of plaque rupture within the first hour of arising from bed in the morning (Porth, 2005).

When atherosclerotic plaque ruptures or erodes, the exposed lipid core of the plaque stimulates platelet aggregation and the extrinsic clotting pathway. Thrombin is generated and fibrin is deposited, forming a clot that severely impairs or obstructs blood flow to tissue distal to the area of plaque rupture. As a result, these cells become ischemic.

Injured myocardial cells contract less effectively, potentially reducing cardiac output if a large area of myocardium is affected. Lactic acid released from ischemic cells stimulates pain receptors, causing chest pain. Ischemia and injury affect electrical impulse conduction, producing inversion of the T wave and possibly elevation of the ST segment on the ECG.

Manifestations

The cardinal manifestation of ACS is chest pain, usually substernal or epigastric. The pain often radiates to the neck, left shoulder, and/or left arm. The pain may occur at rest and typically lasts longer than 10 to 20 minutes. In ACS, the chest pain is more severe and prolonged than that previously experienced by the client. It may be a new onset of pain, or may represent a pattern of increasing frequency and severity of anginal pain. Dyspnea, diaphoresis, pallor, and cool skin may be present. Tachycardia and hypotension may occur. The client may be nauseated or feel light-headed. Table 31–5 compares the features of stable angina, ACS, and acute myocardial infarction.

INTERDISCIPLINARY CARE

The client with ACS generally presents at the emergency department or physician's office with complaints of severe chest pain. The pain may be unrelieved by nitroglycerin or may be more severe and of longer duration than previous anginal episodes. The ECG is used in conjunction with blood levels of cardiac markers to differentiate between unstable angina and acute myocardial infarction. Clients with unstable angina generally are admitted to the acute care unit on bed rest with cardiac monitoring for 12 to 24 hours. Coronary revascularization procedures may be performed within 48 hours if significant CHD is identified.

Diagnosis

The ECG and serum cardiac markers are the primary tests used to establish the diagnosis of ACS. Serum cardiac markers, proteins released from injured and necrotic heart muscle, can be measured. (See the following section on acute myocardial infarction and Table 31–6 for more information about serum cardiac markers.)

■ Cardiac muscle troponins, *cardiac-specific troponin T (cT_nT)* and *cardiac-specific troponin I (cT_nI)*, are sensitive indicators of myocardial damage. Troponins may be elevated in

TABLE 31–5 Comparing Stable Angina, Acute Coronary Syndrome, and Acute Myocardial Infarction

	STABLE ANGINA	ACUTE CORONARY SYNDROME	ACUTE MYOCARDIAL INFARCTION
Pathophysiology	Myocardial ischemia occurs with increased workload (e.g., during exercise) due to stable atherosclerotic plaque narrowing the coronary arteries.	Coronary artery spasm or partial occlusion results from unstable plaque and thrombus formation with increasing myocardial ischemia.	Obstruction of a coronary artery by a thrombus blocks blood supply to a portion of myocardium, resulting in necrosis.
Chest Pain	Stable and predictable, occurring with exertion or emotion Crescendo–decrescendo pattern May radiate to neck, shoulder, arms Usually lasts 2 to 5 minutes, relieved by rest	Occurs at rest; increasing frequency and severity Lasts 10 minutes or longer Radiates to neck, left shoulder, and arm	Begins abruptly, unrelated to rest or exercise Severe, "crushing" Unrelieved by rest or nitroglycerin Radiates to arms, neck, jaw
Other Manifestations	Indigestion, nausea Possible shortness of breath Anxiety	Epigastric pain Dyspnea Tachycardia, hypotension Cool, pale skin	Epigastric pain, nausea Dyspnea Pallor, diaphoresis Tachycardia or bradycardia, hyper- or hypotension
Diagnosis	ECG: T-wave inversion during anginal episodes Cardiac markers: within normal range	ECG: ST-segment depression, T-wave inversion Cardiac markers: within normal range or transient elevation	ECG: ST-segment elevation, possible Q wave Cardiac markers: elevated

ACS or may be within normal limits if chest pain is due to unstable angina.

■ Creatine kinase (CK) and CK-MB (specific to myocardial muscle) levels are likely to be within normal limits or demonstrate transient elevation, returning to normal levels within 12 to 24 hours.

The ECG, particularly when done during the acute episode of chest pain, is a valuable diagnostic tool for ACS. ST-segment changes (elevation or depression) during chest pain that resolve when the pain abates usually indicate acute myocardial ischemia and severe underlying CHD.

Medications

Medications include drugs to reduce myocardial ischemia and those to reduce the risk for blood clotting. Fibrinolytic drugs (that is, drugs that break down the fibrin in blood clots) may be given prior to or on admission to the emergency department. These drugs restore blood flow to ischemic cardiac muscle and can prevent permanent damage. See the section on myocardial infarction for more information about fibrinolytic drugs and their nursing implications.

Nitrates and beta blockers are used to restore blood flow to the ischemic myocardium and reduce the workload of the heart. Nitroglycerin is given by sublingual tablet or buccal spray. If chest pain is unrelieved after three doses 5 minutes apart, an intravenous nitroglycerin infusion is initiated. The infusion may be continued until the chest pain is relieved or for 12 to 24 hours. Topical or oral nitrates are then initiated. Beta-adrenergic blockers are initially given intravenously, followed by oral beta-blockers. See the Medication Administration box on page 973 for the nursing implications of these drugs.

Aspirin, other antiplatelet drugs, and heparin are given to inhibit blood clotting and reduce the risk of thrombus formation. Aspirin and clopidogrel (Plavix) are given to clients with ACS who do not have an excessive bleeding risk. Aspirin and clopidogrel suppress platelet aggregation, interrupting the process of forming a stable blood clot. Both increase the risk of serious hemorrhage; for most clients, however, the benefit outweighs the risk. Intravenous antiplatelet drugs such as abciximab (ReoPro), eptifibatide (Integrilin), or tirofiban (Aggrastat) may be used when an invasive coronary revascularization procedure is anticipated in the immediate or near future. Nursing implications for the antiplatelet drugs are outlined in the Medication Administration box below.

Revascularization Procedures

Several procedures may be used to restore blood flow and oxygen to ischemic tissue. Nonsurgical techniques include translu-

---

MEDICATION ADMINISTRATION Antiplatelet Drugs

ORAL ANTIPLATELET DRUGS
Aspirin
Clopidogrel (Plavix)
Antiplatelet drugs suppress platelet aggregation in arteries, preventing the development of an arterial thrombus. Aspirin and clopidogrel block different platelet activation pathways to inhibit platelet aggregation and clot formation. The dose of aspirin given to achieve antiplatelet effects is low, typically 80 to 325 mg/day.

Nursing Responsibilities
■ Inquire about a history of intracranial hemorrhage, upper gastrointestinal bleeding, peptic ulcer disease, or known bleeding tendency.
■ Observe for and report increased bruising, petechiae, purpura, apparent or occult bleeding (e.g., melena, hematemesis).
■ Do not administer concurrently with warfarin (Coumadin).

Health Education for the Client and Family
■ Take as directed. Take aspirin with food or milk; clopidogrel may be taken at any time of day.
■ Do not use NSAIDs or other over-the-counter drugs that may contain aspirin or an NSAID unless prescribed by your physician.
■ Check with your physician before taking any herbal remedies such as evening primrose oil, feverfew, garlic, ginkgo biloba, or grapeseed extract while taking these medications.
■ Report unusual bruising or excessive bleeding.
■ Inform all care providers (including dental professionals) of use of these drugs.

INTRAVENOUS ANTIPLATELET DRUGS
Abciximab (ReoPro)
Eptifibatide (Integrelin)
Tirofiban (Aggrastat)

The intravenously administered antiplatelet drugs, abciximab, epifibatide, and tirofiban, block the final common pathway of platelet activation, and thus are more effective. However, the risk of bleeding is greater than with the orally administered antiplatelet drugs.

Nursing Responsibilities
■ Determine history of bleeding disorders, intracranial hemorrhage, recent trauma or surgery.
■ Inquire about recent use of oral antiplatelet or anticoagulant drugs.
■ Monitor CBC including hemoglobin, hematocrit, and platelet count; clotting studies, including PT, INR, PTT; vital signs; and ECG during therapy.
■ Maintain a separate intravenous line for blood draws and administration of other drugs during infusion.
■ Closely observe for and immediately report anaphylaxis or bleeding uncontrolled by pressure. Keep resuscitation equipment readily available.
■ Maintain bed rest during infusion.

Health Education for the Client and Family
■ This drug is given to reduce the risk of clotting and myocardial infarction. It helps maintain blood flow through the affected vessel following angioplasty and stent placement.
■ Immediately report any chest tightness, difficulty breathing, shortness of breath, or itching that develops during the infusion.
■ Your risk of bleeding should return to normal within about 2 days following the infusion.
■ Immediately report any unusual bruising or bleeding to your doctor.

minal coronary angioplasty, laser angioplasty, coronary atherectomy, and intracoronary stents. Coronary artery bypass grafting (CABG) is a surgical procedure that may be used.

PERCUTANEOUS CORONARY REVASCULARIZATION *Percutaneous coronary revascularization (PCR)* procedures are used to restore blood flow to the ischemic myocardium in clients with CHD. Approximately 600,000 PCR procedures are done annually in the United States. PCR is used to treat clients with:

- Moderately severe, chronic stable angina unrelieved by medical therapy
- Unstable angina
- Acute myocardial infarction
- Significant stenosis of the left anterior descending coronary artery
- Stenosis of a CABG (Kasper et al., 2005; Tierney et al., 2005).

PCR procedures are similar to the procedure used for coronary angiography. A catheter introduced into the arterial circulation is guided into the opening of the narrowed coronary artery. A flexible guidewire is inserted through the catheter lumen into the affected vessel. The guidewire is then used to thread an angioplasty balloon, arterial stent, or other therapeutic device into the narrowed segment of the artery. The procedure is performed in the cardiac catheterization laboratory using local anesthesia. The hospital stay is short (1 to 2 days), minimizing costs.

In a *percutaneous transluminal coronary angioplasty* (*PTCA*), a balloon-tipped catheter is threaded over the guidewire, with the balloon positioned across the area of narrowing (Figure 31–2 ■). The balloon is inflated in a step-by-step fashion for about 30 seconds to 2 minutes to compress the plaque against the arterial wall, with a goal of reducing the vessel obstruction to less than 50% of the arterial lumen. PTCA typically is accompanied by placement of a stent. *Intracoronary stents* are metallic scaffolds used to maintain an open arterial lumen. Stents reduce the rate of restenosis following angioplasty by about one-third, and are now used in the majority of all PCR procedures (Kasper et al., 2005). The stent is placed over a balloon catheter, guided into position, and expanded as the balloon is inflated. It then remains in the artery as a prop after the balloon is removed. Endothelial cells will completely line the inner wall of the stent to produce a smooth inner lining. Antiplatelet medications (aspirin and ticlopidine) are given following stent insertion to reduce the risk of thrombus formation at the site.

In contrast to stent procedures, which enlarge the artery by displacing plaque, *atherectomy* procedures remove plaque from the identified lesion. The directional atherectomy catheter shaves the plaque off vessel walls using a rotary cutting head, retaining the fragments in its housing and removing them from the vessel. Rotational atherectomy catheters pulverize plaque into particles small enough to pass through the coronary microcirculation. Laser atherectomy devices use laser energy to remove plaque.

Complications following PCR procedures include hematoma at the catheter insertion site, pseudoaneurysm, embolism, hypersensitivity to contrast dye, dysrhythmias, bleeding, vessel perforation, and restenosis, or reocclusion of the treated vessel.

Nursing care of the client undergoing PCR is outlined in the box on the next page.

CORONARY ARTERY BYPASS GRAFTING Surgery for coronary heart disease involves using a section of a vein or an artery to create a connection (or bypass) between the aorta and the coronary artery beyond the obstruction (Figure 31–3 ■). This then allows blood to perfuse the ischemic portion of the heart. The internal mammary artery in the chest and the saphenous vein from the leg are the vessels most commonly used for CABG.

Bypass grafts are safe and effective. Angina is totally relieved or significantly reduced in 90% of clients who undergo

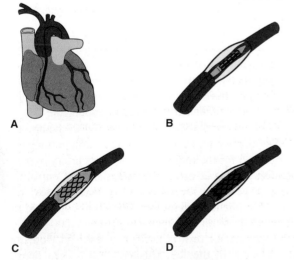

Figure 31–2 ■ Percutaneous coronary revascularization. *A,* The balloon catheter with the stent is threaded into the affected coronary artery. *B, C,* The stent is positioned across the blockage and expanded. *D,* The balloon is deflated and removed, leaving the stent in place.

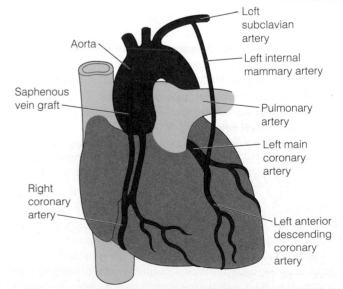

Figure 31–3 ■ Coronary artery bypass grafting using the internal mammary artery and a saphenous vein graft.

NURSING CARE OF THE CLIENT HAVING   PCR

BEFORE THE PROCEDURE

- Assess knowledge of the procedure and expectations of treatment. *This allows information to be tailored to the client's needs and provides an opportunity to clarify misconceptions.*
- Describe the cardiac catheterization laboratory and the planned PCR procedure, including:
  - Preoperative preparation (see Chapter 4 ∞)
  - Planned anesthesia or sedation to be used.
  - Drugs that may be given during the procedure, such as anticoagulants to reduce the risk of thrombus formation, and intravenous nitroglycerin and a calcium channel blocker to dilate coronary arteries and prevent anginal pain.
- Discuss possible sensations during the procedure, including flushing or warmth and a metallic taste in the mouth as the contrast dye is injected, and a feeling of pressure or chest pain during balloon inflation. *Advanced preparation for expected sensations reduces anxiety and improves outcomes.*
- Perform a comprehensive assessment, including hydration status (skin and mucous membrane moisture, turgor) and peripheral circulation (color, warmth, sensation, pulses, and capillary refill).

AFTER THE PROCEDURE

- Complete a head-to-toe assessment. Note any complaints of chest pain, or evidence of decreased cardiac output or myocardial infarction. *Assessment provides a baseline for subsequent assessments and allows early identification of possible complications.*
- Monitor vital signs and cardiac rhythm continuously. Treat dysrhythmias as ordered. Obtain a 12-lead ECG if signs of ischemia develop, and notify physician. *Vital signs reflect cardiac output. Dysrhythmias may develop with reperfusion of the ischemic myocardium. ECG changes may indicate infarction or restenosis of the affected vessel.*
- Maintain intravenous nitroglycerin infusion. Administer anticoagulant and antiplatelet medications, nitrates, and calcium

channel blockers as ordered. *These drugs decrease oxygen demand and increase oxygen supply by dilating the coronary arteries and systemic vasculature. They also reduce the risk of thrombus formation.*
- Monitor for and treat or report chest pain as indicated. *Chest pain may indicate ischemia and possible myocardial infarction.*
- Maintain bed rest as ordered with the head of the bed at 30 degrees or less. Prevent flexion of the leg on the affected side. Following sheath removal, follow protocol for pressure dressing or device or sandbag placement. *A large puncture wound occurs at the insertion site. Immobilization allows the wound to seal; a pressure dressing helps prevent bleeding.*
- Monitor distal pulses, color, movement, sensation, and temperature of the affected leg, and insertion site every 15 minutes for the first hour, every 30 minutes for the next hour, every hour for the next 8 hours, then every 4 hours. *A clot may form at the site, reducing perfusion of the affected leg. The site and dressing are monitored for excessive bleeding, hematoma formation, or pseudoaneurysm. Pseudoaneurysm occurs as a result of inadequate hemostasis after catheter removal.*
- Monitor intake and output, serum electrolytes, blood urea nitrogen (BUN), creatinine, complete blood count (CBC), partial thromboplastin time (PTT), and cardiac enzymes. Report abnormal results to the physician. *Contrast dye causes osmotic diuresis and may cause renal damage or a hypersensitivity reaction. Electrolyte imbalances increase the risk of dysrhythmias. Cardiac enzymes are monitored for indications of possible myocardial damage during the procedure. The PTT monitors the effectiveness of heparin therapy.*
- Monitor for bradycardia, light-headedness, hypotension, diaphoresis, and loss of consciousness during sheath removal. Keep atropine at bedside during sheath removal. *Bradycardia and signs of decreased cardiac output may occur during sheath removal because of a vasovagal reaction. Atropine decreases vagal tone and increases heart rate.*

---

complete revascularization. While anginal pain may recur within 3 years, it rarely is as severe as before surgery. Coronary artery bypass graft has a positive effect on mortality in many cases. It is recommended for clients who have multiple vessel disease and impaired left ventricular function or diabetes, and for clients who have significant obstruction of the left main coronary artery (Kasper et al., 2005).

A median sternotomy commonly is used to access the heart. The heart is usually stopped during surgery. The *cardiopulmonary bypass (CPB) pump* is used to maintain perfusion to the rest of the organs during open-heart surgery. Venous blood is removed from the body through a cannula placed in the right atrium or the superior and inferior venae cavae. Blood then circulates through the CPB pump, where it is oxygenated, its temperature regulated, and it is filtered. Oxygenated blood is returned to the body through a cannula in the ascending aorta (Figure 31–4 ■). Cardiopulmonary bypass enables surgeons to

operate on a quiet heart and a relatively bloodless field. Hypothermia can be maintained to reduce the metabolic rate and decrease oxygen demand during surgery.

Newer techniques have been developed that allow surgeons to perform CABG without cardioplegia (stopping the heart) and CPB. Off-pump coronary artery bypass (OPCAB) allows use of a smaller incision for access. Although cardiopulmonary bypass is employed for the majority of coronary artery bypass procedures, OPCAB is a promising alternative. Controlled studies demonstrate lower mortality and morbidity rates and faster recovery for clients undergoing OPCAB as compared to CABG with cardiopulmonary bypass (Eagle et al., 2004).

When the saphenous vein is used, it is excised from its normal attachments in the leg, flushed with a cold heparinized saline solution, and then reversed so that its valves do not interfere with blood flow. When appropriate, a laparoscopic approach may be used to remove the vein. The vein is

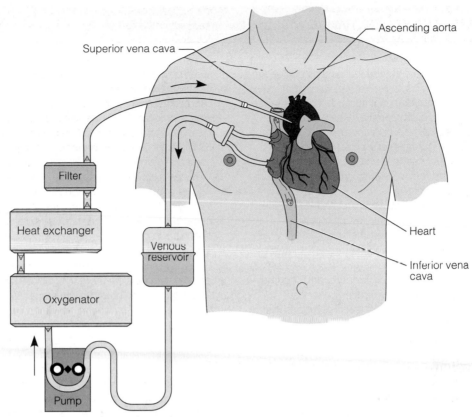

Figure 31–4 ■ A diagrammatic representation of cardiopulmonary bypass. A cannula in the superior and inferior venae cavae removes venous blood, which is then pumped through an oxygenator and heat exchanger. After filtering, oxygenated blood is returned to the ascending aorta.

anastomosed (grafted) to the aorta and the coronary artery, distal to the occlusion (see Figure 31–3). This provides a bridge or conduit for blood flow past the obstruction. If the internal mammary artery (IMA) is used, its distal end is excised and anastomosed to the coronary artery distal to the obstruction. The IMA often is used to revascularize the left coronary artery because of the greater oxygen demand of the left ventricle.

Once grafting is completed, cardiopulmonary bypass is discontinued and the client is rewarmed. Rewarming stimulates the heart to resume beating. Temporary pacing wires are sutured in place and passed through the chest wall in case temporary pacing is necessary. Chest tubes are placed in the pleural space and mediastinum to drain blood and reestablish negative pressure in the thoracic cavity. The sternum is closed using heavy wires and bone wax, the skin is closed with sutures or staples, and sterile dressings are applied over sternal and leg incisions.

Pre- and postoperative nursing care and teaching for the client having a coronary artery bypass graft or other open-heart surgery are outlined on pages 980–982.

MINIMALLY INVASIVE CORONARY ARTERY SURGERY *Minimally invasive coronary artery surgery* is a potential future alternative to CABG. Two approaches may be used: *Port-access coronary artery bypass* uses several small holes, or "ports," in

the chest wall to access vessels for connection to the CPB pump and the surgical site. Alternatively, the femoral artery and femoral vein may be used for CPB (Eagle et al., 2004). CPB is avoided altogether using the *minimally invasive direct coronary artery bypass (MIDCAB)* approach. With MIDCAB, a small surgical incision and several chest wall ports are used to graft a chest wall artery to the affected coronary vessel while the heart continues to beat.

TRANSMYOCARDIAL LASER REVASCULARIZATION A new development in myocardial revascularization techniques is called *transmyocardial laser revascularization (TMLR)*. In this procedure, a laser is used to drill tiny holes into the myocardial muscle itself to provide collateral blood flow to ischemic muscle. Clients whose coronary artery obstructions are too diffuse to bypass are candidates for this new surgical treatment.

NURSING CARE

Health promotion, assessment, nursing diagnoses and interventions for the client with ACS are similar to those identified for clients with angina and with acute myocardial infarction. See the preceding and subsequent sections of this chapter for specific nursing care activities, as well as the Nursing Care Plan that follows.

NURSING CARE OF THE CLIENT HAVING A **Coronary Artery Bypass Graft**

PREOPERATIVE CARE

- Provide routine preoperative care and teaching as outlined in Chapter 4 ∞.
- Verify presence of laboratory and diagnostic test results in the chart, including CBC, coagulation profile, urinalysis, chest x-ray, and coronary angiogram. *These baseline data are important for comparison of postoperative results and values.*
- Type and crossmatch four or more units of blood as ordered. *Blood is made available for use during and after surgery as needed.*
- Provide specific client and family teaching related to procedure and postoperative care. Include the following topics.
  - Cardiac recovery unit; sensory stimuli, personnel; noise and alarms; visiting policies
  - Tubes, drains, and general appearance
  - Monitoring equipment, including cardiac and hemodynamic monitoring systems
  - Respiratory support: ventilator, endotracheal tube, suctioning; communication while intubated
  - Incisions and dressings
  - Pain management

Preoperative teaching reduces anxiety and prepares the client and family for the postoperative environment and expected sensations.

POSTOPERATIVE CARE

- Provide routine postoperative care as outlined in Chapter 4 ∞. In addition to the care needs of all clients having major surgery, the cardiac surgery client has specific care needs related to open-heart and thoracic surgery. These are outlined under the nursing diagnoses identified below.

Decreased Cardiac Output

Cardiac output may be compromised postoperatively due to bleeding and fluid loss; depression of myocardial function by drugs, hypothermia, and surgical manipulation; dysrhythmias; increased vascular resistance; and a potential complication, *cardiac tamponade*, compression of the heart due to collected blood or fluid in the pericardium.

- Monitor vital signs, oxygen saturation, and hemodynamic parameters every 15 minutes. Note trends and report significant changes to the physician. *Initial hypothermia and bradycardia are expected; the heart rate should return to the normal range with rewarming. The blood pressure may fall during rewarming as vasodilation occurs. Hypotension and tachycardia, however, may indicate low cardiac output. Pulmonary artery pressure (PAP), pulmonary artery wedge pressure (PAWP), cardiac output, and oxygen saturation are monitored to evaluate fluid volume, cardiac function, and gas exchange. Hemodynamic monitoring is further discussed in Chapter 32 ∞.*
- Auscultate heart and breath sounds on admission and at least every 4 hours. *A ventricular gallop, or S₃, is an early sign of heart failure; an S₄ may indicate decreased ventricular compliance. Muffled heart sounds may be an early indication of cardiac tamponade. Adventitious breath sounds (wheezes, crackles, or rales) may be a manifestation of heart failure or respiratory compromise.*
- Assess skin color and temperature, peripheral pulses, and level of consciousness with vital signs. *Pale, mottled, or cyanotic coloring, cool and clammy skin, and diminished pulse amplitude are indicators of decreased cardiac output.*
- Continuously monitor and document cardiac rhythm. *Dysrhythmias are common, and may interfere with cardiac filling and contractility, decreasing the cardiac output.*
- Measure intake and output hourly. Report urine output less than 30 mL/h for 2 consecutive hours. *Intake and output measurements help evaluate fluid volume status. A fall in urine output may be an early indicator of decreased cardiac output.*
- Record chest tube output hourly. *Chest tube drainage greater than 70 mL/h or that is warm, red, and free flowing indicates hemorrhage and may necessitate a return to surgery. A sudden drop in chest tube output may indicate impending cardiac tamponade.*
- Monitor hemoglobin, hematocrit, and serum electrolytes. *A drop in hemoglobin and hematocrit may indicate hemorrhage that is not otherwise obvious. Electrolyte imbalances, potassium, calcium, and magnesium in particular, affect cardiac rhythm and contractility.*
- Administer intravenous fluids, fluid boluses, and blood transfusions as ordered. *Fluid and blood replacement helps ensure adequate blood volume and oxygen-carrying capacity.*
- Administer medications as ordered. *Medications ordered in the early postoperative period to maintain the cardiac output include inotropic drugs (e.g., dopamine, dobutamine) to increase the force of myocardial contractions; vasodilators (e.g., nitroprusside or nitroglycerin) to decrease vascular resistance and after-load; and antidysrhythmics to correct dysrhythmias that affect cardiac output.*
- Keep a temporary pacemaker at the bedside; initiate pacing as indicated. *Temporary pacing may be needed to maintain the cardiac output with bradydysrhythmias, such as high-level AV blocks.*

PRACTICE ALERT

Assess for signs of cardiac tamponade: increased heart rate, decreased BP, decreased urine output, increased central venous pressure, a sudden decrease in chest tube output, muffled/distant heart sounds, and diminished peripheral pulses. Notify physician immediately. Cardiac tamponade is a life-threatening complication that may develop postoperatively. Cardiac tamponade interferes with ventricular filling and contraction, decreasing cardiac output. Untreated, cardiac tamponade leads to cardiogenic shock and possible cardiac arrest.

Hypothermia

Hypothermia is maintained during cardiac surgery to reduce the metabolic rate and protect vital organs from ischemic damage. Although rewarming is instituted on completion of the surgery, the client often remains hypothermic on admission to cardiac recovery. Gradual rewarming is necessary to prevent peripheral vasodilation and hypotension.

- Monitor core body temperature (e.g., tympanic membrane, pulmonary artery, bladder) for the first 8 hours following surgery. *Oral and rectal temperature measurements are not reliable indicators of core body temperature during this period.*

NURSING CARE OF THE CLIENT HAVING A Coronary Artery Bypass Graft (continued)

- Institute rewarming measures (e.g., warmed intravenous solutions or blood transfusion, warm blankets, warm inspired gases, radiant heat lamps) as needed to maintain a temperature above 96.8°F (36°C). Administer Thorazine, morphine, or diltiazem as ordered to relieve shivering. *Low body temperature may cause shivering, increasing oxygen demand and consumption. Hypothermia also increases the risk for hypoxia, metabolic acidosis, vasoconstriction and increased cardiac work, altered clotting, and dysrhythmias.*

Acute Pain

Following a CABG, pain is experienced due to both the thoracic incision and removal of the saphenous vein from the leg. Dissection of the internal mammary artery (usually the left IMA) from the chest wall also causes chest pain on the affected side. Chest tube sites are also uncomfortable. The leg from which the saphenous vein graft was obtained may be more painful than the chest incision.

- Frequently assess for pain, including its location and character. Document its intensity using a standard pain scale. Assess for verbal and nonverbal indicators of pain. Validate pain cues with the client. *Pain is subjective, and differs among individuals. Incisional pain is expected; however, anginal pain also may develop. It is important to differentiate the type of pain.*

PRACTICE ALERT

Promptly report anginal or cardiac pain. Cardiac pain may indicate a perioperative or postoperative myocardial infarction.

- Administer analgesics on a scheduled basis, by PCA, or by continuous infusion for the first 24 to 48 hours. *Research demonstrates that adequate pain management in the immediate postoperative period reduces complications from sympathetic stimulation and allows faster recovery. Pain causes muscle tension and vasoconstriction, impairing circulation and tissue perfusion, slowing wound healing, and increasing cardiac work.*
- Premedicate 30 minutes before activities or planned procedures. *Premedication and the subsequent reduction of pain improves client participation and cooperation with care.*

Ineffective Airway Clearance/Impaired Gas Exchange

Atelectasis due to impaired ventilation and airway clearance is a common pulmonary complication of cardiac surgery. Gas exchange may also be affected by blood loss and decreased oxygen-carrying capacity following surgery. Phrenic nerve paralysis is a potential complication of cardiac surgery which may also contribute to impaired ventilation and gas exchange.

- Evaluate respiratory rate, depth, effort, symmetry of chest expansion, and breath sounds frequently. *Pain, anxiety, excess fluid volume, surgical injury, narcotics and anesthesia, and altered homeostasis can affect respiratory rate, depth, and effort postoperatively. Decreased chest expansion or asymmetrical movement may indicate impaired ventilation of one lung, and needs further evaluation.*

- Note endotracheal tube (ETT) placement on chest x-ray. Mark tube position and secure in place. Insert an oral airway if an oral ETT is used. *The chest x-ray documents correct ETT placement above the bifurcation to the right and left mainstem bronchus. Marking its appropriate placement allows evaluation of potential tube movement. Secure the tube firmly in place to prevent slippage or inadvertent removal. An oral airway helps prevent obstruction of an oral ETT by biting.*
- Maintain ventilator settings as ordered. Monitor arterial blood gases (ABGs) as ordered. *Mechanical ventilation promotes optimal lung expansion and oxygenation postoperatively. ABGs are used to evaluate oxygenation and acid–base balance.*
- Suction as needed. *Suctioning is performed only as indicated to clear airway secretions.*
- Prepare for ventilator weaning and extubation, as appropriate. *The client is removed from the ventilator and extubated as soon as possible to reduce complications associated with mechanical ventilation and intubation.*
- After extubation, teach use of the incentive spirometer, and encourage use every 2 hours. Encourage deep breathing; advise against vigorous coughing. Teach use of a "cough pillow" to splint chest incision and decrease pain. Frequently turn and encourage movement. Dangle on postoperative day 1. *Deep breathing, controlled coughing, and position changes improve ventilation and airway clearance and help prevent complications. Vigorous coughing may excessively increase intrathoracic pressure and cause sternal instability.*

Risk for Infection

Following an open chest procedure, a sternal infection may develop that can progress to involve the mediastinum. Incisions for removal of the saphenous vein also may become infected. Clients with IMA grafts, who are diabetic, older, or malnourished, are at high risk: Harvesting of IMA disrupts blood supply to the sternum, and these clients have impaired immune responses and healing.

- Assess sternal incision and leg wounds every shift. Document redness, warmth, swelling, and/or drainage from the site. Note wound approximation. *These assessments provide indicators of inflammation and healing.*
- Maintain a sterile dressing for the first 48 hours, then leave the incision open to air. Use Steri-Strips as needed to maintain approximation of the wound edges. *The sterile dressing prevents early contamination of the wound, whereas exposing the incision after 48 hours promotes healing.*
- Report signs of wound infection: a swollen, reddened area that is hot and painful to the touch; drainage from the wound; impaired healing, or healed areas that reopen. *Evidence of infection or impaired healing requires further evaluation and treatment.*
- Culture wound drainage as indicated. *Identifying the infective organism facilitates appropriate antibiotic therapy.*
- Collaborate with the dietitian to promote nutrition and fluid intake. *Good nutritional status is vital to healing and immune function.*

(continued)

NURSING CARE OF THE CLIENT HAVING A **Coronary Artery Bypass Graft** (continued)

Disturbed Thought Processes

Many factors affect neuropsychologic function after CABG, including the length of cardiopulmonary bypass, age, presurgery organic brain dysfunction, severity of illness, and decreased cardiac output. Sensory overload and deprivation, sleep disruption, and numerous drugs also affect thinking and mental clarity.

- Frequently reorient during initial recovery period. State that surgery is over and that the client is in the recovery area. *Frequent reorientation provides emotional support and reality checks.*
- Explain all procedures before performing them. Speak in a clear, calm voice. Encourage questions, and give honest answers. *These measures provide information, decrease anxiety, and establish trust.*
- Secure all intravenous lines and invasive catheters/tubes (e.g., ETT, Foley catheter, nasogastric tube). *Disoriented clients may tug or pull at invasive equipment, disrupting them and increasing the risk of injury.*
- Note verbal responses to questions. Correct misconceptions immediately (e.g., "Mr. Snow, look at all the special equipment in this room. Does this room look like your bedroom at home?"). *Helping the client recognize differences in the hospital environment offers a basis for continual reality checks.*
- Maintain a calendar and clock within the client's view. *This provides current information regarding day, date, and time.*
- Involve family members in providing reorientation. Place familiar objects and photographs within view. Encourage family presence. *The family provides reassurance and contact with the familiar, assisting with orientation.*
- Promote client participation in care and decision making as appropriate. *This allows the client to maintain a degree of power and control and enables the client to take an active role in recovery.*
- Report signs of hallucinations, delusions, depression, or agitation. *These may indicate progressive deterioration of mental status.*
- Administer sedatives cautiously. *Mild sedation may help prevent injury. Some sedatives may, however, have adverse effects, increasing confusion and disorientation.*
- Reevaluate neurologic status every shift. *These data allow evaluation of the effect of interventions.*

THE CLIENT WITH ACUTE MYOCARDIAL INFARCTION

An **acute myocardial infarction (AMI)**, necrosis (death) of myocardial cells, is a life-threatening event. If circulation to the affected myocardium is not promptly restored, loss of functional myocardium affects the heart's ability to maintain an effective cardiac output. This may ultimately lead to cardiogenic shock and death.

Heart disease remains the leading cause of death in the United States. Of the major heart diseases, myocardial infarction or *heart attack,* and other forms of ischemic heart disease cause the majority of deaths. Annually, approximately 700,000 people in the United States experience their first MI; another 500,000 suffer an MI subsequent to the initial one. Nearly 492,000 people died of coronary heart disease in 2002, with most of these deaths related to MI (NHLBI, 2004).

The majority of deaths from MI occur during the initial period after symptoms begin: approximately 60% within the first hour, and 40% prior to hospitalization. Heightening public awareness of the manifestations of MI, the importance of seeking immediate medical assistance, and training in cardiopulmonary resuscitation (CPR) techniques are vital to decrease deaths due to MI.

Myocardial infarction rarely occurs in clients without preexisting coronary heart disease. While no specific cause has been identified, the risk factors for MI are those for coronary heart disease: age, gender, heredity, race; smoking, obesity, hyperlipidemia, hypertension, diabetes, sedentary lifestyle, diet, and others. See the previous section of this chapter on coronary heart disease for further discussion of these risk factors.

Pathophysiology

Atherosclerotic plaque may form stable or unstable lesions. *Stable* lesions progress by gradually occluding the vessel lumen, whereas *unstable* (or *complicated*) lesions are prone to rupture and thrombus formation. Stable lesions often cause angina (discussed in the previous sections); unstable lesions often lead to acute coronary syndromes, or acute ischemic heart diseases. Acute coronary syndromes include unstable angina, myocardial infarction, and sudden cardiac death (Braunwald et al., 2002).

Myocardial infarction occurs when blood flow to a portion of cardiac muscle is completely blocked, resulting in prolonged tissue ischemia and irreversible cell damage. Coronary occlusion is usually caused by ulceration or rupture of a complicated atherosclerotic lesion. When an atherosclerotic lesion ruptures or ulcerates, substances are released that stimulate platelet aggregation, thrombin generation, and local vasomotor tone. As a result, the vessel constricts and a thrombus (clot) forms, occluding the vessel and interrupting blood flow to the myocardium distal to the obstruction.

Cellular injury occurs when the cells are denied adequate oxygen and nutrients. When ischemia is prolonged, lasting more than 20 to 45 minutes, irreversible hypoxemic damage causes cellular death and tissue necrosis. Oxygen, glycogen, and ATP stores of ischemic cells are rapidly depleted. Cellular metabolism shifts to an anaerobic process, producing hydrogen ions and lactic acid. Cellular acidosis increases cells' vulnerability to further damage. Intracellular enzymes are released through damaged cell membranes into interstitial spaces.

Cellular acidosis, electrolyte imbalances, and hormones released in response to cellular ischemia affect impulse conduction and myocardial contractility. The risk for dysrhythmias increases, and myocardial contractility decreases, reducing stroke volume, cardiac output, blood pressure, and tissue perfusion.

The subendocardium suffers the initial damage, within 20 minutes of injury, because this area is the most susceptible to

NURSING CARE PLAN   A Client with Coronary Artery Bypass Surgery

Six weeks ago, John Clements, age 50, was discharged from the hospital after emergency triple bypass surgery. Despite having emergency surgery, his postoperative recovery was uneventful, and he was discharged 6 days after admission. He returns to the clinic for a postoperative stress test and to discuss his cardiac rehabilitation program. Anne Wagner, RN, CNS, a cardiac clinical nurse specialist and the program coordinator, meets Mr. Clements to obtain specific information regarding his medical status.

ASSESSMENT

Mr. Clements's medical history reveals significant CHD, an anterior wall myocardial infarction that led to his emergency triple bypass, and hyperlipidemia. Current medications include Cardizem, Isordil, Ecotrin, and Transderm-Nitro 5. The ECG reveals sinus rhythm with some ST segment and T wave flattening. Resting heart rate 68, and blood pressure 136/84.

Mr. Clements has a strong family history of CHD. He does not smoke and uses alcohol occasionally in social situations. He enjoys "good Southern-style cooking" and watching television. Mr. Clements states his only regular exercise used to be an evening of dancing with his wife and friends about once a month, "But I get short of breath walking around the block now, so I guess I can't go dancing anymore!"

Mr. Clements owns his own contracting business and states that he typically works about 50 to 60 hours per week. He tells Ms. Wagner, "I don't know what this program is supposed to do for me. I have got to get back to work! You just can't sit around in my business—you have to make sure that the work is getting done on time, and you have to check on supplies and equipment and the like. But I feel like a weakling. I need to get my energy back!"

DIAGNOSES

- *Activity Intolerance* related to general weakness and fatigue
- *Ineffective Role Performance* related to health crisis

EXPECTED OUTCOMES

- Verbalize an understanding of the definition and components of his structured cardiac rehabilitation program.
- Verbalize a desire to make lifestyle changes.
- Identify resources available in the community to assist with lifestyle changes.
- Participate in his activity program without suffering any complications.
- Verbalize an increase in energy after 6 weeks on the program.
- Accept the reality of the temporary change in his usual work responsibilities.

PLANNING AND IMPLEMENTATION

- Define the purpose and components of a cardiac rehabilitation program.
- Enroll in "heart health" classes, including cardiac anatomy, physiology, and coronary heart disease; exercise and activity prescriptions; lifestyle modifications, including diet counseling and stress management; emotional reactions to CAD; sexual activity; use of cardiac medications; and self-responsibility for health.
- Plan an exercise program based on stress test results, physical examination, and interview.
- Encourage to schedule rest periods before and after activity/exercise.
- Review signs and symptoms of overexertion.
- Provide information about community resources for emotional and educational support.
- Assist to identify strategies for dealing with concerns about his business role.

EVALUATION

Mr. Clements decides to "give the rehab program a try." Ms. Wagner and an exercise physiologist work with him to plan an individualized exercise/activity program. A registered dietitian provides dietary counseling. Ms. Wagner emphasizes stress management strategies. Mr. Clements is able to list manifestations of overexertion and states that he realizes the need for gradual activity progression.

After 6 weeks, Mr. Clements has reported a significant increase in energy and strength. "I am feeling much stronger, and have been sleeping better. Mary and I are taking evening walks around the neighborhood. My chest soreness is also gone." He has completed the 12-week cardiac rehabilitation program, and another stress test indicates that his cardiac function is adequate. Mr. Clements has joined the local Mended Hearts support group and states that he is now incorporating "heart-healthy" considerations into his daily routines.

CRITICAL THINKING IN THE NURSING PROCESS

1. Develop a personalized risk factor reduction plan for Mr. Clements.
2. How might denial affect Mr. Clements's ability to (a) accept the need for cardiac rehabilitation, (b) comply with the proposed lifestyle changes, and (c) make permanent adjustments to his daily life?
3. How does spousal support influence a client's compliance with a structured cardiac rehabilitation program?
4. Mr. Clements tells you that since the surgery, his wife has been afraid that sexual activity will induce another heart attack. How would you respond to these concerns?

See Evaluating Your Response in Appendix C.

---

changes in coronary blood flow. If blood flow is restored at this point, the infarction is limited to subendocardial tissue (a *subendocardial* or *non-Q-wave infarction*). The damage progresses to the epicardium within 1 to 6 hours. When all layers of the myocardium are affected, it is known as a *transmural infarction*. A significant Q wave develops with a transmural infarction, so this also may be called a *Q-wave MI*.

Complications such as heart failure are more frequently associated with Q-wave MIs; however, clients with non-Q-wave MIs frequently experience recurrent ischemia or subsequent MI within weeks or months of the event (Woods et al., 2004).

The necrotic, infarcted tissue is surrounded by regions of injured and ischemic tissues. Tissue in this ischemic area is potentially viable; restoration of blood flow minimizes the amount of tissue lost. This surrounding tissue also undergoes metabolic changes. It may be *stunned*, its contractility impaired for hours to days following reperfusion, or *hibernating*, a process that protects myocytes until perfusion is restored. *Myocardial remodeling* also may occur, with cellular hypertrophy and loss of contractility in regions distant from the infarction. Rapid restoration of blood flow limits these changes (McCance & Huether, 2006).

When a larger artery is compromised, *collateral vessels* connecting smaller arteries in the coronary system dilate to maintain blood flow to the cardiac muscle. The degree of collateral circulation helps determine the extent of myocardial damage from ischemia. Acute occlusion of a coronary artery without any collateral flow results in massive tissue damage and possible death. Progressive narrowing of the larger coronary arteries allows collateral vessels to develop and enlarge, meeting the demand for blood flow. Good collateral circulation can limit the size of an MI.

Myocardial infarctions are described by the damaged area of the heart. The coronary artery that is occluded determines the area of damage. Myocardial infarction usually affects the left ventricle because it is the major "workhorse" of the heart; its muscle mass is greater, as are its oxygen demands. Occlusion of the left anterior descending (LAD) artery affects blood flow to the anterior wall of the left ventricle (an *anterior MI*) and part of the interventricular septum. Occlusion of the left circumflex artery (LCA) causes a *lateral MI*. *Right ventricular, inferior,* and *posterior infarcts* involve occlusions of the right coronary artery (RCA) and posterior descending artery (PDA). Occlusion of the left main coronary artery is the most devastating, causing ischemia of the entire left ventricle, and a grave prognosis. Identifying the infarct site helps predict possible complications and determine appropriate therapy.

Cocaine-Induced MI

Acute myocardial infarction may develop due to cocaine intoxication. Cocaine increases sympathetic nervous system activity by both increasing the release of catecholamines from central and peripheral stores and interfering with the reuptake of catecholamines. This increased catecholamine concentration stimulates the heart rate and increases its contractility, increases the automaticity of cardiac tissues and the risk of dysrhythmias, and causes vasoconstriction and hypertension. The client with cocaine-induced MI may present with an altered level of consciousness, confusion and restlessness, seizure activity, tachycardia, hypotension, increased respiratory rate, and respiratory crackles.

Manifestations

Pain is a classic manifestation of myocardial infarction. Chest pain due to MI is more severe than anginal pain. However, it is not the intensity of the chest pain that distinguishes MI from angina or acute coronary syndrome, but its duration and its continuous nature. The onset of pain is sudden and usually is not associated with activity. In fact, most MIs occur in the early morning. Clients with a history of angina may have more frequent anginal attacks in the days or weeks prior to an MI (unstable angina or ACS). Chest pain may be described as crushing and severe; as a pressure, heavy, or squeezing sensation; or as chest tightness or burning. The pain often begins in the center of the chest (*substernal*), and may radiate to the shoulders, neck, jaw, or arms. It lasts more than 15 to 20 minutes and is not relieved by rest or nitroglycerin.

Women and older adults often experience atypical chest pain, presenting with complaints of indigestion, heartburn, nausea, and vomiting (see the box below). Up to 25% of clients with acute MI deny chest discomfort (Woods et al., 2004).

Compensatory mechanisms cause many of the other symptoms of MI. Sympathetic nervous system stimulation causes anxiety, tachycardia, and vasoconstriction. This results in cool, clammy, mottled skin. Pain and blood chemistry changes stimulate the respiratory center, causing tachypnea. The client often has a sense of impending doom and death. Tissue necrosis causes an inflammatory reaction that increases the white blood cell count and elevates the temperature. Serum cardiac enzyme levels rise as enzymes are released from necrotic cardiac cells.

MEETING INDIVIDUALIZED NEEDS **Recognizing Acute Myocardial Infarction in Women and Older Adults**

Women and older adults often present with atypical manifestations of MI. However, heart disease is the number one cause of death in both groups, making early recognition and aggressive treatment vital.

Women are more likely than men to have a "silent" or unrecognized heart attack, or to present in cardiac arrest or with cardiogenic shock. Women often experience epigastric pain and nausea, causing them to blame their discomfort on heartburn. Shortness of breath is common, as is fatigue and weakness of the shoulders and upper arms.

Older people often seek treatment for vague complaints of difficulty breathing, confusion, fainting, dizziness, abdominal pain, or cough. They often attribute their symptoms to a stroke. The prevalence of silent ischemia is greater in older adults.

Stress the importance of seeking medical help promptly for atypical manifestations of MI. Prompt diagnosis and intervention reduces the mortality and morbidity of MI in women and older adults, just as it does in men. Despite this fact, both women and older adults are more likely to delay seeking treatment and are less likely to be accurately diagnosed and aggressively treated for CHD. Younger women are a particularly important group to reach; their mortality rate when MI occurs is twice that of men (Kasper et al., 2005).

Other manifestations may vary, depending on the location and amount of infarcted tissue. Hypertension, hypotension, or signs of heart failure may develop. Vagal stimulation may cause nausea and vomiting, bradycardia, and hypotension. Hiccuping may develop due to diaphragmatic irritation. If a large vessel is occluded, the first sign of MI may be sudden death. Typical manifestations of MI are listed in the box below.

Complications

The risk of complications associated with myocardial infarction is related to the size and location of the MI.

Dysrhythmias

Dysrhythmias, disturbances or irregularities of heart rhythm, are the most frequent complication of MI. Dysrhythmias are discussed in detail in the next section of this chapter.

Infarcted tissue is *arrhythmogenic;* that is, it affects the generation and conduction of electrical impulses in the heart, increasing the risk of dysrhythmias. Premature ventricular contractions (PVCs) are common following an MI, developing in more than 90% of clients with an acute MI. While not dangerous in themselves, they may be predictive of more dangerous dysrhythmias such as ventricular tachycardia or ventricular fibrillation (Woods et al., 2004). The risk of ventricular fibrillation is greatest the first hour after MI; it is a frequent cause of sudden cardiac death associated with acute MI. Its incidence declines with time. If the infarct affects a conduction pathway, electrical conduction may be affected. Any degree of atrioventricular (AV) block may occur following MI, especially when the anterior wall is infarcted. First-degree and Mobitz I (Wenckebach) blocks are most common, although complete heart block may develop. Bradydysrhythmias (abnormal slow rhythms) also may develop, particularly when the inferior wall of the ventricle is affected.

Pump Failure

Myocardial infarction reduces myocardial contractility, ventricular wall motion, and compliance. Impaired contractility and filling may produce heart failure. The risk of heart failure is greatest when large portions of the left ventricle are infarcted. Heart failure may be more severe with an anterior infarction. Loss of 20% to 30% of the left ventricular muscle mass may cause manifestations of left-sided heart failure, including dyspnea, fatigue, weakness, and respiratory crackles on auscultation. Inferior or right ventricular MI may lead to right-sided heart failure with manifestations such as neck vein distention and peripheral edema. Hemodynamic monitoring is often initiated for clients with evidence of heart failure. Heart failure and its manifestations are discussed in greater depth in Chapter 32 ∞.

CARDIOGENIC SHOCK *Cardiogenic shock,* impaired tissue perfusion due to pump failure, results when functioning myocardial muscle mass decreases by more than 40%. The heart is unable to pump enough blood to meet the needs of the body and maintain organ function. Low cardiac output due to cardiogenic shock also impairs perfusion of the coronary arteries and myocardium, further increasing tissue damage. Mortality from cardiogenic shock is greater than 70%, although this can be reduced by prompt intervention with revascularization procedures. See Chapter 11 ∞ for a more extensive discussion of cardiogenic shock.

Infarct Extension

Approximately 10% of clients experience extension or reinfarction in the area of the original infarction during the first 10 to 14 days after an MI. *Extension* of the MI is characterized by increased myocardial necrosis from continued blood flow impairment and ongoing injury. *Expansion* of the MI is described as a permanent expansion of the infarcted area from thinning and dilation of the muscle. Infarct extension and expansion may cause manifestations such as continuing chest pain, hemodynamic compromise, and worsening heart failure.

Structural Defects

Necrotic muscle is replaced by scar tissue that is thinner than the ventricular muscle mass. This can lead to such complications as ventricular aneurysm, rupture of the interventricular septum or papillary muscle, and myocardial rupture. A *ventricular aneurysm* is an outpouching of the ventricular wall. It may develop when a large section of the ventricle is replaced by scar tissue. Because it does not contract during systole, stroke volume decreases. Blood may pool within the aneurysm, causing clots to form. Ischemia of the papillary muscle or chordae tendineae may cause structural damage leading to papillary muscle dysfunction or rupture. This affects AV valve function (usually the mitral valve), causing *regurgitation,* backflow of blood into the atria during systole. The interventricular septum may perforate or rupture due to ischemia and infarction. Myocardial rupture is a risk between days 4 and 7 after MI, when the injured tissue is soft and weak. This potential complication of MI is often fatal.

Pericarditis

Tissue necrosis prompts an inflammatory response. *Pericarditis,* inflammation of the pericardial tissue surrounding the heart, may

---

MANIFESTATIONS **of Acute Myocardial Infarction**

- Chest pain: substernal or precordial (across the entire chest wall); may radiate to neck, jaw, shoulder(s), or left arm
- Tachycardia, tachypnea
- Dyspnea, shortness of breath
- Nausea and vomiting
- Anxiety, sense of impending doom
- Diaphoresis
- Cool, mottled skin; diminished peripheral pulses
- Hypotension or hypertension
- Palpitations, dysrhythmias
- Signs of left heart failure
- Decreased level of consciousness

complicate AMI, usually within 2 to 3 days. Pericarditis causes chest pain that may be aching or sharp and stabbing, aggravated by movement or deep breathing. A *pericardial friction rub* may be heard on auscultation of heart sounds.

Dressler's syndrome, thought to be a hypersensitivity response to necrotic tissue or an autoimmune disorder, may develop days to weeks after AMI. It is a symptom complex characterized by fever, chest pain, and dyspnea. Dressler's syndrome may spontaneously resolve or recur over several months, causing significant discomfort and distress.

> **FAST FACTS**
> ■ Dysrhythmias are the most common complication of AMI.
> ■ Heart failure also is a common complication or consequence of myocardial infarction, developing due to loss of functional muscle tissue.

INTERDISCIPLINARY CARE

Immediate treatment goals for the MI client are to:
- Relieve chest pain.
- Reduce the extent of myocardial damage.
- Maintain cardiovascular stability.
- Decrease cardiac workload.
- Prevent complications.

Slowing the process of coronary heart disease and reducing the risk of future MI is a major long-term management goal for the client.

Rapid assessment and early diagnosis is important in treating AMI. "Time is muscle" is a medical truism for the client with AMI. The evolution of an AMI is dynamic: The quicker the artery is reopened (medically, surgically, or spontaneously), the more myocardium can be salvaged. Survival and long-term outcomes following AMI are improved by rapidly restoring blood flow to the "stunned" myocardium surrounding the infracted tissue, reducing myocardial oxygen demand and limiting the accumulation of toxic by-products of necrosis and reperfusion (Kasper et al., 2005). The AHA recommends initiation of definitive treatment within 1 hour of entry into the healthcare system. A recent study by De Luca et al. (2004) showed that every minute of delay in treating clients with AMI affects the mortality risk during the first year.

The major problem interfering with timely reperfusion is delay in seeking medical care following the onset of symptoms. Up to 44% of clients with symptoms of chest discomfort or pain wait more than 4 hours before seeking treatment. Many factors are cited as reasons for treatment delay, including advanced age, the perception of the seriousness of symptoms, denial, access to medical care, the availability of an emergency response system, and in-hospital delays. Immediate evaluation of the client presenting with manifestations of myocardial infarction is essential to early diagnosis and treatment.

Diagnosis

Diagnostic testing is used to establish the diagnosis of AMI.

Serum cardiac markers are proteins released from necrotic heart muscle. The proteins most specific for diagnosis of MI are the creatine kinase (CK, or creatine phosphokinase, CPK) and cardiac-specific troponins (Table 31–6).

- *Creatine kinase* is an important enzyme for cellular function found principally in cardiac and skeletal muscle and the brain. CK levels rise rapidly with damage to these tissues, appearing in the serum 4 to 6 hours after AMI, peaking within 12 to 24 hours, and then declining over the next 48 to 72 hours. The CK level correlates with the size of the infarction; the greater the amount of infarcted tissue, the higher the serum CK level.

- *CK-MB* (also called MB-bands) is a subset of CK specific to cardiac muscle. This isoenzyme of CK is considered the most sensitive indicator of MI. Elevated CK alone is not specific for MI; elevated CK-MB greater than 5% is considered a positive indicator of MI. CK-MB levels do not normally rise with chest pain from angina or causes other than MI.

- Cardiac muscle troponins, *cardiac-specific troponin T (cT_nT)* and *cardiac-specific troponin I (cT_nI)*, are proteins released during myocardial infarction that are sensitive indicators of myocardial damage. These proteins are part of the actin-myoclin unit in cardiac muscle and normally are not detectable in the blood. With necrosis of cardiac muscle, troponins are released and blood levels rise. The specificity of cT_nT and cT_nI to cardiac muscle necrosis makes these markers particularly useful when skeletal muscle trauma contributes to elevated CK levels (e.g., when CPR has been performed or traumatic injury occurred at the time of the MI). They are sensitive enough to detect very small infarctions that do not cause significant CK elevation. Both cT_nT and cT_nI remain in the blood for 10 to 14 days after an MI, making them useful to diagnose MI when medical treatment is delayed.

Serum levels of cardiac markers are ordered on admission and for 3 succeeding days. Serial blood levels help establish the diagnosis and determine the extent of myocardial damage.

Other laboratory tests may include the following:

- *Myoglobin* is one of the first cardiac markers to be detectable in the blood after an MI. It is released within a few hours of symptom onset. Its lack of specificity to cardiac muscle and rapid excretion (blood levels return to normal within 24 hours) limit its use, however (Kasper et al., 2005).

- *Complete blood count (CBC)* shows an elevated white blood cell (WBC) count due to inflammation of the injured myocardium. The *erythrocyte sedimentation rate (ESR)* also rises because of inflammation.

- *Arterial blood gases (ABGs)* may be ordered to assess blood oxygen levels and acid–base balance.

Electrocardiography, echocardiography, and myocardial nuclear scans are the most common diagnostic tests performed when AMI is suspected. With the exception of the ECG, the timing of these tests depends on the client's immediate condition. Hemodynamic monitoring may be initiated in the unstable client following MI.

- The *electrocardiogram* reflects changes in conduction due to myocardial ischemia and necrosis. Classic ECG changes

TABLE 31-6 Cardiac Markers

MARKER	NORMAL LEVEL	PRIMARY TISSUE LOCATION	SIGNIFICANCE OF ELEVATION	Changes Occurring with MI		
				APPEARS	PEAKS	DURATION
CK (CPK)	Male: 12 to 80 unit/L Female: 10 to 70 unit/L	Cardiac muscle, skeletal muscle, brain	Injury to muscle cells	3 to 6 hours	12 to 24 hours	24 to 48 hours
CK-MB	0% to 3% of total CK	Cardiac muscle	MI, cardiac ischemia, myocarditis, cardiac contusion, defibrillation	4 to 8 hours	18 to 24 hours	72 hours
cT$_n$T	<0.2 mcg/L	Cardiac muscle	Acute MI, unstable angina	2 to 4 hours	24 to 36 hours	10 to 14 days
cT$_n$I	<3.1 mcg/L	Cardiac muscle	Acute MI, unstable angina	2 to 4 hours	24 to 36 hours	7 to 10 days

seen in AMI include T-wave inversion, ST segment elevation, and formation of a Q wave. Ischemic changes in the heart are seen as depression of the ST segment or inversion of the T wave (see Figure 31–2). With myocardial injury, elevation of the ST segment occurs (Figure 31–5A ■). Significant Q-wave development (Figure 31–5B) indicates a transmural, or full-thickness infarction. Myocardial damage can be localized using the 12-lead ECG. See Chapter 30 ∞ for more information about ECGs.

■ *Echocardiography* is done to evaluate cardiac wall motion and left ventricular function. Stunned and infarcted tissue does not contract as effectively (if at all) as healthy myocardium.

■ *Radionuclide imaging* may be done to evaluate myocardial perfusion. These studies cannot differentiate between an acute MI and old scar tissue, but do help identify the specific area of myocardial ischemia and damage.

■ *Hemodynamic monitoring* may be initiated when AMI significantly affects cardiac output and hemodynamic status. These invasive procedures are described in Chapter 32 ∞.

Medications

Aspirin, a platelet inhibitor, is now considered an essential part of treating AMI. A 160- to 325-mg aspirin tablet is given by emergency personnel, with the instruction that it is to be chewed (for buccal absorption). This initial dose is followed by a daily oral dose of 160 to 325 mg of aspirin.

Fibrinolytic agents, analgesics, and antidysrhythmic agents are among the principal classes of drugs used in treating AMI.

ANALGESIA Pain relief is vital in treating the client with AMI. Pain stimulates the sympathetic nervous system, increasing the heart rate and blood pressure and, in turn, myocardial workload. Sublingual nitroglycerin may be given (up to three 0.4-mg doses at 5-minute intervals). Intravenous nitroglycerin may be continued for the first 24 to 48 hours to reduce myocardial work. In addition to pain relief, nitroglycerin decreases myocardial oxygen demand and may increase the supply of oxygen to the myocardium. Nitroglycerin is a peripheral and arterial vasodilator that reduces afterload. It dilates coronary arteries and collateral channels in the heart, increasing coronary blood flow to save myocardial tissue at risk. Nitrates may, however, cause reflex tachycardia or excessive hypotension, so close monitoring is necessary during administration. It also is important to ask the client about use of sildenafil (Viagra) within the previous 24 hours before administering nitroglycerin, as the combination can precipitate a significant drop in blood pressure. See the Medication Administration box on page 973 for the nursing implications of nitroglycerin and other drugs given to reduce myocardial work following AMI.

Morphine sulfate is the drug of choice for pain unrelieved by nitroglycerin and for sedation. Following an initial intravenous dose of 4 to 8 mg, small doses (2 to 4 mg) may be repeated intravenously every 5 minutes until pain is relieved. It is important to assess frequently for pain relief and possible adverse effects of analgesia, such as excessive sedation. Pain unrelieved by expected or usual doses should be reported to the physician as it may indicate a complication such as extension of the infarct. See Chapter 9 ∞ for more details about morphine administration. Antianxiety agents such as diazepam (Valium) may also be administered to promote rest.

FIBRINOLYTIC THERAPY Fibrinolytic agents, drugs that dissolve or break up blood clots, are first-line drugs used to treat acute MI when access to a cardiac catheterization lab for revascularization procedures is not immediately available. Fibrinolytic drugs activate the fibrinolytic system to *lyse* or destroy the clot, restoring blood flow to the obstructed artery. Early fibrinolytic administration (within the first 6 hours of MI onset) limits infarct size, reduces heart damage, and improves outcomes. Activation of the fibrinolytic system can cause multiple complications; approximately 0.5% to 5% of clients receiving fibrinolytic drugs experience serious bleeding complications. Not every client is a candidate for fibrinolytic therapy; for example, it is contraindicated in clients

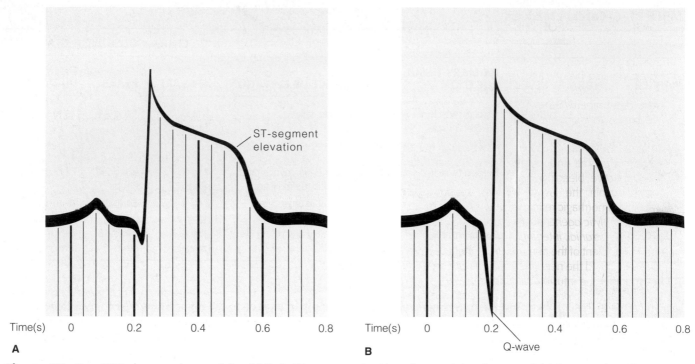

Figure 31–5 ■ ECG changes characteristic of MI. *A*, ST-segment elevation characteristic of myocardial injury. *B*, Clinically significant Q-wave characteristic of a transmural infarction.

with known bleeding disorders, history of cerebrovascular disease, uncontrolled hypertension, pregnancy, or recent trauma or surgery of the head or spine (Tierney et al., 2005).

Several fibrinolytic agents are commonly used today. Among these, little difference in effectiveness has been demonstrated; there are, however, big differences in cost. Streptokinase, a biologic agent derived from group C *Streptococcus* organisms, is the least expensive of the drugs. Its primary drawback is the risk of a severe hypersensitivity reaction, including anaphylaxis. Streptokinase is administered by intravenous infusion. Anisoylated plasminogen streptokinase activator complex (APSAC) is a related drug that can be administered by bolus over 2 to 5 minutes. It has many of the same effects as streptokinase, but is considerably more expensive. Tissue plasminogen activator (t-PA), tenecteplase (TNK), and reteplase (rPA) are more effective in reestablishing myocardial perfusion, especially when the pain developed more than 3 hours previously. These drugs, however, are the most expensive. Nursing care of the client receiving a fibrinolytic agent is outlined on the next page.

ANTIDYSRHYTHMICS Dysrhythmias are a common complication of AMI, particularly in the first 12 to 24 hours. Antidysrhythmic medications are used as needed to treat dysrhythmias. They also may be given prophylactically to prevent dysrhythmias. Ventricular dysrhythmias are treated with a class I or class III antidysrhythmic drug (see the Medication Administration box on page 1006). Symptomatic bradycardia (bradycardia with associated hypotension and other signs of low cardiac output) is treated with intravenous atropine, 0.5 to 1 mg. Intra-

venous verapamil or the short-acting beta blocker esmolol (Brevibloc) may be ordered to treat atrial fibrillation or other supraventricular tachydysrhythmias.

OTHER MEDICATIONS Beta blockers such as propranolol (Inderal), atenolol (Tenormin), and metoprolol (Lopressor) reduce pain, limit infarct size, and decrease the incidence of serious ventricular dysrhythmias in AMI. These drugs decrease the heart rate, reducing cardiac work and myocardial oxygen demand. Initial doses are given intravenously. Oral beta blocker therapy is continued to reduce the risk of reinfarction and death related to cardiovascular causes (Kasper et al., 2005).

ACE inhibitors also reduce mortality associated with AMI. These drugs reduce ventricular remodeling following an MI, reducing the risk for subsequent heart failure. They also may reduce the risk of reinfarction (Kasper et al., 2002).

Anticoagulants and antiplatelet medications often are prescribed to maintain coronary artery patency following thrombolysis or a revascularization procedure. Abciximab (ReoPro) suppresses platelet aggregation and reduces the risk of reocclusion following angioplasty. It also improves vessel opening with fibrinolytic therapy, permitting lower doses of fibrinolytic drugs. Standard or low-molecular-weight heparin preparations often are given to clients with AMI. Heparin helps establish and maintain patency of the affected coronary artery. It also is used, along with long-term warfarin, to prevent systemic or pulmonary embolism in clients with significant left ventricular impairment or atrial fibrillation following AMI. See the Medication Administration box on page 976 for the nursing implications of an-

NURSING CARE OF THE CLIENT RECEIVING Fibrinolytic Therapy

PREINFUSION CARE

- Obtain nursing history, and perform a physical assessment. *Information obtained from the history and physical exam helps determine whether fibrinolytic therapy is appropriate. The goal is to initiate fibrinolytic therapy within 30 minutes of arrival.*
- Evaluate for contraindications to fibrinolytic therapy: recent surgery or trauma (including prolonged CPR), bleeding disorders or active bleeding, cerebral vascular accident, neurosurgery within the last 2 months, gastrointestinal ulcers, diabetic hemorrhagic retinopathy, and uncontrolled hypertension. *Fibrinolytic agents dissolve clots and therefore may precipitate intracranial, internal, or peripheral bleeding.*
- Inform the client of the purpose of the therapy. Discuss the risk of bleeding and the need to keep the extremity immobile during and after the infusion. *Minimal movement of the extremity is necessary to prevent bleeding from the infusion site.*

DURING THE INFUSION

- Assess and record vital signs and the infusion site for hematoma or bleeding every 15 minutes for the first hour, every 30 minutes for the next 2 hours, and then hourly until the intravenous catheter is discontinued. Assess pulses, color, sensation, and temperature of both extremities with each vital sign check. *Vital signs and the site are frequently assessed to detect possible complications.*
- Remind the client to keep the extremity still and straight. Do not elevate head of bed above 15 degrees. *Extremity immobilization helps prevent infusion site trauma and bleeding. Hypotension may develop; keeping the bed flat helps maintain cerebral perfusion.*
- Maintain continuous cardiac monitoring during the infusion. Keep antidysrhythmic drugs and the emergency cart readily available for treatment of significant dysrhythmias. *Ventricular dysrhythmias commonly occur with reperfusion of the ischemic myocardium.*

POSTINFUSION CARE

- Assess vital signs, distal pulses, and infusion site frequently as needed. *The client remains at high risk for bleeding following fibrinolytic therapy.*
- Evaluate response to therapy: normalization of ST segment, relief of chest pain, reperfusion dysrhythmias, early peaking of the CK and CK-MB. *These are signs that the clot has been dissolved and the myocardium is being reperfused.*
- Maintain bed rest for 6 hours. Keep the head of the bed at or below 15 degrees. Reinforce the need to keep the extremity straight and immobile. Avoid any injections for 24 hours after catheter removal. *Precautions such as these are important to prevent bleeding.*
- Assess puncture sites for bleeding. On catheter removal hold direct pressure over the site for at least 30 minutes. Apply a pressure dressing to any venous or arterial sites as needed. Perform routine care in a gentle manner to avoid bruising or injury. *Fibrinolytic therapy disrupts normal coagulation. Peripheral bleeding may occur at puncture sites, and there may not be sufficient fibrin to form a clot. Direct or indirect pressure may be needed to control the bleeding.*
- Assess body fluids, including urine, vomitus, and feces, for evidence of bleeding; frequently assess for changes in level of consciousness and manifestations of increased intracranial pressure, which may indicate intracranial bleeding. Assess surgical sites for bleeding. Monitor hemoglobin and hematocrit levels, prothrombin time (PT), and partial thromboplastin time (PTT). *These provide additional means of assessing for bleeding.*
- Administer platelet-modifying drugs (e.g., aspirin, dipyridamole) as ordered. *Platelet inhibitors decrease platelet aggregation and adhesion and are used to prevent reocclusion of the artery.*
- Report manifestations of reocclusion, including changes in the ST segment, chest pain, or dysrhythmias. *Early recognition of reocclusion is vital to save myocardial tissue.*

---

tiplatelet drugs, and Chapter 34 ∞ for more information about anticoagulant therapy.

Clients with pump failure and hypotension may receive intravenous dopamine, a vasopressor. At low doses (less than 5 mg/kg/min), it improves blood flow to the kidneys, preventing renal ischemia and possible acute renal failure (see Chapter 29 ∞). With increasing doses, dopamine increases myocardial contractility and causes vasoconstriction, improving blood pressure and cardiac output.

Antilipemic agents are used for the client with hyperlipidemia. A stool softener such as docusate sodium is prescribed to maintain normal bowel function and reduce straining.

Treatments

The client with a suspected or confirmed MI is monitored continuously. Care is provided in the intensive coronary care unit for the first 24 to 48 hours, after which time less intensive monitoring (e.g., telemetry) may be required. An intra-

venous line is established to allow rapid administration of emergency medications.

Bed rest is prescribed for the first 12 hours to reduce the cardiac workload. The bedside commode generally is allowed; studies have shown this to be less stressful than using a bedpan. If the client's condition is stable, sitting in a chair at the bedside is permitted after 12 hours. Activities are gradually increased as tolerated. A quiet, calm environment with limited outside stimuli is preferred. Visitors are limited to promote rest. Oxygen is administered by nasal cannula at 2 to 5 L/min to improve oxygenation of the myocardium and other tissues.

A liquid diet may be prescribed for the first 4 to 12 hours to reduce gastric distention and myocardial work. Following that, a low-fat, low-cholesterol, reduced-sodium diet is allowed. Sodium restrictions may be lifted after 2 to 3 days if no evidence of heart failure is present. Small, frequent feedings are often recommended. Drinks containing caffeine, and very hot and cold foods, may also be limited.

Revascularization Procedures

Many clients with AMI are treated with immediate or early percutaneous coronary revascularization such as angioplasty and stent placement. PCR may follow fibrinolytic therapy or be used in place of fibrinolytic therapy to restore blood flow to ischemic myocardium. When compared with fibrinolytic therapy, prompt PCR reduces hospital mortality (Kasper et al., 2005). In some cases, CABG surgery may be performed. The choice of procedure depends on the client's age and immediate condition, the time elapsed from the onset of manifestations, and the extent of myocardial disease and damage. These procedures and related nursing care are covered in more depth in the preceding section on acute coronary syndrome.

Other Invasive Procedures

For clients with large MIs and evidence of pump failure, invasive devices may be used to temporarily take over the function of the heart, allowing the injured myocardium to heal. The intra-aortic balloon pump is widely used to augment cardiac output. Ventricular assist devices are indicated for clients requiring more or longer term artificial support than the intra-aortic balloon pump provides.

INTRA-AORTIC BALLOON PUMP The *intra-aortic balloon pump (IABP)*, also called intra-aortic balloon counterpulsation, is a mechanical circulatory support device that may be used after cardiac surgery or to treat cardiogenic shock following AMI. The IABP temporarily supports cardiac function, allowing the heart gradually to recover by decreasing myocardial workload and oxygen demand and increasing perfusion of the coronary arteries.

A catheter with a 30- to 40-mL balloon is introduced into the aorta, usually via the femoral artery. The balloon catheter is connected to a console that regulates the inflation and deflation of the balloon. The IABP catheter inflates during diastole, increasing perfusion of the coronary and renal arteries, and deflates just prior to systole, decreasing afterload and cardiac workload (Figure 31–6 ■). The inflation–deflation sequence is triggered by the ECG pattern. During the most acute period, the balloon inflates and deflates with each heartbeat (1:1 ratio), providing maximal assistance to the heart. As the client's condition improves, the IABP is weaned to inflate–deflate at varying intervals (e.g., 1:2, 1:4, 1:8). This provides a continually decreasing amount of support as the heart muscle recovers. When mechanical assistance is no longer required, the IABP catheter is removed.

VENTRICULAR ASSIST DEVICES Use of *ventricular assist devices (VADs)* to aid the failing heart is becoming more common with advances in technology. Whereas the IABP can supplement cardiac output by approximately 10% to 15%, the VAD temporarily takes partial or complete control of cardiac function, depending on the type of device used. VADs may be used as temporary or complete assist in AMI and cardiogenic shock when there is a chance for recovery of normal heart function after a period of cardiac rest. The device also may be

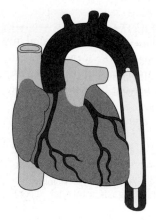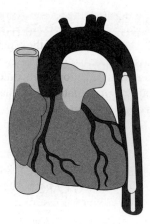

A Diastole   **B** Systole

Figure 31–6 ■ The intra-aortic balloon pump. *A,* When inflated during diastole, the balloon supports cerebral, renal, and coronary artery perfusion. *B,* The balloon deflates during systole, so cardiac output is unimpeded.

used as a bridge to heart transplant. Nursing care for the client with a VAD is supportive and includes assessing hemodynamic status and for complications associated with the device. Clients with VAD are at considerable risk for infection; strict aseptic technique is used with all invasive catheters and dressing changes. Pneumonia also is a risk due to immobility and ventilatory support. Mechanical failure of the VAD is a life-threatening event that requires immediate intervention (Urden et al., 2006).

Cardiac Rehabilitation

Cardiac rehabilitation is a long-term program of medical evaluation, exercise, risk factor modification, education, and counseling designed to limit the physical and psychologic effects of cardiac illness and improve the client's quality of life (Woods et al., 2004). Cardiac rehabilitation begins with admission for a cardiac event such as AMI or a revascularization procedure. Phase 1 of the program is the inpatient phase. A thorough assessment of the client's history, current status, risk factors, and motivation is obtained. During this phase, activity progresses from bed rest to independent performance of activities of daily living (ADLs) and ambulation within the facility. Both subjective and objective responses to increasing activity levels are evaluated. Excess fatigue, shortness of breath, chest pain, tachypnea, tachycardia, or cool, clammy skin indicate activity intolerance. Phase 2, immediate outpatient cardiac rehabilitation, begins within 3 weeks of the cardiac event. The goals for the outpatient program are to increase activity level, participation, and capacity; improve psychosocial status and treat anxiety or depression; and provide education and support for risk factor reduction. Continuation programs, phase 3 of cardiac rehabilitation, are directed at providing a transition to independent exercise and exercise maintenance. During this final phase, the client may "check in" every 3 months to evaluate risk factors, quality of life, and exercise habits (Woods et al., 2004).

NURSING CARE

Nursing care of the client with an acute myocardial infarction focuses on reducing cardiac work, identifying and treating complications in a timely manner, and preparing the client for rehabilitation. See the following Nursing Care Plan for a client with an AMI.

Health Promotion

Health promotion activities to prevent acute myocardial infarction are those outlined for coronary heart disease and angina in previous sections of this chapter. In addition, discuss risk factor management, use of prescribed medications, and cardiac rehabilitation to reduce the risk of complications or future infarctions.

NURSING CARE PLAN   A Client with Acute Myocardial Infarction

Betty Williams, a 62-year-old psychologist, is admitted to the emergency department with complaints of severe substernal chest pain. Mrs. Williams states that the pain began after lunch, about 4 hours ago. She initially attributed the pain to indigestion. She described the pain, which now radiates to her jaw and left arm, as "really severe heartburn." It is accompanied by a "choking feeling," severe shortness of breath, and diaphoresis. The pain is unrelieved by rest, antacids, or three sublingual nitroglycerin tablets (0.4 mg).

Oxygen is started per nasal cannula at 5 L/min. Central and peripheral intravenous lines are inserted. A 12-lead ECG and the following labwork are obtained: cardiac troponins, CK and CK isoenzymes, ABGs, CBC, and a chemistry panel. Morphine sulfate relieves Mrs. Williams's pain.

Mrs. Williams's medical history includes type 2 diabetes, angina, and hypertension. She has a 45-year history of cigarette smoking, averaging 1.5 to 2 packs per day. Family history reveals that Mrs. Williams's father died at age 42 of AMI, and her paternal grandfather died at age 65 of AMI. Mrs. Williams is taking the following medications: tolbutamide (Orinase), hydrochlorothiazide, and isosorbide (Isordil)

Based on ECG changes and cardiac markers, an acute anterior MI is diagnosed. Mrs. Williams has no contraindications to fibrinolytic therapy and is deemed a good candidate. Intravenous alteplase (t-PA, Activase) is given by bolus followed by intravenous infusions of alteplase and heparin. She is transferred to the coronary care unit (CCU).

ASSESSMENT

Dan Morales, RN, is Mrs. Williams's primary care nurse. Mrs. Williams is alert and oriented to person, place, and time. Vital signs are T 99.6°F (37.5°C), P 118, R 24 with adequate depth, and BP 172/92. Auscultation reveals an S_4 and fine crackles in the bases of both lungs. The ECG shows sinus tachycardia with occasional PVCs. Her skin is cool and slightly diaphoretic. Capillary refill is less than 3 seconds, and peripheral pulses are strong and equal. Her nail beds are pink.

A triple-lumen central line is in place. Nitroglycerin is infusing at 200 mcg/min in the distal lumen; the alteplase infusion is in the middle lumen; and a heparin infusion is in the proximal lumen. The peripheral intravenous line has a saline lock. Mrs. Williams states, "The pain is better since the nurse in the ER gave me a shot. But it has been coming and going. I would rate it a 4 right now, but it was terrible before. The doctor told me that this drug I'm getting will quickly open up the artery that is blocked. I hope it works! Do many people get this drug?"

DIAGNOSES

- *Acute Pain* related to ischemic myocardial tissue
- *Anxiety* and *Fear* related to change in health status
- *Ineffective Protection* related to the risk of bleeding secondary to fibrinolytic therapy
- *Risk for Decreased Cardiac Output* related to altered cardiac rate and rhythm

EXPECTED OUTCOMES

- Rate chest pain as 2 or lower on a pain scale of 0 to 10.
- Verbalize reduced anxiety and fear.
- Demonstrate no signs of internal or external bleeding.
- Maintain an adequate cardiac output during and following reperfusion therapy.

PLANNING AND IMPLEMENTATION

The following interventions are planned and implemented during the immediate phase of Mrs. Williams's hospitalization.

- Instruct to report all chest pain. Monitor and evaluate pain using a scale of 0 to 10. Titrate intravenous nitroglycerin infusion for chest pain, stop infusion if systolic BP is below 100 mmHg. Administer 2 to 4 mg morphine intravenously for chest pain unrelieved by nitroglycerin infusion.
- Encourage verbalization of fears and concerns. Respond honestly, and correct misconceptions about the disease, therapeutic interventions, or prognosis.
- Assess knowledge of CHD. Explain the purpose of fibrinolytic therapy to dissolve the fresh clot and reperfuse the heart muscle, limiting heart damage.
- Explain the need for frequent monitoring of vital signs and potential bleeding.
- Assess for manifestations of internal or intracranial bleeding: complaints of back or abdominal pain, headache, decreased level of consciousness, dizziness, bloody secretions or excretions, or pallor. Test all stools, urine, and vomitus for occult blood. Notify physician immediately of any abnormal findings.
- Monitor for signs of reperfusion: decreased chest pain, return of ST segment to baseline, reperfusion dysrhythmias (e.g., PVCs, bradycardia, and heart block).
- Continuously monitor ECG for changes in cardiac rate, rhythm, and conduction. Assess vital signs.
- Treat dangerous dysrhythmias or other cardiac events per protocol. Notify the physician.
- Discuss continuing cardiac care and rehabilitation.

(continued)

NURSING CARE PLAN   A Client with Acute Myocardial Infarction (continued)

EVALUATION

The initial morphine dose reduces Mrs. Williams's chest pain from a rating of 8 to 4. The nitroglycerin infusion and fibrinolytic therapy further reduce her pain to 2. The nitroglycerin infusion is gradually discontinued after 24 hours. As her pain subsides, Mrs. Williams states that she feels "much better now that the pain is gone. I was afraid it would just get worse." She verbalizes an understanding of fibrinolytic therapy to limit myocardial damage. No indication of bleeding problems are noted. Reperfusion is indicated by relief of chest pain, return of the ST segment to baseline on the ECG, early peaking of CK levels, and increased frequency of PVCs but no significant dysrhythmias. Mrs. Williams remains in CCU for 36 hours and is transferred to the floor.

CRITICAL THINKING IN THE NURSING PROCESS

1. How would the initial plan of care have changed if Mrs. Williams were not a candidate for fibrinolytic therapy?
2. Two days after her initial therapy, Mrs. Williams complains of palpitations. You notice frequent PVCs on the ECG monitor. What do you do?
3. What health promotion topics would you teach Mrs. Williams before discharge?
4. Mrs. Williams states, "I've been smoking for over 45 years, and I'm not going to stop now! Besides, it calms me down when I'm anxious." How would you respond to this statement?
See Evaluating Your Response in Appendix C.

Assessment

Nursing assessment for the client with AMI must be both timely and ongoing. Assessment data related to AMI include the following:

- *Health history:* Complaints of chest pain, including its location, intensity, character, radiation, and timing; associated symptoms such as nausea, heartburn, shortness of breath, and anxiety; treatment measures taken since onset of pain; past medical history, especially cardiac related; chronic diseases; current medications and any known allergies to medications; smoking history and use of recreational drugs and alcohol.
- *Physical examination:* General appearance including obvious signs of distress; vital signs; peripheral pulses; skin color, temperature, moisture; level of consciousness; heart and breath sounds; cardiac rhythm (on beside monitor); bowel sounds, abdominal tenderness.

Nursing Diagnoses and Interventions

Priorities of nursing care include relieving chest pain, reducing cardiac work, and promoting oxygenation. Psychosocial support is especially important, because an acute myocardial infarction can be devastating, bringing the client face to face with his or her own mortality for the first time.

Acute Pain

Chest pain occurs when the oxygen supply to the heart muscle does not meet the demand. Myocardial ischemia and infarction cause pain, as does reperfusion of an ischemic area following fibrinolytic therapy or emergent PTCA. Pain stimulates the sympathetic nervous system, increasing cardiac work. Pain relief is a priority of care for the client with AMI.

- Assess for verbal and nonverbal signs of pain. Document characteristics and the intensity of the pain, using a standard pain scale. Verify nonverbal indicators of pain with the client. *Frequent, careful pain assessment allows early intervention to reduce the risk of further damage. Pain is a subjective experience; its expression may vary with location and intensity, previous experiences, and cultural and social background.*

Pain scales provide an objective tool for measuring pain and a way to assess pain relief or reduction.

- Administer oxygen at 2 to 5 L/min per nasal cannula. *Supplemental oxygen increases oxygen supply to the myocardium, decreasing ischemia and pain.*
- Promote physical and psychologic rest. Provide information and emotional support. *Rest decreases cardiac workload and sympathetic nervous system stimulation, promoting comfort. Information and emotional support help decrease anxiety and provide psychologic rest.*
- Titrate intravenous nitroglycerin as ordered to relieve chest pain, maintaining a systolic blood pressure greater than 100 mmHg. *Nitroglycerin decreases chest pain by dilating peripheral vessels, reducing cardiac work, and dilating coronary vessels, including collateral channels, improving blood flow to ischemic tissue.*

PRACTICE ALERT

Intravenous nitroglycerin causes peripheral vasodilation, which may lead to hypotension, reduced coronary blood flow, and tachycardia. Reduce the nitro flow rate and notify the physician if this occurs.

- Administer 2 to 4 mg morphine by intravenous push for chest pain as needed. *Morphine is an effective narcotic analgesic for chest pain. It decreases pain and anxiety, acts as a venodilator, and decreases the respiratory rate. The resulting reduction in preload and sympathetic nervous system stimulation reduces cardiac work and oxygen consumption.*

PRACTICE ALERT

Reassess for relief of chest pain. The goal of care is to achieve pain relief, not simply a reduction in pain to a "manageable" level.

Ineffective Tissue Perfusion

Cardiac muscle damage affects compliance, contractility, and cardiac output. The extent of the effect on tissue perfusion depends on the location and amount of damage. Anterior wall infarcts have a greater effect on cardiac output than do right ventricular infarcts. Infarcted muscle also increases the risk for cardiac dysrhythmias, which can also affect the delivery of blood and oxygen to the tissues.

- Assess and document vital signs. Report increases in heart rate and changes in rhythm, blood pressure, and respiratory rate. *Decreased cardiac output activates compensatory mechanisms that may cause tachycardia and vasoconstriction, increasing cardiac work.*
- Assess for changes in level of consciousness (LOC); decreased urine output; moist, cool, pale, mottled, or cyanotic skin; dusky or cyanotic mucous membranes and nail beds; diminished to absent peripheral pulses; delayed capillary refill. *These are manifestations of impaired tissue perfusion. A change in LOC is often the first manifestation of altered perfusion because brain tissue and cerebral function depend on a continuous supply of oxygen.*
- Auscultate heart and breath sounds. Note abnormal heart sounds (e.g., an S_3 or S_4 gallop or a murmur) or adventitious lung sounds. *Abnormal heart sounds or adventitious lung sounds may indicate impaired cardiac filling or output, increasing the risk for decreased tissue perfusion.*
- Monitor ECG rhythm continuously. *Dysrhythmias can further impair cardiac output and tissue perfusion.*

PRACTICE ALERT
Obtain a 12-lead ECG to assess complaints of chest pain. Report marked changes to the physician. Continued or unrelieved chest pain may indicate further myocardial ischemia and extension of the infarct; an ECG during episodes of chest pain provides a valuable diagnostic tool to assess myocardial perfusion.

- Monitor oxygen saturation levels. Administer oxygen as ordered. Obtain and assess ABGs as indicated. *Oxygen saturation is an indicator of gas exchange, tissue perfusion, and the effectiveness of oxygen administration. ABGs provide a more precise measurement of blood oxygen levels and allow assessment of acid–base balance.*
- Administer antidysrhythmic medications as needed. *Dysrhythmias affect tissue perfusion by altering cardiac output.*
- Obtain serial CK, isoenzyme, and troponin levels as ordered. *Levels of cardiac markers, CK isoenzymes in particular, correlate with the extent of myocardial damage.*
- Plan for invasive hemodynamic monitoring. *Hemodynamic monitoring facilitates AMI management and treatment evaluation by providing a means of assessing pressures in the systemic and pulmonary arteries, the relationship between oxygen supply and demand, cardiac output, and cardiac index.*

PRACTICE ALERT
Continuously evaluate the response to interventions such as fibrinolytic therapy, drugs to improve cardiac output and tissue perfusion, and drugs to reduce cardiac work. Adverse effects of therapy may reduce the effectiveness of treatment. Bleeding due to fibrinolytic therapy may affect vascular volume and cardiac output; reperfusion dysrhythmias also may affect cardiac output. Drugs used to improve cardiac output may also increase cardiac work, whereas those given to reduce cardiac work may significantly affect contractility and cardiac output.

Ineffective Coping
Coping mechanisms help a person deal with a life-threatening event or with acute changes in health. However, certain coping mechanisms may be detrimental to restoring health, particularly if the client relies on them for a prolonged period. Denial, for example, is a common coping mechanism among post–MI clients. In the initial stages, denial can reduce anxiety. Continued denial, however, can interfere with learning and compliance with treatment.

- Establish an environment of caring and trust. Encourage the client to express feelings. *Establishing a trusting nurse–client relationship provides a safe environment for the client to discuss feelings of helplessness, powerlessness, anxiety, and hopelessness. The nurse may then be able to provide additional resources to meet the client's needs.*
- Accept denial as a coping mechanism, but do not reinforce it. *Denial may initially help by diminishing the psychologic threat to health, decreasing anxiety. However, its prolonged use can interfere with acceptance of reality and cooperation, possibly delaying treatment and hindering recovery.*
- Note aggressive behaviors, hostility, or anger. Document any failure to comply with treatments. *These signs can indicate anxiety and denial.*
- Help the client identify positive coping skills used in the past (e.g., problem-solving skills, verbalization of feelings, asking for help, prayer). Reinforce use of positive coping behaviors. *Coping behaviors that have been successful in the past can help the client deal with the current situation. These familiar methods can decrease feelings of powerlessness.*
- Provide opportunities for the client to make decisions about the plan of care, as possible. *This promotes self-confidence and independence. Participating in care planning gives the client a sense of control and the opportunity to use positive coping skills.*
- Provide privacy for the client and significant other to share their questions and concerns. *Privacy provides an opportunity for the client and partner to share their feelings and fears, offer support and encouragement to one another, relieve anxiety, and establish effective coping methods.*

Fear
The fear of death and disability can be a paralyzing emotion that adversely affects the client's recovery from acute myocardial infarction.

- Identify the client's level of fear, noting verbal and nonverbal signs. *This information enables the nurse to plan appropriate interventions. Clients may not voice concerns; attention to nonverbal indicators is important. Controlling fear helps decrease sympathetic nervous system responses and catecholamine release that may increase feelings of fear and anxiety.*
- Acknowledge the client's perception of the situation. Allow to verbalize concerns. *A sudden change in health status causes anxiety and fear of the unknown. Verbalizing these fears may help the client cope with change and allow the healthcare team to provide information and correct misconceptions.*
- Encourage questions and provide consistent, factual answers. Repeat information as needed. *Accurate and consistent information can reduce fear. Honest explanations help*

NURSING CARE OF THE OLDER ADULT   Cardiac Dysrhythmias

Aging affects the heart and the cardiac conduction system, increasing the incidence of dysrhythmias and conduction defects. Older adults may experience dysrhythmias even when no evidence of heart disease is found.

Older adults have a higher incidence of both ventricular and supraventricular dysrhythmias without detrimental effects than younger people. Ectopic beats, including short runs of ventricular tachycardia, occur more commonly during exercise in older adults. These dysrhythmias do not affect cardiac morbidity or mortality. Fibrosis of the bundle branches can lead to atrioventricular blocks; a prolonged PR interval is common in clients over the age of 65. Older adults also have a higher incidence of diseases that may affect heart rhythm. An elderly client with hyperthyroidism, for example, may present with atrial fibrillation, syncope, and confusion instead of the usual manifestations of goiter, tremor, and exophthalmos.

Assessing for Home Care

Assessing older adults for problems related to cardiac dysrhythmias focuses on the effect of the dysrhythmia on functional health status.

- Ask about a history of cardiovascular disease and current medications.
- Inquire about symptoms such as episodes of dizziness, lightheadedness, fainting, palpitations, chest pain, or shortness of breath.

- Ask about relationship of symptoms such as palpitations to intake of certain foods and caffeine-containing beverages.
- Evaluate for other contributing factors such as smoking or alcohol intake.
- Inquire about a history of falls, particularly those occurring without apparent reason.

Teaching for Home Care

Teach measures to reduce the risk of cardiac dysrhythmias and potential adverse consequences of dysrhythmias.

- Emphasize the importance of taking medications as prescribed. Discuss possible effects of over-the-counter medications on the heart.
- Encourage reducing or eliminating caffeine intake. Caffeine increases the risk of ectopic beats and rapid heart rates.
- Encourage participation in a smoking cessation program and to reduce or eliminate alcohol intake if appropriate.
- Encourage engaging in regular exercise. Discuss the beneficial effects of exercise to maintain muscle mass, including cardiac muscle, and cardiovascular health.
- Instruct to contact primary care provider for evaluation of symptoms such as dizziness, fainting, frequent palpitations, shortness of breath, unexplained falls, or chest pain.

---

atria to contract, delivering an extra bolus of blood to the ventricles before they contract (the **atrial kick**). The AV node also controls the number of impulses that reach the ventricles, preventing extremely rapid heart rates.

Pathophysiology

Dysrhythmias arise through disruption of the very properties that stimulate and control the heartbeat: automaticity, excitability, conductivity, and refractoriness.

Dysrhythmias due to altered impulse formation include changes in rate and rhythm and the development of ectopic beats. This category includes *tachydysrhythmias* (rapid heart rates), *bradydysrhythmias* (slow heart rates), and ectopic rhythms. These dysrhythmias result from a change in the automaticity of cardiac cells. The rate of impulse formation may abnormally increase or decrease. Aberrant (abnormal) impulses may originate outside normal conduction pathways, causing **ectopic beats**. Ectopic beats interrupt the normal conduction sequence and may not initiate a normal muscle contraction. Depending on the site and timing of abnormal impulses, they may have little effect on the client or pose a significant threat.

Ischemia, injury, and infarction of myocardial tissue affect its excitability and ability to conduct and respond to an electrical stimulus. Conduction abnormalities cause varying degrees of **heart block**, a block in the normal conduction pathways. Myocardial injury or infarction can obstruct or delay impulse conduction. Bundle branch blocks are common in acute myocardial infarction.

The *reentry phenomenon,* a phenomenon of normal and slow conduction, is a major cause of tachydysrhythmias. A stimulus such as an ectopic beat triggers the reentry phenomenon. The impulse is delayed in one area of the heart (e.g., an area of ischemia or injury) but conducted normally through the rest. Muscle that has been depolarized by the normally conducted impulse is repolarized by the time the impulse traveling through the area of slow conduction reaches it, thus initiating another cycle of depolarization (Porth, 2005). The result is a dysrhythmia that propagates itself.

Several forms of reentry may occur. The impulse may travel through a set pathway to reenter repolarized tissue. Many atrial dysrhythmias follow this pattern, including atrial flutter. In functional reentry, local differences in the conduction of an impulse interrupt the normal wave of depolarization, sending it back upon itself in a spiral pattern and setting up a permanent rotation. This type of pattern suppresses normal pacemaker activity and can lead to atrial fibrillation (Porth, 2005).

Cardiac rhythms are classified according to the site of impulse formation or the site and degree of conduction block. *Supraventricular rhythms* arise above the ventricles. These rhythms usually produce a QRS complex within the normal range. Sinus rhythms, atrial rhythms, and junctional (arising from the AV junction) rhythms are all supraventricular rhythms. *Ventricular rhythms* originate in the ventricles and may prove fatal if left untreated. *AV conduction blocks* result from a defect in impulse transmission from the atria to the ventricles. The major normal and abnormal cardiac rhythms are summarized in Table 31–7.

MEDIALINK   Dysrhythmia Animations

TABLE 31–7 Characteristics of Selected Cardiac Rhythms and Dysrhythmias

RHYTHM/ECG APPEARANCE	ECG CHARACTERISTICS	MANAGEMENT
Supraventricular Rhythms		
Normal sinus rhythm (NSR) 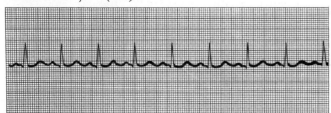	Rate: 60 to 100 beats/min Rhythm: Regular P:QRS: 1:1 PR interval: 0.12 to 0.20 sec QRS complex: 0.06 to 0.10 sec	None; normal heart rhythm.
Sinus arrhythmia 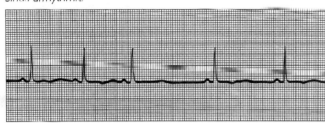	Rate: 60 to 100 beats/min Rhythm: Irregular, varying with respirations P:QRS: 1:1 PR interval: 0.12 to 0.20 sec QRS complex: 0.6 to 0.10 sec	Generally none; considered a normal rhythm in the very young and very old.
Sinus tachycardia 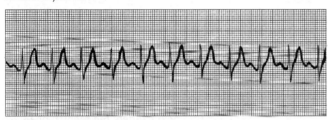	Rate: 101 to 150 beats/min Rhythm: Regular P:QRS: 1:1 (With very fast rates, P wave may be hidden in preceding T wave) PR interval: 0.12 to 0.20 sec QRS complex: 0.6 to 0.10 sec	Treated only if symptomatic or client is at risk for myocardial damage. Treat underlying cause (e.g., hypovolemia, fever, pain). Beta blockers or verapamil may be used.
Sinus bradycardia 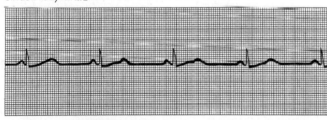	Rate: < 60 beats/min Rhythm: Regular P:QRS: 1:1 PR interval: 0.12 to 0.20 sec QRS complex: 0.6 to 0.10 sec	Treated only if symptomatic. Intravenous atropine or isoproterenol, and/or pacemaker therapy may be used.
Premature atrial contractions (PAC) 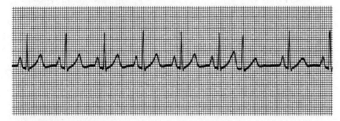	Rate: Variable Rhythm: Irregular, with normal rhythm interrupted by early beats arising in the atria P:QRS: 1:1 PR interval: 0.12 to 0.20 sec, but may be prolonged QRS complex: 0.6 to 0.10 sec	Usually require no treatment. Advise to reduce alcohol and caffeine intake, to reduce stress, and to stop smoking. Beta blocker may be prescribed
Paroxysmal supraventricular tachycardia (PSVT) 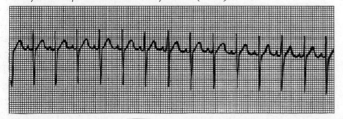	Rate: 100 to 280 beats/min (usually 150 to 200 beats/min) Rhythm: Regular P:QRS: P waves often not identifiable PR interval: Not measured QRS complex: 0.6 to 0.10 sec	Treat if symptomatic. Treatment may include vagal maneuvers (Valsalva, carotid sinus massage); oxygen therapy; adenosine or a beta blocker; temporary pacing, or synchronized cardioversion.

(continued)

TABLE 31–7 **Characteristics of Selected Cardiac Rhythms and Dysrhythmias (continued)**

RHYTHM/ECG APPEARANCE	ECG CHARACTERISTICS	MANAGEMENT
Atrial flutter 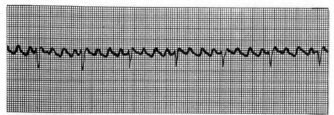	Rate: Atrial 240 to 360 beats/min, ventricular rate depends on degree of AV block and usually is <150 beats/min Rhythm: Atrial regular; ventricular usually regular P:QRS: 2:1, 4:1, 6:1; may vary PR interval: Not measured QRS complex: 0.06 to 0.10 sec	Synchronized cardioversion; medications to slow ventricular response such as a beta blocker or calcium channel blocker, followed by a class I antidysrhythmic agent or amiodarone.
Atrial fibrillation 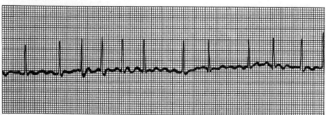	Rate: Atrial 300 to 600 beats/min (too rapid to count); ventricular 100 to 180 beats/min in untreated clients Rhythm: Irregularly irregular P:QRS: Variable PR interval: Not measured QRS complex: 0.06 to 0.10 sec	Synchronized cardioversion; medications to reduce ventricular response rate: metaprolol, diltiazem, or digoxin; anticoagulant therapy to reduce risk of clot formation and stroke.
Junctional escape rhythm 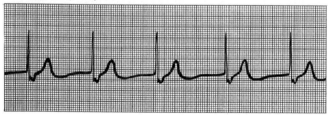	Rate: 40 to 60 beats/min; junctional tachycardia 60 to 140 BPM Rhythm: Regular P:QRS: P waves may be absent, inverted and immediately preceding or succeeding QRS complex, or hidden in QRS complex PR interval: <0.10 sec QRS complex: 0.06 to 0.10 sec	Treat cause if symptomatic.

Ventricular Rhythms

RHYTHM/ECG APPEARANCE	ECG CHARACTERISTICS	MANAGEMENT
Premature ventricular contractions (PVC) 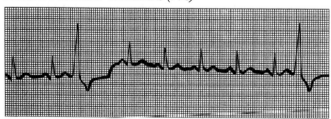	Rate: Variable Rhythm: Irregular, with PVC interrupting underlying rhythm and followed by a compensatory pause P:QRS: No P wave noted before PVC PR interval: Absent with PVC QRS complex: Wide (>0.12 sec) and bizarre in appearance; differs from normal QRS complex	Treat if symptomatic or in presence of severe heart disease. Advise against stimulant use (caffeine, nicotine). Beta blockers, or class I or III antidysrhythmic agents (see the box on page 1006) may be used in clients with severe heart disease who are symptomatic
Ventricular tachycardia (VT, V tach) 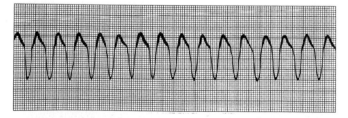	Rate: 100 to 250 beats/min Rhythm: Regular P:QRS: P waves usually not identifiable PR interval: Not measured QRS complex: 0.12 sec or greater; bizarre shape	Treat if VT is sustained, symptomatic, or associated with organic heart disease. Treatment includes DC cardioversion or intravenous procainamide, lidocaine, or a class III antidysrhythmic agent if hemodynamic instability accompanies. Surgical ablation or antitachycardia pacing with an implanted cardioverter/defibrillator (ICD) for repeated episodes.

TABLE 31–7 Characteristics of Selected Cardiac Rhythms and Dysrhythmias (continued)

RHYTHM/ECG APPEARANCE	ECG CHARACTERISTICS	MANAGEMENT
Ventricular fibrillation (VF, V fib) 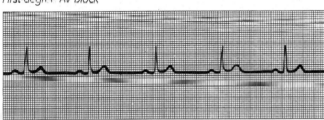	Rate: Too rapid to count Rhythm: Grossly irregular P:QRS: No identifiable P waves PR interval: None QRS: Bizarre, varying in shape and direction	Immediate cardioversion/ defibrillation.
Atrioventricular Conduction Blocks *First-degree AV block*	Rate: Usually 60 to 100 beats/min Rhythm: Regular P:QRS: 1.1 PR interval: >0.21 sec QRS complex: 0.06 to 0.10 sec	None required.
Second-degree AV block, type I (Mobitz I, Wenckebach) 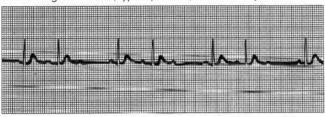	Rate: 60 to 100 beats/min Rhythm: Atrial regular; ventricular irregular P:QRS: 1:1 until P wave blocked with no subsequent QRS complex PR interval: Progressively lengthens in a regular pattern QRS complex: 0.06 to 0.10 sec; sudden absence of QRS complex	Monitoring and observation; rarely progresses to a higher degree of block or requires treatment.
Second-degree AV block, type II (Mobitz II) 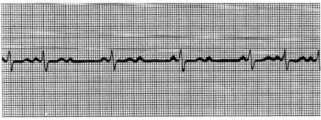	Rate: Atrial 60 to 100 beats/min; Ventricular <60 beats/min Rhythm: Atrial regular; ventricular irregular P:QRS: Typically 2:1, may vary PR interval: Constant PR interval for each conducted QRS complex QRS complex: 0.06 to 0.10 sec	Atropine or isoproterenol; pacemaker therapy.
Third-degree AV block (Complete heart block) 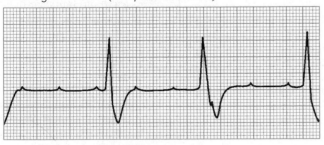	Rate: Atrial 60 to 100 beats/min; ventricular 15 to 60 beats/min Rhythm: Atrial regular; ventricular regular P:QRS: No relationship between P waves and QRS complexes; independent rhythms PR interval: Not measured QRS complex: 0.06 to 0.10 sec if junctional escape rhythm; >0.12 sec if ventricular escape rhythm	Immediate pacemaker therapy.

FAST FACTS

- The normal sinus rate is 60 to 100 beats per minute. Each complex includes a P wave, QRS, and T wave.
- Supraventricular dysrhythmias arise in the sinus node or the atria. A P wave may be present; the QRS appears normal, and a T wave may be seen.
- Junctional dysrhythmias arise in tissue just above or just below the AV node. The P wave may be inverted, and may precede, follow, or be buried in the QRS complex. The QRS usually appears normal and is followed by a T wave.
- Ventricular dysrhythmias arise in ventricular myocardium. They do not reset the SA node or activate the atria. QRS complexes are wide and bizarre.

Supraventricular Rhythms

NORMAL SINUS RHYTHM **Normal sinus rhythm (NSR)** is the normal heart rhythm, in which impulses originate in the SA (sinus) node and travel through all normal conduction pathways without delay. All waveforms are of normal configuration, look alike, and have consistent (fixed) durations. The rate is between 60 and 100 bpm.

SINUS NODE DYSRHYTHMIAS Sinus node dysrhythmias may occur as a normal compensatory response (e.g., to exercise) or because of altered automaticity. In these rhythms, as in NSR, the initiating impulse is from the sinus node. They differ from NSR in rate or regularity of the rhythm. Sinus dysrhythmias include sinus arrhythmia, sinus tachycardia, and sinus bradycardia.

Sinus Arrhythmia *Sinus arrhythmia* is a sinus rhythm in which the rate varies with respirations, causing an irregular rhythm. The rate increases during inspiration and decreases with expiration. Sinus arrhythmia is common in the very young and the very old. It can be caused by an increase in vagal tone, by digitalis toxicity, or by morphine administration.

Sinus Tachycardia *Sinus tachycardia* has all of the characteristics of NSR, except that the rate is greater than 100 bpm. Tachycardia arises from enhanced automaticity in response to changes in the internal environment. Sympathetic nervous system stimulation or blocked vagal (parasympathetic) activity increases the heart rate. Tachycardia is a normal response to any condition or event that increases the body's demand for oxygen and nutrients, such as exercise or hypoxia. In the client on bed rest, tachycardia is an ominous sign. Sinus tachycardia may be an early sign of cardiac dysfunction, such as heart failure. Tachycardia is detrimental in clients with cardiac disease because it increases cardiac work and oxygen use.

Common causes of sinus tachycardia include exercise, excitement, anxiety, pain, fever, hypoxia, hypovolemia, anemia, hyperthyroidism, myocardial infarction, heart failure, cardiogenic shock, pulmonary embolism, caffeine intake, and certain drugs, such as atropine, epinephrine (Adrenalin), or isoproterenol (Isuprel).

Manifestations of sinus tachycardia include a rapid pulse rate. The client may complain of feeling that the heart is "racing," shortness of breath, and dizziness. In the presence of heart disease, sinus tachycardia may precipitate chest pain.

Sinus Bradycardia *Sinus bradycardia* has all of the characteristics of NSR, but the rate is less than 60 beats/min. Sinus bradycardia may result from increased vagal (parasympathetic) activity or from depressed automaticity due to injury or ischemia to the sinus node. Sinus bradycardia may be normal (e.g., in clients with athletic heart syndrome). The heart rate also normally slows during sleep because the parasympathetic nervous system is dominant at this time. Other causes of sinus bradycardia include pain, increased intracranial pressure, sinus node disease, AMI (especially with inferior wall damage), hypothermia, acidosis, and certain drugs.

Sinus bradycardia may be asymptomatic; it is important to assess the client before treating the rhythm. Manifestations of decreased cardiac output, such as decreased level of consciousness, syncope (faintness), or hypotension, indicate a need for intervention.

Sick Sinus Syndrome *Sick sinus syndrome (SSS)* results from sinus node disease or dysfunction that causes problems with impulse formation, transmission, and conduction. Sick sinus syndrome is often found in older adults. It may be caused by direct injury to sinus tissue, fibrosis of conduction fibers associated with aging, and such drugs as digitalis, beta blockers, and calcium channel blockers.

ECG characteristics of SSS include sinus bradycardia, sinus arrhythmia, sinus pauses or arrest, and atrial tachydysrhythmias such as atrial fibrillation, atrial flutter, or atrial tachycardia. Bradycardia-tachycardia syndrome, characterized either by **paroxysmal** (abrupt onset and termination) atrial tachycardia followed by prolonged sinus pauses or alternating periods of bradycardia and tachycardia also may indicate sinus node dysfunction.

Manifestations of sinus node dysfunction often are intermittent, related to a drop in cardiac output caused by the irregular rhythm. Fatigue, dizziness, light-headedness, and syncope are common. The heart rate may not increase in response to stressors such as exercise or fever.

SUPRAVENTRICULAR DYSRHYTHMIAS When an action potential originates in atrial tissue outside the sinus node, the resulting rhythm is classified as a *supraventricular rhythm*. In these dysrhythmias, an ectopic pacemaker takes over, or overrides, the SA node. They may also occur when the SA node fails; an *escape rhythm* develops as a fail-safe mechanism to maintain the heart rate. The most common supraventricular dysrhythmias are premature atrial contractions, paroxysmal supraventricular tachycardia, atrial flutter, and atrial fibrillation. These rhythms may be paroxysmal, that is, occur in bursts with an abrupt beginning and end.

Premature Atrial Contractions A *premature atrial contraction (PAC)* is an ectopic atrial beat that occurs earlier than the next expected sinus beat. PACs can arise anywhere in the atria. They are usually asymptomatic and benign, but they may initiate paroxysmal supraventricular tachycardia in susceptible individuals. PACs are common in older adults, often occurring without an obvious cause. Strong emotions, excessive alcohol intake, tobacco, and stimulants such as caffeine can precipitate PACs. They also may be associated with myocardial infarction, heart failure and other cardiac disorders, hypoxemia, pulmonary embolism, digitalis toxicity, and electrolyte or acid–base imbalances. In clients with underlying heart disease, PACs may precede a more serious dysrhythmia.

The ECG tracing shows interruption of the underlying rhythm by a premature complex that looks similar to the underlying beats. The ectopic impulse of the PAC is usually conducted normally, leading to depolarization of cardiac muscle and a normal QRS complex. Because the impulse arises above the ventricles, it follows normal conduction pathways through the ventricles. The QRS complex is narrow or matches those of the underlying rhythm. The shape of the P wave of a PAC differs from normal P waves because its impulse arises outside the sinus node. A *noncompensatory pause* usually follows, as the PAC resets the SA node rhythm. Occasionally, the ectopic impulse may not be conducted through the heart, resulting in a lone P wave without a QRS, or a nonconducted PAC.

PACs cause few manifestations. If frequent, they may cause palpitations or a fluttering sensation in the chest. Early beats may be noted on auscultating or palpating the pulse.

Paroxysmal Supraventricular Tachycardia *Paroxysmal supraventricular tachycardia (PSVT)* is tachycardia of sudden onset and termination. PSVT is usually initiated by a reentry loop in or around the AV node; that is, an impulse reenters the same section of tissue over and over, causing repeated depolarizations.

PSVT occurs more frequently in women. Sympathetic nervous system stimulation and stressors such as fever, sepsis, and hyperthyroidism may precipitate PSVT. It also may be associated with heart diseases such as CHD, myocardial infarction, rheumatic heart disease, myocarditis, or acute pericarditis. Abnormal conduction pathways associated with Wolff-Parkinson-White (WPW) syndrome may account for PSVT.

PSVT affects ventricular filling and cardiac output, and decreases coronary artery perfusion. Its manifestations include complaints of palpitations and a "racing" heart, anxiety, dizziness, dyspnea, anginal pain, diaphoresis, extreme fatigue, and polyuria (urine output may reach up to 3 L in the first few hours after PSVT onset).

Atrial Flutter *Atrial flutter* is a rapid and regular atrial rhythm thought to result from an intra-atrial reentry mechanism. Causes include sympathetic nervous system stimulation due to anxiety or caffeine and alcohol intake; thyrotoxicosis; coronary heart disease or myocardial infarction; pulmonary embolism; and abnormal conduction syndromes, such as WPW syndrome. Older persons with rheumatic heart disease and/or valvular disease are especially vulnerable.

Two types of atrial flutter have been identified. Type I atrial flutter has an atrial rate of 240 to 340 beats per minute. It develops due to a reentry mechanism in the right atrium. The mechanism leading to type II atrial flutter has not been identified. In this type of flutter, the atrial rate is faster, to 350 beats per minute.

Clients with atrial flutter may complain of palpitations or a fluttering sensation in the chest or throat. If the ventricular rate is rapid, manifestations of decreased cardiac output, such as decreased level of consciousness, hypotension, decreased urinary output, and cool clammy skin, may be noted. The atrial kick

(additional ventricular filling with atrial contraction) is lost because of inadequate atrial filling.

ECG characteristics include a "sawtooth" or "picket fence" appearance of P waves, which are labeled flutter (F) waves. The atrial rate is rapid, often around 300 beats/min. As a protective mechanism, many impulses are blocked at the AV node, and the ventricular rate is rarely greater than 150 to 170 beats/min. Usually, atrial impulses are evenly conducted through the AV node, for example, two impulses to one QRS complex (2:1), four impulses to one QRS complex (4:1), or six impulses to one QRS complex (6:1). A constant conduction ratio results in a regular ventricular rhythm; the ventricular rhythm is irregular if the conduction ratio varies. The ventricular rate usually ranges from 150 to 170 beats/min in 2:1 conduction and 60 to 75 beats/min for lower conduction ratios. The T wave is usually hidden by overriding F waves; some F waves may be hidden in the QRS complex.

Atrial Fibrillation *Atrial fibrillation* is a common dysrhythmia characterized by disorganized atrial activity without discrete atrial contractions. Multiple small reentry circuits develop in the atria. Atrial cells cannot repolarize in time to respond to the next stimulus (Porth, 2005). Extremely rapid atrial impulses bombard the AV node, resulting in an irregularly irregular ventricular response. Atrial fibrillation may occur suddenly and recur, or it may persist as a chronic dysrhythmia. Atrial fibrillation is commonly associated with heart failure, rheumatic heart disease, coronary heart disease, hypertension, and hyperthyroidism.

Manifestations of atrial fibrillation relate to the rate of the ventricular response. With rapid response rates, manifestations of decreased cardiac output such as hypotension, shortness of breath, fatigue, and angina may develop. Clients with extensive heart disease may develop syncope or heart failure. Peripheral pulses are irregular and of variable amplitude (strength).

The specific ECG characteristics of atrial fibrillation include an irregularly irregular rhythm and the absence of identifiable P waves. The atrial rate is so rapid that it is not measurable. The ventricular rate varies.

Atrial fibrillation increases the risk for formation of thromboemboli. Organ infarction may occur as a result; the incidence of stroke is high.

Junctional Dysrhythmias

Rhythms that originate in AV nodal tissue are termed *junctional*. The AV junction includes the AV node and the bundle of His, which branches into the right and left bundle branches. An impulse arising from the AV junction may occur in response to failure of higher pacemakers, as in a *junctional escape rhythm*, or it may result from an abnormal mechanism, such as altered automaticity. An impulse arising from the AV junction may or may not be conducted back up to the atria. This conduction against the normal flow or pattern is called *retrograde conduction*. The resulting atrial wave, called a P′ wave, may be found before, during, or after the QRS complex, depending on the speed of conduction. The P′ wave is inverted in some ECG leads because the impulse moves from the AV node up to the atria instead of from the SA node down toward the AV node. In addition, the P'R interval is shorter than normal (less than 0.12 sec). The QRS complex is typically narrow.

A junctional rhythm may be due to drug toxicity (e.g., digitalis, beta blockers, or calcium channel blockers) or other causes such as hypoxemia, hyperkalemia, increased vagal tone or damage to the AV node, myocardial infarction, and heart failure. Loss of synchronized atrial contraction and the atrial kick may affect cardiac output, leading to manifestations of decreased cardiac output and impaired myocardial tissue perfusion. Heart failure may develop.

Premature junctional contractions (PJCs) occur before the next expected beat of the underlying rhythm. Isolated PJCs may occur in healthy people and are insignificant. *Junctional tachycardia* is a junctional rhythm with a rate greater than 60 beats/min. It is caused by increased automaticity of AV nodal tissue. The ventricular rate is usually less than 140 beats/min. Both rhythms are most commonly associated with digitalis toxicity, hypoxia, ischemia, or electrolyte imbalances.

Ventricular Dysrhythmias

Ventricular dysrhythmias originate in the ventricles. Because the ventricles pump blood into the pulmonary and systemic vasculature, any disruption of their rhythm can affect cardiac output and tissue perfusion. A wide and bizarre QRS complex (greater than 0.12 sec) is a characteristic feature of ventricular dysrhythmias. This occurs because ventricular ectopic impulses begin and travel outside normal conduction pathways. Other characteristics include no relationship of the QRS complex to a P wave, increased amplitude of the QRS complex, an abnormal ST segment, and a T wave deflected in the opposite direction from the QRS complex.

PREMATURE VENTRICULAR CONTRACTIONS *Premature ventricular contractions (PVCs)* are ectopic ventricular beats that occur before the next expected beat of the underlying rhythm. They usually do not reset the atrial rhythm and are followed by a full compensatory pause. PVCs often have no significance in people without heart disease. Frequent, recurrent, or multifocal PVCs may be associated with an increased risk for lethal dysrhythmias. PVCs result from either enhanced automaticity or a reentry phenomenon. They may be triggered by anxiety or stress; tobacco, alcohol, or caffeine use; hypoxia, acidosis, and electrolyte imbalances; sympathomimetic drugs; coronary heart disease; heart failure; and mechanical stimulation of the heart (e.g., the insertion of a cardiac catheter); or reperfusion after fibrinolytic therapy. The incidence and significance of PVCs is greatest after myocardial infarction.

PVCs may be isolated or occur in a specific pattern. Two PVCs in a row are called a *couplet* or *paired* PVCs. Three consecutive PVCs (a *triplet* or *salvo*) is a short run of ventricular tachycardia. *Ventricular bigeminy* is characterized by a PVC following each normal beat; a PVC noted every third beat is called *ventricular trigeminy.* When the ventricular impulse arises from one ectopic site, all PVCs look the same (*monomorphic*) and are called *unifocal* PVCs. *Multifocal* PVCs arise from different ectopic sites and appear different from one another on the ECG (*polymorphic*).

The frequency and patterns of PVCs can be indicative of myocardial irritability and the risk for a lethal dysrhythmia.

The following are considered warning signs in the client with acute heart disease (e.g., an acute MI).

- PVCs that develop within the first 4 hours of an MI
- Frequent PVCs (six or more per minute)
- Couplets or triplets
- Multifocal PVCs
- R-on-T phenomenon (PVCs falling on the T wave).

In people without heart disease, isolated PVCs usually are insignificant and do not require treatment. Clients may complain of feeling their hearts "skip a beat" or of palpitations. In clients with preexisting heart disease, PVCs may indicate a drug toxicity or an increased risk for lethal dysrhythmias and cardiac arrest. The risk is greatest following acute MI.

VENTRICULAR TACHYCARDIA *Ventricular tachycardia (VT, V tach)* is a rapid ventricular rhythm defined as three or more consecutive PVCs. Ventricular tachycardia may occur in short bursts, or "runs," or may persist for more than 30 seconds (sustained ventricular tachycardia). The rate is greater than 100 beats/min, and the rhythm is usually regular. Reentry is the usual electrophysiologic mechanism responsible for VT. Myocardial ischemia and infarction are the most common predisposing factors for VT. It also is associated with cardiac structural disorders such as valvular disease, rheumatic heart disease, or cardiomyopathy. It may occur in the absence of heart disease, and with anorexia nervosa, metabolic disorders, and drug toxicity.

Nonsustained VT may occur paroxysmally and convert back to an effective rhythm spontaneously. The client may experience a fluttering sensation in the chest or complain of palpitations and brief shortness of breath. Clients in sustained VT generally develop signs and symptoms of decreased cardiac output and hemodynamic instability, including severe hypotension, a weak or nonpalpable pulse, and loss of consciousness. Allowed to continue, VT can deteriorate into ventricular fibrillation. Sustained ventricular tachycardia is a medical emergency that requires immediate intervention, particularly in clients with cardiac disease.

Toursades de pointes is a type of ventricular tachycardia associated with *long QT syndrome,* a prolongation of the QT interval. Long QT syndrome may be genetic or acquired, occurring secondarily to electrolyte disruptions, myocardial infarction, cocaine use, liquid protein diets, medications, or other conditions. In toursades de pointes, the QRS complexes vary in size, shape, and amplitude (Figure 31–7 ■). Clients with toursades de pointes may have multiple bursts or episodes of ventricular tachycardia or may develop ventricular fibrillation and sudden cardiac death (Kasper et al., 2005; Porth, 2005).

VENTRICULAR FIBRILLATION *Ventricular fibrillation (VF, V fib)* is extremely rapid, chaotic ventricular depolarization causing the ventricles to quiver and cease contracting; the heart does not pump. This is known as **cardiac arrest**; it is a medical emergency requiring immediate intervention with cardiopulmonary resuscitation (CPR). Death will follow the onset of VF within 4 minutes if the rhythm is not recognized and terminated and an effective perfusing rhythm reestablished.

Ventricular fibrillation is usually triggered by severe myocardial ischemia or infarction. It occurs without warning 50%

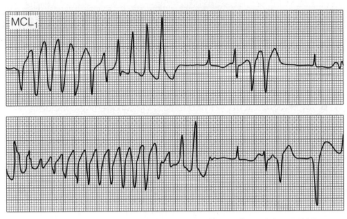

Figure 31–7 ■ Toursades de pointes. Note the wide and bizarre QRS complexes of varying size, shape (morphology), and amplitude.

of the time. It is the terminal event in many disease processes or traumatic conditions. Ventricular fibrillation may be precipitated by a single PVC or may follow VT. Other causes of VF include digitalis toxicity, reperfusion therapy, antidysrhythmic drugs, hypokalemia and hyperkalemia, hypothermia, metabolic acidosis, mechanical stimulation (as with the insertion of cardiac catheters or pacing wires), and electric shock.

Clinically, loss of ventricular contractions results in absence of a palpable or audible pulse. The client loses consciousness and stops breathing as perfusion ceases. The ECG shows grossly irregular, bizarre complexes with no discernible rate or rhythm.

Atrioventricular Conduction Blocks

Conduction defects that delay or block transmission of the sinus impulse through the AV node are called *atrioventricular conduction blocks*. Impaired conduction may result from tissue injury or disease, increased vagal (parasympathetic) tone, drug effects, or a congenital defect. AV conduction blocks vary in severity from benign to severe.

FAST FACTS

- First-degree AV block = delayed conduction through the AV node and a long PR interval.
- Second-degree AV block = complete blockage of *some* impulses through the AV node; some P waves are not followed by a QRS complex.
- Third-degree AV block = complete blockage of *all* impulses through the AV node; no relationship between P waves and QRS complexes.

FIRST-DEGREE AV BLOCK First-degree AV block is a benign conduction delay that generally poses no threat, has no symptoms, and requires no treatment. Impulse conduction through the AV node is slowed, but all atrial impulses are conducted to the ventricles. It may result from injury or infarct of the AV node, other cardiac diseases, or drug effects. The ECG shows all characteristics of NSR, except the PR interval is greater than 0.20 second.

SECOND-DEGREE AV BLOCK Second-degree AV block is characterized by failure to conduct one or more impulses from the atria to the ventricles. Two patterns of second-degree AV block are seen, identified as type I and type II.

Second-Degree AV Block—Type I *Type I second-degree AV block (Mobitz type I or Wenckebach phenomenon)* is characterized by a repeating pattern of increasing AV conduction delays until an impulse fails to conduct to the ventricles. On the ECG, PR intervals progressively lengthen until one QRS complex is not conducted, or dropped. The ventricular rate remains adequate to maintain cardiac output, and the client usually is asymptomatic. Mobitz type I AV block usually is transient, associated with acute MI or drug intoxication (e.g., digitalis, beta blockers, or calcium channel blockers). It rarely progresses to complete heart block.

Second-Degree AV Block—Type II *Type II second-degree AV block (Mobitz type II)* involves intermittent failure of the AV node to conduct an impulse to the ventricles without preceding delays in conduction. The PR interval remains constant, but not all P waves are followed by QRS complexes (e.g., there may be two P waves for every QRS). Conduction through the His-Purkinje system usually is delayed as well, causing a widened QRS complex (Braunwald et al., 2002). Mobitz type II block is frequently associated with acute anterior wall MI and a high rate of mortality (Porth, 2005). Manifestations of Mobitz type II block depend on the ventricular rate. Pacemaker therapy may be required to maintain the cardiac output.

THIRD-DEGREE AV BLOCK Third-degree AV block (complete heart block) occurs when atrial impulses are completely blocked at the AV node, and fail to reach the ventricles. As a result, the atria and ventricles are controlled by different and independent pacemakers, with separate rates and rhythms. The ventricular impulse arises from either junctional fibers (with a rate of 40 to 60 beats/min) or a ventricular pacemaker at a rate of less than 40 beats/min. The width of the QRS complex depends on the location of the escape pacemaker. The QRS is wide and the rate is slow when the rhythm arises distal to the bundle of His.

Third-degree block is frequently associated with an inferior or anteroseptal myocardial infarction. Other causes include congenital conditions, acute or degenerative cardiac disease or damage, drug effects, and electrolyte imbalances. The slow escape rhythm significantly affects cardiac output, causing manifestations such as syncope (known as a *Stokes-Adams attack*), dizziness, fatigue, exercise intolerance, and heart failure. Third-degree AV block is life threatening and requires immediate intervention to maintain adequate cardiac output.

AV DISSOCIATION Complete dissociation of atrial and ventricular rhythms can occur in conditions other than third-degree AV block. The two primary factors leading to AV dissociation are severe sinus bradycardia and a lower pacemaker (junctional or ventricular) that competes with or exceeds the normal sinus rhythm (Braunwald et al., 2002). AV dissociation may result from acute myocardial ischemia or infarction, cardiac surgery, or drug effects. The ECG shows separate and competing atrial (P waves) and ventricular (QRS complexes) rhythms.

Intraventricular Conduction Blocks

Once the impulse enters the ventricles, its conduction through the right and left bundle branches may be impaired (*bundle branch block*). As a result, the impulse is conducted more slowly than normal through the ventricles. On the ECG, the QRS complex is prolonged. Its appearance varies, depending on the affected bundle (right or left). Typically, no clinical manifestations are associated with bundle branch block unless it occurs in conjunction with an AV block.

INTERDISCIPLINARY CARE

Cardiac dysrhythmias may be either benign or critical: Recognizing lethal dysrhythmias is a matter of life and death. Major goals of care include identifying the dysrhythmia, evaluating its effect on physical and psychosocial well-being, and treating underlying causes. This may involve correcting fluid and electrolyte or acid–base imbalances; treating hypoxia, pain, or anxiety; administering antidysrhythmic medications; or mechanical and surgical interventions.

Diagnosis

Diagnostic tests for dysrhythmias include the electrocardiogram, cardiac monitoring, and electrophysiology studies. Laboratory tests such as serum electrolytes, drug levels, and ABGs may be done to help identify the cause of the dysrhythmia.

ELECTROCARDIOGRAM The 12-lead ECG may be required to accurately diagnose a dysrhythmia. It also provides information about underlying disease processes, such as myocardial infarction or other cardiac disease. The ECG may also be used to monitor the effects of treatment. See Chapter 30 ∞ for more information about the 12-lead ECG.

CARDIAC MONITORING Cardiac monitoring allows continuous observation of the cardiac rhythm. It is used in many different circumstances (Box 31–4). Different types of ECG monitoring are employed for different situations.

Continuous Cardiac Monitoring Continuous monitoring of the cardiac rhythm is provided by bedside and central monitoring stations. Electrodes placed on the client's chest attach to cables connected to a monitor. The heart rate and rhythm is visually displayed on a bedside monitor connected to a central monitoring station. The central station allows simultaneous monitoring of multiple clients within a nursing unit. Alarms on both bedside and central monitors warn of potential problems such as very rapid or very slow heart rates. Alarm limits are preset by the nurse for the individual client. Procedure 31–1 describes how to place a client on cardiac monitoring.

Telemetry may be used in acute care settings when the client is ambulatory. Chest electrodes are connected to a portable transmitter worn around the neck or waist; the ECG is transmitted electronically to a central monitoring station for continuous monitoring.

Home Monitoring Clients often complain of palpitations or other heart symptoms but are asymptomatic during evaluation in a hospital or community-based setting. Ambulatory or Holter monitoring may be used to identify intermittent dys-

---

> ### BOX 31–4 **Indications for Cardiac Monitoring**
>
> - Perioperative monitoring of heart rate and rhythm
> - Detecting and identifying dysrhythmias
> - Monitoring the effects of cardiac and noncardiac diseases on the heart
> - Monitoring clients with potentially life-threatening conditions:
>   a. Major trauma (especially cardiac trauma)
>   b. Dissecting aneurysm
>   c. Acute myocardial infarction
>   d. Heart failure
>   e. Shock
>   f. Other emergency conditions
> - Evaluating responses to procedures and interventions:
>   a. Drug therapies
>   b. Diagnostic procedures
>   c. Ablative techniques
>   d. Angioplasty or cardiac catheterization
>   e. Cardiac surgery
>   f. Pacemaker function
>   g. Automatic implantable cardioverter-defibrillator function

rhythmias, to detect silent ischemia, to monitor the effects of treatment, and to assess pacemaker or automatic cardioverter-defibrillator function. Electrodes are applied and the leads attached to the portable telemetry monitor that records and stores all electrical activity. Clients are instructed to leave the electrode pads in place during monitoring, record any cardiac symptoms or events in a journal (such as chest pain, palpitations, syncope), and are told when to return to the clinic. After the prescribed period, usually 48 to 72 hours, the client returns and the monitor is removed. Diary entries are compared to the recorded heart rhythms to identify the effects of dysrhythmias.

ELECTROPHYSIOLOGY STUDIES Diagnostic cardiac *electrophysiology (EP) procedures* are used to identify dysrhythmias and their causes. EP studies are used to analyze components of the conduction system, identify sites of ectopic stimulation, and evaluate the effectiveness of treatment. EP procedures can be used for both diagnosis and as a therapeutic intervention.

In the electrophysiology laboratory, electrode catheters are guided by fluoroscopy into the heart through the femoral or brachial vein. The timing and sequence of electrical activation during normal and abnormal (aberrant) rhythms is observed and measured. Electrical stimulation may be used to induce dysrhythmias similar to the client's clinical dysrhythmia (Woods et al., 2004). Following diagnosis, an EP procedure may be used to treat the dysrhythmia, for example, by overdrive pacing (stimulating the client's heart rate to a rate faster than that of the tachydysrhythmia) to break the dysrhythmia's cycle, or to perform ablative therapy to destroy the ectopic site. See the section on ablative techniques for further information.

Nursing care for the client undergoing an EP procedure is similar to that for a percutaneous coronary revascularization (see the box on page 978). The procedure and expected sensations are explained. The client remains awake during the procedure; antianxiety medications or sedatives are given to reduce

PROCEDURE 31-1 INITIATING CARDIAC MONITORING

GATHER SUPPLIES

- Bedside monitor and cable or telemetry unit with fresh battery
- Electrodes—self-adherent, pregelled, disposable
- Lead wires

- Washcloth, soap, and towel
- Alcohol prep pads
- Dry gauze pads or ECG prep pads

BEFORE THE PROCEDURE

Explain the reason for ECG monitoring. Reassure client that changes in heart rhythm can be noted and immediately treated if necessary. Explain that loose or disconnected lead wires, poor electrode contact, excessive movement, electrical interference, or equipment malfunc-tion may trigger alarms and alert the staff, allowing correction of the problem. Reassure that movement is allowed, within activity restrictions, while on the monitor. Explain skin preparation procedure. Provide for privacy, and drape appropriately.

PROCEDURE

1. Follow standard precautions.

2. Check equipment for damage (i.e., fraying, bent, or broken wires). Connect lead wires to cable, and secure connections.

3. Select electrode sites on the chest wall, avoiding areas of excessive movement, joints, skin creases, scar tissue, or other lesions.

4. Clean sites with soap and water, and dry thoroughly. Alcohol may be used to remove skin oils; allow the skin to dry for 60 seconds after use.

5. Gently rub the site with a dry gauze pad or ECG prep pad to remove dead skin cells, debris, and residue.

6. Open the electrode package; peel the backing from the electrode, and check to ensure that the center of the pad is moist with conductive gel.

7. Apply electrode pads, pressing firmly to ensure contact (see figure).

8. Attach leads and position cable with sufficient slack for comfort. Place the telemetry unit (if used) in gown pouch or pocket.

9. Assess ECG tracing on the monitor, adjusting settings as needed.

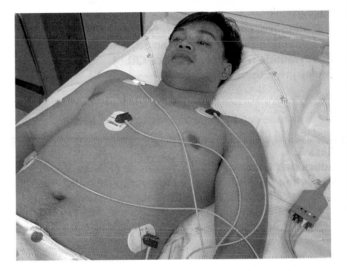

10. Set monitor alarm limits typically at 20 bpm higher and lower than the client's baseline rate. Turn alarms on, and leave on at all times. Assess immediately if an alarm is triggered.

11. Time and date pads with every change.

AFTER THE PROCEDURE

Monitor periodically for comfort. Assess electrode and lead wire connections as needed. Remove and apply new pads every 24 to 48 hours or whenever the pad becomes dislodged or nonadherent. Clean gel residue from previous site, and document skin condition under the pads. Choose an alternative site if the skin appears irritated or blistered. Document ECG strips according to unit policy and/or physician's order, as well when the cardiac rhythm or the client's condition changes (especially with complaints of chest pain, decreased level of consciousness, or changes in vital signs). Note the date, time, client identification, monitor lead, duration of PR and QT intervals, and rhythm interpretation on each ECG strip.

apprehension. Intravenous heparin may be given during the procedure to reduce the risk of thromboembolism.

Complications of EP procedures are infrequent, but include fatal ventricular fibrillation, cardiac perforation, and major venous thrombosis (Woods et al., 2004). Careful postprocedure monitoring is vital.

Medications

The goal of drug therapy is to suppress dysrhythmia formation. No drug has been found to be completely safe and effective. Antidysrhythmic drugs are primarily used for acute treatment of dysrhythmias, although they may also be used to manage chronic conditions. The overall goal of therapy is to maintain an effective cardiac output by stabilizing cardiac rhythm.

It is important to remember that virtually all antidysrhythmic drugs also have *prodysrhythmic* effects; that is, they can worsen existing dysrhythmias and precipitate new ones. Because of this tendency, studies that demonstrate higher mortality rates in clients receiving antidysrhythmic medications, and the increasing safety and availability of interventional techniques, antidysrhythmic medications are used sparingly.

Most antidysrhythmic drugs are classified by their effects on the cardiac action potential. Most are class I drugs, or fast sodium channel blockers. By blocking sodium channels, these

DEFIBRILLATION Unlike carefully synchronized cardioversion, *defibrillation* is an emergency procedure that delivers direct current without regard to the cardiac cycle. Ventricular fibrillation is immediately treated as soon as the dysrhythmia is recognized. Early defibrillation has been shown to improve survival in clients experiencing VF.

Defibrillation can be delivered by external or internal paddles or pads. Conductive gel pads or paste is applied, and external paddles or pads are placed on the chest wall at the apex and base of the heart (Figure 31–8 ■). Internal paddles are applied directly on the heart, and may be used in surgery, the emergency department, or critical care. Internal defibrillation is done only by a physician; external defibrillation may be performed by any healthcare provider who has been trained in the procedure. Automatic external defibrillators (AEDs) are available on most hospital units to allow early defibrillation for cardiac arrest. (See Procedure 31–3.)

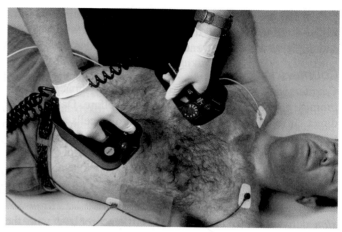

Figure 31–8 ■ Placement of paddles for defibrillation.
Source: Floyd Jackson

Pacemaker Therapy

A **pacemaker** is a pulse generator used to provide an electrical stimulus to the heart when the heart fails to generate or conduct its own at a rate that maintains the cardiac output. The pulse generator is connected to *leads* (insulated wires) passed intravenously into the heart or sutured directly to the epicardium. The leads sense intrinsic electrical activity of the heart and provide an electrical stimulus to the heart when necessary (pacing).

Pacemakers are used to treat both acute and chronic conduction defects such as third-degree AV block. They also may be used to treat bradydysrhythmias and tachydysrhythmias.

Temporary pacemakers use an external pulse generator (Figure 31–9 ■) attached to a lead threaded intravenously into the right ventricle, to temporary pacing wires implanted during cardiac surgery, or to external conductive pads placed on the chest wall for emergency pacing.

PROCEDURE 31-3 EMERGENCY EXTERNAL DEFIBRILLATION

GATHER SUPPLIES

- Automatic external defibrillator or defibrillator with ECG cable and monitor
- Conductive gel pads or paste
- Dry gauze pads
- Emergency medications and cart with pacemaker, airway management equipment, and oxygen supplies.

BEFORE THE PROCEDURE

Verify the lethal dysrhythmia, such as pulseless VT, VF, or asystole. Initiate the cardiac arrest (code) procedure, and obtain the defibrillator. If one is not immediately available, begin CPR until the emergency cart and defibrillator are brought to the bedside. Place client in supine position on a firm surface.

PROCEDURE

1. Turn on the defibrillator. Set it in *defibrillation* mode.
2. Turn ECG recording on for a continuous printout of events during the procedure.
3. Set the energy level and charge the paddles. Initial defibrillation is usually performed at 200 joules.
4. Place conductive pads on the chest, or spread conductive paste evenly on the paddles.
5. Position the paddles, holding them firmly on the chest wall.
6. Ensure that no one is touching the client or the bed. State, "All clear."
7. Depress the button on each paddle simultaneously to discharge the energy.
8. Immediately resume CPR.
9. Evaluate cardiac rhythm and for a pulse after approximately 2 minutes.
10. If the first attempt is unsuccessful, repeat the procedure, increasing the energy level to 300 joules and 360 joules for successive attempts. Reapply conductive paste as necessary.
11. Implement ACLS protocols.

AFTER THE PROCEDURE

If the dysrhythmia is successfully converted, evaluate and support neurologic, cardiovascular, and respiratory status. Monitor and titrate any intravenous infusions as ordered. Maintain ventilatory support as needed. Evaluate skin for burns. Obtain blood for laboratory analysis as ordered. Monitor vital signs and ECG continuously. Transfer to the intensive care unit (ICU) as indicated. Provide support and information to the client and family.

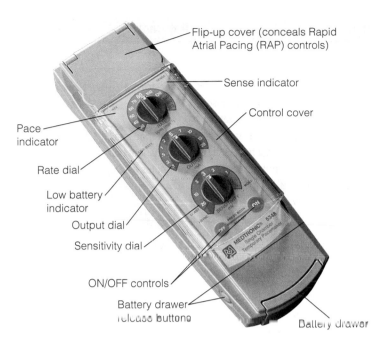

Figure 31–9 ■ Programmable settings on a temporary pacemaker.
Courtesy of Medtronics, Inc.

Permanent pacemakers use an internal pulse generator placed in a subcutaneous pocket in the subclavian space or abdominal wall. The generator connects to leads sewn directly onto the heart (*epicardial*) or passed transvenously into the heart (*endocardial*). Epicardial pacemakers (Figure 31–10 ■) require surgical exposure of the heart. Leads may be placed during cardiac surgery, or using a small subxiphoid incision to expose on the heart. Transvenous pacemaker leads are positioned in the right heart via the cephalic, subclavian, or jugular

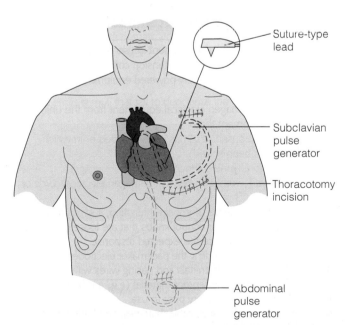

Figure 31–10 ■ A permanent epicardial pacemaker. The pulse generator may be placed in subcutaneous pockets in the subclavian or abdominal regions.

vein (Figure 31–11 ■). Local anesthesia can be used for permanent pacemaker insertion.

Pacemakers are programmed to stimulate the atria or the ventricles (*single-chamber pacing*), or both (*dual-chamber pacing*). Table 31–8 defines terms used to describe pacemaker modes and functions. The most commonly used pacemakers either (1) sense activity in and pace the ventricles only; or (2) sense activity in and pace both the atria and the ventricles. Dual-chamber or *atrioventricular sequential pacing* stimulates both chambers of the heart in sequence. AV pacing imitates the normal sequence of atrial contraction followed by ventricular contraction, improving cardiac output.

Pacing is detected on the ECG strip by the presence of pacing artifact (Figure 31–12 ■). A sharp spike is noted before the P wave with atrial pacing, and before the QRS complex with ventricular pacing. Pacing spikes are seen before both the P wave and QRS complex in AV sequential pacing. Capture is noted if there is a contraction of the chamber immediately following the pacer spike. Problems in sensing, pacing, and capture are noted in Table 31–9.

Care of the client with a temporary or permanent pacemaker focuses on monitoring for pacemaker malfunctioning, maintaining safety (Box 31–5), and preventing infection and postoperative complications. Nursing care for the client having a pacemaker implant is outlined on page 1012.

Implantable Cardioverter-Defibrillator

Sudden cardiac death claims more than 300,000 lives per year in the United States (Woods et al., 2004). The *implantable cardioverter-defibrillator (ICD)* detects life-threatening changes in the cardiac rhythm and automatically delivers an electric shock to convert the dysrhythmia back into a normal

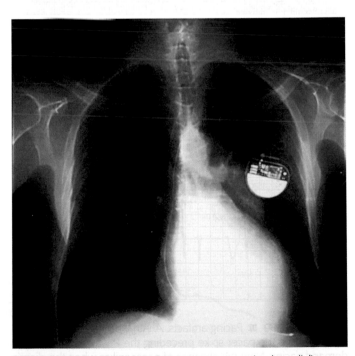

Figure 31–11 ■ A permanent transvenous (endocardial) pacemaker with the lead placed in the right ventricle via the subclavian vein.
Source: Phototake NYC

NURSING CARE OF THE CLIENT HAVING A **Permanent Pacemaker Implant**

Preoperative Care

- Provide routine preoperative care and teaching as outlined in Chapter 4 ∞.
- Assess knowledge and understanding of the procedure, clarifying and expanding on existing knowledge as needed. *Clarifying knowledge, providing information, and conveying emotional support reduces anxiety and fear and allows the client to develop a realistic outlook regarding pacer therapy.*
- Place ECG monitor electrodes away from potential incision sites. *This helps preserve skin integrity.*
- Teach range-of-motion (ROM) exercises for the affected side. *ROM exercises of the affected arm and shoulder prevent stiffness and impaired function following pacemaker insertion.*

Postoperative Care

- Provide postoperative monitoring, analgesia, and care as outlined in Chapter 4 ∞.
- Obtain a chest x-ray as ordered. *A postoperative chest x-ray is used to identify lead location and detect possible complications, such as pneumothorax or pleural effusion.*
- Position for comfort. Minimize movement of the affected arm and shoulder during the initial postoperative period. *Restricting movement minimizes discomfort on the operative side and allows the leads to become anchored, reducing the risk of dislodging.*
- Assist with gentle ROM exercises at least three times daily, beginning 24 hours after pacemaker implantation. *ROM exercises help restore normal shoulder movement and prevent contractures on the affected side.*
- Monitor pacemaker function with cardiac monitoring or intermittent ECGs. Report pacemaker problems to the physician:
  - Failure to pace. *This may indicate battery depletion, damage or dislodgement of pacer wires, or inappropriate sensing.*
  - Failure to capture (the pacemaker stimulus is not followed by ventricular depolarization). *The electrical output of the pacemaker may not be adequate, or the lead may be dislodged.*
  - Improper sensing (the pacemaker is firing or not firing, regardless of the intrinsic rate). *This increases the risk for decreased cardiac output and dysrhythmias.*
  - Runaway pacemaker (a pacemaker firing at a rapid rate). *This may be due to generator malfunction or problems with sensing.*
  - Hiccups. *A lead positioned near the diaphragm can stimulate it, causing hiccups. Hiccups may occur in extremely thin clients or may indicate a medical emergency with perforation of the right ventricle by the pacing electrode tip.*
- Assess for dysrhythmias and treat as indicated. *Until the catheter is "seated" or adheres to the myocardium, its move-*

ment may cause myocardial irritability and dysrhythmias. Fibrotic tissue develops within 2 to 3 days.

- Document the date of pacemaker insertion, the model and type, and settings. *This information is important for future reference.*
- Immediately report signs of potential complications, including myocardial perforation, cardiac tamponade, pneumothorax or hemothorax, emboli, skin breakdown, bleeding, infection, endocarditis, or poor wound healing (see Chapter 32 ∞ for more information about cardiac tamponade and endocarditis, and Chapter 38 ∞ for pneumothorax and hemothorax). *Early identification of complications allows for aggressive intervention.*
- Provide a pacemaker identification card including the manufacturer's name, model number, mode of operation, rate parameters, and expected battery life. *This card provides a reference for the client and future healthcare providers.*

Home Care

Provide appropriate teaching for the client and family about:
- Placement of the pacemaker generator and leads in relation to the heart.
- How the pacemaker works and the rate at which it is set.
- Battery replacement. Most pacemaker batteries last 6 to 12 years. Replacement requires an outpatient surgery to open the subcutaneous pocket and replace the battery.
- How to take and record the pulse rate. Instruct to assess pulse daily before arising and notify the physician if 5 or more bpm slower than the preset pacemaker rate.
- Incision care and signs of infection. Bruising may be present following surgery.
- Signs of pacemaker malfunction to report, including dizziness, fainting, fatigue, weakness, chest pain, or palpitations.
- Activity restrictions as ordered. This usually is limited to contact sports (which may damage the generator) and avoiding heavy lifting for 2 months after surgery.
- Resume sexual activity as recommended by the physician. Avoid positions that cause pressure on the site.
- Avoid tight-fitting clothing over the pacemaker site to reduce irritation and avoid skin breakdown.
- Carry the pacemaker identification card at all times, and wear a Medic-Alert bracelet or tag.
- Notify all care providers of the pacemaker.
- Do not hold or use certain electrical devices over the pacemaker site, including household appliances or tools, garage door openers, antitheft devices, or burglar alarms. Pacemaker will set off airport security detectors; notify security officials of its presence.
- Maintain follow-up care with the physician as recommended.

---

discharge (like a "blow to the chest"). A person in direct contact with the client when the device discharges may experience a tingling sensation.

Cardiac Mapping and Catheter Ablation

Cardiac mapping and catheter ablation are used to locate and destroy an ectopic focus. These diagnostic and therapeutic measures use electrophysiology techniques, and can be per-

formed in the cardiac catheterization laboratory. *Cardiac mapping* is used to identify the site of earliest impulse formation in the atria or the ventricles. Intracardiac and extracardiac catheter electrodes and computer technology are used to pinpoint the ectopic site on a map of the heart. These same catheters can be used to deliver the ablative intervention.

Ablation destroys, removes, or isolates an ectopic focus. In most instances, radio-frequency energy produced by high-frequency alternating current is used to create heat as it passes through tissue. Catheter ablation is used to treat supraventricular tachycardias, atrial fibrillation and flutter, and, in some cases, paroxysmal ventricular tachycardia (Woods et al., 2004).

Anticoagulant therapy may be started after catheter ablation to reduce the risk of clot formation at the ablation site.

Other Therapies

In addition to medications and interventional techniques, other measures may be used to treat selected dysrhythmias. Vagal maneuvers that stimulate the parasympathetic nervous system may be used to slow the heart rate in supraventricular tachycardias. These maneuvers include *carotid sinus massage* and the *Valsalva maneuver.* Carotid sinus massage is performed only by a physi-

cian during continuous cardiac monitoring. Excessive slowing of the heart rate may result. The Valsalva maneuver, forced exhalation against a closed glottis (e.g., bearing down), increases intrathoracic pressure and vagal tone, slowing the pulse rate.

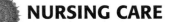

NURSING CARE

Caring for the client with cardiac dysrhythmias requires the ability to recognize, identify, and, in some cases, promptly treat the dysrhythmia. The urgency of intervention is determined by the effects of the dysrhythmia on the client. Nursing care focuses on maintaining cardiac output, monitoring the response to therapy, and teaching. Also see the Nursing Care Plan for a client with a dysrhythmia.

NURSING CARE PLAN   A Client with Supraventricular Tachycardia

Elisa Vasquez, 53 years old, is admitted to the cardiac unit with complaints of palpitations, light-headedness, and shortness of breath. Her history reveals rheumatic fever at age 12 with subsequent rheumatic heart disease and mitral stenosis. An intravenous line is in place and she is receiving oxygen. Marcia Lewin, RN, is assigned to Ms. Vasquez.

ASSESSMENT

Ms. Lewin's assessment reveals that Ms. Vasquez is moderately anxious. Her ECG shows supraventricular tachycardia (SVT) with a rate of 154. Vital signs: T 98.8°F (37.1°C), R 26, BP 95/60. Peripheral pulses weak but equal, mucous membranes pale pink, skin cool and dry. Fine crackles noted in both lung bases. A loud S_3 gallop and a diastolic murmur are noted. Ms. Vasquez is still complaining of palpitations and tells Ms. Lewin, "I feel so nervous and weak and dizzy." Ms. Vasquez's cardiologist orders 2.5 mg of verapamil to be given slowly via intravenous push and tells Ms. Lewin to prepare to assist with synchronized cardioversion if drug therapy does not control the ventricular rate.

DIAGNOSES

- *Decreased Cardiac Output* related to inadequate ventricular filling associated with rapid tachycardia
- *Ineffective Tissue Perfusion: Cerebral/Cardiopulmonary/Peripheral* related to decreased cardiac output
- *Anxiety* related to unknown outcome of altered health state

EXPECTED OUTCOMES

- Maintain adequate cardiac output and tissue perfusion.
- Demonstrate a ventricular rate within normal limits and stable vital signs.
- Verbalize reduced anxiety.
- Verbalize an understanding of the rationale for the treatment measures to control the heart rate.

PLANNING AND IMPLEMENTATION

- Provide oxygen per nasal cannula at 4 L/min.
- Continuously monitor ECG for rate, rhythm, and conduction. Assess vital signs and associated symptoms with changes in ECG. Report findings to physician.
- Explain the importance of rapidly reducing the heart rate. Explain the cardioversion procedure and encourage questions.

- Encourage verbalization of fears and concerns. Answer questions honestly, correcting misconceptions about the disease process, treatment, or prognosis.
- Administer intravenous diazepam as ordered before cardioversion.
- Document pretreatment vital signs, level of consciousness, and peripheral pulses.
- Place emergency cart with drugs and airway management supplies in client unit.
- Assist with cardioversion as indicated.
- Assess LOC, level of sedation, cardiovascular and respiratory status, and skin condition following cardioversion.
- Document procedure and postcardioversion rhythm, and response to intervention.

EVALUATION

Intravenous verapamil lowers Ms. Vasquez's heart rate to 138 for a short time, after which it increases to 164 with BP of 82/64. Her cardiologist, Dr. Mullins, performs carotid sinus massage. The ventricular rate slows to 126 for 2 minutes, revealing atrial flutter waves, and then returns to a rate of 150. Dr. Mullins explains the treatment options, including synchronized cardioversion. Ms. Vasquez agrees to the procedure.

Ms. Vasquez is lightly sedated and synchronized cardioversion is performed. One countershock converts Ms. Vasquez to regular sinus rhythm at 96 beats/min with BP 112/60.

Ms. Vasquez is sleepy from the sedation but recovers without incident. She states that she feels "much better," and her vital signs return to her normal levels. She remains in NSR with a rate of 86 to 92 for the remainder of her hospital stay. Dr. Mullins places Ms. Vasquez on furosemide to treat manifestations of mild heart failure.

CRITICAL THINKING IN THE NURSING PROCESS

1. What is the scientific basis for using carotid massage to treat supraventricular tachycardias? Was this an appropriate maneuver in the case of Ms. Vasquez?
2. What other treatment options might the physician have used to treat Ms. Vasquez's supraventricular tachycardia if she had been asymptomatic with stable vital signs?
3. Develop a teaching plan for Ms. Vasquez related to her prescription for furosemide.

See Evaluating Your Response in Appendix C.

cardiac arrest and cardiogenic shock than with ventricular tachycardia (Kasper et al., 2005).

Pathophysiology

Evidence of coronary heart disease with significant atherosclerosis and narrowing of two or more major coronary arteries is found in 75% of SCD victims. Although most have had prior myocardial infarction, only 20% to 30% have recent acute myocardial infarction. An acute change in cardiovascular status precedes cardiac arrest by up to 1 hour; however, often the onset is instantaneous or abrupt. Tachycardia develops, and the number of PVCs increases. This is followed by a run of ventricular tachycardia that deteriorates into ventricular fibrillation (Kasper et al., 2005).

Abnormalities of myocardial structure or function also contribute. Structural abnormalities include infarction, hypertrophy, myopathy, and electrical anomalies. Functional deviations are caused by such factors as ischemia followed by reperfusion, altered homeostasis, autonomic nervous system and hormone interactions, and toxic effects. The interactions of the two cause myocardial instability and may precipitate fatal dysrhythmias.

Manifestations

SCD may be preceded by typical manifestations of acute coronary syndrome or myocardial infarction, including severe chest pain, dyspnea or orthopnea, and palpitations or light-headedness. The event itself is abrupt, with complete loss of consciousness and death within minutes. If ventricular tachycardia precedes cardiac arrest, consciousness and mentation may be impaired prior to collapse and loss of consciousness.

INTERDISCIPLINARY CARE

The goal of care is to restore cardiac output and tissue perfusion. Treatment measures are initiated as soon as clinical cardiac arrest is verified by the absence of respirations and carotid or femoral pulses. Basic and ACLS measures must be instituted within 2 to 4 minutes of cardiac arrest to prevent permanent neurologic damage and ischemic injury to other organs.

Basic Life Support

Basic life support (BLS) begins with identification of the cardiac arrest and initiation of an emergency response.

Providers trained in use of the *AED* should immediately defibrillate the client in VF. Self-adhesive conductive pads attached to connecting cables are positioned on the chest (Figure 31–13). The AED analyzes the rhythm, and advises the provider to charge the device if VF is detected. After warning all personnel to stand clear, the shock button is depressed to deliver a shock. Following the shock, CPR is immediately initiated. After approximately 2 minutes or five cycles of CPR, the rhythm is evaluated and circulation checked. The sequence of analysis, shock, CPR is continued and ACLS protocols are initiated (AHA, 2005a).

Cardiopulmonary resuscitation is a mechanical attempt to maintain tissue perfusion and oxygenation using oral resuscitation and external cardiac compressions. All healthcare providers need to be proficient in CPR. The technique should be performed according to AHA guidelines and hospital protocol. (See Box 31–7.) Research demonstrates clear benefit from sustained, effective chest compressions, yet compressions often are interrupted for ventilation, assessment of pulses, and other measures. Many clients are excessively ventilated and underperfused during CPR (Sanders & Ewy, 2005). The AHA 2005 guidelines for CPR reflect this research (AHA, 2005a).

CPR carries a high risk for both cardiac and noncardiac trauma. CPR-related complications include injuries to the skin, thorax, upper airway, abdomen, lungs, heart, and great vessels. These complications can be minimized by adhering to accepted CPR techniques.

Advanced Life Support

Advanced life support (ALS), provided by specially trained healthcare personnel, includes advanced airway support (inser-

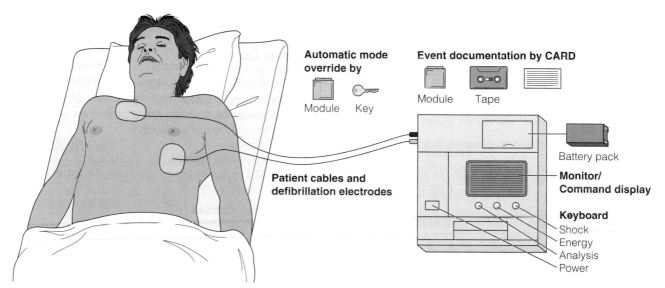

Figure 31–13 ■ Schematic of an automated external defibrillator (AED) attached to a client.

BOX 31-7 Cardiopulmonary Resuscitation

1. Assess for responsiveness; shake the client and shout.
2. Call for help. Dial 911 (if outside the healthcare facility) or initiate the institutional code or cardiac arrest procedure.
3. Open the airway using the head-tilt/chin-lift maneuver. Simultaneously press down on the forehead with one hand while lifting the chin upward with the other (part A of the accompanying figure).
4. Check for breathing; look and listen. Inspect the chest for rise and fall with respirations; listen and feel for air movement through the nose or mouth. This step should take no more than 10 seconds.
5. If not breathing, begin rescue breathing using a pocket mask, mouth shield, or bag-valve mask (see part A of the figure). Administer two breaths (1 second per breath), observing for rise of the chest with each breath.
6. Check the carotid or femoral artery for a pulse (≤10 second).
7. If a pulse is present, continue rescue breathing, administering 8 to 10 breaths per minute, until help arrives or spontaneous respirations resume. Recheck the carotid pulse every 2 minutes.
8. If no pulse is present, analyze rhythm and defibrillate or, if unwitnessed arrest or AED unavailable, initiate external cardiac compressions. Place on a firm surface. Position the heel of one hand in the center of the chest between the nipples (child and adult), with the other hand on top and the fingers either interlocked or extended (see part B of the figure).
9. Initiate hard and fast cardiac compressions, pressing straight down to depress the sternum 1.5 to 2 inches, keeping the elbows locked and positioning the shoulders directly over the hands (part C of the figure). Release pressure completely between compressions but do not lift the hands from the chest.
10. Compress the chest at a rate of approximately 100 times per minute. With one- or two-rescuer CPR, provide two breaths after each 30 compressions. Assess the pulse after five complete cycles of 30 compressions and two breaths; continue CPR until help arrives.

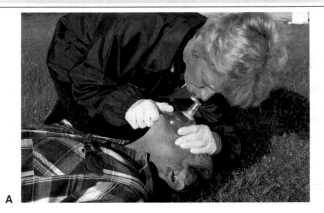

A

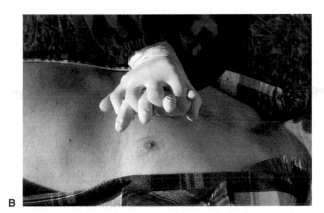

B

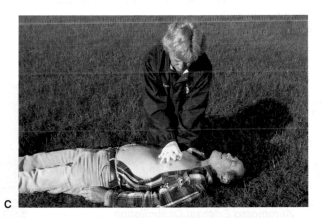

C

A, Head-tilt/chin-lift maneuver and using a bag-valve mask.
B, Placement of hands on the sternum between the nipples.
C, Arm, hand, and shoulder position for cardiac massage.

tion of a laryngeal mask airway, esophageal-tracheal Combitube, or endotracheal intubation) to maintain the airway and oxygenation, use of intravenous drugs following specific protocols, and additional interventions such as repeated defibrillation procedures and cardiac pacing. Epinephrine, vasopressin, sodium bicarbonate, and antidysrhythmic drugs such as amiodarone, bretylium, lidocaine, procainamide, magnesium sulfate, and atropine are used to attempt to restore and maintain an effective cardiac rhythm.

Postresuscitation Care

Clients who experience sudden cardiac death associated with ventricular fibrillation and acute MI have the best prognosis (Kasper et al., 2005). The client is transferred to a coronary care unit and MI treatment measures are instituted. Antidysrhythmic drugs may be continued for 24 to 48 hours to reduce the risk of subsequent episodes of VF.

Because the risk for recurrent SCD is significant in survivors, extensive diagnostic testing and interventions such as

8 In reviewing laboratory results for a client admitted with acute chest pain, the nurse is most concerned about which of the following?
1. hematocrit 35%
2. AST 65 unit/L
3. CK 320 unit/L
4. APTT 35 seconds

9 The nurse recognizes second-degree AV block, type II (Mobitz II), and intervenes appropriately when he:
1. records the finding in the chart.
2. prepares for temporary pacemaker insertion.
3. administers a class IB antidysrhythmic drug.
4. places the client in Fowler's position.

10 On identifying sinus bradycardia at a rate of 45 bpm, the nurse should:
1. assess mental status and blood pressure.
2. assess peripheral pulses on all four extremities.
3. determine if an apical-radial pulse deficit is present.
4. prepare to administer intravenous atropine.

See Test Yourself answers in Appendix C.

BIBLIOGRAPHY

Alber, C. M., Chae, C. U., Grodstein, F., Rose, L. M., Rexrode, K. M., Ruskin, J. N., et al. (2003). Prospective study of sudden cardiac death among women in the United States. *Circulation, 2003*(207), 2096–2101. Retrieved from http://www.circulationaha.org

American Heart Association. (2005a). 2005 Guidelines for CPR and ECC. *Circulation, 112,* IV1–IV205. Retrieved from www.circulationaha.org

_____. (2005b). *Heart disease and stroke statistics—2005 update.* Dallas, TX: Author.

Artinian, N. T. (2001). Perceived benefits and barriers of eating heart healthy. *Medsurg Nursing, 10*(3), 129–138.

Aschcraft, A. S. (2004). Differentiating between pre-arrest and failure-to-rescue. *Medsurg Nursing, 13*(4), 211–215.

Ayers, D. M. M. (2002). EBCT: Beaming in on coronary artery disease. *Nursing, 32*(4), 81.

Blumenthal, R. S., & Margolis, S. (2005). *The Johns Hopkins white papers. Heart attack prevention.* Redding, CT: Medletter Associates.

Braunwald, E., Antman, E. M., Beasley, J. W., Califf, R. M., Cheitlin, M. D., Hochman, J. S., et al. (2002). *ACC/AHA 2002 guideline update for the management of patients with unstable angina and non-ST-segment elevation myocardial infarction: A report of the American College of Cardiology/American Heart Association Task Force on Practice Guidelines (Committee on the Management of Patients with Unstable Angina).* Retrieved from www.acc.org/clinical/guidelines/unstable/unstable.pdf

Chan, D. S., Chan, J. P., & Chang, A. M. (2005). Acute coronary syndromes: Cardiac rehabilitation programmes and quality of life. *Journal of Advanced Nursing, 49*(6), 591–599.

Copstead, L. C., & Banasik, J. L. (2005). *Pathophysiology* (3rd ed.). St. Louis, MO: Saunders.

Crane, P. B., & McSweeney, J. C. (2003). Exploring older women's lifestyle changes after myocardial infarction. *Medsurg Nursing, 12*(3), 170–176.

De Luca, G., Suryapranata, H., Ottervanger, J. P., & Antman, E. M. (2004). Time delay to treatment and mortality in primary angioplasty for acute myocardial infarction: Every minute of delay counts. *Circulation,* March 16, 2004. Retrieved from www.circulationaha.org

DeVon, H. A., & Zerwic, J. J. (2004). Differences in the symptoms associated with unstable angina and myocardial infarction. *Progress in Cardiovascular Nursing, 19*(1) 6–11.

Dochterman, J., & Bulechek, G. (2004). *Nursing Interventions Classification (NIC)* (4th ed.). St. Louis, MO: Mosby.

Eagle, K. A., Guyton, R. A., Davidoff, R., Edwards, F. H., Ewy, G. A., Gardner, T. J., et al. (2004). *ACC/AHA 2004 guideline update for coronary artery bypass graft surgery: A report of the American College of Cardiology/American Heart Association Task Force on Practice Guidelines.* Retrieved from www.acc.org/clinical/guidelines/cabg/cabg.pdf

Engler, M. B. (2004). Familial hypercholesterolemia: Genetic predisposition to atherosclerosis. *Medsurg Nursing, 13*(4), 253–257.

Foley, S. (2005). Update on risk factors for atherosclerosis: The role of inflammation and apolipoprotein E. *Medsurg Nursing, 14*(1), 43–50.

Glessner, T. M., & Walker, M. K. (2001). Standardized measures: Documenting processes and outcomes of care for patients undergoing coronary artery bypass grafting. *Medsurg Nursing, 10*(1), 23–29.

Granger, B. B., & Miller, C. M. (2001). Acute coronary syndrome. *Nursing, 31*(11), 36–43.

Granot, M., Goldstein-Ferber, S., & Azzam, A. S. (2004). Gender differences in the perception of chest pain. *Journal of Pain and Symptom Management, 27*(2), 149–155.

Hart, P. L. (2005). Women's perceptions of coronary heart disease: An integrative review. *Journal of Cardiovascular Nursing, 20*(3), 170–176.

Hummard, J. (2004). Management of atrial fibrillation. *Nursing Times, 100*(6), 42–44.

Kasper, D. L., Braunwald, E., Fauci, A. S., Hauser, S. L., Longo, D. L., & Jameson, J. L. (2005). *Harrison's principles of internal medicine* (16th ed.). New York: McGraw-Hill.

Kellen, J. C. (2004) Implications for nursing care of patients with atrial fibrillation: Lessons learned from the AFFIRM and RACE studies. *Journal of Cardiovascular Nursing, 19*(2), 128–137.

McCance, K. L., & Huether, S. E. (2006). *Pathophysiology: The biologic basis for disease in adults and children* (5th ed.). St. Louis, MO: Mosby.

McSweeney, J. C., & Coon, S. (2004). Women's inhibitors and facilitators associated with making behavioral changes after myocardial infarction. *Medsurg Nursing, 13*(1), 49–56.

Meeker, M. H., & Rothrock, J. C. (1999). *Alexander's care of the patient in surgery* (11th ed.). St. Louis, MO: Mosby.

Miller, K. H., & Grindel, C. G. (2004). Comparison of symptoms of younger and older patients undergoing coronary artery bypass surgery. *Clinical Nursing Research, 13*(3), 179–193.

Milner, K. A., Funk, M., Richards, S., Vaccarino, V., & Krumholz, H. M. (2001). Symptom predictors of acute coronary syndromes in younger and older patients. *Nursing Research, 50*(4), 233–241.

Moorhead, S., Johnson, M., & Maas, M. (2004). *Nursing outcomes classification (NOC)* (3rd ed.). St. Louis, MO: Mosby.

NANDA International. (2005). *NANDA's nursing diagnoses: Definitions & classification 2005–2006.* Philadelphia: Author.

National Cholesterol Education Program. (2002). *Third report of the National Cholesterol Education Program (NCEP) Expert Panel on detection, evaluation, and treatment of high blood cholesterol in adults (Adult Treatment Panel III). Final report.* Bethesda, MD: National Institutes of Health.

National Heart, Lung, and Blood Institute (NHLBI). (2004). *Morbidity & mortality: 2004 chart book of cardiovascular, lung, and blood diseases.* Bethesda, MD: National Institutes of Health.

_____. (2005). Statement from Elizabeth G. Nabel, M.D., director of the National Heart, Lung, and Blood Institute of the National Institutes of Health on the findings of the Women's Health Study. *NIH News,* March 7. Retrieved from www.nhlbi.hih.gov

National High Blood Pressure Education Program. (2004). *The seventh report of the Joint National Committee on Prevention, Detection, Evaluation, and Treatment of High Blood Pressure.* Bethesda, MD: National Heart, Lung, and Blood Institute, National Institutes of Health.

Nicholls, C., & Sani, M. (2004). Antiplatelet therapy. *Nursing of Older People, 16*(8), 35–36.

Obias-Manno, D., & Wijetunga, M. (2004). Risk stratification and primary prevention of sudden cardiac death: Sudden death prevention. *AACN Clinical Issues, 15*(3), 404–418.

Palatnik, A. M. (2001). Critical care. Acute coronary syndrome: New advances and nursing strategies. *Nursing, 31*(5), 32cc1–32cc2, 32cc4, 32cc6.

Paparella, S. (2004). Fibrinolytic therapy: No room for error. *Journal of Emergency Nursing, 30*(4), 348–350.

Pelter, M. M., & Adams, M. G. (2004). Premature beats. *American Journal of Critical Care, 13*(6), 519–520.

Porth, C. M. (2005). *Pathophysiology: Concepts of altered health states* (7th ed.). Philadelphia: Lippincott.

Quigley, M. P. (2004). Promoting cardiac rehabilitation. *Nursing, 34*(8), 24.

Ridker, P. M., Cook, N. R., Lee, I., Gordon, D., Gaziano, J. M., Manson, J. E., et al. (2005). A randomized trial of low-dose aspirin in the primary prevention of cardiovascular disease in women. *New England Journal of Medicine, 352.* Retrieved from http://content.nejm.org/cgi/content/full/352/13/1293

Rosenfeld, A. G. (2004). Treatment-seeking delay among women with acute myocardial infarction: Decision trajectories and their predictors. *Nursing Research, 53*(4), 225–236.

Ryan, C. J., DeVon, H. A., & Zerwic, J. J. (2005). Typical and atypical symptoms: Diagnosing acute coronary syndromes accurately. *American Journal of Nursing, 105*(2), 34–36.

Sanders, A. B., & Ewy, G. A. (2005). Cardiopulmonary resuscitation in the real world: When will the guidelines get the message? *JAMA, 293*(3), 363–365.

Shaffer, R. S. (2002). ICD therapy: The patient's perspective. *American Journal of Nursing, 102*(2), 46–49.

Stewart, S. (2004). Epidemiology and economic impact of atrial fibrillation. *Journal of Cardiovascular Nursing, 19*(2), 94–102.

Tierney, L. M., McPhee, S. J., & Papadakis, M. A. (2005). *Current medical diagnosis & treatment* (44th ed.). New York: McGraw-Hill.

Urden, L. D., Stacy, K. M., & Lough, M. E. (2006). *Thelan's critical care nursing: Diagnosis and management* (5th ed.). St. Louis, MO: Mosby.

U.S. Department of Health & Human Services. (2005). *Dietary guidelines for Americans 2005.* Washington, DC: U.S. Department of Agriculture. Retrieved from www.healthierus.gov/dietaryguidelines

U.S. Preventive Services Task Force. (2002a). Aspirin for the primary prevention of cardiovascular events: Recommendations and rationale. *American Journal of Nursing, 102*(3), 67, 69–70.

_____. (2002b). Screening for lipid disorders in adults: Recommendations and rationale. *American Journal of Nursing, 102*(6), 91, 93, 95.

Way, L. W., & Doherty, G. M. (2003). *Current surgical diagnosis and treatment* (11th ed.). New York: McGraw-Hill.

Wilkinson, J. M. (2005). *Nursing diagnosis handbook with NIC interventions and NOC outcomes* (8th ed.). Upper Saddle River, NJ: Prentice Hall Health.

Wolf, Z. R., Miller, P. A., & Devine, M. (2003). Relationship between nurse caring and patient satisfaction in patients undergoing invasive cardiac procedures. *Medsurg Nursing, 12*(6), 391–396.

Woods, S. L., Froelicher, E. S., Motzer, S. A., & Bridges, E. (2004). *Cardiac nursing* (5th ed.). Philadelphia: Lippincott.

Writing Group for the Women's Health Initiative Investigators. (2002). Risks and benefits of estrogen plus progestin in healthy postmenopausal women. [On-line]. *JAMA, 288*(3). Retrieved from http://jama.ama-assn.org/issues/v288n3/fffull/joc21036.html

Wung, S. (2002). Genetic advances in coronary artery disease. *Medsurg Nursing, 11*(6), 296–300.

Zerwic, J. J., & Ryan, C. J. (2004). Delays in seeking MI treatment. *American Journal of Nursing, 104*(1), 81–83.

CHAPTER 32 Nursing Care of Clients with Cardiac Disorders

LEARNING OUTCOMES

- Compare and contrast the etiology, pathophysiology, and manifestations of common cardiac disorders, including heart failure, structural disorders, and inflammatory disorders.

- Explain risk factors and preventive measures for cardiac disorders such as heart failure, inflammatory disorders, and valve disorders.

- Discuss indications for and management of clients undergoing hemodynamic monitoring.

- Discuss the effects and nursing implications for medications commonly prescribed for clients with cardiac disorders.

- Describe nursing care for the client undergoing cardiac surgery or cardiac transplant.

CLINICAL COMPETENCIES

- Apply knowledge of normal cardiac anatomy and physiology and assessment techniques in caring for clients with cardiac disorders.

- Assess functional health status of clients with cardiac disorders, documenting and reporting deviations for expected findings.

- Based on client assessment and knowledge of the disorder, determine priority nursing diagnoses.

- Plan, prioritize, and provide evidence-based, individualized care for clients with cardiac disorders.

- Safely and knowledgeably administer prescribed medications and treatments to clients with cardiac disorders.

- Actively participate in planning and coordinating interdisciplinary care for clients with cardiac disorders.

- Provide appropriate teaching and community-based care for clients with cardiac disorders and their families.

- Evaluate the effectiveness of nursing care, revising the plan of care as needed to promote, maintain, or restore functional health status of clients with cardiac disorders.

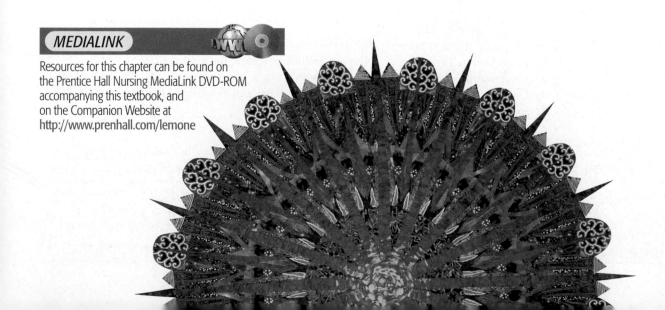

MEDIALINK

Resources for this chapter can be found on the Prentice Hall Nursing MediaLink DVD-ROM accompanying this textbook, and on the Companion Website at http://www.prenhall.com/lemone

Cardiac disorders affect the structure and/or function of the heart. These disorders interfere with the heart's primary purpose: to pump enough blood to meet the body's demand for oxygen and nutrients. Disruptions in cardiac function affect the functioning of other organs and tissues, potentially leading to organ system failure and death.

Heart failure is the most common cardiac disorder. Other cardiac disorders discussed in this chapter include structural cardiac disorders, such as valve disorders and cardiomyopathy, and inflammatory cardiac disorders, such as endocarditis and pericarditis. Before continuing with this chapter, please review the heart's anatomy and physiology, nursing assessment, and diagnostic tests in Chapter 30 ∞.

HEART FAILURE

Heart failure is a complex syndrome resulting from cardiac disorders that impair the ventricles' ability to fill with and effectively pump blood (Hunt et al., 2005). In heart failure, the heart is unable to pump enough blood to meet the metabolic demands of the body. It is the end result of many conditions. Frequently, it is a long-term effect of coronary heart disease (CHD) and myocardial infarction (MI) when left ventricular damage is extensive enough to impair cardiac output (see Chapter 31 ∞). Other diseases of the heart also may cause heart failure, including structural and inflammatory disorders. In normal hearts, failure can result from excessive demands placed on the heart. Heart failure may be acute or chronic.

THE CLIENT WITH HEART FAILURE

As mentioned, heart failure develops when the heart cannot effectively fill or contract with adequate strength to function as a pump to meet the needs of the body. As a result, cardiac output falls, leading to decreased tissue perfusion. The body initially adjusts to reduced cardiac output by activating inherent compensatory mechanisms to restore tissue perfusion. These normal mechanisms may result in vascular congestion—hence, the commonly used term *congestive heart failure (CHF)*. As these

mechanisms are exhausted, heart failure ensues, with increased morbidity and mortality.

Heart failure is a disorder of cardiac function. It frequently is due to *impaired myocardial contraction,* which may result from CHD and myocardial ischemia or infarct or from a primary cardiac muscle disorder such as cardiomyopathy or myocarditis. Structural cardiac disorders, such as valve disorders or congenital heart defects, and hypertension also can lead to heart failure when the heart muscle is damaged by the long-standing *excessive workload* associated with these conditions. Other clients without a primary abnormality of myocardial function may present with manifestations of heart failure due to *acute excess demands* placed on the myocardium, such as volume overload, hyperthyroidism, and massive pulmonary embolus (Table 32–1). Hypertension and coronary heart disease are the leading causes of heart failure in the United States. The high prevalence of hypertension in African Americans contributes significantly to their risk for and incidence of heart failure.

Incidence, Prevalence, and Risk Factors

Nearly 5 million people in the United States are currently living with heart failure; approximately 550,000 new cases of heart failure are diagnosed annually (American Heart Associa-

TABLE 32–1 Selected Causes of Heart Failure

IMPAIRED MYOCARDIAL FUNCTION	INCREASED CARDIAC WORKLOAD	ACUTE NONCARDIAC CONDITIONS
■ Coronary heart disease	■ Hypertension	■ Volume overload
■ Cardiomyopathies	■ Valve disorders	■ Hyperthyroidism
■ Rheumatic fever	■ Anemias	■ Fever, infection
■ Infective endocarditis	■ Congenital heart defects	■ Massive pulmonary embolus

tion [AHA], 2005). Its incidence and prevalence increase with age: Less than 5% of people between ages 55 and 64 have heart failure, whereas 6% to 10% of people older than 65 are affected (see the box below) (AHA, 2005). The prevalence and mortality rate for heart failure is higher in African Americans than in whites. See the accompanying Cultural Diversity box.

Ischemic heart disease (coronary heart disease) is the leading risk factor for heart failure. Cardiomyopathies are the second leading cause of heart failure. Other, less common causes of heart failure are hypertension and congenital and valvular heart disease (Kasper et al., 2005).

The prognosis for a client with heart failure depends on its underlying cause and how effectively precipitating factors can be treated. Most clients with heart failure die within 8 years of the diagnosis. The risk for sudden cardiac death is dramatically increased, occurring at a rate six to nine times that of the general population (AHA, 2005).

Physiology Review

The mechanical pumping action of cardiac muscle propels the blood it receives to the pulmonary and systemic vascular systems for reoxygenation and delivery to the tissues. *Cardiac output (CO)* is the amount of blood pumped from the ventricles in 1 minute. Cardiac output is used to assess cardiac performance, especially left ventricular function. Effective cardiac output depends on adequate functional muscle mass and the ability of the ventricles to work together. Cardiac output normally is regulated by the oxygen needs of the body: As oxygen use increases, cardiac output increases to maintain cellular function. *Cardiac reserve* is the ability of the heart to increase CO to meet metabolic demand. Ventricular damage reduces the cardiac reserve.

Cardiac output is a product of heart rate and stroke volume. *Heart rate (HR)* affects cardiac output by controlling the number of ventricular contractions per minute. It is influenced by the autonomic nervous system, catecholamines, and thyroid hormones. Activation of a stress response (e.g., hypovolemia or fear) stimulates the sympathetic nervous system, increasing the heart rate and its contractility. Elevated heart rates increase cardiac output. Very rapid heart rates, however, shorten ventricular filling time (diastole), reducing stroke volume and cardiac output. On the other hand, a slow heart rate reduces cardiac output simply because of fewer cardiac cycles.

Stroke volume, the volume of blood ejected with each heartbeat, is determined by preload, afterload, and myocardial contractility. *Preload* is the volume of blood in the ventricles at end diastole (just prior to contraction). The blood in the ventricles exerts pressure on the ventricle walls, stretching muscle fibers. The greater the blood volume, the greater the force with which the ventricle contracts to expel the blood. End diastolic volume depends on the amount of blood returning to the ventricles (*venous return*) and the distensibility or stiffness of the ventricles (*compliance*). See Box 32–1.

Afterload is the force needed to eject blood into the circulation. This force must be great enough to overcome arterial pressures

FOCUS ON CULTURAL DIVERSITY

- Up to 5 million Americans have heart failure; of these, about 725,000 (15%) are African Americans.
- In African Americans:
  - Manifestations of heart failure develop at an earlier age.
  - The disease progresses more rapidly.
  - More hospital visits are attributed to heart failure.
  - The mortality rate is higher than in white men and women.

NURSING CARE OF THE OLDER ADULT   Heart Failure

Heart failure is common in older adults, affecting nearly 10% of people over the age of 75 years.

Aging affects cardiac function. Diastolic filling is impaired by decreased ventricular compliance. With aging, the heart is less responsive to sympathetic nervous system stimulation. As a result, maximal heart rate, cardiac reserve, and exercise tolerance are reduced. Concurrent health problems such as arthritis that affect stamina or mobility often contribute to a more sedentary lifestyle, further decreasing the heart's ability to respond to increased stress.

Assessing for Home Care

The older adult with heart failure may not be dyspneic, instead presenting with weakness and fatigue, somnolence, confusion, disorientation, or worsening dementia. Dependent edema and respiratory crackles may or may not indicate heart failure in older adults.

Assess the diet of the older adult. Decreased taste may lead to increased use of salt to bring out food flavors. Limited mobility or visual acuity may cause the older adult to rely on prepared foods that are high in sodium such as canned soups and frozen meals. Discuss normal daily activities and assess sleep and rest patterns. It is also important to assess the environment for:
- Safe roads or neighborhoods for walking
- Access to pharmacy, medical care, and assistive services such as a cardiac rehabilitation program or structured exercise programs designed for older adults.

Health Education for the Client and Family

Teaching for the older adult with heart failure focuses on maintaining function and promptly identifying and treating episodes of heart failure. Teach clients how to adapt to changes in cardiovascular function associated with aging, such as:
- Allowing longer warm-up and cool-down periods during exercise
- Engaging in regular exercise such as walking five or more times a week
- Resting with feet elevated (e.g., in a recliner) when fatigued
- Maintaining adequate fluid intake
- Preventing infection through pneumococcal and influenza immunizations.

BOX 32–1 Explaining Physiologic Terms Using Practical Examples

The concepts of preload, the Frank-Starling mechanism, compliance, and afterload can be difficult to understand and to explain to clients. Use common analogies to make these concepts easier to understand.

■ *Preload:* Think about a new rubber band. As you stretch the rubber band further, it snaps back into shape with greater force.

■ *Frank-Starling mechanism:* When you repeatedly stretch that rubber band beyond a certain limit, it loses some elasticity and fails to return to its original shape and size.

■ *Compliance:* Use a new rubber balloon to illustrate this concept. A new balloon is not very compliant—it takes a lot of work (force) to inflate it. As the balloon is repeatedly inflated and stretched, it becomes more compliant, expanding easily with less force.

■ *Afterload:* When a hose is crimped or plugged, more force is required to eject a stream of water out its end.

within the pulmonary and systemic vascular systems. The right ventricle must generate enough force to open the pulmonary valve and eject its blood into the pulmonary artery. The left ventricle ejects its blood into the systemic circulation by overcoming the arterial resistance behind the aortic valve. Increased systemic vascular resistance (e.g., hypertension) increases afterload, impairing stroke volume and increasing myocardial work.

Contractility is the natural ability of cardiac muscle fibers to shorten during systole. Contractility is necessary to overcome arterial pressures and eject blood during systole. Impaired contractility affects cardiac output by reducing stroke volume. The *ejection fraction (EF)* is the percentage of blood in the ventricle that is ejected during systole. A normal ejection fraction is approximately 60%.

Pathophysiology

When the heart begins to fail, mechanisms are activated to compensate for the impaired function and maintain the cardiac output. The primary compensatory mechanisms are (1) the Frank-Starling mechanism, (2) neuroendocrine responses including activation of the sympathetic nervous system and the renin–angiotensin system, and (3) myocardial hypertrophy. These mechanisms and their effects are summarized in Table 32–2.

Decreased cardiac output initially stimulates aortic baroreceptors, which in turn stimulate the sympathetic nervous system (SNS). SNS stimulation produces both cardiac and vascular responses through the release of norepinephrine. Norepinephrine increases heart rate and contractility by stimulating cardiac beta-receptors. Cardiac output improves as both heart rate and stroke volume increase. Norepinephrine also causes arterial and venous vasoconstriction, increasing venous return to

TABLE 32–2 Compensatory Mechanisms Activated in Heart Failure

MECHANISM	PHYSIOLOGY	EFFECT ON BODY SYSTEMS	COMPLICATIONS
Frank-Starling mechanism	The greater the stretch of cardiac muscle fibers, the greater the force of contraction.	■ Increased contractile force leading to increased CO	■ Increased myocardial oxygen demand ■ Limited by overstretching
Neuroendocrine response	Decreased CO stimulates the sympathetic nervous system and catecholamine release.	■ Increased HR, BP, and contractility ■ Increased vascular resistance ■ Increased venous return	■ Tachycardia with decreased filling time and decreased CO ■ Increased vascular resistance ■ Increased myocardial work and oxygen demand
	Decreased CO and decreased renal perfusion stimulate renin–angiotensin system.	■ Vasoconstriction and increased BP	■ Increased myocardial work ■ Renal vasoconstriction and decreased renal perfusion
	Angiotensin stimulates aldosterone release from adrenal cortex.	■ Salt and water retention by the kidneys ■ Increased vascular volume	■ Increased preload and afterload ■ Pulmonary congestion
	ADH is released from posterior pituitary.	■ Water excretion inhibited	■ Fluid retention and increased preload and afterload ■ Pulmonary congestion
	Atrial natriuretic peptide and brain natriuretic peptide are released.	■ Increased sodium excretion ■ Diuresis ■ Vasodilation	
	Blood flow is redistributed to vital organs (heart and brain).	■ Decreased perfusion of other organ systems ■ Decreased perfusion of skin and muscles	■ Renal failure ■ Anaerobic metabolism and lactic acidosis
Ventricular hypertrophy	Increased cardiac workload causes myocardial muscle to hypertrophy and ventricles to dilate.	■ Increased contractile force to maintain CO	■ Increased myocardial oxygen demand ■ Cellular enlargement

the heart. Increased venous return increases ventricular filling and myocardial stretch, increasing the force of contraction (the Frank-Starling mechanism). Overstretching the muscle fibers past their physiologic limit results in an ineffective contraction.

Blood flow is redistributed to the brain and the heart to maintain perfusion of these vital organs. Decreased renal perfusion causes renin to be released from the kidneys. Activation of the renin–angiotensin system produces additional vasoconstriction and stimulates the adrenal cortex to produce aldosterone and the posterior pituitary to release antidiuretic hormone (ADH). Aldosterone stimulates sodium reabsorption in renal tubules, promoting water retention. ADH acts on the distal tubule to inhibit water excretion and also causes vasoconstriction. The effect of these hormones is significant vasoconstriction and salt and water retention, with a resulting increase in vascular volume. Increased ventricular filling increases the force of contraction, improving cardiac output. The effects of the renin–angiotensin–aldosterone system and ADH release are counterbalanced to a certain extent by two additional hormones. The increased vascular volume and venous return prompted by vasoconstriction and sodium and water retention increase the volume and pressures in the heart. Stimulation of stretch receptors in the atria and ventricles lead to the release of *atrial natriuretic peptide (ANP)* and *brain natriuretic peptide (BNP)* from stores in the atria (ANP and BNP) and ventricles (BNP). These hormones promote sodium and water excretion and inhibit the release of norepinephrine, renin, and ADH, with resulting vasodilation. Although beneficial, the effects of these hormones are too weak to completely counteract the vasoconstriction and sodium and water retention that occurs in heart failure.

Ventricular remodeling occurs as the heart chambers and myocardium adapt to fluid volume and pressure increases. The chambers dilate to accommodate excess fluid resulting from increased vascular volume and incomplete emptying. Initially, this additional stretch causes more effective contractions. *Ventricular hypertrophy* occurs as existing cardiac muscle cells enlarge, increasing their contractile elements (actin and myosin) and force of contraction.

Although these responses may help in the short-term regulation of cardiac output, it is now recognized that they hasten the deterioration of cardiac function. The onset of heart failure is heralded by *decompensation*, the loss of effective compensation. Heart failure progresses due to the very mechanisms that initially maintained circulatory stability.

The rapid heart rate shortens diastolic filling time, compromises coronary artery perfusion, and increases myocardial oxygen demand. Resulting ischemia further impairs cardiac output. Beta-receptors in the heart become less sensitive to continued SNS stimulation, decreasing heart rate and contractility. As the beta-receptors become less sensitive, norepinephrine stores in the cardiac muscle become depleted. In contrast, alpha-receptors on peripheral blood vessels become increasingly sensitive to persistent stimulation, promoting vasoconstriction and increasing afterload and cardiac work.

Initially, ventricular hypertrophy and dilation increase cardiac output, but chronic distention causes the ventricular wall eventually to thin and degenerate. The purpose of hypertrophy is thus defeated. In addition, chronic overloading of the dilated ventricle eventually stretches the fibers beyond the optimal point for effective contraction. The ventricles continue to dilate to accommodate the excess fluid, but the heart loses the ability to contract forcefully. The heart muscle may eventually become so large that the coronary blood supply is inadequate, causing ischemia.

Chronic distention exhausts stores of ANP and BNP. The effects of norepinephrine, renin, and ADH prevail, and the renin–angiotensin pathway is continually stimulated. This mechanism ultimately raises the hemodynamic stress on the heart by increasing both preload and afterload. As heart function deteriorates, less blood is delivered to the tissues and to the heart itself. Ischemia and necrosis of the myocardium further weaken the already failing heart, and the cycle repeats.

In normal hearts, the cardiac reserve allows the heart to adjust its output to meet metabolic needs of the body, increasing the cardiac output by up to five times the basal level during exercise. Clients with heart failure have minimal to no cardiac reserve. At rest, they may be unaffected; however, any stressor (e.g., exercise, illness) taxes their ability to meet the demand for oxygen and nutrients. Manifestations of activity intolerance when the person is at rest indicate a critical level of cardiac decompensation.

Classifications and Manifestations of Heart Failure

Heart failure is commonly classified in several different ways, depending on the underlying pathology. Classifications include systolic versus diastolic failure, left-sided versus right-sided failure, high-output versus low-output failure, and acute versus chronic failure.

FAST FACTS

Terms used to describe or classify heart failure:
- Systolic or diastolic failure
- Left ventricular (or sided) or right ventricular (or sided) failure
- Low-output or high-output failure
- Acute or chronic failure
- Forward or backward effects.

Systolic versus Diastolic Failure

Systolic failure occurs when the ventricle fails to contract adequately to eject a sufficient blood volume into the arterial system. Systolic function is affected by loss of myocardial cells due to ischemia and infarction, cardiomyopathy, or inflammation. The manifestations of systolic failure are those of decreased cardiac output: weakness, fatigue, and decreased exercise tolerance.

Diastolic failure results when the heart cannot completely relax in diastole, disrupting normal filling. Passive diastolic filling decreases, increasing the importance of atrial contraction to preload. Diastolic dysfunction results from decreased ventricular compliance due to hypertrophic and cellular changes and impaired relaxation of the heart muscle. Its manifestations result from increased pressure and congestion behind the ventricle:

shortness of breath, tachypnea, and respiratory crackles if the left ventricle is affected; distended neck veins, liver enlargement, anorexia, and nausea if the right ventricle is affected. Many clients have components of both systolic and diastolic failure.

Left-Sided versus Right-Sided Failure

Depending on the pathophysiology involved, either the left or the right ventricle may be primarily affected. In chronic heart failure, however, both ventricles typically are impaired to some degree. Coronary heart disease and hypertension are common causes of *left-sided heart failure*, whereas *right-sided heart failure* often is caused by conditions that restrict blood flow to the lungs, such as acute or chronic pulmonary disease. Left-sided heart failure also can lead to right-sided failure as pressures in the pulmonary vascular system increase with congestion behind the failing left ventricle.

As left ventricular function fails, cardiac output falls. Pressures in the left ventricle and atrium increase as the amount of blood remaining in the ventricle after systole increases. These increased pressures impair filling, causing congestion and increased pressures in the pulmonary vascular system. Increased pressures in this normally low-pressure system increase fluid movement from the blood vessels into interstitial tissues and the alveoli (Figure 32–1 ■).

The manifestations of left-sided heart failure result from pulmonary congestion (*backward effects*) and decreased cardiac output (*forward effects*). Fatigue and activity intolerance are common early manifestations. Dizziness and syncope also may result from decreased cardiac output. Pulmonary congestion causes dyspnea, shortness of breath, and cough. The client may develop **orthopnea** (difficulty breathing while lying down), prompting use of two or three pillows or a recliner for sleeping. Cyanosis from impaired gas exchange may be noted. On auscultation of the lungs, inspiratory crackles (rales) and wheezes may be heard in lung bases. An S_3 gallop may be present, reflecting the heart's attempts to fill an already distended ventricle.

In right-sided heart failure, increased pressures in the pulmonary vasculature or right ventricular muscle damage impair the right ventricle's ability to pump blood into the pulmonary circulation. The right ventricle and atrium become distended, and blood accumulates in the systemic venous system. Increased venous pressures cause abdominal organs to become congested and peripheral tissue edema to develop (Figure 32–2 ■).

Dependent tissues tend to be affected because of the effects of gravity; edema develops in the feet and legs, or if the client

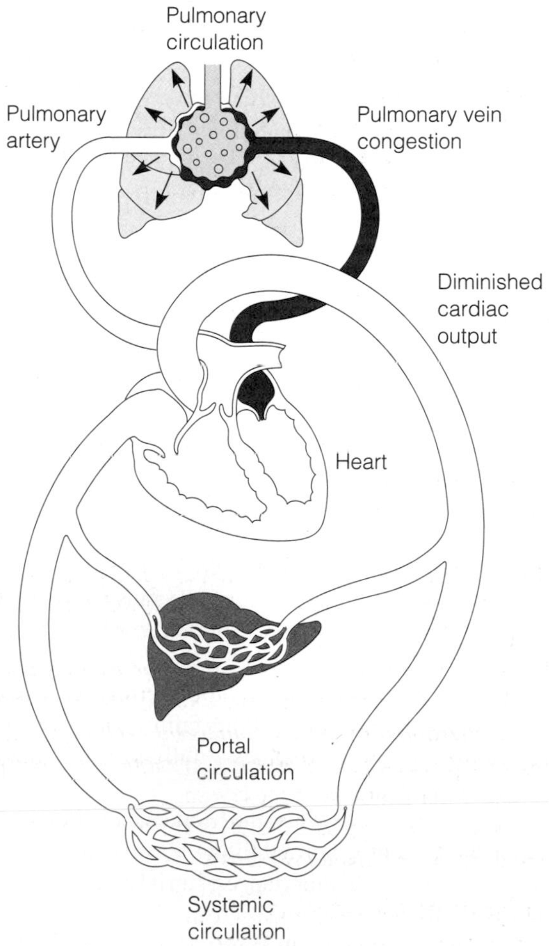

Pulmonary circulation

Pulmonary artery

Pulmonary vein congestion

Diminished cardiac output

Heart

Portal circulation

Systemic circulation

Figure 32–1 ■ The hemodynamic effects of left-sided heart failure.

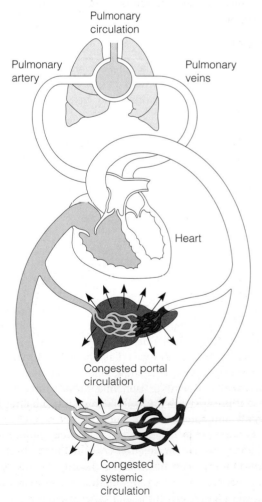

Pulmonary circulation

Pulmonary artery

Pulmonary veins

Heart

Congested portal circulation

Congested systemic circulation

Figure 32–2 ■ The hemodynamic effects of right-sided heart failure.

is bedridden, in the sacrum. Congestion of gastrointestinal tract vessels causes anorexia and nausea. Right upper quadrant pain may result from liver engorgement. Neck veins distend and become visible even when the client is upright, due to increased venous pressure.

Low-Output versus High-Output Failure

Clients with heart failure due to coronary heart disease, hypertension, cardiomyopathy, and other primary cardiac disorders develop *low-output failure* and manifestations such as those previously described. Clients in hypermetabolic states (e.g., hyperthyroidism, infection, anemia, or pregnancy) require increased cardiac output to maintain blood flow and oxygen to the tissues. If the increased blood flow cannot meet the oxygen demands of the tissues, compensatory mechanisms are activated to further increase cardiac output, which in turn further increases oxygen demand. Thus, even though cardiac output is high, the heart is unable to meet increased oxygen demands. This condition is known as *high-output failure*.

Acute versus Chronic Failure

Acute failure is the abrupt onset of a myocardial injury (such as a massive MI) resulting in suddenly decreased cardiac function and signs of decreased cardiac output. *Chronic failure* is a progressive deterioration of the heart muscle due to cardiomyopathies, valvular disease, or CHD.

Other Manifestations

In addition to the previous manifestations for the various classifications of heart failure, other signs and symptoms commonly are seen.

A fall in cardiac output activates mechanisms that cause increased salt and water retention. This causes weight gain and further increases pressures in the capillaries, resulting in edema. *Nocturia,* voiding more than one time at night, develops as edema fluid from dependent tissues is reabsorbed while the client is supine. **Paroxysmal nocturnal dyspnea (PND)**, a frightening condition in which the client awakens at night acutely short of breath, also may develop. Paroxysmal nocturnal dyspnea occurs when edema fluid that has accumulated during the day is reabsorbed into the circulation at night, causing fluid overload and pulmonary congestion. Severe heart failure may cause dyspnea at rest as well as with activity, signifying little or no cardiac reserve. Both an S_3 and an S_4 gallop may be heard on auscultation.

See page 1028 for the *Multisystem Effects of Heart Failure.*

Complications

The compensatory mechanisms initiated in heart failure can lead to complications in other body systems. Congestive hepatomegaly and splenomegaly caused by engorgement of the portal venous system result in increased abdominal pressure, ascites, and gastrointestinal problems. With prolonged right-sided heart failure, liver function may be impaired. Myocardial distention can precipitate dysrhythmias, further impairing cardiac output. Pleural effusions and other pulmonary problems may develop. Major complications of severe heart failure are cardiogenic shock (described in Chapter 11) and acute pulmonary edema, a medical emergency described in the next section of this chapter.

INTERDISCIPLINARY CARE

The main goals for care of heart failure are to slow its progression, reduce cardiac workload, improve cardiac function, and control fluid retention. Treatment strategies are based on the evolution and progression of heart failure (Table 32–3).

Diagnosis

Diagnosis of heart failure is based on the history, physical examination, and diagnostic findings.

- *Atrial natriuretic peptide (ANP),* also called *atrial natriuretic hormone (ANH),* and *brain natriuretic peptide (BNP)* are hormones released by the heart muscle in response to changes in blood volume. Blood levels of these hormones increase in heart failure. BNP levels, in particular, have been shown to positively correlate with pressures in the left ventricle and the pulmonary vascular system. As the severity of left ventricular failure increases, BNP levels increase (White, 2005). It is important to remember, however, that BNP levels may be elevated in women and in people over age 60 who do not have heart failure. Therefore, an elevated BNP cannot be used alone to diagnosis heart failure (Hunt et al., 2005).
- *Serum electrolytes* are measured to evaluate fluid and electrolyte status. Serum osmolarity may be low due to fluid retention. Sodium, potassium, and chloride levels provide a baseline for evaluating the effects of treatment; serum calcium and magnesium are measured as well.
- *Urinalysis, blood urea nitrogen (BUN),* and *serum creatinine* are obtained to evaluate renal function.
- *Liver function tests* including ALT, AST, LDH, serum bilirubin, and total protein and albumin levels are obtained to evaluate possible effects of heart failure on liver function.
- Thyroid function tests, including TSH and TH levels, are obtained because both hyperthyroidism and hypothyroidism can be either a primary or a contributing cause of heart failure (Hunt et al., 2005).
- In acute heart failure, *arterial blood gases (ABGs)* are drawn to evaluate gas exchange in the lungs and tissues.
- *Chest x-ray* may show pulmonary vascular congestion and cardiomegaly in heart failure.
- *Electrocardiography* is used to identify ECG changes associated with ventricular enlargement and to detect dysrhythmias, myocardial ischemia, or infarction.
- *Echocardiography with Doppler flow studies* are performed to evaluate left ventricular function. Either *transthoracic echocardiography* or *transesophageal echocardiography* may be used. See Chapter 30 for more information and the nursing implications of these tests.
- *Radionuclide imaging* is used to evaluate ventricular function and size (see Chapter 30).

Hemodynamic Monitoring

Hemodynamics is the study of forces involved in blood circulation. Hemodynamic monitoring is used to assess cardiovascular function in the critically ill or unstable client. The main

MULTISYSTEM EFFECTS OF **Heart Failure**

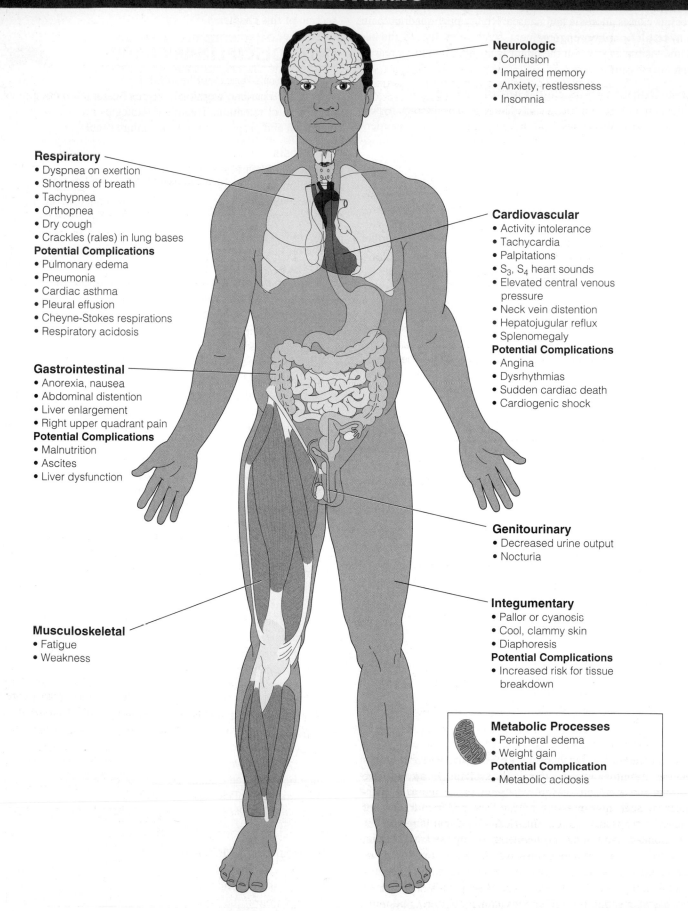

Neurologic
- Confusion
- Impaired memory
- Anxiety, restlessness
- Insomnia

Respiratory
- Dyspnea on exertion
- Shortness of breath
- Tachypnea
- Orthopnea
- Dry cough
- Crackles (rales) in lung bases

Potential Complications
- Pulmonary edema
- Pneumonia
- Cardiac asthma
- Pleural effusion
- Cheyne-Stokes respirations
- Respiratory acidosis

Cardiovascular
- Activity intolerance
- Tachycardia
- Palpitations
- S_3, S_4 heart sounds
- Elevated central venous pressure
- Neck vein distention
- Hepatojugular reflux
- Splenomegaly

Potential Complications
- Angina
- Dysrhythmias
- Sudden cardiac death
- Cardiogenic shock

Gastrointestinal
- Anorexia, nausea
- Abdominal distention
- Liver enlargement
- Right upper quadrant pain

Potential Complications
- Malnutrition
- Ascites
- Liver dysfunction

Genitourinary
- Decreased urine output
- Nocturia

Integumentary
- Pallor or cyanosis
- Cool, clammy skin
- Diaphoresis

Potential Complications
- Increased risk for tissue breakdown

Musculoskeletal
- Fatigue
- Weakness

Metabolic Processes
- Peripheral edema
- Weight gain

Potential Complication
- Metabolic acidosis

TABLE 32-3 Stages of Heart Failure

STAGE	DESCRIPTION	RECOMMENDED TREATMENT MEASURES
A	Clients at high risk for developing heart failure, but without structural heart disease or symptoms of heart failure (clients with hypertension, CHD, diabetes, obesity, metabolic syndrome, or who have a family history of cardiomyopathy, or who are taking cardiotoxic drugs)	Treat underlying risk factors (e.g., hypertension) including lipid disorders ACE inhibitor or angiotensin-receptor blocker (ARB) therapy as appropriate Exercise Salt restriction Smoking cessation Discourage alcohol, illicit drug use Control blood glucose in clients with metabolic syndrome
B	Clients with structural heart disease but no manifestations of heart failure (clients with previous MI, asymptomatic valve disease, or left ventricular dysfunction)	As for stage A ACE inhibitor or ARB therapy as appropriate Beta-blocker therapy if indicated
C	Clients with structural heart disease and current or prior symptoms of heart failure (shortness of breath, fatigue, decreased exercise tolerance)	As for stages A and B Drug therapy with a diuretic, ACE inhibitor, and/or beta-blocker Additional drugs as indicated, such as an aldosterone antagonist, ARB, digitalis, hydralazine, nitrates Ventricular pacing or an implantable defibrillator (ICD) as indicated
D	Refractory heart failure (clients with manifestations of heart failure at rest despite aggressive treatment)	As for stages A, B, and C as appropriate Hospice care Hemodynamic monitoring Continual infusion of positive inotropic agents Valve replacement, cardiac transplant as indicated Permanent mechanical support; experimental surgery or drug therapy

Source: Adapted from "ACC/AHA 2005 Guideline Update for the Diagnosis and Management of Chronic Heart Failure in the Adult: Executive Summary: A Report of the American College of Cardiology/American Heart Association Task Force on Practice Guidelines (Writing Committee to Update the 2001 Guidelines for the Evaluation and Management of Heart Failure)" by S. A. Hunt, W. T. Abraham, M. H. Chin, A. M. Feldman, G. S. Francis, T. G. Ganiats, M. Jessup, M. A. Konstam, D. M. Mancini, K. Michl, M. A. Silver, L. W. Stevenson, and C. W. Yancy, 2005, American College of Cardiology Web Site. Available at http://www.acc.org/clinical/guidlines/failure/index/pdf

goals of invasive hemodynamic monitoring are to evaluate cardiac and circulatory function and the response to interventions.

Hemodynamic parameters include heart rate, arterial blood pressure, central venous or right atrial pressure, pulmonary pressures, and cardiac output. *Direct* hemodynamic parameters are obtained straight from the monitoring device (e.g., heart rate, arterial and venous pressures). *Indirect* or *derived* measurements are calculated using the direct data (e.g., the cardiac index, mean arterial blood pressure, and stroke volume). Invasive hemodynamic monitoring is routinely used in critical care units.

Hemodynamic monitoring systems measure the pressure within a vessel and convert this signal into an electrical waveform that is amplified and displayed. The electrical signal may be graphically recorded on graph paper and displayed digitally on the monitor. System components include an invasive catheter threaded into an artery or vein connected to a transducer by stiff, high-pressure tubing. The pressure transducer translates pressures into an electrical signal that is relayed to the monitor. Additional components of the system include stopcocks and a continuous flush system with normal saline or heparinized saline and an infusion pressure bag to prevent clots from forming in the catheter. Figure 32–3 ■ illustrates a pressure transducer and typical hemodynamic monitoring system.

Hemodynamic pressure monitoring may be used to measure peripheral arterial pressures, or central pressures, such as central venous pressure or right atrial pressure and pulmonary artery pressure. Although the information obtained from invasive monitoring is valuable, the procedure is not without risk. Nursing care of the client undergoing hemodynamic monitoring is outlined on page 1031. Box 32–2 lists potential complications of central pressure monitoring.

INTRA-ARTERIAL PRESSURE MONITORING Intra-arterial pressure monitoring is commonly used in intensive and coronary care units. An indwelling arterial line, commonly called an *art line* or an *A line*, allows direct and continuous monitoring of systolic,

BOX 32-2 Potential Complications of Central Catheters

- Bleeding
- Hematoma
- Pneumothorax
- Hemothorax
- Arterial puncture
- Dysrhythmias
- Venospasm
- Infection
- Air embolism
- Thromboembolism
- Brachial nerve injury
- Thoracic duct injury

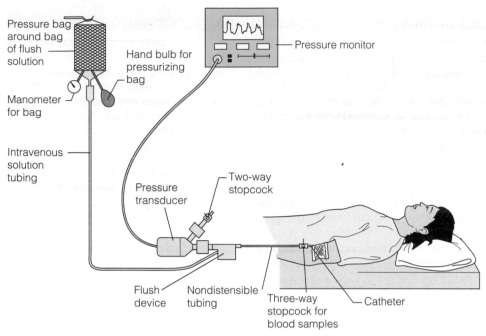

Figure 32–3 ■ A hemodynamic monitoring setup.

diastolic, and mean arterial blood pressure and provides easy access for arterial blood sampling. Arterial lines are used to assess blood volume, to monitor the effects of vasoactive drugs, and to obtain frequent ABG determinations. Because the invasive catheter is inserted directly into the artery, it offers immediate access for blood gas measurements and blood testing.

The arterial blood pressure reflects the cardiac output and the resistance to blood flow created by the elastic arterial walls (*systemic vascular resistance, SVR*). Cardiac output is determined by the blood volume and the ability of the ventricles to fill and effectively pump that blood. Systemic vascular resistance is primarily determined by vessel diameter and distensibility (compliance). Factors such as SNS input, circulating hormones (e.g., epinephrine, norepinephrine, ANP, and vasopressin), and the renin–angiotensin system affect SVR.

The systolic blood pressure, normally about 120 mmHg in healthy adults, reflects the pressure generated during ventricular systole. During diastole, elastic arterial walls keep a minimum pressure within the vessel (diastolic blood pressure) to maintain blood flow through the capillary beds. The average diastolic pressure in a healthy adult is 80 mmHg. The **mean arterial pressure (MAP)** is the average pressure in the arterial circulation throughout the cardiac cycle. It reflects the driving pressure, or perfusion pressure, an indicator of tissue perfusion. The formula MAP = CO × SVR often is used to show the relationships between factors determining the blood pressure. Mean arterial pressure can be calculated by adding one-third of the pulse pressure (PP) to the diastolic pressure (MAP = DBP + PP/3). For example, a blood pressure of 120/80 results in a MAP of 93. Mean arterial pressures of 70 to 90 mmHg are desirable. Perfusion to vital organs is severely jeopardized at MAPs of 50 or less; MAPs greater than 105 mmHg may indicate hypertension or vasoconstriction.

VENOUS PRESSURE MONITORING Central venous pressure (CVP) and *right atrial pressure (RAP)* are measures of blood volume and venous return. They also reflect right heart filling pressures. Pressures are elevated in right-sided heart failure. CVP and RAP are primarily used to monitor fluid volume status. To measure venous and atrial pressures, a catheter is inserted in the internal jugular or subclavian vein. The distal tip of the catheter is positioned in the superior vena cava just above or just inside the right atrium. CVP may be measured in either centimeters of water (cm H$_2$O) or in millimeters of mercury (mmHg). A water manometer is a clear tube with calibrated markings that is attached between a central catheter and the intravenous fluid bag. Pressure in the venous system causes fluid in the manometer to rise or fall. The CVP is recorded by noting the fluid level in the manometer. If the central line is connected to a pressure transducer, venous pressure is displayed digitally in millimeters of mercury.

The normal range for CVP is 2 to 8 cm H$_2$O or 2 to 6 mmHg, but CVP varies in individual clients. Hypovolemia and shock decrease the CVP; fluid overload, vasoconstriction, and cardiac tamponade increase CVP.

PULMONARY ARTERY PRESSURE MONITORING The pulmonary artery (PA) catheter is a flow-directed, balloon-tipped catheter first used in the early 1970s. The PA catheter is often called a *Swan-Ganz catheter,* after the physicians who developed it. The PA catheter is used to evaluate left ventricular and overall cardiac function. The PA catheter is inserted into a central vein, usually the internal jugular or subclavian vein, and threaded into the right atrium. A small balloon at the tip of the catheter allows the catheter to be drawn into the right ventricle and from there into the pulmonary artery (Figure 32–4 ■). The inflated balloon carries the catheter forward until the balloon wedges in a small branch of pulmonary vasculature. Once in

NURSING CARE OF THE CLIENT UNDERGOING   Hemodynamic Monitoring

- Calibrate and level the system at least once a shift using the right atrium as a constant reference level. Relevel the transducer after a change in position. Mark the right atrial position (at the fourth intercostal space, midaxillary line) on the chest wall, and use this as a reference point for all readings. *Calibration and leveling ensure that accurate pressures are recorded. Marking the right atrial level provides a consistent reference point for all caregivers.*
- Measure all pressures between breaths. *This ensures that intrathoracic pressure does not influence pressure readings.*
- Maintain 300 mmHg of pressure on the flush solution at all times. *This ensures a continuous flow of flush solution through the pressure tubing and catheter to prevent clot formation and catheter occlusion.*
- Monitor pressure trends rather than individual readings. *Individual readings may not reflect the client's true status. Trends in pressure readings along with clinical observations provide a better overall picture of the client's status.*
- Obtain a chest x-ray before infusing intravenous fluid into any newly placed central line. *Chest x-ray verifies the location of the catheter and helps prevent pulmonary complications of incorrect catheter placement such as pneumothorax.*
- Set alarm limits for monitored hemodynamic variables. Turn alarms on. *Alarms warn of hemodynamic instability. Always investigate alarms. They may be temporarily silenced to change tubing or draw blood but should never be turned off.*
- Use aseptic technique during catheter insertion and site care. *Aseptic technique is important to prevent infection.*
- Assess and document appearance of the insertion site at least every shift; observe for signs of infiltration, infection, or phlebitis. *Frequent assessment allows early detection and prompt treatment of complications.*
- Change intravenous solutions every 24 hours, site dressing every 48 hours, and tubing to the insertion site every 72 hours. Label solution, tubing, and dressing with date and time of change. *These measures help prevent infection.*
- Thoroughly flush stopcock ports after drawing blood samples from the pressure line. *Flushing prevents colonization of bacteria and occlusion of the catheter.*
- Assess pulse and perfusion distal to the monitoring site. *Frequent assessment is vital to ensure perfusion of the distal extremity.*
- When discontinuing the pressure line, apply manual pressure to the insertion site as soon as the catheter tip is out. Hold pressure for 5 to 15 minutes or until the bleeding stops. *This is particularly important for arterial lines to prevent bleeding and hematoma formation.*
- Secure all connections and stopcocks. *This is done to prevent disconnection of the invasive line and potential hemorrhage.*
- Ensure that electrical equipment is grounded, intact, and operating as expected. *This helps prevent electrical injury.*
- Loosely restrain the affected extremity if the client pulls on the catheter or connections. *Restraints may be necessary to prevent injury from accidental or intentional disconnection or discontinuation of invasive lines (i.e., if the client has dementia or is agitated).*
- Keep tubing free of kinks and tension. *This prevents the catheter from becoming clotted or inadvertently dislodged.*

---

place, the balloon is deflated, and multiple lumens of the catheter allow measurement of pressures in the right atrium, pulmonary artery, and left ventricle. The normal PA pressure is around 25/10 mmHg; normal mean pulmonary artery pressure is about 15 mmHg (Figure 32–5A ■). Pulmonary artery pressure is increased in left-sided heart failure.

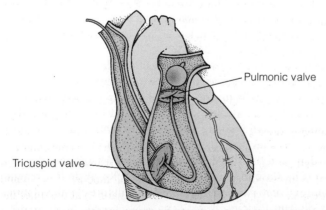

Figure 32–4 ■ Inflation of the balloon on the flow-directed catheter allows it to be carried through the pulmonic valve into the pulmonary artery.

Pulmonic valve

Tricuspid valve

Inflation of the balloon effectively blocks pressure from behind the balloon and allows measurement of pressures generated by the left ventricle. This is known as pulmonary artery wedge pressure (PAWP or PWP) and is used to assess left ventricular function. The normal PAWP is 8 to 12 mmHg (Figure 32–5B). PAWP is increased in left ventricular failure and pericardial tamponade, and decreased in hypovolemia.

Cardiac output also can be measured with the PA catheter using a technique called *thermodilution*. Cardiac output and the cardiac index are used to assess the heart's ability to meet the body's oxygen demands. Because body size affects overall cardiac output, the cardiac index is a more precise measure of heart function. The *cardiac index* is a calculation of cardiac output per square meter of body surface area. The normal cardiac index is 2.8 to 4.2 $L/min/m^2$.

Medications

Clients with heart failure often receive multiple medications to reduce cardiac work and improve cardiac function. The main drug classes used to treat heart failure are the angiotensin-converting enzyme (ACE) inhibitors, angiotensin II receptor blockers (ARBs), beta-blockers, diuretics, inotropic medications (including digitalis, sympathomimetic agents, and phosphodiesterase inhibitors), direct vasodilators, and antidysrhythmic drugs. Nursing implications for ACE inhibitors and ARBs,

Pulmonary Artery Pressure (PAP)

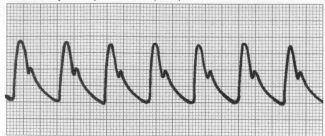

Pulmonary Capillary Wedge Pressure (PCWP)

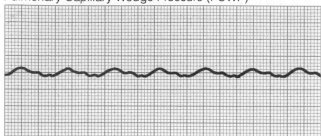

Figure 32–5 ■ Typical waveforms seen when measuring (*A*) pulmonary artery pressure and (*B*) pulmonary wedge pressure.

diuretics, and inotropic medications are found in the Medication Administration box on the following page.

ACE inhibitors, ARBs, and beta-blockers interfere with the neurohormonal mechanisms of sympathetic activation and the renin–angiotensin system. ACE inhibitors interrupt the conversion of angiotensin I to angiotensin II by inhibiting the enzyme that mediates the conversion (angiotensin-converting enzyme). Angiotensin II causes intense vasoconstriction, increasing afterload and ventricular wall stress and increasing preload and ventricular dilation. It also stimulates aldosterone and ADH production, causing fluid retention. ACE inhibitors block this renin–angiotensin system activity, decreasing cardiac work and increasing cardiac output. They reduce the progression and manifestations of heart failure, thus reducing the number and frequency of hospital admissions, decreasing mortality rates, and preventing cardiac complications (Kasper et al., 2005).

In contrast to ACE inhibitors, ARBs do not block the production of angiotensin II; instead, they block its action. The pharmacologic effect is similar, and they also are used in heart failure to slow its progression, reduce manifestations, and prevent cardiac complications.

Beta-blockers improve cardiac function in heart failure by inhibiting SNS activity. This prevents the long-term deleterious effects of sympathetic stimulation. Because beta-blockers reduce the force of myocardial contraction and may actually worsen symptoms, they are used in low doses. The combination of ACE inhibitors and beta-blockers improves client outcomes. Beta-blockers are discussed on pages 973–974.

Clients with symptomatic heart failure often are treated with diuretics as well. Diuretics relieve symptoms related to fluid retention. They may, however, cause significant electrolyte imbal-

ances and rapid fluid loss. Clients with severe heart failure are often treated with a loop, or high-ceiling, diuretic such as furosemide (Lasix), bumetanide (Bumex), torsemide (Demadex), or ethacrynic acid (Edecrin). These drugs have a rapid onset of action, inhibiting chloride reabsorption in the ascending loop of Henle, prompting sodium and water excretion. Their major drawback is their efficacy in promoting diuresis; loss of vascular volume can stimulate the SNS. Thiazide diuretics may be used for clients with less severe manifestations of heart failure. These agents promote fluid excretion by blocking sodium reabsorption in the terminal loop of Henle and the distal tubule.

Vasodilators relax smooth muscle in blood vessels, causing dilation. Arterial dilation reduces peripheral vascular resistance and afterload, reducing myocardial work. Venous dilation reduces venous return and preload. Pulmonary vascular relaxation reduces pulmonary capillary pressure, allowing reabsorption of fluid from interstitial tissues and the alveoli. Vasodilators include nitrates, hydralazine, and prazosin, an alpha-adrenergic blocker. See Chapter 35 ∞ for more information about vasodilators.

Nitrates produce both arterial and venous vasodilation. They may be given by nasal spray or the sublingual, oral, or intravenous route. Sodium nitroprusside is a potent vasodilator that may be used to treat acute heart failure. It can cause excessive hypotension, so it is often given along with dopamine or dobutamine to maintain the blood pressure. Isosorbide or nitroglycerin ointment may be used in long-term management of heart failure. See pages 973–974.

In 2005, the U.S. Food and Drug Administration (FDA) approved a new drug for treatment of heart failure in African Americans. This drug, known as BiDil, is a combination of two vasodilators, hydralazine and isosorbide, in fixed doses. In a study of African Americans with severe heart failure, BiDil improved symptoms and significantly reduced the number of hospitalizations and deaths attributed to heart failure (U.S. FDA, 2005). The Cultural Diversity box on page 1035 discusses the nursing implications for BiDil.

Digitalis glycosides are used judiciously in symptomatic heart failure. Digitalis has a *positive inotropic effect* on the heart, increasing the strength of myocardial contraction by increasing the intracellular calcium concentrations. Digitalis also decreases sinoatrial (SA) node automaticity and slows conduction through the atrioventricular (AV) node, increasing ventricular filling time.

Digitalis has a narrow therapeutic index; in other words, therapeutic levels are very close to toxic levels. Early manifestations of digitalis toxicity include anorexia, nausea and vomiting, headache, altered vision, and confusion. A number of cardiac dysrhythmias are also associated with digitalis toxicity, including sinus arrest, supraventricular and ventricular tachycardias, and high levels of AV block. Low serum potassium levels increase the risk of digitalis toxicity, as do low magnesium and high calcium levels. Older adults are at particular risk for digitalis toxicity.

Digitalis levels may be affected by a number of other drugs; check for potential interactions.

MEDICATION ADMINISTRATION Heart Failure

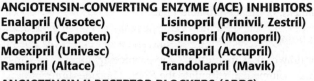

ANGIOTENSIN-CONVERTING ENZYME (ACE) INHIBITORS

Enalapril (Vasotec)	Lisinopril (Prinivil, Zestril)
Captopril (Capoten)	Fosinopril (Monopril)
Moexipril (Univasc)	Quinapril (Accupril)
Ramipril (Altace)	Trandolapril (Mavik)

ANGIOTENSIN II RECEPTOR BLOCKERS (ARBS)

Candesartan (Atacand)	Irbesartan (Avapro)
Losartan (Cozaar)	Telmisartan (Micardis)
Valsartan (Diovan)	

ACE inhibitors and ARBs prevent acute coronary events and reduce mortality in heart failure. ACE inhibitors interfere with production of angiotensin II, resulting in vasodilation, reduced blood volume, and prevention of its effects in the heart and blood vessels. In heart failure, ACE inhibitors reduce afterload and improve cardiac output and renal blood flow. They also reduce pulmonary congestion and peripheral edema. ACE inhibitors suppress myocyte growth and reduce ventricular remodeling in heart failure. While the pharmacologic effect of ARBs is similar, they block the action of angiotensin II at the receptor rather than interfering with its production.

Nursing Responsibilities

- Do not give these drugs to women in the second and third trimesters of pregnancy.
- Carefully monitor clients who are volume depleted or who have impaired renal function.
- Use an infusion pump when administering ACE inhibitors intravenously.
- Monitor blood pressure closely for 2 hours following first dose and as indicated thereafter.
- Monitor serum potassium levels; ACE inhibitors can cause hyperkalemia (this is less of a concern with ARBs).
- Monitor white blood cell (WBC) count for potential neutropenia. Report to the physician.

Health Education for the Client and Family

- Take the drug at the same time every day to ensure a stable blood level.
- Monitor your blood pressure and weight weekly. Report significant changes to your doctor.
- Avoid making sudden position changes; for example, rise from bed slowly. Lie down if you become dizzy or light-headed, particularly after the first dose.
- Report any signs of easy bruising and bleeding, sore throat or fever, edema, or skin rash. Immediately report swelling of the face, lips, or eyelids, and itching or breathing problems.
- A persistent, dry cough may develop if you are taking an ACE inhibitor. Contact your doctor if this becomes a problem.
- Take captopril or moexipril 1 hour before meals.

DIURETICS

Chlorothiazide (Diuril)	Spironolactone (Aldactone)
Furosemide (Lasix)	Triamterene (Dyrenium)
Ethacrynic acid (Edecrin)	Amiloride (Midamor)
Bumetanide (Bumex)	Acetazolamide (Diamox)
Hydrochlorothiazide (HydroDIURIL)	

Diuretics act on different portions of the kidney tubule to inhibit the reabsorption of sodium and water and promote their excretion. With the exception of the potassium-sparing diuretics—spironolactone, triamterene, and amiloride—diuretics also promote potassium excretion, increasing the risk of hypokalemia. Spironolactone, an al-

dosterone receptor blocker, reduces symptoms and slows progression of heart failure. Aldosterone receptors in the heart and blood vessels promote myocardial remodeling and fibrosis, activate the sympathetic nervous system, and promote vascular fibrosis (which decreases compliance) and baroreceptor dysfunction.

Nursing Responsibilities

- Obtain baseline weight and vital signs.
- Monitor blood pressure, intake and output, weight, skin turgor, and edema as indicators of fluid volume status.
- Assess for volume depletion, particularly with loop diuretics (furosemide, ethacrynic acid, and bumetanide): dizziness, orthostatic hypotension, tachycardia, muscle cramping.
- Report abnormal serum electrolyte levels to the physician. Replace electrolytes as indicated.
- Do not administer potassium replacements to clients receiving a potassium-sparing diuretic.
- Evaluate renal function by assessing urine output, BUN, and serum creatinine.
- Administer intravenous furosemide slowly, no faster than 20 mg/minute. Evaluate for signs of ototoxicity. Do not administer this drug or ethacrynic acid concurrently with aminoglycoside antibiotics (e.g., gentamicin), which are also ototoxic.

Health Education for the Client and Family

- Drink at least 6 to 8 glasses of water per day.
- Take your diuretic at times that will be the least disruptive to your lifestyle, usually in the morning and early afternoon If a second dose is ordered. Take with meals to decrease gastric upset.
- Monitor your blood pressure, pulse, and weight weekly. Report significant weight changes to your doctor.
- Report any of the following to your doctor: severe abdominal pain, jaundice, dark urine, abnormal bleeding or bruising, flu-like symptoms, signs of hypokalemia, hyponatremia, and dehydration (thirst, salt craving, dizziness, weakness, rapid pulse). See Chapter 10 ∞ for manifestations of electrolyte imbalances.
- Avoid sudden position changes. You may experience dizziness, light-headedness, or feelings of faintness.
- Unless you are taking a potassium-sparing diuretic, integrate foods rich in potassium into your diet (see Chapter 10 ∞). Limit sodium use.

POSITIVE INOTROPIC AGENTS

Digitalis Glycosides
Digoxin (Lanoxin)

Digitalis improves myocardial contractility by interfering with ATPase in the myocardial cell membrane and increasing the amount of calcium available for contraction. The increased force of contraction causes the heart to empty more completely, increasing stroke volume and cardiac output. Improved cardiac output improves renal perfusion, decreasing renin secretion. This decreases preload and afterload, reducing cardiac work. Digitalis also has electrophysiologic effects, slowing conduction through the AV node. This decreases the heart rate and reduces oxygen consumption.

Nursing Responsibilities

- Assess apical pulse before administering. Withhold digitalis and notify the physician if heart rate is below 60 bpm and/or

(continued)

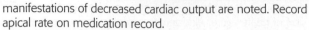

MEDICATION ADMINISTRATION Heart Failure (continued)

manifestations of decreased cardiac output are noted. Record apical rate on medication record.

- Evaluate ECG for scooped (spoon-shaped) ST segment, AV block, bradycardia, and other dysrhythmias (especially PVCs and atrial tachycardias).
- Report manifestations of digitalis toxicity: anorexia, nausea, vomiting, abdominal pain, weakness, vision changes (diplopia, blurred vision, yellow-green or white halos seen around objects), and new-onset dysrhythmias.
- Assess potassium, magnesium, calcium, and serum digoxin levels before giving digitalis. Hypokalemia can precipitate toxicity even when the serum digitalis level is in the "normal" range.
- Monitor clients with renal insufficiency or renal failure and older adults carefully for digitalis toxicity.
- Prepare to administer digoxin immune fab (Digibind) for digoxin toxicity.

Health Education for the Client and Family

- Take your pulse daily before taking your digoxin. Do not take the digoxin if your pulse is below 60 bpm or if you are weak, fatigued, light-headed, dizzy, short of breath, or having chest pain. Notify your physician immediately.
- Contact your doctor if you develop manifestations of digitalis toxicity: palpitations, weakness, loss of appetite, nausea, vomiting, abdominal pain, blurred or colored vision, double vision.
- Avoid using antacids and laxatives; they decrease digoxin absorption.
- Notify your physician immediately if you develop manifestations of potassium deficiency: weakness, lethargy, thirst, depression, muscle cramps, or vomiting.
- Incorporate foods high in potassium into your diet: fresh orange or tomato juice, bananas, raisins, dates, figs, prunes, apricots, spinach, cauliflower, and potatoes.

Sympathomimetic Agents
Dopamine (Inotropin)
Dobutamine (Dobutrex)

Sympathomimetic agents stimulate the heart, improving the force of contraction. Dobutamine is preferred in managing heart failure because it does not increase the heart rate as much as dopamine, and it has a mild vasodilatory effect. These drugs are given by intravenous infusion and may be titrated to obtain their optimal effects.

Phosphodiesterase Inhibitors
Amrinone (Inocor)
Milrinone (Primacor)

Phosphodiesterase inhibitors are used in treating acute heart failure to increase myocardial contractility and cause vasodilation. The net effects are an increase in cardiac output and a decrease in afterload.

Nursing Responsibilities

- Use an infusion pump to administer these agents. Monitor hemodynamic parameters carefully.
- Avoid discontinuing these drugs abruptly.
- Change solutions and tubing every 24 hours.
- Amrinone is given as an intravenous bolus over 2 to 3 minutes, followed by an infusion of 5 to 10 mg/kg/min.
- Amrinone may be infused full strength or diluted in normal saline or half-strength saline. Do not mix this drug with dextrose solutions. After dilution, amrinone can be piggybacked into a line containing a dextrose solution.
- Monitor liver function and platelet counts; amrinone may cause hepatotoxicity and thrombocytopenia.

Health Education for the Client and Family

- Notify the nursing staff if you experience abdominal pain or notice a skin rash or bruising.

Dysrhythmias are common in clients with heart failure. Although premature ventricular contractions (PVCs) may be frequent, they are often not associated with an increased risk of ventricular tachycardia and fibrillation. Because many antidysrhythmic medications depress left ventricular function, PVCs are frequently left untreated in heart failure. Amiodarone is the drug of choice to treat nonsustained ventricular tachycardia, which is associated with a poor prognosis. See page 1006.

Nutrition and Activity

A sodium-restricted diet is recommended to minimize sodium and water retention. Intake is generally limited to 1.5 to 2 g of sodium per day, a moderate restriction. Box 10–4 lists high-sodium foods to avoid; Box 10–5 includes client teaching regarding sodium-restricted diet.

Exercise intolerance, decreased ability to participate in activities using large skeletal muscles due to fatigue or dyspnea, is a common early manifestation of heart failure. Activity may be restricted to bed rest during acute episodes of heart failure to reduce cardiac workload and allow the heart to recompen-

sate. Prolonged bed rest and continued activity limitations, however, are not recommended. A moderate, progressive activity program is prescribed to improve myocardial function. Exercise should be performed 3 to 5 days per week, and each session should include a 10- to 15-minute warm-up period, 20 to 30 minutes of exercise at the recommended intensity, and a cool-down period. Walking is encouraged on nontraining days (Piña et al., 2003).

Other Treatments

In end-stage heart failure, devices to provide circulatory assistance or surgery may be required. Surgery may be used to treat the underlying cause of failure (e.g., replacement of diseased valves) or to improve quality of life. Valve replacement is discussed later in this chapter. Heart transplant is currently the only clearly effective surgical treatment for end-stage heart failure; its use is limited by the availability of donor hearts.

CIRCULATORY ASSISTANCE Devices such as the intra-aortic balloon pump or a left-ventricular assist device may be used when the client is expected to recover or as a bridge to trans-

FOCUS ON CULTURAL DIVERSITY BiDil for Treating Heart Failure in African Americans

BiDil, a fixed-dose combination of two vasodilators (hydralazine and isosorbide), is indicated as an adjunctive treatment in African Americans with heart failure. It has been shown to reduce symptoms, decrease the number of hospitalizations, and prolong life in blacks. The recommended dose is 1 to 2 tablets three times per day, although the dose may be as low as 1/2 tablet three times a day if side effects are intolerable.

Nursing Implications
- Assess vital signs and fluid volume status before administering this drug, because hypotension (orthostatic hypotension in particular) is a common effect.
- Notify the physician if manifestations of systemic lupus erythematosus, glomerulonephritis, or peripheral neuropathy develop.
- Use caution when administering concurrently with monoamine oxidase inhibitors.
- Closely monitor for hypotension when administered concurrently with any potent parenteral antihypertensive agent.

Health Education for the Client and Family
- Take this drug as prescribed.
- Headache is a common adverse effect of this drug, particularly when first starting therapy. Headaches tend to subside with continued treatment.
- Notify your doctor if headaches continue after the first few weeks of therapy, or if you develop chest pain or palpitations while taking this drug.
- This drug can cause a drop in blood pressure, particularly when changing positions from lying to sitting or sitting to standing. Change positions slowly and use caution to prevent falls.
- Do not use drugs such as sildenafil (Viagra, Revatio), vardenafil (Levitra), or tadalafil (Cialis) while taking this medication because the combination may cause an extreme drop in blood pressure leading to fainting, chest pain, or a heart attack.

plant. (See Chapter 31∞.) Newer devices that will allow longer term support outside the hospital are in the developmental stages. These devices will serve either as a bridge to transplant or allow the myocardium to heal over an extended period of time.

CARDIAC TRANSPLANTATION Heart transplant is the treatment of choice for end-stage heart disease. Survival rates are good: 83% at 1 year and 76% at 3 years. More than 90% of clients return to normal, unrestricted functional abilities following transplant (Kasper et al., 2005). The most frequently used transplant procedure leaves posterior walls of the atria, the superior and inferior venae cavae, and pulmonary veins of the recipient intact (Figure 32–6A ■). The atrial walls of the donor heart are then anastomosed to the recipient's atria (Figure 32–6B). The donor pulmonary artery and aorta are anastomosed to the recipient vessels (Figure 32–6C). Care is taken to avoid damaging the sinus node of the donor heart and to ensure integrity of the suture line to prevent postoperative bleeding. Donor organs typically

are obtained from young accident victims with no evidence of cardiac trauma.

Nursing care of the heart transplant client is similar to care of any cardiac surgery client (see pages 980–982). Bleeding is a major concern in the early postoperative period. Chest tube drainage is frequently monitored (initially every 15 minutes), as are the cardiac output, pulmonary artery pressures, and CVP. Cardiac tamponade (compression of the heart) can develop, presenting as either a sudden event or a gradual process. Chest tubes are gently milked (not stripped) as needed to maintain patency. Atrial dysrhythmias are relatively common following cardiac transplant. Temporary pacing wires are placed during surgery as the conduction system may be disrupted by surgical manipulation or postoperative swelling. Hypothermia is induced during surgery; postoperatively, the client is gradually rewarmed over a 1- to 2-hour period. Prevention of rapid rewarming and shivering are important to maintain hemodynamic stability and reduce oxygen consumption. Cardiac function is impaired in up to 50% of transplanted hearts during

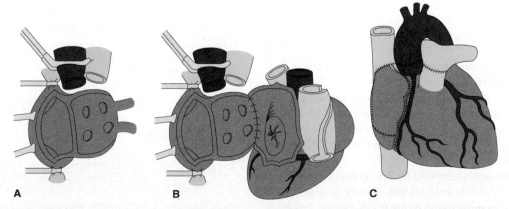

A   **B**   **C**

Figure 32–6 ■ Cardiac transplantation. *A,* The heart is removed, leaving the posterior walls of the atria intact. The donor heart is anastomosed to the atria, *B,* and the great vessels, *C.*

the early postoperative period. Inotropic agents such as low-dose dopamine, dobutamine, or milrinone may be required to support cardiac function and circulation (Wade et al., 2004).

Infection and rejection are major postoperative concerns; these are the chief causes of mortality in transplant clients. Rejection may develop immediately after transplant (a rare occurence), within weeks to months, or years after the transplant. Acute rejection usually presents within weeks of the transplant, developing when the transplanted organ is recognized by the immune system as foreign. Lymphocytes infiltrate the organ, and myocardial cell necrosis can be detected on biopsy. Acute rejection often can be treated using immunosuppressive drugs (Wade et al., 2004). These drugs also are given to prevent rejection of the transplanted organ, even when the tissue match is good (see Chapter 13 ∞). Although immunosuppressive medications help prevent organ rejection, they impair the client's defenses against infection. Early postoperative infections commonly are bacterial or fungal (*candida*). Multiple invasive lines, prolonged ventilator support, and immunosuppressive therapy contribute to the transplant recipient's risk for infection. Aggressive nursing care directed at prevention of infection is vital: limiting visitors with communicable diseases, pulmonary hygiene measures, early ambulation, and strict aseptic technique (Wade et al., 2004).

The donor heart is denervated during the transplant procedure. Lack of innervation by the autonomic nervous system affects the heart rate (usually between 90 and 110 bpm in transplanted hearts), its response to position changes, stress, exercise, and certain drugs.

OTHER PROCEDURES Other surgical procedures such as cardiomyoplasty and ventricular reduction surgery do not improve the prognosis or quality of life in clients with end-stage heart failure. *Cardiomyoplasty* involves wrapping the latissimus dorsi muscle around the heart to support the failing myocardium. The muscle is stimulated in synchrony with the heart, providing a more forceful contraction and increasing cardiac output. In ventricular reduction surgery (or *partial ventriculectomy*), a portion of the anterolateral left ventricular wall is resected to improve cardiac function (Tierney et al., 2005).

Complementary Therapies

Strong evidence supports the use of several complementary therapies for heart failure. Hawthorn, a shrubby tree, contains natural cardiotonic ingredients in its blossoms, leaves, and fruit. It increases the force of myocardial contraction, dilates blood vessels, and has a natural ACE inhibitor. Hawthorn should never be used without consulting an experienced herb practitioner and advising the physician (Fontaine, 2005). Nutritional supplements of coenzyme Q10, magnesium, and thiamine may be used in conjunction with other treatments. Coenzyme Q10 improves mitochondria function and energy production.

End-of-Life Care

Unless a cardiac transplant is performed, chronic heart failure is ultimately a terminal disease. The client and family need honest discussions about the anticipated course of the disease and treatment options. It is important to discuss advance directives such as the living will and medical power of attorney, differentiating

potential acute events from which recovery would be anticipated (e.g., reversible exacerbation of heart failure, sudden cardiac arrest) from prolonged life support without reasonable expectation of functional recovery. Hospice services are available for clients with heart failure, and should be offered when appropriate. Severe dyspnea is common in the final stages of the disease. It may be managed with narcotic analgesics or with frequent intravenous diuretics and continuous infusion of a positive inotropic agent (Hunt et al., 2005).

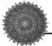 **NURSING CARE**

Health Promotion

Health promotion activities to reduce the risk for and incidence of heart failure are directed at the risk factors. Teach clients about coronary heart disease, the primary underlying cause of heart failure. Discuss CHD risk factors and ways to reduce those risk factors (see Chapter 31 ∞).

Hypertension also is a major cause of heart failure. Routinely screen clients for elevated blood pressure, and refer clients to a primary care provider as indicated. Discuss the importance of effectively managing hypertension to reduce the future risk for heart failure. Likewise, stress the relationship between effective diabetes management and reduced risk of heart failure.

Assessment

Obtain both subjective and objective data when assessing the client with heart failure:

- *Health history:* Complaints of increasing shortness of breath, dyspnea with exertion, decreasing activity tolerance, or paroxysmal nocturnal dyspnea; number of pillows used for sleeping; recent weight gain; presence of a cough; chest or abdominal pain; anorexia or nausea; history of cardiac disease, previous episodes of heart failure; other risk factors such as hypertension or diabetes; current medications; usual diet and activity and recent changes.
- *Physical examination:* General appearance; ease of breathing, conversing, changing positions; apparent anxiety; vital signs including apical pulse; color of skin and mucous membranes; neck vein distention, peripheral pulses, capillary refill, presence and degree of edema; heart and breath sounds; abdominal contour, bowel sounds, tenderness; right upper abdominal tenderness, liver enlargement.
- *Diagnostic tests:* BNP, serum electrolyte, BUN, creatinine, and digitalis levels; ABG results; ECG, echocardiogram, and chest x-ray reports.

Nursing Diagnoses and Interventions

Heart failure impacts quality of life, interfering with such daily activities as self-care and role performance. Reducing the oxygen demand of the heart is a major nursing care goal for the client in acute heart failure. This includes providing rest and carrying out prescribed treatment measures to reduce cardiac work, improve contractility, and manage symptoms. See also the accompanying Nursing Care Plan for additional nursing diagnoses and interventions for the client with heart failure.

NURSING CARE PLAN   A Client with Heart Failure

One year ago, Arthur Jackson, 67 years old, had a large anterior wall MI and underwent subsequent coronary artery bypass surgery. On discharge, he was started on a regimen of enalapril (Vasotec), digoxin, furosemide (Lasix), warfarin (Coumadin), and a potassium chloride supplement. He is now in the cardiac unit complaining of severe shortness of breath, hemoptysis, and poor appetite for 1 week. He is diagnosed with acute heart failure.

ASSESSMENT

Mr. Jackson refuses to settle in bed, preferring to sit in the bedside recliner in high Fowler's position. He states, "Lately, this is the only way I can breathe." Mr. Jackson states that he has not been able to work in his garden without getting short of breath. He complains of his shoes and belt being too tight.

When Ms. Takashi, RN, Mr. Jackson's nurse, obtains his nursing history, Mr. Jackson insists that he takes his medications regularly. He states that he normally works in his garden for light exercise. In his diet history, Mr. Jackson admits fondness for bacon and Chinese food and sheepishly admits to snacking between meals "even though I need to lose weight."

Mr. Jackson's vital signs are: BP 95/72 mmHg, HR 124 and irregular, R 28 and labored, and T 97.5°F (36.5°C). The cardiac monitor shows atrial fibrillation. An S_3 is noted on auscultation; the cardiac impulse is left of the midclavicular line. He has crackles and diminished breath sounds in the bases of both lungs. Significant jugular venous distention, 3+ pitting edema of feet and ankles, and abdominal distention are noted. Liver size is within normal limits by percussion. Skin cool and diaphoretic. Chest x-ray shows cardiomegaly and pulmonary infiltrates.

DIAGNOSES

- *Excess Fluid Volume* related to impaired cardiac pump and salt and water retention
- *Activity Intolerance* related to impaired cardiac output
- *Impaired Health Maintenance* related to lack of knowledge about diet restrictions

EXPECTED OUTCOMES

- Demonstrate loss of excess fluid by weight loss and decreases in edema, jugular venous distention, and abdominal distention.
- Demonstrate improved activity tolerance.
- Verbalize understanding of diet restrictions.

PLANNING AND IMPLEMENTATION

- Hourly vital signs and hemodynamic pressure measurements.
- Administer and monitor effects of prescribed diuretics and vasodilators.
- Weigh daily; strict intake and output.
- Enforce fluid restriction of 1500 mL/24 hours: 600 mL day shift, 600 mL evening shift, 300 mL at night.

- Auscultate heart and breath sounds every 4 hours and as indicated.
- Administer oxygen per nasal cannula at 2 L/min. Monitor oxygen saturation continuously. Notify physician if less than 94%.
- High Fowler's or position of comfort.
- Notify physician of significant changes in laboratory values.
- Teach about all medications and how to take and record pulse. Provide information about anticoagulant therapy and signs of bleeding.
- Design an activity plan with Mr. Jackson that incorporates preferred activities and scheduled rest periods.
- Instruct about sodium-restricted diet. Allow meal choices within allowed limits.
- Consult dietitian for planning and teaching Mr. and Mrs. Jackson about low-sodium diet.

EVALUATION

Mr. Jackson is discharged after 3 days in the cardiac unit. He has lost 8 pounds during his stay and states it is much easier to breathe and his shoes fit better. He is able to sleep in semi-Fowler's position with only one pillow. His peripheral edema has resolved. Mr. and Mrs. Jackson met with the dietitian, who helped them develop a realistic eating plan to limit sodium, sugar, and fats. The dietitian also provided a list of high-sodium foods to avoid. Mr. Jackson is relieved to know that he can still enjoy Chinese food prepared without monosodium glutamate (MSG) or added salt. Ms. Takashi and the physical therapist designed a progressive activity plan with Mr. Jackson that he will continue at home. He remains in atrial fibrillation, a chronic condition. His knowledge of digoxin and Coumadin has been assessed and reinforced. Ms. Takashi confirms that he is able to accurately check his pulse and can list signs of digoxin toxicity and excessive bleeding.

CRITICAL THINKING IN THE NURSING PROCESS

1. Mr. Jackson's medication regimen remains the same after discharge. What specific teaching does he need related to potential interactions of these drugs?
2. Mr. Jackson tells you, "Talk to my wife about my medications—she's Tarzan and I'm Jane now." How would you respond?
3. Design an exercise plan for Mr. Jackson to prevent deconditioning and conserve energy.
4. Mr. Jackson tells you, "Sometimes I forget whether I have taken my aspirin, so I'll take another just to be sure. After all, they are only baby aspirin. One or two extra a day shouldn't hurt, right?" What is your response?
5. Mr. Jackson is admitted to the neuro unit 6 months later with a cerebral vascular accident (CVA). What is the probable cause of his stroke?

See Evaluating Your Response in Appendix C.

Decreased Cardiac Output

As the heart fails as a pump, stroke volume and tissue perfusion decrease.

- Monitor vital signs and oxygen saturation as indicated. *Decreased cardiac output stimulates the SNS to increase the heart rate in an attempt to restore CO. Tachycardia at rest is*

common. Diastolic blood pressure may initially be elevated because of vasoconstriction; in late stages, compensatory mechanisms fail, and BP falls. Oxygen saturation levels provide a measure of gas exchange and tissue perfusion.

- Monitor BNP levels, reporting trends. *BNP levels indicate the severity of heart failure: as the cardiac index decreases* and left ventricular pressures increase, BNP levels increase. Noting trends provides additional information about cardiac output and effectiveness of the cardiac pump.

■ Auscultate heart and breath sounds regularly. S_1 and S_2 may be diminished if cardiac function is poor. A ventricular gallop (S_3) is an early sign of heart failure; atrial gallop (S_4) may also be present. Crackles are often heard in the lung bases; increasing crackles, dyspnea, and shortness of breath indicate worsening failure.

PRACTICE ALERT

Report manifestations of decreased cardiac output and tissue perfusion: changes in mentation; decreased urine output; cool, clammy skin; diminished pulses; pallor or cyanosis; dysrhythmias. These are manifestations of decreased tissue perfusion to organ systems.

■ Administer supplemental oxygen as needed. *This improves oxygenation of the blood, decreasing the effects of hypoxia and ischemia.*

■ Administer prescribed medications as ordered. *Drugs are used to decrease the cardiac workload and increase the effectiveness of contractions.*

■ Encourage rest, explaining the rationale. Elevate the head of the bed to reduce the work of breathing. Provide a bedside commode, and assist with activities of daily living (ADLs). Instruct to avoid the Valsalva maneuver. *These measures reduce cardiac workload.*

PRACTICE ALERT

Promote psychologic rest and decrease anxiety. Maintain a quiet environment, and encourage expression of fears and feelings. Explain care measures and their purpose. Psychologic rest decreases oxygen consumption and improves cardiac function.

Excess Fluid Volume

As cardiac output falls, compensatory mechanisms cause salt and water retention, increasing blood volume. This increased fluid volume places additional stress on the already failing ventricles, making them work harder to move the fluid load.

■ Assess respiratory status and auscultate lung sounds at least every 4 hours. Notify the physician of significant changes in condition. *Declining respiratory status indicates worsening left heart failure.*

PRACTICE ALERT

Immediately notify the physician if the client develops air hunger, an overwhelming sense of impending doom or panic, tachypnea, severe orthopnea, or a cough productive of large amounts of pink, frothy sputum. Acute pulmonary edema, a medical emergency, can develop rapidly, necessitating immediate intervention to preserve life.

■ Monitor intake and output. Notify the physician if urine output is less than 30 mL/h. Weigh daily. *Careful monitoring of fluid volume is important during treatment of heart failure. Diuretics may reduce circulating volume, producing hypo-*

volemia despite persistent peripheral edema. *A fall in urine output may indicate significantly reduced cardiac output and renal ischemia. Weight is an objective measure of fluid status: 1 L of fluid is equal to 2.2 lb of weight.*

■ Record abdominal girth every shift. Note complaints of a loss of appetite, abdominal discomfort, or nausea. *Venous congestion can lead to ascites and may affect gastrointestinal function and nutritional status.*

■ Monitor and record hemodynamic measurements. Report significant changes and negative trends. *Hemodynamic measurements provide a means of monitoring condition and response to treatment.*

■ Restrict fluids as ordered. Allow choices of fluid type and timing of intake, scheduling most fluid intake during morning and afternoon hours. Offer ice chips and frequent mouth care; provide hard candies if allowed. *Providing choices increases the client's sense of control. Ice chips, hard candies, and mouth care relieve dry mouth and thirst and promote comfort.*

Activity Intolerance

Clients with heart failure have little or no cardiac reserve to meet increased oxygen demands. As the disease progresses and cardiac function is further compromised, activity intolerance increases. The low cardiac output and inability to participate in activities may hinder self-care.

PRACTICE ALERT

Monitor vital signs and cardiac rhythm during and after activities. Tachycardia, dysrhythmias, increasing dyspnea, changes in blood pressure, diaphoresis, pallor, complaints of chest pain, excessive fatigue, or palpitations indicate activity intolerance. Instruct to rest if manifestations are noted. The failing heart is unable to increase cardiac output to meet increased oxygen demands associated with activity. Assessing response to activities helps evaluate cardiac function. Decreasing activity tolerance may signal deterioration of cardiac function, not overexertion.

■ Organize nursing care to allow rest periods. *Grouping activities together allows adequate time to "recharge."*

■ Assist with ADLs as needed. Encourage independence within prescribed limits. *Assisting with ADLs helps ensure that care needs are met while reducing cardiac workload. Involving the client promotes a sense of control and reduces helplessness.*

■ Plan and implement progressive activities. Use passive and active range-of-motion (ROM) exercises as appropriate. Consult with physical therapist on activity plan. *Progressive activity slowly increases exercise capacity by strengthening and improving cardiac function without strain. Activity also helps prevent skeletal muscle atrophy. ROM exercises prevent complications of immobility in severely compromised clients.*

■ Provide written and verbal information about activity after discharge. *Written information provides a reference for important information. Verbal information allows clarification and validation of the material.*

Deficient Knowledge: Low-Sodium Diet

Diet is an important part of long-term management of heart failure to manage fluid retention.

- Discuss the rationale for sodium restrictions. *Understanding fosters compliance with the prescribed diet.*
- Consult with dietitian to plan and teach a low-sodium and, if necessary for weight control, low-kilocalorie diet. Provide a list of high-sodium, high-fat, high-cholesterol foods to avoid. Provide American Heart Association materials. *Dietary planning and teaching increase the client's sense of control and participation in disease management. Food lists are useful memory aids.*

PRACTICE ALERT
Teach how to read food labels for nutritional information. Many processed foods contain "hidden" sodium, which can be identified by careful label reading.

- Assist the client to construct a 2-day meal plan choosing foods low in sodium. *This allows learning assessment, clarification of misunderstandings, and reinforcement of teaching.*
- Encourage small, frequent meals rather than three heavy meals per day. *Small, frequent meals provide continuing energy resources and decrease the work required to digest a large meal.*

NANDA, NIC, and NOC Linkages

Chart 32–1 shows links between NANDA nursing diagnoses, NIC, and NOC for the client with heart failure.

Community-Based Care

Heart failure is a chronic condition requiring active participation by the client and family for effective management. In teaching for home care, include the following topics:

- The disease process and its effects on the client's life
- Warning signals of cardiac decompensation that require treatment
- Desired and adverse effects of prescribed drugs; monitoring for effects; importance of compliance with drug regimen to prevent acute and long-term complications of heart failure
- Prescribed diet and sodium restriction; practical suggestions for reducing salt intake; recommend American Heart Association materials and recipes
- Exercise recommendations to strengthen the heart muscle and improve aerobic capacity (Box 32–3)
- The importance of keeping scheduled follow-up appointments to monitor disease progression and effects of therapy.

Provide referrals for home health care and household assistance (shopping, transportation, personal needs, and housekeeping) as indicated. Referrals to community agencies, such as local cardiac rehabilitation programs, heart support groups, or the AHA, can provide the client and family with additional materials and psychosocial support.

THE CLIENT WITH PULMONARY EDEMA

Pulmonary edema is an abnormal accumulation of fluid in the interstitial tissue and alveoli of the lung. Both cardiac and noncardiac disorders can cause pulmonary edema. Cardiac causes

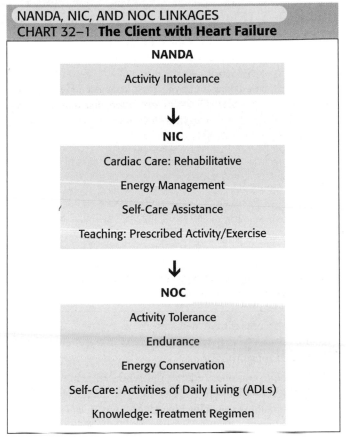

NANDA, NIC, AND NOC LINKAGES
CHART 32–1 **The Client with Heart Failure**

NANDA

Activity Intolerance

↓

NIC

Cardiac Care: Rehabilitative

Energy Management

Self-Care Assistance

Teaching: Prescribed Activity/Exercise

↓

NOC

Activity Tolerance

Endurance

Energy Conservation

Self-Care: Activities of Daily Living (ADLs)

Knowledge: Treatment Regimen

Data from *NANDA's Nursing Diagnoses: Definitions & Classification 2005–2006* by NANDA International (2005), Philadelphia; *Nursing Interventions Classification (NIC)* (4th ed.) by J. M. Dochterman & G. M. Bulechek (2004), St. Louis, MO: Mosby; and *Nursing Outcomes Classification (NOC)* (3rd ed.) by S. Moorhead, M. Johnson, and M. Maas (2004), St. Louis, MO: Mosby.

include acute myocardial infarction, acute heart failure, and valvular disease. *Cardiogenic pulmonary edema,* the focus of this section, is a sign of severe cardiac decompensation. Noncardiac causes of pulmonary edema include primary pulmonary disorders, such as acute respiratory distress syndrome (ARDS), trauma, sepsis, drug overdose, or neurologic sequelae. Pulmonary edema due to ARDS is discussed in Chapter 39 ∞.

FAST FACTS
- Cardiogenic pulmonary edema is a severe form of heart failure. Risk factors are those associated with heart failure, and treatment focuses on maintaining oxygenation and improving cardiac function.
- Noncardiogenic pulmonary edema is a primary or secondary lung disorder. It usually occurs secondarily to a critical event such as major trauma, shock, or disseminated intravascular coagulation (DIC). Treatment focuses on maintaining oxygenation and the primary, underlying disorder.

Pulmonary edema is a medical emergency: The client is literally drowning in the fluid in the alveolar and interstitial pulmonary spaces. Its onset may be acute or gradual, progressing to severe respiratory distress. Immediate treatment is necessary.

BOX 32–3 Home Activity Guidelines for the Client with Heart Failure

- Perform as many activities as independently as you can.
- Space your meals and activities.
  a. Eat six small meals a day.
  b. Allow time during the day for periods of rest and relaxation.
- Perform all activities at a comfortable pace.
  a. If you get tired during any activity, stop what you are doing and rest for 15 minutes.
  b. Resume activity only if you feel up to it.
- Stop any activity that causes chest pain, shortness of breath, dizziness, faintness, excessive weakness, or sweating. Rest. Notify your physician if your activity tolerance changes and if symptoms continue after rest.
- Avoid straining. Do not lift heavy objects. Eat a high-fiber diet and drink plenty of water to prevent constipation. Use laxatives or stool softeners, as approved by your physician, to avoid constipation and straining during bowel movements.
- Begin a graded exercise program. Walking is good exercise that does not require any special equipment (except a good pair of

walking shoes). Plan to walk twice a day at a comfortable, slow pace for the first couple of weeks at home, and then gradually increase the distance and pace. Below is a suggested schedule—but progress at your own speed. Take your time. Aim for walking at least 3 times per week (every other day).

Week 1	200 to 400 ft	Twice a day, slow leisurely pace
Week 2	1/4 mile	15 min, minimum of 3 times per week
Weeks 2 to 3	1/2 mile	30 min, minimum of 3 times per week
Weeks 3 to 4	1 mile	30 min, minimum of 3 times per week
Weeks 4 to 5	1 1/2 mile	30 min, minimum of 3 times per week
Weeks 5 to 6	2 miles	40 min, minimum of 3 times per week

Pathophysiology

In cardiogenic pulmonary edema, the contractility of the left ventricle is severely impaired. The ejection fraction falls because the ventricle is unable to eject the blood that enters it, causing a sharp rise in end-diastolic volume and pressure. Pulmonary hydrostatic pressures rise, ultimately exceeding the osmotic pressure of the blood. As a result, fluid leaking from the pulmonary capillaries congests interstitial tissues, decreasing lung compliance and interfering with gas exchange. As capillary and interstitial pressures increase further, the tight junctions of the alveolar walls are disrupted, and the fluid enters the alveoli, along with large red blood cells (RBCs) and protein molecules. Ventilation and gas exchange are severely disrupted, and hypoxia worsens.

Manifestations

The client with acute pulmonary edema presents with classic manifestations (see box below). Dyspnea, shortness of breath, and labored respirations are acute and severe, accompanied by orthopnea (inability to breathe when lying down). Cyanosis is present, and the skin is cool, clammy, and diaphoretic. A productive cough with pink, frothy sputum develops due to fluid, RBCs, and plasma proteins in the alveoli and airways. Crackles are heard throughout the lung fields on auscultation. As the condition worsens, lung sounds become harsher. The client often is restless and highly anxious, although severe hypoxia may cause confusion or lethargy.

As noted earlier, pulmonary edema is a medical emergency. Without rapid and effective intervention, severe tissue hypoxia and acidosis will lead to organ system failure and death.

INTERDISCIPLINARY CARE

Immediate treatment for acute pulmonary edema focuses on restoring effective gas exchange and reducing fluid and pressure in the pulmonary vascular system. The client is placed in an upright sitting position with the legs dangling to reduce venous return by trapping some excess fluid in the lower extremities. This position also facilitates breathing.

Diagnostic testing is limited to assessment of the acute situation. *ABGs* are drawn to assess gas exchange and acid–base balance. Oxygen tension (PaO_2) is usually low. Initially, carbon dioxide levels ($PaCO_2$) may also be reduced because of rapid respirations. As the condition progresses, the $PaCO_2$ rises and respiratory acidosis develops (see Chapter 10 ∞). *Oxygen saturation* levels also are continuously monitored. The *chest x-ray* shows pulmonary vascular congestion and alveolar edema. Provided the client's condition allows, *hemodynamic monitoring* is instituted. In cardiogenic pulmonary edema, the PAWP is elevated, usually over 25 mmHg. Cardiac output may be decreased.

Morphine is administered intravenously to relieve anxiety and improve the efficacy of breathing. It also is a vasodilator that reduces venous return and lowers left atrial pressure. Although morphine is very effective for clients with cardiogenic

MANIFESTATIONS of Pulmonary Edema

RESPIRATORY
- Tachypnea
- Labored respirations
- Dyspnea
- Orthopnea
- Paroxysmal nocturnal dyspnea
- Cough productive of frothy, pink sputum
- Crackles, wheezes

CARDIOVASCULAR
- Tachycardia
- Hypotension
- Cyanosis
- Cool, clammy skin
- Hypoxemia
- Ventricular gallop

NEUROLOGIC
- Restlessness
- Anxiety
- Feeling of impending doom

pulmonary edema, naloxone, its antidote, is kept readily available in case respiratory depression occurs.

Oxygen is administered using a positive pressure system that can achieve a 100% oxygen concentration. A continuous positive airway pressure (CPAP) mask system may be used, or the client may be intubated and mechanical ventilation employed (see Chapter 39 ∞). Positive pressure increases alveolar pressures and gas exchange while decreasing fluid diffusion into the alveoli.

Potent loop diuretics such as furosemide, ethacrynic acid, or bumetanide are administered intravenously to promote rapid diuresis. Furosemide is also a venous dilator, reducing venous return to the heart. Vasodilators such as intravenous nitroprusside are given to improve cardiac output by reducing afterload. Dopamine or dobutamine and possibly digoxin are administered to improve the myocardial contractility and cardiac output. Intravenous aminophylline may be used cautiously to reduce bronchospasm and decrease wheezing.

When the client's condition has stabilized, further diagnostic tests may be done to determine the underlying cause of pulmonary edema, and specific treatment measures directed at the cause instituted.

NURSING CARE

Nursing care of the client with acute pulmonary edema focuses on relieving the pulmonary effects of the disorder. Interventions are directed toward improving oxygenation, reducing fluid volume, and providing emotional support.

The nurse often is instrumental in recognizing early manifestations of pulmonary edema and initiating treatment. As with many critical conditions, emergent care is directed toward the ABCs: airway, breathing, and circulation.

Nursing Diagnoses and Interventions

Promoting effective gas exchange and restoring an effective cardiac output are the priorities for nursing and interdisciplinary care of the client with cardiogenic pulmonary edema. The experience of acute dyspnea and shortness of breath is terrifying for the client; the nurse is instrumental in providing emotional support and reassurance.

Impaired Gas Exchange

Accumulated fluid in the alveoli and airways interferes with ventilation of the lungs. As a result, alveolar oxygen levels fall and carbon dioxide levels may rise. Reduced alveolar oxygen decreases diffusion of the gas into pulmonary capillaries. In addition, pulmonary edema increases the distance over which gases must diffuse to cross the alveolar–capillary membrane, further reducing oxygen levels in the blood and oxygen delivery to the tissues.

- Ensure airway patency. *A patent airway is absolutely vital for pulmonary function, including ventilation and gas exchange.*

PRACTICE ALERT
Assess the effectiveness of respiratory efforts and airway clearance. Pulmonary edema increases the work of breathing. This increased effort can lead to fatigue and decreased respiratory effort.

- Assess respiratory status frequently, including rate, effort, use of accessory muscles, sputum characteristics, lung sounds, and skin color. *The status of a client in acute pulmonary edema can change rapidly for the better or worse.*
- Place in high-Fowler's position with the legs dangling. *The upright position facilitates breathing and decreases venous return.*
- Administer oxygen as ordered by mask, CPAP mask, or ventilator. *Supplemental oxygen promotes gas exchange; positive pressure increases the pressure within the alveoli, airways, and thoracic cavity, decreasing venous return, pulmonary capillary pressure, and fluid leak into the alveoli.*
- Encourage to cough up secretions; provide nasotracheal suctioning if necessary. *Coughing moves secretions from smaller airways into larger airways where they can be suctioned out if necessary.*

PRACTICE ALERT
Have emergency equipment readily available in case of respiratory arrest. Be prepared to assist with intubation and initiation of mechanical ventilation. Fatigue, impaired gas exchange, and respiratory acidosis can lead to respiratory and cardiac arrest.

Decreased Cardiac Output

Cardiogenic pulmonary edema usually is caused by either an acute decrease in myocardial contractility or increased workload that exceeds the ability of the left ventricle. The significant decrease in cardiac output increases pressure within the pulmonary vascular system and triggers compensatory mechanisms that increase the heart rate and blood volume. These compensatory mechanisms further increase the workload of the failing heart.

- Monitor vital signs, hemodynamic status, and rhythm continuously. *Acute pulmonary edema is a critical condition, and cardiovascular status can change rapidly.*
- Assess heart sounds for possible S_3, S_4, or murmurs. *These abnormal heart sounds may be due to excess work or may indicate the cause of the acute pulmonary edema.*
- Initiate an intravenous line for medication administration. Administer morphine, diuretics, vasodilators, bronchodilators, and positive inotropic medications (e.g., digoxin) as ordered. *These drugs reduce cardiac work and improve contractility.*

PRACTICE ALERT
Insert an indwelling catheter; record output hourly. Urine output of less than 30 mL/h indicates impaired renal perfusion due to severely impaired cardiac output and a risk for renal failure or other complications.

- Keep accurate intake and output records. Restrict fluids as ordered. *Fluids may be restricted to reduce vascular volume and cardiac work.*

Fear

Acute pulmonary edema is a very frightening experience for everyone (including the nurse).

MEDIALINK Care Plan Activity: Acute Pulmonary Edema

- Provide emotional support for the client and family members. *Fear and anxiety stimulate the sympathetic nervous system, which can lead to ineffective respiratory patterns and interfere with cooperation with care measures.*
- Explain all procedures and the reasons they are performed to the client and family members. Keep information brief and to the point. Use short sentences and a reassuring tone. *Anxiety and fear interfere with the ability to assimilate information; brief, factual information and reassurance reduce anxiety and fear.*
- Maintain close contact with the client and family, providing reassurance that recovery from acute pulmonary edema is often as dramatic as its onset.

- Answer questions, and provide accurate information in a caring manner. *Knowledge reduces anxiety and psychologic stress associated with this critical condition.*

Community-Based Care

During the acute period, teaching is limited to immediate care measures. Once the acute episode of pulmonary edema has resolved, teach the client and family about its underlying cause and prevention of future episodes. If pulmonary edema follows an acute MI, include information related to CHD and the acute AMI, as well as information related to heart failure. Review the teaching and home care for clients with these disorders for further information.

INFLAMMATORY HEART DISORDERS

Any layer of cardiac tissue—the endocardium, myocardium, or pericardium—can become inflamed, thus damaging the heart valves, heart muscle, or pericardial lining. Manifestations of inflammatory heart disorders range from very mild to life threatening. This section discusses the causes and management of rheumatic heart disease, endocarditis, myocarditis, and pericarditis.

THE CLIENT WITH RHEUMATIC FEVER AND RHEUMATIC HEART DISEASE

Rheumatic fever is a systemic inflammatory disease caused by an abnormal immune response to pharyngeal infection by group A beta-hemolytic streptococci. Rheumatic fever usually is a self-limiting disorder, although it may become recurrent or chronic. Although the heart commonly is involved in the acute inflammatory process, only about 10% of people with rheumatic fever develop rheumatic heart disease (Porth, 2005). Rheumatic heart disease frequently damages the heart valves and is a major cause of mitral and aortic valve disorders discussed in the next section of this chapter.

Incidence, Prevalence, and Risk Factors

In the United States and other industrialized nations, rheumatic fever and its sequelae are rare. The peak incidence of rheumatic fever is between ages 5 and 15; although it is rare after age 40, it may affect people of any age. About 3% of people with untreated group A streptococcal pharyngitis develop rheumatic fever (Kasper et al., 2005). Rheumatic fever and rheumatic heart disease remain significant public health problems in many developing countries. Highly virulent strains of group A streptococci have caused scattered outbreaks in the United States in recent years (McCance & Huether, 2006).

Risk factors for streptococcal infections of the pharynx include environmental and economic factors such as crowded living conditions, malnutrition, immunodeficiency, and poor access to health care. Evidence also suggests an unknown genetic factor in susceptibility to rheumatic fever.

FAST FACTS
- The peak incidence of rheumatic fever is in children ages 5 to 15.
- Young adults (in late adolescence and the early 20s) are the primary adult population affected by rheumatic fever.
- People past age 40 rarely develop the disease, unless it is a case of recurrent rheumatic fever.
- Although crowded living conditions and lower socioeconomic status are risk factors, a relatively recent outbreak in the United States occurred in people with ready access to health care. Mucoid strains of *streptococcus pyogenes* have been associated with this outbreak (Veasy et al, 2004).

Pathophysiology

The pathophysiology of rheumatic fever is not yet totally understood. It is thought to result from an abnormal immune response to M proteins on group A beta-hemolytic streptococcal bacteria. These antigens can bind to cells in the heart, muscles, and brain. They also bind with receptors in synovial joints, provoking an autoimmune response (McCance & Huether, 2006). The resulting immune response to the bacteria also leads to inflammation in tissues containing these M proteins. Inflammatory lesions develop in connective tissues on the heart, joints, and skin. The antibodies may remain in the serum for up to 6 months following the initiating event. See Chapters 12 ∞ and 13 ∞ for more information about the immune system and inflammatory response.

Carditis, inflammation of the heart, develops in about 50% of people with rheumatic fever. The inflammatory process usually involves all three layers of the heart—the pericardium, myocardium, and endocardium. *Aschoff bodies,* localized areas of tissue necrosis surrounded by immune cells, develop in cardiac tissues. Pericardial and myocardial inflammation tends to be mild and self-limiting. Endocardial inflammation, however, causes swelling and erythema of valve structures and small vegetative lesions on valve leaflets. As the inflammatory process resolves, fibrous scarring occurs, causing deformity.

Rheumatic heart disease (RHD) is a slowly progressive valvular deformity that may follow acute or repeated attacks of rheumatic fever. Valve leaflets become rigid and deformed; commissures (openings) fuse, and the chordae tendineae fibrose and shorten. This results in stenosis or regurgitation of the valve. In **stenosis**, a narrowed fused valve obstructs forward blood flow. **Regurgitation** occurs when the valve fails to close properly (an *incompetent* valve), allowing blood to flow back through it. Valves on the left side of the heart are usually affected; the mitral valve is most frequently involved.

Manifestations

Manifestations of rheumatic fever typically follow the initial streptococcal infection by about 2 to 3 weeks. Fever and migratory joint pain are often initial manifestations. The knees, ankles, hips, and elbows are common sites of swelling and inflammation. *Erythema marginatum* is a temporary nonpruritic skin rash characterized by red lesions with clear borders and blanched centers usually found on the trunk and proximal extremities. Neurologic symptoms of rheumatic fever, although rare in adults, may range from irritability and an inability to concentrate to clumsiness and involuntary muscle spasms.

Manifestations of carditis include chest pain, tachycardia, a pericardial friction rub, or evidence of heart failure. On auscultation, an S_3, S_4, or a heart murmur may be heard. Cardiomegaly or pericardial effusion may develop. Other manifestations of rheumatic fever are listed in the box below.

INTERDISCIPLINARY CARE

Management of the client with rheumatic heart disease (RHD) focuses on eradicating the streptococcal infection and managing the manifestations of the disease. Carditis and resulting heart failure are treated with measures to reduce the inflammatory process and manage the heart failure. Activities are limited, but bed rest is not generally ordered.

MANIFESTATIONS of Rheumatic Fever

CARDIAC
- Chest pain
- Friction rub
- Heart murmur

MUSCULOSKELETAL
- *Migratory polyarthritis:* redness, heat, swelling, pain, and tenderness of more than one joint
- Usually affects large joints of extremities

SKIN
- *Erythema marginatum:* transitory pink, nonpruritic, macular lesions on trunk or inner aspect of upper arms or thighs
- *Subcutaneous nodules* over extensors of wrist, elbow, ankle, and knee joints

NEUROLOGIC
- *Sydenham's chorea:* irritability, behavior changes; sudden, jerky, involuntary movements

---

Diagnosis

In addition to the history and physical examination, a number of laboratory and diagnostic tests may be ordered for the client with suspected rheumatic fever. Table 32–4 identifies tests and values indicative of carditis associated with rheumatic fever.

- *Complete blood count (CBC)* and *erythrocyte sedimentation rate (ESR)* are indicators of the inflammatory process. The WBC count is elevated, and the number of RBCs may be low due to the inflammatory inhibition of erythropoiesis. The ESR, a general indicator of inflammation, is elevated.
- *C-reactive protein (CRP)* is positive in an active inflammatory process.
- *Antistreptolysin (ASO) titer* is a test for streptococcal antibodies. It rises within 2 months of the onset and is positive in most clients with rheumatic fever.
- Throat culture is positive for group A beta-hemolytic streptococcus in only 25% to 40% of clients with acute rheumatic fever (Kasper et al., 2005).

Medications

As soon as rheumatic fever is diagnosed, antibiotics are started to eliminate the streptococcal infection. Penicillin is the antibiotic of choice to treat group A streptococci. Antibiotics are prescribed for at least 10 days. Erythromycin or clindamycin is used if the client is allergic to penicillin. Prophylactic antibiotic therapy is continued for 5 to 10 years to prevent recurrences. Recurrences after 5 years or age 25 are rare (Tierney et al., 2005). Penicillin G, 1.2 million units injected intramuscularly every 3 to 4 weeks, is the prophylaxis of choice. Oral penicillin, amoxicillin, sulfadiazine, or erythromycin may also be used.

TABLE 32–4 Diagnostic Tests for Rheumatic Heart Disease

TEST	VALUES CHARACTERISTIC OF RHEUMATIC HEART DISEASE
White blood cell (WBC) count	Greater than 10,000/mm³
Red blood cell (RBC) count	Less than 4 million/mm³
Erythrocyte sedimentation rate (ESR)	More than 20 mm/h
C-reactive protein	Positive
Antistreptolysin (ASO) titer	Above 250 international unit/mL
Throat culture	Usually positive for group A beta-hemolytic streptococci
Cardiac enzymes	Elevated in severe carditis
ECG changes	Prolonged PR interval
Chest x-ray	May show cardiac enlargement
Echocardiogram	May show valvular damage, enlarged chambers, decreased ventricular function, or pericardial effusion

Joint pain and fever are treated with salicylates (e.g., aspirin), ibuprofen, or another nonsteroidal anti-inflammatory drug (NSAID); corticosteroids may be used for severe pain due to inflammation or carditis. See Chapter 13 ∞ for information about the use of these anti-inflammatory medications.

 ## NURSING CARE

Health Promotion

Rheumatic fever is preventable. Prompt identification and treatment of streptococcal throat infections help decrease spread of the pathogen and the risk for rheumatic fever. Characteristics of streptococcal sore throat; include a red, fiery-looking throat; pain with swallowing; enlarged and tender cervical lymph nodes; fever range of 101° to 104°F (38.3° to 40.0°C); and headache. Emphasize the importance of finishing the complete course of medication to eradicate the pathogen.

Assessment

Assess clients at risk for rheumatic fever (prolonged, untreated, or recurrent pharyngitis) for possible manifestations.

- *Health history:* Complaints of recent sore throat with fever, difficulty swallowing, and general malaise; treatment measures; previous history of strep throat or rheumatic fever; history of heart murmur or other cardiac problems; current medications.
- *Physical examination:* Vital signs including temperature; skin color, presence of rash on trunk or proximal extremities; mental status; evidence of inflamed joints; heart and lung sounds.
- *Diagnostic tests:* WBC and differential, ESR, CRP results; ASO titer and throat culture results; ECG and echocardiogram reports.

Nursing Diagnoses and Interventions

The nursing care focus for the client with RHD is on providing supportive care and preventing complications. Teaching to prevent recurrence of rheumatic fever is extremely important. *Pain* and *Activity Intolerance* are priority nursing diagnoses for the client with rheumatic fever and RHD.

Acute Pain

Joint and chest pain due to acute inflammation is common in rheumatic fever. Pain and inflammation may interfere with rest and healing.

- Administer anti-inflammatory drugs as ordered. Promptly report manifestations of aspirin toxicity, including tinnitus, vomiting, and gastrointestinal bleeding. Give aspirin and other NSAIDs with food, milk, or antacids to minimize gastric irritation. *Joint pain and fever may be treated with anti-inflammatory agents such as aspirin and NSAIDs. When used for its anti-inflammatory effect, aspirin doses may be high, and it is given around the clock (e.g., every 4 hours). Steroids may be prescribed for severe carditis.*

- Provide warm, moist compresses for local pain relief of acutely inflamed joints. *Moist heat helps relieve pain associated with inflamed joints by reducing inflammation.*
- Auscultate heart sounds as indicated (every shift or each home visit). Notify the physician if a pericardial friction rub or a new murmur develops. *A friction rub is produced as inflamed pericardial surfaces rub against each other. This also stimulates pain receptors, and may increase discomfort.*

Activity Intolerance

The client with acute carditis or RHD may develop heart failure if the heart is unable to supply enough oxygen to meet the body's demand. Manifestations of fatigue, weakness, and dyspnea on exertion may result.

- Explain the importance of activity limitations and reinforce teaching as needed. *Activities are limited during the acute phase of carditis to reduce the workload of the heart. Understanding the rationale improves cooperation with the limitations.*
- Encourage social and diversional activities such as visits with friends and family, reading, playing cards or board games, watching television, and listening to music or talking books. *Diversional activities provide a focus for the client whose physical activities must be limited.*
- Encourage gradual increases in activity, monitoring for evidence of intolerance or heart failure. Consult a cardiac rehabilitation specialist to help design an activity progression schedule. *Gradual activity progression is encouraged as the client's condition improves. Activity tolerance is monitored and activities modified as needed.*

Community-Based Care

Most clients with rheumatic fever and carditis do not require hospitalization. Teaching for home care focuses on both acute care and preventing recurrences and further tissue damage. Include the following topics:

- The importance of completing the full course of antibiotic therapy and continuing antibiotic prophylaxis as prescribed. For the client with chronic RHD, include the importance of antibiotic prophylaxis for invasive procedures (e.g., dental care, endoscopy, or surgery) to prevent bacterial endocarditis. Pamphlets on endocarditis prevention are helpful reminders, and are available from the American Heart Association.
- Preventive dental care and good oral hygiene to maintain oral health and prevent gingival infections, which can lead to recurrence of the disease.
- Early recognition of streptococcal sore throat and appropriate treatment for both the client and family members.
- Early manifestations of heart failure to report to the physician.
- Prescribed medications, including their dosage, route, intended and potential adverse effects, and manifestations to report to the physician.
- Dietary sodium restriction if ordered or recommended. A high-carbohydrate, high-protein diet may be recommended to facilitate healing and combat fatigue.

Refer for home health services or household assistance as indicated.

THE CLIENT WITH INFECTIVE ENDOCARDITIS

Endocarditis, inflammation of the endocardium, can involve any portion of the endothelial lining of the heart. The valves usually are affected. Endocarditis is usually infectious in nature, characterized by colonization or invasion of the endocardium and heart valves by a pathogen.

FAST FACTS

- Subacute bacterial endocarditis develops more slowly and usually occurs in people with previous heart valve damage.
- Acute bacterial endocarditis has an abrupt onset and typically affects people with no previous history of heart problems.

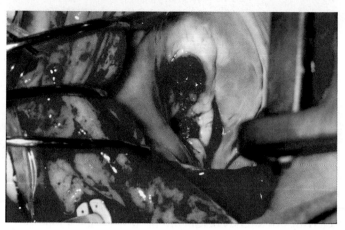

Figure 32–7 ■ A vegetative lesion of bacterial endocarditis.
Source: M. English/Custom Medical Stock Photo, Inc.

Incidence and Risk Factors

Endocarditis is relatively uncommon, with an incidence of 1.5 to 6.2 cases per 100,000 people in developed countries (Kasper et al., 2005). The greatest risk factor for endocarditis is previous heart damage. Lesions develop on deformed valves, on valve prostheses, or in areas of tissue damage due to congenital deformities or ischemic disease. The left side of the heart, the mitral valve in particular, is usually affected. Intravenous drug use also is a significant risk factor. The right side of the heart usually is affected in these clients. Other risk factors include invasive catheters (e.g., a central venous catheter, hemodynamic monitoring, or an indwelling urinary catheter), dental procedures or poor dental health, and recent heart surgery.

Prosthetic valve endocarditis (PVE) may occur in clients with a mechanical or tissue valve replacement. This infection may develop in the early postoperative period (within 2 months after surgery) or late. Prosthetic valve endocarditis accounts for 10% to 20% of endocarditis cases. It usually affects males over the age of 60, and is more frequently associated with aortic valve prostheses than with mitral valve replacements. Early PVE is usually due to prosthetic valve contamination during surgery or perioperative bacteremia. Its course often is rapid, and mortality is high. Late-onset PVE more closely resembles subacute endocarditis.

Pathophysiology

Entry of pathogens into the bloodstream is required for infective endocarditis to develop. Bacteria may enter through oral lesions, during dental work or invasive procedures, such as intravenous catheter insertion, surgery, or urinary catheterization; during intravenous drug use; or as a result of infectious processes such as urinary tract or upper respiratory infection.

The initial lesion is a sterile platelet-fibrin vegetation formed on damaged endothelium (Figure 32–7 ■). In acute infective endocarditis, these lesions develop on healthy valve structures, although the mechanism is unknown. In subacute endocarditis, they usually develop on already damaged valves or in endocardial tissue that has been damaged by abnormal pressures or blood flow within the heart.

Organisms that have invaded the blood colonize these vegetations. The vegetation enlarges as more platelets and fibrin are attracted to the site and cover the infecting organism. This covering "protects" the bacteria from quick removal by immune defenses such as phagocytosis by neutrophils, antibodies, and complement. Vegetations may be singular or multiple. They expand while loosely attached to edges of the valve. Friable vegetations can break or shear off, embolizing and traveling through the bloodstream to other organ systems. When they lodge in small vessels, they may cause hemorrhages, infarcts, or abscesses. Ultimately, the vegetations scar and deform the valves and cause turbulence of blood flowing through the heart. Heart valve function is affected, either obstructing forward blood flow, or closing incompletely.

Endocarditis is classified by its acuity and disease course (Table 32–5). *Acute infective endocarditis* has an abrupt onset and is a rapidly progressive, severe disease. Although almost any organism can cause infective endocarditis, virulent organisms such as *Staphylococcus aureus* cause a more abrupt onset and destructive course. *S. aureus* is commonly the infective organism in acute endocarditis. In contrast, *subacute infective endocarditis* has a more gradual onset, with predominant systemic manifestations. It is more likely to occur in clients with preexisting heart disease. *Streptococcus viridans,* enterococci, other gram-negative and gram-positive bacilli, yeasts, and fungi tend to cause the subacute forms of endocarditis (Porth, 2005).

Manifestations

The manifestations of infective endocarditis often are nonspecific (see the box on page 1046). A temperature above 101.5°F (39.4°C) and flulike symptoms develop, accompanied by cough, shortness of breath, and joint pain. The presentation of acute staphylococcal endocarditis is more severe, with a sudden onset, chills, and a high fever. Heart murmurs are heard in 90% of persons with infective endocarditis. An existing murmur may worsen, or a new murmur may develop.

Splenomegaly is common in chronic disease. Peripheral manifestations of infective endocarditis result from microemboli or circulating immune complexes. These manifestations include:

- *Petechiae:* small, purplish-red hemorrhagic spots on the trunk, conjunctiva, and mucous membranes

TABLE 32–5 Classifications of Infective Endocarditis

	ACUTE INFECTIVE ENDOCARDITIS	SUBACUTE INFECTIVE ENDOCARDITIS
Onset	Sudden	Gradual
Usual organism	*Staphylococcus aureus*	*Streptococcus viridans*, enterococci, gram-negative and gram-positive bacilli, fungi, yeasts
Risk factors	Usually occurs in previously normal heart; intravenous drug use, infected intravenous sites	Usually occurs in damaged or deformed hearts; dental work, invasive procedures, and infections
Pathologic process	Rapid valve destruction	Valve destruction leading to regurgitation; embolization of friable vegetations
Presentation	Abrupt onset with spiking fever and chills; manifestations of heart failure	Gradual onset of febrile illness with cough, dyspnea, arthralgias, abdominal pain

MANIFESTATIONS of Infective Endocarditis

- Chills and fever
- General malaise, fatigue
- Arthralgias
- Cough, dyspnea
- Heart murmur
- Anorexia, abdominal pain
- Petechiae, splinter hemorrhages
- Splenomegaly

- *Splinter hemorrhages:* hemorrhagic streaks under the fingernails or toenails
- *Osler's nodes:* small, reddened, painful raised growths on finger and toe pads
- *Janeway lesions:* small, nontender, purplish-red macular lesions on the palms of the hands and soles of the feet
- *Roth's spots:* small, whitish spots (cotton-wool spots) seen on the retina.

Complications

Embolization of vegetative fragments may affect any organ system, particularly the lungs, brain, kidneys, and the skin and mucous membranes, with resulting organ infarction. Other common complications of infective endocarditis include heart failure, abscess, and aneurysms due to infiltration of the arterial wall by organisms. Without treatment, endocarditis is almost universally fatal; fortunately, antibiotic therapy is usually effective to treat this disease.

INTERDISCIPLINARY CARE

Eradicating the infecting organism and minimizing valve damage and other adverse consequences of infective endocarditis are the priorities of care.

Diagnosis

There are no definitive tests for infective endocarditis, but diagnostic tests help establish the diagnosis.

- *Blood cultures* usually are positive for bacteria or other pathogens. Blood cultures are considered positive when a

typical infecting organism is identified from two or more separate blood cultures (drawn from different sites and/or at different times, e.g., 12-hour intervals).

- *Echocardiography* (either transthoracic or transesophageal) to visualize vegetations can be diagnostic for infective endocarditis when combined with positive blood cultures. See Chapter 30 ∞ for more information about echocardiography.
- *Serologic immune testing* for circulating antigens to typical infective organisms may be done.

Other diagnostic tests may include the CBC, ESR, serum creatinine, chest x-ray, and an electrocardiogram.

Medications

Preventing endocarditis in clients at high risk is important. Antibiotics are commonly prescribed for clients with preexisting valve damage or heart disease prior to high-risk procedures (Table 32–6).

Antibiotic therapy effectively treats infective endocarditis in most cases. The goal of therapy is to eradicate the infecting organism from the blood and vegetative lesions in the heart. The fibrin covering that protects colonies of organisms from immune defenses also protects them from antibiotic therapy. Therefore, an extended course of multiple intravenous antibiotics is required.

Following blood cultures, antibiotic therapy is initiated with drugs known to be effective against the most common infecting organisms: staphylococci, streptococci, and enterococci. The initial regimen may include nafcillin or oxacillin, penicillin or ampicillin, and gentamicin. Once the organism has been identified, therapy is tailored to that organism. Streptococcal and enterococcal infections are treated with a combination of penicillin and gentamicin. If the client is allergic to penicillin, ceftriaxone, cefazolin, or vancomycin may be used. Staphylococcal infections are treated with nafcillin or oxacillin and gentamicin; cefazolin or vancomycin may be used if penicillin allergy is present. Intravenous drug therapy is continued for 2 to 8 weeks, depending on the infecting organism, the drugs used, and the results of repeat blood cultures. See Chapter 12 ∞ for the nursing implications for antibiotic therapy.

The client with prosthetic valve endocarditis requires extended treatment, usually 6 to 8 weeks. Combination therapy

TABLE 32–6 Antibiotic Prophylaxis for Infective Endocarditis

INDICATIONS FOR PROPHYLAXIS	SELECTED PROCEDURES FOR WHICH PROPHYLAXIS IS RECOMMENDED	SUGGESTED ANTIBIOTICS
Prosthetic valves	Dental procedures in which bleeding is likely, including cleaning	Amoxicillin
Previous episode(s) of infective endocarditis		Erythromycin
Rheumatic heart disease	Most surgeries	Ampicillin
Hypertrophic cardiomyopathy	Bronchoscopy	Clindamycin
Mitral valve prolapse with regurgitation and murmur	Cystoscopy	Vancomycin
	Urinary catheterization when infection is present	(*Note:* Choice of antibiotic depends on procedure.)
Sclerotic aortic valve	Incision and drainage of infected tissue	
Most congenital heart malformations	Vaginal delivery if infection is present	

using vancomycin, rifampin, and gentamicin is used to treat these resistant infections.

Surgery

Some clients with infective endocarditis require surgery to:
- Replace severely damaged valves.
- Remove large vegetations at risk for embolization.
- Remove a valve that is a continuing source of infection that does not respond to antibiotic therapy.

The most common indication for surgery is valvular regurgitation that causes heart failure and does not respond to medical therapy. When the infection has not responded to antibiotic therapy within 7 to 10 days, the infected valve may be replaced to facilitate eradication of the organism. Clients with fungal endocarditis usually require surgical intervention. More information on valve replacement surgery is provided in the section on valve disorders.

 NURSING CARE

Health Promotion

Prevention of endocarditis is vital in susceptible people. Education is a key part of prevention. Use every opportunity to educate individuals and the public about the risks of intravenous drug use, including endocarditis. Discuss preventive measures with all clients with specific risk factors, such as a heart murmur or known heart disease.

Assessment

Assessment related to ineffective endocarditis includes identifying risk factors and manifestations of the disease.
- *Health history:* Complaints of persistent flulike symptoms, fatigue, shortness of breath, and activity intolerance; history of recent dental work or other invasive procedures; known heart murmur, valve or other heart disorder; recent intravenous drug use.
- *Physical examination:* Vital signs including temperature; apical pulse and heart sounds; rate and ease of respirations, lung sounds; skin color, temperature, and presence of petechiae or splinter hemorrhages.
- *Diagnostic tests:* WBC and differential, ESR; blood culture and sensitivity results; echocardiogram reports.

Nursing Diagnoses and Interventions

Nursing care focuses on managing the manifestations of endocarditis, administering antibiotics, and teaching the client and family members about the disorder. In addition to the diagnoses identified below, nursing diagnoses and interventions for heart failure also may be appropriate for clients with infective endocarditis.

Risk for Imbalanced Body Temperature

Fever is common in clients with infective endocarditis. It may be acutely elevated and accompanied by chills, particularly with acute infective endocarditis. The inflammatory process initiates a cycle of events that affects the regulation of temperature and causes discomfort.
- Record temperature every 2 to 4 hours. Report temperature above 101.5°F (39.4°C). Assess for complaints of discomfort. *Fever is usually low grade (below 101.5°F [39.4°C]) in infective endocarditis; higher temperatures may cause discomfort. The temperature usually returns to normal within 1 week after initiation of antibiotic therapy. Continued fever may indicate a need to modify the treatment regimen.*
- Obtain blood cultures as ordered, before initial antibiotic dose. *Initial blood cultures are obtained before antibiotic therapy is started to obtain adequate organisms to culture and identify. Follow-up cultures are used to assess the effectiveness of therapy.*
- Provide anti-inflammatory or antipyretic agents as prescribed. *Fever may be treated with anti-inflammatory or antipyretic agents such as aspirin, ibuprofen, or acetaminophen.*
- Administer antibiotics as ordered; obtain peak and trough drug levels as indicated. *Intravenous antibiotics are given to eradicate the pathogen. Peak and trough levels are used to evaluate the dose effectiveness in maintaining a therapeutic blood level.*

Risk for Ineffective Tissue Perfusion

Embolization of vegetative lesions can threaten tissue and organ perfusion. Vegetations from the left heart may lodge in arterioles or capillaries of the brain, kidneys, or peripheral tissues, causing infarction or abscess. A large embolism can cause manifestations of stroke or transient ischemic attack, renal failure, or tissue ischemia. Emboli from the right side of the heart become entrapped in pulmonary vasculature, causing manifestations of pulmonary embolism.

- Assess for, document, and report manifestations of decreased organ system perfusion:
  a. *Neurologic:* changes in level of consciousness, numbness or tingling in extremities, hemiplegia, visual disturbances, or manifestations of stroke
  b. *Renal:* decreased urine output, hematuria, elevated BUN or creatinine
  c. *Pulmonary:* dyspnea, hemoptysis, shortness of breath, diminished breath sounds, restlessness, sudden chest or shoulder pain
  d. *Cardiovascular:* chest pain radiating to jaw or arms, tachycardia, anxiety, tachypnea, hypotension.

  All major organs and tissues, and the microcirculation, may be affected by emboli when vegetations break off due to turbulent blood flow. Emboli may cause manifestations of organ dysfunction. The most devastating effects of emboli are in the brain and the myocardium, with resulting infarctions. Intravenous drug users have a high risk of pulmonary emboli as a result of right-sided endocardial fragments.

- Assess and document skin color and temperature, quality of peripheral pulses, and capillary refill. *Peripheral emboli affect tissue perfusion, with a risk for tissue necrosis and possible extremity loss.*

Ineffective Health Maintenance

The client with endocarditis often is treated in the community. Teaching about disease management and prevention of possible recurrences of endocarditis is vital.

- Demonstrate intravenous catheter site care and intermittent antibiotic administration if the client and family will manage therapy. Have the client and/or significant other redemonstrate appropriate techniques. *Intermittent antibiotic infusions may be managed by the client or family members, or the client may go to an outpatient facility to receive the infusions. Appropriate site care is necessary to reduce the risk of trauma and infection.*
- Explain the actions, doses, administration, and desired and adverse effects of prescribed drugs. Identify manifestations to be reported to the physician. Provide practical information about measures to reduce the risk of superinfection (e.g., consuming 8 oz of yogurt or buttermilk containing live bacterial cultures daily). *Careful compliance with prescribed drug therapy is vital to eradicate the infecting organism. Antibiotic therapy can, however, cause superinfections such as candidiasis due to elimination of normal body flora.*
- Teach about the function of heart valves and the effects of endocarditis on heart function. Include a simple definition of endocarditis, and explain the risk for its recurrence. *Information helps the client and family understand endocarditis, its treatment, and its effects. Understanding increases compliance.*
- Describe the manifestations of heart failure to be reported to the physician. *Evidence of heart failure may necessitate modification of the treatment regimen or replacement of infected valves.*

PRACTICE ALERT

Stress the importance of notifying all care providers of valve disease, heart murmur, or valve replacement before undergoing invasive procedures. Invasive procedures provide a portal of entry for bacteria. A history of valve disease increases the risk for the development or recurrence of endocarditis.

- Encourage good dental hygiene and mouth care and regular dental checkups. Teach how to prevent bleeding from the gums and avoid developing mouth ulcers (e.g., gentle toothbrushing, ensuring that dentures fit properly, and avoiding toothpicks, dental floss, and high-flow water devices). *The oropharynx harbors streptococci, which are common causes of endocarditis. Bleeding gums offer an opportunity for bacteria to enter the bloodstream.*
- Encourage the client to avoid people with upper respiratory infections. *Streptococci are normal pathogens in the upper respiratory tract; exposure to people with upper respiratory infections may increase the risk of infection.*
- If anticoagulant therapy is ordered, explain its actions, administration, and major side effects. Identify manifestations of bleeding to be promptly reported to the physician. *Clients with valve disease or a prosthetic valve following infective endocarditis may require continued anticoagulant therapy to prevent thrombi and emboli. Knowledge is vital for appropriate management of anticoagulant therapy and prevention of complications.*

Community-Based Care

When preparing the client with infective endocarditis for home care, provide teaching as outlined for the nursing diagnosis *Ineffective Health Maintenance.* In addition, discuss the following topics:

- Although serious and frightening, infective endocarditis can usually be treated effectively with intravenous antibiotics.
- The importance of promptly reporting any unusual manifestation, such as a change in vision, sudden pain, or weakness, so that interventions to control complications can be promptly implemented.
- The rationale for all treatments and procedures.
- Preventing recurrences of infective endocarditis.
- The importance of maintaining contact with the physician for follow-up care and monitoring for long-term effects such as progressive valve damage and dysfunction.
- If appropriate, explain the risks associated with intravenous drug use.

Provide educational materials on infective endocarditis from the American Heart Association. Refer as appropriate to home health or home intravenous therapy services. Refer the client and family members or significant others as appropriate to a drug or substance abuse treatment program or facility. Provide follow-up care to ensure compliance with the referral and treatment plan.

THE CLIENT WITH MYOCARDITIS

Myocarditis is inflammation of the heart muscle. It usually results from an infectious process, but also may occur as an immunologic response, or due to the effects of radiation, toxins, or drugs. In the United States, myocarditis is usually viral, caused by coxsackievirus B. Approximately 10% of people with HIV disease develop myocarditis due to infiltration of the myocardium by the virus. Bacterial myocarditis, much less common, may be associated with endocarditis caused by *S. aureus,* or with diphtheria. Parasitic infections caused by *Trypanosoma cruzi* (Chagas' disease) are common in Central and South America (Kasper et al., 2005).

Incidence and Risk Factors

Myocarditis may occur at any age, and it is more common in men than women. Factors that alter immune response (e.g., malnutrition, alcohol use, immunosuppressive drugs, exposure to radiation, stress, and advanced age) increase the risk for myocarditis. It also is a common complication of rheumatic fever and pericarditis.

Pathophysiology

In myocarditis, myocardial cells are damaged by an inflammatory process that causes local or diffuse swelling and damage. Infectious agents infiltrate interstitial tissues, forming abscesses. Autoimmune injury may occur when the immune system destroys not only the invading pathogen but also myocardial cells. The extent of damage to cardiac muscle ultimately determines the long-term outcome of the disease. Viral myocarditis usually is self-limited; it may progress, however, to become chronic, leading to dilated cardiomyopathy (see the section of this chapter that follows). Severe myocarditis may lead to heart failure.

Manifestations

The manifestations of myocarditis depend on the degree of myocardial damage. The client may be asymptomatic. Nonspecific manifestations of inflammation such as fever, fatigue, general malaise, dyspnea, palpitations, and arthralgias may be present. A nonspecific febrile illness or upper respiratory infection often precedes the onset of myocarditis symptoms. Abnormal heart sounds such as muffled S_1, an S_3, murmur, and pericardial friction rub may be heard. In some cases, manifestations of myocardial infarction, including chest pain, may occur.

INTERDISCIPLINARY CARE

Myocarditis treatment focuses on resolving the inflammatory process to prevent further damage to the myocardium.

Diagnostic studies may be ordered to help diagnose myocarditis:
- *Electrocardiography* may show transient ST-segment and T-wave changes, as well as dysrhythmias and possible heart block.
- *Cardiac markers,* such as the creatinine kinase, troponin T, and troponin I, may be elevated, indicating myocardial cell damage.
- *Endomyocardial biopsy* to examine myocardial cells is necessary to establish a definitive diagnosis; patchy cell necrosis and the inflammatory process can be identified.

If appropriate, antimicrobial therapy is used to eradicate the infecting organism. Antiviral therapy with interferon alpha may be instituted. Immunosuppressive therapy with corticosteroids or other immunosuppressive agents (see Chapter 13 ∞) may be used to minimize the inflammatory response. Heart failure is treated as needed, using ACE inhibitors and drugs. Clients with myocarditis often are particularly sensitive to the effects of digitalis, so it is used with caution. Other medications used in treating myocarditis include antidysrhythmic agents to control dysrhythmias and anticoagulants to prevent emboli.

Bed rest and activity restrictions are ordered during the acute inflammatory process to reduce myocardial work and prevent myocardial damage. Activities may be limited for as long as 6 months to a year (Porth, 2005).

NURSING CARE

Nursing care is directed at decreasing myocardial work and maintaining cardiac output. Both physical and emotional rest are indicated, because anxiety increases myocardial oxygen demand. Hemodynamic parameters and the ECG are monitored closely, especially during the acute phase of the illness. Activity tolerance, urine output, and heart and breath sounds are frequently assessed for manifestations of heart failure. Consider the following nursing diagnoses for the client with myocarditis:
- *Activity Intolerance* related to impaired cardiac muscle function
- *Decreased Cardiac Output* related to myocardial inflammation
- *Fatigue* related to inflammation and impaired cardiac output
- *Anxiety* related to possible long-term effects of the disorder
- *Excess Fluid Volume* related to compensatory mechanisms for decreased cardiac output.

Community-Based Care

Include the following topics when preparing the client with myocarditis for home care:
- Activity restrictions and other prescribed measures to reduce cardiac workload
- Early manifestations of heart failure to report to the physician
- The importance of following the prescribed treatment regimen
- Any recommended dietary modifications (such as a low-sodium diet for heart failure)
- Prescribed medications, their purpose, doses, and possible adverse effects
- The importance of adhering to the treatment plan and recommended follow-up appointments to reduce the risk of long-term consequences such as cardiomyopathy.

THE CLIENT WITH PERICARDITIS

The pericardium is the outermost layer of the heart. It is a two-layered membranous sac with a thin layer of serous fluid (normally no more than 30 to 50 mL) separating the layers. It protects and cushions the heart and the great vessels, provides a barrier to infectious processes in adjacent structures, prevents displacement of the myocardium and blood vessels, and prevents sudden distention of the heart.

Pericarditis is the inflammation of the pericardium. Pericarditis may be a primary disorder or develop secondarily to another cardiac or systemic disorder. Some possible causes of pericarditis are listed in Box 32–4. Acute pericarditis is usually viral and affects men (usually under the age of 50) more frequently than women (Tierney et al., 2005). Pericarditis affects 40% to 50% of clients with end-stage renal disease and uremia. Postmyocardial infarction pericarditis and postcardiotomy (following open-heart surgery) pericarditis also are common.

Pathophysiology

Pericardial tissue damage triggers an inflammatory response. Inflammatory mediators released from the injured tissue cause vasodilation, hyperemia, and edema. Capillary permeability increases, allowing plasma proteins, including fibrinogen, to escape into the pericardial space. White blood cells amass at the site of injury to destroy the causative agent. Exudate is formed, usually fibrinous or serofibrinous (a mixture of serous fluid and fibrinous exudate). In some cases, the exudate may contain red blood cells or, if infectious, purulent material. The inflammatory process may resolve without long-term effects, or scar tissue and adhesions may form between the pericardial layers.

Fibrosis and scarring of the pericardium may restrict cardiac function. Pericardial effusions may develop as serous or purulent exudate (depending on the causative agent) collects in the pericardial sac. Pericardial effusion may be recurrent. Chronic inflammation causes the pericardium to become rigid.

Manifestations

Classic manifestations of acute pericarditis include chest pain, a pericardial friction rub, and fever. Chest pain, the most common symptom, has an abrupt onset. It is caused by inflammation of nerve fibers in the lower parietal pericardium and pleura covering the diaphragm. The pain is usually sharp, may be steady or intermittent, and may radiate to the back or neck. The pain can mimic myocardial ischemia; careful assessment is important to rule out myocardial infarction. Pericardial pain is aggravated by respiratory movements (i.e., deep inspiration and/or coughing), changes in body position, or swallowing. Sitting upright and leaning forward reduces the discomfort by moving the heart away from the diaphragmatic side of the lung pleura.

Although not always present, a *pericardial friction rub* is the characteristic sign of pericarditis. A pericardial friction rub is a leathery, grating sound produced by the inflamed pericardial layers rubbing against the chest wall or pleura. It is heard most clearly at the left lower sternal border with the client sitting up or leaning forward. The rub is usually heard on expiration and may be constant or intermittent.

A low-grade fever (below 100°F [38.4°C]) often develops due to the inflammatory process. Dyspnea and tachycardia are common.

Complications

Pericardial effusion, cardiac tamponade, and constrictive pericarditis are possible complications of acute pericarditis.

Pericardial Effusion

A *pericardial effusion* is an abnormal collection of fluid between the pericardial layers that threatens normal cardiac function. The fluid may consist of pus, blood, serum, lymph, or a combination. The manifestations of a pericardial effusion depend on the rate at which the fluid collects. Although the pericardium normally contains about 30 to 50 mL of fluid, the sac can stretch to accommodate a gradual accumulation of fluid. Over time, the pericardial sac can accommodate up to 2 L of fluid without immediate adverse effects. Conversely, a rapid buildup of pericardial fluid (as little as 100 mL) does not allow the sac to stretch and can compress the heart, interfering with myocardial function. This compression of the heart is known as **cardiac tamponade**. Slowly developing pericardial effusion is often painless and has few manifestations. Heart sounds may be distant or muffled. The client may have a cough or mild dyspnea.

Cardiac Tamponade

Cardiac tamponade is a medical emergency that must be aggressively treated to preserve life. Cardiac tamponade may result from pericardial effusion, trauma, cardiac rupture, or hemorrhage. Rapid collection of fluid in the pericardial sac interferes with ventricular filling and pumping, critically reducing cardiac output.

Classic manifestations of cardiac tamponade result from rising intracardiac pressures, decreased diastolic filling, and decreased cardiac output. A hallmark of cardiac tamponade is a paradoxical pulse, or *pulsus paradoxus*. A paradoxical pulse markedly decreases in amplitude during inspiration. Intrathoracic pressure normally drops during inspiration, enhancing venous return to the right heart. This draws more blood into the right side of the heart than the left, causing the interventricular septum to bulge slightly into the left ventricle. When ventricular filling is impaired by excess fluid in the pericardial sac, this bulging of the interventricular septum decreases cardiac output during inspiration (see Figure 32–8). On palpation of the carotid or femoral artery, the pulse is diminished or absent during inspiration. A drop in systolic blood pressure of more than 10 mmHg during inspiration also indicates pulsus paradoxus.

Other manifestations of cardiac tamponade include muffled heart sounds, dyspnea and tachypnea, tachycardia, a nar-

---

BOX 32–4 Selected Causes of Pericarditis

Infectious
- Viruses
- Bacteria
- Tuberculosis
- Fungi
- Syphilis
- Parasites

Noninfectious
- Myocardial and pericardial injury
- Uremia
- Neoplasms
- Radiation
- Trauma or surgery
- Myxedema
- Autoimmune disorders
- Rheumatic fever
- Connective tissue diseases
- Prescription and nonprescription drugs
- Postcardiac injury

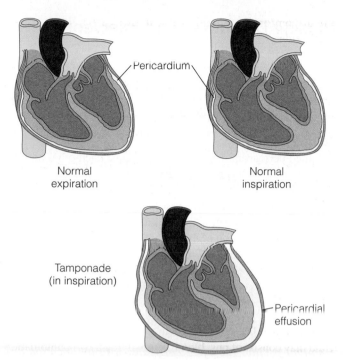

Figure 32–8 ■ Cardiac tamponade. Note increased volume in the right ventricle during inspiration in both the normal heart and the heart affected by a pericardial effusion. In tamponade, fluid in the pericardial sac and the distended right ventricle restrict filling of the left ventricle and consequently, cardiac output.

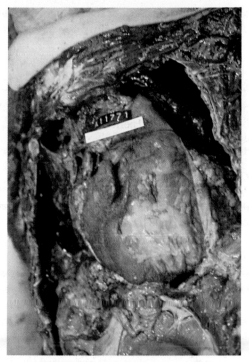

Figure 32–9 ■ Constrictive pericarditis.
Source: Custom Medical Stock Photo, Inc.

rowed pulse pressure, and distended neck veins (see the box below).

Chronic Constrictive Pericarditis

Chronic pericardial inflammation can lead to scar tissue formation between the pericardial layers. This scar tissue eventually contracts, restricting diastolic filling and elevating venous pressure. Constrictive pericarditis may follow viral infection, radiation therapy, or heart surgery. Its manifestations include progressive dyspnea, fatigue, and weakness. Ascites is common; peripheral edema may develop. Neck veins are distended, and may be particularly noticeable during inspiration (*Kussmaul's sign*). This occurs because the right atrium is unable to dilate to accommodate increased venous return during inspiration. See Figure 32–9 ■.

MANIFESTATIONS of Cardiac Tamponade

- Paradoxical pulse
- Narrowed pulse pressure, hypotension
- Tachycardia
- Weak peripheral pulses
- Distant, muffled heart sounds
- Jugular venous distention
- High central venous pressure
- Decreased level of consciousness
- Low urine output
- Cool, mottled skin

INTERDISCIPLINARY CARE

Care for the client with pericarditis focuses on identifying its cause if possible, reducing inflammation, relieving symptoms, and preventing complications. The client is closely monitored for early manifestations of cardiac tamponade so that it can be treated promptly.

Diagnosis

There are no specific laboratory tests to diagnose pericarditis, but tests are often performed to differentiate pericarditis from myocardial infarction.

- *CBC* shows elevated WBCs and an ESR greater than 20 mm/h, indicating acute inflammation.
- *Cardiac enzymes* may be slightly elevated because the inflammatory process extends to involve the epicardial surface of the heart. Cardiac enzymes are typically much lower in pericarditis than in myocardial infarction.
- *Electrocardiography* shows typical changes associated with pericarditis, such as diffuse ST-segment elevation in all leads. This resolves more quickly than changes of acute MI and is not associated with the QRS-complex and T-wave changes typically seen in MI. With a large pericardial effusion, the QRS amplitude may be decreased. Atrial dysrhythmias may occur in acute pericarditis.
- *Echocardiography* is used to assess heart motion, for pericardial effusion, and the extent of restriction.
- *Hemodynamic monitoring* may be used in acute pericarditis or pericardial effusion to assess pressures and cardiac output. Elevated pulmonary artery pressures and venous pressures occur with impaired filling due to pericardial effusion or constrictive pericarditis.
- *Chest x-ray* may show cardiac enlargement if a pericardial effusion is present.

- *Computed tomography (CT) scan* or *magnetic resonance imaging (MRI)* may be used to identify pericardial effusion or constrictive pericarditis.

Medications

Drug treatment for pericarditis addresses its manifestations. Aspirin and acetaminophen may be used to reduce fever. NSAIDs are used to reduce inflammation and promote comfort. In severe cases or with recurrent pericarditis, corticosteroids may be given to suppress the inflammatory response.

Pericardiocentesis

Pericardiocentesis may be done to remove fluid from the pericardial sac for diagnostic or therapeutic purposes (see Figure 30–15 ∞). The physician inserts a large (16- to 18-gauge) needle into the pericardial sac and withdraws excess fluid. The needle is attached to an ECG monitoring lead to help determine if the needle is touching the epicardial surface, which helps prevent piercing the myocardium. Pericardiocentesis may be an emergency procedure for the client with cardiac tamponade. Nursing implications for pericardiocentesis are outlined in Chapter 30 ∞.

Surgery

For recurrent pericarditis or recurrent pericardial effusion, a rectangular piece of the pericardium, or "window," may be excised to allow collected fluid to drain into the pleural space. Constrictive pericarditis may necessitate a partial or total *pericardiectomy,* removal of part or all of the pericardium, to relieve the ventricular compression and allow adequate filling.

 NURSING CARE

Health Promotion

While it may not yet be possible to identify many clients at risk for and to prevent acute pericarditis, early identification and treatment of the disorder can reduce the risk of complications. Promptly report a pericardial friction rub or other manifestations of pericarditis in clients with recent acute AMI, cardiac surgery, or systemic diseases associated with a risk for pericarditis.

Assessment

Assessment data to collect from the client with suspected pericarditis includes:

- *Health history:* Complaints of acute substernal or precordial chest pain, effect of movement and breathing on discomfort, pain radiation, associated symptoms; recent acute AMI, heart surgery, or other cardiac disorder; current medications; chronic conditions such as renal failure or a connective tissue or autoimmune disorder.
- *Physical examination:* Vital signs including temperature, variation in systolic BP with respirations; strength of peripheral pulses, variations with respiratory movement; apical pulse, clarity, changes with respiratory movement, presence of a friction rub; neck vein distention; level of consciousness, skin color, and other indicators of cardiac output.
- *Diagnostic tests:* WBC and differential, ESR; cardiac enzyme levels; ECG and echocardiogram reports.

Nursing Diagnoses and Interventions

Nursing care for the client with pericarditis may occur in the acute or community setting. Closely observe for early manifestations of increasing effusion or cardiac tamponade. Priority nursing diagnoses relate to comfort, the risk for tamponade, and effects of the acute inflammatory process.

Acute Pain

Inflamed pericardial layers rubbing against each other and the lung pleura stimulate phrenic nerve pain fibers in the lower portion of the parietal pericardium. Pain is usually acute and may be severe until inflammation resolves.

- Assess chest pain using a standard pain scale and noting the quality and radiation of the pain. Note nonverbal cues of pain (grimacing, guarding behaviors), and validate with the client. *Careful assessment helps identify the cause of pain. The pain of pericarditis may radiate to the neck or back and is aggravated by movement, coughing, or deep breathing. A pain scale allows evaluation of the effectiveness of interventions.*
- Auscultate heart sounds every 4 hours. *Presence of a pericardial friction rub often correlates with the location and severity of the pain.*
- Administer NSAIDs on a regular basis as prescribed with food. Document effectiveness. *NSAIDs reduce fever, inflammation, and pericardial pain. They are most effective when administered around the clock on a consistent basis. Administering the medications with food helps decrease gastric distress.*
- Maintain a quiet, calm environment, and position of comfort. Offer back rubs, heat/cold therapy, diversional activity, and emotional support. *Supportive interventions enhance the effects of the medication, may decrease pain perception, and convey a sense of caring.*

Ineffective Breathing Pattern

Respiratory movement intensifies pericardial pain. In an effort to decrease pain, the client often breathes shallowly, increasing the risk for pulmonary complications.

> **PRACTICE ALERT**
> Document respiratory rate, effort, and breath sounds every 2 to 4 hours. Report adventitious or diminished breath sounds. Shallow, guarded respirations may lead to increased respiratory rate and effort. Poor ventilation of peripheral alveoli may lead to congestion or atelectasis.

- Encourage deep breathing and use of the incentive spirometer. Provide pain medication before respiratory therapy, as needed. *Deep breathing and an incentive spirometer promote alveolar ventilation and prevent atelectasis. Administration of analgesia prior to respiratory treatments improves their effectiveness by decreasing guarding.*
- Administer oxygen as needed. *Supplementary oxygen promotes optimal gas exchange and tissue oxygenation.*
- Place in Fowler's or high-Fowler's position. Assist to a position of comfort. *Appropriate positioning reduces the work of breathing and decreases chest pain due to pericarditis.*

Risk for Decreased Cardiac Output

The acute inflammatory process of pericarditis can lead to significant pericardial effusion and cardiac tamponade. This potentially fatal complication can also occur with chronic pericardial effusion if the amount of fluid exceeds the ability of the pericardial sac to expand. Constrictive pericarditis increases the risk for decreased cardiac output because of restricted cardiac filling.

- Document vital signs hourly during the acute inflammatory processes. *Frequent assessment allows early recognition of manifestations of decreased cardiac output, such as tachycardia, hypotension, or changes in pulse pressure.*

PRACTICE ALERT
Assess heart sounds and peripheral pulses, and observe for neck vein distention and paradoxical pulse hourly. Promptly report distant, muffled heart sounds, new murmurs or extra heart sounds, decreasing quality of peripheral pulses, and distended neck veins. Acute pericardial effusion interferes with normal cardiac filling and pumping, causing venous congestion and decreased cardiac output. As the amount of fluid increases in the pericardial sac, heart sounds are obscured. A drop in systolic blood pressure of more than 10 mmHg on inspiration signifies an abnormal response to changes in intrathoracic pressure.

- Report significant changes or trends in hemodynamic parameters and dysrhythmias. *Compression of the heart interferes with venous return, increasing CVP and right atrial pressures; dysrhythmias may also occur.*
- Promptly report other signs of decreased cardiac output: decreased level of consciousness; decreased urine output; cold, clammy, mottled skin; delayed capillary refill; and weak peripheral pulses. *These signs of decreased organ and tissue perfusion indicate a significant drop in cardiac output.*
- Maintain at least one patent intravenous access site. *The client in cardiac tamponade may require rapid intravenous fluid infusion to restore blood volume and administration of emergency drugs to support the circulation.*
- Prepare for emergency pericardiocentesis and/or surgery as necessary. Provide appropriate explanations and reassurance. Observe for adverse responses during pericardiocentesis. *Excess pericardial fluid must be rapidly evacuated to prevent further compromise of cardiac output and death. Emotional support and explanations reduce the client's and family's anxiety and promote a caring atmosphere.*

Activity Intolerance

In chronic constrictive pericarditis, pericardial adhesions and scarring restrict pericardial compliance, restricting heart filling and movement. Restricted filling and ineffective cardiac contraction decrease the cardiac output. The heart cannot compensate for increased metabolic demands by increasing cardiac output, and cardiac reserve falls significantly.

- Document vital signs, cardiac rhythm, skin color, and temperature before and after activity. Note any subjective complaints of fatigue, shortness of breath, chest pain, palpitations, or other symptoms with activity. *These parameters help determine the response to increased cardiac work. Increased heart rate and respiratory rate and effort, decreased blood pressure, and dysrhythmias are indicators of activity intolerance. Pallor or cyanosis and cool, clammy, mottled skin are signs of decreased tissue perfusion. Complaints of weakness, shortness of breath, fatigue, dizziness, or palpitations are further evidence of activity intolerance.*
- Work with the client and physical therapist to develop a realistic, progressive activity plan. Monitor response. Encourage independence, but provide assistance as needed. *Client involvement in planning increases the likelihood of success, as well as the client's self-esteem and sense of control. Promoting self-care provides additional control and independence and enhances self-image. Activity that significantly increases the heart rate (more than 20 beats/min over resting) should be stopped and reassessed for intensity.*
- Plan interventions and care activities to allow uninterrupted rest and sleep. *This supports healing and restoration of physical and emotional health.*

Community-Based Care

Include the following topics when teaching the client and family in preparation for home care:

- The importance of continuing anti-inflammatory medications as ordered. Advise to take NSAIDs with food, milk, or antacids to minimize gastric distress, and to notify the physician if unable to tolerate the drug. Instruct to avoid aspirin or preparations containing aspirin while taking NSAIDs because it may interfere with activity.
- Prescribed medications, including dose, desired and possible adverse effects, and interactions with other drugs or food.
- Monitoring weight twice weekly because NSAIDs may cause fluid retention.
- Maintaining fluid intake of at least 2500 mL/day to minimize the risk of renal toxicity due to NSAID use.
- Measures to maintain activity restriction if ordered. Activity will be gradually increased once the inflammatory process has resolved.
- Manifestations of recurrent pericarditis, and the importance of reporting these manifestations promptly to the physician.

DISORDERS OF CARDIAC STRUCTURE

THE CLIENT WITH VALVULAR HEART DISEASE

Proper heart valve function ensures one-way blood flow through the heart and vascular system. **Valvular heart disease** interferes with blood flow to and from the heart. Acquired valvular disorders can result from acute conditions, such as infective endocarditis, or from chronic conditions, such as rheumatic heart disease. Rheumatic heart disease is the most common cause of valvular disease (McCance & Huether,

2006). Acute myocardial infarction also can damage heart valves, causing tearing, ischemia, or damage to the papillary muscles that affects valve leaflet function. Congenital heart defects may affect the heart valves, often with no manifestations until adulthood. Aging affects heart structure and function, and also increases the risk for valvular disease.

Physiology Review

The heart valves direct blood flow within and out of the heart. The valves are fibroelastic tissue supported by a ring of fibrous tissue (the annulus) that provides support.

The AV valves, the **mitral** (or *bicuspid*) **valve** on the left and the **tricuspid valve** on the right, separate the atria from the ventricles. These valves normally are fully open during diastole, allowing blood to flow freely from the atria into the ventricles. Rising pressure within the ventricles at the onset of systole (contraction) closes the AV valves, creating the S_1 heart sound ("lub"). The leaflets of the AV valves are connected to ventricular papillary muscles by fibrous *chordae tendineae*. The chordae tendineae prevent the valve leaflets from bulging back into the atria during systole.

The semilunar valves, the **aortic** and **pulmonic valves**, separate the ventricles from the great vessels. They open during systole, allowing blood to flow out of the heart with ventricular contraction. As the ventricle relaxes and intraventricular pressure falls at the beginning of diastole, the higher pressure within the great vessels (the aorta and pulmonary artery) closes these valves, creating the S_2 heart sound ("dup").

Pathophysiology

Valvular heart disease occurs as two major types of disorders: stenosis and regurgitation. Stenosis occurs when valve leaflets fuse together and cannot fully open or close. The valve opening narrows and becomes rigid (Figure 32–10A ■). Scarring of the valves from endocarditis or infarction, and calcium deposits can lead to stenosis. Stenotic valves impede the forward flow of blood, decreasing cardiac output because of impaired ventricular filling or ejection and stroke volume. Because stenotic

valves also do not close completely, some backflow of blood occurs when the valve should be fully closed.

Regurgitant valves (also called *insufficient* or *incompetent* valves) do not close completely (Figure 32–10B). This allows regurgitation, or backflow of blood, through the valve into the area it just left. Regurgitation can result from deformity or erosion of valve cusps caused by the vegetative lesions of bacterial endocarditis, by scarring or tearing from myocardial infarction, or by cardiac dilation. As the heart enlarges, the valve *annulus* (supporting ring of the valve) is stretched, and the valve edges no longer meet to allow complete closure.

Valvular disease causes hemodynamic changes both in front of and behind the affected valve. Blood volume and pressures are reduced in front of the valve, because flow is obstructed through a stenotic valve and backflow occurs through a regurgitant valve. By contrast, volumes and pressures characteristically increase behind the diseased valve. These hemodynamic changes may lead to pulmonary complications or heart failure. Higher pressures and compensatory changes to maintain cardiac output lead to remodeling and hypertrophy of the heart muscle.

Stenosis increases the work of the chamber behind the affected valve as the heart attempts to move blood through the narrowed opening. Excess blood volume behind regurgitant valves causes dilation of the chamber. In mitral stenosis, for example, the left atrium hypertrophies to generate enough pressure to open and deliver its blood through the narrowed mitral valve. Not all of the blood is delivered before the valve closes, leaving blood to accumulate in the left atrium. This chamber dilates to accommodate the excess volume.

Eventually, cardiac output falls as compensatory mechanisms become less effective. The normal balance of oxygen supply and demand is upset, and the heart begins to fail. Increased muscle mass and size increase myocardial oxygen consumption. The size and workload of the heart exceed its blood supply, causing ischemia and chest pain. Eventually, necrosis occurs and functional muscle is lost. Contractile force, stroke volume, and cardiac output decrease. High pressures on the left side of the heart are reflected backward into the pulmonary system, causing pulmonary edema, pulmonary hypertension, and, eventually, right ventricular failure.

Valvular disorders interfere with the smooth flow of blood through the heart. The flow becomes turbulent, causing a **murmur**, a characteristic manifestation of valvular disease. Table 32–7 describes the murmurs associated with various types of valvular disorders.

Blood forced through the narrowed opening of a stenotic valve or regurgitated from a higher pressure chamber through an incompetent valve creates a jet stream effect (much like water spurting out of a partially occluded hose opening). The physical force of this jet stream damages the endocardium of the receiving chamber, increasing the risk for infective endocarditis.

The higher pressures on the left side of the heart subject its valves (the mitral and aortic valves) to more stress and damage than those on the right side of the heart (the tricuspid and pulmonic). Pulmonic valve disease is the least common of the valvular disorders.

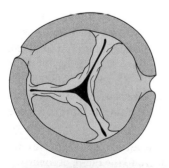 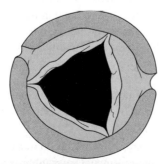

A. Thickened and stenotic valve leaflets

B. Retracted fibrosed valve openings

Figure 32–10 ■ Valvular heart disorders. *A,* Stenosis of a heart valve. *B,* An incompetent or regurgitant heart valve.

TABLE 32-7 Heart Murmur Timing and Characteristics

MURMUR	CARDIAC CYCLE TIMING	AUSCULTATION SITE	CONFIGURATION OF SOUND	CONTINUITY
Mitral stenosis	Diastole	Apical	S_2 —— S_1	Rumble that increases in sound toward the end, continuous
Mitral regurgitation	Systole	Apex	S_1 —— S_2	Holosystolic (occurs throughout systole), continuous
Aortic stenosis	Midsystolic	Right sternal border (RSB) 2nd intercostal space (ICS)	S_1 —— S_2	Crescendo–decrescendo, continuous
Aortic regurgitation	Diastole (early)	3rd ICS, left sternal border (LSB)	S_2 —— S_1	Decrescendo, continuous
Tricuspid stenosis	Diastole	Lower LSB	S_2 —— S_1	Rumble that increases in sound toward the end, continuous
Tricuspid regurgitation	Systole	4th ICS, LSB	S_1 —— S_2	Holosystolic, continuous

Mitral Stenosis

Mitral stenosis narrows the mitral valve, obstructing blood flow from the left atrium into the left ventricle during diastole. It is usually caused by rheumatic heart disease or bacterial endocarditis; it rarely results from congenital defects. It affects females more frequently (66%) than males (Kasper et al., 2005). Mitral stenosis is chronic and progressive.

In mitral valve stenosis, fibrous tissue replaces normal valve tissue, causing valve leaflets to stiffen and fuse. Resulting changes in blood flow through the valve lead to calcification of the valve leaflets. As calcium is deposited in and on the valve, the leaflets become more rigid and narrow the opening further. As the valve leaflets become less mobile, the chordae tendineae fuse, thicken, and shorten. Thromboemboli may form on the calcified leaflets.

The narrowed mitral opening impairs blood flow into the left ventricle, reducing end-diastolic volume and pressure, and decreasing stroke volume. The narrowed opening also forces the left atrium to generate higher pressure to deliver blood to the left ventricle. This leads to left atrial hypertrophy. The left atrium also dilates as obstructed blood flow increases its volume. As the resistance to blood flow increases, high atrial pressures are reflected back into the pulmonary vessels, increasing pulmonary pressures (Figure 32–11 ■). Pulmonary hypertension increases the workload of the right ventricle, causing it to dilate and hypertrophy. Eventually, heart failure occurs.

MANIFESTATIONS Mitral stenosis may be asymptomatic or cause severe impairment. Its manifestations depend on cardiac output and pulmonary vascular pressures. Dyspnea on exertion is typically the earliest manifestation. Others include cough, hemoptysis, frequent pulmonary infections such as bronchitis and pneumonia, paroxysmal nocturnal dyspnea, orthopnea, weakness, fatigue, and palpitations. As the stenosis worsens, manifestations of right heart failure, including jugular venous distention, hepatomegaly, ascites, and peripheral edema, develop. Crackles may be heard in the lung bases. In severe mitral stenosis, cyanosis of the face and extremities may be noted. Chest pain is rare but may occur.

On auscultation, a loud S_1, a split S_2, and a mitral opening snap may be heard. The opening snap reflects high left atrial pressure. The murmur of mitral stenosis occurs during diastole, and is typically low pitched, rumbling, crescendo–decrescendo. It is heard best with the bell of the stethoscope in the apical region. It may be accompanied by a palpable thrill (vibration).

COMPLICATIONS Atrial dysrhythmias, particularly atrial fibrillation, are common due to chronic atrial distention. Thrombi may form and subsequently embolize to the brain, coronary arteries, kidneys, spleen, and extremities—potentially devastating complications.

Women with mitral stenosis may be asymptomatic until pregnancy. As the heart tries to compensate for increased circulating volume (30% more in pregnancy) by increasing cardiac output,

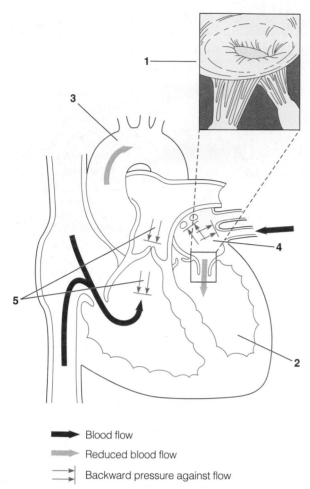

Blood flow

Reduced blood flow

Backward pressure against flow

Figure 32–11 ■ Mitral stenosis. Narrowing of the mitral valve orifice (1) reduces blood volume to left ventricle (2) reducing cardiac output (3). Rising pressure in the left atrium (4) causes left atrial hypertrophy and pulmonary congestion. Increased pressure in pulmonary vessels (5) causes hypertrophy of the right ventricle and right atrium.

left atrial pressures rise, tachycardia reduces ventricular filling and stroke volume, and pulmonary pressures increase. Sudden pulmonary edema and heart failure may threaten the lives of the mother and fetus.

Mitral Regurgitation

Mitral regurgitation or *insufficiency* allows blood to flow back into the left atrium during systole because the valve does not close fully. Rheumatic heart disease is a common cause of mitral regurgitation. Men develop mitral regurgitation more frequently than women. Degenerative calcification of the mitral annulus may cause mitral regurgitation in older women. Processes that dilate the mitral annulus or affect the supporting structures, papillary muscles, or the chordae tendineae may cause mitral regurgitation (e.g., left ventricular hypertrophy and MI). Congenital defects also may cause mitral regurgitation.

In mitral regurgitation, blood flows into both the systemic circulation and back into the left atrium through the deformed valve during systole. This increases left atrial volume (Figure 32–12 ■). The left atrium dilates to accommodate its extra volume, pulling

the posterior valve leaflet further away from the valve opening and worsening the defect. The left ventricle dilates to accommodate its increased preload and low cardiac output, further aggravating the problem.

MANIFESTATIONS Mitral regurgitation may be asymptomatic or cause symptoms such as fatigue, weakness, exertional dyspnea, and orthopnea. In severe or acute regurgitation, manifestations of left-sided heart failure develop, including pulmonary congestion and edema. High pulmonary pressures may lead to manifestations of right-sided heart failure.

The murmur of mitral regurgitation is usually loud, high pitched, rumbling, and holosystolic (occurring throughout systole). It is often accompanied by a palpable thrill and is heard most clearly at the cardiac apex. It may be characterized as a cooing or gull-like sound or have a musical quality (Kasper et al., 2005).

MITRAL VALVE PROLAPSE *Mitral valve prolapse (MVP)* is a type of mitral insufficiency that occurs when one or both mitral valve cusps billow into the atrium during ventricular systole.

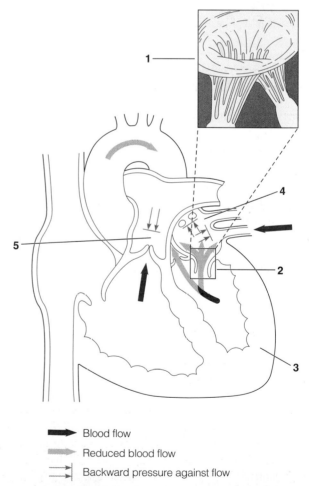

Blood flow

Reduced blood flow

Backward pressure against flow

Figure 32–12 ■ Mitral regurgitation. The mitral valve closes incompletely (1), allowing blood to regurgitate during systole from the left ventricle to the left atrium (2). Cardiac output falls; to compensate, the left ventricle hypertrophies (3). Rising left atrial pressure (4) causes left atrial hypertrophy and pulmonary congestion. Elevated pulmonary artery pressure (5) causes slight enlargement of the right ventricle.

MVP is more common in young women between ages 14 and 30; its incidence declines with age. Its cause often is unclear. It also can result from acute or chronic rheumatic damage, ischemic heart disease, or other cardiac disorders. It commonly affects people with inherited connective tissue disorders such as Marfan syndrome (see the Genetic Considerations box below). Mitral valve prolapse usually is benign, but about 0.01% to 0.02% of people with MVP have thickened mitral leaflets and a significant risk of morbidity and sudden death.

Excess collagen tissue in the valve leaflets and elongated chordae tendineae impair closure of the mitral valve, allowing the leaflets to billow into the left atrium during systole. Some ventricular blood volume regurgitates into the left atrium (Figure 32–13 ■).

MANIFESTATIONS AND COMPLICATIONS Mitral valve prolapse usually is asymptomatic. A midsystolic ejection click or murmur may be audible. A high-pitched late systolic murmur, sometimes described as a "whoop" or "honk," due to the regurgitation of blood through the valve, may develop in MVP. Atypical chest pain is the most common symptom of MVP. It may be left sided or substernal and is frequently related to fatigue, not exertion. Tachydysrhythmias may develop with MVP, causing palpitations, light-headedness, and syncope. Increased sympathetic nervous system tone may cause a sense of anxiety (Woods et al., 2004).

Mitral valve prolapse increases the risk for bacterial endocarditis. Progressive worsening of regurgitation can lead to heart failure. Thrombi may form on prolapsed valve leaflets; embolization may cause transient ischemic attacks (TIAs).

Aortic Stenosis

Aortic stenosis obstructs blood flow from the left ventricle into the aorta during systole. Aortic stenosis is more common in males (80%) than females (Kasper et al., 2005). Aortic stenosis may be idiopathic, or due to a congenital defect, rheumatic damage, or degenerative changes. When rheumatic heart disease is the cause, mitral valve deformity is also often present. RHD destroys aortic valve leaflets, with fibrosis and calcification causing rigidity and scarring. In the older adult, calcific aortic stenosis may result from degenerative changes associ-

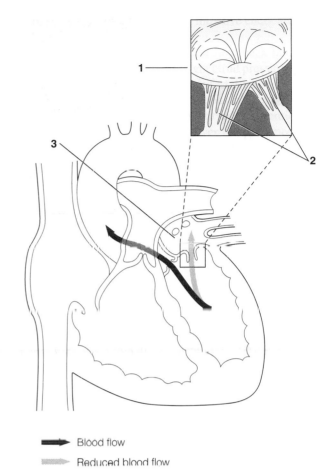

Blood flow

Reduced blood flow

Figure 32–13 ■ Mitral valve prolapse. Excess tissue in the valve leaflets *(1)* and elongated chordae tendineae *(2)* impair mitral valve closure during systole. Some ventricular blood regurgitates into the left atrium *(3)*.

ated with aging. Constant "wear and tear" on this valve can lead to fibrosis and calcification. Idiopathic calcific stenosis generally is mild and does not impair cardiac output.

As aortic stenosis progresses, the valve annulus decreases in size, increasing the work of the left ventricle to eject its volume through the narrowed opening into the aorta. To compensate, the ventricle hypertrophies to maintain an adequate stroke volume and cardiac output (Figure 32–14 ■). Left ventricular compliance also decreases. The additional workload increases myocardial oxygen consumption, which can precipitate myocardial ischemia. Coronary blood flow may also decrease in aortic stenosis. As left ventricular end-diastolic pressure increases because of reduced stroke volume, left atrial pressures increase. These pressures also affect the pulmonary vascular system; pulmonary vascular congestion and pulmonary edema may result.

COURSE AND MANIFESTATIONS Aortic stenosis may be asymptomatic for many years. As the disease progresses and compensation fails, usually between age 50 and 70 years, obstructed cardiac output causes manifestations of left ventricular failure. Dyspnea on exertion, angina pectoris, and exertional syncope are classic manifestations of aortic stenosis. Pulse pressure, an indicator of stroke volume, narrows to 30 mmHg

GENETIC CONSIDERATIONS
Clients with Marfan Syndrome

Marfan syndrome is a genetic (autosomal dominant) connective tissue disorder that affects the skeleton, eyes, and cardiovascular system. Skeletal characteristics include a long, thin body, with long extremities and long, tapering fingers, sometimes called *arachnodactyly* (spider fingers) (Copstead & Banasik, 2005). Joints are hyperextensible, and skeletal deformities such as kyphosis, scoliosis, pigeon chest, or pectus excavatum are common. The potentially life-threatening cardiovascular effects of Marfan syndrome include mitral valve prolapse, progressive dilation of the aortic valve ring, and weakness of arterial walls. People with Marfan syndrome frequently die young, between 30 and 40 years, often due to dissection and rupture of the aorta (Porth, 2005).

- *Echocardiography* is used routinely to diagnose valvular disease. Thickened valve leaflets, vegetations or growths on valve leaflets, myocardial function, and chamber size can be determined, and pressure gradients across valves and pulmonary artery pressures can be estimated. Either transthoracic or transesophageal echocardiography may be used.
- *Chest x-ray* can identify cardiac hypertrophy, chamber and great vessel enlargement, and dilation of the pulmonary vasculature. Calcification of the valve leaflets and annular openings may also be visible.
- *Electrocardiography* can demonstrate atrial and ventricular hypertrophy, conduction defects, and dysrhythmias associated with valvular disease.
- *Cardiac catheterization* may be used to assess contractility and to determine the pressure gradients across the heart valves, in the heart chambers, and in the pulmonary system.

Medications

Heart failure resulting from valvular disease is treated with diuretics, ACE inhibitors, vasodilators, and possibly digitalis glycosides. Digitalis increases the force of myocardial contraction to maintain cardiac output. Diuretics, ACE inhibitors, and vasodilators reduce preload and afterload. (See the Medication Administration box on pages 1033–1034.)

In clients with valvular disorders, atrial distention often causes atrial fibrillation. Digitalis or small doses of beta-blockers are given to slow the ventricular response. (See Chapter 31 ∞ for more information about atrial fibrillation and its treatment.) Anticoagulant therapy is added to prevent clot and embolus formation, a common complication of atrial fibrillation as blood pools in the noncontracting atria. Anticoagulant therapy also is required following insertion of a mechanical heart valve. See Chapter 35 ∞ for more information about anticoagulant therapy.

Valvular damage increases the risk for infective endocarditis as altered blood flow allows bacterial colonization. Antibiotics are prescribed prophylactically prior to any dental work, invasive procedures, or surgery to minimize the risk of bacteremia (bacteria in the blood) and subsequent endocarditis.

Percutaneous Balloon Valvuloplasty

Percutaneous balloon valvuloplasty is an invasive procedure performed in the cardiac catheterization laboratory. A balloon catheter similar to that used in coronary angioplasty procedures is inserted into the femoral vein or artery. Guided by fluoroscopy, the catheter is advanced into the heart and positioned with the balloon straddling the stenotic valve. The balloon is then inflated for approximately 90 seconds to divide the fused leaflets and enlarge the valve orifice (Figure 32–16 ■). Balloon valvuloplasty is the treatment of choice for symptomatic mitral valve stenosis. It is used to treat children and young adults with aortic stenosis, and may be indicated for older adults who are poor surgical risks, and as a "bridge to surgery" when heart function is severely compromised (Kasper et al., 2005). Nursing care of the client with a balloon valvuloplasty is similar to that of the client following percutaneous coronary revascularization (see page 978).

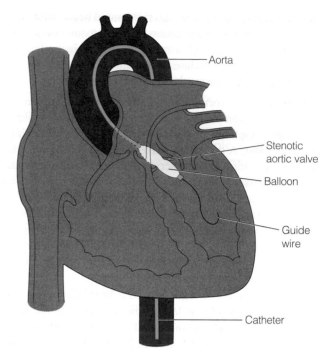

Figure 32–16 ■ Balloon valvuloplasty. The balloon catheter is guided into position straddling the stenosed valve. The balloon is then inflated to increase the size of the valve opening.

Surgery

Surgery to repair or replace the diseased valve may be done to restore valve function, alleviate symptoms, and prevent complications and death. Ideally, diseased valves are repaired or replaced before cardiopulmonary function is severely compromised. The diseased valve is repaired when possible, because the risk for surgical mortality and complications is lower than with valve replacement.

RECONSTRUCTIVE SURGERY *Valvuloplasty* is a general term for reconstruction or repair of a heart valve. Methods include "patching" the perforated portion of the leaflet, resecting excess tissue, debriding vegetations or calcification, and other techniques. Valvuloplasty may be used for stenotic or regurgitant mitral and tricuspid valves, mitral valve prolapse, and aortic stenosis. Common valvuloplasty procedures include the following:

- *Open commissurotomy,* surgical division of fused valve leaflets, is done to open stenotic valves. Fused commissures (junctions between valve leaflets or cusps) are incised, and calcium deposits are debrided as needed.
- *Annuloplasty* repairs a narrowed or an enlarged or dilated valve annulus, the supporting ring of the valve. A prosthetic ring may be used to resize the opening, or stitches and purse-string sutures may be used to reduce and gather excess tissue. Annuloplasty may be used for either stenotic or regurgitant valves.

VALVE REPLACEMENT Valve replacement is indicated when manifestations of valve dysfunction develop, preferably before left heart function is seriously impaired. In general, three factors determine the outcome of valve replacement surgery: (1) heart function at the time of surgery, (2) intraoperative and

TABLE 32–8 Advantages and Disadvantages of Prosthetic Heart Valves

CATEGORY	TYPES	ADVANTAGES	DISADVANTAGES
Mechanical valves	Ball-and-cage Tilting disk	Long-term durability Good hemodynamics	Lifetime anticoagulation Audible click Risk of thromboembolism Infections are harder to treat
Biologic tissue valves	Porcine heterograft Bovine heterograft Human aortic homograft	Low incidence of thromboembolism No long-term anticoagulation Good hemodynamics Quiet Infections are easier to treat	Prone to deterioration Frequent replacement is required

postoperative care, and (3) characteristics and durability of the replacement valve.

Many different prosthetic heart valves are available, including mechanical and biologic tissue valves. Selection depends on the valve hemodynamics, resistance to clot formation, ease of insertion, anatomic suitability, and client acceptance (Rothrock, 2003). The client's age, underlying condition, and contraindications to anticoagulation (such as a desire to become pregnant) also are considered in selecting the appropriate prosthesis. Table 32–8 lists the advantages and disadvantages of biologic and mechanical valves.

Biologic tissue valves may be *heterografts*, excised from a pig (Figure 32–17A) or made of calf pericardium, or *homografts* from a human (obtained from a cadaver or during heart transplant). Biologic valves allow more normal blood flow and have a low risk of thrombus formation. As a result, long-term anticoagulation rarely is necessary. They are less durable, however, than mechanical valves. Up to 50% of biologic valves must be replaced by 15 years.

Mechanical prosthetic valves have the major advantage of long-term durability. These valves are frequently used when life expectancy exceeds 10 years. Their major disadvantage is

the need for lifetime anticoagulation to prevent the development of clots on the valve.

Most mechanical valves are either a tilting-disk (Figure 32–17B) or a ball-and-cage design. The tilting-disk valve designs are frequently used because they have a lower profile than the caged-ball types, allowing blood to flow through the valve with less obstruction. The St. Jude bileaflet design has good hemodynamics and low risk for clot formation. Both biologic and mechanical valves increase the risk of endocarditis, although its incidence is fairly low.

NURSING CARE

Health Promotion

Preventing rheumatic heart disease is a key element in preventing heart valve disorders. Rheumatic heart disease is a consequence of rheumatic fever (see the previous section of this chapter), an immune process that may be a sequela to beta-hemolytic streptococcal infection of the pharynx (strep throat). Early treatment of strep throat prevents rheumatic fever. Teach individual clients, families, and communities

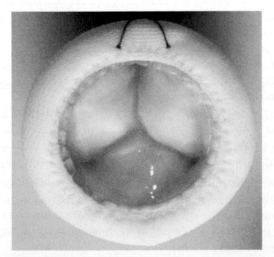
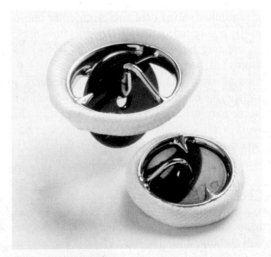

Figure 32–17 ■ Prosthetic heart valves. *A,* Mosaic tissue valve. *B,* Medtronic Hall Prosthetic valve.
Courtesy of Medtronic, Inc.

about the importance of timely and effective treatment of strep throat. Emphasize the importance of completing the full prescription of antibiotics to prevent development of resistant bacteria. Prophylactic antibiotic therapy before invasive procedures to prevent infectious endocarditis is an important health promotion measure for clients with preexisting heart disease.

Assessment

Assessment data related to valvular heart disease include the following:

- *Health history:* Complaints of decreasing exercise tolerance, dyspnea on exertion, palpitations; history of frequent respiratory infections; previous history of rheumatic heart disease, endocarditis, or a heart murmur.
- *Physical examination:* Vital signs; skin color and temperature, evidence of clubbing or peripheral edema; neck vein distention; breath sounds; heart sounds and presence of S_3, S_4, or murmur; timing, grade, and characteristics of any murmur; palpate for cardiac heave and thrills; abdominal contour, liver and spleen size.
- *Diagnostic tests:* Echocardiogram and cardiac catheterization reports; cardiac index and cardiac output.

Nursing Diagnoses and Interventions

Nursing priorities include maintaining cardiac output, managing manifestations of the disorder, teaching about the disease process and its management, and preventing complications. Nursing care of the client undergoing valve surgery is similar to that of the client having other types of open-heart surgery, with increased attention to anticoagulation and preventing endocarditis.

Decreased Cardiac Output

Nearly all valve disorders affect ventricular filling and/or emptying, reducing cardiac output. Stenosis of the AV valves impairs ventricular filling and increases atrial pressures. Regurgitation of these valves reduces cardiac output as a portion of the blood in the ventricle regurgitates into the atria during systole. Stenosis of the semilunar valves obstructs ventricular outflow to the great vessels; regurgitation allows blood to flow back into the ventricles, creating higher filling pressures. When compensatory measures fail, heart failure develops.

- Monitor vital signs and hemodynamic parameters, reporting changes from the baseline. *A fall in systolic blood pressure and tachycardia may indicate decreased cardiac output. Increasing pulmonary artery and pulmonary wedge pressures may also indicate decreased cardiac output, causing increased congestion and pressure in the pulmonary vascular system.*

PRACTICE ALERT

Promptly report changes in level of consciousness; distended neck veins; dyspnea or respiratory crackles; urine output less than 30 mL/h; cool, clammy, or cyanotic skin; diminished peripheral pulses; or slow capillary refill. These findings indicate decreased cardiac output and impaired tissue and organ perfusion.

- Monitor intake and output; weigh daily. Report weight gain of 3 to 5 lb within 24 hours. *Fluid retention is a compensatory mechanism that occurs when cardiac output decreases; 2.2 lb (1 kg) of weight equals 1 L of fluid.*
- Restrict fluids as ordered. *Fluid intake may be restricted to reduce cardiac workload and pressures within the heart and pulmonary circuit.*
- Monitor oxygen saturation continuously and arterial blood gases as ordered. Report oxygen saturation less than 95% (or as specified) and abnormal ABG results. *Oxygen saturation levels and ABGs allow assessment of oxygenation.*
- Elevate the head of the bed. Administer supplemental oxygen as ordered. *These measures improve alveolar ventilation and oxygenation.*
- Provide for physical, emotional, and mental rest. *Physical and psychologic rest decrease the cardiac workload.*
- Administer prescribed medications as ordered to reduce cardiac workload. *Diuretics, ACE inhibitors, and direct vasodilators may be prescribed to reduce fluid volume and afterload, reducing cardiac work.*

Activity Intolerance

Altered blood flow through the heart impairs delivery of oxygen and nutrients to the tissues. As the heart muscle fails and is unable to compensate for altered blood flow, tissue perfusion is further compromised. Dyspnea on exertion is often an early symptom of valvular disease.

- Monitor vital signs before and during activities. *A change in heart rate of more than 20 bpm, a change of 20 mmHg or more in systolic BP, and complaints of dyspnea, shortness of breath, excessive fatigue, chest pain, diaphoresis, dizziness, or syncope may indicate activity intolerance.*
- Encourage self-care and gradually increasing activities as allowed and tolerated. Provide for rest periods, uninterrupted sleep, and adequate nutritional intake. *Gradual progression of activities avoids excessive cardiac stress. Encouraging self-care increases the client's self-esteem and sense of power. Adequate rest and nutrition facilitate healing, decrease fatigue, and increase energy reserves.*
- Provide assistance as needed. Suggest use of a shower chair, sitting while brushing hair or teeth, and other energy-saving measures. *Reducing energy expenditure helps maintain a balance of oxygen supply and demand.*
- Consult with cardiac rehabilitation specialist or physical therapist for in-bed exercises and an activity plan. *In-bed exercises may help improve strength.*
- Discuss ways to conserve energy at home. *Information provides practical ways to deal with activity limitations and empowers the client to manage these limitations.*

Risk for Infection

Damaged and deformed valve leaflets and turbulent blood flow through the heart significantly increase the risk of infective endocarditis. Invasive diagnostic and monitoring lines (e.g., cardiac catheterization, hemodynamic monitoring) and disrupted skin with surgery also increase the risk of infection.

- Use aseptic technique for all invasive procedures. *Invasive procedures breach the body's protective mechanisms, poten-*

tially allowing bacteria to enter. Aseptic technique reduces this risk.

- Assess wounds and catheter sites for redness, swelling, warmth, pain, or evidence of drainage. *These signs of inflammation may signal infection.*
- Administer antibiotics as ordered. Ensure completion of the full course. *Antibiotics are used to prevent and treat infection. Completion of the full course of therapy prevents drug-resistant organisms from multiplying.*
- Monitor WBC and differential. Notify physician of leukocytosis or leukopenia. *A high WBC count and increased percentage of immature WBCs (bands) may indicate bacterial infection; a low WBC count may indicate an impaired immune response and increased susceptibility to infection.*

Ineffective Protection

Anticoagulant therapy commonly is prescribed for clients with chronic atrial fibrillation, a history of emboli, and following valve replacement surgery. Although chronic anticoagulant therapy decreases the risk of clots and emboli, it increases the risk for bleeding and hemorrhage.

- Test stools and vomitus for occult blood. *Bleeding due to excessive anticoagulation may not be apparent.*
- Instruct to avoid using aspirin or other NSAIDs. Encourage reading ingredient labels on over-the-counter drugs; many contain aspirin. *Aspirin and other NSAIDs interfere with clotting and may potentiate the effects of the anticoagulant therapy.*
- Advise using a soft-bristled toothbrush, electric razor, and gentle touch when cleaning fragile skin. *These measures decrease the risk of skin or gum trauma and bleeding.*

Community-Based Care

For most clients, valvular disease is a chronic condition. The client has the primary responsibility for managing effects of the disorder. To prepare the client and family for home care, discuss the following topics:
- Management of symptoms, including any necessary activity restrictions or lifestyle changes
- The importance of adequate rest to prevent fatigue
- Diet restrictions to reduce fluid retention and symptoms of heart failure
- Information about prescribed medications, including purpose, desired and possible adverse effects, scheduling, and possible interactions with other drugs
- The importance of keeping follow-up appointments to monitor the disease and its treatment
- Notifying all healthcare providers about valve disease or surgery to facilitate prescription of prophylactic antibiotics before invasive procedures or dental work
- Manifestations to immediately report to the healthcare provider: increasing severity of symptoms, especially of worsening heart failure or pulmonary edema; signs of transient ischemic attacks or other embolic events; evidence of bleeding, such as joint pain, easy bruising, black and tarry stools, bleeding gums, or blood in the urine or sputum.

Provide referrals to community resources such as home maintenance services, home health services, and structured cardiac rehabilitation programs. Refer the client and family (especially the primary food preparer) to a dietitian or nutritionist for teaching and assistance with menu planning. See the accompanying Nursing Care Plan for additional nursing care and teaching for a client with mitral valve prolapse.

THE CLIENT WITH CARDIOMYOPATHY

The **cardiomyopathies** are disorders that affect the heart muscle itself. They are a diverse group of disorders that affect both systolic and diastolic functions. Cardiomyopathies may be either primary or secondary in origin. Primary cardiomyopathies are idiopathic; their cause is unknown. Secondary cardiomyopathies occur as a result of other processes, such as ischemia, infectious disease, exposure to toxins, connective tissue disorders, metabolic disorders, or nutritional deficiencies. In many cases, the cause of cardiomyopathy is unknown. Close to 27,000 deaths annually are directly attributed to cardiomyopathy. Mortality associated with cardiomyopathy is higher in older adults, men, and African Americans (AHA, 2005).

Pathophysiology

The cardiomyopathies are categorized by their pathophysiology and presentation into three groups: dilated, hypertrophic, and restrictive. Table 32–9 compares the causes, pathophysiology, manifestations, and management of the cardiomyopathies.

Dilated Cardiomyopathy

Dilated cardiomyopathy is the most common type of cardiomyopathy, accounting for 87% of cases (AHA, 2005). Dilated cardiomyopathy also is a common cause of heart failure, accounting for about one in three cases. It is primarily a disease of middle age males; African American males have a higher risk than whites (Kasper et al., 2005).

NURSING CARE PLAN   A Client with Mitral Valve Prolapse

Julie Snow, a 22-year-old college student, sees a nurse practitioner at the college health clinic for a physical examination after experiencing palpitations, fatigue, and a headache during midterm examinations. Ms. Snow tells Lakisha Johnson, FNP, "I'm scared that something is wrong with me."

Over the last few months, Ms. Snow has had occasional palpitations that she describes as "feeling like my heart is doing flip-flops." Rarely, these palpitations have been accompanied by a sharp, stabbing pain in her chest that lasts only a few seconds. She initially attributed her symptoms to stress, but she is increasingly concerned because the "attacks" are becoming more frequent. Ms. Snow states that she has "always been healthy," does not smoke, uses alcohol socially, and exercises, albeit intermittently. Ms. Snow admits that she has been drinking a lot of coffee and cola and eating a lot of "junk food" lately.

ASSESSMENT

Ms. Johnson's assessment of Ms. Snow documents the following: height 66 in. (168 cm), weight 140 lb (63.6 kg), T 99.3, BP 118/64, P 82, and R 18. Slightly anxious but in no acute distress. Systolic click and soft crescendo murmur grade II/VI noted on auscultation. Apical impulse at fifth ICS left MCL. Lungs clear to auscultation. Review of remaining systems reveals no apparent abnormalities. An ECG shows sinus rhythm with occasional PACs. Based on the admission history, manifestations, and physical assessment, Ms. Johnson suspects mitral valve prolapse (MVP).

DIAGNOSES

- *Anxiety* related to fear of heart disease and implications for lifestyle
- *Powerlessness* related to unpredictability of symptoms
- *Risk of Infection (Endocarditis)* related to altered valve function

EXPECTED OUTCOMES

- Verbalize an understanding of MVP and its management.
- Discuss ways to decrease or relieve MVP symptoms.
- Acknowledge the risk for endocarditis and identify precautions to prevent it.

PLANNING AND IMPLEMENTATION

- Consult with and refer to cardiologist for continued monitoring and follow-up.
- Teach about MVP, including heart valve anatomy, physiology, and function, common manifestations of MVP, and treatment rationale.
- Discuss symptoms of progressive mitral regurgitation, and the need to report these to the cardiologist.
- Discuss recommended follow-up care and its rationale.

- Allow to verbalize feelings and share concerns about MVP. Encourage to attend an MVP support group meeting.
- Discuss the prognosis for MVP, emphasizing that most clients live normal lives using diet and lifestyle management.
- Instruct to keep a weekly record of symptoms and their frequency for 1 month.
- Discuss lifestyle changes to manage symptoms: aerobic exercise with warm-up and cooldown periods; maintaining adequate fluid intake, especially during hot weather or exercise; relaxation techniques (e.g., meditation, deep-breathing exercises, music therapy, yoga, guided imagery, heat therapy, or progressive muscle relaxation) to perform daily; avoiding caffeine and crash diets; forming healthy eating habits.
- Teach about infective endocarditis risk and prevention with prophylactic antibiotics. Encourage notifying dentist and other healthcare providers of MVP before dental or any invasive procedure.

EVALUATION

After several educational sessions at the college health clinic, Ms. Snow verbalizes an understanding of MVP by explaining heart valve function, listing common manifestations of MVP, and describing indications of deteriorating heart function. She states she will report these manifestations to her cardiologist if they occur. She is given a booklet on MVP for additional reading. She also verbalizes understanding of the risk of endocarditis, and states that she will notify her doctors of her MVP and the need for antibiotics before invasive procedures. Ms. Snow is attending a monthly MVP support group (led by a cardiology clinical nurse specialist) on campus and states, "I am so glad to know I'm not alone! It really helps to know that others are living well with MVP." Her weekly symptom log shows her symptoms are associated with late-night studying and drinking large amounts of coffee and cola. Ms. Snow has moderated her caffeine intake and increased her fluids, relieving her symptoms. In addition, Ms. Snow is taking a relaxation music therapy class. Ms. Snow states that she realizes that she has "the ability to control my life through the choices I make."

CRITICAL THINKING IN THE NURSING PROCESS

1. Develop an action plan for Ms. Snow that outlines specific activities she can use to manage symptoms of MVP.
2. Why are clients with symptomatic MVP encouraged to include regular exercise in their health habits?
3. How does the support of family, friends, and other people with MVP assist MVP clients in managing their condition?
4. What manifestations would indicate a progressive worsening of Ms. Snow's mitral regurgitation?

See Evaluating Your Response in Appendix C.

The cause of dilated cardiomyopathy is unknown, although it appears to frequently result from toxins, metabolic conditions, or infection. Reversible dilated cardiomyopathy may develop due to alcohol and cocaine abuse, chemotherapeutic drugs, pregnancy, and systemic hypertension. Up to 20% of cases of dilated cardiomyopathy may be genetic in origin, most commonly transmitted in an autosomal dominant pattern, although autosomal recessive, X-linked, and mitochondrial

patterns of inheritance also are seen (Kasper et al., 2005; Porth, 2005).

In dilated cardiomyopathy, heart chambers dilate and ventricular contraction is impaired. Both end-diastolic and end-systolic volumes increase, and the left ventricular ejection fraction is substantially reduced, decreasing cardiac output. Left ventricular dilation is prominent; left ventricular hypertrophy is usually minimal. The right ventricle also may be enlarged. Ex-

TABLE 32–9 Classifications of Cardiomyopathy

	DILATED	HYPERTROPHIC	RESTRICTIVE
Causes	Usually idiopathic; may be secondary to chronic alcoholism or myocarditis	Hereditary; may be secondary to chronic hypertension	Usually secondary to amyloidosis, radiation, or myocardial fibrosis
Pathophysiology	Scarring and atrophy of myocardial cells Thickening of ventricular wall Dilation of heart chambers Impaired ventricular pumping Increased end-diastolic and end-systolic volumes Mural thrombi common	Hypertrophy of ventricular muscle mass Small left ventricular volume Septal hypertrophy may obstruct left ventricular outflow Left atrial dilation	Excess rigidity of ventricular walls restricts filling Myocardial contractility remains relatively normal
Manifestations	Heart failure Cardiomegaly Dysrhythmias S_3 and S_4 gallop; murmur of mitral regurgitation	Dyspnea, anginal pain, syncope Left ventricular hypertrophy Dysrhythmias Loud S_4 Sudden death	Dyspnea, fatigue Right-sided heart failure Mild to moderate cardiomegaly S_3 and S_4 Mitral regurgitation murmur
Management	Management of heart failure Implantable cardioverter-defibrillator (ICD) as needed Cardiac transplantation	Beta-blockers Calcium channel blockers Antidysrhythmic agents ICD, dual-chamber pacing Surgical excision of part of the ventricular septum	Management of heart failure Exercise restriction

tensive interstitial fibrosis (scarring) is evident; necrotic my-ocardial cells also may be seen (Kasper et al., 2005).

MANIFESTATIONS AND COURSE Manifestations of dilated cardiomyopathy develop gradually. Heart failure often presents years after the onset of dilation and pump failure. Both right- and left-sided failure occur, with dyspnea on exertion, orthopnea, paroxysmal nocturnal dyspnea, weakness, fatigue, peripheral edema, and ascites. Both S_3 and S_4 heart sounds are commonly heard, as well as an AV regurgitation murmur. Dysrhythmias are common, including supraventricular tachycardias, atrial fibrillation, and complex ventricular tachycardias. Untreated dysrhythmias can lead to sudden death (Porth, 2005). Mural thrombi (blood clots in the heart wall) may form in the left ventricular apex and embolize to other parts of the body.

The prognosis of dilated cardiomyopathy is grim; most clients get progressively worse and 50% die within 5 years after the diagnosis; 75% die within 10 years (AHA, 2005).

Hypertrophic Cardiomyopathy

Hypertrophic cardiomyopathy is characterized by decreased compliance of the left ventricle and hypertrophy of the ventricular muscle mass. This impairs ventricular filling, leading to small end-diastolic volumes and low cardiac output. About half of all clients with hypertrophic cardiomyopathy have a family history of the disease. It is genetically transmitted in an autosomal dominant pattern (Kasper et al., 2005).

The pattern of left ventricular hypertrophy is unique in that the muscle may not hypertrophy "equally." In a majority of clients, the interventricular septal mass, especially the upper portion, increases to a greater extent than the free wall of the ventricle. The enlarged upper septum narrows the passageway of blood into the aorta, impairing ventricular outflow. For this reason, this disorder is also known as *idiopathic hypertrophic subaortic stenosis (IHSS)* or *hypertrophic obstructive cardiomyopathy (HOCM)*.

MANIFESTATIONS AND COURSE Hypertrophic cardiomyopathy may be asymptomatic for many years. Symptoms typically occur when increased oxygen demand causes increased ventricular contractility. They may develop suddenly during or after physical activity; in children and young adults, sudden cardiac death may be the first sign of the disorder. Hypertrophic cardiomyopathy is the probable or definite cause of death in 36% of young athletes who die suddenly (AHA, 2005). It is hypothesized that sudden cardiac death is due to ventricular dysrhythmias or hemodynamic factors. Predictors of sudden cardiac death in this population include age of less than 30 years, a family history of sudden death, syncopal episodes, severe ventricular hypertrophy, and ventricular tachycardia seen on ambulatory ECG monitoring (Kasper et al., 2005). (For a brief synopsis of a nursing research study regarding family presence during CPR and invasive procedures, see the box below.)

The usual manifestations of hypertrophic cardiomyopathy are dyspnea, angina, and syncope. Angina may result from ischemia due to overgrowth of the ventricular muscle, coronary artery abnormalities, or decreased coronary artery perfusion. Syncope may occur when the outflow tract obstruction severely decreases cardiac output and blood flow to the brain. Ventricular dysrhythmias are common; atrial fibrillation also may develop. Other manifestations of hypertrophic cardiomyopathy include fatigue, dizziness, and palpitations. A harsh, crescendo–decrescendo systolic murmur of variable intensity heard best at the lower left sternal border and apex is characteristic in hypertrophic cardiomyopathy. An S_4 may also be noted on auscultation.

Restrictive Cardiomyopathy

The least common form of cardiomyopathy, *restrictive cardiomyopathy*, is characterized by rigid ventricular walls that impair diastolic filling. Causes of restrictive cardiomyopathy include myocardial fibrosis and infiltrative processes, such as amyloidosis. Fibrosis of the myocardium and endocardium causes excessive stiffness and rigidity of the ventricles. Decreased ventricular compliance impairs filling, with decreased ventricular size, elevated end-diastolic pressures, and decreased cardiac output. Contractility is unaffected, and the ejection fraction is normal.

MANIFESTATIONS AND COURSE The manifestations of restrictive cardiomyopathy are those of heart failure and decreased tissue perfusion. Dyspnea on exertion and exercise intolerance are common. Jugular venous pressure is elevated, and S_3 and S_4 are common. The prognosis for restrictive cardiomyopathy is poor. Most clients die within 3 years, and the systemic nature of the underlying disease process precludes effective treatment.

INTERDISCIPLINARY CARE

With the exception of treating an underlying cause, little can be done to treat either dilated or restrictive cardiomyopathies. For these disorders, treatment focuses on managing heart failure and treating dysrhythmias. Refer to the section of this chapter

---

NURSING RESEARCH   Evidence-Based Practice: Sudden Cardiac Death

When cardiac arrest occurs or invasive procedures are performed, family members typically are asked to leave the client's care unit. The traditional rationale for this practice is fear of disrupted clinical interventions, trauma of the witnesses, and risk for increased hospital liability. However, in 1995, the Emergency Nurses Association (ENA) adopted a position supporting family presence during invasive procedures, including resuscitation efforts (CPR), as a means of "preserving the wholeness, dignity, and integrity of the family unit from birth to death" (Myers et al., 2000, p. 33). This study evaluated the responses of families, nurses, and physicians to family presence during invasive procedures and CPR.

Results of the study showed that families saw their presence as a positive experience and their right. They viewed themselves as active care partners, and being present met their needs for information and providing comfort and connection with the client. Nurses overwhelmingly supported family presence; attending physicians also demonstrated a positive response. Physician residents were the least supportive of family presence.

IMPLICATIONS FOR NURSING

Family members often are asked to leave the client's side during invasive procedures and CPR with the intention of protecting them from the trauma of witnessing painful or distressing events.

This study clearly showed being present as a positive experience, even when the ultimate outcome was the client's death.

Offering the opportunity to be present and providing information as well as psychologic and emotional support to an appropriate family member during invasive procedures and CPR supports the family unit and the client during times of crisis. Screening is important: People who are combative, emotionally unstable, or have altered mental status (e.g., dementia, alcohol intoxication) probably are not appropriate. It also is important to allow families to decline the invitation without guilt.

CRITICAL THINKING IN CLIENT CARE

1. Identify procedures and situations in which family members are often asked to leave the client's side. When would it be appropriate to allow at least one significant other to remain with the client?
2. How would you present the option and prepare a family member for being present during a traumatic event such as CPR following the sudden death of a young adult with undiagnosed hypertrophic cardiomyopathy?
3. You support family presence during traumatic events and procedures, but your charge nurse does not. What steps might you use to effect a change in policy on your unit?

on heart failure and Chapter 31 ∞ for specific treatment strategies. Treatment of hypertrophic cardiomyopathy focuses on reducing contractility and preventing sudden cardiac death. Strenuous physical exertion is restricted, because it may precipitate dysrhythmias or sudden cardiac death. Dietary and sodium restrictions may help diminish the manifestations.

Diagnosis

Diagnosis begins with a history and physical assessment to rule out known causes of heart failure. Other tests may include the following:

- *Echocardiography* is done to assess chamber size and thickness, ventricular wall motion, valvular function, and systolic and diastolic function of the heart.
- *Electrocardiography* and *ambulatory ECG monitoring* demonstrate cardiac enlargement and detect dysrhythmias.
- *Chest x-ray* shows cardiomegaly, enlargement of the heart, and any pulmonary congestion or edema.
- *Hemodynamic studies* are used to assess cardiac output and pressures in the cardiac chambers and pulmonary vascular system.
- *Radionuclear scans* help identify changes in ventricular volume and mass, as well as perfusion deficits.
- *Cardiac catheterization* and *coronary angiography* may be done to evaluate coronary perfusion, the cardiac chambers, valves, and great vessels for function and structure, pressure relationships, and cardiac output.
- *Myocardial biopsy* uses the transvenous route to obtain myocardial tissue for biopsy. The cells are examined for infiltration, fibrosis, or inflammation.

Medications

The drug regimen used to treat heart failure also is used for dilated or restrictive cardiomyopathy. This includes ACE inhibitors, vasodilators, and digitalis (see the previous section of this chapter). Beta-blockers also may be used with caution in clients with dilated cardiomyopathy. Anticoagulants are given to reduce the risk of thrombus formation and embolization. Antidysrhythmic drugs are avoided if possible due to their tendency to precipitate further dysrhythmias (Kasper et al., 2005).

Beta-blockers are the drugs of choice to reduce anginal symptoms and syncopal episodes associated with hypertrophic cardiomyopathy. The negative inotropic effects of beta-blockers and calcium channel blockers decrease the myocardial contractility, decreasing obstruction of the outflow tract. Beta-blockers also decrease heart rate and increase ventricular compliance, increasing diastolic filling time and cardiac output. Vasodilators, digitalis, nitrates, and diuretics are contraindicated. Amiodarone may be used to treat ventricular dysrhythmias (Kasper et al., 2005).

Surgery

Without definitive treatment, clients with cardiomyopathy develop end-stage heart failure. Cardiac transplant is the definitive treatment for dilated cardiomyopathy. Ventricular assist devices may be used to support cardiac output until a donor heart is available. Transplantation is not a viable option for restrictive cardiomyopathy, because transplantation does not eliminate the underlying process causing infiltration or fibrosis, and eventually the transplanted organ is affected as well. See the section on heart failure for more information about cardiac transplantation.

In severely symptomatic clients with obstructive hypertrophic cardiomyopathy, excess muscle may be surgically resected from the aortic valve outflow tract. The septum is incised, and tissue is removed. This procedure provides lasting improvement in about 75% of clients (Kasper et al., 2005).

An implantable cardioverter-defibrillator (ICD) often is inserted to treat potentially lethal dysrhythmias, reducing the need for antidysrhythmic medications. A dual-chamber pacemaker also may be used to treat hypertrophic cardiomyopathy.

NURSING CARE

Nursing assessment and care for clients with dilated and restrictive cardiomyopathy are similar to those for clients with heart failure. Teaching about the disease process and its management is vital. Some degree of activity restriction often is necessary; assist to conserve energy while encouraging self-care. Support coping skills and adaptation to required lifestyle changes. Provide information and support for decision making about cardiac transplantation if that is an option. Discuss the toxic and vasodilator effects of alcohol, and encourage abstinence. See the nursing care section for heart failure for nursing diagnoses and suggested interventions.

The client with hypertrophic cardiomyopathy requires care similar to that provided for myocardial ischemia; nitrates and other vasodilators, however, are avoided. If surgery is performed, nursing care is similar to that for any client undergoing open-heart surgery or cardiac transplant. Discuss the genetic transmission of hypertrophic cardiomyopathy, and suggest screening of close relatives (parents and siblings).

Provide pre- and postoperative care and teaching as appropriate for clients undergoing invasive procedures or surgery for cardiomyopathy.

Nursing diagnoses that may be appropriate for clients with cardiomyopathy include:

- *Decreased Cardiac Output* related to impaired left ventricular filling, contractility, or outflow obstruction
- *Fatigue* related to decreased cardiac output
- *Ineffective Breathing Pattern* related to heart failure
- *Fear* related to risk for sudden cardiac death
- *Ineffective Role Performance* related to decreasing cardiac function and activity restrictions
- *Anticipatory Grieving* related to poor prognosis.

Community-Based Care

Cardiomyopathies are chronic, progressive disorders generally managed in home and community care settings unless surgery or transplant is planned or end-stage heart failure develops. When teaching the client and family for home care, include the following topics:

- Activity restrictions and dietary changes to reduce manifestations and prevent complications

- Prescribed drug regimen, its rationale, intended and possible adverse effects
- The disease process, its expected ultimate outcome, and treatment options
- Cardiac transplantation, including the procedure, the need for lifetime immunosuppression to prevent transplant rejection, and the risks of postoperative infection and long-term immunosuppression

- Symptoms to report to the physician or for which immediate care is needed.
- Cardiopulmonary resuscitation procedures and available training sites.

Refer the client and family for home and social services and counseling as indicated. Provide community resources such as support groups or the AHA.

EXPLORE MediaLink

Prentice Hall Nursing MediaLink DVD-ROM
Audio Glossary
NCLEX-RN® Review

Animations
Digoxin
Hemodynamics

COMPANION WEBSITE www.prenhall.com/lemone
Audio Glossary
NCLEX-RN® Review
Care Plan Activity: Acute Pulmonary Edema
Case Study: Rheumatic Fever
MediaLink Applications
Beta Blockers
Heart Failure
Links to Resources

CHAPTER HIGHLIGHTS

- All of the disorders discussed in this chapter can lead to heart failure, a condition in which the heart is unable to pump effectively to meet the body's needs for blood and oxygen to the tissues.
- Coronary heart disease (myocardial ischemia) and cardiomyopathies are the leading causes of heart failure.
- When the heart starts to fail, compensatory mechanisms are activated to help maintain tissue perfusion. While these mechanisms, including increased contractile force, vasoconstriction, sodium and water retention, and remodeling of the heart, effectively maintain cardiac output in the short term, in the long term they hasten deterioration of heart function.
- The goals of heart failure management are to reduce the workload of the heart and improve its function. Medical management includes administration of drugs such as ACE inhibitors, beta blockers, diuretics, and vasodilators to reduce the workload of the heart, and inotropic medications such as digitalis to improve the strength of cardiac muscle contraction.
- Nursing care of the client with heart failure is primarily supportive and educative, providing the client and family with necessary knowledge and resources to manage this chronic condition.
- Cardiogenic pulmonary edema, a manifestation of severe cardiac decompensation, is a medical emergency, requiring immediate and effective treatment to preserve life. The nurse's role in managing pulmonary edema focuses on supporting respiratory

and cardiac function, administering prescribed medications, and providing reassurance to the client and family.
- Inflammatory and infectious processes, such as rheumatic fever, endocarditis, myocarditis, and pericarditis, can affect any layer of the heart. While some, such as myocarditis and pericarditis, typically are mild and self-limiting, others can have long-term effects on cardiac structure and function.
- Processes such as rheumatic heart disease, endocarditis, and congenital conditions can affect the structure and function of the heart valves, resulting in either stenosis (narrowing) of the valve and restricted flow through it, or regurgitation, backflow of blood through a valve that does not fully close. The mitral and aortic valves are commonly affected due to the higher pressures and increased workload of the left side of the heart.
- Valve disorders may be mild, producing a heart murmur but no functional impairment for the client, or severe, causing symptoms of heart failure even at rest. Repair or replacement of the valve may ultimately be required.
- Cardiomyopathies affect the heart muscle and its ability to stretch during filling and contract effectively. Dilated cardiomyopathy, the most common type, is progressive, ultimately necessitating heart transplant. Hypertrophic cardiomyopathy affects both ventricular filling and outflow through the aortic valve. Surgical resection of excess tissue may relieve its manifestations.

TEST YOURSELF NCLEX-RN® REVIEW

1 In reviewing the physician's admitting notes for a client with heart failure, the nurse notes that the client has an ejection fraction of 25%. The nurse recognizes this as meaning:
1. ventricular function is severely impaired.
2. the amount of blood being ejected from the ventricles is within normal limits.
3. 25% of the blood entering the ventricle remains in the ventricle after systole.
4. cardiac output is greater than normal, overtaxing the heart.

2 In assessing a client admitted 24 hours previously with heart failure, the nurse notes that the client has lost 2.5 lb (1 kg) of weight, his heart rate is 88 (HR was 105 on admission), and he now has crackles in the bases of his lung fields only. The nurse correctly interprets these data as indicating:
1. the client's condition is unchanged from admission.
2. a need for more aggressive treatment.
3. the treatment regimen is achieving the desired effect.
4. no further treatment is required at this time as the failure has resolved.

3 The nurse assessing a client admitted with left ventricular failure would recognize which of the following findings as consistent with the diagnosis? (Select all that apply.)
1. 5 cm jugular vein distention at 30°
2. complaints of shortness of breath with minimal exertion
3. substernal chest pain during exercise
4. bilateral inspiratory crackles to midscapula
5. fatigue

4 The nurse caring for a client undergoing pulmonary artery pressure monitoring provides appropriate care when he
1. secures the intravenous line to the bed linens.
2. maintains flush solution flow by gravity.
3. reports waveform dampening during wedge pressure measurements.
4. calibrates and levels the system every shift.

5 Morphine 2 to 5 mg IV as needed for pain and dyspnea is ordered for a client in acute pulmonary edema. The nurse appropriately:
1. questions this order because no time intervals have been specified.
2. administers the drug as ordered, monitoring respiratory status.
3. withholds the drug until the client's respiratory status improves.
4. administers the drug only when the client complains of chest pain.

6 The nurse notes a grating heart sound when auscultating the apical pulse of a client with pericarditis. The most appropriate response is to

1. note the finding in the client's medical record.
2. obtain an electrocardiogram.
3. immediately notify the physician.
4. initiate resuscitation measures.

7 An appropriate goal of nursing care for the client with acute infective endocarditis would be:
1. "Will resume usual activities within 1 week of treatment."
2. "Will relate the benign and self-limiting nature of the disease."
3. "Will consider cardiac transplantation as a viable treatment option."
4. "Will state the importance of continuing intravenous antibiotic therapy as ordered."

8 An expected assessment finding in a client with mitral stenosis being admitted for a valve replacement would be:
1. muffled heart sounds.
2. S_3 and S_4 heart sounds.
3. diastolic murmur heard at the apex.
4. cardiac heave.

9 A client facing heart valve replacement asks the nurse which type of valve is the best, biologic or mechanical. An appropriate response would be:
1. the need to take drugs to prevent rejection of biologic tissue is a major consideration.
2. clotting is a risk with mechanical valves, necessitating anticoagulant drug therapy after insertion.
3. biologic valves tend to be more durable than mechanical valves.
4. endocarditis is a risk following valve replacement; it is more easily treated with mechanical valves.

10 The parents of a young athlete who collapsed and died due to hypertrophic cardiomyopathy ask the nurse how it is possible that their son had no symptoms of this disorder before experiencing sudden cardiac death. The nurse responds:
1. "Exercise causes the heart to contract more forcefully, and can lead to changes in the heart's rhythm or the outflow of blood from the heart in people with hypertrophic cardiomyopathy."
2. "It is likely that your son had symptoms of the disorder before he died, but he may not have thought them important enough to tell someone about."
3. "In this type of cardiomyopathy, the ventricle does not fill normally. During exercise, the heart may not be able to meet the body's needs for blood and oxygen."
4. "Cardiomyopathy results in destruction and scarring of cardiac muscle cells. As a result, the ventricle may rupture during strenuous exercise, leading to sudden death."

See Test Yourself answers in Appendix C.

BIBLIOGRAPHY

Albert, N. M. (2004a). A "current" choice for hemodynamic monitoring. *Nursing, 34*(10), 58–60.

Albert, N. M. (2004b). Ventricular dysrhythmias in heart failure. *Journal of Cardiovascular Nursing, 19*(6S), S11–S26.

Aldred, H., Gott, M., & Gariballa, S. (2005). Advanced heart failure: Impact on older patients and informal carers. *Journal of Advanced Nursing, 49*(2), 116–124.

American Heart Association. (2005). *Heart disease and stroke statistics–2005 update.* Dallas, TX: Author.

Artinian, N. T. (2003). The psychosocial aspects of heart failure. *American Journal of Nursing, 103*(12), 32–42.

Benton, M. J. (2005). Safety and efficacy of resistance training in patients with chronic heart failure: Research-based evidence. *Progressive Cardiovascular Nursing, 20*(1), 17–23.

Bixby, M. (2005). Turn back the tide of cardiogenic pulmonary edema. *Nursing, 35*(5), 56–61.

Bolton, M. M., & Wilson, B. A. (2005). The influence of race on heart failure in African-American women. *Medsurg Nursing, 14*(1), 8–15.

Bond, A. E., Nelson, K., Germany, C. L., & Smart, A. N. (2003). The left ventricular assist device. *American Journal of Nursing, 103*(1), 32–40.

Brodie, D. A., & Inoue, A. (2005). Motivational interviewing to promote physical activity for people with chronic heart failure. *Journal of Advanced Nursing, 50*(5), 518–527.

Brown, H. (2005). Action stat. Cardiac tamponade. *Nursing, 35*(3), 88.

Brown, P. A., Launius, B. K., Mancini, M. C., & Cush, E. M. (2004). Depression and anxiety in the heart transplant patient: A case study. *Critical Care Nursing Quarterly, 27*(1), 92–95.

Bruce, J. (2005). Getting to the heart of cardiomyopathies. *Nursing, 35*(8), 44–47.

Vessel Spasm

When a blood vessel is damaged, thromboxane A_2 (TXA_2) is released from platelets and cells, causing vessel spasm. This spasm constricts the damaged vessel for about 1 minute, reducing blood flow.

Formation of the Platelet Plug

Platelets attracted to the damaged vessel wall change from smooth disks to spiny spheres. Receptors on the activated platelets bind with von Willebrand's factor, a protein molecule, and exposed collagen fibers at the site of injury to form the platelet plug (Figure 33–5 ■). The platelets release adenosine diphosphate (ADP) and TXA_2 to activate nearby platelets, adhering them to the developing plug. Activation of the clotting pathway on the platelet surface converts fibrinogen to fibrin.

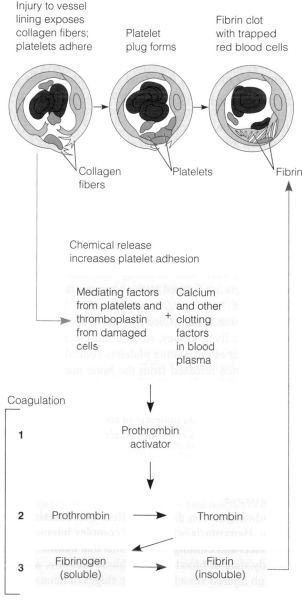

Figure 33–5 ■ Platelet plug formation and blood clotting. The flow diagram summarizes the events leading to fibrin clot formation.

Fibrin, in turn, forms a meshwork that binds the platelets and other blood cells to form a stable plug (Figure 33–6 ■).

Development of the Fibrin Clot

The process of coagulation creates a meshwork of fibrin strands that cements the blood components to form an insoluble clot. Coagulation requires many interactive reactions and two clotting pathways (Figure 33–7 ■). The slower intrinsic pathway is activated when blood contacts collagen in the injured vessel wall; the faster extrinsic pathway is activated when blood is exposed to tissues. The final outcome of both pathways is fibrin clot formation. Each procoagulation substance is activated in sequence; the activation of one coagulation factor activates another in turn. Table 33–2 lists known factors, their origin, and their function or pathway. A deficiency of one or more factors or inappropriate inactivation of any factor alters normal coagulation.

Clot Retraction

After the clot is stabilized (within about 30 minutes), trapped platelets contract, much like muscle cells. Platelet contraction squeezes the fibrin strands, pulling the broken portions of the ruptured blood vessel closer together. Growth factors released by the platelets stimulate cell division and tissue repair of the damaged vessel.

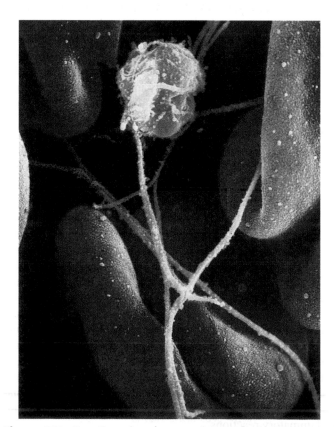

Figure 33–6 ■ Scanning electron micrograph of a RBC trapped in a fibrin mesh. The spherical gray object at top is a platelet.

Source: Copyright © Boehniger Ingelheim; photo Lennart Nilsson, Albert Bonniers Förlog AB.

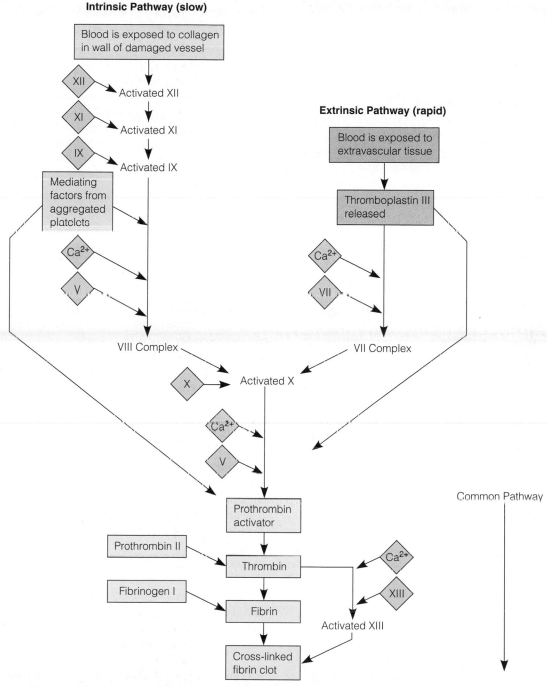

Figure 33–7 ■ Clot formation. Both the slower intrinsic pathway and the more rapid extrinsic pathway activate factor X. Factor X then combines with other factors to form prothrombin activator. Prothrombin activator transforms prothrombin into thrombin, which then transforms fibrinogen into long fibrin strands. Thrombin also activates Factor XIII, which draws the fibrin strands together into a dense meshwork. The complete process of clot formation occurs within 3 to 6 minutes after blood vessel damage.

Clot Dissolution

Fibrinolysis, the process of clot dissolution, begins shortly after the clot has formed, restoring blood flow and promoting tissue repair. Like coagulation, fibrinolysis requires a sequence of interactions between activator and inhibitor substances. Plasminogen, an enzyme that promotes fibrinolysis, is con-

verted into plasmin, its active form, by chemical mediators released from vessel walls and the liver. Plasmin dissolves the clot's fibrin strands and certain coagulation factors. Stimuli such as exercise, fever, and vasoactive drugs promote plasminogen activator release. The liver and endothelium also produce fibrinolytic inhibitors.

TABLE 33–2 Blood Coagulation Factors

FACTOR	NAME	FUNCTION OR PATHWAY
I	Fibrinogen	Converted to fibrin strands
II	Prothrombin	Converted to thrombin
III	Thromboplastin	Catalyzes conversion of thrombin
IV	Calcium ions	Needed for all steps of coagulation
V	Proaccelerin	Extrinsic/intrinsic pathways
VII	Serum prothrombin conversion accelerator	Extrinsic pathway
VIII	Antihemophilic factor	Intrinsic pathway
IX	Plasma prothrombin componcnt	Intrinsic pathway
X	Stuart factor	Extrinsic/intrinsic pathways
XI	Plasma prothrombin antecedent	Intrinsic pathway
XII	Hageman factor	Intrinsic pathway
XIII	Fibrin stabilizing factor	Cross-links fibrin strands to form insoluble clot

ANATOMY, PHYSIOLOGY, AND FUNCTIONS OF THE PERIPHERAL VASCULAR SYSTEM

The two main components of the peripheral vascular system are the arterial network and the venous network. The arterial network begins with the major arteries that branch from the aorta. The major arteries of the systemic circulation are illustrated in Figure 33–8 ■. These major arteries branch into successively smaller arteries, which in turn subdivide into the smallest of the arterial vessels, called *arterioles*. The smallest arterioles feed into beds of hairlike capillaries in the body's organs and tissues.

In the capillary beds, oxygen and nutrients are exchanged for metabolic wastes, and deoxygenated blood begins its journey back to the heart through venules, the smallest vessels of the venous network. Venules join the smallest of veins, which in turn join larger and larger veins. The blood transported by the veins empties into the superior and inferior venae cavae entering the right side of the heart. The major veins of the systemic circulation are shown in Figure 33–9 ■.

Structure of Blood Vessels

The structure of blood vessels reflects their different functions within the circulatory system (Figure 33–10 ■). Except for the tiniest vessels, blood vessel walls have three layers: the tunica intima, the tunica media, and the tunica adventitia. The tunica intima, the innermost layer, is made of simple squamous epithelium (the endothelium); this provides a slick surface to facilitate the flow of blood. In arteries, the middle layer, or tunica media, is made of smooth muscle and is thicker than the tunica media of veins. This makes arteries more elastic than veins and allows the arteries to alternately expand and recoil as the heart contracts and relaxes with each beat, producing a pressure wave, which can be felt as a **pulse** over an artery. The smaller arterioles are less elastic than arteries but contain more smooth muscle, which promotes their constriction (narrowing) and dilation (widening). In fact, arterioles exert the major control over arterial blood pressure. The tunica adventitia, or outermost layer, is made of connective tissue and serves to protect

and anchor the vessel. Veins have a thicker tunica adventitia than do arteries.

Blood in the veins travels at a much lower pressure than blood in the arteries. Veins have thinner walls, a larger lumen, and greater capacity, and many are supplied with valves that help blood flow against gravity back to the heart (see Figure 33–10). The "milking" action of skeletal muscle contraction (called the muscular pump) also supports venous return. When skeletal muscles contract against veins, the valves proximal to the contraction open, and blood is propelled toward the heart. The abdominal and thoracic pressure changes that occur with breathing (called the respiratory pump) also propel blood toward the heart.

The tiny capillaries, which connect the arterioles and venules, contain only one thin layer of tunica intima that is permeable to the gases and molecules exchanged between blood and tissue cells. Capillaries typically are found in interwoven networks. They filter and shunt blood from precapillary arterioles to postcapillary venules.

Physiology of Arterial Circulation

The factors that affect arterial circulation are blood flow, peripheral vascular resistance, and blood pressure. **Blood flow** refers to the volume of blood transported in a vessel, in an organ, or throughout the entire circulation over a given period of time. It is commonly expressed as liters or milliliters per minute or cubic centimeters per second.

Peripheral vascular resistance (PVR) refers to the opposing forces or impedance to blood flow as the arterial channels become more and more distant from the heart. Peripheral vascular resistance is determined by three factors:

- *Blood viscosity:* The greater the viscosity, or thickness, of the blood, the greater its resistance to moving and flowing.
- *Length of the vessel:* The longer the vessel, the greater the resistance to blood flow.

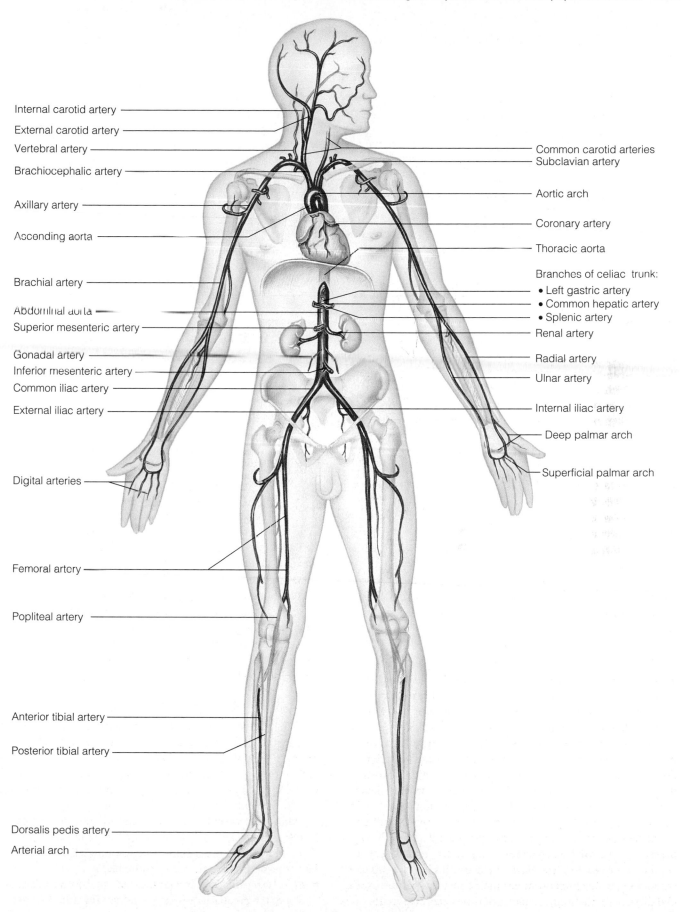

Internal carotid artery
External carotid artery
Vertebral artery
Brachiocephalic artery
Axillary artery
Ascending aorta
Brachial artery
Abdominal aorta
Superior mesenteric artery
Gonadal artery
Inferior mesenteric artery
Common iliac artery
External iliac artery
Digital arteries
Femoral artery
Popliteal artery
Anterior tibial artery
Posterior tibial artery
Dorsalis pedis artery
Arterial arch

Common carotid arteries
Subclavian artery
Aortic arch
Coronary artery
Thoracic aorta
Branches of celiac trunk:
• Left gastric artery
• Common hepatic artery
• Splenic artery
Renal artery
Radial artery
Ulnar artery
Internal iliac artery
Deep palmar arch
Superficial palmar arch

Figure 33–8 ■ Major arteries of the systemic circulation.

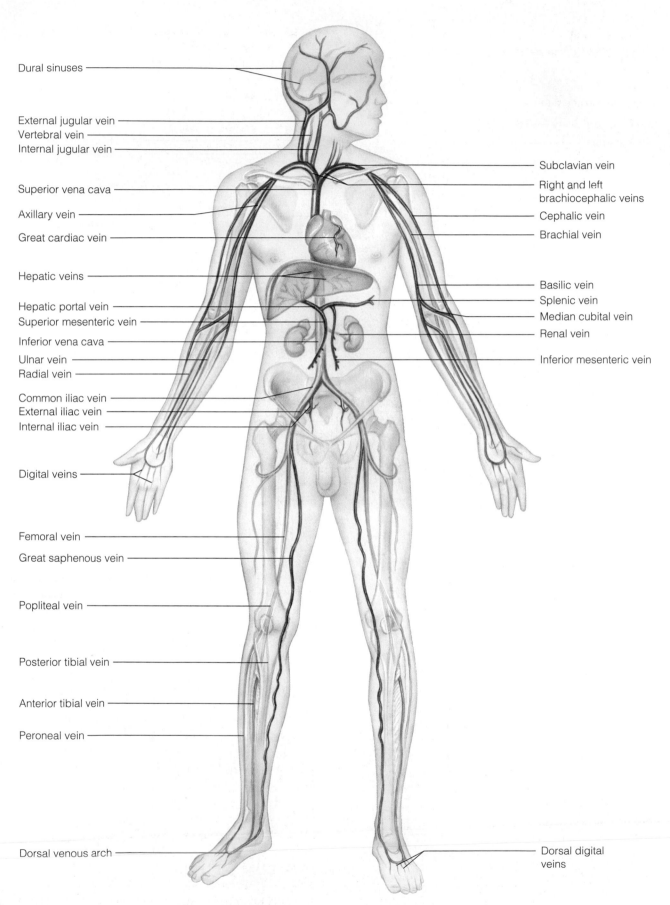

Dural sinuses

External jugular vein
Vertebral vein
Internal jugular vein

Superior vena cava

Axillary vein

Great cardiac vein

Hepatic veins

Hepatic portal vein
Superior mesenteric vein

Inferior vena cava

Ulnar vein
Radial vein

Common iliac vein
External iliac vein
Internal iliac vein

Digital veins

Femoral vein

Great saphenous vein

Popliteal vein

Posterior tibial vein

Anterior tibial vein

Peroneal vein

Dorsal venous arch

Subclavian vein
Right and left
brachiocephalic veins
Cephalic vein
Brachial vein

Basilic vein
Splenic vein
Median cubital vein
Renal vein

Inferior mesenteric vein

Dorsal digital
veins

Figure 33–9 ■ Major veins of the systemic circulation.

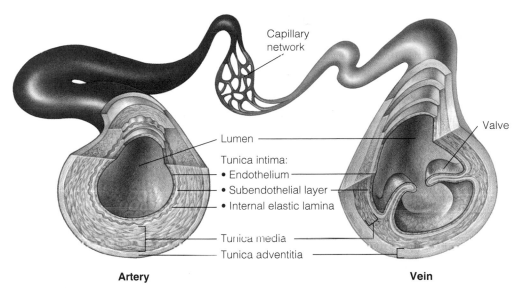

Figure 33–10 ■ Structure of arteries, veins, and capillaries. Capillaries are composed of only a fine tunica intima. Notice that the tunica media is thicker in arteries than in veins.

- *Diameter of the vessel:* The smaller the diameter of a vessel, the greater the friction against the walls of the vessel and, thus, the greater the impedance to blood flow.

Blood pressure is the force exerted against the walls of the arteries by the blood as it is pumped from the heart. It is most accurately referred to as **mean arterial pressure (MAP)**. The highest pressure exerted against the arterial walls at the peak of ventricular contraction (systole) is called the systolic blood pressure. The lowest pressure exerted during ventricular relaxation (diastole) is the diastolic blood pressure.

Mean arterial blood pressure is regulated mainly by cardiac output (CO) and peripheral vascular resistance (PVR), as represented in this formula: $MAP = CO \times PVR$. For clinical use, the MAP may be estimated by calculating the diastolic blood pressure plus one-third of the pulse pressure (the difference between the systolic and diastolic blood pressure).

Factors Influencing Arterial Blood Pressure

Blood flow, peripheral vascular resistance, and blood pressure, which influence arterial circulation, are in turn influenced by various factors, as follows:

- The sympathetic and parasympathetic nervous systems are the primary mechanisms that regulate blood pressure. Stimulation of the sympathetic nervous system exerts a major effect on peripheral resistance by causing vasoconstriction of the arterioles, thereby increasing blood pressure. Parasympathetic stimulation causes vasodilation of the arterioles, lowering blood pressure.
- Baroreceptors and chemoreceptors in the aortic arch, carotid sinus, and other large vessels are sensitive to pressure and chemical changes and cause reflex sympathetic stimulation, resulting in vasoconstriction, increased heart rate, and increased blood pressure.
- The kidneys help maintain blood pressure by excreting or conserving sodium and water. When blood pressure decreases, the kidneys initiate the renin–angiotensin mechanism. This stimulates vasoconstriction, resulting in the release of the hormone aldosterone from the adrenal cortex, increasing sodium ion reabsorption and water retention. In addition, pituitary release of antidiuretic hormone (ADH) promotes renal reabsorption of water. The net result is an increase in blood volume and a consequent increase in cardiac output and blood pressure.
- Temperatures may also affect peripheral resistance: Cold causes vasoconstriction, whereas warmth produces vasodilation. Many chemicals, hormones, and drugs influence blood pressure by affecting CO and/or PVR. For example, epinephrine causes vasoconstriction and increased heart rate; prostaglandins dilate blood vessel diameter (by relaxing vascular smooth muscle); endothelin, a chemical released by the inner lining of vessels, is a potent vasoconstrictor; nicotine causes vasoconstriction; and alcohol and histamine cause vasodilation.
- Dietary factors, such as intake of salt, saturated fats, and cholesterol elevate blood pressure by affecting blood volume and vessel diameter.
- Race, gender, age, weight, time of day, position, exercise, and emotional state may also affect blood pressure. These factors influence the arterial pressure. Systemic venous pressure, though it is much lower, is also influenced by such factors as blood volume, venous tone, and right atrial pressure.

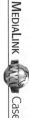

ANATOMY, PHYSIOLOGY, AND FUNCTIONS OF THE LYMPHATIC SYSTEM

The structures of the lymphatic system include the lymphatic vessels and several lymphoid organs (Figure 33–11 ■). The organs of the lymphatic system are the lymph nodes, the spleen, the thymus, the tonsils, and the Peyer's patches of the small intestine. Lymph nodes are small aggregates of specialized cells that assist the immune system by removing foreign

5 An older client is severely dehydrated and, as a result, has increased blood viscosity. How will this affect the peripheral vascular resistance (PVR)?
1. increased PVR
2. decreased PVR
3. no change
4. depends on gender

6 What is the source of lymph?
1. the respiratory system
2. the cardiovascular system
3. the central nervous system
4. the integumentary system

7 What method would be most appropriate to assess the carotid arteries?
1. Inspect for absence of movement.
2. Auscultate with the bell of the stethoscope.
3. Palpate with firm pressure.
4. Percuss lightly over each artery.

8 When auscultating the abdominal aorta, you hear a murmuring or blowing sound. You would document this sound as a:

1. hypokinetic pulse.
2. bigeminal pulse.
3. bruit.
4. dysrhythmia.

9 Swelling of a body part as a result of lymphatic obstruction is labeled:
1. lymphedema.
2. lymphadenopathy.
3. atrophic change.
4. central cyanosis.

10 You are assessing a man who has severe leg pain. The leg is cool and cyanotic. You are unable to palpate a femoral pulse. What would be your priority intervention based on these assessments?
1. Document your findings.
2. Ask the family about this problem.
3. Teach the man relaxation techniques.
4. Notify the physician immediately.

See Test Yourself answers in Appendix C.

BIBLIOGRAPHY

Amella, E. (2004). Presentation of illness in older adults: If you think you know what you're looking for, think again. *American Journal of Nursing, 104*(10), 40–52.

Benbow, M. (2004). Doppler readings and leg ulceration. *Practice Nurse, 28*(4), 16, 18, 21.

Bench, S. (2004). Clinical skills: Assessing and treating shock. A nursing perspective. *British Journal of Nursing, 13*(12), 715–721.

Bickley, L., & Szilagyi, P. (2007). *Bates' guide to physical examination and history taking* (9th ed.). Philadelphia: Lippincott.

Board, J., & Harlow, W. (2002). Lymphoedema 1: Components and function of the lymphatic system. *British Journal of Nursing, 11*(5), 304–309.

Day, M. (2004). Action stat. Hypertensive emergency. *Nursing, 34*(7), 88.

Eliopoulos, E. (2005). *Gerontological nursing* (6th ed.). Philadelphia: Lippincott Williams & Wilkins.

Jarvis, C. (2004). *Physical examination & health assessment.* St. Louis, MO: Mosby.

Kee, J. (2005). *Prentice Hall handbook of laboratory & diagnostic tests with nursing implications.* Upper Saddle River, NJ: Prentice Hall.

Millard, F. (2004). The lymphatic system: Applied anatomy. *AAO Journal, 14*(1), 9–15.

Murrary, J. (2004). Leg ulceration part 2: Patient assessment. *Nursing Standard, 19*(2), 45–54.

National Institutes of Health. (2003). *Genes and disease. Blood and lymph diseases.* Retrieved from http://www.ncbi.nlm.nih.gov/books/bv.fcgi?rid=gnd.section98

Porth, C., (2005). *Pathophysiology: Concepts of altered health states* (7th ed.). Philadelphia: Lippincott.

Reilly, P. (2004). How to check perfusion lickety-split. *Nursing, 34*(4), 64.

Rice, K. (2005). How to measure ankle/brachial index. *Nursing, 35*(1), 56–57.

Rushing J. (2004). Taking blood pressure accurately. *Nursing, 43*(11), 26.

_____. (2005). Assessing for orthostatic hypotension. *Nursing, 35*(1), 30.

Tanabe, P., Steinmann, R., Kippenhan, M., Stehman, C., & Beach, C. (2004). Undiagnosed hypertension in the ED setting—an unrecognized opportunity by emergency nurses. *Journal of Emergency Nursing, 30*(3), 225–229, 292–297.

Weber, J., & Kelley, J. (2006). *Health assessment in nursing* (3rd ed.). Philadelphia: Lippincott.

Willis, K. (2001). Gaining perspective on peripheral vascular disease. *Nursing, 31*(2), Hospital Nursing, 32hn1–4.

Woodrow, P. (2003). Assessing pulse in older people. *Nursing Older People, 15*(6), 38–40.

Young, T. (2001). Leg ulcer assessment. *Practice Nurse, 21*(7), 50, 52.

CHAPTER 34

Nursing Care of Clients with Hematologic Disorders

LEARNING OUTCOMES

- Relate the physiology and assessment of the hematologic system and related systems to commonly occurring hematologic disorders.

- Describe the pathophysiology of common hematologic disorders.

- Explain nursing implications for medications and other treatments prescribed for clients with hematologic disorders.

- Discuss indications for and complications of bone marrow or stem cell transplantation, as well as related nursing care.

- Compare and contrast the pathophysiology, manifestations, and management of bleeding disorders.

- Describe the major types of leukemia and the most common treatment modalities and nursing interventions.

- Differentiate Hodgkin's disease from non-Hodgkin's lymphomas.

CLINICAL COMPETENCIES

- Assess effects of hematologic disorders and prescribed treatments on clients' functional health status.

- Monitor and document continuing assessment data, including laboratory test results, subjective and objective information, reporting data outside the normal or expected range.

- Based on knowledge of pathophysiology, prescribed treatment, and assessed data, identify and prioritize nursing diagnoses for clients with hematologic disorders.

- Use nursing research and evidence-based practice to identify and implement individualized nursing interventions for the client with a hematologic disorder.

- Safely and knowledgeably administer prescribed medications and treatments for clients with hematologic disorders.

- Collaborate with the interdisciplinary care team to plan and provide coordinated, effective care for clients with hematologic disorders.

- Provide appropriate teaching for clients with hematologic disorders, evaluating learning and the need for continued reinforcement of information.

- Use continuing assessment data to revise the plan of care as needed to restore, maintain, or promote functional health in the client with a hematologic disorder.

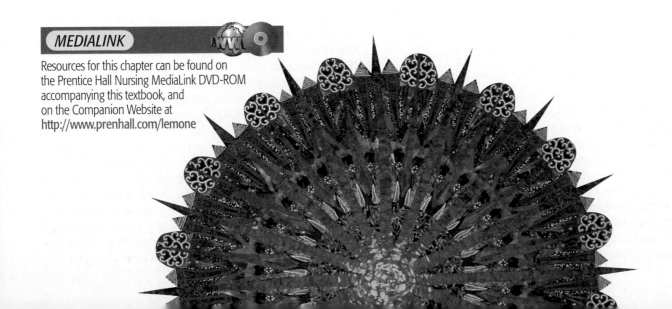

MEDIALINK

Resources for this chapter can be found on the Prentice Hall Nursing MediaLink DVD-ROM accompanying this textbook, and on the Companion Website at
http://www.prenhall.com/lemone

anemia, *1102*
aplastic anemia, *1109*
bone marrow transplant (BMT), *1124*
disseminated intravascular
  coagulation (DIC), *1146*
hemolytic anemias, *1106*
hemophilia, *1142*

hemostasis, *1139*
iron deficiency anemia, *1103*
leukemia, *1118*
lymphoma, *1129*
multiple myeloma, *1136*
pernicious anemia, *1105*
polycythemia, *1117*

sickle cell anemia, *1106*
sickle cell crisis, *1107*
stem cell transplant
  (SCT), *1124*
thalassemia, *1109*
thrombocytopenia, *1139*

Disorders affecting the blood and blood-forming organs have effects that range from minor disruptions in daily activities to major life-threatening crises. Clients with hematologic disorders need holistic nursing care, including emotional support and care for problems involving major body systems.

This chapter focuses on health changes resulting from changes in red cells, white cells, platelets, and clotting factors. Before proceeding with this chapter, read Chapter 33 ∞, which provides a review of the physiology of blood and its formation, as well as important information about assessing clients with hematologic disorders.

RED BLOOD CELL DISORDERS

Red blood cells (RBCs) transport oxygen to body tissues and help return carbon dioxide to the lungs for excretion. Alterations in the number, size, shape, or composition of RBCs affect their ability to effectively carry out these functions. Anemia, the most common RBC disorder, is an abnormally low RBC count or reduced hemoglobin content. Polycythemia is an abnormally high RBC count.

THE CLIENT WITH ANEMIA

Anemia is an abnormally low number of circulating RBCs, low hemoglobin concentration, or both. Decreased numbers of circulating RBCs is the usual cause of anemia. This may result from blood loss, inadequate RBC production, or increased RBC destruction. Insufficient or defective hemoglobin within RBCs contributes to anemia. Depending on its severity, anemia may affect all major organ systems.

FAST FACTS
- Iron deficiency anemia, a nutritional anemia, is the most common type of anemia.
- Blood loss anemia may be either acute, resulting from hemorrhage, or chronic, resulting from chronic blood loss (e.g., menstrual flow, slow GI bleeding).

Physiology Review

As blood flows through the pulmonary vascular system, oxygen diffuses from alveoli into capillary blood. The majority of the oxygen binds reversibly with the hemoglobin in red blood cells; only about 3% of the oxygen remains in solution in the blood. When the blood reaches the capillaries serving body tissues, oxygen is released from the hemoglobin molecule, and diffuses out of the capillary to reach the cells. The amount of oxygen that reaches the tissues depends on a number of factors, including:
- Available oxygen in the alveoli
- The diffusing surface and capacity of the lungs

- The number of red blood cells and the amount and type of hemoglobin they contain
- The ability of the cardiovascular system to transport blood and oxygen to the tissues.

For more information about red blood cells, hemoglobin, and their production and function, see Chapter 33 ∞ .

Physiology and Manifestations

A number of different pathologic mechanisms can lead to anemia (Box 34–1). Regardless of the cause, every type of anemia reduces the oxygen-carrying capacity of the blood due to a deficiency of RBCs or hemoglobin, leading to tissue hypoxia. The resulting manifestations depend on the severity of the anemia, how quickly it develops, and other factors such as age and health status.

When anemia develops gradually and the RBC reduction is moderate, successful compensatory mechanisms may result in few symptoms except when the oxygen needs of the body increase due to exercise or infection. Symptoms develop as RBCs and hemoglobin levels are further reduced. Pallor of the skin, mucous membranes, conjunctiva, and nail beds develops as a result of blood redistribution to vital organs and lack of hemoglobin (Figure 34–1 ■). As tissue oxygenation decreases, the heart and respiratory rates rise in an attempt to increase cardiac output and tissue perfusion. Tissue hypoxia may cause angina, fatigue, dyspnea on exertion, and night cramps. It also stimulates erythropoietin release; increased erythropoietin activity stimulates RBC production in the bone marrow, and may lead to bone pain. Cerebral hypoxia can lead to headache, dizziness, and dim vision. Heart failure may develop in severe anemia.

With rapid blood loss, blood volume is decreased as well as the oxygen-carrying capacity of the blood. Initial manifestations include tachycardia and tachypnea; the skin may be pale, cool, and clammy as peripheral vessels constrict to maintain blood flow to the heart and brain. With significant blood loss, signs of circulatory shock may occur, including hypotension,

---

BOX 34–1 Pathophysiologic Mechanisms of Anemia

Decreased RBC Production
- Altered hemoglobin synthesis
  - Iron deficiency
  - Thalassemias
  - Chronic inflammation
- Altered DNA synthesis
  - Vitamin B_{12} or folic acid malabsorption or deficiency
- Bone marrow failure
  - Aplastic anemia (stem cell dysfunction)
  - Red cell aplasia
  - Myeloproliferative leukemias
  - Cancer metastasis, lymphoma
  - Chronic infection or inflammation, physical and emotional fatigue

Increased RBC Loss or Destruction
- Acute or chronic blood loss
  - Hemorrhage or trauma
  - Chronic gastrointestinal bleeding, menorrhagia
- Increased hemolysis
  - Hereditary cell membrane disorders
  - Defective hemoglobin—sickle cell anemia or trait
  - Pyruvate kinase (PK) or G6PD deficiency affecting glycolysis or cell oxidation
  - Immune mechanisms and disorders (e.g., blood reaction, hypersensitivity responses, autoimmune disorders)
  - Splenomegaly and hypersplenism
  - Infection
  - Erythrocyte trauma (e.g., due to cardiopulmonary bypass, hemolytic uremic syndrome)

---

tachycardia, decreased level of consciousness, and oliguria. With chronic bleeding, fluid shifts from the interstitial spaces into the vessels, maintaining blood volume. Blood viscosity is reduced, which may result in a systolic heart murmur. See page 1104 for *Multisystem Effects of Anemia*.

Anemia is categorized by cause: blood loss, nutritional, hemolytic, and bone marrow suppression. The pathophysiology and specific manifestations of these types of anemias follow.

Blood Loss Anemia

When anemia results from acute or chronic bleeding, RBCs and other blood components (such as iron) are lost from the body. With acute blood loss, circulating volume decreases. As a result, the cardiac output falls. Compensatory mechanisms are activated to maintain the cardiac output: the heart rate increases, and peripheral blood vessels constrict. Vessels in the liver, a blood storage organ, also constrict, increasing circulating volume. Fluid shifts from the interstitial spaces into the vascular compartment to maintain blood volume, diluting the cellular components of the blood and reducing its viscosity. If

hemorrhage continues, compensatory mechanisms become less effective, increasing the risk for shock and circulatory failure (see Chapter 11 ∞).

In acute blood loss, circulating RBCs are of normal size and shape (*normocytic*). Early in the hemorrhage, the RBC count, hemoglobin, and hematocrit may be normal; as fluid shifts from the interstitial space into the vascular space to maintain circulating volume, the RBC count, hemoglobin, and hematocrit fall. If sufficient iron is available, the number of circulating RBCs and hemoglobin levels return to normal within 3 to 4 weeks after the bleeding episode. Chronic blood loss, on the other hand, depletes iron stores as RBC production attempts to maintain the RBC supply. The resulting RBCs are *microcytic* (small) and *hypochromic* (pale).

Nutritional Anemias

A number of different nutrients are required for normal red blood cell development (erythropoiesis). Iron is a key nutrient necessary for hemoglobin synthesis. In addition, adequate supplies of protein (and its building blocks, amino acids), vitamins, and other minerals are required. The B vitamins, particularly B_{12} (cobalamin) and folate, play a key role in RBC development. Vitamins C and E also are necessary. Nutritional anemias result from nutrient deficits that affect RBC formation or hemoglobin synthesis. The nutrient deficit may be caused by inadequate diet, malabsorption of the nutrient, or an increased need for the nutrient. The most common types of nutritional anemias are iron deficiency anemia, vitamin B_{12} anemia, and folic acid deficiency anemia. Vitamin B_{12} and folic acid anemias are sometimes called *megaloblastic* anemias, because enlarged nucleated RBCs called megaloblasts are seen in these anemias.

***IRON DEFICIENCY ANEMIA* Iron deficiency anemia** is the most common type of anemia. It develops when the supply of iron is inadequate for optimal RBC formation. The body cannot synthesize hemoglobin without iron. Normally, the body efficiently recycles and stores iron, reusing much of the iron contained in RBCs that are removed from circulation due to age or damage. However, small amounts of iron continually are lost

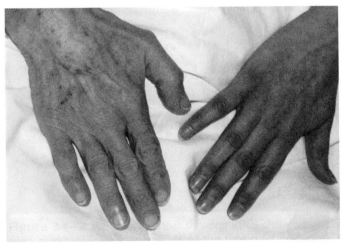

Figure 34–1 ■ The skin of the client with anemia appears pale beside that of a person with a normal hemoglobin and hematocrit.

Source: Westminster Hospital, Photo Researchers, Inc.

Sickle Cell Anemia

Hemoglobin S and Red Blood Cell Sickling

Sickle cell anemia is caused by an inherited autosomal recessive defect in Hb synthesis. Sickle cell hemoglobin (HbS) differs from normal hemoglobin only in the substitution of the amino acid valine for glutamine in both beta chains of the hemoglobin molecule.

When HbS is oxygenated, it has the same globular shape as normal hemoglobin. However, when HbS off-loads oxygen, it becomes insoluble in intracellular fluid and crystallizes into rodlike structures. Clusters of rods form polymers (long chains) that bend the erythrocyte into the characteristic crescent shape of the sickle cell.

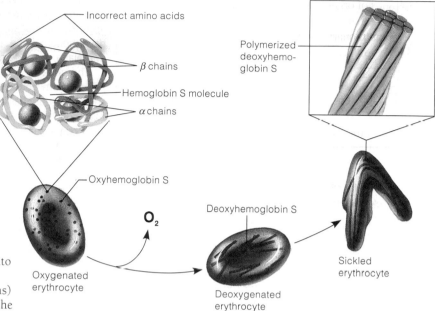

The Sickle Cell Disease Process

Sickle cell disease is characterized by episodes of acute painful crises. Sickling crises are triggered by conditions causing high tissue oxygen demands or that affect cellular pH. As the crisis begins, sickled erythrocytes adhere to capillary walls and to each other, obstructing blood flow and causing cellular hypoxia. The crisis accelerates as tissue hypoxia and acidic metabolic waste products cause further sickling and cell damage.

Sickle cell crises cause microinfarcts in joints and organs, and repeated crises slowly destroy organs and tissues. The spleen and kidneys are especially prone to sickling damage.

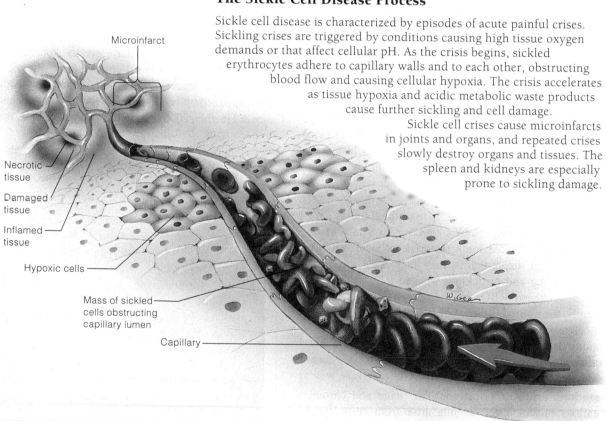

occluded vessels supplying the dermis. Repeated infarcts associated with sickling can affect the structure and function of nearly every organ system. People with sickle cell disease may develop an enlarged spleen and liver, renal insufficiency, gallstones, and other manifestations of organ dysfunction. *Acute chest syndrome*, a symptom complex that includes fever, chest pain, an increasing WBC count, and pulmonary infiltrates, may develop, as well as other pulmonary complications such as pneumonia, pulmonary infarction, and pulmonary embolism (Porth, 2005).

The shortened RBC life span and compromised erythropoiesis can lead to profound *aplastic anemia* in sickle cell disease. *Sequestration crises* are marked by pooling of large amounts of blood in the liver and spleen. This sickle cell crisis only occurs in children, but is thought to be the cause of sickle cell disease-related deaths in early childhood (Porth, 2005).

THALASSEMIA The **thalassemias** are inherited disorders of hemoglobin synthesis in which either the alpha or beta chains of the hemoglobin molecule are missing or defective. This leads to deficient hemoglobin production and fragile hypochromic, microcytic RBCs called *target cells* because of their distinctive bull's-eye appearance.

Thalassemia usually affects certain populations. People of Mediterranean descent (southern Italy and Greece) are more likely to have beta-defect thalassemias (often called *Cooley's anemia* or Mediterranean anemia). People of Asian ancestry, especially from Thailand, the Philippines, and China, more often have alpha-defect thalassemia. Africans and African Americans may have both alpha- and beta-defect thalassemia. As with sickle cell anemia, only one defective beta chain forming gene may be present (*beta thalassemia minor*), causing mild symptoms, or both may be defective (*beta-thalassemia major*), leading to more severe symptoms. Children with thalassemia major rarely reach adulthood, although repeated blood transfusions may extend their life span (McCance & Huether, 2006). Four genes are responsible for alpha chain formation; one, two, three, or all four may be defective. In the latter case (*alpha-thalassemia major*), death is inevitable and usually occurs *in utero*. Genetic studies and counseling are recommended for people at risk for this illness.

Manifestations and Complications People with thalassemia minor often are asymptomatic. When manifestations do occur, they include mild to moderate anemia, mild splenomegaly, bronze skin coloring, and bone marrow hyperplasia. The major form of the disease causes severe anemia, heart failure, and liver and spleen enlargement from increased red cell destruction. Fractures of the long bones, ribs, and vertebrae may result from bone marrow expansion and thinning due to increased hematopoiesis. Jaundice may develop due to hemolysis, as well as hepatomegaly and splenomegaly. Accumulation of iron in the heart, liver, and pancreas following repeated transfusions for treatment may eventually cause failure of these organs.

ACQUIRED HEMOLYTIC ANEMIA *Acquired hemolytic anemia* results from hemolysis due to factors outside of the RBC. Causes of acquired hemolytic anemias include:

- Mechanical trauma to RBCs produced by prosthetic heart valves, severe burns, hemodialysis, or radiation
- Autoimmune disorders

- Bacterial or protozoal infection
- Immune-system-mediated responses, such as transfusion reactions
- Drugs, toxins, chemical agents, or venoms.

The manifestations of acquired hemolytic anemia depend on the extent of hemolysis and the body's ability to replace destroyed RBCs. The anemia itself often is mild to moderate as erythropoiesis increases to replace the destroyed RBCs. The spleen enlarges as it removes damaged or destroyed RBCs. If the breakdown of heme units exceeds the liver's ability to conjugate and excrete bilirubin, jaundice develops. When the condition is severe, bone marrow expands, and bones may be deformed or may develop pathologic fractures. The severity of generalized manifestations of anemia (tachycardia, pallor, etc.) depends on the degree of anemia and deficiency of tissue oxygenation.

GLUCOSE-6-PHOSPHATE DEHYDROGENASE (G6PD) ANEMIA *Glucose-6-phosphate dehydrogenase (G6PD) anemia* is caused by a hereditary defect in RBC metabolism. It is relatively common in people of African and Mediterranean descent. The defective gene is located on the X chromosome and therefore affects more males than females. There are many variations of this genetic defect.

G6PD is an enzyme that catalyzes glycolysis, the process in which an RBC derives cellular energy. A defect in G6PD action causes direct oxidation of hemoglobin, damaging the RBC. Hemolysis usually occurs only when the affected person is exposed to stressors (e.g., drugs such as aspirin, sulfonamides, or vitamin K derivatives) that increase the metabolic demands on RBCs. The G6PD deficiency impairs the necessary compensatory increase in glucose metabolism and causes cellular damage. Damaged RBCs are destroyed over a period of 7 to 12 days.

When exposed to a stressor triggering G6PD anemia, symptoms develop within several days. These may include pallor, jaundice, hemoglobinuria (hemoglobin in the urine), and an elevated reticulocyte count. As new RBCs develop, counts return to normal.

Aplastic Anemia

In **aplastic anemia**, the bone marrow fails to produce all three types of blood cells, leading to *pancytopenia*. Normal bone marrow is replaced by fat. Fortunately, aplastic anemia is rare. *Fanconi anemia* is a rare aplastic anemia caused by defects of DNA repair. The underlying cause of about 50% of acquired aplastic anemia is unknown (*idiopathic aplastic anemia*). Other cases follow stem cell damage caused by exposure to radiation or certain chemical substances such as benzene, arsenic, nitrogen mustard, certain antibiotics (especially chloramphenicol), and chemotherapeutic drugs (McCance & Huether, 2006). Aplastic anemia also may occur with viral infections such as mononucleosis, hepatitis C, and HIV disease (Porth, 2005).

In aplastic anemia, the number of stem cells in the bone marrow is significantly reduced. The stem cell pool may be less than 1% of normal when the disease is recognized. Anemia develops as the bone marrow fails to replace RBCs that have reached the end of their life span. Remaining RBCs may be normochromic and normocytic or may be large with increased mean corpuscular volume.

Manifestations Manifestations of aplastic anemia vary with the severity of the pancytopenia. Its onset usually is insidious, but may be sudden. Manifestations include fatigue, pallor, progressive weakness, exertional dyspnea, headache, and ultimately tachycardia and heart failure. Platelet deficiency leads to bleeding problems; bleeding gums, excessive bruising, and nosebleeds may be the initial symptoms. A deficiency of white blood cells increases the risk of infection, causing manifestations such as sore throat and fever.

INTERDISCIPLINARY CARE

Ensuring adequate tissue oxygenation is the priority of care in treating anemia. Specific therapy is determined by the underlying cause of the disorder. Usual treatments include medications, dietary modifications, blood replacement, or supportive interventions. Table 34–1 outlines interdisciplinary care measures for selected types of anemia.

Diagnosis

When anemia is suspected, the following laboratory and diagnostic tests may be ordered:

- *Complete blood count (CBC)* is done to determine blood cell counts, hemoglobin, hematocrit, and red blood cell indices. The severity of the anemia, shape, volume, and iron content of the RBCs can help determine the cause of anemia.
- *Iron levels* and *total iron-binding capacity* are performed to detect iron deficiency anemia. A low serum iron concentration and elevated total iron-binding capacity are indicative of iron deficiency anemia.
- *Serum ferritin* is low due to depletion of the total iron reserves available for hemoglobin synthesis. Ferritin is an iron-storage protein produced by the liver, spleen, and bone marrow. Ferritin mobilizes stored iron when metabolic needs are higher than dietary intake.
- *Sickle cell test* is a screening test to evaluate hemolytic anemia and detect HbS.
- *Hemoglobin electrophoresis* separates normal hemoglobin from abnormal forms. It is used to evaluate hemolytic ane-

TABLE 34–1 Interdisciplinary Care Focus for Major Anemias

TYPE OF ANEMIA	INTERDISCIPLINARY CARE
Iron deficiency anemia	■ Increased dietary intake of iron-rich foods ■ Oral or parenteral iron supplements
Vitamin B_{12} deficiency	■ Increased dietary intake of foods containing vitamin B_{12} (e.g., meats, eggs, and dairy products) ■ Oral or parenteral vitamin B_{12} supplements ■ Parenteral vitamin B_{12} for deficiency due to malabsorption or lack of intrinsic factor
Folic acid deficiency	■ Increased dietary intake of foods rich in folic acid (folate) ■ Oral folic acid supplements ■ Folic acid supplements recommended for women who are pregnant or may become pregnant to prevent neural tube defects

Sickle cell anemia	■ Treatment is primarily supportive
	■ Hydroxyurea 10–30 mg/kg per day
	■ Sickle cell crisis:
	  ■ Rest
	  ■ Oxygen therapy to maintain SaO_2
	  ■ Narcotic analgesia
	  ■ Vigorous hydration
	  ■ Treatment of precipitating factors
	■ Acute chest syndrome:
	  ■ Careful hydration; hemodynamic monitoring
	  ■ Oxygen therapy
	  ■ Transfusion
	■ Folic acid supplements
	■ Blood transfusions during surgery or pregnancy as necessary
	■ Genetic counseling recommended

Thalassemia	■ Regular blood transfusions ■ Folic acid supplements ■ Possible splenectomy ■ Genetic counseling
Aplastic anemia	■ Withdrawal of the causative agent, if known ■ Blood transfusions ■ Bone marrow transplant as indicated

NURSING CARE PLAN   A Client with Folic Acid Deficiency Anemia

Sheri Matthews is a 76-year-old widow who lives alone. She tells Lisa Apana, RN, the nurse in her care provider's office, that she liked to cook when her husband was alive, but preparing an entire meal just for herself seems senseless. She relates that her typical day's menu includes coffee for breakfast, a bologna sandwich and coffee for lunch, and a hot dog or two, a few cookies, and a glass of milk for dinner.

ASSESSMENT

Mrs. Matthews's nursing history includes a 20-lb (9-kg) weight loss since her husband died 8 months ago. She states that she sometimes has heart palpitations and always feels weak. Physical assessment shows: T 99.0°F (37.1°C), P 110, R 22, BP 90/52. Skin warm, pale, and dry. Diagnostic tests indicate folic acid deficiency anemia, and Mrs. Matthews is started on an oral folic acid supplement and instructed about foods containing folic acid.

DIAGNOSES

- *Activity Intolerance* related to weakness secondary to decreased tissue oxygenation
- *Imbalanced Nutrition: Less than Body Requirements* related to lack of motivation to cook and understanding of nutritional needs, as manifested by weight loss of 20 lb and folic acid deficiency
- *Deficient Knowledge* related to lack of information about a well-balanced diet and foods containing folic acid

EXPECTED OUTCOMES

- Verbalize the importance of taking folic acid supplements and eating a balanced diet.
- Gain at least 1 lb (0.45 kg) per week.
- Return to previous level of physical energy.
- Consume a balanced diet, including foods containing folic acid.

PLANNING AND IMPLEMENTATION

- Discuss foods required for a well-balanced diet, as well as dietary sources of folic acid.
- Develop a dietary plan with Mrs. Matthews that includes food preferences and foods that are easy and quick to prepare.
- Discuss the importance of taking the folic acid supplement. Advise to continue taking it even after she begins to feel better.
- Help Mrs. Matthews develop a schedule of activities that provides adequate rest and energy for cooking.

EVALUATION

Mrs. Matthews gained 1 lb (0.45 kg) during the first week of treatment. She has met with a nutritionist and has a better understanding of nutritional needs. She states that she can prepare hot meals when she schedules a rest period before and after lunch. Ms. Apana has provided written and verbal information about the folic acid supplement and diet. Mrs. Matthews verbalizes understanding, stating, "I will continue to take the folic acid until the doctor tells me to stop. I'm beginning to enjoy cooking again, now that I have a reason to cook!" Ms. Apana contacts the local senior services representative to determine if Mrs. Matthews is able to participate in the local Meals-on-Wheels program.

CRITICAL THINKING IN THE NURSING PROCESS

1. What is the pathophysiologic basis for Mrs. Matthews's abnormal vital signs during her initial assessment?
2. Design a week's menu that includes foods high in folic acid.
3. Why was Mrs. Matthews placed on a folic acid supplement in addition to dietary modifications?
4. Why is the older adult at increased risk for developing folic acid deficiency anemia? Consider physiologic, economic, and social factors.

See Evaluating Your Response in Appendix C.

- *Diagnostic tests:* CBC, hemoglobin, and hematocrit; bone marrow studies; specialized tests (e.g., hemoglobin electrophoresis, Schilling test).

Nursing Diagnoses and Interventions

Anemia affects circulating oxygen levels and tissue oxygenation. Priority nursing diagnoses include activity intolerance, altered oral mucous membranes, and self-care deficits. With acute blood-loss anemia, risk for insufficient cardiac output also is a priority. Clients with sickle cell disease have specific needs related to the effects of the disease on tissue perfusion; see the section on disseminated intravascular coagulation later in this chapter for nursing interventions appropriate to ineffective tissue perfusion, associated pain, and maintaining oxygenation.

Activity Intolerance

Anemia causes weakness and shortness of breath on exertion. These symptoms are due to decreased circulating oxygen levels secondary to low hemoglobin levels. Weakness, fatigue, and/or vertigo may occur even during activities of daily living, including those associated with self-care, home life, job performance, and social roles.

- Help identify ways to conserve energy when performing necessary or desired activities. *Modifying the approach to a particular activity may reduce cardiorespiratory symptoms and activity-related fatigue. Alternative ways of performing tasks (e.g., sitting when performing hygiene care and kitchen tasks) may reduce oxygen demands. In some cases, assistance from others is necessary to conserve energy and reduce symptoms.*
- Help the client and family establish priorities for tasks and activities. *Because family members may need to assume responsibility for additional tasks, the plan's success depends on mutually established goals.*
- Assist to develop a schedule of alternating activity and rest periods throughout the day. *Rest periods decrease oxygen needs, reducing strain on the heart and lungs, and allowing restoration of homeostasis before further activities.*
- Encourage 8 to 10 hours of sleep at night. *Rest decreases oxygen demands and increases available energy for morning activities.*
- Monitor vital signs before and after activity. *Vital signs provide a measure of activity tolerance. Increased heart and respiratory rates or a change in blood pressure may indicate intolerance of the activity.*

- Discontinue activity if any of the following occurs:
  a. Complaints of chest pain, breathlessness, or vertigo
  b. Palpitations or tachycardia that does not return to normal within 4 minutes of resting
  c. Bradycardia
  d. Tachypnea or dyspnea
  e. Decreased systolic blood pressure.
  These changes may signify cardiac decompensation due to insufficient oxygenation. The intensity, duration, or frequency of the activity needs to be reduced.
- Instruct the client not to smoke. *Smoking causes vasoconstriction and increases carbon monoxide levels in the blood, interfering with tissue oxygenation.*

Impaired Oral Mucous Membrane

Glossitis and cheilosis may occur with nutritional deficiencies of iron, folate, and vitamin B_{12}. The tongue and lips become very red, and fissures or cracks may form at the corners of the mouth.

- Monitor condition of lips and tongue daily. *Glossitis and cheilosis increase the risk for bleeding and infection and may require medical treatment. Pain and discomfort may interfere with oral intake, further worsening the nutritional deficiency.*
- Use a mouthwash of saline, saltwater, or half-strength peroxide and water to rinse the mouth every 2 to 4 hours. Avoid alcohol-based mouthwashes. *This cleanses and soothes oral mucous membranes. Alcohol-based mouthwashes further irritate and dry oral tissues.*
- Provide frequent oral hygiene (after each meal and at bedtime) with a soft bristle toothbrush or sponge. *Removing food debris from painful fissures promotes comfort. A soft toothbrush reduces irritation or bleeding of oral mucosa. Keeping the oral cavity clean also reduces the risk of infection.*
- Apply a petroleum-based lubricating jelly or ointment to the lips after oral care. *Lubricating ointment helps to retain moisture, facilitate healing, and protect the lips from other drying agents.*
- Instruct to avoid hot, spicy, or acidic foods. *Such foods may further irritate and dry mucous membranes.*
- Encourage soft, cool, bland foods. *Foods that are soothing to the mucous membranes promote comfort and help maintain adequate food and fluid intake. Minimizing oral pain may also promote compliance with oral care routines.*
- Encourage eating four to six small meals daily with high protein and vitamin content. *Small, frequent meals may be better tolerated, increasing intake. Nutrient-rich meals promote healing of the mucous membranes.*

Risk for Decreased Cardiac Output

Cardiac output may be affected by acute bleeding and volume loss or by heart failure resulting from severe anemia. In addition, impaired tissue oxygenation leads to an increased respiratory rate and dyspnea.

- Monitor vital signs, breath sounds, and apical pulse. *Increased cardiac workload can affect the blood pressure, heart, and respiratory rates. Increased blood flow can lead to heart murmur or abnormal heart sounds such as S_3 or S_4. Tachypnea and dyspnea may affect the depth of respirations, alveolar ventilation, and blood and tissue oxygenation.*

- Assess for pallor, cyanosis, and dependent edema. *Blood is shunted to the vital organs, causing vasoconstriction of skin vessels. This, in addition to lower levels of hemoglobin, causes pallor. Cyanosis, especially of the lips and nail beds, indicates inadequate oxygenation of blood. Dependent edema occurs in response to right ventricular failure.*

PRACTICE ALERT
Report signs of decreased cardiac output to the physician. Severe anemia can lead to heart failure, necessitating additional treatment.

- Closely monitor for manifestations of anaphylaxis (urticaria, erythema or flushing, edema, wheezing, dyspnea, nausea and vomiting, anxiety) when administering parenteral iron preparations, particularly iron dextran. Immediately notify the physician, and prepare to administer prescribed drugs such as diphenhydramine (Benadryl) or epinephrine as ordered. Institute cardiopulmonary resuscitation measures as necessary. *Anaphylaxis, a systemic type I hypersensitivity (allergic) reaction, is a risk when administering parenteral iron preparations, iron dextran in particular. Anaphylaxis can lead to severe cardiopulmonary compromise, necessitating emergency measures to preserve life.*

Self-Care Deficit

Energy expenditures for activities of daily living (ADLs) may cause oxygen demands to exceed supply in the client with severe anemia.

- Assist with ADLs, such as bathing, grooming, and eating, as needed. *Assistance decreases energy expenditures and tissue requirements for oxygen, reducing cardiac workload.*
- Discuss the importance of rest periods prior to such activities as dressing. *Rest reduces oxygen demand and cardiac workload. The person who is able to perform self-care in activities of daily living maintains independence, self-esteem, and morale.*

NANDA, NIC, and NOC Linkages

See Chart 34–1 for linkages between NANDA nursing diagnoses, nursing interventions, and nursing outcomes for the client with anemia.

Community-Based Care

With the exception of anemia resulting from acute hemorrhage, most clients with anemia are treated in the home and community setting. Include the following topics when preparing the client and family for home care:

- Nutritional strategies to address deficiencies
- Prescribed medications, vitamins, or mineral supplements and their appropriate use, intended effect, possible adverse effects, and interactions with food or other medications
- Energy conservation strategies
- Other recommended treatment measures and follow-up
- If the anemia is genetically transmitted, such as sickle cell anemia, include inheritance patterns of the disorder, symptoms of crisis, and manifestations to report to the physician.

Provide referrals for counseling to facilitate decisions about pregnancy as indicated. Also refer for nutritional assistance and

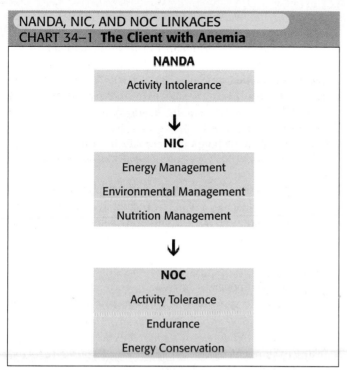

NANDA, NIC, AND NOC LINKAGES
CHART 34–1 **The Client with Anemia**

NANDA

Activity Intolerance

↓

NIC

Energy Management

Environmental Management

Nutrition Management

↓

NOC

Activity Tolerance

Endurance

Energy Conservation

Data from *NANDA's Nursing Diagnoses: Definitions & Classification 2005–2006* by NANDA International (2005), Philadelphia; *Nursing Interventions Classification (NIC)* (4th ed.) by J. M. Dochterman & G. M. Bulechek (2004), St. Louis, MO: Mosby; and *Nursing Outcomes Classification (NOC)* (3rd ed.) by S. Moorhead, M. Johnson, and M. Mass (2004), St. Louis, MO: Mosby.

teaching, home health care, or assistance with self-care and home maintenance activities as indicated. Older adults with nutritional anemias may benefit from community services such as senior meals or Meals-on-Wheels.

THE CLIENT WITH MYELODYSPLASTIC SYNDROME

Myelodysplastic syndrome (MDS) is a group of blood disorders characterized by abnormal-appearing bone marrow and cytopenia (low numbers of circulating blood cells). MDS is not a single disease; at least five variations of the disorder have been identified. Anemia that does not respond to treatment (*refractory anemia*) is a characteristic of most forms of myelodysplasia.

Idiopathic MDS primarily affects older adults; men have a slightly higher incidence of the disorder than women. Risk factors for secondary MDS include exposure to environmental toxins such as cigarette smoke, benzene, radiation, radiation therapy or chemotherapy for cancer treatment, and other anemias such as aplastic anemia or Fanconi's anemia (Demakos & Linebaugh, 2005; Kasper et al., 2005).

FAST FACTS

- Idiopathic or primary MDS accounts for 70% to 80% of all identified cases.
- Twenty percent to 30% of MDS cases occur as a secondary condition, related to factors such as smoking or exposure to environmental toxins, radiation, chemotherapy, or other risk factors (Demakos & Linebaugh, 2005).

Pathophysiology

MDS is a stem cell disorder in which stem cells fail to reproduce and differentiate into the various types of blood cells. The genetic components of stem cells (nuclear DNA and/or mitochondrial DNA) are altered. The bone marrow loses its ability to produce normal blood cells, instead producing abnormal (*dysplastic*) cells. With significant alterations, leukemia (proliferation of abnormal white blood cells) may develop in people with MDS.

Manifestations

Anemia is the predominant early manifestation of MDS. The client may develop symptoms of the anemia with increasing fatigue, weakness, dyspnea and pallor. In many cases, the disorder is asymptomatic, identified when a routine blood count shows anemia. Splenomegaly may develop, leading to discomfort and a feeling of fullness in the left upper quadrant of the abdomen. Hepatomegaly also may develop, leading to right upper quadrant discomfort. Thrombocytopenia can lead to abnormal bleeding tendencies, and neutropenia increases the risk for infection (Demakos & Linebaugh, 2005).

INTERDISCIPLINARY CARE

Clients with MDS require long-term supportive care and therapy to maintain their quality of life. Stem cell transplant offers the only real hope for cure in MDS. See the Interdisciplinary Care section of the client with leukemia later in this chapter for more information about stem cell transplant and associated nursing care.

Diagnosis

- The *CBC* reveals anemia. Although anemia may be the only abnormality of the blood count, the white blood cell (WBC) count also may be low, as may be the platelet count. Abnormalities of size and shape may be noted in all blood cells.
- The *bone marrow* often appears normal, although precursor cells may have an abnormal appearance. Increased numbers of myeloblasts (granulocyte precursor cells) may be present in the bone marrow.
- *Serum erythropoietin, vitamin B_{12}, serum iron, total iron-binding capacity, ferritin levels,* and *RBC folate levels* are drawn to help guide supportive therapy.

Treatment

Management of MDS is based on the severity of the disease. Several classification systems are available, including the French-American-British (FAB) classification system, the International Prognostic Scoring System (IPSS), and the World Health Organization (WHO) classification system (National Comprehensive Cancer Network [NCCN], 2006). These systems are used to guide therapy for the client with MDS.

All clients with MDS require monitoring, with regular physician visits and laboratory evaluations. Psychosocial support is provided to assist the client and family dealing with a chronic, progressive, and ultimately fatal disease.

Clients with MDS may require frequent red blood cell transfusions to treat the predominant anemia. Each unit of packed

RBCs contains 250 to 300 mg of iron. The body is unable to excrete this excess iron, so it accumulates, leading to problems such as endocrine dysfunction, cirrhosis, pericarditis, and heart failure. *Iron chelation therapy* is used to remove excess iron from the body. Desferrioxamine (Desferal) is administered by slow intravenous infusion or continuous subcutaneous infusion using an infusion pump to maintain a normal or negative iron balance. This drug is relatively safe, although local skin reactions such as rash and urticaria may develop. An oral form of the drug, deferasirox, is available, but not widely used.

Blood cell growth factors may be administered to stimulate stem cell development in MDS, although the response rate is low. Platelet transfusions are given when bleeding occurs due to low platelet levels. Antibiotic therapy is initiated for bacterial infections (NCCS, 2006). Chemotherapy regimens similar to those employed to treat leukemia may be used, but rarely are effective in treating MDS. Azacitidine (Vidaza), an antileukemic agent that acts on abnormal blood-forming cells in the bone marrow, may be more effective in treating MDS than standard chemotherapy regimens (Demakos & Linebaugh, 2005). As previously noted, stem cell transplant offers the only hope for cure. This high-risk therapy, however, is reserved for higher risk clients. Factors such as age, functional ability, and other existing disease conditions help guide the decision to undergo stem cell transplant (NCCN, 2006).

 NURSING CARE

Nursing Diagnoses and Interventions

Activity intolerance and the need for education about this disorder are the priorities of nursing care for the client with MDS being managed in a community-based setting. Although neutropenia and thrombocytopenia may accompany the anemia of MDS, these problems are less common. See the section of this chapter on leukemia for additional potential nursing diagnoses and interventions for the client with MDS.

Activity Intolerance

The client with MDS experiences fatigue, weakness, and shortness of breath on exertion related to the lack of RBCs and ineffective oxygen transport. These symptoms may affect the client's ability to maintain self-care, home life, job performance, and social roles.

- Monitor vital signs, breath sounds, and apical pulse. *Increased cardiac workload due to anemia and impaired oxygen transport can affect the blood pressure, heart, and respiratory rates. Increased blood flow can lead to heart murmur or abnormal heart sounds such as S_3 or S_4. Accumulated iron can lead to pericarditis and a pericardial friction rub.*
- Help identify energy-conserving ways of performing necessary or desired activities. *Alternative ways of performing tasks (e.g., sitting while performing hygiene measures) may reduce oxygen demands and fatigue.*
- Help the client and family establish priorities for tasks and activities. *Because family members may need to assume responsibility for additional tasks, the plan's success depends on mutually established goals.*
- Suggest planning recreational activities following a transfusion and adjusting activity level between transfusions to match energy and minimize fatigue. *The client with MDS will have more energy and activity tolerance following a transfusion when RBC counts, hemoglobin, and hematocrit approach normal levels and oxygen transport is optimal.*
- Encourage 8 to 10 hours of sleep at night. *Rest decreases oxygen demands and increases available energy for morning activities.*
- Discontinue activity if any of the following occurs:
  a. Complaints of chest pain, breathlessness, or vertigo
  b. Palpitations or tachycardia that does not return to normal within 4 minutes of resting
  c. Bradycardia
  d. Tachypnea or dyspnea
  e. Decreased systolic blood pressure.
  These changes may signify cardiac decompensation due to insufficient oxygenation. The intensity, duration, or frequency of the activity needs to be reduced.
- Instruct the client not to smoke. *Smoking causes vasoconstriction and increases carbon monoxide levels in the blood, interfering with tissue oxygenation.*

Risk for Ineffective Health Maintenance

MDS is a chronic, usually progressive disorder, requiring active management to maintain functional status and quality of life. Regular visits to the physician or clinic may be necessary. In addition, the client or family members may need to learn to administer iron chelation therapy or chemotherapy drugs and measures to prevent complications. The chronic nature of the disorder and the often advanced age of the client and family caregivers may interfere with effective management of the disorder.

- Assess knowledge of the disorder and the related treatments. *Assessment allows identification of knowledge gaps and provides a basis on which to provide additional information. Impaired disease management may be due to lack of knowledge or an inability to learn and perform psychomotor skills (e.g., administration of parenteral drug therapy).*
- Provide information about the disorder, its effects, and prescribed medications and treatments. *Individualized instruction is more effective than general, possibly irrelevant information. The client and caregivers need to be able to identify and manage possible adverse effects of drug therapy, as well as recognize potential complications to be reported to the physician.*
- Provide emotional support, expressing confidence in the client's and caregivers' abilities to manage care. *Emotional support helps the client and family caregivers incorporate the care regimen into their lifestyle.*
- Provide supervised learning and practice opportunities for administering parenteral medications if ordered. *Successful practice sessions instill confidence in the ability to manage care and provide an opportunity for questions and exploring alternatives.*

Community-Based Care

The client with myelodysplastic syndrome needs information about this chronic and ultimately fatal disease. Provide information about treatment options, including management of the infusion pump if ordered. Discuss the timing of and options for stem cell transplant, and assist the client to evaluate the potential benefits and risks of this treatment option.

THE CLIENT WITH POLYCYTHEMIA

Polycythemia, or *erythrocytosis,* is an excess of red blood cells characterized by a hematocrit higher than 55%. The two major types of polycythemia are primary and secondary. A third type of polycythemia, relative polycythemia, results from a fluid volume deficit, not excess RBCs.

FAST FACTS

- *Primary polycythemia (polycythemia vera)* is uncommon.
  - In primary polycythemia, RBC production is increased.
  - Primary polycythemia more commonly affects men of European Jewish ancestry between age 40 and 70.
- *Secondary polycythemia (erythrocytosis)* is the most common form of polycythemia.
  - Secondary polycythemia occurs when erythropoietin levels are elevated.
  - It may affect clients of any age or origin.
  - It usually develops in response to hypoxia (living at a high altitude, smoking, or chronic lung disease).
- *Relative polycythemia* occurs due to fluid deficit, not excess RBCs.
  - In relative polycythemia the total RBC count is normal.
  - The hematocrit is elevated because of increased cell concentration.
  - It is corrected by rehydration.

Pathophysiology

Primary Polycythemia

Primary polycythemia, or polycythemia vera (PV), is a neoplastic stem cell disorder characterized by overproduction of RBCs and, to a lesser extent, white blood cells and platelets. It is classified as a myeloproliferative disorder. Its cause is unknown. In PV, colonies of endogenous erythroid stem cells develop. These colonies produce RBCs in the absence of erythropoietin, leading to excess RBC production.

MANIFESTATIONS Initially, PV is asymptomatic, and the diagnosis may be made during routine blood tests. Its manifestations are caused by increased blood volume and viscosity. Hypertension is common, and may lead to complaints of headaches, dizziness, and vision and hearing disruptions. Venous stasis causes *plethora,* a ruddy, red color of the face, hands, feet, and mucous membranes. This often is accompanied by severe, painful itching of the fingers and toes. Retinal and cerebral vessels may be engorged. Hypermetabolism develops, causing weight loss and night sweats. Mental status may be altered, leading to drowsiness or delirium.

Thrombosis and hemorrhage are potential complications of PV. Thrombosis may cause transient ischemic attacks, angina, or manifestations of peripheral vascular disease. Gastrointestinal bleeding may occur, and portal hypertension may develop.

Secondary Polycythemia

Secondary polycythemia, or erythrocytosis, is increased numbers of RBCs in response to excess erythropoietin secretion or prolonged hypoxia. Secondary polycythemia is the most common form of polycythemia.

Abnormally high erythropoietin levels can result from kidney disease or erythropoietin-secreting tumors (e.g., renal cell carcinoma). Chronic hypoxia that stimulates erythropoietin release is a more common cause of secondary polycythemia. People living at high altitudes where the atmospheric oxygen pressure is lower develop a degree of polycythemia, as do people with chronic heart or lung disease and smokers. Abnormal hemoglobin that forms tighter bonds with oxygen also may lead to secondary polycythemia.

MANIFESTATIONS The manifestations of secondary polycythemia are similar to those of primary polycythemia. Splenomegaly, however, does not develop. Early symptoms often are overshadowed by the manifestations of the underlying disorder. For the manifestations of polycythemia see the box below.

INTERDISCIPLINARY CARE

Diagnosis

In PV, serum erythropoietin levels are low. Bone marrow studies show hyperplasia of all hematopoietic elements. With secondary polycythemia, serum erythropoietin levels usually are high, and bone marrow studies show only red stem cell hyperplasia.

Treatments

For secondary polycythemia, treatment focuses on the underlying cause of the disorder. It is a physiologic response in people living at high altitudes, and unless the hematocrit is too high or oxygen saturation levels are low, no treatment is usually necessary. Smokers are urged to quit. Measures to raise oxygen saturation levels and reduce tissue hypoxia often will relieve the polycythemia. Clients with both primary and secondary polycythemia benefit from periodic phlebotomy, removing 300 to 500 mL of blood, to keep blood volume and viscosity within normal levels. For PV, chemotherapeutic agents such as hydroxyurea may be used to suppress marrow function but may

---

MANIFESTATIONS of Polycythemia

- Hypertension
- Headache, tinnitus, blurred vision
- Plethora: dark redness of the lips, feet, ears, fingernails, and mucous membranes
- Splenomegaly (polycythemia vera)
- Severe pruritus, extremity pain
- Weight loss, night sweats
- Gastrointestinal bleeding
- Intermittent claudication
- Symptoms from thrombosis within various organs

increase the risk of developing leukemia (discussed later in this chapter). Pruritus may be relieved by antihistamines, or may require more aggressive treatment with interferon alpha or other treatments. One 325-mg aspirin tablet daily may be ordered to control thrombosis without increasing the risk of bleeding.

NURSING CARE

Preventing polycythemia begins with educating children and adults about the dangers of smoking. Measures to reduce risk factors for cardiovascular disease also may be beneficial.

This chronic condition is managed in community-based settings unless a complication develops. Teach the client and family the importance of maintaining adequate hydration, and increasing fluid intake during hot weather and when exercising. Discuss measures to prevent blood stasis: elevating legs and feet when sitting, using support stockings, and continuing treatment measures. Instruct to report manifestations of thrombosis (leg or calf pain, chest pain, neurologic symptoms) or bleeding (black, tarry stools, vomiting of blood or coffee-grounds emesis) immediately. Monitor the hematocrit and cell counts throughout treatment.

Examples of nursing diagnoses appropriate for the client with polycythemia follow:
- *Decisional Conflict Regarding Smoking Cessation* related to addictive effects
- *Pain* related to effects of altered blood flow in distal extremities
- *Risk for Ineffective Tissue Perfusion* related to sluggish blood flow and increased risk for thrombosis.

WHITE BLOOD CELL AND LYMPHOID TISSUE DISORDERS

Disorders of the white blood cells and lymphoid tissue include infectious mononucleosis, the leukemias, multiple myeloma, and malignant lymphomas (Hodgkin's disease and non-Hodgkin's lymphoma). Review the physiology of WBCs and lymphoid tissues and assessment of their function in Chapter 33 ∞ before proceeding with this section.

THE CLIENT WITH LEUKEMIA

Leukemia (literally, "white blood") is a group of chronic malignant disorders of white blood cells and white blood cell precursors. In leukemia, the usual ratio of red to white blood cells is reversed. Leukemias are characterized by replacement of bone marrow by malignant immature white blood cells, abnormal immature circulating WBCs, and infiltration of these cells into the liver, spleen, and lymph nodes throughout the body.

Incidence and Risk Factors

Although leukemia is often thought of as a childhood disease, it is diagnosed 10 times more often in adults than in children. An estimated 34,810 new cases of leukemia occur annually; slightly more than half are acute leukemia and less than half are chronic leukemia. In 2005, the ACS (2005) estimated that approximately 22,570 people died of leukemia. The highest incidence of leukemia is found in the United States, Canada, Sweden, and New Zealand (McCance & Huether, 2006).

Although the cause of most leukemias is unknown, certain risk factors have been identified. Men are affected more frequently than are women. People with certain genetic disorders such as Down syndrome have a higher incidence of leukemia. Environmental risk factors play a role as well. Risk factors for myeloid leukemia include cigarette smoking and chemicals such as benzene (present in cigarette smoke and gasoline). Exposure to ionizing radiation increases the risk for several types of leukemia. Clients who have undergone treatment for cancer have an increased risk. The human T-cell leukemia/lymphoma virus-1, a retrovirus, is known to cause certain leukemias and lymphomas (ACS, 2005).

Physiology Review

White blood cells are the most diverse of the cellular components of the blood. White blood cells arise from three different precursor cells: myeloblasts, which further differentiate into the granular leukocytes (granulocytes), neutrophils, eosinophils, and basophils; monoblasts, which mature into circulating monocytes, and ultimately into macrophages; and lymphoblasts, which become lymphocytes and mature in lymphoid tissue to B cells and T cells.

As a whole, the primary function of WBCs is to help maintain the body's immune defenses. Neutrophils, the most numerous WBC in circulation, are active phagocytes, the first cells to arrive to injured tissue. Monocytes and macrophages also are phagocytic cells that dispose of foreign and waste material from tissues. Eosinophils and basophils are more specialized. Eosinophils are primarily involved in allergic responses and parasitic infections. Basophils are actively involved in the inflammatory response, releasing substances such as histamine and heparin into inflamed tissues. Lymphocytes, the smallest of the WBCs, are an integral part of the immune system. B cells are part of the humoral immune response, producing antibodies to specific antigens. T cells are part of the cell-mediated immune response. For more information about the inflammatory and immune responses, see Chapter 12 ∞. The normal WBC count and differential are presented in Table 34–2.

TABLE 34–2 Normal White Blood Cell Count and Differential

LABORATORY TEST	VALUE
WBC count	5000–10,000/mm³
Differential WBC count	
Neutrophils	60–70% or 3000–7000/mm³
Eosinophils	1–3% or 50–400/mm³
Basophils	0.3–0.5% or 25–200/mm³
Lymphocytes	20–30% or 1000–4000/mm³
Monocytes	3–8% or 100–600/mm³

Pathophysiology

Leukemia begins with malignant transformation of a single stem cell. Leukemic cells proliferate slowly, but do not differentiate normally. They have a prolonged life span and accumulate in the bone marrow. As they accumulate, they compete with the proliferation of normal cells. Leukemic cells do not function as mature WBCs, and are ineffective in the inflammatory and immune processes. Leukemic cells replace normal hematopoietic elements in the marrow. Because erythrocyte- and platelet-producing cells are crowded out, severe anemia, splenomegaly, and bleeding difficulties result.

Leukemic cells leave the bone marrow and travel through the circulatory system, infiltrating other body tissues such as the CNS, testes, skin, gastrointestinal tract, and the lymph nodes, liver, and spleen. Death usually is due to internal hemorrhage and infections.

Manifestations

The general manifestations of leukemia (regardless of type) result from anemia, infection, and bleeding. These include pallor, fatigue, tachycardia, malaise, lethargy, and dyspnea on exertion. Infection may cause fever, night sweats, oral ulcerations, and frequent or recurrent respiratory, urinary, integumentary, or other infections. Increased bleeding due to thrombocytopenia leads to bruising, petechiae, bleeding gums, and bleeding within specific organs and tissues. *Multisystem Effects of Leukemia* can be seen on page 1120.

Other manifestations result from leukemic cell infiltration, increased metabolism, and increased leukocyte destruction. Infiltration of the liver, spleen, lymph nodes, and bone marrow causes pain and tissue swelling in the involved areas. Meningeal infiltration may cause manifestations of increased intracranial pressure, such as headache, altered level of consciousness, cranial nerve impairment, nausea, and vomiting. Infiltration of the kidneys may affect renal function, with decreased urine output and increased blood urea nitrogen and creatinine. Increased metabolism causes heat intolerance, weight loss, dyspnea on exertion, and tachycardia. Destruction of large numbers of WBCs releases substantial amounts of uric acid into the circulation; uric acid crystals may obstruct renal tubules, causing renal insufficiency.

Without treatment, leukemia is invariably fatal, usually due to complications of leukemic cell infiltration of bone marrow or vital organs. With treatment, prognosis varies. The overall 5-year survival rate is 46%. Survival rates differ by type of leukemia: People with acute myeloid leukemia have a 20% 5-year survival rate, whereas the rate is 73% for people with chronic lymphocytic leukemia (American Cancer Society, [ACS], 2005). The types, pathology, manifestations, and treatment for the major leukemias are outlined in Table 34–3.

Classifications

Leukemias are classified by their acuity and by the predominant cell type involved. The *acute* leukemias are characterized by an acute onset, rapid disease progression, and immature or undifferentiated blast cells. *Chronic* leukemias, on the other hand, have a gradual onset, prolonged course, and abnormal mature-appearing cells. *Lymphocytic* (or *lymphoblastic*) leukemias involve immature lymphocytes and their precursor cells in the bone marrow. Lymphocytic leukemias infiltrate the spleen, lymph nodes, CNS, and other tissues. *Myeloid* (also called *myelogenous, myelocytic,* or *myeloblastic*) leukemias involve myeloid stem cells in the bone marrow, interfering with the maturation of all types of blood cells, including granulocytes, RBCs, and thrombocytes (Porth, 2005). Acute lymphoblastic leukemia is the most common type of leukemia in children. In adults, acute myeloid leukemia and chronic lymphocytic leukemia are the most common types (McCance &

TABLE 34–3 Major Types of Leukemia

CLASSIFICATION	CHARACTERISTICS	MANIFESTATIONS	TREATMENT
Acute lymphoblastic leukemia (ALL)	Primarily affects children and young adults; leukemic cells may infiltrate CNS	Recurrent infections; bleeding; pallor, bone pain, weight loss, sore throat, fatigue, night sweats, weakness	Chemotherapy; bone marrow transplant (BMT), or stem cell transplant (SCT)
Chronic lymphocytic leukemia (CLL)	Primarily affects older adults; insidious onset and slow, chronic course	Fatigue; exercise intolerance; lymphadenopathy and splenomegaly; recurrent infections, pallor, edema, thrombophlebitis	Often requires no treatment; chemotherapy; BMT
Acute myeloid leukemia (AML)	Common in older adults, may affect children and young adults. Strongly associated with toxins, genetic disorders, and treatment of other cancers	Fatigue, weakness, fever; anemia; headache; bone and joint pain; abnormal bleeding and bruising; recurrent infection; lymphadenopathy, splenomegaly, and hepatomegaly	Chemotherapy; SCT
Chronic myeloid leukemia (CML)	Primarily affects adults; early course slow and stable, progressing to aggressive phase in 3–4 years	*Early:* weakness, fatigue, dyspnea on exertion; possible splenomegaly; *Later:* fever, weight loss, night sweats	Interferon alpha; chemotherapy with imatinib mesylate (Gleevec), SCT

MULTISYSTEM EFFECTS of Leukemia

Neurologic
- Headache
- Altered LOC
- Cranial nerve impairment

Potential complications
- Subarachnoid hemorrhage
- Retinal hemorrhage
- Seizures, coma

Respiratory
- Dyspnea on exertion
- Pharyngitis, sore throat
- Frequent respiratory infections

Potential complication
- Pulmonary bleeding

Gastrointestinal
- Anorexia, nausea
- Oral ulcerations, infection
- Bleeding gums
- Gingival hyperplasia
  (gum overgrowth)
- Abdominal pain
- Hepatomegaly
- Occult GI bleeding

Urinary
- Urinary tract infection
- Hematuria

Potential complication
- Renal insufficiency or failure

Musculoskeletal
- Weakness
- Bone tenderness, pain
- Joint pain

Metabolic Processes
- Malaise, lethargy
- Heat intolerance
- Diaphoresis
- Chills, fever
- Night sweats
- Weight loss

Cardiovascular
- Tachycardia, palpitations
- Orthostatic hypotension
- Heart murmurs
- Hematomas
- Edema

Potential complications
- Hemorrhage
- Thrombophlebitis

Hematologic
- Anemia
- Thrombocytopenia
- Leukopenia
- Bleeding (epistaxis)
- Splenomegaly

Potential complication
- DIC

Immunologic
- Frequent or recurrent infections
- Lymphadenopathy

Potential complications
- Abscesses
- Septicemia

Integumentary
- Skin and mucous membrane pallor
- Petechiae
- Bruising, purpura
- Ulcerations
- *Chloromas* (skin infiltrations near
  bony prominences)

Huether, 2006). In summary, the general types of leukemia are as follows:

- Acute lymphocytic (lymphoblastic) leukemia (ALL)
- Chronic lymphocytic leukemia (CLL)
- Acute myeloid (myeloblastic) leukemia (AML)
- Chronic myeloid (myelogenous) leukemia (CML).

This general system of classifying leukemias does not differentiate subtypes of acute leukemias. The FAB system for classifying acute leukemias further differentiates acute leukemias by the predominant cell involved and the degree of cell differentiation (Table 34–4).

Acute Myeloid Leukemia

Acute myeloid leukemia is characterized by uncontrolled proliferation of myeloblasts (the precursors of granulocytes) and hyperplasia of the bone marrow and spleen (Figure 34–5 ■). AML accounts for 80% of acute leukemia cases in adults (Copstead & Banasik, 2005). Treatment induces complete remission in 66% of clients, although only about 30% to 40% achieve cure or long-term remission (Porth, 2005).

The manifestations of AML result from neutropenia and thrombocytopenia. Decreased neutrophils lead to recurrent severe infections, such as pneumonia, septicemia, abscesses, and mucous membrane ulceration. The manifestations of thrombocytopenia include petechiae, purpura, ecchymoses (bruising), epistaxis (nosebleeds), hematomas, hematuria, and gastrointestinal bleeding. Bone infarctions or subperiosteal infiltrates of leukemic cells may cause bone pain. Anemia is a late manifestation, causing fatigue, headaches, pallor, and dyspnea on exertion. Death usually results from infection or hemorrhage.

Bone marrow aspiration shows a proliferation of immature WBCs. The CBC shows thrombocytopenia and normocytic, normochromic anemia.

Chronic Myeloid Leukemia

Chronic myeloid leukemia is characterized by abnormal proliferation of all bone marrow elements. This type of leukemia constitutes approximately 15% of adult leukemias. It affects men more frequently than women. The onset of CML typically is between ages 30 or 40 and 50, although it is seen in children and adolescents as well (Copstead & Banasik, 2005; Porth 2005).

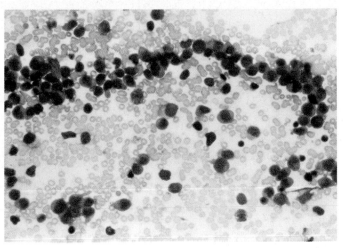

Figure 34–5 ■ A blood smear from the bone marrow of a client with acute myeloid leukemia. Note the abnormally large number of myelocyte WBCs (stained purple) among the small RBCs.

Source: Dr. Gopal Murti. Photo Researchers, Inc.

CML is usually associated with a chromosome abnormality called the Philadelphia chromosome, a balanced translocation of chromosome 22 to chromosome 9 (Figure 34–6 ■). The fusion gene produced by this translocation, known as *bcr/abl*, is an *oncogene* capable of initiating a malignancy. Very large doses of ionizing radiation also may induce CML in some clients (Kasper et al., 2005).

People with CML are often asymptomatic in the early stages and, in fact, are often diagnosed when a routine blood test reveals abnormal cell counts. Anemia causes weakness, fatigue, and dyspnea on exertion. The spleen often is enlarged, causing abdominal discomfort. Within 3 to 4 years, disease progresses to a more aggressive phase. Rapid cell proliferation and hypermetabolism cause fatigue, weight loss, sweating, and heat intolerance. The spleen enlarges, leading to a sensation of abdominal fullness and discomfort. Platelet function is affected in this stage, leading to bleeding and increased bruising. Finally, the disease evolves to acute leukemia, with blast cell proliferation. This stage, known as the *terminal blast crisis phase,* is characterized by significant constitutional manifestations, splenomegaly, and infiltration of leukemic cells into the skin, lymph nodes, bones, and CNS

TABLE 34–4 FAB Classification of Acute Leukemia

TYPE	CLASS	PREDOMINANT CELLS	PROGNOSIS
Acute lymphocytic	L_1	Immature lymphoblasts	>90% remission rate in children
leukemia	L_2	Mature lymphoblasts	Relapse common after 2 or more years of remission
Acute myeloid	M_0	Undifferentiated cells	Poor
leukemia	M_1	Immature myeloblasts	Good; complete response in 65% or more
	M_2	Mature myeloblasts	Good for 2 or more years of remission
	M_3	Promyelocytes	Good in adults
	M_4	Myelocytes and monocytes	Poorest in adults
	M_5	Poorly or well-differentiated monocytes	Poor
	M_6	Predominant erythroblasts	Variable
	M_7	Megakaryocytes	

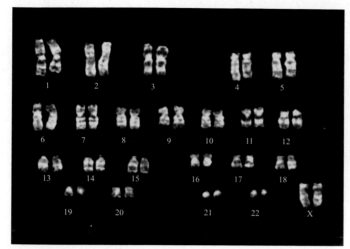

Figure 34–6 ■ The Philadelphia chromosome. Note the chromosomes of pairs 9 and 22. In each instance, the left-hand chromosome of the pair is normal, whereas an exchange of material between chromosomes has made the right-hand chromosome 9 larger and the right-hand chromosome 22 smaller. In stem cells within the bone marrow, the chromosome 22 defect leads to chronic myeloid leukemia.

Source: Addenbrookes Hospital, Photo Researchers, Inc.

(Porth, 2005). Survival following the onset of this final stage averages only 2 to 4 months.

Acute Lymphocytic Leukemia

Acute lymphocytic leukemia is the most common type of leukemia in children and young adults. In adults, ALL is rarely seen until late middle age, and then its incidence increases with aging. Genetic factors may play a role in its development, particularly the *bcr/abl* translocation also implicated in CML (Copstead & Banasik, 2005).

Most (80%) cases of ALL result from malignant transformation of B cells, with the remaining 20% arising from T cells. The malignant cells resemble immature lymphocytes (*lymphoblasts*); however, they do not mature or function effectively to maintain immunity. These lymphoblasts accumulate in the bone marrow, lymph nodes, and spleen, as well as in circulating blood. Some types of lymphoma (discussed later in this chapter) are thought to represent a later stage of the same disease.

The onset of ALL is usually rapid. Lymphoblasts proliferating in bone marrow and peripheral tissues crowd the growth of normal cells (Figure 34–7 ■). Normal hematopoiesis is suppressed, leading to thrombocytopenia, leukopenia, and anemia. Manifestations of infections, bleeding, and anemia develop. Bone pain resulting from rapid generation of marrow elements, lymphadenopathy, and liver enlargement are also common. Infiltration of the CNS causes headaches, visual disturbances, vomiting, and seizures.

The CBC shows an elevated WBC count with increased lymphocytes on the differential. RBC and platelet counts are decreased. Bone marrow studies reveal a hypercellular marrow with growth of lymphoblasts. Combination chemotherapy produces complete remission in 80% to 90% of adults with ALL.

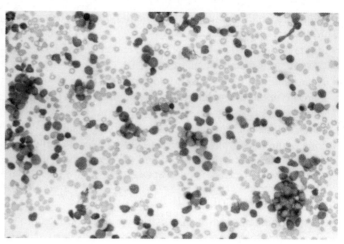

Figure 34–7 ■ ■ A blood smear from the bone marrow of a client with acute lymphocytic leukemia. Note the abnormally large number of lymphocytes (stained purple) crowding the bone marrow. As a result, normal production of RBCs, functional WBCs, and platelets is suppressed.

Source: Dr. Gopal Murti, Photo Researchers, Inc.

Chronic Lymphocytic Leukemia

Chronic lymphocytic leukemia is characterized by proliferation and accumulation of small, abnormal, mature lymphocytes in the bone marrow, peripheral blood, and body tissues. The abnormal cells are usually B lymphocytes that are unable to produce adequate antibodies to maintain normal immune function. Only about 5% of CLL involves T cells (Copstead & Banasik, 2005). CLL occurs more commonly in adults, especially in older adults (median age 65). CLL is the least common type of the major leukemias.

CLL has a slow onset and is often diagnosed during a routine physical examination. If symptoms are present, they usually include vague complaints of weakness or malaise. Possible clinical findings include anemia, infection, and enlarged lymph nodes, spleen, and liver. As in other leukemias, bone marrow hyperplasia is present. Erythrocyte and platelet counts are reduced. Leukocyte counts may either be elevated or reduced, but abnormal cells are always present. In CLL, years may elapse before treatment is required. Survival of this disease averages approximately 7 years.

INTERDISCIPLINARY CARE

Treatment for leukemia focuses on achieving remission or cure and relieving symptoms. The methods of treatment may include chemotherapy, radiation therapy, and bone marrow or stem cell transplantation. Cure is more often achieved in children with acute leukemia than in adults, although long-term remissions (disease-free periods with no signs or symptoms) often can be achieved.

Diagnosis

The following diagnostic tests are ordered when leukemia is suspected:

■ *CBC* with differential is done to evaluate cell counts, hemoglobin and hematocrit levels, and the number, distribution, and morphology (size and shape) of WBCs.

TABLE 34–5 Diagnostic Findings by Type of Leukemia

TEST	AML	CML	ALL	CLL
RBC count	Low	Low	Low	Low
Hemoglobin	Low	Low	Low	Low
Hematocrit	Low	Low	Low	Low
Platelet count	Very low	High early, low late	Low	Low
WBC count	Varies	Increased	Varies	Increased
Myeloblasts	Present			
Neutrophils	Decreased	Increased	Decreased	Normal
Lymphocytes		Normal		Increased
Monocytes		Normal/low		
Blasts	Present	Present (crisis)	Present	
Bone Marrow	Hypercellular		Hypercellular	
Myeloblasts	Present			
Lymphoblasts			Present	
Lymphocytes				Present

- *Platelets* are measured to identify possible thrombocytopenia secondary to the leukemia and the risk of bleeding.
- *Bone marrow examination* provides information about cells within the marrow, the type of erythropoiesis, and the maturity of erythropoietic and leukopoietic cells.

Table 34–5 outlines usual diagnostic test results in the various forms of leukemia.

Chemotherapy

Single agent or combination chemotherapy is the treatment of choice for most types of leukemia, with the goal of eradicating leukemic cells and producing remission. Table 34–6 outlines typical chemotherapy regimens for different types of leukemia. Combination chemotherapy reduces drug resistance and toxicity, and interrupts cell growth at various stages of the cell cycle, producing a complementary effect of the drugs used. Cancer treatment with chemotherapy is discussed in detail in Chapter 14 ∞.

Chemotherapy for leukemia generally is divided into the induction phase and postremission therapy. During *induction*, drug doses are high to eradicate leukemic cells from the bone marrow. These high doses often also damage stem cells and interfere with production of normal blood cells. Circulating mature blood cells are not affected because they are no longer dividing. The degree of bone marrow suppression is influenced by a number of factors, including age, nutritional status, concurrent chronic diseases such as impaired liver or renal function, the drug and drug dose, and prior treatment.

Colony-stimulating factors (CSFs), also called hematopoietic growth factors, often are administered to "rescue" the bone marrow following induction chemotherapy. CSFs are cytokines that regulate the growth and differentiation of blood cells. Factors that support neutrophil maturation, *granulocyte-macrophage CSF (GM-CSF)* and *granulocyte CSF (G-CSF)*, are commonly used. Bone pain is a common side effect of therapy with these agents. Clients also may experience fevers, chills, anorexia, muscle aches, and lethargy (Kasper et al., 2005).

Once remission has been achieved, postremission chemotherapy is continued to eradicate any additional leukemic cells, prevent relapse, and prolong survival. A single chemotherapeutic agent, combination therapy, or bone marrow transplant may be used for postremission treatment.

Radiation Therapy

Radiation therapy damages cellular DNA. While the cell continues to function, it cannot divide and multiply. Cells that divide rapidly, such as bone marrow and cancer cells (radiosensitive cells), respond quickly to radiation therapy.

TABLE 34–6 Chemotherapeutic Regimens Used to Treat Leukemia

Acute myeloid leukemia	■ Cytarabine (Cytoxan, an alkylating agent), *with* daunorubicin (Cerubidine, an antitumor antibiotic) *or* idarubicin (Idamycin, an antitumor antibiotic) ■ All-*trans* retinoic acid (ATRA) added for clients with promyelocytic leukemia
Chronic myeloid leukemia	■ Imatinib mesylate (Gleevec), a *bcr/abl* tyrosine kinase (enzyme) inhibitor ■ Hydroxyurea (a DNA inhibitor) *or* homoharringtonine (HHT, a plant alkaloid) if imatinib not tolerated
Acute lymphocytic leukemia	■ Daunorubicin (Cerubidine, an antitumor antibiotic) *with* vincristine (Oncovin, a plant alkaloid) *with* prednisone *with* asparaginase (Elspar)
Chronic lymphocytic leukemia	■ Fludarabine (Fludara, an antimetabolite) *or* chlorambucil (Chloromycetin, an antitumor antibiotic) ■ Cyclophosphamide (Cytoxan, an alkylating agent), vincristine, and prednisone ■ Cyclophosphamide, doxorubicin (Adriamycin, an antitumor antibiotic), vincristine, and prednisone

Although normal cells are affected, they are better able to recover from the damage caused by the radiation than are cancer cells. The types of delivery, effects, and toxicities of radiation are discussed in greater detail in Chapter 14 ∞.

Bone Marrow Transplant

Bone marrow transplant (BMT) is the treatment of choice for some types of leukemia (see Table 34–3). BMT often is used in conjunction with or following chemotherapy or radiation. There are two major categories of BMT: In allogeneic BMT, the bone marrow of a healthy donor is infused into the client with the illness; in autologous BMT, the client is infused with his or her own bone marrow.

ALLOGENEIC BMT *Allogeneic BMT* uses bone marrow cells from a donor (often from a sibling with closely matched tissue antigens; closely matched unrelated donors also may be used). Prior to allogeneic BMT, high doses of chemotherapy and/or total body irradiation are used to destroy leukemic cells in the bone marrow. The donor's bone marrow is aspirated (Figure 34–8 ■) and infused through a central venous line into the recipient. Prior to BMT and reestablishment of bone marrow function, the client is critically ill and at significant risk for infection and bleeding due to depletion of WBCs and platelets.

AUTOLOGOUS BMT *Autologous BMT* uses the client's own bone marrow to restore bone marrow function after chemotherapy or radiation. This procedure is often called *bone marrow rescue*. In autologous BMT, about 1 L of bone marrow is aspirated (usually from the iliac crests) during a period of disease remission. The bone marrow is then frozen and stored for use after treatment. If relapse occurs, lethal doses of chemotherapy or radiation are given to destroy the immune

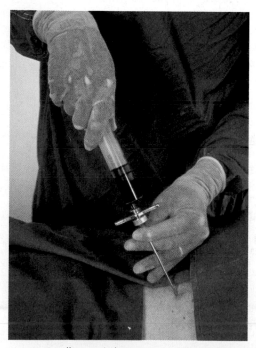

Figure 34–8 ■ Allogeneic bone marrow transplant. Bone marrow from the donor is aspirated, then filtered and infused into the recipient.
Source: Simon Fraser, Photo Researchers, Inc.

system and malignant cells, and to prepare space in the bone marrow for new cells. The filtered bone marrow is then thawed and infused intravenously through a central line. The infused marrow cells slowly become a part of the client's bone marrow, the neutrophil count increases, and normal hematopoiesis takes place.

As in allogeneic BMT, the client is critically ill during the period of bone marrow destruction and immunosuppression. The client is hospitalized in a private room for 6 to 8 weeks or more. Potential complications include malnutrition, infection, and bleeding.

Stem Cell Transplant

Allogeneic **stem cell transplant (SCT)** is an alternative to bone marrow transplant. SCT results in complete and sustained replacement of the recipient's blood cell lines (WBCs, RBCs, and platelets) with cells derived from the donor stem cells.

Donors must have tissue that is closely matched with that of the recipient. Prior to harvesting, hematopoietic growth factors, including G-CSF and GM-CSF, are administered to the donor for 4 to 5 days. This increases the concentration of stem cells in peripheral blood, allowing it to be used for the transplant instead of bone marrow. Peripheral blood is removed and white cells are separated from the plasma, then administered via a large central venous catheter. Large concentrations of stem cells also are present in umbilical cord blood. This may be stored and used in some cases (Kasper et al., 2005).

The recipient undergoes similar treatment prior to SCT as for BMT. The risks for infection and other complications, as well as graft-versus-host disease, are similar.

Graft-Versus-Host Disease

Allogeneic BMT or SCT may precipitate *graft-versus-host disease (GVHD)*, which develops in up to 60% of all clients receiving an allogeneic BMT or SCT (Kasper et al., 2005). In GVHD, immune cells of the donated bone marrow identify the recipient's body tissue as foreign. Consequently, T lymphocytes in the donated marrow attack the liver, skin, and GI tract, causing skin rashes progressing to desquamation (loss of skin), diarrhea, GI bleeding, and liver damage. *Acute GVHD* develops within days or weeks of the transplant and is usually marked by a pruritic, maculopapular rash that begins on the palms and soles of the feet, and may extend over the entire body. Vaso-occlusive disease of the liver affects up to 25% of allogeneic bone marrow transplant recipients, with jaundice and elevated liver function tests (Porth, 2005). *Chronic GVHD* develops later, 100 or more days after the transplant, affecting 20% to 50% of clients who survive 6 months or more following allogeneic BMT or SCT (Kasper et al., 2005). It may follow acute GVHD or develop in clients with no prior symptoms. GVHD is treated with antibiotics and steroids; immunosuppressant drugs such as thalidomide and immunotoxin (XomaZyme) may be used if necessary.

Biologic Therapy

Cytokines such as interferons and interleukins are biologic agents that may be used to treat some leukemias. These agents modify the body's response to cancer cells; in some cases they are cytotoxic as well. Interferons are a complex group of messenger proteins normally produced in response to antigens such as viruses (see Chapter 12 ∞). They have multiple effects, including moderating immune function and inhibiting abnormal cell proliferation and growth. Interferon alpha may be used to treat some leukemias, particularly CML. Side effects commonly associated with interferon therapy include flulike symptoms, persistent fatigue and lethargy, weight loss, and muscle and joint pain.

Complementary Therapies

Although many complementary and alternative medicine therapies have been purported to treat cancer in general, at this time none have been shown to have sustained benefit in treating leukemia. Clinical trials have demonstrated the efficacy of both

coping skills training (relaxation and imagery) and hypnosis to significantly reduce oral discomfort associated with leukemia and its treatment (Spencer & Jacobs, 2003).

NURSING CARE

For nursing care specific to the client undergoing diagnostic testing for leukemia, see the accompanying Nursing Care Plan.

Health Promotion

Health promotion activities related to leukemia include teaching about leukemia risk factors, particularly those that can be controlled. Discuss the potential dangers of exposure to ionizing

---

NURSING CARE PLAN A Client with Acute Myelocytic Leukemia

Catherine Cole is a 37-year-old secretary who lives with her husband, Ray, and teenage daughter, Amy, in an apartment in a large metropolitan area. About 2 months ago, Mrs. Cole began to tire easily and experience night sweats several times a week. She also noted that she was pale, bruised easily, and was having heavier menstrual periods. Blood tests ordered by her primary care provider are abnormal. She is admitted for a bone marrow biopsy.

ASSESSMENT

Mary Losapio, RN, obtains a nursing history and physical assessment for Mrs. Cole. Mrs. Cole tells her, "I'm so tired, and I have these bruises all over me. I'm so afraid of the results of the bone marrow examination. I don't know what we will do if I have cancer." Mrs. Cole clutches her husband's hand and then begins to cry. Physical assessment data include height, 64 inches (156 cm); weight, 106 lb (48.1 kg), vital signs: T 100°F, P 102, R 22, BP 130/82. Numerous petechiae scattered over trunk and arms; ecchymoses noted on lower right arm and right calf. Oral mucosa is red, with several small ulcerations in buccal areas.

Blood count shows reduced RBCs, hemoglobin, and hematocrit levels. The WBC is high, with myeloblasts seen on differential. The platelet count is very low. A tentative diagnosis of acute myelogenous leukemia is made.

DIAGNOSES

- *Risk for Infection* related to altered WBC production and immune function
- *Ineffective Protection* related to reduced platelet count and risk for bleeding
- *Impaired Oral Mucous Membrane* secondary to anemia and reduced platelets
- *Fatigue* related to anemia
- *Anxiety* related to fear of leukemia diagnosis

EXPECTED OUTCOMES

- Remain free of infection.
- Experience no significant bleeding.
- Have intact oral mucous membranes.
- Manage self-care activities despite fatigue.
- Verbalize decreased anxiety.

PLANNING AND IMPLEMENTATION

- Place in a private room.
- Limit visitors to immediate family for the present.

- Instruct all staff, the family, and client to carefully wash hands. Post a sign over the washbasin in the room as a reminder.
- Record vital signs every 4 hours.
- Avoid invasive procedures unless absolutely necessary.
- Monitor for bleeding every 4 hours, including skin, oral mucosa, abdominal assessment, body fluids, and menstrual pad count.
- Instruct to perform oral hygiene every 2 to 4 hours, using a soft-bristle toothbrush.
- Ask the dietitian to work with Mrs. Cole to identify preferred foods. Instruct to avoid foods that may damage oral mucosa, such as very hot, very cold, or highly acidic or spicy foods.
- Provide for periods of rest alternating with activity.
- Teach about the bone marrow biopsy. Allow time for questions and to verbalize fears.
- Refer to the oncology nurse specialist for further teaching and support.

EVALUATION

The bone marrow biopsy confirms the diagnosis of acute myelogenous leukemia. Mrs. Cole is very upset, but calms as the physician and the oncology nurse discuss treatment plans and the possibility of remission. She decides to have outpatient chemotherapy. During her hospital stay, Mrs. Cole remained free of infection or further bleeding. She tells Ms. Losapio that her mouth feels better, although it is still painful. During routine assessment, Mrs. Cole remarks, "You know, I was so scared when I came here, but I think I am a little less so now. Sometimes not knowing what is wrong is worse than knowing."

CRITICAL THINKING IN THE NURSING PROCESS

1. Describe how alterations in WBCs can increase a person's susceptibility to infection.
2. List sources of potential infection for the hospitalized client.
3. What is the rationale for having the client do her own oral and physical hygiene?
4. Outline a teaching plan for this client and her family for home care to prevent infection.
5. Develop a care plan for Mrs. Cole for the nursing diagnosis *Activity Intolerance*.

See Evaluating Your Response in Appendix C.

radiation and certain chemicals such as benzene. Encourage all clients to avoid smoking cigarettes. Discuss genetic counseling with clients at high risk for having a child with Down syndrome (over age 35).

Assessment

Focused assessment data related to leukemia include:

- *Health history:* Complaints of fatigue, weakness, dyspnea on exertion, frequent infections, sore throat, night sweats, bleeding gums, or nose bleeds; recent weight loss; exposure to ionizing radiation (multiple x-rays, residence near a site of radiation or atomic testing) or chemicals (occupational); prior treatment for cancer; history of an immune disorder.
- *Physical examination:* Skin and mucous membranes for bruising, purpura, petechiae, ulcers or lesions; pallor; vital signs including orthostatic vitals; heart and lung sounds; abdominal examination; stool for occult blood.
- *Diagnostic tests:* Blood count with differential; bone marrow studies.

Nursing Diagnoses and Interventions

When caring for the client with leukemia, the nurse considers the chronic and life-threatening nature of the disease as well as the effects of treatment. See the Nursing Research box below. Priority nursing problems may include *Risk for Infection, Imbalanced Nutrition: Less than Body Requirements, Impaired Oral Mucous Membranes, Ineffective Protection (Bleeding),* and *Anticipatory Grieving.*

Risk for Infection

Changes in white blood cell function impair the immune and inflammatory responses in leukemia, increasing the risk for infection. WBCs may be immature and ineffective or, in some cases, deficient. Chemotherapy or radiation therapy further depresses bone marrow function and increases the risk for infection.

- Promptly report manifestations of infection: fever, chills, throat pain, cough, chest pain, burning on urination, purulent drainage, and itching and burning in vaginal or rectal areas. *Prompt reporting allows timely intervention to prevent overwhelming infection and sepsis.*
- Institute infection protection measures:
  a. Maintain protective isolation as indicated.
  b. Ensure meticulous hand washing among all people in contact with the client.
  c. Assist as needed with appropriate hygiene measures.
  d. Restrict visitors with colds, flu, or infections.
  e. Provide oral hygiene after every meal.
  f. Avoid invasive procedures when possible, including injections, intravenous catheters, catheterizations, and rectal and vaginal procedures. When necessary, use strict aseptic technique for all invasive procedures and monitor carefully for infection.

These precautions minimize exposure to bacterial, viral, and fungal pathogens. Infection is the major cause of death in clients with leukemia. Mucous membranes are especially susceptible to breakdown and infection as a result of tissue damage from chemotherapy or radiation.

NURSING RESEARCH Evidence-Based Practice for Clients with Acute Leukemia and Lymphoma

Clients with acute leukemia and malignant lymphoma experience a number of distressing manifestations of their disease, including malaise and fatigue, fever, night sweats, infections, and possible hemorrhage. Treatments such as radiation therapy and chemotherapy often have numerous adverse effects as well, including anorexia and nausea, stomatitis, lethargy, malaise, and fatigue. In these studies, clients in remission from acute leukemia or malignant lymphoma were surveyed regarding physical problems, their view of help they received and who was of most help during treatment, and the impact of the disease and treatment on their current life (Persson, Hallberg, & Ohlsson, 1997; Persson & Hallberg, 2004).

Clients identified energy loss and nutritional problems as being most troublesome during disease treatment. In general, clients with more physical problems were less satisfied with the nursing care they received, suggesting that nurses were less effective in meeting the needs of the sickest clients. Clients continued to experience reduced psychologic and sexual energy and a significant need for intimate help and counseling during remission. While family relationships improved, work and finances were negatively impacted by their disease.

IMPLICATIONS FOR NURSING

This study points out the need for nurses to actively focus their care on the physical problems experienced during treatment, es-

pecially energy loss and nutritional problems. Overwhelming fatigue interferes with the client's ability to provide self-care, but its effects may not be readily apparent to nurses. The long-term effects of reduced psychologic and sexual energy, as well as continued susceptibility to infections, indicate a need for continued follow-up care, teaching, and possibly referral to counseling services.

CRITICAL THINKING IN CLIENT CARE

1. Explain the physiologic responses to malignancies and cancer treatments that cause fatigue, malaise, and nutritional problems.
2. Clients undergoing treatment for leukemia, malignant lymphoma, and other cancers may have few outward manifestations of their disease or responses to treatment. Discuss how this apparent well-being may affect the nurses' perception of care needs.
3. How may continued problems of fatigue and lack of psychologic and sexual energy affect family relations?
4. Develop a nursing care plan for a client with acute leukemia to address the nursing diagnosis *Ineffective Sexuality Patterns* related to fatigue and lack of energy.

- Monitor vital signs including temperature and oxygen saturation every 4 hours. Report temperature spikes with chilling, tachypnea, tachycardia, restlessness, change in PaO_2, and hypotension. *The inflammatory response may be impaired in leukemia, masking signs of infection until sepsis develops, indicated by manifestations such as those above.*
- Monitor neutrophil levels (measured in cubic millimeters) for relative risk for infection:
  2000 to 2500: no risk
  1000 to 2000: minimal risk
  500 to 1000: moderate risk
  Below 500: severe risk.
  Neutrophils are the first line of defense against infection. As levels decrease, the risk for infection increases.
- Explain infection precautions and restrictions and their rationale; explain that these measures are usually temporary. *Client and family understanding increases compliance and lowers the risk of infection.*

Imbalanced Nutrition:
Less than Body Requirements

The client with leukemia may have difficulty meeting nutritional needs due to increased metabolism, fatigue, loss of appetite from radiation, nausea and vomiting from chemotherapy, or painful oral mucous membranes that make chewing and swallowing difficult and/or painful.

- Weigh regularly and evaluate weight loss over time to determine degree of malnutrition. A weight loss of 10% to 20% may indicate malnutrition. *A minimum intake of nutrients is necessary for health and tissue repair; cancer increases metabolic needs over this basal requirement. Weight loss occurs when metabolic requirements are not met. Both the disease process and its treatment can interfere with nutrient intake.*
- Address causative or contributing factors to inadequate food and fluid intake.
  a. Provide mouth care before and after meals; use a soft toothbrush or sponges as necessary.
  b. Provide liquids with different textures and tastes.
  c. Increase liquid intake with meals.
  d. Reduce intake of milk and milk products, which makes mucus more tenacious.
  e. Assist to a sitting position for eating.
  f. Ensure that the environment is clean and odor free.
  g. Provide medications for pain or nausea 30 minutes before meals, if prescribed.
  h. Provide rest periods before meals.
  i. Offer small, frequent meals including low-fat, high-kilocalorie foods throughout the day.
  j. Provide commercial supplements, such as Ensure.
  k. Avoid painful or unpleasant procedures immediately before or after meals.
  l. Suggest measures to improve food tolerance, such as eating dry foods when arising, consuming salty foods if allowed, and avoiding very sweet, rich, or greasy foods.

Anorexia, nausea and vomiting, diarrhea, stomatitis, taste changes, and dysphagia often make eating difficult during cancer treatment when good nutrition is most important.

Maintaining nutritional status decreases morbidity and mortality by preventing weight loss, improving the response to treatment, minimizing adverse effects, and improving quality of life. Small, frequent meals are often better tolerated, especially high-protein, high-kilocalorie foods.

Impaired Oral Mucous Membrane

Stomatitis, inflammation and ulceration of the oral mucous membrane, is common in leukemia. Chemotherapy can further impair the integrity of constantly dividing oral tissues.

- Inspect the buccal region, gums, sublingual area, and the throat daily for swelling or lesions. Ask about oral pain or burning. *Breakdown of the oral mucous membrane increases the risk of infection and bleeding, causes pain and discomfort with eating and swallowing, and may cause swelling that interferes with the airway.*
- Culture any oral lesions. *Herpes simplex virus and* Candida *(yeast) are more common in clients with neutropenia. Herpes lesions are usually red, raised, fluid-filled blisters;* Candida *causes a white coating and patches of white plaque.*
- Assist with mouth care and oral rinses with saline or a solution of hydrogen peroxide and water (1:1 or 1:3 hydrogen peroxide and water) every 2 to 4 hours. Apply petroleum jelly to the lips to prevent dryness and cracking. *These measures help prevent infection and increase comfort.*
- Encourage use of soft-bristle toothbrush or sponge to clean teeth and gums. *Toothbrushes with hard bristles may abrade inflamed mucosa, causing bleeding and increasing the risk of infection.*
- Administer medications as ordered to treat infection or relieve pain. *Topical antifungal agents such as nystatin may be prescribed to treat* Candida *infections. Topical anesthetics such as lidocaine may be prescribed to relieve comfort and facilitate good oral care.*
- Instruct to avoid alcohol-based mouthwashes, citrus fruit juices, spicy foods, very hot or very cold foods, alcohol, and crusty foods. Suggest bland, cool foods and cool liquids at least every 2 hours. *Avoiding mucosa-traumatizing foods and liquids increases comfort; bland, cool foods and liquids cause the least pain. Intake of adequate fluids is necessary to prevent dehydration.*

Ineffective Protection

Bleeding is the second most common cause of leukemia deaths. As platelet counts decrease, the risk of bleeding increases (see the section later in this chapter on thrombocytopenia). Tumor lysis syndrome also is a risk in clients with leukemia who are undergoing their initial treatment with chemotherapy. Tumor lysis syndrome develops when a large number of malignant cells are destroyed by treatment with chemotherapy or radiation. The resultant by-products of cell lysis can overwhelm the body's ability to effectively eliminate them, leading to hyperkalemia, hyperphosphatemia with secondary hypocalcemia, and hyperuricemia (Cantril & Haylock, 2004).

- Assess vital signs every 4 hours and body systems every shift for bleeding:
  a. Skin and mucous membranes for petechiae, ecchymoses, and purpura

b. Gums, nasal membranes, and conjunctiva for bleeding

c. Vomitus, stool, and urine for visible or occult blood

d. Vaginal bleeding

e. Prolonged bleeding from puncture sites

f. Neurologic changes such as headache, visual changes, altered mentation, decreased level of consciousness, seizures

g. Abdomen for complaints of epigastric pain, diminished bowel sounds, increasing abdominal girth, rigidity or guarding.

Early identification of bleeding helps prevent significant blood loss and potential shock. Internal hemorrhage may lead to tachycardia, hypotension, pallor, and diaphoresis. Bleeding into the lungs may cause dyspnea; bleeding into the abdomen causes increased girth, pain, and guarding. Intracranial bleeding affects mental status and level of consciousness.

- Avoid invasive procedures such as rectal temperatures and suppositories, vaginal douches, suppositories, tampons, urinary catheterization, and parenteral injections if possible. Diagnostic procedures such as biopsy or lumbar puncture should not be done if the platelet count is less than 50,000. *Invasive procedures can cause tissue trauma and bleeding. Procedures that use large-bore needles should be delayed until the platelet count is increased.*

- Apply pressure to injection sites for 3 to 5 minutes, and to arterial punctures for 15 to 20 minutes. *Pressure prevents prolonged bleeding by prompting hemostasis and clot formation.*

- Instruct to avoid forcefully blowing or picking the nose, forceful coughing or sneezing, and straining to have a bowel movement. *These activities can damage mucous membranes, increasing the risk for bleeding.*

- Monitor and promptly report abnormal blood levels of electrolytes, uric acid, urea nitrogen, and creatinine, or manifestations of tumor lysis syndrome. *Significant alterations in electrolyte levels can lead to complications such as cardiac dysrhythmias, muscle weakness or tetany, paresthesias, and mental status changes. Excess uric acid can compromise renal function, and lead to metabolic acidosis and gout.*

- Maintain adequate hydration and administer prescribed medications such as allopurinol and diuretics as ordered. *Hydration is vital to maintain renal function and promote elimination of tumor lysis by-products. Allopurinol reduces the risk of uric acid crystallization in the kidneys and other tissues* (Cantril & Haylock, 2004).

Anticipatory Grieving

The diagnosis of cancer and a potentially life-threatening illness causes actual or perceived losses, such as loss of function, independence, normal appearance, friends, self-esteem, and self. Grieving is the emotional response to those losses. The adaptive process of mourning a loss and resolving grief is called grief work; grief work cannot begin until a loss is acknowledged. See Chapter 5 ∞ for a detailed discussion of grief and loss.

- Discuss roles of the client and family and ways in which they managed stressful situations in the past. Assess coping strategies and their effectiveness. Help identify sources of strength and support. Discuss changing roles resulting from leukemia diagnosis, and its effect on spiritual, social, and economic status and usual lifestyle. Evaluate cultural or ethnic factors that affect grief reactions. *Grieving is a normal response to a real or potential loss that begins at the time of diagnosis. The timing, duration, and intensity of grief and responses to grief may differ among family members. Share information on diagnosis, role change, and physical loss among all family members to build the foundation for mutual understanding and trust.*

- Use therapeutic communication skills to facilitate open discussion of losses and provide permission to grieve. *Encouraging discussion of the meaning of the loss helps decrease some of the anxiety associated with loss. This in turn allows the client and family to examine the current situation and compare it with past situations that they have coped with successfully.*

- Provide information about agencies that may help in resolving grief, and make referrals as indicated. Consider self-help groups, cancer support groups, and bereavement groups. *Participating in support groups with others who are anticipating or experiencing a similar loss can decrease feelings of isolation.*

Linking NANDA, NIC, and NOC

Chart 34–2 shows links between NANDA nursing diagnoses, NIC, and NOC for the client with leukemia.

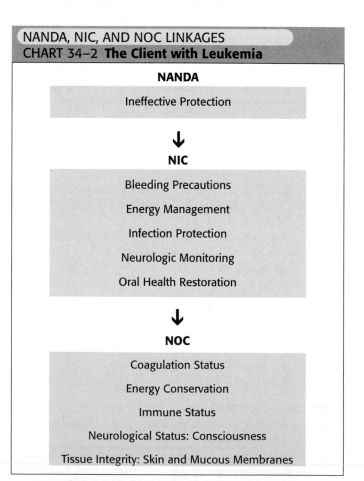

NANDA, NIC, AND NOC LINKAGES
CHART 34–2 The Client with Leukemia

NANDA

Ineffective Protection

↓

NIC

Bleeding Precautions

Energy Management

Infection Protection

Neurologic Monitoring

Oral Health Restoration

↓

NOC

Coagulation Status

Energy Conservation

Immune Status

Neurological Status: Consciousness

Tissue Integrity: Skin and Mucous Membranes

Data from *NANDA's Nursing Diagnoses: Definitions & Classification 2005–2006* by NANDA International (2005), Philadelphia; *Nursing Interventions Classification (NIC)* (4th ed.) by J. M. Dochterman & G. M. Bulechek (2004), St. Louis, MO: Mosby; and *Nursing Outcomes Classification (NOC)* (3rd ed.) by S. Moorhead, M. Johnson, and M. Mass (2004), St. Louis, MO: Mosby.

Community-Based Care

Client and family teaching for home care after treatment for leukemia focuses on encouraging self-care, providing information about the disease and the treatment, preventing infection and injury, and promoting nutrition. Teaching topics for each of these areas are as follows.

Encouraging Self-Care

- Hygiene measures and energy conservation during self-care activities
- Oral hygiene including using a soft-bristle toothbrush several times daily; avoiding flossing
- Reporting lesions, bleeding, or signs of infection promptly
- Maintaining a balance of rest and activity.

Information about Leukemia and Treatment

- Bone marrow function, the pathophysiology of leukemia, and potential complications of leukemia
- Prognosis for the specific type of leukemia
- Treatment measures such as chemotherapy, radiation, bone marrow or stem cell transplant, their purpose and effects, where treatment is available, and potential adverse effects or risks
- Community, regional, and national resources for people with leukemia.

Preventing Infection and Injury

- Hand washing and other measures to reduce exposure to pathogens such as avoiding people who are ill and avoiding crowds
- Avoiding foodborne illnesses by washing fruits and vegetables, proper food storage
- Dental hygiene measures
- Avoiding immunizations
- Manifestations to report: fever, chills, burning on urination, foul-smelling urine, vaginal or rectal discharge, skin lesions
- Avoiding contact sports or strenuous exercise if platelet count is low
- Using an electric razor for shaving, avoiding rectal or vaginal suppositories, vaginal tampons, or enemas
- Increasing dietary fiber and using a bulk-forming laxative as needed to prevent straining
- Avoiding over-the-counter or prescription drugs that interfere with platelet function (see Box 34–6 on page 1140)
- The importance of reporting any bleeding (nosebleeds, rectal bleeding, vomiting blood, excessive menstrual periods, blood in the urine, bleeding gums, bruises, or collections of blood under the skin) or changes in behavior to the healthcare provider.

Promoting Nutrition

- Eating several small, low-fat, high-calorie meals and drinking five to eight glasses of water daily
- Reporting continued weight loss, loss of appetite, or inability to eat for 24 hours
- Discussing dietary needs with the dietitian.

Assistance with physical care, finances, and transportation may be required following discharge. Refer the client and family to social services, support groups, home care services as needed, and other agencies that can provide needed services (such as local chapters of the American Cancer Society, which can provide hospital beds and transportation for outpatient cancer treatment).

THE CLIENT WITH MALIGNANT LYMPHOMA

Lymphomas are malignancies of lymphoid tissue. They are characterized by the proliferation of lymphocytes, histiocytes (resident monocytes or macrophages), and their precursors or derivatives. Lymphomas are closely related to lymphocytic leukemias. Some experts consider them to be different forms or stages of the same disease processes.

Although there are many types of malignant lymphoid cells, at this time lymphomas commonly are identified as Hodgkin's disease or non-Hodgkin's lymphoma.

Incidence and Risk Factors

Malignant lymphomas are the seventh leading cause of cancer deaths in the United States. Approximately 63,740 new cases of lymphoma were diagnosed in 2005, and 20,600 deaths were attributed to the disease. The incidence of non-Hodgkin's lymphoma has nearly doubled since 1970, but currently has stabilized, primarily due to a fall in its incidence related to HIV infection and AIDS. The incidence of Hodgkin's disease has significantly declined since 1990 (ACS, 2005).

While the cause of lymphoma is unknown, some risk factors have been identified. See the accompanying Genetics Considerations box for information about identified genetic links for lymphoma development. Immunosuppression due to drug therapy following organ transplant or to HIV disease increases the risk for non-Hodgkin's lymphoma. Infectious agents such as HTLV-1 and EBV also have been identified as risk factors. Others may include occupational herbicide or chemical exposure (ACS, 2005).

Pathophysiology

Hodgkin's Disease

Hodgkin's disease is a lymphatic cancer, occurring most often in people between the ages of 15 and 35 or over age 50. It is somewhat more common in men than women. Approximately

---

GENETIC CONSIDERATIONS
Focus on Lymphoma

Although specific genetic alterations have not been identified for all types of lymphoma, recurring genetic abnormalities associated with lymphomas point to a genetic link in disease development. Three distinct genetic abnormalities have been identified in non-Hodgkin's lymphomas: gross chromosomal changes such as translocations, rearrangements of specific genes, and altered expression of specific oncogenes (overexpression, underexpression, or mutation). Consistent genetic changes are associated with some lymphomas; in other cases, several genetic abnormalities may be seen. Hodgkin's disease is unique from other lymphomas in that no specific genetic abnormalities have been identified (Kasper et al., 2005). For more information about genetics and disease, see Chapter 8 ∞ .

7350 new cases of Hodgkin's disease were diagnosed in 2005 (ACS, 2005). The exact cause of Hodgkin's disease is unknown, but both Epstein-Barr virus (EBV) infection and genetic factors appear to play a role in its development. Hodgkin's disease is one of the most curable cancers. As many as 60% to 90% of people with localized disease achieve cure with a normal life span (Porth, 2005).

Hodgkin's disease develops in a single lymph node or chain of nodes, spreading to adjoining nodes. Involved lymph nodes contain *Reed-Sternberg cells* (malignant cells) surrounded by host inflammatory cells. These malignant cells secrete inflammatory mediator substances, attracting inflammatory cells to the tumor site. They may invade almost any tissue in the body. The spleen often is involved; as the disease progresses, the liver, lungs, digestive tract, and CNS may be affected (Porth, 2005). Rapid proliferation of abnormal lymphocytes impairs the immune response, especially cell-mediated immune responses. Infections are common.

Hodgkin's disease is classified as classic Hodgkin's disease or as nodular lymphocyte-predominant Hodgkin's disease. The classic form of the disease accounts for 95% of all cases; nodular lymphocyte-predominant Hodgkin's is rare. Classic Hodgkin's can be further divided into four subtypes by cells identified within the tumor, but the subtype does not affect the prognosis (Copstead & Banasik, 2005; Kasper et al., 2005).

MANIFESTATIONS The most common symptom of Hodgkin's disease is one or more painlessly enlarged lymph nodes, usually in the cervical or subclavicular region. Systemic manifestations such as persistent fever, night sweats, fatigue, and weight loss are associated with a poorer prognosis for the disease. Late symptoms such as malaise, pruritus, and anemia indicate spread of the disease (Porth, 2005). The spleen may be enlarged, and other organ systems such as the lungs and gastrointestinal tract are occasionally involved.

Non-Hodgkin's Lymphoma

Non-Hodgkin's lymphoma is a diverse group of lymphoid tissue malignancies that do not contain Reed-Sternberg cells. Non-Hodgkin's lymphomas tend to arise in peripheral lymph nodes and spread early to tissues throughout the body. Non-Hodgkin's lymphoma is more common than Hodgkin's disease, affecting an estimated 56,390 people annually and causing about 19,200 deaths in 2005 (ACS, 2005). Older adults are more often affected, and it occurs more frequently in men than in women. Like Hodgkin's disease, its cause is unknown, although both genetic and environmental factors (e.g., viral infections such as EBV, human T-cell leukemia/lymphoma virus-1 [HTLV-1] and HTLV-2, and HIV) are thought to play a role.

As in most malignancies, non-Hodgkin's lymphoma begins as a single transformed cell; it may arise from T cells, B cells, or tissue macrophages (histocytes). The primary types of non-Hodgkin's lymphoma are identified in Table 34–7. Although non-Hodgkin's lymphoma usually arises in a lymph node, it can originate in any lymphoid tissue. It tends to spread early and unpredictably to other lymphoid tissues and organs. Extra-

TABLE 34–7 Subtypes of Non-Hodgkin's Lymphoma

SUBTYPE	INCIDENCE	COURSE AND PROGNOSIS
B-Cell Lymphomas		
Diffuse large B-cell lymphomas	Most common adult type (40%–50% of adult lymphomas) More common in males Incidence increases with aging	Aggressive tumor 45%–50% cure rate
Follicular lymphoma	Accounts for 40% of adult lymphomas, rare in children Incidence increases with aging	Bone marrow frequently involved Course slow, indolent; 72% 5-year survival
Extranodal marginal zone lymphoma (MALT lymphoma)	Accounts for about 5% of adult lymphomas, rare in children Incidence increases with aging More common in Italy	Presents with tumors outside lymphatic system: GI tract, lung, thyroid, urinary tract, skin, CNS Slow, indolent course; 74% 5-year survival
Mantle cell lymphoma	Accounts for 3% to 4% of adult lymphomas, rare in children Predominantly affects older men (74%)	Aggressive, difficult to cure 27% 5-year survival
Burkitt lymphoma	Rare in adults (<1% of lymphomas), more common in children (~30% NHL)	Rapidly progressive but responds well to therapy 45% 5-year survival
T-Cell Lymphomas		
Precursor T-cell lymphoblastic leukemia/lymphoma	More common in children and young adults More common in males than females	Can present either as ALL or lymphoma Aggressive disease; 26% 5-year survival
Peripheral T-cell lymphoma	Most common T-cell lymphoma in adults	Often presents as disseminated disease 25% 5-year survival
Mycosis fungoides/cutaneous T-cell lymphoma	Onset typically during mid-50s; more common in African Americans	Cutaneous lymphoma Slow course, progressing from patchy skin lesions to plaque to cutaneous tumors

nodal spread may involve the nasopharynx, gastrointestinal tract, bone, CNS, thyroid, testes, and soft tissue.

The prognosis for non-Hodgkin's lymphoma ranges from excellent to poor, depending on the identified cell type and grade of differentiation. Low-grade tumors (better differentiated) tend to be less aggressive and more curable. Higher grade tumors often are disseminated at the time of diagnoses, and have a poorer prognosis (Copstead & Banasik, 2005).

MANIFESTATIONS The early manifestations of non-Hodgkin's lymphoma are similar to those for Hodgkin's disease. Painless lymphadenopathy may be localized or widespread (Figure 34–9 ■). Systemic manifestations such as fever, night sweats, fatigue, and weight loss may be present, but are less common in non-Hodgkin's lymphoma. Organ system involvement may cause symptoms such as abdominal pain, nausea, and vomiting. Headaches, peripheral or cranial nerve symptoms, altered mental status, or seizures may signal CNS involvement.

The manifestations and clinical features of Hodgkin's disease and non-Hodgkin's lymphoma are compared in Table 34–8.

Course

In both Hodgkin's disease and non-Hodgkin's lymphoma, the stage of the disease, the presence of systemic manifestations, and factors such as age help determine the prognosis. The prognosis is good when the disease is localized to one or two node regions. Factors such as anemia, thrombocytopenia, and older age reduce the likelihood of disease cure.

INTERDISCIPLINARY CARE

Chemotherapy and radiation therapy, either alone or in combination, are the primary treatments for Hodgkin's and non-Hodgkin's lymphomas. Use of monoclonal antibodies to target lymphoma cells, and bone marrow and peripheral stem cell transplants are under investigation for treating lymphomas as well. See the previous section on treatment of leukemia for more information about these transplants.

Diagnosis

The following diagnostic tests may be ordered for lymphomas:
- *CBC* often shows a mild normochromic, normocytic anemia in Hodgkin's disease; other findings in Hodgkin's disease

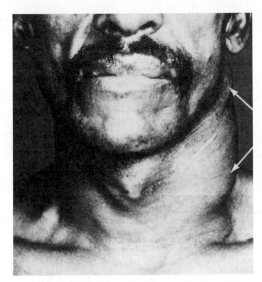

Figure 34–9 ■ Cervical lymphadenopathy in a client with lymphoma of the neck.

Source: Centers for Disease Control and Prevention (CDC)

may include leukocytosis with high neutrophil and eosinophil counts, and an elevated erythrocyte sedimentation rate (ESR). In non-Hodgkin's lymphoma, the CBC typically remains normal until late in the disease, when pancytopenia may develop.
- An ESR is done to identify possible inflammatory causes of lymph node enlargement.
- *Chemistry studies* of major organ function (including liver function tests and renal function studies) are performed to identify possible organ involvement. *Serum LDH levels* and *protein electrophoresis* also may be done when Hodgkin's disease is suspected.
- *Chest x-ray* is done to identify possible enlarged mediastinal lymph nodes and pulmonary involvement.
- *CT scans* of the chest, abdomen, and pelvis are performed to identify abnormal or enlarged nodes.
- *Positron emission tomography (PET or gallium scans)* may be performed in diagnosing the disease, as well as to evaluate the effectiveness of treatment.
- *Biopsy* of the largest, most central enlarged lymph node and of the bone marrow is done to establish the diagnosis for both

---

TABLE 34–8 Features and Manifestations of Hodgkin's Disease and Non-Hodgkin's Lymphoma

FEATURE OR MANIFESTATION	HODGKIN'S DISEASE	NON-HODGKIN'S LYMPHOMA
Lymphadenopathy	Localized to a single node or chain, often cervical, subclavicular, or mediastinal	Multiple peripheral nodes, nodes of the mesentery often involved
Spread	Orderly and continuous	Diffuse and unpredictable
Extranodal involvement	Rare	Early and common
Bone marrow involvement	Uncommon	Common
Fever, night sweats, weight loss	Common	Uncommon until disease is extensive
Other manifestations	Fatigue, pruritus, splenomegaly; anemia, neutrophilia	Abdominal pain, nausea, vomiting; dyspnea, cough; CNS symptoms; lymphocytopenia

Hodgkin's disease and non-Hodgkin's lymphoma. The presence of Reed-Sternberg cells confirms the diagnosis of Hodgkin's disease.

Staging

Staging is used to determine the extent of the disease and appropriate treatment. The Ann Arbor Staging System is used to assess the extent and severity of lymphomas. The stages are:

Stage I: involvement of a single lymph node region or lymphoid structure (e.g., spleen, thymus, lymphoid tonsillar tissue)

Stage II: involvement of two or more lymph node regions on the same side of the diaphragm

Stage III: involvement of lymph node regions or structures on both sides of the diaphragm

- III_1: limited to upper abdomen (spleen, splenic, celiac, or portal nodes)
- III_2: involvement of lower abdominal nodes (para-aortic, iliac, or mesenteric)

Stage IV: involvement of an extranodal site (not proximal or contiguous with an involved node) such as the liver, lung or pleura, bone or bone marrow, or skin.

The presence or absence of systemic symptoms is indicated by either an A (no systemic symptoms) or B (systemic symptoms of fever, night sweats, weight loss).

Chemotherapy

Combination chemotherapy is used to treat both Hodgkin's disease and non-Hodgkin's lymphoma. In both cases, chemotherapy often is followed by radiation therapy to involved lymph node regions. The choice of drug combination depends on the stage of the disease as well as the client's age and general condition. Combination regimens used in the United States include CHOP (cyclophosphamide, doxorubicin, vincristine, and prednisone); ABVD (doxorubicin, bleomycin, vinblastine, and dacarbazine); MOPP (nitrogen mustard, vincristine, procarbazine, and prednisone); and ChlVPP (chlorambucil, vinblastine, procarbazine, and prednisone). These regimens also may be combined in alternating months to reduce the adverse effects and improve tumor cell kill. More than 75% of clients with Hodgkin's disease who do not have systemic symptoms achieve complete remission with treatment. The prognosis for clients with non-Hodgkin's lymphoma varies by the type and stage of the disease. For more information about nursing care of the client receiving combination chemotherapy, see Chapter 14 ∞.

Radiation Therapy

Radiation therapy may be the primary treatment for early-stage Hodgkin's disease, although early chemotherapy is becoming more common. In later stages and in non-Hodgkin's lymphoma it usually is combined with chemotherapy. Many lymphomas are highly responsive to radiation. The involved lymph node region is treated, with careful shielding to protect unaffected areas and minimize the extent of radiation burn and normal cell destruction (Figure 34–10 ■). If the disease is advanced, total nodal irradiation may be done. See Chapter 14 ∞ for nursing care of the client receiving radiation therapy.

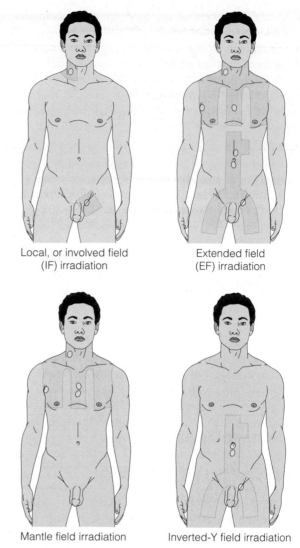

Local, or involved field (IF) irradiation

Extended field (EF) irradiation

Mantle field irradiation

Inverted-Y field irradiation

Figure 34–10 ■ Patterns of radiation therapy used to treat lymphoma based on the location and extent of the disease.

Stem Cell Transplant

Autologous peripheral blood stem cell transplant (PBSCT) is a treatment option for clients who experience remission of malignant lymphoma. Autologous PBSCT uses the client's own stem cells to restore bone marrow function after chemotherapy or radiation. In autologous PBSCT, stem cells are obtained from peripheral blood following chemotherapy and treatment with colony-stimulating factors to promote development of normal blood cells. The blood containing these normal stem cells is then frozen and stored for use after treatment. If relapse occurs, lethal doses of chemotherapy or radiation are given to destroy the immune system and malignant cells. The blood is then thawed and infused intravenously through a peripheral line. The infused stem cells become a part of the client's bone marrow and normal hematopoiesis takes place.

The client is critically ill during the period of bone marrow destruction and immunosuppression. The client is hospitalized in a private room for 6 to 8 weeks or more. See the accompanying nursing research box for discussion of fatigue related to autologous PBSCT.

NURSING RESEARCH **Evidence-Based Practice: Client Undergoing Stem Cell Transplant**

Fatigue and depression are common adverse effects of chemotherapy and radiation therapy in clients undergoing cancer treatment. Fatigue is prevalent, affecting 80% to 100% of people undergoing standard chemotherapy and often leading to lost work time and difficulty maintaining functional roles within the family and society. A study by El-Banna and colleagues (2004) sought to describe patterns of fatigue and depression and their relationship to one another among clients undergoing autologous PBSCT. Three time periods during therapy were selected for evaluation: prior to the initiation of chemotherapy, during chemotherapy just prior to transplant, and following the transplant. The setting for this study allowed transplant clients to reside in a hotel-like suite with a designated caregiver (family member or friend).

This study revealed that, among study participants, total fatigue and all its identified dimensions (behavioral, cognitive/mood, sensory, and affective) increased sharply at the time of the transplant, peaking at 7 days post-transplant. Depression followed the same pattern as fatigue, peaking at post transplant day 7. Peak depression scores were indicative of major depression using the tool employed in this study.

IMPLICATIONS FOR NURSING

This study suggests that nurses should assess for fatigue and depression in clients following stem cell transplant. Nursing measures to help conserve the client's energy are appropriate to manage fatigue. Early detection and intervention for fatigue may actually reduce the intensity of fatigue at its peak. Nurses can use this information to prepare clients for common symptom patterns following SCT, thus reducing anxiety and concern that their condition may be declining rather than improving after SCT. Additionally, assessment tools to measure fatigue and depression among clients undergoing SCT should be incorporated into nursing care.

CRITICAL THINKING IN CLIENT CARE

1. The average age of participants ($N=27$) in this study was 49 years (range: 19 to 71 years); 56% were male, 44% female. Does this sample reflect the demographic of clients with malignant lymphoma and those undergoing autologous PBSCT? How can information about the sample be used to guide application of study findings to the general population of clients undergoing this treatment? To older adults? To adolescents and young adults?
2. In this study, participants resided in a hotel-like setting with a family member or friend who participated in care. How might you expect the results to differ had the clients been unable to closely interact with a caregiver of their own choosing?
3. Can the results of this study be applied when caring for clients undergoing allogeneic BMT or SCT? Why or why not?

Complications of Treatment

Both chemotherapy and radiation therapy may have long-term effects. Permanent sterility is common, especially in older adults. Bone marrow depression can lead to immunosuppression, anemia, and bleeding. Secondary cancers and cardiac injury are the most serious late adverse effects of treatment. Chemotherapy regimens using the MOPP or a related protocol carry a risk of acute leukemia. Cancers such as breast or lung cancer may develop 10 or more years after thoracic radiation. Thoracic radiation also increases the risk for coronary heart disease and hypothyroidism (Kasper et al., 2005).

NURSING CARE

Assessment and priority nursing care for the client with lymphoma follows. See also the Nursing Care Plan at the end of this section for application of nursing care strategies for a specific client with Hodgkin's disease.

Assessment

Focused assessment of the client with Hodgkin's disease or non-Hodgkin's lymphoma includes:

- *Health history:* Complaints of enlarged lymph node(s), fever, night sweats, weight loss, fatigue or general malaise, abdominal pain, respiratory symptoms, numbness or tingling of extremities, visual changes, or changes in mentation; history of infectious mononucleosis, HIV disease, or other immunosuppressive disorders.
- *Physical examination:* Mental status exam; inspect and palpate lymph nodes (cervical, subclavicular, axillary, and inguinal) for enlargement, tenderness; heart and lung sounds;

abdominal examination for tenderness, masses, liver or spleen enlargement.
- *Diagnostic tests:* CBC, hemoglobin and hematocrit, ESR; serum chemistry results; x-ray, scan, and biopsy results.

Nursing Diagnoses and Interventions

Nursing care of the client with malignant lymphoma involves both physical and emotional support during diagnosis and treatment. Common nursing care problems include impaired protection due to bone marrow suppression, fatigue, nausea, and altered body image. See the nursing care section for leukemia for specific nursing interventions for *Ineffective Protection*.

Fatigue

General malaise and fatigue may accompany malignant lymphoma and are side effects of chemotherapy. In addition, the physical and psychologic stress of dealing with a chronic, debilitating disease and its treatment may cause fatigue.

- Inquire about feelings of malaise (a vague feeling of body weakness or discomfort) and fatigue (a pervasive, drained feeling that cannot be eliminated). *Both malaise and fatigue are subjective experiences with physiologic, situational, and psychologic components.*
- Encourage verbalization of feelings about the impact of the disease and fatigue on lifestyle. *Discussion of feelings helps the client clarify values and may assist in identifying priorities.*
- Encourage enjoyable but quiet activities, such as reading, listening to music, or hobbies. *Enjoyable activities help decrease feelings of fatigue. Quiet activities conserve energy while yielding a sense of accomplishment.*

NURSING CARE PLAN   A Client with Hodgkin's Disease

Albin Quito, age 28, is the nurse manager of a thoracic intensive care unit in a large teaching hospital. Lately he has been more tired than usual, often wakes up at night covered with sweat, and just does not feel well. He had thought that his symptoms were due to a viral illness and his busy work schedule. However, yesterday morning Albin noticed a large swollen area on the right side of his neck. He made an appointment with his primary health provider who found a large cervical lymph node. A biopsy of the node and a CT scan of the chest were scheduled.

ASSESSMENT

David Herzog, the nurse in charge of the outpatient clinic, obtains a nursing history and assessment on Mr. Quito. His physical examination is essentially normal, with the exception of the enlarged node, which is not tender to palpation. When Mr. Quito is weighed, he tells Mr. Herzog that he has lost 7 lb (3.2 kg) in the past 2 months. In reviewing the results of the blood studies, Mr. Herzog notes mild anemia and an increased neutrophil count. The lymph node biopsy shows Reed-Sternberg cells. The clinic physician and Mr. Herzog tell Mr. Quito that the findings indicate stage 1-B Hodgkin's disease but that the prognosis is very good. The physician recommends a short course of combination chemotherapy followed by radiation therapy to involved sites.

DIAGNOSES

- *Anxiety* related to the diagnosis of Hodgkin's disease and effects of treatment on job performance
- *Risk for Infection* related to potential bone marrow depression due to chemotherapy
- *Fatigue* related to effects of cancer, chemotherapy, and radiation therapy

EXPECTED OUTCOMES

- Verbalize reduced anxiety.
- Remain free of infection.
- Identify and use methods to preserve energy.

PLANNING AND IMPLEMENTATION

- Encourage to consider a leave of absence from work during course of treatment.
- Discuss joining a support group for people with cancer.
- Provide information about the illness, combination chemotherapy, and radiation therapy.
- Reinforce knowledge of actions to decrease the risk of infection.
- Discuss ways to decrease fatigue and maintain energy:
  - Take a 1- to 2-hour nap once or twice a day.
  - Avoid overexertion during weekends and time off.
  - Maintain a well-balanced diet.

EVALUATION

When Mr. Quito returns the following week to begin chemotherapy, he brings his friend Nancy to meet Mr. Herzog and asks him to discuss his treatment with her. Mr. Quito says, "I am still really scared, but being able to talk about this with Nancy will help a lot." Mr. Quito has made arrangements to take a 4-month leave from work, with the understanding that his job will be held for him. He states that he will have some problems with money but is working them out. He also says he feels that taking a nap is silly but that he will rest to maintain his energy level. Mr. Quito and Nancy express confidence that he will be cured and say they plan to be active members of the cancer support group—even after recovery.

CRITICAL THINKING IN THE NURSING PROCESS

1. Discuss the rationale for treating Hodgkin's disease with chemotherapy and radiation.
2. Design a teaching plan to help Mr. Quito prevent infection while he is at home.
3. What effect does the diagnosis of cancer have on the developmental tasks of a young adult?
4. Develop a care plan for Mr. Quito for the nursing diagnosis *Ineffective Role Performance.*
   See Evaluating Your Response in Appendix C.

- Encourage to establish priorities and include rest periods or naps when scheduling daily activities. *This provides a sense of control over activities and helps maintain self-esteem. Scheduled rest periods help restore energy and decrease fatigue.*
- Encourage delegation of some responsibilities to family members. *Delegation helps maintain the client's involvement and role in family decisions and responsibilities, while conserving energy for those activities identified as high priority by the client.*
- Identify and encourage the client to use energy-saving equipment. *Performing tasks with less exertion and in less time helps conserve energy.*
- Encourage a diet high in carbohydrates and fluids. *A high-carbohydrate diet helps maintain muscle glycogen stores. A liberal fluid intake promotes excretion of metabolic by-products that may contribute to malaise and fatigue.*

Nausea

The effects of malignant lymphoma and its treatment with chemotherapy and/or radiation therapy can contribute to nausea and interfere with nutritional status. Nausea, a sensation of abdominal fullness, and fear of vomiting often limit food intake. See also the nursing diagnosis *Imbalanced Nutrition* in the section on leukemia for additional interventions.

- Assess precipitating factors for nausea and/or vomiting, the frequency of vomiting, and relief measures used by the client. *Careful assessment allows development of interventions tailored to the client's situation and needs.*

PRACTICE ALERT

Provide ordered antiemetics before chemotherapy is started. Administering prescribed antiemetics before chemotherapy helps prevent nausea and the psychologic association of nausea with chemotherapy.

- Teach measures to prevent or relieve nausea and vomiting.
  a. Eat soda crackers and suck on hard candy.
  b. Eat soft, bland foods that are cold or at room temperature.
  c. Avoid unpleasant odors, and get fresh air.
  d. Eat prior to but not immediately before chemotherapy.

e. Use distraction or progressive muscle relaxation when nauseated.

f. If vomiting occurs, gradually resume oral intake with frequent sips of clear liquids or ice, progressing to bland foods.

Crackers and hard candy often relieve queasiness, whereas hot, spicy, sweet, or strong smelling foods may increase nausea. Alternative nausea relief measures may be effective.

- Provide small feedings of high-kilocalorie, high-protein foods and fluids. *This increases nutritional intake.*

- Assist with oral care, general hygiene, and environmental control of temperature, appearance, and odors. *These measures enhance appetite.*

- Identify and provide preferred foods. *This promotes nutritional intake.*

- Assist to a sitting position during and immediately after meals. *The sitting position helps decrease early feelings of fullness.*

Disturbed Body Image

The diagnosis of cancer is often devastating to the sense of trust in and the perception of one's body. Radiation and chemotherapy lead to changes in appearance and body function (e.g., hair loss, reduced libido, and infertility), further altering body image. Reactions to this diagnosis vary and may include refusal to look in a mirror or discuss the effects of the disease or treatment, unwillingness to participate in rehabilitation, inappropriate treatment decisions, increasing dependence on others or refusal to provide self-care, hostility, withdrawal, and signs of grieving.

- Assess perception of body image through subjective information such as:

  a. What the client likes most and least about his or her body

  b. Preillness perception of people who are sick or have a disability

  c. Current understanding of health and limitations imposed by illness or treatment

  d. Feelings about the illness and its effect on perception of self and others.

Body image is one's mental idea or picture of the body. It is based on past and present experiences and includes components of one's actual body and emotional responses to that body. Body image changes constantly. There is often a time lag between an actual body change and the changed body image; during this time, the diagnosis, teaching, and treatment may be rejected.

- Discuss the risk for and measures to cope with alopecia. Suggest wearing wigs, scarves, hats, or caps. Teach proper scalp care using baby shampoo or mild soap, a soft brush, sunscreen, and mineral oil to reduce itching. If eyelashes and eyebrows are lost, teach eye protection, such as wearing eyeglasses and caps with wide brims. *Chemotherapeutic agents attack rapidly dividing cells such as those responsible for hair growth. Hair loss usually begins 1 to 2 weeks after initiation of chemotherapy, with maximum loss 1 to 2 months later. Alopecia may range from thinning to total hair loss. Regrowth depends on the treatment schedule and doses; however, it usually begins 2 to 3 months after treatment ends. New hair may be softer, more curly, and slightly different in color. Teaching and emotional support help the client antic-ipate hair loss, discuss its potential effect on body image, and learn self-care techniques.*

- Discuss available resources for financial assistance with purchase of wigs, including local American Cancer Society chapters and insurance plans. *A well-matched wig (or one the color the client has always wished for!) can help maintain a positive body image.*

Sexual Dysfunction

Sexual dysfunction may result from the malignancy and the effects of radiation and chemotherapy. Reproductive tissues are made of rapidly dividing cells, and cancer treatment may cause temporary or permanent sterility, changes in menstruation, and changes in libido.

- Encourage discussion of actual or potential sexual dysfunction or sterility with the client and significant other. *Clients may be reluctant to discuss this unintended effect of treatment unless encouraged.*

- Assess knowledge, provide information, and clarify misconceptions. Discuss realistic measures for coping (e.g., sperm banking prior to chemotherapy or radiation therapy). *Clients and their partners may be unclear about expected effects on sexuality, reproduction, and the permanency of these effects.*

- Refer for counseling as indicated. *Sexual counseling can help the client and partner develop alternative strategies for expressing their sexuality.*

Risk for Impaired Skin Integrity

Malignant lymphomas may cause significant pruritus and drenching night sweats. As a result, skin integrity may be impaired. In addition, radiation therapy can cause superficial burns, which also may affect skin integrity.

- Frequently assess skin, especially in areas undergoing radiation. *Early identification of lesions allows timely treatment and can prevent further disruption of this important line of defense against infection.*

- Provide and teach measures to promote comfort and relieve itching: Use cool water and a mild soap to bathe; blot (rather than rub) dry skin; apply plain cornstarch or nonperfumed lotion or powder to the skin unless contraindicated; use lightweight blankets and clothing; maintain adequate humidity and a cool room temperature; wash bedding and clothes in mild detergent, and put them through second rinse cycle. *Pruritus is aggravated by excessive warmth, excessive dryness, rough fabrics, fatigue, and stress. Lotions and some powders may be contraindicated during radiation therapy.*

Linking NANDA, NIC, and NOC

Chart 34–3 shows linkages between nursing diagnoses, nursing interventions, and nursing outcomes for the client with malignant lymphoma.

Community-Based Care

When teaching the client and family for home care, include the following topics in addition to those previously identified for specific nursing diagnoses:

- Information about the illness, planned treatment, and anticipated side effects of treatment

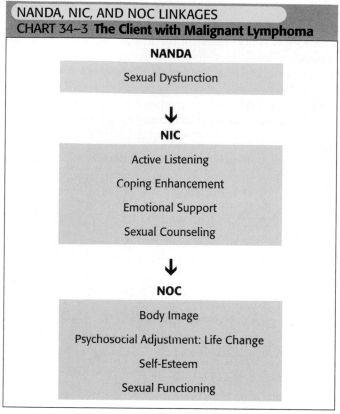

NANDA, NIC, AND NOC LINKAGES
CHART 34–3 **The Client with Malignant Lymphoma**

NANDA

Sexual Dysfunction

↓

NIC

Active Listening

Coping Enhancement

Emotional Support

Sexual Counseling

↓

NOC

Body Image

Psychosocial Adjustment: Life Change

Self-Esteem

Sexual Functioning

Data from *NANDA's Nursing Diagnoses: Definitions & Classification 2005–2006* by NANDA International (2005), Philadelphia; *Nursing Interventions Classification (NIC)* (4th ed.) by J. M. Dochterman & G. M. Bulechek (2004), St. Louis, MO: Mosby; and *Nursing Outcomes Classification (NOC)* (3rd ed.) by S. Moorhead, M. Johnson, and M. Mass (2004), St. Louis, MO: Mosby.

- Skin care and measures to relieve itching and protect areas of radiation
- Symptoms to report to the physician, including those of vertebral compression (decreased sensation or strength in lower extremities)
- Use of analgesics and alternative relief strategies for abdominal pain and peripheral neuropathies
- Respiratory care if mediastinal nodes are enlarged or lungs or pleurae are involved
- Planning activities of daily living to ensure adequate rest and exercise
- Measures to relieve nausea and maintain adequate nutrition.

Refer clients and family members to the local chapter of the American Cancer Society for information, assistance, and counseling. A list of state and local agencies that offer information about malignant lymphoma and financial assistance can be obtained from the Leukemia Society of America.

THE CLIENT WITH MULTIPLE MYELOMA

Multiple myeloma is a malignancy in which plasma cells multiply uncontrollably and infiltrate the bone marrow, lymph nodes, spleen, and other tissues. *Plasma cells* are B-cell lymphocytes that develop to produce antibodies (immunoglobins).

Incidence and Risk Factors

The incidence of multiple myeloma is increasing slightly, with an estimated 15,980 cases diagnosed and 11,300 deaths due to the disease in 2005 (ACS, 2005). It affects blacks nearly twice as often as whites, and men slightly more frequently than women. The incidence of multiple myeloma increases with age, rarely occurring before age 40 (Kasper et al., 2005). Its cause is unknown. Possible contributing factors include genetic alterations, radiation exposure, oncogenic virus, inflammatory stimuli, and chronic antigenic stimulation. The risk for developing multiple myeloma is higher in people of lower socioeconomic status. This increased risk may relate to environmental factors such as poor housing, occupational hazards, poor nutritional status, and other physical and psychosocial stressors such as exposure to infectious agents (Mangan, 2005).

Pathophysiology

Malignant plasma cells arise from one clone (*monoclonal*) of B cells that produce abnormally large amounts of a particular immunoglobin called the *M protein*. This abnormal protein interferes with normal antibody production and impairs the humoral immune response. It also increases blood viscosity and may damage kidney tubules. As myeloma cells proliferate, they replace the bone marrow and infiltrate the bone itself. Cortical bone is progressively destroyed by tumor growth and enzymes produced by myeloma cells. These enzymes facilitate bone destruction, its infiltration by tumor cells, development of new blood vessels to sustain the tumor, and growth of myeloma cells (McCance & Huether, 2006). Affected bones (primarily the vertebrae, ribs, skull, pelvis, femur, clavicle, and scapula) are weakened and may break without trauma (*pathologic fracture*). With disease progression, malignant cells spread via the bloodstream to invade other organs (Figure 34–11 ■).

Manifestations

The disease develops slowly, with up to 30% of clients diagnosed during evaluation for unrelated problems (Mangan, 2005). Manifestations of multiple myeloma are due to its effects on the bone and the impaired immune response due to M-protein production. Bone pain is the most common presenting symptom. With progression of the disease, the pain may increase in severity and become more localized. Rapid bone destruction releases calcium from the bone, leading to hypercalcemia and manifestations of neurologic dysfunction, such as lethargy, confusion, and weakness.

As functional antibody formation decreases and the humoral immune response is suppressed, recurrent infections develop. Cell-mediated immunity remains intact. *Bence Jones proteins* are found in the urine in multiple myeloma. These proteins are toxic to the renal tubules, and may lead to renal failure with azotemia and uremia. (See Chapter 29 ∞ for more information about renal failure.)

About 15% of clients with multiple myeloma die within 3 months of the diagnosis. More frequently, the disease course is chronic, progressing more rapidly with each relapse after remission. The acute terminal stage of the disease is marked by pancytopenia and widespread organ infiltration by myeloma cells (Kasper et al., 2005).

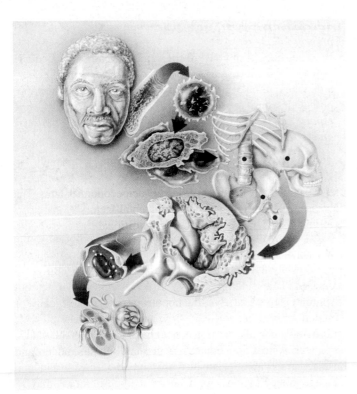

Figure 34-11 ■ An illustration of the progress of multiple myeloma in an African American male. Abnormal plasma cells proliferate uncontrollably, gradually replacing bone marrow and infiltrating bone itself. As the disease progresses, these cells spread to other organs via the bloodstream.

Source: Kevin A. Somerville, Phototake NYC

INTERDISCIPLINARY CARE

Diagnosis and Staging

Diagnostic tests for multiple myeloma include the following:

- *X-rays* and other radiologic studies of the bone may reveal multiple punched-out lesions.
- *Bone marrow examination* shows an abnormal number of immature plasma cells.
- *CBC* shows moderate to severe anemia, and the *ESR* usually is elevated.
- *Protein electrophoresis* shows a spike of one type of antibody, usually IgG.
- *Serum calcium, creatinine, uric acid,* and *BUN* levels often are elevated.
- *Urinalysis* shows Bence Jones protein in the urine.
- *Biopsy* of myeloma lesions confirms the diagnosis of multiple myeloma.

Staging of multiple myeloma is based on the hemoglobin and serum calcium levels, the amount of abnormal protein present, and the degree of bone involvement.

Treatment

There is no cure for multiple myeloma. In some clients, active observation is indicated, as the disease may continue with a slow, *indolent* (sluggish, not developing or progressing) course for many years (Mangan, 2005). When indicated by disease stage or progression, standard treatment includes induction

chemotherapy followed by stem cell transplant and maintenance chemotherapy to control progression of the disease. Supportive care is provided to reduce complications of the disease and their effects.

Combination chemotherapy with an alkylating agent (melphalan [Alkeran], cyclophosphamide [Cytoxan], or chlorambucil [Chloromycetin]) and prednisone administered for 4 to 7 days every 4 to 6 weeks is commonly used. Chemotherapy typically reduces bone pain, hypercalcemia, anemia, and the number of infections (Kasper et al., 2005). Localized radiation therapy may be used to treat painful bone lesions. High-dose chemotherapy followed by peripheral allogeneic stem cell transplant may be more effective in achieving a cure, but is associated with a high mortality rate. When autologous SCT is used, granulocyte colony-stimulating factor is administered prior to harvesting and preserving peripheral stem cells for transplant.

Supportive care may include treatment of hypercalcemia with hydration, possible bisphosphonate therapy to reduce bone loss (see Chapter 42), and calcium, vitamin D, and fluoride supplements to support bone structure. Plasma exchange therapy (plasmapheresis) to remove circulating M proteins is used as needed to treat acute renal failure. Infections are treated promptly when they develop.

NURSING CARE

Assessment

Focused assessment data for the client with multiple myeloma include the following:

- *Health history:* Complaints of back or bone pain, onset, duration, and intensity; complaints of weakness, fatigue, anorexia; history of frequent or recurrent infections; neurologic symptoms such as numbness and tingling or clumsiness.
- *Physical examination:* Level of consciousness and mental status; mobility, gait; localized tenderness or pain, bony crepitus with movement or palpation; movement and sensation in extremities.

Nursing Diagnoses and Interventions

Nursing care of the client with multiple myeloma focuses on problems of chronic pain, impaired mobility, and the risk for injury. Risk for infection is a major nursing care focus; see the previous section on leukemia for specific interventions to reduce this risk. Other nursing care needs are similar to those of clients with other cancers and chronic pain. See Chapters 9 and 14 for additional specific nursing interventions for these problems.

Chronic Pain

Clients with multiple myeloma typically experience chronic back pain and deep bone pain as myeloma cells saturate the bone marrow and invade the bone structure. Pathologic fractures are a common and reoccurring problem.

- Assess pain, including intensity (use a standard pain scale), onset, duration, precipitating factors, and effective relief measures. *Identifying the intensity, causes, and precipitating factors of pain helps determine and evaluate effective pain relief measures.*

- Determine position of greatest comfort, and assist as needed into this position. *The client is best able to identify positions that minimize pain, but may need assistance with repositioning.*
- Support position with pillows. *Bony prominences may be painful due to infiltrates. Pillows can help relieve pressure on these prominences, thus reducing pain.*
- Provide uninterrupted rest periods. *Adequate rest facilitates pain relief and improves pain tolerance.*
- Teach adjunctive pain relief strategies such as relaxation or guided imagery. *A combination of pharmacologic and non-pharmacologic methods provides better management of chronic pain, especially bone pain.*
- Teach effective analgesic use, including the family in instruction. *Analgesics are most effective when taken before pain becomes severe. Clients and their families may be reluctant to use prescription analgesics on a regular basis.*
- Report unrelieved pain to the physician. *A different analgesic or addition of an adjunctive medication such as a nonsteroidal anti-inflammatory drug (NSAID) may be needed to effectively control pain.*

Impaired Physical Mobility

Painful bony infiltrates and pathologic fractures may limit mobility. A brace or splint may be used to protect extremities or support the back. In addition, persistent weakness associated with the cancer and anemia may limit the client's ability to participate in usual activities.

- Assist to change position at least every 2 hours. *Assistance with repositioning is necessary due to weakness. Frequent repositioning improves comfort and reduces the risk for impaired skin and tissue integrity.*

PRACTICE ALERT

Gently support extremities during repositioning. Weakened extremities due to infiltration of bone by myeloma cells and muscle atrophy from lack of use increase the risk for pathologic fractures.

- Provide a trapeze to assist in repositioning. *A trapeze provides better leverage, allowing the client to assist with repositioning and providing a degree of independence. The ability to participate in self-care improves self-esteem.*

Risk for Injury

The bone involvement of multiple myeloma places the client at high risk for pathologic and traumatic fractures. Pathologic fractures can occur with simple activities such as turning or reaching for an item. The spine usually is affected; the ribs and bones of the extremities also may be at risk for fracture.

- Place needed items close at hand. *Straining to reach objects increases the risk of falling or sustaining other injury.*
- Provide safety measures to prevent falls from bed: Place the bed in a low position, use side rails as indicated, and place the call bell within reach. *Safety measures help prevent acci-*

dental injury. *A secure environment minimizes risk and helps prevent falls.*

- Provide shoes with nonskid soles, a clear pathway, adequate lighting, and a level surface free of scatter rugs or other hazards when ambulating. Provide a walker as needed for support and security. *Weight-bearing exercise promotes bone repair. Safety measures, such as an unobstructed pathway and a firm walking surface, help prevent falls.*

Community-Based Care

When teaching clients and their families for home care, include the following topics:

- Strategies for home maintenance management
- Signs and symptoms of complications to be reported to the physician (e.g., symptoms of vertebral and extremity fractures)
- Manifestations of infection to report: fever and chills; increased malaise, fatigue, or weakness; cough with or without sputum; sore throat; dysuria, nocturia, frequency, urgency, or malodorous urine.

Provide referrals for home health and home maintenance services, physical or occupational therapy, social services, and hospice care as appropriate.

THE CLIENT WITH NEUTROPENIA

Leukopenia is a decrease in the total circulating white blood cell count. Although any type of WBC may be affected, neutrophils, which make up the majority of WBCs, are affected most often. *Neutropenia* is a decrease in circulating neutrophils, usually less than 1500 cells/mm^3. Neutropenia may be either congenital or acquired, developing secondarily to prolonged infection, hematologic disorders, starvation, or autoimmune disorders (such as rheumatoid arthritis). Chemotherapy and other drugs can suppress the bone marrow. Neutropenia develops in approximately half of clients undergoing chemotherapy to treat cancer (Eggenberger et al., 2004). *Agranulocytosis* is severe neutropenia, with less than 200 cells/µm. Numbers of other granulocytes also are reduced. It is usually due to impaired leukocyte formation in the bone marrow or increased cell destruction in circulating blood. Agranulocytosis significantly increases the risk for infection. *Aplastic anemia* affects production of all blood cells, resulting in anemia, thrombocytopenia, and agranulocytosis.

Pathophysiology and Manifestations

Neutrophils are an integral component of the immune response. They are phagocytes, drawn to and activated by infection and inflammation to engulf and degrade invading microorganisms. Their life span in peripheral blood is short, less than 1 day. When *granulopoiesis* (the development and maturation of granulocytes) in the bone marrow is suppressed, the number of circulating neutrophils falls rapidly. As a result, the body's ability to defend itself against infection is significantly reduced.

The manifestations of neutropenia reflect the resulting impaired immunity and inflammatory response. Opportunistic bacterial, fungal, and protozoal infections develop, commonly affecting the respiratory tract and mucosa of the mouth, GI tract, and vagina. Malaise, chills, and fever with extreme weakness and fatigue are common manifestations.

INTERDISCIPLINARY CARE

The diagnosis of neutropenia is made based on the client's manifestations, risk factors, and the CBC. The total white blood count is low, often less than 1000/mm³.

Hematopoietic growth factors such as GM-CSF are administered to stimulate granulocyte maturation and differentiation. Infections are treated with antibiotic therapy. Protective isolation procedures may be initiated to prevent exposure to pathogens. When neutropenia is related to chemotherapy, cancer treatment often must be halted, at least temporarily, to allow the bone marrow to recover.

NURSING CARE

The primary nursing care focus is early identification of neutropenia and protecting the client from infection. The WBC count is monitored on a regular basis, and any decline reported to the physician. Protective isolation may be indicated, including restricting the number of visitors and people with apparent illness. See *Risk for Infection* in the earlier section on leukemia for specific nursing interventions for the client with neutropenia.

THE CLIENT WITH INFECTIOUS MONONUCLEOSIS

Infectious mononucleosis is characterized by invasion of B cells in the oropharyngeal lymphoid tissues by the Epstein-Barr virus. This disease is usually benign and self-limiting. It often affects young adults between the ages of 15 and 30. Although many children are infected with EBV, symptomatic infectious mononucleosis is uncommon in early childhood. The virus is present in saliva, which appears to be the primary mode of transmission. As a result, infectious mononucleosis is often called the "kissing disease."

EBV also is associated with some cancers, including Burkitt's lymphoma and Hodgkin's disease, B-cell lymphoma, and nasopharyngeal carcinoma (Kasper et al., 2005).

Pathophysiology and Manifestations

When the virus enters the body, unaffected B cells produce antibodies against the virus, and T cells directly attack the virus. Infected B cells are destroyed as the virus replicates. The proliferation of B and T cells, as well as the removal of dead and damaged leukocytes, is responsible for the swelling of lymphoid tissues.

The incubation period for infectious mononucleosis is 4 to 8 weeks. Its onset is insidious, with headache, malaise, and fatigue. Fever, sore throat, and cervical lymphadenopathy (lymph node enlargement and pain) lasting 1 to 3 weeks is common. Symptom severity varies from person to person. Lymph node involvement may be generalized; about 50% of people with infectious mononucleosis develop an enlarged spleen (splenomegaly).

INTERDISCIPLINARY CARE

Laboratory findings include increased lymphocytes and monocytes, with about 20% of the cells atypical in form. Early in the infection, the WBC count usually is normal or low, but by the second week it increases and remains elevated for 4 to 8 weeks. Platelet counts are often low during the illness.

Recovery occurs in 2 to 3 weeks; however, debility and lethargy may last for up to 3 months. The treatment includes bed rest and analgesic agents to alleviate the symptoms. Nursing care is primarily educational to prevent further spread of the disease.

PLATELET AND COAGULATION DISORDERS

Platelet and coagulation disorders affect **hemostasis**, control of bleeding. Hemostasis maintains a relatively steady state of blood volume, blood pressure, and blood flow through injured vessels. Bleeding disorders result from deficient platelets, disruption of the clotting cascade, or a combination of factors

THE CLIENT WITH THROMBOCYTOPENIA

Thrombocytopenia is a platelet count of less than 100,000 per milliliter of blood. It can lead to abnormal bleeding. A continuing decline in circulating platelets to less than 20,000/mL can lead to spontaneous bleeding and hemorrhage from minor trauma (Figure 34–12 ■). Bleeding due to platelet deficiency usually occurs in small vessels, causing manifestations such as *petechiae* and *purpura*. The mucous membranes of the nose, mouth, GI

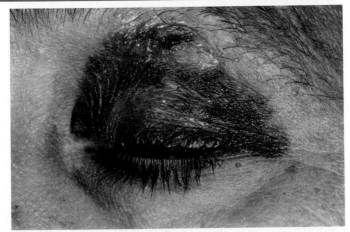

Figure 34–12 ■ Significant ecchymosis of the eyelid associated with minor trauma in a client with thrombocytopenia.

Source: Scott Camazine, Photo Researchers, Inc.

tract, and vagina often bleed. Serious and potentially fatal bleeding occurs when the platelet count is less than 10,000/mL.

Thrombocytopenia results from one of three mechanisms: decreased production, increased sequestration in the spleen, or accelerated destruction. Primary thrombocytopenia that leads to increased platelet destruction is discussed below. Secondary thrombocytopenia may be caused by aplastic anemia, bone marrow malignancy, infection, radiation therapy, or drug therapy (Box 34–6). Heparin therapy is the most common drug-induced thrombocytopenia; it is included in the discussion that follows. Platelet sequestration usually is due to an enlarged spleen. Up to 80% of platelets may be removed from circulation with significant splenomegaly (Porth, 2005). Finally, thrombocytopenia may result from premature platelet destruction associated with disseminated intravascular coagulation (DIC).

Physiology Review

Effective control of bleeding requires a series of complex interactions between the damaged tissue and blood vessel, platelets, clotting factors, and processes to dissolve clots once bleeding has been controlled (see Figures 33–5, 33–6, and 33–7 ∞). Platelets are formed in the bone marrow under control of thrombopoietin, a protein produced by the liver, kidney, smooth muscle, and bone marrow. Platelets are attracted to the damaged vessel wall, where they aggregate and release mediators that activate the clotting process. See Chapter 33 ∞ for a more complete discussion about platelets, clotting, and hemostasis.

Pathophysiology

The two types of primary thrombocytopenia are immune thrombocytopenic purpura and thrombotic thrombocytopenic purpura.

Immune Thrombocytopenic Purpura

Immune thrombocytopenic purpura (ITP), also known as *idiopathic thrombocytopenic purpura*, is an autoimmune disorder in which platelet destruction is accelerated. In ITP, proteins on the platelet cell membrane stimulate autoantibody production, usually IgG antibodies. These autoantibodies adhere to the platelet membrane. Although the platelets function normally, the spleen reacts to them as being foreign and destroys the altered platelets after only 1 to 3 days of circulation.

MANIFESTATIONS The manifestations of ITP are due to bleeding from small vessels and mucous membranes. Petechiae and purpura develop, often on the anterior chest, arms, neck, and oral mucous membranes. Bruising also may be apparent. As bleeding progresses, epistaxis (nosebleed), hematuria, excess menstrual bleeding, and bleeding gums occur. Spontaneous intracranial bleeding is rare but does occur. Associated symptoms include weight loss, fever, and headache.

INCIDENCE AND COURSE Acute ITP affects people of any age following a viral illness (Copstead & Banasik, 2005). Acute ITP typically lasts only 1 to 2 months, resolving without long-term consequences. In its chronic form, ITP typically affects adults between ages 20 and 50; women are affected more often than men. Its onset is insidious. Chronic (or adult) ITP often occurs in people with other immune-associated disorders such as systemic lupus erythematosus or HIV disease (Copstead & Banasik, 2005).

Thrombotic Thrombocytopenic Purpura

Thrombotic thrombocytopenic purpura (TTP) is a rare disorder in which thrombi occlude arterioles and capillaries of the microcirculation. Many organs are affected, including the heart, kidneys, and brain. The incidence of TTP is increasing (McCance & Huether, 2006). Its cause is unknown. Platelet aggregation is a key feature of the disorder. As RBCs circulate through partially occluded vessels, they fragment, leading to hemolytic anemia (Porth, 2005).

MANIFESTATIONS TTP may be acute, the more common and severe form, or chronic. Acute idiopathic TTP may be fatal within months if untreated. The manifestations of TTP include purpura and petechiae, and neurologic symptoms such as headache, seizures, and altered consciousness.

Heparin-Induced Thrombocytopenia

Heparin-induced thrombocytopenia (HIT) develops as a result of an abnormal response to heparin therapy. Unfractionated heparin carries a greater potential to precipitate HIT; it can, however, develop in clients receiving low-molecular-weight heparin who have previously been treated with unfractionated heparin. See Chapter 35 ∞ for further discussion of heparin therapy and the forms of heparin.

Heparin is a protein that occurs naturally in human tissues and inflammatory cells. It can react directly with platelets, causing them to agglutinate (clump) and be removed from circulation by phagocytosis. This form of HIT, called type I HIT, typically causes mild thrombocytopenia. The more severe form, type II HIT, results from an immune reaction to heparin. In type II HIT, heparin forms an immune complex with a platelet protein known as platelet factor 4 (PF4). This complex acts as a foreign antigen in some clients, stimulating antibody production. The antibody binds with the heparin-PF4 complex, and these antibody-heparin-PF4 complexes subsequently bind with circulating

---

BOX 34–6 Selected Causes of Secondary Thrombocytopenia

Diseases

- Vitamin B$_{12}$ anemia
- Folic acid anemia
- Aplastic anemia
- Leukemia
- Alcoholism
- DIC
- Infectious mononucleosis
- Viral infections
- HIV disease

Drugs

- Thiazide diuretics
- Aspirin
- Ibuprofen
- Indomethacin
- Naproxen
- Sulfonamides
- Phenytoin
- Cimetidine
- Digoxin
- Furosemide
- Heparin
- Morphine

Treatments

- Radiation therapy
- Chemotherapy
- Massive transfusion of stored blood

platelets, causing them to aggregate. As affected platelets aggregate, they are removed from circulation, leading to thrombocytopenia. In addition, small pieces of platelets can break loose, stimulating the clotting cascade and the development of thrombosis (clotting) (Francis & Drexler, 2005). The thrombocytopenia and the thrombosis can be reversed by prompt withdrawal of heparin therapy (Kasper et al., 2005).

MANIFESTATIONS Despite thrombocytopenia, bleeding is usually a manifestation of HIT, probably because of the increased tendency to form clots that deplete clotting factors. The client may develop manifestations of an arterial thrombosis (severe pain, paresthesias, pallor and cool skin temperature, and pulselessness distal to the arterial occlusion) or of venous thrombosis (edema, redness, and warmth of the affected area). On rare occasion, an intravenous bolus of unfractionated heparin can precipitate an acute inflammatory response with manifestations that may mimic an acute pulmonary embolism: fever, chills, hypertension, tachycardia, dyspnea, chest pain, and cardiopulmonary arrest (Francis & Drexler, 2005).

INTERDISCIPLINARY CARE

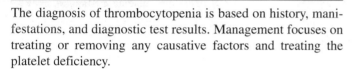

The diagnosis of thrombocytopenia is based on history, manifestations, and diagnostic test results. Management focuses on treating or removing any causative factors and treating the platelet deficiency.

Diagnosis

The following diagnostic tests are used to identify thrombocytopenia:

- *CBC with platelet count* is done to evaluate blood cell counts, hemoglobin, and hematocrit.
- *Antinuclear antibodies (ANA)* are measured to assess for autoantibodies and identify possible contributing disorders such as systemic lupus erythematosus.
- *Serologic studies* for hepatitis viruses, cytomegalovirus (CMV), EBV, toxoplasma, and HIV may be done. Serologic testing also may be performed when HIT is suspected.
- *Bone marrow examination* evaluates for aplastic anemia and megakaryocyte production.

Medications

Oral glucocorticoids, such as prednisone, are prescribed to suppress the autoimmune response. Many clients who respond to glucocorticoid treatment relapse when the drug is withdrawn, however. Immunosuppressive drugs such as azathioprine, cyclophosphamide, and cyclosporine may be used.

Prompt withdrawal of heparin therapy is vital when HIT is the cause of thrombocytopenia. All sources of heparin are removed, including heparin used to flush intravenous or other catheters and heparin-coated catheters (Francis & Drexler, 2005). A non-heparin anticoagulant such as lepirudin (Refludan) or argatroban may be substituted. Lepirudin is a thrombin inhibitor. It is a recombinant form of hirudin, originally isolated from the salivary glands of leeches. Its primary adverse effect is bleeding; as a protein, it also can stimulate antibody development, resulting in rare instances of anaphylaxis. Argatroban is a synthetic direct thrombin inhibitor with a short half-life. It clears quickly when the infusion is discontinued, an advantage if excessive bleeding develops or invasive procedures must be performed (Rice et al., 2002).

Treatments

Platelet transfusions may be required to treat acute bleeding due to thrombocytopenia. Platelets are prepared from fresh whole blood; one unit contains 30 to 60 mL of platelet concentrate. The expected increase in platelets after one unit is infused is 10,000/mL. *Plasmapheresis,* or *plasma exchange therapy,* is the primary treatment for acute thrombotic thrombocytopenic purpura. The client's plasma is removed and replaced with fresh frozen plasma to remove autoantibodies, immune complexes, and toxins.

Surgery

A *splenectomy* (surgical removal of the spleen) is the treatment of choice if the client with ITP relapses when glucocorticoids are discontinued. The spleen is the site of platelet destruction and antibody production. This surgery often cures the disorder, although relapse may occur years after splenectomy.

NURSING CARE

Assessment

- *Health history:* Complaints of bruising with minor or no trauma, bleeding gums, nosebleed, heavy or prolonged menstrual periods, black, tarry, or bloody stools, hematemesis, headache, fever, or neurologic symptoms; recent weight loss; recent viral or other illness; current and recent medications; exposure to toxins; previous exposure to heparin.
- *Physical examination:* Skin and mucous membranes for color, temperature, petechiae, purpura, or bruises; vital signs; weight; mental status and level of consciousness; heart and breath sounds; abdominal exam; body fluids for occult blood.
- *Diagnostic tests:* CBC, hemoglobin and hematocrit, platelet count; serologic and ANA test results; bone marrow examination results.

Nursing Diagnoses and Interventions

Inadequate platelets impair hemostasis, placing the client at risk for bleeding. Bleeding gums, an early sign of the disorder, affects oral mucous membrane integrity as well.

Ineffective Protection

Bleeding is a serious complication associated with thrombocytopenia. As platelet counts (measured in cubic millimeters) decrease, the risk of bleeding increases. The risk is minimal with counts greater than 50,000 mm^3; moderate when the count is between 20,000 and 50,000 mm^3; and significant when the count falls below 20,000 mm^3.

- Monitor vital signs, heart and breath sounds every 4 hours. Frequently assess for other manifestations of bleeding:
  a. Skin and mucous membranes for petechiae, ecchymoses, and hematoma formation
  b. Gums, nasal membranes, and conjunctiva for bleeding
  c. Overt or occult blood in emesis, urine, or stool

d. Vaginal bleeding
e. Prolonged bleeding from puncture sites
f. Neurologic changes: headache, visual changes, altered mental status, decreasing level of consciousness, seizures
g. Abdominal: epigastric pain, absence of bowel sounds, increasing abdominal girth, abdominal guarding or rigidity.
Early identification of bleeding is important to prevent serious blood loss and shock.

PRACTICE ALERT

Avoid invasive procedures such as rectal temperatures, urinary catheterization, and parenteral injections to the extent possible. Diagnostic procedures such as biopsy or lumbar puncture should be avoided if the platelet count is less than 50,000 mm^3. Invasive procedures can cause tissue trauma and bleeding. Procedures that use large-bore needles should be delayed until the platelet count is increased.

- Apply pressure to puncture sites for 3 to 5 minutes; apply pressure to arterial puncture sites for 15 to 20 minutes. *Pressure promotes hemostasis and clot formation.*
- Instruct to avoid forcefully blowing the nose or picking crusts from the nose, straining to have a bowel movement, and forceful coughing or sneezing. *These activities increase the risk of external and internal bleeding.*

Impaired Oral Mucous Membranes

Thrombocytopenia frequently leads to bleeding of the gums and oral mucosa. As a result, risk for infection and impaired nutrition increases.

- Frequently assess the mouth for bleeding. Inquire about oral pain or tenderness. *Breakdown of oral mucous membranes increases the risk of infection and bleeding, and causes discomfort with eating.*
- Encourage use of a soft-bristle toothbrush or sponge to clean teeth and gums. *Hard bristles may abrade oral mucosa, causing bleeding and increasing the risk of infection.*
- Instruct to rinse the mouth with saline every 2 to 4 hours. Apply petroleum jelly to lips as needed to prevent dryness and cracking. *Saline mouth rinses and petroleum jelly help maintain oral tissue integrity and promote cleansing and healing.*
- Instruct to avoid alcohol-based mouthwashes, very hot foods, alcohol, and crusty foods. Teach to drink cool liquids at least every 2 hours. *Avoiding foods and liquids that traumatize oral mucosa increases comfort; fluid intake prevents dehydration and helps maintain mucous membrane integrity.*

Community-Based Care

In the adult, ITP often is a chronic disorder that the client and family must learn to manage. Secondary thrombocytopenia may be either acute or chronic. Discuss the following topics when preparing the client and family for home care:

- Nature of the disorder, its usual course, and the treatment plan
- Use of and desired and potential adverse effects of prescribed medications
- Risks and benefits of surgery or treatments such as plasma replacement therapy

- The importance of follow-up tests and visits for care
- Measures to reduce the risk of bleeding: safety measures such as a soft-bristle toothbrush, electric razor, avoidance of contact sports and hazardous activities, and avoiding medications that further interfere with platelet function (Box 34–7)

Refer for home health or other community services (e.g., housekeeping, shopping) as indicated.

THE CLIENT WITH HEMOPHILIA

Hemophilia is a group of hereditary clotting factor disorders that lead to persistent and sometimes severe bleeding (see the accompanying Genetic Considerations box). Although often considered a disease of children, hemophilia may be diagnosed in adults. Deficiencies of three clotting factors, VIII, IX, and XI, account for 90% to 95% of the bleeding disorders collectively called hemophilia (McCance & Huether, 2006).

Physiology Review

When tissue injury occurs, platelets collect at the site, adhering to the damaged vessel wall (the platelet plug). Activation of the clotting cascade, a sequential process of interactive reactions of clotting factors, is vital to form a stable clot. Clotting factors are plasma proteins primarily produced by the liver. A number of these factors require the presence of vitamin K for synthesis and activation. Once the clot has been formed and stabilized, it begins to retract, pulling together the edges of the damaged blood vessel to initiate the healing process.

Pathophysiology

Hemophilia A (or *classic hemophilia*) is the most common type of hemophilia, caused by deficiency or dysfunction of clotting factor VIII. It is transmitted as an X-linked recessive disorder from mothers to sons (Figure 34–13 ■). The genetic defect of hemophilia A on the X chromosome may cause deficient factor VIII production or a defective form of the pro-

---

BOX 34–7 Medications That May Interfere with Platelet Function

Over-the-Counter Medications

- Aspirin and salicylates, including:
  - Alka-Seltzer
  - Bufferin
  - Doan's pills
  - Ecotrin
  - Excedrin
  - Midol
  - Pepto-Bismol
  - Vanquish
- NSAIDs such as
  - Advil
  - Aleve
  - Nuprin
  - Pamprin IB

Prescription Medications

- Aspirin-containing analgesics
- Chemotherapy drugs
- Antibiotics such as penicillin
- Carbamazepine (Tegretol)
- Colchicine
- Dipyridamole (Persantine)
- Gold salts
- Heparin
- Quinine derivatives
- Sulfonamides
- Thiazide diuretics

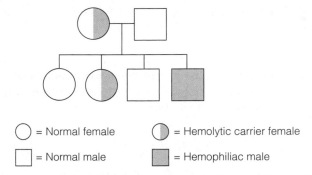

○ = Normal female   ◐ = Hemolytic carrier female

□ = Normal male   ■ = Hemophiliac male

Figure 34–13 ■ The inheritance pattern of hemophilia A and B. Both are transmitted as X-linked recessive disorders. Females may be carriers, but males develop these disorders.

GENETIC CONSIDERATIONS
Focus on Hemophilia

The incidence and pattern of inheritance for the forms of hemophilia differ.

- Hemophilia A occurs in about 1 in 10,000 male births, transmitted on the X chromosome: Each male offspring has a 50% risk of inheriting the defective gene; each female offspring has a 50% risk of becoming a carrier.
- Hemophilia B occurs in about 1 in 100,000 male births, transmitted on the X chromosome.
- Von Willebrand's disease affects about 1 in 100 to 500 people, usually inherited as an autosomal dominant trait: Offspring of an affected person have a 50% risk of inheriting the trait and the disorder.
- Factor XI deficiency inherited as an autosomal recessive trait: Each offspring of a carrier and an unaffected individual has as 50% risk of inheriting the trait; each offspring of two carriers has a 50% risk of being a carrier and a 25% risk of having the disorder. This deficiency is common in Ashkenazi Jews.

tein. When the concentration of the clotting factor is 5% to 35% of normal, the disease is *mild*. Bleeding is infrequent, and usually associated with trauma. Concentrations of 1% to 5% of normal result in *moderate* disease. Again, bleeding usually occurs secondarily to trauma. *Severe* hemophilia occurs when concentrations are less than 1% of normal. Bleeding is frequent, often occurring without trauma (Kasper et al., 2005; McCance & Huether, 2006).

Hemophilia B (also called *Christmas disease*) accounts for about 15% of cases, and is caused by a deficiency in Factor IX. Despite the difference in clotting factor deficits, hemophilia A and B are clinically identical.

Von Willebrand's disease, often considered a type of hemophilia, is the most common hereditary bleeding disorder (Porth, 2005). It is caused by a deficit of or defective von Willebrand (vW) factor, a protein that mediates platelet adhesion (Tierney et al., 2005). Reduced levels of Factor VIII often also are present, because vW factor carries Factor VIII. This clotting disorder affects men and women equally. Bleeding associ-

ated with von Willebrand's disease rarely is severe. It often is diagnosed when prolonged bleeding follows surgery or a dental extraction.

Factor XI deficiency (or *hemophilia C*) is usually a mild disorder, identified when postoperative bleeding is prolonged. A comparison of the types of hemophilia is found in Table 34–9.

People with hemophilia form a platelet plug at the site of bleeding, but the clotting factor deficit impairs formation of a stable fibrin clot. The effect of vW factor deficiency is somewhat different, in that platelet aggregation at the site of injury is impaired. In either case, prolonged or extensive bleeding may result. Often bleeding occurs in response to injury or as a result of surgery. However, a severe clotting factor deficit can lead to spontaneous bleeding into the joints (*hemarthrosis*), deep tissues, and CNS. Hemarthrosis often causes joint deformity and disability, usually of the elbows, hips, knees, and ankles.

Manifestations

The following are manifestations of hemophilia:

- Hemarthrosis
- Easy bruising and cutaneous hematoma formation with minor trauma (e.g., an injection)
- Bleeding from the gums and prolonged bleeding following minor injuries or cuts

TABLE 34–9 Types of Hemophilia

TYPE/NAME	DEFICIENCY	CHARACTERISTICS	TREATMENT
Hemophilia A (classic hemophilia)	Factor VIII	Transmitted by females; occurs primarily in males; bleeding time normal; coagulation time prolonged	Factor VIII concentrate or cryoprecipitate
Hemophilia B	Factor IX	Transmitted by females; occurs primarily in males; bleeding time normal; coagulation time prolonged	Factor IX (Christmas disease concentrate)
Von Willebrand's disease	vW factor Factor VIII	Occurs in both females and males; bleeding time and coagulation time are both prolonged	Cryoprecipitate and DDAVP
Factor XI deficiency	Factor XI	Occurs in both males and females; the activated partial thromboplastin time is prolonged	Fresh frozen plasma

- Gastrointestinal bleeding, with hematemesis (vomiting blood), occult blood in the stools, gastric pain, or abdominal pain
- Spontaneous hematuria or epistaxis (nosebleed)
- Pain or paralysis due to the pressure of hematomas on nerves
- Intracranial hemorrhage is a potentially life-threatening manifestation of hemophilia.

INTERDISCIPLINARY CARE

Treatment of hemophilia focuses on preventing and/or treating bleeding, primarily by replacing deficient clotting factors. Specific treatment depends on the severity of the disorder and the specific factor deficiency. Care may be complicated by hepatitis or HIV disease in people with hemophilia treated with clotting factor concentrates prepared from multiple units of donated blood. Today, routine testing of all blood, improved blood donor screening, and current methods of treating hemophilia have significantly reduced the risk for these bloodborne diseases.

Diagnosis

The following laboratory tests may be ordered:
- *Serum platelet levels* are measured and are usually normal.
- *Coagulation studies* such as APTT, bleeding time, and prothrombin time are used to screen for hemophilia when abnormal bleeding occurs. APTT is increased in all types of hemophilia. Prothrombin time is unaffected in these disorders but may be measured to rule out other disorders. Bleeding time is prolonged in von Willebrand's disease but normal in hemophilia A and B.
- *Factor assays* are performed; Factor VIII is decreased in hemophilia A and often in von Willebrand's disease, Factor IX is decreased in hemophilia B, and Factor XI in hemophilia C.
- *Amniocentesis* or *chorionic villus sampling* is used to identify the genetic defect of hemophilia when there is a known family history of the disease.

Medications

Deficient clotting factors are replaced regularly, as a prophylactic measure before surgery and dental procedures, and to control bleeding. Clotting factors may be given as fresh-frozen plasma, cryoprecipitates, or concentrates. Factor levels are measured on a regular basis to determine whether the treatment is adequate. Clotting factors are often self-administered and may be taken either on a regular or intermittent schedule.

Fresh-frozen plasma replaces all clotting factors (including both Factor VIII and Factor IX) except platelets. When the cause of bleeding is not yet determined, fresh-frozen plasma may be administered intravenously until a definitive diagnosis is made.

Hemophilia A is usually treated with either heat-treated Factor VIII concentrate (heat treating reduces the risk of transmitting disease) or recombinant Factor VIII. Although recombinant Factor VIII, produced using recombinant DNA technology, eliminates the risk of viral disease transmission, its use is limited by cost. The dose of Factor VIII is determined by the severity of the deficit and the presence or prospect of active bleeding (e.g., planned surgery).

Desmopressin acetate (DDAVP, Stimate) may be given to people with mild hemophilia A or von Willebrand's disease prior to minor surgeries. This drug causes release of Factor VIII and will raise blood levels by two- or threefold for several hours, reducing the risk of bleeding and the need for clotting factor concentrate (Tierney et al., 2005).

Factor IX concentrate (administered intravenously) is used to treat hemophilia B. Because Factor IX concentrates also contain a number of other proteins, there is risk of thrombosis with recurrent use. They are used judiciously, only when needed. Products produced by recombinant technology or that are monoclonally purified carry a lower risk of stimulating thrombus formation (Kasper et al., 2005). Fresh-frozen plasma replaces Factor XI and is used when necessary. It may be given daily until the risk for bleeding decreases.

Factor VIII concentrates contain functional vW factor, and may be used to treat von Willebrand's disease. Aspirin is avoided in all types of hemophilia.

NURSING CARE

Although primary responsibility for care falls to the client and family, nursing care presents challenges. For additional assessment and nursing care strategies, see the accompanying Nursing Care Plan.

Health Promotion

Encourage clients with a family history of hemophilia or bleeding disorders to seek genetic counseling during their family planning process. Although tests are available for the hemophilia gene, the technology to correct the disorder *in utero* does not yet exist. See Chapter 8 ∞.

Assessment

While severe hemophilia usually is diagnosed in childhood, milder cases may not be identified until surgery, invasive dental work, or a traumatic injury causes extensive or prolonged bleeding. Focused assessment related to hemophilia includes the following:
- *Health history:* Previous bleeding episodes with or without trauma; history of easy bruising, hematomas, epistaxis, bleeding gums, hematuria, vomiting blood, or joint pain; aspirin use; family history of hemophilia or bleeding disorders.
- *Physical examination:* Vital signs; bruising or bleeding of skin or mucous membranes; mental status; abdominal assessment; presence of joint deformity, decreased range of motion.
- *Diagnostic tests:* CBC including hemoglobin, hematocrit, and platelet count; clotting factor assays; tests for occult blood (urine, stool, emesis); x-ray and scan results for evidence of bleeding.

Nursing Diagnoses and Interventions

Impaired blood clotting, the need for continuing care and disease management, and the risk for genetic transmission of hemophilia are priority problems for the client with hemophilia.

NURSING CARE PLAN   A Client with Hemophilia

Jenniel Cruise is a 20-year-old student at the community college. He is admitted to the emergency department with a nosebleed that began when he fell during a touch football game. It has continued to bleed for over an hour.

ASSESSMENT

Mr. Cruise states that he has hemophilia and realizes that playing contact sports "is probably a dumb thing to do." He adds that he has not had any recent bleeding episodes. An icebag and manual pressure are applied in the emergency department. The physician orders Factor VIII concentrate to be administered. Physical assessment findings are T 97.2°F (36.2°C), BP 118/64, R 18. Skin pale but warm. Laboratory tests reveal a prolonged APTT and a normal bleeding time and PT. Following treatment, Mr. Cruise's bleeding subsides.

DIAGNOSES

- *Risk for Aspiration* related to uncontrolled nosebleed
- *Noncompliance* with activity recommendations
- *Ineffective Protection* related to lack of clotting factor VIII

EXPECTED OUTCOMES

- Exhibit no further signs of bleeding.
- Maintain vital signs within his usual range.
- Maintain an open airway.
- Identify sports and recreation activities in which he can safely participate.
- Verbalize self-care measures to control bleeding.

PLANNING AND IMPLEMENTATION

- Monitor vital signs and for further signs of bleeding.
- Assess airway and auscultate breath sounds.

- Review emergency measures to help stop bleeding.
- Reiterate the importance of seeking prompt medical attention if bleeding should occur.
- Advise regarding the importance of wearing a Medic-Alert bracelet identifying him as a hemophiliac.
- Discuss alternative noncontact sports and recreational activities.

EVALUATION

On discharge, Mr. Cruise has no further signs of bleeding, shock, or aspiration. He is able to verbalize methods to help stop local bleeding and the importance of seeking medical attention promptly when bleeding continues. Mr. Cruise agrees to stop at a local drug store on the way home to order a Medic-Alert bracelet. In addition, Mr. Cruise verbalizes an understanding of the importance of avoiding contact sports and has identified swimming and golf as alternative leisure activities that he might enjoy.

CRITICAL THINKING IN THE NURSING PROCESS

1. What is the pathophysiologic basis for the bleeding that occurs in hemophilia A and B?
2. What was Mr. Cruise's priority nursing diagnosis? Why?
3. Why is family planning a special consideration with a client who has hemophilia?
4. Outline a plan to teach the family of a client diagnosed with hemophilia how to administer an intravenous infusion.
5. Develop a care plan for Mr. Cruise for the nursing diagnosis *Impaired Social Interaction*. Consider Mr. Cruise's age and developmental level in creating the plan.

See Evaluating Your Response in Appendix C.

Ineffective Protection

The inability to form stable clots and stem bleeding from injured blood vessels creates a significant risk for the client with hemophilia. Nursing care measures focus on preventing injury and protecting the skin from damage.

- Monitor for signs of bleeding, including hematomas, ecchymoses, and purpura, as well as surface oozing or bleeding. Check emesis and stool for occult blood. *Bleeding may occur in cutaneous tissues as well as internal organs. Bleeding in the upper gastrointestinal tract may not be readily apparent in the stool.*
- Notify the physician of any apparent bleeding. *Prompt intervention with administration of clotting factor concentrate decreases the risk of hemorrhage and subsequent hypovolemia.*
- Avoid intramuscular injections, rectal temperatures, and enemas. *These can pose a risk of tissue and vascular trauma, which can precipitate bleeding.*
- Use safety measures in personal care. For example, use an electric razor rather than a razor blade to shave. *Use of an electric razor minimizes the opportunity to develop superficial cuts that may result in bleeding.*
- If bleeding occurs, control blood loss using gentle pressure, ice, or a topical hemostatic agent, such as an absorbable gelatin sponge, microfibrillar collagen hemostat, or topical thrombin. *Direct pressure occludes bleeding vessels. Ice, a*

vasoconstrictor, may facilitate bleeding control, as do topical hemostatic agents.

- Instruct to avoid activities that increase the risk of trauma, including contact sports, physical exertion associated with job performance, and to eliminate safety hazards in the home. *Depending on the severity of the clotting factor deficit, even minor trauma can lead to serious bleeding episodes. Safer activities such as noncontact sports (e.g., swimming, golf) and occupations that do not require physical labor may be substituted.*

Risk for Ineffective Health Maintenance

Hemophilia is a chronic disorder, requiring active management to prevent and control bleeding and complications. Frequent visits to the physician or clinic may be necessary. In addition, the client may need to learn to self-administer clotting factors and measures to prevent complications. The lifelong nature of the disorder may interfere with compliance, especially during early adulthood.

- Assess knowledge of disorder and the related treatments. *Assessment allows identification of knowledge gaps and provides a basis on which to provide additional information. Impaired disease management may be due to lack of knowledge or a conscious decision not to follow the recommendations of the healthcare provider.*

- Provide information about the bleeding disorder and prescribed medications and treatments. *Individualized instruction is more effective than general, possibly irrelevant information.*
- Provide emotional support, expressing confidence in the client's self-care abilities. *Emotional support helps the client incorporate the care regimen into his or her lifestyle.*
- Provide supervised learning and practice opportunities for administering clotting factors and topical hemostatic agents. *Successful practice sessions instill confidence in the ability to manage care and provide an opportunity for questions and exploring alternatives.*

Linking NANDA, NIC, and NOC

Linkages between NANDA nursing diagnoses, nursing interventions, and nursing outcomes for the client with hemophilia are illustrated in Chart 34–4.

Community-Based Care

Discuss the following topics when preparing the client with a bleeding disorder and the family for home care:

- Recognizing the manifestations of internal bleeding: pallor, weakness, restlessness, headache, disorientation, pain, swelling. These manifestations require emergency medical care and should be reported immediately.
- Applying cold packs and immobilizing the joint for 24 to 48 hours if hemarthrosis occurs.
- Using analgesics for pain; avoiding prescription and over-the-counter drugs containing aspirin.

NANDA, NIC, AND NOC LINKAGES
CHART 34–4 The Client with Hemophilia

NANDA

Ineffective Health Maintenance

NIC

Health Education

Self-Responsibility Facilitation

Teaching: Procedure/Treatment

NOC

Health-Seeking Behavior

Knowledge: Health Behaviors

Knowledge: Treatment Regimen

Data from *NANDA's Nursing Diagnoses: Definitions & Classification 2005–2006* by NANDA International (2005), Philadelphia; *Nursing Interventions Classification (NIC)* (4th ed.) by J. M. Dochterman & G. M. Bulechek (2004), St. Louis, MO: Mosby; and *Nursing Outcomes Classification (NOC)* (3rd ed.) by S. Moorhead, M. Johnson, and M. Mass (2004), St. Louis, MO: Mosby.

- Ensuring a safe home environment (e.g., padding sharp edges of furniture, using transition lighting or a night light; avoiding scatter rugs, and wearing protective gloves when working in the house or yard).
- Using safe grooming practices such as electric razors.
- Wearing a Medic-Alert bracelet in case of accident.
- Practicing good dental hygiene to decrease potential tooth decay and extractions. If dental procedures are necessary, discuss the need for prophylactic factor administration with the dentist and physician.
- Following safer sex practices.
- Preparing and administering intravenous medications.

    Refer the client and family to a local hemophilia or bleeding disorders support group. Provide contact information for national organizations and information clearinghouses, such as the National Hemophilia Foundation.

THE CLIENT WITH DISSEMINATED INTRAVASCULAR COAGULATION

Disseminated intravascular coagulation (DIC) is a disruption of hemostasis characterized by widespread intravascular clotting and bleeding. It may be acute and life threatening or relatively mild. DIC is a clinical syndrome that develops as a complication of a wide variety of other disorders (Box 34–8). Sepsis is the most common cause of DIC. Gram-negative and gram-positive bacteria as well as viruses, fungi, and protozoal infections may lead to DIC (McCance & Huether, 2006).

Pathophysiology

DIC is triggered by endothelial damage, release of tissue factors into the circulation, or inappropriate activation of the clotting cascade by an endotoxin. Both the intrinsic and the extrinsic clotting cascade may be activated, although the extrinsic cascade usually is the one activated. Extensive thrombin

---

BOX 34–8 Conditions That May Precipitate Disseminated Intravascular Coagulation

Tissue Damage
- Trauma: burns, gunshot wounds, frostbite, head injury
- Obstetric complications: septic abortion, abruptio placentae, amniotic fluid embolus, retained dead fetus
- Neoplasms: acute leukemia, adenocarcinomas
- Hemolysis
- Fat embolism

Vessel Damage
- Aortic aneurysm
- Acute glomerulonephritis
- Hemolytic uremic syndrome

Infections
- Bacterial infection or sepsis
- Viral or mycotic infections
- Parasitic or rickettsial infection

entering the systemic circulation overwhelms natural anticoagulants, leading to unrestricted clot formation (McCance & Huether, 2006). Clotting may be localized to an individual organ, or widespread with deposition of small thrombi and emboli throughout the microvasculature (Kasper et al., 2005). The widespread clotting consumes clotting factors (prothrombin, platelets, factor V, and factor VIII in particular) and activates fibrinolytic processes with anticoagulant production. As a result, hemorrhage occurs (Figure 34–14 ■).

The sequence of DIC follows:

1. Endothelial damage, tissue factors, or toxins stimulate the clotting cascade.
2. Excess thrombin within the circulation overwhelms naturally occurring anticoagulants.
3. Widespread clotting occurs within the microvasculature.
4. Thrombi and emboli impair tissue perfusion, leading to ischemia, infarction, and necrosis.
5. Clotting factors and platelets are consumed faster than they can be replaced.
6. Clotting activates fibrinolytic processes, which begin to break down clots.
7. Fibrin degradation products (FDPs, potent anticoagulants) are released, contributing to bleeding.
8. Clotting factors are depleted, the ability to form clots is lost, and hemorrhage occurs.

Manifestations

The manifestations of DIC result from both clotting and bleeding, although bleeding is more obvious, especially in acute DIC. Bleeding ranges from oozing blood following an injection to frank hemorrhage from every body orifice (see box below). Chronic DIC may be asymptomatic, or may present with peripheral cyanosis, thrombosis, and pregangrenous changes in the fingers and toes, nose, and genitalia (Kasper et al., 2005).

MANIFESTATIONS of DIC

- Frank hemorrhage from incisions
- Oozing of blood from punctures, intravenous catheter sites
- Purpura, petechiae, bruising
- Cyanosis of extremities
- Gastrointestinal bleeding or hemorrhage
- Dyspnea, tachypnea, bloody sputum
- Tachycardia, hypotension
- Hematuria, oliguria, acute renal failure
- Manifestations of increased intracranial pressure: decreased level of consciousness, papillary, motor, and sensory changes
- Mental status changes

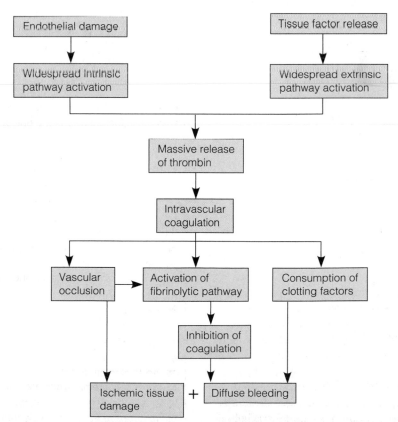

Figure 34–14 ■ Disseminated intravascular coagulation (DIC). Endothelial cell injury or release of tissue factors activate the intrinsic or extrinsic clotting pathway (or both). As a result, numerous microthrombi form throughout the vasculature, causing ischemic tissue damage. Simultaneously, rapid consumption of clotting factors and activation of fibrinolytic mechanisms trigger widespread bleeding.

INTERDISCIPLINARY CARE

Treatment of DIC is directed toward treating the underlying disorder and preventing further bleeding or massive thrombosis. Treatment stabilizes the client, reduces complications, and allows recovery to occur; it does not cure DIC (Kasper et al., 2005).

Diagnosis

Diagnostic tests are used to confirm the diagnosis of DIC and evaluate the risk for hemorrhage.

- *CBC* and *platelet count* are used to evaluate the hemoglobin, hematocrit, and number of circulating platelets. *Schistocytes*, fragmented RBCs, may be noted due to cell trapping and damage within fibrin thrombi. The platelet count is decreased.
- *Coagulation studies* show prolonged *prothrombin time (PT), partial thromboplastin time (PTT)*, and *thrombin time*, and a low *fibrinogen level* due to depletion of clotting factors. The fibrinogen level helps predict bleeding in DIC: As it falls, the risk of bleeding increases (Kasper et al., 2005).
- *Fibrin degradation products (FDPs)* or *fibrin split products (FSPs)* are increased due to the fibrinolysis that occurs with DIC.

Treatments

When bleeding is the major manifestation of DIC, fresh frozen plasma and platelet concentrates are given to restore clotting factors and platelets. Heparin, although controversial, may be administered. Heparin interferes with the clotting cascade and may prevent further clotting factor consumption due to uncontrolled thrombosis. It is used when bleeding is not controlled by plasma and platelets, as well as when the client has manifestations of thrombotic problems such as acrocyanosis and possible gangrene. Long-term heparin therapy (administered by injection or continuous infusion using a portable pump) may be necessary for clients with chronic DIC.

NURSING CARE

Assessment

Nurses can be instrumental in identifying early manifestations of DIC, facilitating timely intervention. Focused nursing assessment for DIC includes:

- *Health history:* Recent abortion (spontaneous or therapeutic) or current pregnancy; presence of a known malignant tumor; history of abnormal bleeding episodes or a hematologic disorder.
- *Physical examination:* Bleeding from puncture wounds (e.g., injections), IV sites, incisions; hematuria, obvious or occult blood in emesis or stool, epistaxis, other abnormal bleeding; vital signs; heart and breath sounds; abdominal assessment including girth, contour, bowel sounds, tenderness or guarding to palpation; color, temperature, skin condition of hands, feet, and digits; petechiae or purpura of skin, mucous membranes.

- *Diagnostic tests:* CBC with hemoglobin, hematocrit; platelet count; coagulation studies; evaluations of organ system function (e.g., liver and renal function tests); CT scans of the head and abdomen.

Nursing Diagnoses and Interventions

Clients with acute DIC often are critically ill, with multiple nursing care needs. Priority nursing diagnoses discussed in this section focus on impaired tissue perfusion and gas exchange, pain, and fear. Septic shock may precipitate DIC; hemorrhagic shock may occur as a complication of DIC. See Chapter 11 ∞ for nursing diagnoses and interventions related to these problems.

Ineffective Tissue Perfusion

Thrombi and emboli forming throughout the microcirculation affect the perfusion of multiple organs and tissues. Additionally, bleeding due to clotting factor consumption affects cardiac output and blood flow to these tissues.

- Assess extremity pulses, warmth, and capillary refill. Monitor level of consciousness (LOC) and mental status. *Monitoring central and peripheral tissue perfusion facilitates early treatment of impaired perfusion.*

PRACTICE ALERT

Promptly report complaints of chest pain, changes in mental status, LOC, tissue perfusion, respirations, gastrointestinal function, and urinary output. Chest pain or respiratory changes (tachypnea, dyspnea, orthopnea) may be due to angina, pulmonary embolism, or bleeding into lung tissue. Changes in mentation or LOC can indicate cerebral ischemia. A painful, pale, and cold extremity with no or diminished pulses indicates arterial occlusion. Prompt intervention is critical to save the extremity. Acute abdominal pain, decreased bowel sounds, and GI bleeding may indicate mesenteric occlusion, a surgical emergency. Decreased urine output may signify renal artery thrombosis; renal failure may develop.

- Carefully reposition at least every 2 hours. *Position changes facilitate circulation and tissue perfusion and also provide an opportunity to assess for purpura, pallor, and bleeding.*
- Discourage crossing the legs, and do not elevate the knees on the bed or with a pillow. *These positions may impair arterial and venous flow to the lower legs and feet, increasing vascular stasis and the risk for thrombosis.*
- Minimize use of tape on the skin, using binders, nonadhesive dressings, and other devices as needed. *Preventing skin trauma reduces the risk for bleeding and potential infection.*

Impaired Gas Exchange

Microclots in the pulmonary vasculature are likely to interfere with gas exchange in the client with DIC.

- Monitor oxygen saturation continuously. Administer oxygen as ordered. *Oxygen saturation levels are a noninvasive means of assessing gas exchange. Supplemental oxygen promotes gas exchange and reduces cardiac work, relieving dyspnea.*

- Place in Fowler's or high-Fowler's position as tolerated. *Elevating the head of the bed improves diaphragmatic excursion and alveolar ventilation.*
- Maintain bed rest. *Bed rest reduces oxygen demands and cardiac work.*
- Encourage deep breathing and effective coughing. *Increased respiratory depth and clearance of secretions from airways improves alveolar ventilation and oxygenation.*
- Cautious nasotracheal suctioning may be instituted if cough is ineffective or an endotracheal tube is in place. *Removal of secretions facilitates ventilation and oxygenation. However, care must be used to minimize suction-induced hypoxia and airway trauma.*
- Administer analgesics and antianxiety drugs as needed to control pain and anxiety. Provide reassurance and comfort measures. *Pain and anxiety increase the respiratory rate and decrease the depth of respirations, reducing effective ventilation and gas exchange.*

Pain

Both the underlying cause of DIC and tissue ischemia from microvascular clots can cause pain. Identifying the etiology of pain is important to identify potential complications or harmful effects of DIC and to institute effective treatment.

- Use a standard pain scale to evaluate and monitor pain and analgesic effectiveness. *Monitoring pain and response to medication facilitates development of an appropriate and effective treatment plan.*

- Handle extremities gently. *Gentle handling reduces the risk of further injury to and pain in ischemic tissues.*
- Apply cool compresses to painful joints. *Application of cold decreases pain through the gate-control mechanism, inhibiting the dorsal horn of the spinal cord and reducing the sensation of pain.*

Fear

The underlying serious illness and a complication such as DIC result in an uncertain prognosis, often accompanied by fear.

- Encourage the client and family to verbalize concerns. *This helps the client and family identify their concerns and frame questions.*
- Answer questions truthfully. *Providing honest answers is vital to developing a therapeutic nurse–client relationship. Accurate responses allow the client and family to set priorities as they plan for an uncertain future.*
- Help the client and family identify coping strategies to manage this significant situational stressor. *Implementing past effective coping methods may provide the skills to manage the current crisis.*
- Provide emotional support. *The presence of a caring nurse helps reduce the fear and anxiety associated with a crisis.*
- Maintain a calm environment. *A calm environment provides reassurance that the situation is in control, reduces anxiety, and promotes rest.*
- Respond promptly when the client calls for help. *Prompt response to expressed needs helps develop a trusting relationship and a sense of security that assistance is readily available.*
- Teach relaxation techniques. *Relaxation techniques can reduce muscle tension and other signs of anxiety. Gaining control over physical responses can help the client gain a sense of control over the situation.*

Community-Based Care

Although the immediate crisis of acute DIC is resolved prior to discharge, the client may have some continuing effects of the disorder, such as impaired tissue integrity of distal extremities. Teach the client and family about specific care needs, such as foot care (see Box 35–4 ∞) or dressing changes. Provide instruction about any continuing medications and follow-up care.

Clients with chronic DIC may require continuing heparin therapy, using either intermittent subcutaneous injections or a portable infusion pump. Teach the client and family members how to administer the injection or manage the infusion pump. Provide a referral to home health care or a home intravenous management service for assistance. Discuss the manifestations of excessive bleeding or recurrent clotting that need to be reported to the physician.

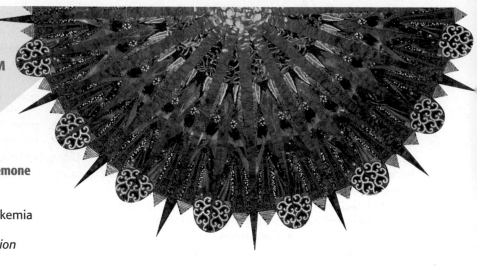

EXPLORE MediaLink

Prentice Hall Nursing MediaLink DVD-ROM
Audio Glossary
NCLEX-RN® Review

Animation/Video
Sickle Cell Anemia

COMPANION WEBSITE www.prenhall.com/lemone
Audio Glossary
NCLEX-RN® Review
Care Plan Activity: Acute Myelocytic Leukemia
Case Studies
Disseminated Intravascular Coagulation
Immune Thrombocytopenic Purpura
MediaLink Applications
Blood Alternatives
Sickle Cell Anemia
Stem Cell Transplant
Synthetic Blood Products
Links to Resources

CHAPTER HIGHLIGHTS

- Anemia is the most common disorder of the red blood cells; nutritional deficiencies are the most common causes of anemia. Its manifestations relate to the function of RBCs and hemoglobin, transporting oxygen to the cells: fatigue, increased respiratory and heart rates, shortness of breath with activity, and pallor.

- Genetically transmitted disorders such as sickle cell disease and thalassemia can cause significant anemia and associated problems in affected populations. These clients require teaching and episodic acute care for crises such as vaso-occlusive crisis in sickle cell disease.

- Nursing care related to anemia is primarily educational to prepare the client for effective self-care, including diet, prescribed medications, and measures to prevent sickling episodes (for clients with sickle cell disease).

- Leukemia and lymphomas are the primary disorders of white blood cells and lymphoid tissues.

- Manifestations of the leukemias reflect the altered ability of abnormal WBCs to perform effective immune surveillance and crowding of the bone marrow and other organs by rapidly proliferating cells. Frequent sore throats, increased risk for infection, and manifestations of anemia and thrombocytopenia are seen, as well as an enlarged spleen and abdominal pain.

- Four major subgroups of leukemia are identified, acute and chronic myeloid leukemias, and acute and chronic lymphocytic (or lymphoblastic) leukemias. The primary population affected differs for each of these leukemias, as does their course.

- Genetic alterations and certain viruses are linked to the development of leukemia, as are exposure to chemotherapy drugs, environmental toxins, and ionizing radiation.

- Lymphocytic leukemias and lymphomas are closely related disorders.

- Nursing care for clients with leukemia and lymphoma focuses on reducing the risk for infection and bleeding, managing the effects of chemotherapy and radiation therapy, and, in some cases, caring for clients before and after bone marrow or stem cell transplant.

- The major risks associated with bone marrow and stem cell transplant are infection prior to and immediately following the transplant and graft-versus-host disease, a potentially fatal condition. A pruritic rash and desquamation of the palms and soles; abdominal pain, nausea, and diarrhea; and jaundice and elevated liver enzymes are common early manifestations of GVHD.

- The treatment of and nursing care for clients with lymphomas (including Hodgkin's lymphoma and non-Hodgkin's lymphomas) is similar to that provided for clients with leukemia.

- Multiple myeloma is a malignancy of plasma cells, B lymphocytes that produce antibodies. Circulating M proteins and Bence Jones proteins in the urine are seen in multiple myeloma. The usual presenting manifestation is bone pain. Pathologic fractures and hypercalcemia are common complications of multiple myeloma as bone is destroyed.

- Bleeding and clotting disorders can result from either inadequate platelets (thrombocytopenia) or disruption of the clotting mechanisms (hemophilia, DIC). Petechiae and purpura are common manifestations of bleeding/clotting disorders.

- Hemophilias are genetically transmitted disorders. Hemophilia A and B are transmitted on the X chromosome (sex-linked) from mother to son. Von Willebrand's disease, the most common bleeding disorder, is transmitted as an autosomal dominant disorder and affects men and women equally.

- Hemophilias are treated by replacement of the missing clotting factor and measures to prevent injury and bleeding.

- Disseminated intravascular coagulation is a disorder of widespread microvascular clotting. It commonly is precipitated by sepsis, but also may occur with conditions such as major trauma, malignancy, or as an obstetric emergency.

- In DIC, platelets and clotting factors are consumed by the abnormal clotting processes, leading the manifestations of bleeding, including frank hemorrhage, hematuria, oozing blood from parenteral and intravenous injection sites, and GI bleeding. Blood flow to organs and tissues is compromised by clot formation, leading to manifestations such as cyanosis of extremities, abdominal pain, renal failure, and changes in mental status and level of consciousness. Nursing care is

supportive, focusing on administering prescribed treatments and monitoring and supporting cardiovascular, respiratory, and renal function.

TEST YOURSELF NCLEX-RN® REVIEW

1 In assessing a female client with moderate anemia, the nurse would expect to find which of the following?
1. hematocrit 45%
2. pulse rate 140
3. complaints of shortness of breath with exercise
4. WBC 14,000/µL

2 The nurse following a client after gastric resection observes carefully for evidence of nutritional deficiency anemia related to malabsorption, including:
1. numbness and tingling of extremities.
2. steatorrhea.
3. dark yellow or bronze skin color.
4. bone pain.

3 Which of the following nursing diagnoses would be of highest priority for the client hospitalized for a bone marrow transplant to treat relapse of acute myelocytic leukemia?
1. *Disturbed Body Image*
2. *Ineffective Protection*
3. *Anxiety*
4. *Imbalanced Nutrition, Less than Body Requirements*

4 The nurse caring for a client with acute myeloid leukemia plans which of the following nursing interventions during hospitalization? (Select all that apply.)
1. Place in a private room.
2. Implement airborne infection control precautions.
3. Assist with oral hygiene after meals.
4. Monitor rectal temperature q4h.
5. Request soft, bland diet.

5 A client with non-Hodgkin's lymphoma tells the nurse, "I might as well give up on dating. No woman will want me now." What is the most appropriate response?
1. "It sounds like you are concerned about the effects of this disease and the proposed treatment plan."
2. "Don't worry. Malignant lymphomas are very treatable when caught in an early stage of the disease."
3. "Well, you may never be able to have children all right, but there are other ways to have a satisfying relationship with a woman."
4. "Lots of women find bald men attractive; besides, your hair may grow back soft and curly."

6 The nurse caring for a client with lymphoma who is being started on the CHOP chemotherapy regimen understands that chemotherapy drugs are used in combination to:

1. target malignant cells in different organs.
2. prevent the development of adverse effects.
3. target different phases of the cell cycle.
4. support growth and development of normal cells.

7 A client with multiple myeloma calls the home health nurse complaining of severe back pain of new onset. The appropriate response by the nurse is to:
1. reassure the client that bone pain is expected with this disease.
2. inquire about the client's use of NSAIDs and analgesics to manage pain.
3. suggest use of a back brace to reduce pain.
4. notify the physician of the onset of new pain.

8 The nurse observes reddish-purple spots and areas of purple bruising on a newly admitted client. Which laboratory results support this assessment finding?
1. hematocrit 28%
2. platelets 6000/mm^3
3. INR 4.0
4. WBC 4500/mm^3

9 A client whose husband has hemophilia asks if her newborn baby girl could have the disease. The nurse's response is based on the knowledge that:
1. the most common forms of hemophilia are transmitted as sex-linked recessive disorders; her daughter is at risk for carrying the defective gene.
2. because hemophilia is a sex-linked recessive disorder carried on the Y chromosome, her daughter has no risk of having or carrying the disease.
3. hemophilia is an autosomal dominant disorder; therefore, her daughter has a 50% chance of having the disorder.
4. although hemophilia is genetically transmitted, its pattern of inheritance is unknown, and her daughter will need to be tested for the defective gene.

10 The nurse administering platelets to a client with disseminated intravascular coagulation (DIC) understands that the intended effect of this treatment is to:
1. replace specific clotting factors.
2. promote intravascular clotting.
3. restore tissue oxygenation.
4. replace depleted platelets.

See Test Yourself answers in Appendix C.

BIBLIOGRAPHY

American Cancer Society. (2002). *Gleevec's new successes show growing promise of targeted therapies.* Retrieved from http://www.cancer.org/eprise/main/docroot/NWS/content/NWS_1_1x_Gleevec
_____. (2005). *Cancer facts and figures 2005.* Atlanta: Author.
Barcelona, R. (2001). Type II heparin-induced thrombocytopenia: New treatment options. Retrieved from http://www.cleavelandclinicmeded.com/medical_info/pharmacy/septoct2001

Bennett, L. (2005). Understanding sickle cell disorders. *Nursing Standard, 19*(32), 52–63.
Beser, N. G., & Öz, F. (2005). Quality of life in lymphoma patients. *Clinical Excellence for Nurse Practitioners, 9*(3), 153–161.
Blackhouse, R. (2004). Understanding disseminated intravascular coagulation. *Nursing Times, 100*(36), 38–42.
Breed, C. D. (2003). Diagnosis, treatment, and nursing care of patients with chronic leukemia. *Seminars in Oncology Nursing, 19*(2), 109–117.

Brewster, B. (2003). Achieving optimal patient outcomes with intravenous iron. *Nursing Times, 99*(29), 30–32.
Burruss, N., & Holz, S. (2005). Managing the risks of thrombocytopenia. *Nursing, 35*(6), 32hn1–32hn2, 32hn4–32hn5.
Cantril, C. A., & Haylock, P. J. (2004). Tumor lysis syndrome. *American Journal of Nursing, 104*(4), 49–52.
Cashion, A. (2002) Genetics in transplantation. *Medsurg Nursing, 11*(2), 91–94.
Coleman, E. A., Coon, S., Hall-Barrow, J., Richards, K., Gaylor, D., & Stewart, B. (2004). Feasibility of exercise during

treatment for multiple myeloma. *Cancer Nursing, 26*(5), 410–419.

Coleman, E. A., Hutchins, L., & Goodwin, J. (2004). An overview of cancer in the older adult. *Medsurg Nursing, 13*(2), 75–80, 109.

Colfer, M. (2003). Achieving optimal patient outcomes with intravenous iron. *Nephrology Nursing, 30*(4), 449–453.

Coon, S. K., & Coleman, E. A. (2004). Exercise decisions within the context of multiple myeloma, transplant, and fatigue. *Cancer Nursing, 27*(2), 108–118.

Cope, D. (2004). Tumor lysis syndrome. *Clinical Journal of Oncology Nursing, 8*(4), 415–416.

Copstead, L. C., & Banasik, J. L. (2005). *Pathophysiology* (3rd ed.). St. Louis, MO: Elsevier/Saunders.

_____. (2004a). Chronic myelogenous leukemia. *Clinical Journal of Oncology Nursing, 9*(5), 535–538, 561–563.

D'Antonio, J. (2004b). You can lessen leukemia's toll. *Nursing, 34*(7), 32hn1–32hn2, 32hn4.

Demakos, E. P., & Linebaugh, J. A. (2005). Advances in myelodysplastic syndrome: Nursing implications of azacitidine. *Clinical Journal of Oncology Nursing, 9*(4), 417–423.

Devenney, B., & Erickson, C. (2004). Multiple myeloma: An overview. *Clinical Journal of Oncology Nursing, 8*(4), 401–405.

Devine, H., & DeMeyer, E. (2003) Hematopoietic cell transplantation in the treatment of leukemia. *Seminars in Oncology Nursing, 19*(2), 118–132.

Dochterman, J., & Bulechek, G. (2004). *Nursing interventions classification (NIC)* (4th ed.). St. Louis, MO: Mosby.

Dolan, S., Crombez, P., & Mumoz, M. (2005). Neutropenia management with granulocyte colony-stimulating factors: From guidelines to nursing practice protocols. *European Journal of Oncology Nursing, 9*(Suppl 1), S14–S23.

Dowsett, C. (2005). Managing leg ulceration in patients with sickle cell disorder. *Nursing Times, 101*(16), 48–49.

Dressler, D. K. (2004). DIC: Coping with a coagulation crisis. *Nursing, 34*(5), 58–62.

Druker, B. J., Sawyers, C. L., Capdeville, R., Ford, J. M., Baccarani, M., & Goldman, J. M. (2001). Chronic myelogenous leukemia. *Hematology (American Society of Hematology Education Program)*, pp. 87–113. Abstract from National Cancer Institute. Retrieved from http://www.nci.nih.gov/cancerinformation/doc_cit.aspx?args= 22; 11722980

Dyson, S. (2005). Sickle cell and thalassaemia screening. *Practice Nurse, 29*(10), 17–18, 20.

Eggenberger, S. K., Krumwiede, N., Meiers, S. J., Bliesmer, M., & Earle, P. (2004). Family caring strategies in neutropenia. *Clinical Journal of Oncology Nursing, 8*(6), 617–621, 638–640.

El-Banna, M. M., Berger, A. M., Farr, L., Foxall, M. J., Friesth, B., & Schreiner. E. (2004). Fatigue and depression in patients with lymphoma undergoing autologous peripheral blood stem cell transplantation. *Oncology Nursing Forum, 31*(5), 937–944.

Fischbach, F. (2002). *Nurses' quick reference to common laboratory and diagnostic tests* (3rd ed.). Philadelphia: Lippincott.

Fontaine, K. L. (2005). *Healing practices: Alternative therapies for nursing* (2nd ed.). Upper Saddle River, NJ: Prentice Hall Health.

Francis. J. L., & Drexler, A. J. (2005). Striking back at heparin-induced thrombocytopenia. *Nursing, 35*(9), 48–51.

Gever, M. P. (2005). Lepirudin: Test your drug IQ. *Nursing, 35*(11), 32cc4.

Holcomb, S. S. (2005). Anemia. *Nursing, 35*(3), 53.

Iovino, C. S., & Camacho, L. H. (2003). Acute myeloid leukemia: A classification and treatment update. *Clinical Journal of Oncology Nursing, 7*(5), 535–540.

Kasper, D. L., Braunwald, E., Fauci, A. S., Hauser, S. L., Longo, D. L., & Jameson, J. L. (Eds.). (2005). *Harrison's principles of internal medicine* (16th ed.). New York: McGraw-Hill.

Krimmel, T. (2003). Disseminated intravascular coagulation. *Clinical Journal of Oncology Nursing, 7*(4), 479–481.

Lea, D. H., & Williams, J. K. (2002). Genetic testing and screening. *American Journal of Nursing, 102*(7), 36–43.

Mangan, P. (2005). Recognizing multiple myeloma. *Nurse Practitioner, 30*(3), 14–18, 23–24, 26–29.

Maningo, J. (2002). Peripheral blood stem cell transplant: Easier than getting blood from a bone. *Nursing, 32*(12), 52–55,

McCance, K. L., & Huether, S. E. (2006). *Pathophysiology: The biologic basis for disease in adults & children* (4th ed.). St. Louis, MO: Mosby.

McCloskey, J. C., & Bulechek, G. M. (Eds.). (2000). *Nursing interventions classification (NIC)* (3rd ed.). St. Louis, MO: Mosby.

McGrath, P. (2004). Positive outcomes for survivors of haematological malignancies from a spiritual perspective. *International Journal of Nursing Practice, 10*(6), 280–291.

Meduff, E. (2000). Oncology today: Leukemia. *RN, 63*(9), 42–49.

Moorhead, S., Johnson, M., & Maas, M. (2004). *Nursing Outcomes Classification (NOC)* (3rd ed.). St. Louis, MO: Mosby.

NANDA International. (2005). *Nursing Diagnoses: Definitions and Classification 2005–2006.* Philadelphia: Author.

National Comprehensive Cancer Network. (2006). *Clinical practice guidelines in oncology. Myelodysplastic syndromes* (Version 3). Retrieved from http://www.nccn.org/professionals/physician_gls/PDF/mds.pdf

National Heart, Lung, and Blood Institute, National Institutes of Health. (2002). *Morbidity & mortality: 2002 chart book of cardiovascular, lung, and blood diseases.* Bethesda, MD: Author.

Navuluri, R. (2001). Understanding hemostasis. *American Journal of Nursing, 101*(9), Hospital extra: 24B, 24C.

Persson, L., & Hallberg, I. R. (2004). Lived experience of survivors of leukemia or malignant lymphoma. *Cancer Nursing, 27*(4), 303–313.

_____ , Hallberg, I. R., & Ohlsson, O. (1997). Survivors of acute leukemia and highly malignant lymphoma— retrospective views of daily life problems during treatment and when in remission. *Journal of Advanced Nursing, 25*(1), 68–78.

Porth, C. M. (2005). *Pathophysiology: Concepts of altered health states* (7th ed.). Philadelphia: Lippincott.

Redaelli, A., Laskin, B. L., Stephens, J. M., Botteman, M. F., & Pashos, C. L. (2004). The clinical and epidemiological burden of chronic lymphocytic leukaemia. *European Journal of Cancer Care, 13*(3), 279–289.

_____, (2005). A systematic literature review of the clinical and epidemiological burden of acute lymphoblastic leukaemia (ALL). *European Journal of Cancer Care, 14*(1), 53–62.

Rempher, K. J., & Little, J. (2004). Assessment of red blood cell and coagulation laboratory data. *AACN Clinical Issues, 15*(4), 622–637.

Rice, L., Nguyen, P. H., & Vann, A. R. (2002). Preventing complications in heparin-induced thrombocytopenia. *Postgraduate Medicine online.* Retrieved from http://www.postgradmed.com/issues/2002/09_02/rice.htm

Rogers, B. (2005). Looking at lymphoma & leukemia. *Nursing, 35*(7), 56–64.

Sadler, G. R., Wasserman, L., Fullerton, J. T., & Romero, M. (2004). Supporting patients through genetic screening for cancer risk. *Medsurg Nursing, 13*(4), 233–246.

Shelton, B. K. (2003). Evidence-based care for the neutropenic patient with leukemia. *Seminars in Oncology Nursing, 19*(2), 133–141.

Simmons, P. (2003). A primer for nurses who administer blood products. *Medsurg Nursing, 12*(3), 184–190.

Spahis, J. (2002). Human genetics: Constructing a family pedigree. *American Journal of Nursing, 102*(7), 44–49.

Spencer, J. W., & Jacobs, J. J. (2003). *Complementary and alternative medicine: An evidence-based approach* (2nd ed.). St. Louis, MO: Mosby.

Tariman, J. D., & Estrella, S. M. (2005). The changing treatment paradigm in patients with newly diagnosed multiple myeloma: Implications for nursing. *Oncology Nursing Forum, 32*(6), Online Exclusive: E127–38.

Tierney, L. M., Jr., McPhee, S. J., & Papadakis, M. A. (Eds.). (2005). *Current medical diagnosis & treatment* (44th ed.). New York: McGraw-Hill.

Treating the older patient with leukemia, lymphoma, and myeloma. (2004). *ONS News, 19*(9 Suppl), 77–78.

U.S. Food and Drug Administration, Center for Drug Evaluation and Research. (2001). *Drug information. Gleevec (imatinib mesylate) questions and answers.* Retrieved from http://www.fda.gov/cder/drug/infopage/gleevec/qa.htm

Viele, C. S. (2003). Diagnosis, treatment and nursing care of acute leukemia. *Seminars in Oncology Nursing, 19*(2), 109–117.

Waldman, A. R. (2003). Understanding non-Hodgkin's lymphomas. *Clinical Journal of Oncology Nursing, 7*(1), 93–96.

Wilkinson, J. M. (2005). *Nursing diagnosis handbook* (8th ed.). Upper Saddle River, NJ: Prentice Hall.

Wilson, C., & Sylvanus, T. (2005). Graft failure following allogeneic blood and marrow transplant: Evidence based nursing care study review. *Clinical Journal of Oncology Nursing, 9*(2), 151–159.

Wuicik, D. (2003). Molecular biology of leukemia. *Seminars in Oncology Nursing, 19*(2), 83–89.

CHAPTER 35 Nursing Care of Clients with Peripheral Vascular Disorders

LEARNING OUTCOMES

- Describe the etiology, pathophysiology, and manifestations of common peripheral vascular and lymphatic disorders.

- Compare and contrast the manifestations and effects of disorders affecting large and small vessels, arteries and veins.

- Explain risk factors for and measures to prevent peripheral vascular disorders and their complications.

- Explain the nursing implications for medications and other interdisciplinary treatments used for clients with peripheral vascular disorders.

- Describe preoperative and postoperative nursing care of clients having vascular surgery.

CLINICAL COMPETENCIES

- Assess clients with peripheral vascular disorders, using data to select and prioritize appropriate nursing diagnoses and identify desired outcomes of care

- Identify the effects of peripheral vascular disorders on the functional health status of assigned clients.

- Use research and an evidence-based plan to provide individualized care for clients with peripheral vascular disorders.

- Collaborate with the interdisciplinary care team in planning and providing care for clients with peripheral vascular disorders.

- Safely and knowledgeably administer medications and prescribed treatments for clients with peripheral vascular disorders.

- Provide client and family teaching to promote, maintain, and restore health in clients with common peripheral vascular disorders.

MEDIALINK

Resources for this chapter can be found on the Prentice Hall Nursing MediaLink DVD-ROM accompanying this textbook, and on the Companion Website at http://www.prenhall.com/lemone

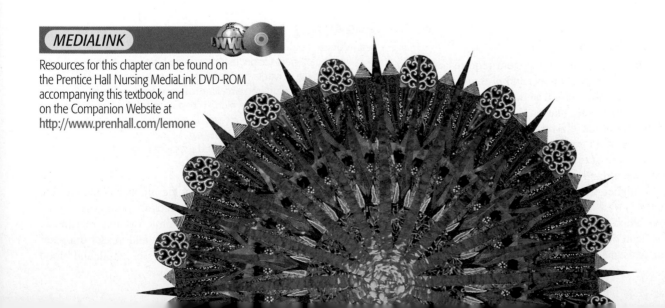

KEY TERMS

aneurysm, *1170*
atherosclerosis, *1176*
blood pressure, *1154*
chronic venous insufficiency, *1194*
deep venous thrombosis (DVT), *1186*
diastolic blood pressure, *1154*
dissection, *1172*
embolism, *1184*
hypertension, *1154*
intermittent claudication, *1172*

lymphedema, *1199*
mean arterial pressure (MAP), *1154*
peripheral vascular disease
   (PVD), *1176*
primary hypertension, *1155*
pulse pressure, *1154*
Raynaud's disease/phenomenon,
   1182
secondary hypertension, *1167*
systolic blood pressure, *1154*

thromboangiitis obliterans,
   1180
thromboembolus, *1184*
thrombus, *1184*
varicose veins, *1195*
vasoconstriction, *1176*
vasodilation, *1176*
venous thrombosis, *1186*

The major processes that interfere with peripheral blood flow and that of lymphatic fluid include constriction, obstruction, inflammation, and vasospasm. These conditions lead to disorders of blood pressure regulation, peripheral artery function, aortic structure, venous circulation, and lymphatic circulation.

A holistic approach is important when caring for clients with disorders of the peripheral vascular and lymphatic systems. The focus of care is on teaching long-term care measures, pain relief, improving peripheral blood and lymphatic circulation, preventing tissue damage, and promoting healing. The prescribed treatment may have emotional, social, and economic effects on the client and family.

DISORDERS OF BLOOD PRESSURE REGULATION

Blood flows through the circulatory system from areas of higher pressure to areas of lower pressure. The amount of pressure in any portion of the vascular system is affected by a number of factors, including blood volume, vascular resistance, and cardiac output. The **blood pressure** is the tension or pressure exerted by blood against arterial walls. A certain amount of pressure within the system is necessary to maintain open vessels, capillary perfusion, and oxygenation of all body tissues. Excess pressure, however, has harmful effects, increasing the workload of the heart, altering the structure of the vessels, and affecting sensitive body tissues such as the kidneys, eyes, and central nervous system (CNS).

This section focuses on **hypertension**, or excess pressure in the arterial portion of systemic circulation. Excessively low blood pressure, *hypotension,* is discussed in the shock section of Chapter 11 ∞. Altered pulmonary vascular pressures are discussed in Chapter 39 ∞.

Physiology Review

Blood flow through the circulatory system requires *sufficient blood volume* to fill the blood vessels and *pressure differences* within the system that allow blood to move forward. The arterial, or supply, side of the circulation has relatively high pressures created by the thick elastic walls of the arteries and arterioles. The venous, or return, side of the system, on the other hand, is a low-pressure system of thin-walled, distensible veins. Blood flows through the capillaries linking these two systems from the higher pressure arterial side to the lower pressure venous side.

The arterial blood pressure is created by the ejection of blood from the heart during systole (*cardiac output* or *CO*) and the tension, or resistance to blood flow, created by the elastic arterial walls (*systemic vascular resistance* or *SVR*). The blood pressure rises as the heart contracts during systole, ejecting its blood. This pressure wave, or the **systolic blood pressure**, is felt as the peripheral pulse and heard as the Korotkoff's sounds during blood pressure measurement. In healthy adults the average systolic pressure is less than 120 mmHg. During diastole, or cardiac relaxation and filling, elastic arterial walls maintain a minimum pressure, the **diastolic blood pressure**, to maintain blood flow through the capillary beds. The average diastolic pressure in a healthy adult is less than 80 mmHg. The difference between the systolic and diastolic pressure, normally about 40 mmHg, is known as the **pulse pressure**. The **mean arterial pressure (MAP)** is the average pressure in the arterial circulation throughout the cardiac cycle. It can be calculated using the formula [systolic BP + 2 (diastolic BP)] / 3.

PRACTICE ALERT
- Cardiac output and systemic (or peripheral) vascular resistance are the primary factors that determine blood pressure.
- A decrease in cardiac output (e.g., due to hemorrhage) or decreased peripheral vascular resistance (e.g., systemic vasodilation) cause the blood pressure to fall.
- Increased cardiac output (e.g., during exercise) or increased peripheral vascular resistance (e.g., vasoconstriction due to drug administration) cause the blood pressure to rise.

Cardiac output is determined by the blood volume and the ability of the ventricles to fill and effectively pump that blood. A number of factors contribute to systemic vascular resistance, including vessel length, blood viscosity, and vessel diameter and distensibility (compliance). While vessel length and blood viscosity remain relatively constant, vessel diameter and compliance are subject to normal regulatory activities and disease.

The arterioles normally determine the SVR as their diameter changes in response to a variety of stimuli:

- *Sympathetic nervous system (SNS)* stimulation. Baroreceptors in the aortic arch and carotid sinus signal the SNS via the cardiovascular control center in the medulla when the MAP changes. A drop in MAP stimulates the SNS, increasing the heart rate and cardiac output, and constricting arterioles (except in skeletal muscle). As a result, BP rises. A rise in MAP has the opposite effect, decreasing the heart rate and cardiac output, and causing arteriolar vasodilation.
- *Circulating epinephrine and norepinephrine* from the adrenal cortex (e.g., the fight-or-flight response) have the same effect as SNS stimulation.
- *Renin–angiotensin–aldosterone system* responds to renal perfusion. A drop in renal perfusion stimulates renin release. Renin converts angiotensinogen to angiotensin I, which is subsequently converted to angiotensin II in the lungs by angiotensin-converting enzyme (ACE). Angiotensin II is a potent vasoconstrictor. It also promotes sodium and water retention both directly and by stimulating the adrenal medulla to release aldosterone. Both SVR and CO increase, raising BP.
- *Atrial natriuretic peptide (ANP)* and *brain natriuretic peptide (BNP)* are released from atrial cells in response to stretching by excess blood volume. These hormones promote vasodilation and sodium and water excretion, lowering BP.
- *Adrenomedullin* is a peptide synthesized and released by endothelial and smooth muscle cells in blood vessels. It is a potent vasodilator.

- *Vasopressin* or *antidiuretic hormone* (from the posterior pituitary gland) promotes water retention and vasoconstriction, raising BP.
- *Local factors* such as inflammatory mediators and various metabolites can promote vasodilation, affecting BP.

In addition to the preceding, the primary factor affecting vessel compliance is the extent of arteriosclerosis (hardening of the arteries) and atherosclerosis (plaque accumulation). Figure 35–1 ■ summarizes the interrelationships of major factors regulating blood pressure.

FAST FACTS

- Sympathetic nervous system stimulation, epinephrine and norepinephrine, and the hormones angiotensin II and vasopressin (antidiuretic hormone or ADH) are *vasoconstrictors*, increasing the blood pressure.
- Parasympathetic nervous system stimulation and the hormones ANP, BNP, and adrenomedullin are *vasodilators*, decreasing the blood pressure.
- The hormones aldosterone and ADH promote sodium and water retention, increasing the blood pressure.

THE CLIENT WITH PRIMARY HYPERTENSION

Primary hypertension, also known as *essential hypertension*, is a persistently elevated systemic blood pressure. About 50 to 65 million people in the United States have hypertension (American Heart Association [AHA], 2005; National Heart, Lung, and Blood Institute [NHLBI], 2004b). More than 90% of these have primary hypertension, which has no identified cause.

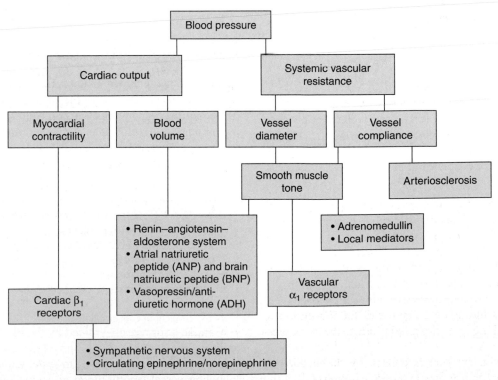

Figure 35–1 ■ Factors affecting blood pressure.

Hypertension is defined as systolic blood pressure of 140 mmHg or higher, or diastolic pressure of 90 mmHg or higher, based on the average of three or more readings taken on separate occasions (NHLBI, 2004b). Exceptions include clients being treated for hypertension and an initial reading of a systolic pressure of 210 mmHg or higher and/or a diastolic blood pressure of 120 mmHg or higher. Table 35–1 identifies classifications of blood pressure for adults age 18 and older as defined by the Joint National Committee.

Hypertension is an important public health issue: While it rarely causes symptoms or noticeably limits the client's functional health, hypertension is a major risk factor for coronary heart disease, heart failure, stroke, and renal failure. Hypertension and its consequences are not unique to the United States. The World Health Organization identifies blood pressure above optimal levels (a systolic BP > 115 mmHg) as responsible for 62% of cerebrovascular disease and 49% of ischemic heart disease worldwide (NHLBI, 2004b).

While the identification and treatment of hypertension in the United States has improved significantly in the past 25 years, approximately 30% of hypertensive adults remain unaware of their condition. Although 59% of hypertensive adults are being treated for the disorder, effective blood pressure control is achieved in only about 34% (NHLBI, 2004b).

Incidence and Risk Factors

Hypertension primarily affects middle-aged and older adults: More than 50% of people ages 60 to 69 and about 75% of those age 70 and older are hypertensive (NHLBI, 2004b). An age-related increase in the systolic blood pressure is the primary factor leading to the high incidence of hypertension in older adults. Unlike the diastolic blood pressure, which tends to rise until approximately age 50, then level off, the systolic blood pressure continues to rise with aging (NHLBI, 2004b).

The prevalence of hypertension is significantly higher in blacks than in whites and Hispanics. Nearly 40% of black adults are hypertensive, whereas less than 30% of adult white and Hispanic people are affected. In whites and Hispanics, more males than females are hypertensive; in blacks, more women than men are affected (NHLBI, 2004a). Essential hypertension affects people of all income groups, having great financial effects because of its effects on other body systems.

FAST FACTS

- Almost one-third of the adult population in the United States has hypertension.
- The prevalence of hypertension is highest in African American females and lowest in people of Asian ancestry.
- The prevalence of hypertension is higher among people who live in the southeastern United States.
- Up until age 55, more men than women are affected by hypertension; after that it affects more women than men.
- Hypertension increases the risk of stroke to about four times that of people with normal blood pressure, and the risk for heart failure by two to three times that of people with normal blood pressure (AHA, 2005).

A number of risk factors have been identified for primary hypertension (Box 35–1). Genetics plays a role, as do environmental factors.

- *Family history.* Studies show a genetic link in about 30% of people with primary hypertension (Kasper et al., 2005). Genes involved in the renin–angiotensin–aldosterone system and others that affect vascular tone, salt and water transportation in the kidney, obesity, and insulin resistance are likely involved in the development of hypertension, although no consistent genetic linkages have been found.

- *Age.* The incidence of hypertension rises with increasing age. Aging affects baroreceptors involved in blood pressure regulation as well as arterial compliance. As the arteries become less compliant, pressure within the vessels increases. This is often most apparent as a gradual increase in the systolic pressure with aging. See the Nursing Care of the Older Adult box on page 1157.

- *Race.* Essential hypertension is more common and more severe in blacks than in people of other ethnic backgrounds (see the accompanying Focus on Cultural Diversity box). It also tends to develop at an earlier age, and is associated with more cardiovascular and renal damage. More African Americans with hypertension have low renin levels and altered re-

TABLE 35–1 Classification of Blood Pressure for Adults[a]

CATEGORY	SYSTOLIC (mmHG)		DIASTOLIC (mmHG)
Normal	<120	and	<80
Prehypertension	120–139	or	80–89
Hypertension[b]			
Stage 1	140–159	or	90–99
Stage 2	≥160	or	≥100

[a]When systolic and diastolic blood pressures fall into different categories, the higher category is used to classify blood pressure status.
[b]Based on the average of two or more readings taken at each of two or more visits after an initial screening.
Source: Adapted from *The Seventh Report of the Joint National Committee on Prevention, Detection, Education, and Treatment of High Blood Pressure,* NIH Publication No. 04-5250 by NHLBI, 2004b, Bethesda, MD. National Institutes of Health. Retrieved from http://www.nhlbi.nih.gov/guidelines/hypertension.

BOX 35–1 Factors Contributing to Hypertension

Modifiable Factors
- High sodium intake
- Low potassium, calcium, and magnesium intake
- Obesity
- Excess alcohol consumption
- Insulin resistance

Nonmodifiable Factors
- Genetic factors
- Family history
- Age
- Race

NURSING CARE OF THE OLDER ADULT   Hypertension

Controlling high blood pressure is as important in the older adult as in younger adults. In the United States, the lifetime risk of hypertension is about 90% in men and women who live to age 80 to 85 (NHLBI, 2004b). Systolic hypertension is common, as is an elevated pulse pressure (systolic BP minus diastolic BP), indicating decreased compliance of large arteries. Despite this fact, less than two-thirds of people over age 80 who have high blood pressure are being treated and only 38% of men and 23% of women undergoing treatment had blood pressures that met established targets (NHLBI, 2005).

The Framingham Heart Study shows that cardiovascular deaths are two to five times more common in older adults with isolated systolic hypertension than in people with normal blood pressures. Stroke also is more common in older adults with sys-

tolic hypertension. These findings appear to relate to changes in blood vessels associated with aging: decreased compliance and decreased baroreceptor sensitivity. Decreased compliance impairs the ability of the vessels to expand and contract with varying amounts of blood, increasing peripheral vascular resistance and decreasing renal blood flow.

To obtain accurate blood pressure readings for older clients, slightly different procedures may be required. Palpation of the artery during cuff inflation is recommended to prevent inaccurate systolic readings due to an auscultatory gap, present in many older adults. The reflexes that maintain blood pressure during position changes diminish with aging. Allow the older client to sit upright or stand for 2 to 5 minutes before evaluating the blood pressure for true orthostatic readings.

---

nal excretion of sodium at normal blood pressure levels. This genetic tendency to conserve salt may have developed as an adaptation to working in a warm environment, when salt and water conservation are beneficial (Porth, 2005).

- *Mineral intake.* High sodium intake often is associated with fluid retention. Hypertension related to sodium intake involves a number of different physiologic mechanisms, including the renin–angiotensin–aldosterone system, nitric oxide, catecholamines, endothelin, and ANP (Copstead & Banasik, 2005). Low potassium, calcium, and magnesium intakes also contribute to hypertension by unknown mechanisms. The ratio of sodium to potassium intake appears to play a role, possibly through the effects of increased potassium intake on sodium excretion. Potassium also promotes vasodilation by reducing responses to catecholamines and angiotensin II. Calcium also has a vasodilator effect. While magnesium has been shown to reduce the blood pressure, the mechanism of action is unclear.

- *Obesity.* Central obesity (fat cell deposits in the abdomen), determined by an increased waist-to-hip ratio, has a stronger correlation with hypertension than body mass index or skinfold thickness. Although a clear correlation exists between obesity and hypertension, the relationship may be one of com-

mon cause: Genetic factors appear to play a role in the common triad of obesity, hypertension, and insulin resistance.

- *Insulin resistance.* Insulin resistance with resulting hyperinsulinemia is linked with hypertension by its effects of excess circulating insulin on the sympathetic nervous system, vascular smooth muscle, renal regulation of sodium and water, and ion transport across cell membranes. Insulin resistance may be a genetic or an acquired trait. Although it is more commonly seen in obese individuals, insulin resistance also has been found in people of normal weight.

- *Excess alcohol consumption.* Regular consumption of three or more drinks a day increases the risk of hypertension. Decreasing or discontinuing alcohol consumption reduces the blood pressure, particularly systolic readings. Lifestyle factors associated with excessive alcohol intake (obesity and lack of exercise) may contribute to hypertension as well.

- *Stress.* Physical and emotional stress cause transient elevations of blood pressure, but the role of stress in primary hypertension is less clear. Blood pressure normally fluctuates throughout the day, increasing with activity, discomfort, or emotional responses such as anger. Frequent or continued stress may cause vascular smooth muscle hypertrophy or affect central integrative pathways of the brain (Porth, 2005).

Pathophysiology

Primary hypertension is thought to develop from complex interactions among factors that regulate cardiac output and systemic vascular resistance. These interactions may include:

- Excess sympathetic nervous system with overstimulation of α- and β-adrenergic receptors, resulting in vasoconstriction and increased cardiac output.
- Altered function of the renin–angiotensin–aldosterone system and its responsiveness to factors such as sodium intake and overall fluid volume. The renin–angiotensin–aldosterone system affects vasomotor tone and salt and water excretion. Chronically high levels of angiotensin II lead to arteriolar remodeling, which permanently increases SVR. In approximately 20% of people with primary hypertension, renin levels are lower

FOCUS ON CULTURAL DIVERSITY
Hypertension in African Americans

- The prevalence of hypertension among African Americans living in the United States is among the highest in the world: in African American adults, 41.8% of males and 45.4% of females are hypertensive.
  - African Americans with the highest risk for hypertension tend to be:
    - Middle aged or older
    - Less educated
    - Overweight or obese
    - Physically inactive
    - Affected by diabetes (AHA, 2005).

BOX 35–3 DASH Diet Recommendations

- Grains—7 to 8 servings per day
- Vegetables—4 to 5 servings per day
- Fruits—4 to 5 servings per day
- Nonfat/low-fat dairy products—2 to 3 servings per day
- Meats, poultry, and fish—2 or less 3-oz servings per day
- Nuts, seeds, and dry beans—4 to 5 servings per week
- Fats and oils—2 to 3 servings per day
- Sweets—5 servings per week (should be low in fat)

well-being. Previously sedentary clients are encouraged to engage in aerobic exercise for 30 to 45 minutes per day most days of the week (5 to 6 days). Isometric exercise (such as weight training) may not be appropriate, because it can raise the systolic blood pressure.

ALCOHOL AND TOBACCO USE The recommended alcohol intake for clients with hypertension is no more than 1 oz of ethanol or two drinks per day. A drink is 12 oz of beer, 5 oz of wine, or 1.5 oz of 80-proof whiskey. Women and lighter weight people should reduce this limit by half. Although alcohol withdrawal may increase blood pressure, this is usually temporary and diminishes as abstinence or restricted intake continues.

Although nicotine is a vasoconstrictor, substantial data linking smoking to hypertension are lacking. A definitive link exists between smoking and heart disease, however. Clients who smoke are strongly urged to quit. Smoking also reduces the ef-

fect of some antihypertensive medications such as propranolol (Inderal). Smoking cessation aids such as nicotine patches and gum contain lower amounts of nicotine and usually do not raise blood pressure.

STRESS REDUCTION Stress stimulates the sympathetic nervous system, increasing vasoconstriction, systemic vascular resistance, cardiac output, and the blood pressure. Regular, moderate exercise is the treatment of choice for reducing stress in hypertensive clients. Relaxation techniques such as biofeedback, therapeutic touch, yoga, and meditation to relax both mind and body may also lower blood pressure, although their effect has not been proven in hypertension management.

Medications

Current pharmacologic treatment of hypertension involves using one or more of the following drug classes: diuretics, beta-adrenergic blockers, centrally acting sympatholytics, vasodilators, ACE inhibitors, angiotensin II receptor blockers (ARBs), and calcium channel blockers. For most clients, two or more antihypertensive drugs selected from different drug classes are necessary to achieve effective control. These drug classes have different sites of action (Figure 35–3 ■). Nursing implications for administration of antihypertensive drugs (other than diuretics) are outlined on pages 1161–1162.

DRUG CLASSES Diuretics are the preferred treatment for systolic hypertension in older adults. Diuretics are relatively safe and well-tolerated drugs; in addition, most are relatively inexpensive. Thiazide diuretics, such as hydrochlorothiazide (HydroDIURIL),

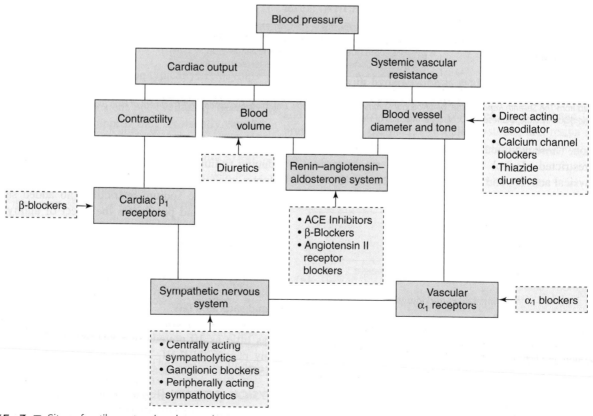

Figure 35–3 ■ Sites of antihypertensive drug action.

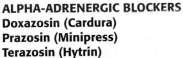

MEDICATION ADMINISTRATION Antihypertensive Drugs

ALPHA-ADRENERGIC BLOCKERS
Doxazosin (Cardura)
Prazosin (Minipress)
Terazosin (Hytrin)
Alpha-adrenergic blocking agents block alpha-receptors in vascular smooth muscle, decreasing vasomotor tone and vasoconstriction. They also reduce serum levels of low-density lipoproteins (LDL) and very low-density lipoproteins (VLDL). However, vasodilation may cause orthostatic hypotension and reflex stimulation of the heart, resulting in tachycardia and palpitations. A beta-blocker may be ordered to minimize this effect.

Nursing Responsibilities
- Give the first dose at bedtime to minimize risk of fainting (called "first-dose syncope"). If the first dose is given in the daytime (or if the dose is increased), instruct to remain in bed for 3 to 4 hours.
- Assess blood pressure and apical pulse before each dose and as indicated thereafter.

Health Education for the Client and Family
- There is a risk of fainting after taking the first dose of this drug. Take the drug at bedtime to reduce this risk, and do not drive or engage in other hazardous activities for 12 to 24 hours after the first dose.
- This drug may cause dizziness or light-headedness. Change positions slowly, and sit down if you become dizzy or light-headed.
- Notify your primary care provider if you develop nasal congestion or impotence while taking this drug.
- Notify your primary care provider before discontinuing this medication.

ANGIOTENSIN-CONVERTING ENZYME (ACE) INHIBITORS
Benazepril (Lotensin) **Moexipril (Univasc)**
Captopril (Capoten) **Perindopril (Aceon)**
Enalapril (Vasotec) **Quinapril (Accupril)**
Fosinopril (Monopril) **Ramipril (Altace)**
Lisinopril (Prinivil, Zestril) **Trandolapril (Mavik)**

ANGIOTENSIN II RECEPTOR BLOCKERS (ARBS)
Candesartan (Atacand) **Olmesartan (Benicar)**
Eprosartan (Teveten) **Telmisartan (Micardis)**
Irbesartan (Avapro) **Valsartan (Diovan)**
Losartan (Cozaar)
The ACE inhibitors lower blood pressure by preventing conversion of angiotensin I to angiotensin II. This in turn prevents vasoconstriction and sodium and water retention. ARBs have the same effect, but they act by blocking the effect of angiotensin II on receptors. Both ACE inhibitors and ARBs are less effective in black clients and are contraindicated in pregnancy (Lehne, 2004). Their primary adverse effects are persistent cough, first-dose hypotension, and hyperkalemia.

Nursing Responsibilities
- Assess blood pressure and WBC before giving the first dose. Monitor blood pressure for 2 hours after the first dose and regularly thereafter.
- Administer PO 1 hour before meals; tablets may be crushed.
- Report changes in WBC or differential, hyperkalemia, or changes in BUN or serum creatinine to the primary care provider.

- Do not administer to clients with renal artery stenosis or who are pregnant.
- Immediately report and treat manifestations of angioedema (giant wheals and edema of the tongue, glottis, and pharynx). Initiate resuscitation measures as needed. Discontinue drug immediately and do not use in the future.

Health Education for the Client and Family
- Report peripheral edema, signs of infection, or difficulty breathing to your primary care provider.
- Change position (lying to sitting and sitting to standing) slowly to prevent dizziness; sit down if dizziness or light-headedness develops.
- Do not take a potassium supplement or use a potassium-based salt substitute while taking this drug unless prescribed by your physician.
- Notify your physician if you become pregnant while taking this drug. Although it is safe early in pregnancy, taking the drug during the second and third trimesters may harm the fetus.

BETA-ADRENERGIC BLOCKING AGENTS
Acebutolol (Sectral) **Nadolol (Corgard)**
Atenolol (Tenormin) **Penbutolol (Levatol)**
Betaxolol (Kerlone) **Pindolol (Visken)**
Bisoprolol (Zebeta) **Propranolol (Inderal)**
Metoprolol tartrate (Lopressor) **Timolol (Blocadren)**
Combined with an alpha-blocker:
Carvedilol (Coreg) **Labetalol (Normodyne)**
Beta-adrenergic blockers are commonly used to control hypertension. Beta-blockers reduce blood pressure by preventing beta-receptor stimulation in the heart, thereby decreasing heart rate and cardiac output. Beta-blockers also interfere with renin release by the kidneys, decreasing the effects of angiotensin and aldosterone. Potential adverse effects of beta-blockers include bronchospasm, fatigue, sleep disturbances, nightmares, bradycardia, heart block, worsening of heart failure, gastrointestinal disturbances, impotence, and increased triglyceride levels.

Nursing Responsibilities
- Before giving initial dose, assess for contraindications to beta-blockers such as asthma, chronic lung disease, bradycardia, or heart block.
- Assess blood pressure and apical pulse before giving; notify primary care provider if vital signs are outside established parameters.
- Report adverse effects such as bradycardia, decreased cardiac output (fatigue, dyspnea with exertion, hypotension, decreased level of consciousness), heart failure, heart block, bronchoconstriction (wheezing, dyspnea), or altered blood glucose levels (in diabetic clients).
- Carefully monitor responses of the older client.

Health Education for the Client and Family
- Monitor blood pressure and pulse daily as instructed.
- Change position (lying to sitting and sitting to standing) slowly to prevent dizziness and possible falls.
- Report effects such as fatigue, lethargy, and impotence to your primary care provider.
- Notify your physician if you become short of breath or develop a cough or swelling of your extremities.

(continued)

MEDICATION ADMINISTRATION Antihypertensive Drugs (continued)

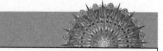

- If you have diabetes, check blood glucose levels more frequently because hypoglycemia may develop with few symptoms.
- Talk to your primary care provider before taking any over-the-counter medications.
- Carry an adequate supply of the drug when traveling. Do not stop taking this drug without notifying your primary care provider.

CALCIUM CHANNEL BLOCKERS

Amlodipine (Norvasc)	Nicardipine (Cardene)
Diltiazem (Cardizem)	Nifedipine (Procardia)
Felodipine (Plendil)	Nisoldipine (Sular)
Isradipine (DynaCirc)	Verapamil (Isoptin)

Calcium channel blockers inhibit the flow of calcium ions across the cell membrane of vascular tissue and cardiac cells. In doing so, they relax arterial smooth muscle, lowering peripheral resistance through vasodilation. Calcium channel blockers can cause reflex tachycardia, and some (e.g., verapamil and diltiazem) may impair cardiac function, worsening heart failure.

Nursing Responsibilities
- Assess blood pressure, apical pulse, and liver and renal function tests prior to giving these drugs.
- Calcium channel blockers may be given orally or intravenously.
- Do not administer verapamil or diltiazem to clients with severe hypotension, sinus, or atrioventricular blocks. Administer with caution to clients also taking digoxin or a beta-blocker.
- Periodically monitor blood pressure and apical pulse during therapy. Promptly report signs of bradycardia, AV block, or heart failure to the physician.

Health Education for the Client and Family
- Take blood pressure and pulse daily as taught. Notify your physician if your pulse is less than 60 bpm or your blood pressure is not within the specified range.
- This drug may cause constipation. Drink six to eight glasses of water each day, and increase fiber in diet.
- Report shortness of breath, weight gain, or swelling in feet or ankles to your primary care provider.

CENTRALLY ACTING SYMPATHOLYTICS

Clonidine (Catapres)	Methyldopa (Aldomet)
Guanfacine (Tenex)	Reserpine (generic)

The centrally acting sympatholytics stimulate the α_2-receptors in the CNS to suppress sympathetic outflow to the heart and blood vessels. A fall in cardiac output and vasodilation result, reducing blood pressure. Dry mouth and sedation are common adverse effects. Severe reflex hypertension may occur if abruptly discontinued. Clonidine is contraindicated during pregnancy; methyldopa is contraindicated for clients with active liver disease.

Nursing Responsibilities
- Assess for contraindications to therapy. Obtain baseline blood pressure, CBC, Coombs' test, and liver function studies.
- Administer oral doses at bedtime to minimize effects of sedation.
- Methyldopa may be given intravenously for hypertensive emergencies.

- Apply transdermal clonidine patch to dry, hairless area of intact skin on the chest or upper arm. Assess for rash, which indicates allergy, at area of application.
- Promptly report changes in laboratory values to the physician. Discontinue methyldopa if manifestations of liver dysfunction develop.

Health Education for the Client and Family
- Relieve dry mouth by sipping water or chewing sugarless gum.
- Take with meals if gastric upset or nausea develop.
- Change position (lying to sitting and sitting to standing) slowly to prevent dizziness and possible falls.
- Do not suddenly discontinue medication or skip doses; this could cause serious hypertension.
- Report mental depression or decreased mental acuity to your healthcare provider.
- Side effects (such as dry mouth, nausea, and dizziness) tend to diminish over time.
- Do not drive a car if the medications cause drowsiness.

VASODILATORS

Hydralazine (Apresoline)	Minoxidil (Loniten)

Vasodilators reduce blood pressure by relaxing vascular smooth muscle (especially in the arterioles), and decreasing peripheral vascular resistance. These drugs are often prescribed in combination with a diuretic or beta-blocker, because they can cause reflex tachycardia and fluid retention. Because these drugs can have significant toxic effects, they are not routinely used to manage chronic hypertension.

Nursing Responsibilities
- Hydralazine may be given orally or intravenously; minoxidil is given orally.
- Assess blood pressure and pulse before giving the drug and monitor during therapy as indicated. Report tachycardia or hypotension to the physician.
- Report peripheral edema and manifestations of volume overload and heart failure.
- Immediately report muffled heart sounds or paradoxical pulse because pericardial effusion and possible cardiac tamponade may develop during minoxidil therapy.
- Discontinue hydralazine and report manifestations of a systemic lupus erythematosus (SLE) like syndrome: muscle or joint pain, fever, or symptoms of nephritis or pericarditis.

Health Education for the Client and Family
- Change position (lying to sitting and sitting to standing) slowly to prevent dizziness and possible falls.
- Report muscle, joint aches, and fever to your healthcare provider.
- Headache, palpitations, and rapid pulse may develop but should abate in about 10 days.
- Do not discontinue the medication without talking to your healthcare provider.
- Minoxidil may cause excessive hair growth. Contact your physician if this becomes troublesome.

are widely used. In major clinical studies, treatment with a single diuretic controlled blood pressure in about 50% of the clients and reduced hypertension-linked morbidity and mortality related to coronary heart disease. Diuretics control hypertension primarily by preventing tubular reabsorption of sodium, thus promoting sodium and water excretion and reducing blood volume. Thiazide diuretics also reduce systemic vascular resistance through an unknown mechanism. Diuretics are particularly effective in blacks and in clients who are obese, older, or who have increased plasma volume or low renin activity. The adverse effects of diuretics generally are dose related. In addition to hypokalemia, diuretics may affect serum levels of glucose, triglycerides, uric acid, LDLs, and insulin. More information about diuretics can be found in Chapters 10 and 29 ∞.

Clients with heart failure, coronary heart disease (CHD), or diabetes may initially be treated with a beta-blocker. These drugs lower blood pressure, apparently by reducing peripheral vascular resistance. They may also reduce the amount of renin released by the kidneys by blocking beta$_1$-receptors in the kidney. Beta-blockers reduce the risk of complications such as heart failure and stroke. They are, however, relatively contraindicated for clients with asthma or chronic obstructive pulmonary disease, because they promote bronchial constriction.

ACE inhibitors and ARBs also are commonly used in initial treatment of hypertension, particularly for clients who are diabetic or who have heart failure, a history of myocardial infarction (MI), or chronic kidney disease. ACE inhibitors block formation of angiotensin II by inhibiting the action of angiotensin-converting enzyme. Angiotensin II is a potent vasoconstrictor that also stimulates aldosterone release from the adrenal gland; blocking its action prevents vasoconstriction and sodium and water retention resulting from aldosterone release. ARBs have a very similar effect, although their action is to block angiotensin II receptors, thus preventing its vasoconstrictive and volume expansion effects.

Several drug classes work through their ability to promote vasodilation and reduce peripheral vascular resistance. Alpha-blockers such as prazosin and terazosin block stimulation of alpha$_1$-receptors on arterioles and veins, preventing vasoconstriction. Because of their ability to dilate both arterioles and veins, alpha-blockers can cause significant orthostatic hypotension, particularly following the initial dose. Calcium channel blockers promote dilation of arterioles, the primary regulators of peripheral vascular resistance. These drugs can cause reflex tachycardia. Some calcium channel blockers, verapamil and diltiazem in particular, also suppress heart function, reducing stroke volume and cardiac output. Reflex tachycardia is minimal with these calcium channel blockers. Direct-acting vasodilators such as hydralazine and minoxidil also directly affect the arterioles, reducing peripheral vascular resistance. These drugs have little effect on veins, so the risk of orthostatic hypotension is minimal. They are, however, associated with reflex tachycardia and fluid retention, so rarely are administered as in single-drug treatment regimens.

Other factors considered in selecting drugs for treating hypertension include demographic characteristics of the client, concurrent conditions, quality of life, cost, and possible interactions among prescribed drugs. In general, diuretics and calcium channel blockers are more effective for treating hypertension in blacks than beta-blockers or ACE inhibitors. Beta-blockers are preferred to treat hypertension with concurrent coronary heart disease and angina, but are contraindicated for clients who have asthma or depression. Beta-blockers also reduce exercise tolerance and may adversely affect lifestyle for some clients.

DRUG REGIMENS Treatment usually is initiated using a single antihypertensive drug at a low dose. Unless otherwise indicated, a diuretic is recommended as the initial drug of choice. The dose is slowly increased until optimal blood pressure control is achieved. If the drug does not effectively lower the blood pressure or has troubling side effects, a different drug from another class of antihypertensive medications is substituted. If, on the other hand, the drug is tolerated well but has not lowered blood pressure to the desired level, a second drug from another class may be added to the treatment regimen.

Treatment of clients with stage 2 hypertension generally is more aggressive to minimize the risk of MI, heart failure, or stroke. When the average blood pressure is greater than 200/120, immediate therapy, and possible hospitalization, is vital.

After a year of effective hypertension control, an effort may be made to reduce the dosage and number of drugs. This is known as step-down therapy. It is more successful in clients who have made lifestyle modifications. Careful blood pressure monitoring is necessary during and after step-down therapy, because the blood pressure often rises again to hypertensive levels.

Complementary Therapies

Behavioral and mind–body therapies may be helpful for some clients in lowering blood pressure (see the Nursing Research box on page 1164). The blood pressure increases in response to physiologic and psychologic stress and anxiety. Mind–body therapies such as yoga and t'ai chi, meditation, and guided imagery are designed to modify both physiologic and cognitive aspects of the stress response. In a study of older African American men and women with moderate hypertension, transcendental mediation was shown to reduce the blood pressure. Eastern exercises such as yoga and t'ai chi, which often combine imagery, meditation, and physical exercise, have been shown to reduce sympathetic nervous system activity, blood pressure, and heart and respiratory rates (Spencer & Jacobs, 2003). A nursing research study of hypertensive clients in Thailand demonstrated the effectiveness of yoga to reduce blood pressure, heart rate, and body mass index (McCaffrey et al., 2005).

NURSING CARE

Health Promotion

Health promotion teaching and activities focus on the modifiable risk factors for hypertension. Advise all clients (as well as children and adolescents) to stop or never start smoking. Discuss the risks of obesity, excess alcohol intake, and a sedentary lifestyle with clients. Encourage all clients to eat a diet rich in fruits and vegetables and low in total and saturated fat. Discuss the potential benefits of following the DASH diet or a similar

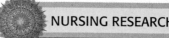

NURSING RESEARCH   Evidence-Based Practice: The Client with Primary Hypertension

Standard therapies for hypertension include lifestyle changes and medications. Clients often are advised to reduce stress levels in their lives, but rarely are provided with the tools to do so. A study by Yucha and colleagues (2005) sought to identify those clients who were most likely to benefit (reduced blood pressure in both clinic and ambulatory settings) from biofeedback-assisted relaxation training. Participants, all of whom had stage 1 or 2 hypertension, received 8 weeks of relaxation training with biofeedback provided by measurements of finger temperature, muscle tension, and respiratory sinus arrhythmia. The most benefit (greatest reduction in BP) occurred in participants who were not taking antihypertensive medication, had lower starting finger temperatures, had less daytime blood pressure variation, and who had a more external health locus of control.

IMPLICATIONS FOR NURSING

Predicting which clients would benefit from biofeedback-assisted relaxation training to lower blood pressure could potentially reduce the risk that these clients will go on to develop stage 1 or 2 hypertension. While biofeedback-assisted relaxation training is expensive and may not be covered by insurance, its benefits in reducing the overall costs of treating hypertension and its potential consequences are significant.

Nurses are in a position to identify clients with prehypertension through blood pressure screening. It is very appropriate to suggest mind–body therapies such as relaxation training with biofeedback to these clients, most of whom do not require medication.

CRITICAL THINKING IN CLIENT CARE

1. This study found that clients who were not taking antihypertensive medications were more likely to benefit from training in biofeedback-assisted relaxation. Think about the different ways in which antihypertensive medications work. Why do you think more benefit was seen in those clients who were not taking drugs?
2. Another finding of the study showed more benefit in clients with a more external health locus of control. Compare characteristics of clients with an internal health locus of control and those with an external health locus. What differences in these clients might account for this finding?
3. While you are discussing lifestyle modifications and the use of mind–body therapies with a client with prehypertension, he tells you that he thinks all this is nonsense. How would you respond?

eating plan. Advise all clients to remain active and engage in aerobic exercise 5 or more days a week. Discuss the stress-reducing benefits of exercise.

Offer blood pressure screening, and refer clients for follow-up as indicated (Table 35–2).

Assessment

Focused assessment of the client with hypertension includes:

- *Health history:* Complaints of morning headache, cervical pain; cardiovascular or central nervous system manifestations; history of hypertension, renal disease, diabetes; family history of high blood pressure, heart failure, or kidney disease; current medications.
- *Physical examination:* Vital signs including blood pressure in both arms, apical and peripheral pulses; ophthalmologic exam of retinal fundus as appropriate.
- *Diagnostic tests:* Serum electrolytes, glucose, and creatinine; cholesterol and lipoprotein profile; urinalysis.

Nursing Diagnoses and Interventions

All clients with primary hypertension and their families need significant teaching to manage this chronic condition. Health maintenance is a high-priority problem. Depending on the stage of hypertension and concurrent illnesses, other appropriate nursing diagnoses may include *Imbalanced Nutrition, Fluid Volume Excess,* and *Risk for Noncompliance.*

Ineffective Health Maintenance

Unhealthy lifestyle and behaviors can contribute to health problems such as hypertension. When hypertension has been identified, knowledge of the disease and its management is vital for the client. Willingness to take responsibility for hypertension management is central to effective blood pressure control. Adopting healthy lifestyle changes enhances drug therapy; in some cases, the need for medications may be eliminated or reduced. Because hypertension is often an asymptomatic disease and many antihypertensive drugs have unpleasant side effects, it

TABLE 35–2 Recommended Blood Pressure Follow-Up

CATEGORY	BLOOD PRESSURE (mmHG)	RECOMMENDED FOLLOW-UP
Normal	<120/80	Recheck in 2 years.
Prehypertension	120–139/80–89	Recheck in 1 year.
Stage 1 hypertension	140–159/90–99	Confirm within 2 months.
Stage 2 hypertension	≥160/≥100	Evaluate or refer to care provider within 1 month; for higher pressures (e.g., ≥180/≥110), evaluate or refer to care provider immediately or within 1 week as indicated.

Source: Adapted from *The Seventh Report of the Joint National Committee on Prevention, Detection, Education, and Treatment of High Blood Pressure,* NIH Publication No. 04-5250, by NHLBI, 2004b, Bethesda, MD: National Institutes of Health. Retrieved from http://www.nhlbi.nih.gov/guidelines/hypertension.

is vital that the client understand the chronic progressive nature of the disease and its long-term consequences.

- Assist with identifying current behaviors that contribute to hypertension. *The client must first identify contributory behaviors before he or she can change them. Using knowledge of hypertension risk factors, the nurse can help identify behaviors and factors contributing to hypertension that can be changed. Including the family in this process is important to reduce potential sabotage of the client's efforts to adopt healthier behaviors.*
- Assist in developing a realistic health maintenance plan. *Preparing a health maintenance plan for the client does little to encourage personal responsibility for health. However, nurses can guide clients in developing realistic goals and expectations for the treatment plan and modifying risk factors such as smoking, exercise, diet, and stress.*
- Help the client and family identify strengths and weaknesses in maintaining health. *Discussing areas of the health maintenance plan that are working well and those that present difficulties can help to identify necessary changes in the plan and additional strategies for implementing it.*

Risk for Noncompliance

Noncompliance, or failure to follow the identified treatment plan, is a continuing risk for any client with a chronic disease. Recommended lifestyle changes such as diet, exercise, restricted alcohol intake, stress reduction, and smoking cessation often are difficult to maintain on a continuing basis. In addition, prescribed medications may have undesirable effects whereas hypertension itself often has no symptoms or noticeable effects.

- Inquire about reasons for noncompliance with recommended treatment plan. Listen openly and without judging. *Nonthreatening discussion of factors contributing to noncompliance validates the client's self-esteem and partnership in the treatment plan.*

> **PRACTICE ALERT**
> Assess factors contributing to noncompliance, such as adverse drug effects. Suggest measures to manage adverse effects or, if indicated, contact the primary care provider about possible alternative drugs. Some adverse effects of antihypertensive drugs, such as gastric upset, light-headedness, or nocturia, may be easily managed by changing the timing of the drug dose. Others, such as fatigue, decreased exercise tolerance, or impotence may interfere with lifestyle and life roles to the extent that the client finds them intolerable.

- Evaluate knowledge of hypertension, its long-term effects, and treatment. Provide additional information and reinforce teaching as needed. *Knowledge increases the sense of control, which also increases the likelihood of compliance with treatment.*
- Assist to develop realistic short-term goals for lifestyle changes. *Attempting to lose weight, exercise daily, stop smoking, and dramatically change the diet all at the same time may be overwhelming, leading to a sense of failure. Smaller, gradual changes are more easily incorporated into lifestyle and daily activities, improving compliance.*

> **PRACTICE ALERT**
> Work with the client to develop mutual outcomes for the treatment plan. Discuss measures to improve compliance. The client has absolute control over compliance with the treatment plan. Demonstrating respect and involving the client in decision making and planning can improve compliance.

- Help the client identify cues and develop reminders (e.g., written notes, a medication box filled weekly) to assist with maintaining a schedule for exercise and medications. *Cues and other devices provide helpful reminders of activities and schedules until they are incorporated into habits.*
- Reassure the client that relapse into old habits and behaviors is common. Encourage avoiding feelings of guilt associated with relapse, and use the circumstance to renew efforts to comply with treatment. *Guilt and feelings of failure can lead to further noncompliance unless the event is used to identify reasons for noncompliance and ways to prevent it from recurring in the future.*

Imbalanced Nutrition: More than Body Requirements

The relationship between obesity, excess alcohol intake, and hypertension is well documented. Hypertension is particularly associated with central obesity, identified by waist circumference greater than hip circumference. Although weight loss is difficult and takes commitment to changing eating and exercise habits, it is possible for most clients to achieve.

- Assess usual daily food intake, and discuss possible contributing factors to excess weight, such as sedentary lifestyle, or using food as a reward or stress reliever. Inquire about diversional activities, exercise patterns, and previous weight reduction efforts (e.g., participation in weight reduction programs or using fad or crash diets). *Assessment data provide clues about contributing factors to obesity, the client's knowledge base about the relationship between eating and exercise habits and weight, and safe weight loss strategies. This provides direction for further teaching and for developing a realistic weight reduction plan.*
- Mutually determine with the client a realistic target weight (e.g., loss of 10% of current body weight over a 6-month period). Regularly monitor weight. Encourage a system of nonfood rewards for achieving small, incremental goals. *Setting weight loss goals helps formalize the process and provides motivation for continued progress. Developing realistic goals may be difficult; unrealistic goals, however, set the client up for failure. Continuous incremental weight loss provides reassurance that it can be achieved and promotes permanent weight reduction.*
- Refer to a dietitian for information about low-fat, low-calorie foods and eating plans. Focus on changing eating habits as opposed to "following a diet." *Focusing on changing eating habits promotes the sense that low-fat, low-calorie eating patterns should become a part of lifestyle rather than a short-term measure to be endured until the weight loss goal is achieved.*

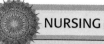

NURSING CARE PLAN   A Client with Hypertension

Margaret Spezia is a married, 49-year-old Italian American with eight children whose ages range from 3 to 18 years. For the past 2 months, Mrs. Spezia has had frequent morning headaches, and occasional dizziness and blurred vision. At her annual physical examination 1 month ago, her blood pressure was 168/104 and 156/94. She was instructed to reduce her fat and cholesterol intake, to avoid using salt at the table, and to start walking for 30 to 45 minutes daily. Mrs. Spezia returns to the clinic for follow-up.

ASSESSMENT

While escorting Mrs. Spezia to the exam room and obtaining her weight, blood pressure, and history, Lisa Christos, RN, notices that Mrs. Spezia seems restless and upset. Ms. Christos says, "You look upset about something. Is everything OK?" Mrs. Spezia responds, "Well, my head is throbbing, and I'm sort of dizzy. I think I'm just overdoing it and not getting enough rest. You know, raising eight children is a lot of work and expense. I just started working part time so we wouldn't get behind in our bills. I thought the extra money might relieve some of my stress, but I'm not so sure that's really happening. I'm not getting any better and I'm worried that I'll lose my job or become disabled and that my husband won't be able to manage the children by himself. I really need to go home, but first, I want to get rid of this awful headache. Would you please get me a couple of aspirin or something?"

Mrs. Spezia's history shows a steady weight gain during the past 18 years. She has no known family history of hypertension. Physical findings include height 63 inches (160 cm), weight 225 lb (102 kg), T 99°F (37.2°C), P 100 regular, R 16, BP 180/115 (lying), 170/110 (sitting), 165/105 (standing), average 10-point difference in readings between right and left arm (lower on left). Skin cool and dry, capillary refill 4 seconds right hand, 3 seconds left hand. Mrs. Spezia's total serum cholesterol is 245 mg/dL (normal <200 mg/dL). All other blood and urine studies are within normal limits. Based on analysis of the data, Mrs. Spezia is started on enalapril 5 mg and hydrochlorothiazide 12.5 mg in a combination drug (Vaseretic), and placed on a low-fat, low-cholesterol, no-added-salt diet.

DIAGNOSES

- *Fatigue* related to effects of hypertension and stresses of daily life
- *Imbalanced Nutrition: More than Body Requirements* related to excessive food intake
- *Ineffective Health Maintenance* related to inability to modify lifestyle
- *Deficient Knowledge* related to effects of prescribed treatment

EXPECTED OUTCOMES

- Reduce blood pressure readings to less than 150 systolic and 90 diastolic by return visit next week.
- Incorporate low-sodium and low-fat foods from a list provided into her diet.

- Develop a plan for regular exercise.
- Verbalize understanding of the effects of prescribed drug, dietary restrictions, exercise, and follow-up visits to help control hypertension.

PLANNING AND IMPLEMENTATION

- Teach to take own blood pressure daily and record it, bringing the record to scheduled clinic visits.
- Teach name, dose, action, and side effects of her antihypertensive medication.
- Instruct to walk for 15 minutes each day this week, and to investigate swimming classes at the local pool.
- Discuss strategies for achieving a realistic weight loss goal.
- Refer for a dietary consultation for further teaching about fat and sodium restrictions.
- Discuss stress-reducing techniques, helping identify possible choices.

EVALUATION

Mrs. Spezia returns to the clinic 1 week later. Her average blood pressure is now 148/88 mmHg. She has lost 1.5 lb, and states that her oldest daughter has suggested that they join a weight reduction program together. Mrs. Spezia is walking for an average of 20 minutes at a local mall each day. She verbalizes an understanding of her medication, and is taking it in the morning and before dinner each day. She met with the dietitian and discussed ways to reduce the sodium and fat in her diet. The dietitian provided a list of low-fat, low-sodium foods and recommended cookbooks to help Mrs. Spezia modify her cooking. Mrs. Spezia tells Ms. Christos, "I just can't believe how much better I feel already. My headaches are gone, and I've actually lost some weight—and I feel motivated to keep going. If I had only known how much better I could feel! I don't expect I'll ever go back to my old habits again; it's just not worth it!"

CRITICAL THINKING IN THE NURSING PROCESS

1. Identify the factors that contributed to Mrs. Spezia's hypertension. Which were modifiable and which were not?
2. What is the rationale for reducing sodium and fat in Mrs. Spezia's diet?
3. Suppose your hypertensive client is homeless and has no source of income. How could you help ensure your client would follow the treatment plan? What would you do if the client did not follow it?
4. Discuss the role of stress in hypertension. What factors in Mrs. Spezia's life contribute to her stress level?
5. Develop a plan of care for the nursing diagnosis *Low Self-Esteem* related to obesity.
See Evaluating Your Response in Appendix C.

THE CLIENT WITH HYPERTENSIVE CRISIS

Some clients with hypertension may, for reasons not clearly understood, develop rapid, significant elevations in systolic and/or diastolic pressures. In a *hypertensive emergency* (or *malignant hypertension*), the systolic pressure is greater than 180 mmHg and the diastolic pressure higher than 120 mmHg. Immediate treatment (within 1 hour) is vital to prevent cardiac, renal, and vascular damage, and reduce morbidity and mortality. Intense cerebral artery spasms help protect the brain from excess pressure; however, cerebral edema often develops. Prolonged severe hypertension damages walls of the arterioles and renal blood vessels, and may lead to intravascular coagulation and acute renal failure.

Clients presenting with a hypertensive emergency may have manifestations such as headache, confusion, swelling of the optic nerve (papilledema), blurred vision, restlessness, and motor and sensory deficits. Manifestations of hypertensive emergencies are listed in the accompanying box.

Most hypertensive emergencies occur when clients suddenly stop taking their medications or their hypertension is poorly controlled. Younger clients (30 to 50 years old), African American men, pregnant women with preeclampsia, and people with collagen and/or renal disease also are at higher risk for a hypertensive emergency (Porth, 2005).

The goal of care in hypertensive emergencies is to reduce the blood pressure by no more than 25% within minutes to 1 hour, then toward 160/100 within 2 to 6 hours. It is important to avoid rapid or excessive blood pressure decreases that may lead to renal, cerebral, or cardiac ischemia (NHLBI, 2004b). Blood pressure is monitored frequently (every 5 to 30 minutes)

MANIFESTATIONS of Hypertensive Emergencies

- Rapid onset
- Blurred vision, papilledema
- Systolic pressure > 180 mmHg
- Diastolic pressure > 120 mmHg
- Headache
- Confusion
- Motor and sensory deficits

during a hypertensive emergency. The BUN, serum creatinine, calcium, and total protein levels are carefully monitored to help determine the prognosis for recovery. Drug treatment for malignant hypertension includes parenteral administration of a rapidly acting antihypertensive, such as the potent vasodilator sodium nitroprusside (Nipride). Other medications that may be used are outlined in Table 35–3. Management also focuses on

TABLE 35–3 Intravenous Drugs Used to Treat Hypertensive Emergencies

CLASS/DRUG	ONSET	DURATION	NURSING IMPLICATIONS
Vasodilator			
Sodium nitroprusside (Nipride)	seconds	1 to 2 min	■ Effective, easy to titrate ■ May cause nausea, vomiting, muscle twitching, sweating ■ Use with caution in increased intracranial pressure
Nitroglycerin	2 to 5 min	5 to 10 min	■ Used when coronary ischemia accompanies hypertension ■ May cause headache, vomiting ■ Tolerance may develop with prolonged use
Diazoxide (Hyperstat)	1 to 2 min	4 to 24 h	■ Avoided in clients with coronary artery disease ■ Used with beta-blockers and diuretics ■ Painful if it enters tissues
Fenoldopam (Corlopam)	<5 min	30 min	■ Use with caution in clients with glaucoma ■ May cause tachycardia, headache, nausea, flushing ■ Do not use concurrently with beta-blockers ■ Monitor for heart failure, ischemic heart disease
Hydralazine (Apresoline)	10 to 30 min	2 to 6 h	■ May be used for hypertension associated with eclampsia ■ Avoided in clients with CHD ■ May cause tachycardia, flushing, headache, vomiting, angina
Calcium Channel Blocker			
Nicardipine (Cardene)	5 to 10 min	15 to 30 min; up to 4 h	■ Use with caution in CHD ■ Avoid in clients with heart failure ■ May cause tachycardia, headache, flushing, local phlebitis
ACE Inhibitor			
Enalaprilat (Vasotec)	15 to 30 min	6 to 12 h	■ Monitor for hypotension ■ Used in acute left heart failure ■ Avoid in acute myocardial infarction
Adrenergic Blockers			
Labetalol (Trandate)	5 to 10 min	3 to 6 h	■ Avoid in clients with acute heart failure and asthma ■ May cause nausea, vomiting, dizziness ■ Monitor for dyspnea, wheezing, heart block, orthostatic hypotension
Esmolol (Brevibloc)	1 to 2 min	10 to 30 min	■ Avoided in clients with heart failure and asthma ■ May cause nausea ■ Monitor for hypotension, dyspnea, wheezing, heart failure, first-degree heart block
Phentolamine (Regitine)	1 to 2 min	10 to 30 min	■ May cause tachycardia, flushing, headache

treating any underlying or coexisting heart, kidney, and CNS disorders.

Nursing care for the client with a hypertensive emergency focuses on continuous monitoring of the blood pressure and titrating drugs (administered by intravenous bolus or infusion) as ordered to achieve desired blood pressure. Avoiding excessive or very rapid blood pressure reductions is as important as achieving the desired blood pressure readings. Reassure the client and family of the rapid effect of prescribed drugs. Provide psychologic and emotional support as needed. Maintain an attitude of confidence that the treatment will achieve the desired effect. Following resolution of the hypertensive crisis, review causes of the crisis. Teach the client and family measures to effectively manage hypertension and prevent future hypertensive emergencies.

DISORDERS OF THE AORTA AND ITS BRANCHES

The aorta and its branches may be affected by occlusions, aneurysms, and inflammations. These disorders may be chronic or acute and life threatening (e.g., a thoracic dissection). This section focuses on aneurysms of the aorta and its branches.

THE CLIENT WITH AN ANEURYSM

An **aneurysm** is an abnormal dilation of a blood vessel, commonly at a site of a weakness or tear in the vessel wall. Aneurysms commonly affect the aorta and peripheral arteries, because of the high pressure in these vessels. An aneurysm also may develop in the ventricular wall, usually affecting the left ventricle. Most arterial aneurysms are caused by arteriosclerosis or atherosclerosis; trauma also may lead to aneurysm formation.

Arterial aneurysms are most common in men over age 50, most of whom are asymptomatic at the time of diagnosis. Hypertension is a major contributing factor in the development of some types of aortic aneurysms.

FAST FACTS

- The incidence of aortic aneurysm is an estimated 5.9 per 100,000 persons per year.
- Aortic dissection affects an estimated 5 to 30 per 1 million people per year.
- Although aortic aneurysm and aortic dissection can occur concurrently, this is rare (Wung & Aouizerat, 2004).

Pathophysiology and Manifestations

Aneurysms form due to weakness of the arterial wall. The major structural proteins of the aorta are collagen and elastin. Collagen provides tensile strength of the vessel, preventing excessive dilation. Elastin allows vessel recoil, during which the vessel returns to its original size following systole. This recoil provides continued propulsion of the bolus of blood expelled from the ventricle. Elastin is a primary component of internal elastic lamina, which separates the intimal and medial layers of the aorta, and of the media, the smooth muscle layer of the aorta. Destruction of elastin can lead to abnormal dilation of the vessel; collagen destruction can allow the vessel to rupture (Wung & Aouizerat, 2004).

True aneurysms are caused by slow weakening of the arterial wall due to the long-term, eroding effects of atherosclerosis and hypertension. True aneurysms affect all three layers of the vessel wall, and most are fusiform and circumferential. *Fusiform aneurysms* are spindle shaped and taper at both ends. *Circumferential aneurysms* involve the entire diameter

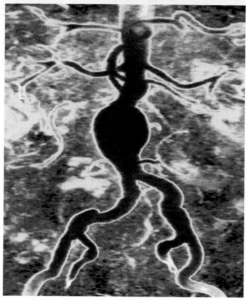

Figure 35–4 ■ A magnetic resonance angiogram (MRA) showing a circumferential aneurysm of the lower abdominal aorta.
Source: Zephyr, Photo Researchers, Inc.

of the vessel (Figure 35–4 ■). They generally grow slowly but progressively. Their length and diameter vary considerably among clients. A large fusiform aneurysm may affect most of the ascending aorta as well as a large portion of the abdominal aorta.

False aneurysms, also known as traumatic aneurysms, are caused by a traumatic break in the vessel wall rather than weakening of the vessel. They often are *saccular,* shaped like small outpouchings (sacs) on a portion of the vessel wall (Figure 35–5 ■). A *berry aneurysm* is a type of saccular aneurysm. They are often small (less than 2 cm in diameter), caused by congenital weakness in the tunica media of the artery. Berry aneurysms are commonly found in the circle of Willis in the brain.

Dissecting aneurysms are unique, developing when a break or tear in the tunica intima and media allows blood to invade or *dissect* the layers of the vessel wall. The blood usually is contained by the adventitia, forming a saccular or longitudinal aneurysm).

Aneurysms affect different segments of the aorta and its branches. Their manifestations generally are due to pressure of the aneurysm on adjacent structures. Table 35–4 summarizes the manifestations and complications of various types of aortic aneurysms.

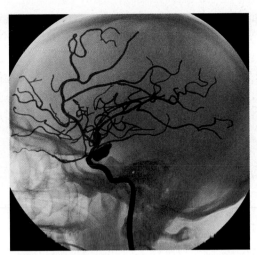

Figure 35–5 ■ An angiogram showing a saccular (berry) aneurysm in the carotid artery of a 50-year-old man.

Source: Simon Fraser/RNC, Newcastle, Photo Researchers, Inc.

Thoracic Aortic Aneurysms

Thoracic aortic aneurysms account for about 10% of aortic aneurysms, with an annual incidence of about 6 per 100,000 people (Klein, 2005). See Figure 35–6 ■. They usually result from weakening of the aortic wall by arteriosclerosis and hypertension (Tierney et al., 2005). Other causes include trauma, coarctation of the aorta, tertiary syphilis, fungal infections, and Marfan syndrome. The syphilis spirochete can invade and weaken aortic smooth muscle, causing an aneurysm to develop as long as 20 years after the primary infection. Marfan syndrome fragments elastic fibers of the aortic media, weakening the vessel wall. The box on page 1172 discusses genetic links associated with thoracic aortic aneurysms.

Thoracic aneurysms frequently are asymptomatic. When present, manifestations are caused by the effects of the aneurysm on blood flow (e.g., to the coronary arteries and

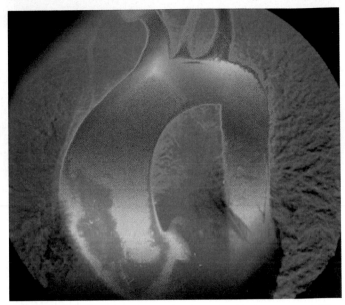

Figure 35–6 ■ An angiogram showing a large aneurysm of the ascending aorta and aortic arch.

great vessels of the head and upper body) and pressure placed by distended aorta on surrounding structures. Consequently, manifestations vary by the location, size, and growth rate of the aneurysm. Substernal, neck, or back pain may occur. Pressure on the trachea, esophagus, laryngeal nerve, or superior vena cava may cause dyspnea, stridor, cough, difficult or painful swallowing, hoarseness, edema of the face and neck, and distended neck veins.

Aneurysms of the ascending aorta typically cause angina due to disruption of blood flow into the coronary arteries. Heart failure may develop as a result of disruption of the aortic valve and

TABLE 35–4 Manifestations and Complications of Aortic Aneurysms

TYPE OR LOCATION	MANIFESTATIONS	COMPLICATIONS
Thoracic	■ May be asymptomatic ■ Back, neck, or substernal pain ■ Dyspnea, stridor, or brassy cough if pressing on trachea ■ Hoarseness and dysphagia if pressing on esophagus or laryngeal nerve ■ Edema of the face and neck ■ Distended neck veins	■ Rupture and hemorrhage
Abdominal	■ Pulsating abdominal mass ■ Aortic calcification noted on x-ray ■ Mild to severe midabdominal or lumbar back pain ■ Cool, cyanotic extremities if iliac arteries are involved ■ Claudication (ischemic pain with exercise, relieved by rest)	■ Peripheral emboli to lower extremities ■ Rupture and hemorrhage
Aortic dissection	■ Abrupt, severe, ripping or tearing pain in area of aneurysm ■ Mild or marked hypertension early ■ Weak or absent pulses and blood pressure in upper extremities ■ Syncope	■ Hemorrhage ■ Renal failure ■ MI, heart failure, cardiac tamponade ■ Sepsis ■ Weakness or paralysis of lower extremities

GENETIC CONSIDERATIONS
Thoracic Aortic Aneurysms

About 20% of clients with aortic aneurysms have a family history of the disorder.

A condition known as *cystic medial necrosis* is prevalent in clients with Marfan syndrome and Ehlers-Danlos syndrome, inherited disorders involving connective tissues. In cystic medial necrosis, collagen and elastic fibers of the tunica media of the aorta degenerate. This loss of collagen and elastic tissues weakens the wall of the proximal aorta, leading to circumferential dilation of the ascending aorta and development of a fusiform aneurysm. In many other clients with thoracic aortic aneurysm (up to 20%), genetic syndromes affecting collagen and elastin are not recognized, but a strong family history of the disorder is present (Wung & Aouizerat, 2004).

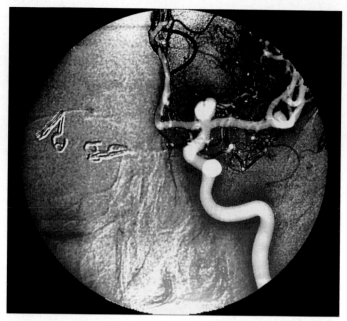

Figure 35–7 ■ An angiogram showing several popliteal aneurysms.
Source: Zephyr, Photo Researchers, Inc.

regurgitation of blood back into the left ventricle. Aneurysms of the aortic arch often cause dysphagia, dyspnea, hoarseness, confusion, and dizziness (due to disrupted cerebral blood flow). Thrombi that form within a thoracic aneurysm can embolize, causing a stroke, renal or mesenteric ischemia, or ischemia of the lower extremities (Klein, 2005). Aneurysms of the thoracic aorta tend to enlarge progressively and may rupture, causing death.

Abdominal Aortic Aneurysms

Abdominal aortic aneurysms are associated with arteriosclerosis and hypertension. Increasing age and smoking are believed to contribute as well. Most abdominal aortic aneurysms are found in adults over age 70. The vast majority (over 90%) develop below the renal arteries, usually where the abdominal aorta branches to form the iliac arteries (see Figure 35–4).

Most abdominal aneurysms are asymptomatic, but a pulsating mass in the mid and upper abdomen and a bruit over the mass are found on exam. When pain is present, it may be constant or intermittent, usually felt in the midabdominal region or lower back. Its intensity may range from mild discomfort to severe pain. Pain intensity often correlates with the size and severity of the aneurysm. Severe pain may indicate impending rupture.

Sluggish blood flow within the aneurysm may cause thrombi (blood clots) to form. These can become emboli (circulating clots), traveling to the lower extremities and occluding peripheral arteries. The aneurysm may also rupture, with hemorrhage and hypovolemic shock. The risk of rupture increases as the size of the aneurysm increases; 20% to 40% of aneurysms more than 5 cm in diameter rupture. After acute rupture, the mortality rate is greater than 50%, even when emergency surgery is performed (Kasper et al., 2005).

Popliteal and Femoral Aneurysms

Most popliteal and femoral aneurysms are due to arteriosclerosis. They are often bilateral and usually affect men.

Popliteal aneurysms may be asymptomatic (Figure 35–7 ■). Manifestations, if any, are due to decreased blood flow to the lower extremity and include **intermittent claudication** (cramping or pain in the leg muscles brought on by exercise and relieved by rest), rest pain, and numbness. A pulsating mass may be palpable in the popliteal fossa (behind the knee). Thrombo-

sis and embolism are complications; gangrene may result, often necessitating amputation.

A *femoral aneurysm* usually is detected as a pulsating mass in the femoral area. The manifestations are similar to those of popliteal aneurysms, resulting from impaired blood flow. Femoral aneurysms may rupture.

Aortic Dissections

Dissection is a life-threatening emergency caused by a tear in the intima of the aorta with hemorrhage into the media. The hemorrhage dissects or splits the vessel wall, forming a blood-filled channel between its layers. Dissection can occur anywhere along the aorta. *Type A dissection* (also called *proximal dissection*) affects the ascending aorta; *type B dissection* (*distal dissection*) is limited to the descending aorta.

Hypertension is a major predisposing factor for aortic dissection, accounting for 70% of aortic dissections. Cystic medial necrosis (see the Genetic Considerations box above) also is a major risk factor. Other risk factors include male gender, advancing age, pregnancy, congenital defects of the aortic valve, coarctation of the aorta, and inflammatory aortitis (Kasper et al., 2005).

Dissection of the thoracic aortic walls progresses along the length of the vessel, moving both proximally and distally. As the aneurysm expands, pressure may prevent the aortic valve from closing or may occlude the branches of the aorta. Descending aortic dissection may extend into the renal, iliac, or femoral arteries.

The primary symptom of an aortic dissection is sudden, excruciating pain. The pain, often described as a ripping or tearing sensation, is usually over the area of dissection. Thoracic dissections cause chest or back pain. Other symptoms may include syncope, dyspnea, and weakness. The blood pressure may initially be increased, but rapidly falls and is often inaudible as the dissection occludes blood flow. Peripheral pulses are absent for the same reason.

Complications develop if major arteries are affected. Obstruction of the carotid artery causes neurologic symptoms such as weakness or paralysis. The myocardium, kidneys, or bowel may become ischemic or infarct if blood flow to the coronary arteries, renal arteries, or mesenteric artery is affected. Acute aortic regurgitation may develop with dissection of the ascending aorta. With treatment, the long-term prognosis is generally good, although the in-hospital mortality rate following surgery is 15% to 20% (Kasper et al., 2005).

INTERDISCIPLINARY CARE

Most aneurysms are asymptomatic, detected through a routine physical examination. Treatment depends on the size of the aneurysm. Small, asymptomatic aneurysms may not be treated or are medically managed; large aneurysms (>5 cm) at risk for rupture require surgery.

Diagnosis

Diagnostic studies done to establish the diagnosis and determine the size and location of the aneurysm may include:

- *Chest x-ray* to visualize thoracic aortic aneurysms.
- *Abdominal ultrasonography* to diagnose abdominal aortic aneurysms.
- *Transesophageal echocardiography* to identify the specific location and extent of a thoracic aneurysm and to visualize a dissecting aneurysm.
- *Contrast-enhanced CT* or *MRI* allows precise measurements of aneurysm size.
- *Angiography* uses contrast solution injected into the aorta or involved vessel to visualize the precise size and location of the aneurysm.

Medications

Thoracic aortic aneurysms may be treated with long-term beta-blocker therapy and additional antihypertensive drugs as needed to control heart rate and blood pressure.

Clients with aortic dissection are initially treated with intravenous beta-blockers such as propranolol (Inderal), metoprolol (Lopressor), or esmolol (Brevibloc) to reduce the heart rate to about 60 bpm. Sodium nitroprusside (Nipride) infusion is started concurrently to reduce the systolic pressure to 120 mmHg or less. Calcium channel blockers (verapamil and diltiazem) also may be used. Direct vasodilators such as diazoxide (Hyperstat) and hydralazine (Apresoline) are avoided because they may actually worsen the dissection (Kasper et al., 2005). Constant monitoring of vital signs, hemodynamic pressures (via Swan-Ganz catheter; see Chapter 32 ∞ for more information about hemodynamic pressure monitoring), and urine output are vital to ensure adequate perfusion of vital organs.

Following surgical correction of an aneurysm, anticoagulant therapy may be initiated. Heparin therapy is used initially, with conversion to oral anticoagulation prior to discharge. Many clients are maintained indefinitely on anticoagulant therapy; others may use lifelong, low-dose aspirin therapy to reduce the risk of clot formation.

Surgery

Operative repair of aortic aneurysms is indicated when the aneurysm is symptomatic or expanding rapidly. Thoracic aneurysms more than 6 cm in diameter are surgically repaired; asymptomatic abdominal aneurysms greater than 5 cm in diameter may be repaired, depending on the client's operative risk factors. Type A dissections are repaired as soon as feasible; type B dissections may be surgically repaired, depending on the extent of involvement and risk for rupture (Kasper et al., 2005).

Endovascular stent grafts (EVSGs) are increasingly being used to treat abdominal and thoracic aortic aneurysms. The use of EVSG to treat aortic dissections is in investigational stages. The stent, which consists of a metal sheath covered with polyester fabric or a woven polyester tube, usually is placed percutaneously via the femoral artery. Fluoroscopy is used to guide its placement. Both straight and bifurcated grafts are available. Endovascular stent placement results in a shorter hospital stay and lower treatment cost. EVSG is associated with fewer pulmonary, renal, and cardiovascular complications than open surgical aneurysm repair (Jones, 2005). This option generally is preferred for clients who have a high surgical risk. The most common complication of endovascular aneurysm repair is persistent perfusion of the aneurysm (*endoleak*) caused by an ineffective seal at the proximal or distal end of the graft (Way & Doherty, 2003). Regular follow-up with abdominal CT scans is necessary to detect this complication, which can develop at any time postoperatively. Because stent grafts are handcrafted to fit the individual, repeated CT scans with contrast media are required preoperatively, increasing the risk for kidney damage and renal failure. On rare occasions, the graft may be malpositioned or may migrate from the desired location (Jones, 2005).

An open surgical procedure in which the aneurysm is excised and replaced with a synthetic fabric graft is the standard treatment for expanding abdominal aortic aneurysms (Figure 35–8 ■). Although the aneurysm walls may be excised, they usually are left intact and used to cover the graft. Surgical repair of thoracic aneurysms is similar but more complex due to major vessels exiting at the aortic arch. Cardiopulmonary bypass is required if the ascending aorta is involved. The aortic valve also may be replaced during surgery. See the box on page 1174 for nursing care of the client having surgery of the aorta.

NURSING CARE

Assessment

Focused assessment for the client with a suspected aortic aneurysm includes:

- *Health history:* Complaints of chest, back, or abdominal pain; extremity weakness; shortness of breath, cough, difficult or painful swallowing, hoarseness; history of hypertension, coronary heart disease, heart failure, or peripheral vascular disease.
- *Physical examination:* Vital signs including blood pressure in upper and lower extremities; peripheral pulses; skin color

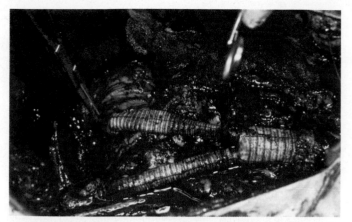

Figure 35–8 ■ Repair of an abdominal aortic aneurysm. The aorta is exposed and clamped between the renal and iliac arteries. Atherosclerotic plaque and thrombotic material are removed. A synthetic graft is used to replace the aneurysm. The aneurysm walls are then sutured around the graft.

Source: Stevie Grand, Photo Researchers, Inc.

and temperature; neck veins; abdominal exam including gentle palpation for masses and auscultation for bruits; neurologic exam including level of consciousness (LOC), sensation, and movement of extremities.

Nursing Diagnoses and Interventions

Nursing care for clients with an aneurysm of the aorta or its branches focuses on monitoring and maintaining tissue perfusion, relieving pain, and reducing anxiety. Nursing care usually is acute, precipitated by a complication or surgical repair of the aneurysm.

Risk for Ineffective Tissue Perfusion

Clients with aortic aneurysms are at risk for impaired tissue perfusion due to aneurysm rupture with resulting hemorrhage and lack of blood flow to tissues distal to the rupture. In addition, thrombi often form within the aneurysm and may become emboli, obstructing distal arterial blood flow.

NURSING CARE OF THE CLIENT HAVING   Surgery of the Aorta

PREOPERATIVE CARE
- As time permits, provide routine preoperative care and teaching as outlined in Chapter 4 ∞. *Clients having vascular surgery have similar preoperative nursing care needs to other clients having major abdominal or thoracic surgery. If emergent surgery is required, time for preoperative care and teaching may be limited.*
- Implement measures to reduce fear and anxiety:
  a. Orient to the intensive care unit, if appropriate.
  b. Describe and explain the reason for all equipment and tubes, such as cardiac monitors, ventilators, nasogastric tubes, urinary catheters, intravenous lines and fluids, and intra-arterial lines.
  c. Explain what to expect following surgery (sights, sounds, frequency of taking vital signs, dressings, pain relief measures, communication strategies).
  d. Allow time for questions and expression of fears and concerns.
  These explanations provide a sense of control for the client and family.
- Monitor for and implement care to reduce the risk of aneurysm rupture (see the following section). *Clients with a rapidly expanding or symptomatic aneurysm are at risk for rupture prior to surgical repair.*

POSTOPERATIVE CARE
- Provide routine postoperative care and specific measures as ordered by the physician. *Clients undergoing aneurysm repair require nursing care similar to that provided to all clients with major thoracic or abdominal surgery, in addition to specific measures related to vascular surgery.*
- Maintain fluid replacement and blood or volume expanders as ordered. Promptly report changes in vital signs, level of consciousness, and urine output. *Hypovolemic shock may develop due to blood loss during surgery, third spacing, inadequate fluid replacement, and/or hemorrhage if graft separation or leakage occurs.*

PRACTICE ALERT
Monitor for and report manifestations of graft leakage:
  a. Ecchymoses of the scrotum, perineum, or penis; a new or expanding hematoma
  b. Increased abdominal girth
  c. Weak or absent peripheral pulses; tachycardia; hypotension
  d. Decreased motor function or sensation in the extremities
  e. Fall in hemoglobin and hematocrit
  f. Increasing abdominal, pelvic, back, or groin pain
  g. Decreasing urinary output (less than 30 mL/h)
  h. Decreasing CVP, pulmonary artery pressure, or pulmonary artery wedge pressure.
These manifestations may signal graft leakage and possible hemorrhage. Pain may be due to pressure from an expanding hematoma or bowel ischemia. Decreased renal perfusion causes the glomerular filtration rate and urine output to fall.

- Report manifestations of lower extremity embolism: pain and numbness in lower extremities, decreasing pulses, and pale, cool, or cyanotic skin. *Pulses may be absent for 4 to 12 hours postoperatively due to vasospasm; however, absent pulses with pain, changes in sensation, and a pale, cool extremity are indicative of arterial occlusion.*
- Report manifestations of bowel ischemia or gangrene: abdominal pain and distention, occult or fresh blood in stools, and diarrhea. *Bowel ischemia may result from an embolism or occur as a complication of surgery.*
- Report manifestations of impaired renal function: urine output less than 30 mL/h, fixed specific gravity, increasing BUN and serum creatinine levels. *Hypovolemia or clamping of the aorta during surgery may impair renal perfusion, leading to acute renal failure.*
- Report manifestations of spinal cord ischemia: lower extremity weakness or paraplegia. *Impaired spinal cord perfusion may lead to ischemia and impaired function.*

PRACTICE ALERT

Immediately report manifestations of impending rupture, expansion, or dissection of the aneurysm: increased pain; discrepancy between upper and lower extremity blood pressures and peripheral pulses; increased mass size; change in LOC or motor or sensory function; laboratory results. Rapid expansion may indicate increased risk for rupture, with resulting hemorrhage, shock, and possible death. Elective or planned surgery may rapidly become emergency surgery to prevent complications.

■ Implement interventions to reduce the risk of aneurysm rupture:
  a. Maintain bed rest with legs flat.
  b. Maintain a calm environment, implementing measures to reduce psychologic stress.
  c. Prevent straining during defecation and instruct to avoid holding the breath while moving.
  d. Administer beta-blockers and antihypertensives as prescribed.

Activity, stress, and the Valsalva maneuver increase blood pressure, increasing the risk of rupture. Elevating or crossing the legs restricts peripheral blood flow and increases pressure in the aorta or iliac arteries. Beta-blockers and antihypertensives often are ordered to reduce pressure in the dilated vessel.

PRACTICE ALERT

Report manifestations of arterial thrombosis or embolism: absent peripheral pulses; a pale or cyanotic, cool extremity; severe, diffuse abdominal pain with guarding; or increased groin, lumbar, or lower extremity pain. Sluggish blood flow within the aneurysm often causes thrombi to form. These thrombi can break loose, becoming emboli that can occlude peripheral arteries or arteries to the kidneys or mesentery. Arterial occlusion may necessitate emergency surgery to restore blood flow and prevent tissue infarct or gangrene.

■ Continuously monitor cardiac rhythm. Report complaints of chest pain or changes in ECG tracing. Administer oxygen as indicated. *Aortic dissection and repair place the client at significant risk for MI, a major cause of postoperative mortality and morbidity (Kasper et al., 2005). Rapid identification and treatment of this complication can reduce the risk of death or long-term adverse effects of MI.*

PRACTICE ALERT

Immediately report changes in mental status or symptoms of peripheral neurologic impairment (weakness, paresthesias, paralysis). The expanding aneurysm or dissection can affect carotid and cerebral blood flow or spinal cord perfusion, leading to neurologic symptoms. Immediate restoration of blood flow is vital to prevent permanent neurologic deficits.

Risk for Injury

Potent antihypertensive drugs often are given intravenously to reduce the pressure on an expanding or dissecting aneurysm. Continuous monitoring of infusions and hemodynamic param-

eters such as arterial pressure, pulmonary pressures, and cardiac output is vital to ensure that adequate tissue perfusion is maintained during infusions of these potent drugs.

PRACTICE ALERT

Use an infusion control device for all drug infusions. These devices prevent accidental or inadvertent changes in the rate of the infusion and dose of the drug.

■ Continuously monitor arterial pressure and hemodynamic parameters as indicated. Promptly report results outside the specified parameters to the physician. *Many of the drugs used are effective within minutes. Responses vary among individuals, particularly in the older adult, necessitating continuous monitoring.*
■ Monitor urine output hourly. Report output less than 30 mL/h. *The kidneys are very sensitive to reduced perfusion pressure; inadequate renal blood flow can lead to acute renal failure.*

Anxiety

Clients with aortic aneurysms often are highly anxious because of the urgent nature of the disorder. The nurse must manage the anxiety levels of both the client and family members to effectively address physiologic care needs. Stress reduction also is necessary to help maintain the blood pressure within desired limits.

■ Explain all procedures and treatments, using simple and understandable terms. *Simplified explanations are necessary when anxiety levels interfere with learning and understanding.*
■ Respond to all questions honestly, using a calm, empathetic, but matter-of-fact manner. *Honesty with the client and family promotes trust and provides reassurance that the true nature of the situation is not being "hidden" from them.*
■ Provide care in a calm, efficient manner. *Using a calm manner even during preparations for emergency surgery reassures the client and family that although the situation is critical, the staff is prepared to handle things effectively.*
■ Spend as much time as possible with the client. Allow supportive family members to remain with the client when possible. *The presence of a health professional and supportive family member reassures the client that he or she is not alone in facing this crisis.*

Community-Based Care

Topics to discuss when preparing clients and their families for home care or care in a community-based setting depend on the treatment plan. Discuss the following topics when surgical repair is not immediately planned and the aneurysm will be monitored:
■ Measures to control hypertension, including lifestyle and prescribed drugs
■ The benefits of smoking cessation
■ Manifestations of increasing aneurysm size or complications to report to the physician.

Following surgery, discuss the following topics in preparing the client and family for home care:
■ Wound care and preventing infection; manifestations of impaired healing or infection to be reported
■ Prescribed antihypertensive and anticoagulant medications and their expected and unintended effects

- The importance of adequate rest and nutrition for healing
- Measures to prevent constipation and straining at stool (such as increasing fluid and fiber in the diet)
- The importance of avoiding prolonged sitting, lifting heavy objects, engaging in strenuous exercise, and having sexual intercourse until approved by the physician (usually 6 to 12 weeks)

- Signs and symptoms of complications to report to the physician.

   Provide referrals to a home health agency or community health service as necessary. Referrals are especially important for older adults and their caregivers, who may require additional assistance with the complex care needs.

DISORDERS OF THE PERIPHERAL ARTERIES

Disorders that impair peripheral arterial blood flow may be *acute* (e.g., arterial thrombosis) or *chronic* (e.g., peripheral arteriosclerosis). Chronic occlusive disorders may be due to structural defects of the arterial walls or spasm of affected arteries. Impaired peripheral arterial circulation limits the availability of oxygen and nutrients to the tissues, and can have significant adverse effects. This section focuses on acute and chronic disorders affecting peripheral arteries. The nurse's role in caring for clients with peripheral arterial disorders focuses on maintaining tissue perfusion and educating the client and family about the disorder and its management.

Physiology Review

Peripheral arteries are the part of the systemic circulation that delivers oxygen and nutrients to the skin and the extremities. Arterial walls have three layers: the intima, which includes the endothelium and a layer of connective tissue and the basement membrane; the media, composed of smooth muscle and elastic fibers; and the adventitia, a thin layer of connective tissue that contains collagen and elastic fibers. The smooth muscle of peripheral arteries controls blood flow as it contracts and relaxes. Contraction narrows the vessel lumen (**vasoconstriction**), whereas smooth muscle relaxation expands the vessel (**vasodilation**). Peripheral arteries become progressively smaller; arterioles are less than 0.5 mm in diameter and are composed primarily of smooth muscle. The arterioles control blood flow through the capillary beds where gas, nutrient, and waste product exchange occurs. Capillary walls are very thin, consisting of a single layer of endothelial cells surrounded by a thin basement membrane.

   Blood flows from an area of higher pressure to an area of lower pressure. *Resistance* opposes blood flow. Resistance is created by friction of the blood itself, although the primary determinants of vascular resistance are the diameter and length of the blood vessel. See the physiology review section earlier in this chapter under "Disorders of Blood Pressure Regulation" for more information about factors that determine vessel resistance.

THE CLIENT WITH PERIPHERAL VASCULAR DISEASE

Arteriosclerosis is the most common chronic arterial disorder, characterized by thickening, loss of elasticity, and calcification of arterial walls. **Atherosclerosis** is a form of arteriosclerosis in which deposits of fat and fibrin obstruct and harden the arteries. In the peripheral circulation, these pathologic changes impair the blood supply to peripheral tissues, particularly the lower extremities. This is known as **peripheral vascular disease (PVD)** or peripheral artery disease (PAD).

Incidence and Risk Factors

PVD usually affects people in their 60s and 70s; men are more often affected than women. Deaths attributed to peripheral arterial disease are about the same for black and white males, but are higher among black women than white women (NHLBI, 2004a).

   Risk factors for PVD are similar to those for atherosclerosis and CHD (see Chapter 30 ∞). Diabetes mellitus, hypercholesterolemia, hypertension, cigarette smoking, and high homocystine levels are risk factors for PVD (Kasper et al., 2005).

> **FAST FACTS**
> - PVD is a common manifestation of atherosclerosis, particularly in older men.
> - PVD interferes with arterial blood flow to the lower extremities, increasing the risk for neuropathy and paresthesias, ulcers that do not heal, necrosis, gangrene, and amputation.
> - Regular daily exercise is a primary intervention for all types of peripheral arterial disease to promote development of collateral circulation and maintain tissue perfusion.

Pathophysiology

The pathophysiology of atherosclerosis is detailed in Chapter 31 ∞ . Atherosclerotic lesions involve both the intima and the media of the involved arteries. Lesions typically develop in large and midsize arteries, particularly the abdominal aorta and iliac arteries (30% of symptomatic clients), the femoral and popliteal arteries (80% to 90% of clients), and more distal arteries (40% to 50% of clients) (Kasper et al., 2005). Arteriosclerosis in the abdominal aorta leads to the development of aneurysms as plaque erodes the vessel wall.

   Plaque tends to form at arterial bifurcations. The vessel lumen is progressively obstructed, decreasing blood flow to the lower extremities. Tissue hypoxia or anoxia results. With gradual obstruction of the vessel, collateral circulation often develops. However, it is usually not adequate to supply tissue needs, especially when metabolic demand increases (e.g., during exercise). Manifestations typically develop only when the vessel is occluded by 60% or more.

Manifestations and Complications

Pain is the primary symptom of peripheral atherosclerosis. **Intermittent claudication,** a cramping or aching pain in the calves of the legs, the thighs, and the buttocks that occurs with a predictable level of activity, is characteristic of PVD. The pain is often accompanied by weakness and is relieved by rest.

Rest pain, in contrast, occurs during periods of inactivity. It is often described as a burning sensation in the lower legs. Rest pain increases when the legs are elevated and decreases when the legs are dependent (e.g., hanging over the side of the bed). The legs also may feel cold or numb along with the pain. Sensation is diminished and the muscles may atrophy.

Peripheral pulses may be decreased or absent. A bruit may be heard over large affected arteries, such as the femoral artery and the abdominal aorta. The legs are pale when elevated, but often are dark red (*dependent rubor*) when dependent. The skin often is thin, shiny, and hairless, with discolored areas. Toenails may be thickened. Areas of skin breakdown and ulceration may be evident. Edema may develop with severe PVD. See the box below for manifestations of peripheral atherosclerosis.

Complications of peripheral atherosclerosis include gangrene and extremity amputation, rupture of abdominal aortic aneurysms, and possible infection and sepsis.

INTERDISCIPLINARY CARE

Management of peripheral vascular disease focuses on slowing the atherosclerotic process and maintaining tissue perfusion.

Diagnosis

Although PVD often can be diagnosed by the history and physical examination, diagnostic tests may be ordered to evaluate its extent. Noninvasive studies often are sufficient.

- *Segmental pressure measurements* use sphygmomanometer cuffs and a Doppler device to compare blood pressures between the upper and lower extremities (normally similar) and within different segments of the affected extremity. In PVD, the BP may be lower in the legs than in the arms.
- *Stress testing* using a treadmill provides functional assessment of limitations. In PVD, pressure at the ankle may decline even further with exercise, confirming the diagnosis. Evaluation for coronary heart disease may be done simultaneously during exercise testing (Kasper et al., 2005).
- *Doppler ultrasound* uses sound waves reflected off moving red blood cells within a vessel to evaluate blood flow. The impulses may be translated into an audible signal or a graphic waveform. With significant PVD, the waveform becomes progressively flatter as the transducer is moved distally along the affected vessel. Segmental pressures may be used to locate the site of obstruction.

MANIFESTATIONS of Peripheral Atherosclerosis

- Intermittent claudication
- Rest pain
- Paresthesias (numbness, decreased sensation)
- Diminished or absent peripheral pulses
- Pallor with extremity elevation, dependent rubor when dependent
- Thin, shiny, hairless skin; thickened toenails
- Areas of discoloration or skin breakdown

- *Duplex Doppler ultrasound* combines the audible or graphic Doppler ultrasound with ultrasound imaging to identify arterial or venous abnormalities. Ultrasonic imaging provides views of the affected vessel while Doppler ultrasound evaluates blood flow. *Color-flow Doppler ultrasound (CDU)* provides color images of the vessel and blood flow.
- *Transcutaneous oximetry* evaluates oxygenation of tissues.
- *Angiography* or *magnetic resonance angiography* is done before revascularization procedures to locate and evaluate the extent of arterial obstruction. For angiography, a contrast medium is injected and vessels are visualized using fluoroscopy and x-rays. MRA does not require injection of a contrast medium and may replace angiography.

See Chapter 33 ∞ for more information on diagnostic testing for PVD.

Medications

Drug treatment of peripheral atherosclerosis is less effective than with coronary heart disease. Medications to inhibit platelet aggregation, such as aspirin or clopidogrel (Plavix), are ordered to reduce the risk of arterial thrombosis. Cilostazol (Pletal), a platelet inhibitor with vasodilator properties, improves claudication. Pentoxifylline (Trental) decreases blood viscosity and increases red blood cell flexibility, increasing blood flow to the microcirculation and tissues of the extremities. Parenteral vasodilator prostaglandins may be given on a long-term basis to decrease pain and facilitate healing in clients with severe limb ischemia (Kasper et al., 2005).

Treatments

Smoking cessation is vital. Nicotine not only promotes atherosclerosis, but also causes vasospasm, further reducing blood flow to the extremities.

Meticulous foot care is vital to prevent ulceration and infection (Box 35–4). Elastic support hose, which reduce circulation to the skin, are avoided. Elevating the head of the bed on blocks may help relieve rest pain. Regular, progressively strenuous exercise, such as 30 to 45 minutes of walking daily, is important. The client is taught to rest at the onset of claudication, resuming activity when the pain resolves.

Other measures to slow the process of atherosclerosis, such as controlling diabetes and hypertension, lowering cholesterol levels, and weight loss, also are recommended (see Chapter 30 ∞). See the box on page 1178 for care of the older adult.

Revascularization

Revascularization may be performed if symptoms are progressive, severe, or disabling. Other indications for surgery include symptoms that significantly interfere with activities of daily living (ADLs), rest pain, and pregangrenous or gangrenous lesions. Either nonsurgical revascularization procedures or surgery may be performed.

Nonsurgical procedures include percutaneous transluminal angioplasty (PTA), stent placement, or atherectomy. Techniques may include balloon angioplasty to dilate the narrowed lumen, mechanical atherectomy to remove plaque, or laser or thermal angioplasty to vaporize the occluding material. In either case, a stent typically is placed at the time of PTA to maintain vessel

---

BOX 35–4 Foot Care for the Client with Peripheral Atherosclerosis

1. Keep legs and feet clean, dry, and comfortable.
   - Wash legs and feet daily in warm water, using mild soap.
   - Pat dry using a soft towel; be sure to dry between the toes.
   - Apply moisturizing cream to prevent drying.
   - Use powder on the feet and between the toes.
   - Buy shoes in the afternoon (when feet are largest); never buy shoes that are uncomfortable. Be sure toes have adequate room.
   - Wear a clean pair of cotton socks each day.
2. Prevent accidents and injuries to the feet.
   - Always wear shoes or slippers when getting out of bed.
   - Walk on level ground and avoid crowds, if possible.
   - Do not go barefoot.

- Inspect legs and feet daily; use a mirror to examine backs of legs and bottoms of feet.
- Have a professional foot care provider trim toenails and care for corns, calluses, ingrown toenails, or athlete's foot.
- Always check the temperature of the water before stepping into the tub.
- Do not get the legs or tops of the feet sunburned.
- Report leg or foot problems (increased pain, cuts, bruises, blistering, redness, or open areas) to your healthcare provider.

3. Improve blood supply to the legs and feet.
   - Do not cross legs.
   - Do not wear garters or knee stockings.
   - Do not swim or wade in cold water.

---

patency. Iliac and femoral-popliteal PTA initially reestablish good blood flow and relieve symptoms in more than 80% of clients. While the 3-year success rate is lower, stent placement improves the duration of symptom relief (Kasper et al., 2005). See Chapter 31 ∞ for more information about revascularization procedures.

Surgical options include endarterectomy to remove occlusive plaque from the artery and bypass grafts. Knitted Dacron bypass grafts are commonly used. Both immediate and long-term graft patency is better with bypass grafting than with non-surgical revascularization procedures, but the risk for operative complications such as myocardial infarction, stroke, infection, and peripheral embolization is higher (Kasper et al., 2005). Nursing care for the client having revascularization surgery is similar to that provided for clients having an aortic aneurysm repair (see the box on page 1174).

Complementary Therapies

Complementary therapies for peripheral vascular disease include interventions to improve circulation and to reduce stress. A number of complementary therapies may improve peripheral circulation, including aromatherapy with rosemary or vetiver; biofeedback; healing or therapeutic touch and massage;

herbals such as ginkgo, garlic, cayenne, hawthorn, and bilberry; and exercise including yoga. Aromatherapy and yoga also may reduce stress, as can breathing exercises, meditation, and counseling. In addition, complementary therapies to reduce atherosclerosis and lower cholesterol levels may slow the progress of PVD. Measures such as a very low-fat or vegetarian diet, including antioxidant nutrients or using vitamin C, vitamin E, or garlic supplements, and traditional Chinese medicine may be useful.

 NURSING CARE

Health Promotion

Discuss healthy lifestyle habits with community and religious groups, schoolchildren (grades K through 12), and through the print media to reduce the incidence and slow the progression of atherosclerosis.

Strongly encourage all clients to avoid smoking in the first place, and to stop all forms of tobacco use. Discuss the adverse effects of smoking and the benefits of quitting. Provide information about dietary recommendations to maintain a healthy weight and optimal cholesterol levels. Discuss the benefits and importance of regular exercise. Finally, encourage clients with cardiovascular risk factors to undergo regular screening for hypertension, diabetes, and hyperlipidemia.

Assessment

Focused assessment related to peripheral atherosclerosis includes the following:

- *Health history:* Complaints of pain, its relationship to exercise or rest, timing, associated symptoms, and relief measures; history of coronary heart disease, peripheral vascular disease, hyperlipidemia, hypertension, or diabetes; current medications; smoking history; usual diet and activity patterns.
- *Physical examination:* Vital signs; strength and equality of peripheral pulses of all extremities; capillary refill; skin color, temperature, hair distribution, presence of any discolorations or lesions; movement and sensation of lower extremities.

NURSING CARE OF THE OLDER ADULT
Peripheral Vascular Disease

With aging, blood vessels thicken and become less compliant. These changes reduce oxygen delivery to the tissues and impair carbon dioxide and waste product removal from the tissues. When normal effects of aging combine with an increased risk of atherosclerosis, the risk of peripheral vascular disease is high.

The older adult with peripheral vascular disease requires the same care and teaching as other clients. However, visual deficits and osteoarthritis may make foot care more difficult. Long-standing smoking habits are difficult to break. Mobility may be impaired by arthritis or the effects of neurologic disorders. The client who lives alone may resist walking. Periodic visits by a community or home health nurse may be helpful, as may be encouraging the client to join a support group for stopping smoking, changing eating habits, and taking part in regular activity.

Nursing Diagnoses and Interventions

Impaired tissue perfusion is an obvious problem in peripheral atherosclerosis. Acute and chronic pain may interfere with ADLs, and ambulation may be limited. The possibility of losing a lower extremity is frightening.

Ineffective Tissue Perfusion: Peripheral

Impaired blood flow to the lower extremities affects gas, nutrient, and waste product exchange between the capillaries and cells. Oxygen and nutrient deprivation impairs cell function and tissue integrity, causing pain and impaired healing. Pain develops with exercise and when extremities are elevated.

- Assess peripheral pulses, pain, color, temperature, and capillary refill every 4 hours and as needed. Use a Doppler device if pulses are not palpable. Mark pulse locations with an indelible marker. *Assessment data provide a baseline for evaluating the effectiveness of interventions and identifies changes in arterial blood flow.*
- Position with extremities dependent. *Gravity promotes arterial flow to the dependent extremity, increasing tissue perfusion and relieving pain.*

PRACTICE ALERT

Instruct to avoid smoking. If necessary, obtain an order for a nicotine patch or gum from the physician. Nicotine is a potent vasoconstrictor that further impairs arterial blood flow. Smoking cessation is a vital component of care. Nicotine patches and gum contain less nicotine than cigarettes, and can help reduce the stress of smoking cessation.

- Discuss the benefits of regular exercise. *Exercise promotes development of collateral circulation to ischemic tissues and slows the process of atherosclerosis.*
- Use a foot cradle and lightweight blankets, socks, and slippers to keep extremities warm. Avoid electric heating pads or hot water bottles. *Keeping extremities warm conserves heat, prevents vasospasm, and promotes arterial flow. External heating devices are avoided to reduce the risk of burns in the client with impaired sensation. The foot cradle protects tissues from compression by linens.*
- Encourage frequent position changes. Instruct to avoid crossing legs or using a pillow under the knees. *Position changes promote blood flow and reduce damage caused by pressure. Leg crossing and excessive flexion of the hip or knee joints can compress partially obstructed arteries and impair blood flow to distal tissues.*

Pain

Impaired blood flow results in tissue ischemia. Metabolism shifts from an efficient aerobic process to an anaerobic process. Lactic acid and metabolic waste products accumulate in tissues, causing pain. Severe and cramping pain generally occurs with exercise early in the disease. Rest initially produces relief, similar to the process of angina (see Chapter 31 ∞). As the disease progresses, pain develops with less exercise and often occurs even at rest. Rest pain disrupts sleep, the sense of well-being, and has significant disruptive effects on life roles.

- Assess pain at least every 4 hours, using a standard pain scale. *Pain is a subjective experience. Using a standard pain scale allows evaluation of treatment measures in relieving pain and restoring blood flow.*
- Keep extremities warm. *Cooling leads to vasoconstriction, increasing pain. Warming the extremities promotes vasodilation and improves arterial flow, reducing pain.*
- Teach pain relief and stress reduction techniques such as relaxation, meditation, and guided imagery. *Pain increases stress. The stress response leads to vasoconstriction, increasing pain. Stress reduction techniques, when combined with other measures to promote blood flow, can help reduce pain.*

Impaired Skin Integrity

Clients with PVD are at risk for impaired skin integrity as a result of oxygen and nutrient deprivation. Chronic tissue ischemia leads to dry, scaly, and atrophied skin. Pruritus can lead to scratching; minor injuries may go unnoticed due to impaired sensation. Impaired tissue healing can lead to ulceration, infection, and potential gangrene.

PRACTICE ALERT

Assess and document skin condition at least every 8 hours or with each home visit; more frequently as indicated. Tissue ischemia increases the risk for damage, even with minor trauma such as pressure from poorly fitting shoes or bed linens. Frequent inspection and documentation of skin condition is vital to identify early indicators of impaired skin integrity and reduce the risk of complications such as infection.

- Provide meticulous daily skin care, keeping the skin clean and dry. Apply a moisturizing cream to dry or scaly areas. *Intact skin is the body's first defense against bacterial invasion. Ischemic tissues of the injured extremity provide an excellent medium for microorganism growth. Clean, dry, supple skin decreases the risk of breakdown.*
- Apply a bed cradle. *The bed cradle suspends bed linens over the legs, preventing them from placing pressure on extremities and injured tissues. Minimizing pressure on the tissues promotes capillary blood flow.*
- Provide an egg-crate mattress, flotation pad, sheepskin, or heel protectors. *Ischemic tissues may be damaged by minor trauma such as that created by the shearing forces of skin against bed linens.*

Activity Intolerance

Pain and impaired perfusion of peripheral tissues may limit the client's ability to engage in desired activities, even impairing self-care.

- Assist with care activities as needed. *Severe claudication or rest pain may limit activities. Muscle atrophy of affected extremities is common, leading to fatigue and weakness.*
- Unless contraindicated, encourage gradual increases in duration and intensity of exercise. Teach to rest with extremities dependent when claudication develops, resuming activity after pain has abated. *Gradual increases in the duration and intensity of exercise promote development of collateral circulation,*

improve exercise tolerance, provide a sense of well-being, and support self-esteem.

- Provide diversional activities during periods of prescribed bed rest. Encourage relaxation techniques to reduce muscle tension. *Diversional activities help prevent boredom and stress associated with enforced rest. Relaxation techniques reduce vasoconstriction induced by stress, improving peripheral circulation.*
- Encourage frequent position changes and active range-of-motion exercises. Encourage self-care to the extent possible. *Position changes relieve pressure on tissues, improving capillary circulation and reducing tissue ischemia. Range-of-motion exercises help prevent muscle atrophy and joint contractures. Self-care supports self-esteem.*

Using NANDA, NIC, and NOC

Chart 35–2 shows links between NANDA nursing diagnoses, NIC, and NOC for the client with peripheral vascular disease.

Community-Based Care

Discuss the following topics when preparing the client and family for home and community-based care. See the accompanying Nursing Care Plan for additional community-based nursing interventions.

- Smoking cessation strategies and ways to avoid second-hand smoke

---

NANDA, NIC, AND NOC LINKAGES
CHART 35–2 The Client with Peripheral Vascular Disease

NANDA

Ineffective Tissue Perfusion: Peripheral

↓

NIC

Circulatory Care: Arterial Insufficiency

Exercise Promotion

Positioning

Skin Surveillance

↓

NOC

Tissue Integrity: Skin and Mucous Membranes

Activity Tolerance

Tissue Perfusion: Peripheral

Data from *NANDA's Nursing Diagnoses: Definitions & Classification 2005–2006* by NANDA International (2005), Philadelphia; *Nursing Interventions Classification (NIC)* (4th ed.) by J. M. Dochterman & G. M. Bulechek (2004), St. Louis, MO: Mosby; and *Nursing Outcomes Classification (NOC)* (3rd ed.) by S. Moorhead, M. Johnson, and M. Maas (2004), St. Louis, MO: Mosby.

- Prescribed medications and anticoagulants, their purpose, doses, desired and adverse effects
- Signs of excess bleeding to report to the physician
- Skin surveillance and foot care (see Box 35–4)
- Recommended diet and exercise
- Weight loss strategies if appropriate.

If revascularization or surgery has been performed, include the following topics as appropriate:

- Incision care
- Manifestations of complications (e.g., infection, graft leakage, or thrombosis) to be reported to the physician
- Activity limitations.

Provide referrals to home health services, physical or occupational therapy, and home maintenance assistance services as indicated. Consider resources such as Meals-on-Wheels for clients who are severely limited by their disease.

THE CLIENT WITH THROMBOANGIITIS OBLITERANS

Thromboangiitis obliterans (also called *Buerger's disease*) is an occlusive vascular disease in which small and midsize peripheral arteries become inflamed and spastic, causing clots to form. This disease may affect either the upper or lower extremities; it often affects a leg or foot. Its exact etiology is unknown.

Incidence and Risk Factors

Thromboangiitis obliterans primarily affects men under age 40 who smoke. Cigarette smoking is the single most significant cause of the disease. The disease is more prevalent in Asians and people of Eastern European descent. The incidence of HLA-B5 and 2A9 antigens is higher in people with thromboangiitis obliterans, suggesting a genetic link.

Pathophysiology and Course

Inflammatory cells infiltrate the wall of small and midsize arteries in the feet and possibly the hands. This inflammatory process is accompanied by thrombus formation and vasospasms of arterial segments that impair blood flow. Adjacent veins and nerves also may be affected. As the disease progresses, affected vessels become scarred and fibrotic.

The course of the disease is intermittent with dramatic exacerbations and marked remissions. The disease may remain dormant for periods of weeks, months, or years. As the disease progresses, collateral vessels are more extensively involved. Consequently, subsequent episodes are more intense and prolonged. Prolonged periods of tissue hypoxia increase the risk for tissue ulceration and gangrene.

Manifestations and Complications

Pain in the affected extremities is the primary manifestation of thromboangiitis obliterans. Both claudication, cramping pain in calves and feet or the forearms and hands, and rest pain in

NURSING CARE PLAN   A Client with Peripheral Vascular Disease

William Duffy, age 69, is retired. His wife convinces him to see his primary care provider for increasing leg pain with walking and other exercise.

ASSESSMENT

Katie Kotson, RN, obtains Mr. Duffy's history before he sees his physician. He states that he can only walk about a block before the pain in his calves gets so bad that he has to stop and rest. As a result, he has been less and less active, spending most of his time the past few months watching sports on television. He denies rest pain. He was diagnosed with type 2 diabetes about 15 years ago, which he manages with daily glyburide (DiaBeta), an oral hypoglycemic. He also has stable angina, for which he takes atenolol (Tenormin) and an occasional nitroglycerin tablet. His alcohol intake is moderate, averaging one to two beers per day, and he smokes about a pack of cigarettes per day. He states he tried to quit smoking after developing angina, but "after nearly 50 years of smoking, I think that's impossible!"

Physical exam findings include height 68 inches (173 cm), weight 235 lb (107 kg), BP 160/78, P 66, R 16, T 97.6°F (36.5°C); upper extremities warm and pink, normal hair distribution, pulses strong and equal; lower extremities below knees cool and ruddy when dependent, pale to pink when elevated, skin shiny, scant hair; posterior tibial pulses weak bilaterally; weak pedal pulse on R, unable to palpate on L; 1+ to 2+ edema both feet and ankles.

The physician finds that Mr. Duffy's systolic blood pressure in his legs is an average of 28 mmHg lower than in his arms. He makes the diagnosis of peripheral atherosclerosis, and schedules Mr. Duffy for an exercise stress test with ankle pressure measurements before and after exercise and a color-flow Doppler ultrasound. Mr. Duffy is to return in 3 weeks after these studies have been completed.

DIAGNOSES

- *Activity Intolerance* related to poor blood flow to lower extremities
- *Ineffective Health Maintenance* related to smoking and lack of information about disease management
- *Risk for Impaired Skin Integrity* related to ischemic tissues of legs and feet
- *Risk for Peripheral Neurovascular Dysfunction* related to impaired peripheral blood flow to lower extremities

EXPECTED OUTCOMES

- Walk for at least 15 minutes three to four times per day, gradually increasing his pace and duration of exercise.
- Relate the benefits of smoking cessation.
- Identify strategies to improve chances for success in stopping smoking.
- Meet with dietitian before next visit to discuss dietary measures to promote weight loss and slow atherosclerosis.

- Verbalize an understanding of appropriate foot care measures.
- Identify measures to prevent inadvertent injury of feet and legs.

PLANNING AND IMPLEMENTATION

- Teach about peripheral atherosclerosis and its relationship to Mr. Duffy's symptoms.
- With Mr. and Mrs. Duffy, plan strategies to start and maintain a program of regular exercise.
- Instruct to warm up slowly, and to stop exercise and rest for 3 minutes (or until pain is relieved) when claudication develops, then resume exercising.
- Discuss the effects of smoking on blood vessels.
- Help Mr. Duffy identify smoking cessation strategies such as support groups, clinics, and nicotine patches.
- Schedule an appointment with the dietitian to develop a low-calorie, low-fat, and low-cholesterol ADA diet that includes preferred foods and considers usual eating patterns.
- Reinforce and supplement previous foot care teaching.
- Discuss effects of impaired circulation on sensation in feet and legs and measures to prevent injury.

EVALUATION

When Mr. Duffy returns to the office 3 weeks later, his diagnosis has been confirmed by the diagnostic studies. The physician decides to continue conservative therapy, now prescribing atorvastatin (Lipitor) to lower Mr. Duffy's serum cholesterol level, and cilostazol (Pletal) to reduce the risk of thrombosis and improve symptoms of claudication. Mr. Duffy also asks his physician for a prescription for nicotine patches, saying he is ready to quit smoking, but thinks he needs help to be successful. Mr. and Mrs. Duffy tell Miss Kotson that they are walking before every meal and really enjoying being outside more. They plan to walk in the local shopping mall when the weather gets worse. Mrs. Duffy has bought an American Heart Association cookbook, and is carefully planning their meals. Both Mr. and Mrs. Duffy have lost 5 lb since the previous visit. Mr. Duffy's skin on his legs and feet remains intact, and he identifies the measures he is using to protect his lower extremities from injury.

CRITICAL THINKING IN THE NURSING PROCESS

1. What additional lifestyle changes related to peripheral atherosclerosis might be appropriate to suggest to Mr. Duffy at this time? Why?
2. Explain the relationship between physical exercise and pain in the client with peripheral atherosclerosis. Compare this relationship to that between exercise and angina.
3. Mr. Duffy uses a beta-blocker, atenolol, to prevent angina. Why is this drug not effective in preventing claudication?
4. Develop a nursing care plan for the nursing diagnosis *Imbalanced Nutrition: More than Body Requirements.*
   See Evaluating Your Response in Appendix C.

---

the fingers and toes may occur. Sensation is diminished. Eventually, the skin becomes thin and shiny and the nails are thickened and malformed. On examination, the involved digits and/or extremities are pale, cyanotic, or ruddy, and cool or cold to touch. Distal pulses (e.g., the dorsalis pedis, posterior tibial,

ulnar, or radial) are either difficult to locate or absent, even with a Doppler device.

Painful ulcers and gangrene may develop in the fingers and toes as a result of severely impaired blood flow. Amputation may be necessary to remove necrotic tissue.

INTERDISCIPLINARY CARE

Thromboangiitis obliterans usually is diagnosed by the history and physical examination. Doppler studies may be used to locate and determine the extent of the disease. Angiography and magnetic resonance imaging may also be used to evaluate the extent of the disease, but usually are unnecessary.

The one most important component in managing this disease is smoking cessation. While stopping smoking does not cure the disease, it may slow its extension to other vessels. With continued smoking, attacks become increasingly intense and last much longer, significantly increasing the risk for ulcerations and gangrene.

Additional conservative measures are used to prevent vasoconstriction, improve peripheral blood flow, and prevent complications of chronic ischemia. These measures include keeping extremities warm, managing stress, keeping affected extremities in a dependent position, preventing injury to affected tissues, and regular exercise. Walking for 20 or more minutes several times a day is recommended.

There are no specific drugs for thromboangiitis obliterans. A calcium channel blocker such as diltiazem (Cardizem) or verapamil (Isoptin), or pentoxifylline (Trental), which decreases blood viscosity and increases red blood cell flexibility to improve peripheral blood flow, may provide some symptom relief.

Surgical approaches for thromboangiitis obliterans include sympathectomy or arterial bypass graft. Sympathectomy interrupts sympathetic nervous system input to affected vessels, reducing vasoconstriction and spasm. Arterial bypass grafts may be useful when larger vessels are affected by the disease. Amputation of an affected digit or extremity may be necessary if gangrene develops (see Chapter 41 ∞ for more information about amputation). Only portions of digits or of limbs (e.g., below the knee) are usually amputated, to preserve as much healthy tissue as possible.

The prognosis for thromboangiitis obliterans depends significantly on the client's ability and willingness to stop smoking. With smoking cessation and good foot care, the prognosis for saving the extremities is good, even though no cure is available.

NURSING CARE

Health promotion activities to prevent thromboangiitis obliterans focus on preventing smoking, especially in high-risk populations. Nursing assessment and care for clients with this disease are similar to those provided for clients with other arterial occlusive diseases. Nursing care focuses on promoting arterial circulation and preventing prolonged tissue hypoxia. Because inflammatory, spastic episodes may be unpredictable, care focuses on smoking cessation and relieving acute manifestations. In addition, postsurgical care is necessary if surgery has been performed. See the nursing care section for peripheral atherosclerosis as well as nursing care of the postsurgical client (Chapter 4 ∞) and following amputation (Chapter 41 ∞).

Community-Based Care

Discuss the following topics when preparing clients with thromboangiitis obliterans and their families for home or community-based care:
- Absolute necessity of smoking cessation
- Foot care
- Protecting affected extremities from injury
- Purpose, dose, desired and adverse effects, interactions, and any precautions associated with prescribed medications
- Signs and symptoms to report to the physician.

THE CLIENT WITH RAYNAUD'S DISEASE

Raynaud's disease and **phenomenon** are characterized by episodes of intense vasospasm in the small arteries and arterioles of the fingers and sometimes the toes (Porth, 2005). Raynaud's disease and phenomenon differ only in terms of cause. Raynaud's disease has no identifiable cause; Raynaud's phenomenon occurs secondarily to another disease (such as collagen vascular diseases such as scleroderma and rheumatoid arthritis), other known causes of vasospasm, or long-term exposure to cold or machinery (McCance & Huether, 2006; Porth, 2005).

Raynaud's disease primarily affects young women between the ages of 20 and 40. Genetic predisposition may play a role in its development, although the actual cause is unknown. Table 35–5 compares thromboangiitis obliterans and Raynaud's disease.

Pathophysiology and Manifestations

Raynaud's disease and phenomenon are characterized by spasms of the small arteries in the digits. The arterial spasms limit arterial blood flow to the fingers and possibly the toes. Initial attacks may involve only the tips of one or two fingers; with disease progression, the entire finger and all fingers may be affected.

The manifestations of Raynaud's occur intermittently when spasms develop. Raynaud's disease has been called the "blue-white-red disease," because affected digits initially turn blue as blood flow is reduced due to vasospasm, then white as circulation is more severely limited, and finally very red as the fingers are warmed and the spasm resolves (Figure 35–9 ■). Sensory changes may occur during attacks, including numbness, stiffness, decreased sensation, and aching pain.

The attacks tend to become more frequent and prolonged over time. With repeated attacks (and resultant decrease in oxygenation), the fingertips thicken and the nails become brittle. Ulceration and gangrene are serious complications that rarely occur.

INTERDISCIPLINARY CARE

Raynaud's disease and phenomenon are primarily diagnosed by the history and physical examination. There are no specific diagnostic tests for these disorders.

Vasodilators may be prescribed to provide symptomatic relief. Low doses of a sustained release calcium channel blocker

TABLE 35–5   Comparison of Raynaud's Disease and Thromboangiitis Obliterans

TOPIC	RAYNAUD'S DISEASE	THROMBOANGIITIS OBLITERANS
Etiology	■ Unknown ■ Possible genetic predisposition	■ Cigarette smoking most probable single cause ■ Possible autoimmune response
Incidence/course of the disease	■ Onset commonly between 15 and 45 years of age ■ Usually affects young women ■ Becomes progressively worse over time	■ Occurs predominantly in men under age 40 ■ More common in Asians and people of European heritage ■ Intermittent course with exacerbations and remissions ■ Increased severity and duration of attacks over time
Triggering stimuli	■ Emotional stress ■ Exposure to cold	■ Cigarette smoking
Assessment findings	■ Usually affects hands, sometimes toes ■ Pain becomes more severe and prolonged as disease progresses ■ "Blue-white-red" changes in color of hands with accompanying changes in skin temperature	■ Claudication and pain ■ Numbness or diminished sensation ■ Cool, pale, or cyanotic skin ■ Shiny, thin skin and white, malformed nails in affected extremities ■ Distal pulses difficult to find or absent ■ Trophic changes to nail beds ■ Ulceration and gangrene in later stages ■ Small, red, tender vascular cords in affected extremities
Management	■ Avoid unnecessary cold exposure ■ Emphasize smoking cessation ■ Medications such as calcium channel or alpha-adrenergic blockers as indicated ■ Teach stress management	■ Stop smoking (crucial) ■ Regular exercise ■ Protect extremities from cold injury ■ Teach stress management

such as nifedipine (Procardia) or diltiazem (Cardizem) may be prescribed. The alpha-adrenergic blocker prazosin (Minipress) also may reduce the frequency and severity of attacks. Transdermal nitroglycerin (or longer acting oral nitrates) helps some clients by decreasing the amount of time necessary for the hands to return to normal following an attack (Tierney et al., 2005).

Conservative measures are a mainstay of treatment. Clients are instructed to keep their hands warm, wearing gloves when outside in cold weather and kitchen gloves when handling cold items (for instance, when preparing and serving cold foods and cleaning the refrigerator). Measures to avoid injury to the hands

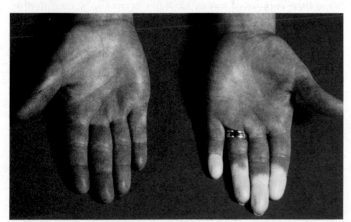

Figure 35–9 ■ Hands of a client with Raynaud's phenomenon. Note cyanosis of fingers on the right hand and the left thumb and the extreme pallor of the other digits of the left hand.
Source: Bart's Medical Library, Phototake NYC.

are taught. Sometimes attacks can be stopped by swinging the arms back and forth, increasing perfusion pressure in the small arteries by centrifugal force.

Smoking cessation is important. Stress reduction measures such as exercise, relaxation techniques, massage therapy, hobbies, aroma therapy, and counseling are taught or suggested. Additional lifestyle habits that contribute to vascular health are encouraged, such as reducing dietary fat, increasing activity level, and maintaining normal body weight.

NURSING CARE

Nursing care for the client with Raynaud's disease or phenomenon is primarily educative and supportive. Protecting the hands and feet from exposure to cold and trauma is the major teaching topic. Nursing diagnoses and interventions previously outlined for peripheral atherosclerosis also are appropriate for clients with Raynaud's.

Community-Based Care

Reassure clients with Raynaud's phenomenon that most people with the disorder experience only mild, infrequent episodes. Discuss the following topics in preparing the client for managing the disorder:
- Dress warmly, keeping the trunk and hands warm.
- Avoid unnecessary exposure to cold.
- Stop smoking or do not start.
- The use, purpose, desired and potential adverse effects of prescribed medications, if any.

THE CLIENT WITH ACUTE ARTERIAL OCCLUSION

A peripheral artery may be acutely occluded by development of a thrombus (blood clot) or by an embolism. Blood flow to tissues supplied by the artery is impaired, resulting in acute tissue ischemia and a risk for necrosis and gangrene.

Pathophysiology

Arterial Thrombosis

A **thrombus** is a blood clot that adheres to the vessel wall. Thrombi tend to develop in areas where intravascular factors stimulate coagulation (e.g., where a vessel lumen is partially obstructed and its wall is damaged and roughened by atherosclerosis). Other disorders, such as infection or inflammation of the vessel wall or pooling of blood (e.g., in an aneurysm) also can prompt coagulation and thrombus formation (McCance & Huether, 2006). A developing thrombus can occlude arterial blood flow through the vessel, leading to ischemia of tissues supplied by that artery. The extent of ischemia depends on the size of the affected artery and the degree of collateral circulation. In gradual processes of arterial occlusion such as atherosclerosis, collateral vessels often develop to compensate for impaired arterial flow. The extent of collateral circulation affects the degree of tissue ischemia distal to the thrombus.

Arterial Embolism

An **embolism** is sudden obstruction of a blood vessel by debris. A thrombus can break loose from the arterial wall to become a **thromboembolus**. Other substances also can become emboli: atherosclerotic plaque, masses of bacteria, cancer cells, amniotic fluid, bone marrow fat, and foreign objects such as air bubbles or broken intravenous catheters. Regardless of cause, an embolus eventually lodges in a vessel that is too small to allow it to pass.

Arterial emboli often originate in the left side of the heart. They are associated with myocardial infarction, valvular heart disease, left-sided heart failure, atrial fibrillation, or infectious heart diseases. Emboli from the left heart often enter the carotid arteries and become trapped in the cerebral circulation, causing neurologic deficits (see Chapter 43 ∞). Thromboemboli that develop in the aorta or peripheral arterial circulation tend to lodge in areas where the arterial lumen is narrowed by atherosclerotic plaque and at arterial bifurcations.

Manifestations

The manifestations of arterial thrombosis and embolism are those of tissue ischemia. Ischemic tissues are painful, pale, and cool or cold. Distal pulses are absent. Paresthesias (numbness and tingling) develop in the extremity. Cyanosis and mottling are common. Paralysis and muscle spasms may develop in the affected extremity. A line of demarcation between normal and ischemic tissue may be seen, particularly with embolism. Tissue below the line is cool or cold, and pale, cyanotic, or mottled. See the Manifestations box that follows.

Arterial occlusion can result in permanent vessel and limb damage. Complete arterial occlusion leads to tissue necrosis and gangrene unless blood flow is promptly restored.

> ### MANIFESTATIONS of Acute Arterial Occlusion
>
> - Pain
> - Pallor or mottling
> - Paresthesias (numbness and tingling)
> - Cool or cold skin
> - Pulselessness distal to the blockage
> - Possible paralysis, weakness, or muscle spasms
> - Possible line of demarcation; with pallor, cyanosis, and cooler skin distal to the blockage (especially with arterial embolism)

INTERDISCIPLINARY CARE

Acute arterial occlusions may require emergency treatment to preserve the limb if the obstructed vessel is large or collateral circulation is minimal. If the limb is not in jeopardy, more conservative management may be initiated.

Diagnosis

The diagnosis of acute arterial occlusion often is apparent by the signs and symptoms. *Arteriography* is used to confirm the diagnosis, locate the occlusion, and determine its extent.

Medications

Anticoagulation with intravenous heparin is initiated to prevent further clot propagation and recurrent embolism. Anticoagulation is continued with oral anticoagulants after discharge. See the section on venous thrombosis later in this chapter for more information about anticoagulant therapy.

Arterial thrombosis may be treated with intra-arterial fibrinolytic therapy using streptokinase, urokinase, or tissue plasminogen activator (t-PA) (see Chapter 31 ∞). Lysis of the thrombus or embolus is achieved in 50% to 80% of the cases (Tierney et al., 2005). Local intra-arterial injection of the fibrinolytic drug allows use of lower doses and reduces the bleeding risk associated with fibrinolytic drugs.

Surgery

Immediate *embolectomy* (within 4 to 6 hours) is the treatment of choice for acute arterial occlusion by an embolus to prevent tissue necrosis and gangrene. When the involved vessel is in an extremity, local anesthesia and a special balloon-tipped catheter known as a Fogarty catheter may be used for high surgical risk clients (Tierney et al., 2005). An embolus in the mesenteric circulation necessitates emergency laparotomy. The risk of complications and limb loss increases significantly if surgery is delayed by 12 or more hours. Potential major complications include compartment syndrome (see Chapter 41 ∞), acute respiratory distress syndrome (Chapter 39 ∞), or acute renal failure (Chapter 28 ∞).

Arterial thrombosis also may be treated surgically, although the required surgery may be more extensive due to the length of the vessel involved. *Thromboendarterectomy* is done to remove the thrombus and plaque in the artery. An arterial graft may be required. Nursing care for clients who have undergone embolectomy or thrombus removal is discussed in the nursing care section that follows.

NURSING CARE

Assessment

Nursing assessment for the client with an acute arterial occlusion is highly focused due to the emergency nature of the problem.

- *Health history:* Complaints of pain, numbness, tingling, or weakness in the involved extremity; history of atherosclerotic vessel disease, heart disease, or recent invasive procedure (e.g., angiography, percutaneous revascularization procedure).
- *Physical examination:* Vital signs; peripheral pulses in both extremities; color, temperature, sensation, and movement of involved extremity; skin condition; presence of a line of demarcation.

Nursing Diagnoses and Interventions

Nursing care related to acute arterial occlusion focuses on protecting the affected extremity, managing anxiety, and reducing the risk of complications related to anticoagulant therapy.

Ineffective Tissue Perfusion: Peripheral

Protecting ischemic tissue from injury prior to surgery or medical thrombolysis is vital. Following surgery, there is a risk for thrombosis at the graft site or impaired perfusion due to edema of the surgical site.

PRACTICE ALERT

Monitor extremity perfusion, comparing affected and unaffected extremities. Assess peripheral pulses (using the Doppler stethoscope as needed), skin temperature and color, capillary refill, movement, and sensation every 1 to 4 hours. Promptly report changes or complaints of increased or unrelieved pain. Propagation of a thrombus can further obstruct arterial flow, increasing tissue ischemia. Following surgery, arterial spasms may cause a cyanotic, pulseless extremity; normal color and pulses should return within 12 hours. A thrombus may form at the surgical site or within a graft, causing tissue ischemia with pain and other manifestations of arterial occlusion. Further measures to restore circulation may be necessary.

- Maintain intravenous fluids as ordered. *Adequate circulating blood volume is necessary to maintain cardiac output and tissue perfusion.*
- Protect the extremity, keeping it horizontal or lower than the heart. Use a cradle to keep bedclothes off the extremity and sheepskin or foam pad to protect it from hard or abrasive surfaces. Do not apply heat or cold. *Keeping the extremity lower than the heart promotes collateral blood flow. Ischemic tissue is easily damaged by minimal trauma such as shearing by bed linens, or heat or cold application.*
- Following surgery, avoid raising the knee gatch, placing pillows under the knees, or sitting with 90-degree hip flexion. *These activities may impair blood flow through the affected vessel.*

Anxiety

Clients with an acute arterial occlusion often are very anxious. The rapid and intense nature of preoperative activities can be overwhelming, increasing anxiety about the disorder and its out-

come. Manifestations of anxiety may include trembling, palpitations, restlessness, dry mouth, helplessness, inability to relax, irritability, forgetfulness, and lack of awareness of surroundings. Nursing measures focus on establishing trust and minimizing the effects of anxiety to decrease surgical risk and improve recovery.

- Spend as much time as possible with the client. Provide opportunities to verbalize anxiety; offer reassurance and support. Support adaptive coping mechanisms. *The presence of a caring nurse provides a safe environment for expressing fears and anxieties. Coping mechanisms reduce the immediate perceived threat and increase the ability to deal with the situational crisis.*
- Perform required measures in an expedient but calm manner. *Calm, confident performance of treatment measures reassures the client and family that appropriate care is being given to treat the problem at hand.*
- Assess anxiety level at least every 8 hours; more often as needed. Intervene as indicated to reduce anxiety. *Assessment helps determine the intensity of anxiety, the client's ability to control it, and directs interventions to reduce it.*
- Decrease sensory stimuli as much as possible. *Reducing environmental stimuli provides the client a degree of control over anxiety.*
- Speak slowly and clearly and avoid unnecessary interruptions when listening. Give concise directions, focusing on the present. Involve the client in simple tasks and decisions to the extent possible. *High levels of anxiety interfere with learning. Keeping interactions focused on the present situation directs the client's focus and provides reassurance that it is the most important focus of the nurse as well. Providing opportunities for self care and decision making reinforces the client's importance and power to control the situation.*

Altered Protection

Fibrinolytic and/or anticoagulant therapy used to dissolve existing clots and prevent further clot formation increase the risk for bleeding. Close monitoring of physical status and laboratory data is vital, as are measures to reduce the risk for injury and bleeding.

PRACTICE ALERT

Assess for and report manifestations of impaired clotting, including excessive incisional bleeding; prolonged oozing from injection sites; bleeding gums, nosebleed, or hematuria; petechiae, bruising, or purpura. Anticoagulants and fibrinolytics interfere with the clotting cascade and may cause abnormal bleeding.

- Monitor activated partial thromboplastin time (aPTT) during heparin therapy and prothrombin time (PT) or International Normalized Ratio (INR) during oral anticoagulant therapy. Report values outside desired range. *The APTT, PT, and INR are prolonged by anticoagulant therapy. Values higher than the desired range may indicate an increased risk for bleeding; values below the target may indicate inadequate anticoagulation.*
- Protect from injury: Use side rails or other measures as needed to prevent falls; avoid parenteral injections and other invasive procedures as much as possible; hold firm pressure over injection and intravenous sites for 5 minutes and over

occludes. See Chapter 39 ∞ for more information about pulmonary emboli.

Superficial Venous Thrombosis

Venous catheters and infusions are the primary risk factors for superficial venous thrombosis. Superficial venous thrombosis also may develop in conjunction with thromboangiitis obliterans, varicose veins, or DVT. It may develop spontaneously in pregnant women or following delivery. In some cases, superficial venous thrombosis of the long saphenous vein is the earliest sign of an abdominal cancer such as pancreatic cancer (Tierney et al., 2005).

Superficial venous thrombosis is marked by pain and tenderness at the site of the thrombus. A reddened, warm, tender cord extending along the affected vein can be palpated. The area surrounding the vein may be swollen and red (see the Manifestations box).

INTERDISCIPLINARY CARE

It is important to differentiate venous thrombosis from other causes of extremity pain, such as cellulitis, muscle strain, contusion, and lymphedema. The history, physical examination, and diagnostic tests are used to establish the diagnosis. Treatment focuses on preventing further clotting or extension of the clot and addressing underlying causes.

Diagnosis

- *Duplex venous ultrasonography* is a noninvasive test used to visualize the vein and measure the velocity of blood flow in the veins. Although the clot often cannot be visualized directly, its presence can be inferred by an inability to compress the vein during the examination.
- *Plethysmography* is a noninvasive test that measures changes in blood flow through the veins. It is often used in conjunction with Doppler ultrasonography. Plethysmography is most valuable in diagnosing thromboses of larger or more superficial veins.
- *Magnetic resonance imaging (MRI)* is another noninvasive means of detecting DVT. It is particularly useful when thrombosis of the venae cavae or pelvic veins is suspected.
- *Ascending contrast venography* uses an injected contrast medium to assess the location and extent of venous thrombosis. Although invasive, expensive, and uncomfortable, contrast venography is the most accurate diagnostic tool for venous thrombosis. It is used when the results of less invasive tests leave the diagnosis unclear (Tierney et al., 2005).

Prophylaxis

Medications and other measures are used to prevent venous thrombosis when the risk is high. Low-molecular-weight (LMW) heparins prevent DVT in clients who are undergoing general or orthopedic surgery, experiencing acute medical illness, or on prolonged bed rest. Oral anticoagulation also may be used as a prophylactic measure in clients with fractures or who are undergoing orthopedic surgery.

Elevating the foot of the bed with the knees slightly flexed promotes venous return. Early mobilization and leg exercises

such as ankle flexion and extension assist venous flow by muscle compression. Intermittent pneumatic compression devices applied to the legs are effective to prevent DVT. They also are used when anticoagulation is contraindicated due to the increased risk for bleeding (Kasper et al., 2005). Elastic stockings are also used to prevent venous thrombosis in clients at risk.

Medications

Anticoagulants to prevent clot propagation and enable the body's own lytic system to dissolve the clot are the mainstay of treatment for venous thrombosis. Fibrinolytic drugs such as streptokinase or t-PA may accelerate the process of clot lysis and prevent damage to venous valves. There is, however, no evidence that fibrinolytic therapy is more effective in preventing pulmonary embolism in clients with existing DVT than anticoagulants (Kasper et al., 2005). It also significantly increases the risk for bleeding and hemorrhage.

Nonsteroidal anti-inflammatory agents (NSAIDs) such as indomethacin (Indocin) or naproxen (Naprosyn) may be ordered to reduce inflammation in the veins and provide symptomatic relief, particularly for clients with superficial venous thrombosis.

ANTICOAGULANTS Anticoagulants are given to prevent clot extension and reduce the risk of subsequent pulmonary embolism. See the Medication Administration box on pages 1189–1190 for the nursing implications for anticoagulant therapy.

Anticoagulation is initiated with unfractionated heparin or LMW heparin. Following an initial intravenous bolus of 7500 to 10,000 units of unfractionated heparin, a continuous heparin infusion of 1000 to 1500 international units per hour is started. The dosage is calculated to maintain the aPTT at approximately twice the control or normal value. An infusion pump is used to deliver the prescribed dosage. Frequent monitoring of the infusion is an important nursing responsibility. Subcutaneous heparin injections may be used as an alternative to intravenous infusion in some instances.

LMW heparins are increasingly used to prevent and treat venous thrombosis. They do not require the close laboratory monitoring of unfractionated heparins. LMW heparin is administered subcutaneously in fixed doses once or twice daily, allowing the option of outpatient treatment. LMW heparins have additional advantages, in that they are more effective and carry lower risks for bleeding and thrombocytopenia than conventional, unfractionated heparins.

Oral anticoagulation with warfarin may be initiated concurrently with heparin therapy. Overlapping heparin and warfarin therapy for 4 to 5 days is important because the full anticoagulant effect of warfarin is delayed, and it may actually promote clotting during the first few days of therapy (Tierney et al., 2005). Warfarin doses are adjusted to maintain the INR at 2.0 to 3.0 (Kasper et al., 2005).

Once this level is achieved, the heparin is discontinued and a maintenance dose of warfarin is prescribed to prevent recurrent thrombosis. Anticoagulation generally is continued for at least 3 months. When DVT is recurrent or risk factors such as altered coagulability or cancer are present, anticoagulant therapy may be prolonged. Regular follow-up is necessary to

MEDICATION ADMINISTRATION Anticoagulant Therapy

HEPARIN

Heparin interferes with the clotting cascade by inhibiting the effects of thrombin and preventing the conversion of fibrinogen to fibrin. This prevents the formation of a stable fibrin clot. At therapeutic levels, heparin prolongs the thrombin time, clotting time, and activated partial thromboplastin time. When given intravenously, its effect is immediate. Given subcutaneously, its onset of action is within 1 hour. When heparin is discontinued, clotting times return to normal within 2 to 6 hours (Spratto & Woods, 2003). *Heparin-induced thrombocytopenia (HIT)* is a potential complication of therapy with unfractionated heparin. See Chapter 34 for more information about HIT and nursing responsibilities in monitoring for this dangerous potential complication.

Nursing Responsibilities

- Assess for history of unexplained or active bleeding. Assess laboratory results for abnormal clotting profile or evidence of active bleeding.
- Give a test dose as indicated to clients with a history of multiple allergies or a history of asthma.
- Administer by deep subcutaneous injection; abdominal sites are preferred. Avoid injecting within 2 inches of the umbilicus. Rotate sites. Do not aspirate prior to injecting or massage after the injection.
- Intravenous solutions may be diluted with dextrose, normal saline, or Ringer's solution. Use an infusion pump.
- Keep protamine sulfate, a heparin antagonist, available to treat excessive bleeding.
- Monitor and report abnormal laboratory results and aPTT values outside the desired range.
- Promptly report evidence of bleeding such as hematemesis, hematuria, bleeding gums, or unexplained abdominal or back pain.

Health Education for the Client and Family

- Report unusual bleeding or excessive menstrual flow.
- Use an electric razor and a soft-bristle toothbrush; prevent injury by clearing pathways, using a night light, and other measures. Do not consume alcohol.
- Avoid contact sports while on anticoagulant therapy.
- Do not consume large amounts of food rich in vitamin K (yellow and dark green vegetables).
- Do not use aspirin or NSAIDs while on heparin therapy unless advised to do so by your physician.
- Wear a Medic-Alert tag and advise all healthcare providers (including dentists and podiatrists) of therapy.

LOW-MOLECULAR-WEIGHT HEPARINS
Ardeparin (Normiflo)
Dalteparin (Fragmin)
Enoxaparin (Lovenox)
Tinzaparin (Innohep)

LMW heparins are the most bioavailable fraction of heparin. They provide a more precise and predictable anticoagulant effect than unfractionated heparins. Like unfractionated heparin, LMW heparin prevents conversion of prothrombin to thrombin, liberation of thromboplastin from platelets, and formation of a stable clot. LMW heparins cannot be used interchangeably with each other or with unfractionated heparin. Although the risk of heparin-induced thrombocytopenia is significantly lower with LMW heparin, clients who were previously treated with unfractionated heparin may develop HIT when treated with LMW heparin.

Nursing Responsibilities

- Assess for evidence of active bleeding, a history of bleeding disorders or thrombocytopenia, or sensitivity to heparin, sulfites, or pork products.
- Monitor for unusual or masked bleeding. PT and aPTT levels may be within normal levels even in the presence of hemorrhage.
- Administer by deep subcutaneous injection into abdominal wall, thigh, or buttocks. Rotate sites. Do not aspirate or massage.

Health Education for the Client and Family

- Subcutaneous self-administration technique, timing of doses, and site rotation. Do not rub site after administering to minimize bruising.
- Do not take aspirin, NSAIDs, or other over-the-counter drugs unless recommended by your physician.
- Promptly report excessive bruising or bleeding, chest pain, difficulty breathing, itching, rash, or swelling to your healthcare provider.
- Keep follow-up appointments as scheduled.

ORAL ANTICOAGULANT
Warfarin (Coumadin)

Warfarin interferes with synthesis of vitamin K–dependent clotting factors by the liver, leading to depletion of these factors. It has no effect on already circulating clotting factors or on existing clots. Warfarin inhibits extension of existing thrombi and the formation of new clots. Its action is cumulative and more prolonged than that of heparin.

Nursing Responsibilities

- Assess laboratory results and history for evidence of abnormal bleeding.
- Multiple drugs affect the metabolism and protein binding of warfarin; note all medications and assess for interactions with warfarin.
- Do not give during pregnancy because warfarin may cause congenital malformations.
- Oral tablets may be crushed and given without regard to meals.
- Dilute intravenous warfarin with supplied diluent; administer within 4 hours by direct intravenous injection at a rate of 25 mg/min.
- Keep vitamin K available to reverse effects of warfarin in the event of excessive bleeding or hemorrhage.
- Monitor PT or INR; report values outside the desired range.

Health Education for the Client and Family

- If bleeding occurs (hematemesis, bright red or black tarry feces, hematuria, bleeding gums, excessive bruising, etc.), do not take your prescribed dose and notify your physician immediately. Report rash or manifestations of hepatitis (dark urine, malaise, yellow skin or sclera).
- Take your warfarin at the same time every day; do not change brands because their effects may differ.

(continued)

MEDICATION ADMINISTRATION **Anticoagulant Therapy (continued)**

■ Menstrual bleeding may be slightly increased; contact your healthcare provider if it increases significantly. Use reliable birth control to prevent pregnancy while taking warfarin. Immediately contact your healthcare provider if you think you may be pregnant.

■ Take precautions to prevent injury and bleeding: use a soft-bristle toothbrush and electric razor, wear shoes, and use a night light. Avoid participating in contact sports.

■ Do not smoke, use alcohol, or take any over-the-counter drugs unless specifically recommended by your healthcare provider. Notify all healthcare providers, including dentists and podiatrists, of therapy. Wear a Medic-Alert tag.

■ Obtain lab tests as scheduled and keep all scheduled follow-up appointments.

be sure prothrombin times (INR) remain within the desirable range for anticoagulation.

Treatments

Treatment of venous thrombosis also includes measures to relieve symptoms and reduce inflammation. With superficial venous thrombosis, applying warm, moist compresses over the affected vein, extremity rest, and anti-inflammatory agents usually provide relief of symptoms.

Bed rest may be ordered for deep venous thrombosis. The duration of bed rest typically is determined by the extent of leg edema. The legs are elevated 15 to 20 degrees, with the knees slightly flexed, above the level of the heart to promote venous return and discourage venous pooling. Elastic antiembolism stockings (TEDS) or pneumatic compression devices are also frequently ordered to stimulate the muscle-pumping mechanism that promotes the return of blood to the heart. When permitted, walking is encouraged while avoiding prolonged standing or sitting. Crossing the legs also is avoided, as are tight-fitting garments or stockings that bind.

Surgery

Venous thrombosis usually is effectively treated with conservative measures and anticoagulation. In some cases, however, surgery is required to remove the thrombus, prevent its extension into deep veins, or prevent the effects of embolization.

Venous thrombectomy is done when thrombi lodge in the femoral vein and their removal is necessary to prevent pulmonary embolism or gangrene. Successful thrombus removal rapidly improves venous circulation. The duration of this effect varies.

When venous thrombosis is recurrent and anticoagulant therapy is contraindicated, a filter may be inserted into the vena cava to capture emboli from the pelvis and lower extremities, preventing pulmonary embolism. Several different filters are available (Figure 35–11 ■). The Greenfield filter is widely used for its ability to trap emboli within its apex while maintaining patency of the vena cava. The filter can be inserted under fluoroscopy with local anesthesia. Mortality and morbidity associated with the filter are very low.

Extensive thrombosis of the saphenous vein may necessitate ligation and division of the saphenous vein where it joins the femoral vein to prevent clot extension into the deep venous system. A vein affected by septic venous thrombosis

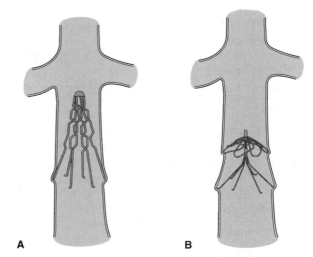

Figure 35–11 ■ Venal caval filters. *A,* Greenfield filter. *B,* Nitinol filter.

is excised to control the infection. Antibiotic therapy also is initiated.

NURSING CARE

Health Promotion

Prevention of venous thrombosis is an important component of nursing care for all at-risk clients. Position clients to promote venous blood flow from the lower extremities, with the feet elevated and the knees slightly bent. Avoid placing pillows under the knees and positions in which the hips and knees are sharply flexed. Use a recliner chair or footstool when sitting. Ambulate clients as soon as possible, and maintain a regular schedule of ambulation throughout the day. Teach ankle flexion and extension exercises, and frequently remind clients to perform them. Apply elastic hose and pneumatic compression devices when appropriate. Instruct clients to avoid crossing legs when in bed or sitting. Inquire about possible prophylactic heparin or warfarin therapy for clients undergoing orthopedic surgery or other high-risk procedures. Frequently assess intravenous sites. Change the site and catheter as dictated by agency protocol and if evidence of local inflammation is noted.

Assessment

Assess clients at risk for venous thrombosis for manifestations and risk factors.

- *Health history:* Complaints of leg or calf pain, its duration and characteristics, and the effect of walking on the pain; history of venous thrombosis or other clotting disorders; current medications.
- *Physical examination:* Inspect affected extremity for redness, edema; palpate for tenderness, warmth, cordlike structures; body temperature.
- *Diagnostic tests:* Clotting studies (aPTT, protime, INR).

See the accompanying Nursing Care Plan for an example of an assessment of a client with deep venous thrombosis.

Nursing Diagnoses and Interventions

In addition to the preventive measures identified earlier, priority nursing diagnoses for the client with venous thrombosis relate to pain, maintenance of tissue perfusion and integrity, and the potential adverse effects of prescribed treatments.

Pain

The pain associated with venous thrombosis results from inflammation of the involved vein. It may be aggravated by use

---

NURSING CARE PLAN A Client with Deep Venous Thrombosis

Mrs. Opal Hipps, age 75, lives alone with her dog, Chester, in her family home in the suburbs. She retired from her job as a postal clerk 10 years ago and now spends a lot of time reading and watching television. Over the past week she has developed a vague aching pain in her right leg. She ignored the pain until last night when it developed into a much more severe pain in her right calf. She noticed that her right lower leg seemed larger than the left, and it was very tender to the touch. After seeing her physician and undergoing Doppler ultrasound studies, Mrs. Hipps is admitted to the hospital with the diagnosis of deep venous thrombosis in the right leg. She is placed on bed rest, and intravenous heparin. Michael Cookson, RN, is assigned to admit and care for Mrs. Hipps.

ASSESSMENT

Mr. Cookson notices that Mrs. Hipps was admitted 14 months ago for repair of a fractured femur. Mrs. Hipps says, "This business about a blood clot really has me worried." She also tells Mr. Cookson that she is worried about who will care for her dog while she is in the hospital. Physical findings include height 62 inches (157 cm), weight 149 lb (68 kg), T 99.2°F (37.3°C); vital signs within normal limits otherwise. Her left leg is warm and pink, with strong peripheral pulses and good capillary refill. Her right calf is dark red, very warm, and dry to touch. It is tender to palpation. The right femoral and popliteal pulses are strong, but the pedal and posterior tibial pulses are difficult to locate. The right calf diameter is 0.5 inch (1.27 cm) larger than the left.

DIAGNOSES

- *Pain* related to inflammatory response in affected vein
- *Anxiety* related to unexpected hospitalization and uncertainty about the seriousness of her illness
- *Ineffective Tissue Perfusion: Peripheral* related to decreased venous circulation in the right leg
- *Risk for Impaired Skin Integrity* related to pooling of venous blood in the right leg

EXPECTED OUTCOMES

- Verbalize relief of right leg pain by day of discharge.
- Verbalize reduced anxiety by the second day of her hospitalization.
- Demonstrate reduced right leg diameter by 0.25 inch (0.64 cm) by the fifth day of hospitalization.
- Maintain intact skin in the right foot throughout the hospital stay.

PLANNING AND IMPLEMENTATION

- Elevate legs, maintaining slight knee flexion, while in bed.
- Apply warm, moist compresses to right leg using a 2-hour-on, 2-hour-off schedule around the clock.
- Administer prescribed analgesics and evaluate effectiveness.
- Spend time with Mrs. Hipps to explain venous thrombosis and its treatment.
- Arrange for a friend or neighbor to care for Mrs. Hipps's dog.
- Apply antiembolism stockings as ordered; remove for 30 minutes every 8 hours.
- Monitor laboratory values to assess effect of anticoagulant therapy; report values outside desired range.
- Assist with progressive ambulation when allowed.
- Inspect legs and feet and record findings every 8 hours.

EVALUATION

Seven days after admission, the pain in Mrs. Hipps's right leg has subsided and the diameter of her right calf is equal to that of her left calf. Mrs. Hipps admits to Mr. Cookson that her fears really relate to a cousin who was hospitalized for a similar problem and had his leg amputated. After talking about her condition and the steps she can take to prevent its recurrence, she is much less anxious. Before discharge, Mr. Cookson reviews instructions for antiembolism stockings, daily walking, warfarin schedule, and scheduled follow-up appointment. Her neighbor, Kate, came to pick her up. As Mr. Cookson was helping Mrs. Hipps into the car, Kate handed her a small brown dog and said, "I took good care of Chester for you, but he's missed you." Mrs. Hipps smiled, and assured Mr. Cookson that she would call the number he provided if she had any questions.

CRITICAL THINKING IN THE NURSING PROCESS

1. Describe the pathophysiologic reasons for the pain in Mrs. Hipps's right leg.
2. How would you respond if Mrs. Hipps tells you she does not have the money to buy the prescribed anticoagulant when she goes home?
3. How would you change your teaching and discharge planning if Mrs. Hipps had difficulty caring for herself?
4. Design a plan of care for Mrs. Hipps for the nursing diagnosis *Activity Intolerance*.

See Evaluating Your Response in Appendix C.

of the involved extremity. Associated edema and swelling may contribute to discomfort. Measures to reduce the inflammation often help relieve the pain.

- Regularly assess pain location, characteristics, and level using a standardized pain scale. Report increasing pain or changes in its location or characteristics. *Tissue substances released during the inflammatory process can stimulate pain receptors. In addition, localized swelling presses on pain-sensitive structures in the area of the inflammation, contributing to discomfort. As inflammation and swelling are reduced, pain should abate. Continued or increasing pain may indicate extension of the thrombosis. Sudden chest pain may indicate a pulmonary embolism, necessitating immediate intervention.*
- Measure calf and thigh diameter of the affected extremity on admission and daily thereafter. Report increases promptly. *The inflammatory process causes vasodilation and increases vessel permeability, causing edema of the affected extremity. Baseline and subsequent measurements provide a measure of treatment effectiveness.*
- Apply warm, moist heat to affected extremity at least four times daily, using warm, moist compresses or an aqua-K pad. *Moist heat penetrates tissues to a greater depth. Warmth promotes vasodilation, allowing reabsorption of excess fluid into the circulation. Vasodilation also reduces resistance within the affected vessel, reducing pain. As edema subsides, pressure on surrounding tissues is relieved, thereby reducing pain.*
- Maintain bed rest as ordered. *Using leg muscles during walking exacerbates the inflammatory process and increases edema. This, in turn, increases venous compression and pain.*

Ineffective Tissue Perfusion: Peripheral

As thrombi develop, they occlude the lumen of the vein and obstruct blood flow. In addition, the accompanying inflammatory response may precipitate vessel spasms, further impairing arterial and venous blood flow and tissue perfusion. Impaired tissue perfusion, in turn, deprives tissues of nutrients and oxygen. As a result, distal tissues of the affected extremity are at risk for ulceration and infection.

PRACTICE ALERT

Assess peripheral pulses, skin integrity, capillary refill times, and color of extremities at least every 8 hours. Report changes promptly. Assessment of both extremities allows comparison of the affected and unaffected limbs. Weak or absent pulses, impaired capillary refill, or significant color changes in the affected extremity may indicate extension of the thrombus or a possible complication.

- Assess skin of the affected lower leg and foot at least every 8 hours; more often as indicated. *Frequent assessment is important to rapidly detect early signs of tissue breakdown and implementation of measures to protect vulnerable tissues. Early intervention allows healing and restoration of tissue integrity; allowed to continue, the process can lead to necrosis and potential gangrene.*

- Elevate extremities at all times, keeping knees slightly flexed and legs above the level of the heart. *Elevation of the extremities promotes venous return and reduces peripheral edema. Knee flexion promotes muscle relaxation.*

PRACTICE ALERT

Remove antiembolic stockings or pneumatic compression device for 30 to 60 minutes during daily hygiene. Antiembolic stockings (e.g., TED hose) and pneumatic compression devices exert pressure on the extremity and promote venous return. They can, however, impair perfusion of the dermis. Removing them periodically allows assessment of the underlying tissue and restores perfusion of the dermis, reducing the risk for skin breakdown. Their use may be continued following discharge to reduce the risk of recurrent venous thrombosis.

- Use mild soaps, solutions, and lotions to clean the affected leg and foot daily. Pat dry after washing, and apply a non-alcohol-based lotion or moisturizing cream. *Daily hygiene with nondrying soaps and solutions removes potential pathogens from the skin surface, and maintains skin integrity and the first line of defense against infection. Caustic or harsh soaps or solutions can dry and crack the skin. Dry, cracked skin permits bacteria and other microorganisms to enter and infect the tissue, potentially leading to ulceration and venous gangrene.*
- Use egg-crate mattress or sheepskin on the bed as needed. *Egg-crate mattresses and sheepskins distribute weight more evenly, preventing excess pressure on affected tissues.*
- Encourage frequent position changes, at least every 2 hours while awake. *Frequent position changes reduce pressure on bony prominences and edematous tissue, reducing the risk of tissue breakdown.*

Ineffective Protection

Anticoagulant therapy interferes with the body's normal clotting mechanisms, increasing the risk for bleeding and hemorrhage.

PRACTICE ALERT

Assess for and promptly report evidence of bleeding, such as petechiae, bruising, bleeding gums, obvious or occult blood in vomitus, stool, or urine, unexplained back or abdominal pain. Anticoagulants interfere with the ability to form a stable clot and prevent excessive bleeding. Even minor trauma such as toothbrushing or bumping into furniture can result in bleeding.

- Monitor laboratory results, including the INR (prothrombin time), aPTT, hemoglobin, and hematocrit as indicated. Report values outside the normal or desired range. *Coagulation studies are used to monitor the effect of anticoagulant medications. Values within the desired range prevent further clot development while carrying a low risk for bleeding and hemorrhage. A fall in the hemoglobin and hematocrit may indicate undetected bleeding.*

Impaired Physical Mobility

Although prolonged bed rest rarely is required, it is associated with many problems, including constipation, joint contractures, muscle atrophy, and boredom. Nursing care goals include maintaining joint range of motion, minimizing muscle atrophy, and reducing boredom.

- Encourage active range-of-motion (ROM) exercises at least every 8 hours. Provide passive range of motion as needed. *ROM exercises maintain joint mobility and prevent contractures. Active range of motion (performed by the client) also helps prevent muscle atrophy and preserve function. While passive ROM exercises do not prevent muscle atrophy, they do maintain joint mobility.*
- Encourage frequent position changes, deep breathing, and coughing. *Prolonged immobility can lead to impaired airway clearance and respiratory complications, such as atelectasis or pneumonia. Turning, coughing, and deep breathing facilitate expulsion of secretions from the respiratory tract, airway clearance, and alveolar ventilation.*
- Encourage increased fluid and dietary fiber intake. *Constipation is a frequent complication of immobility due to decreased gastrointestinal motility and loss of abdominal muscle strength. Increasing fluid and fiber intake helps maintain soft, easily expelled stools.*
- Assist with and encourage ambulation as allowed. *Ambulation promotes venous blood flow, helps maintain muscle tone and joint mobility, and increases the sense of well-being.*
- Encourage diversional activities such as reading, handiwork or other hobbies, television or video games, and socializing. *Boredom may lead to dozing and inertia, with little physical movement or mental stimulation, increasing the risk for complications of immobility.*

Risk for Ineffective Tissue Perfusion: Cardiopulmonary

A thrombus that forms in the deep veins of the legs or pelvis may break loose or fragment, becoming an embolism. Emboli that originate in the venous system usually become trapped in the pulmonary circulation (pulmonary embolism). Gas exchange in the affected area is impaired as blood flow ceases or is reduced to an area of the lungs that is well ventilated (see Chapter 38 ∞).

- Frequently assess respiratory status, including rate, depth, ease, and oxygen saturation levels. *A mismatch of ventilation and perfusion can significantly affect gas exchange, leading to rapid, shallow respirations, dyspnea and air hunger, and a fall in oxygen saturation levels.*

PRACTICE ALERT
Immediately report complaints of chest pain and shortness of breath, anxiety, or a sense of impending doom. The manifestations of pulmonary embolism are similar to those of myocardial infarction. Prompt intervention to restore pulmonary blood flow can reduce the risk of significant adverse effects.

- Initiate oxygen therapy, elevate the head of the bed, and reassure the client who is experiencing manifestations of pulmonary embolism. *Oxygen therapy and elevating the head of*

the bed promote ventilation and gas exchange in those alveoli that are well perfused, helping maintain tissue oxygenation. Reassurance helps reduce anxiety and slow the respiratory rate, promoting greater respiratory depth and alveolar ventilation.

Using NANDA, NIC, and NOC

Chart 35–3 illustrates linkages between nursing diagnoses, nursing interventions, and nursing outcomes for the client with deep venous thrombosis.

Community-Based Care

Treatment measures for venous thrombosis may be initiated and carried out on an outpatient basis or continued for an extended period of time following hospital discharge. Include the following topics when teaching for home care:

- Explanation of the disease process
- Treatment measures, including laboratory tests and their purposes, medications and adverse effects that should be reported
- Appropriate methods of heat application
- Prescribed activity restrictions
- Measures to prevent future episodes of venous thrombosis
- The importance of follow-up visits and laboratory tests as scheduled.

Refer clients for community nursing services for continued assessment and reinforcement of teaching. Provide referrals for assistance with ADLs and home maintenance services as indicated. Consider referral for physical therapy if needed.

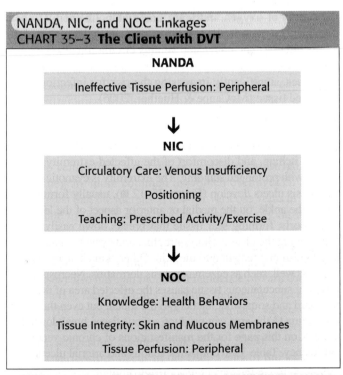

NANDA, NIC, and NOC Linkages
CHART 35–3 The Client with DVT

NANDA

Ineffective Tissue Perfusion: Peripheral

↓

NIC

Circulatory Care: Venous Insufficiency

Positioning

Teaching: Prescribed Activity/Exercise

↓

NOC

Knowledge: Health Behaviors

Tissue Integrity: Skin and Mucous Membranes

Tissue Perfusion: Peripheral

Data from *NANDA's Nursing Diagnoses: Definitions & Classification 2005–2006* by NANDA International (2005), Philadelphia; *Nursing Interventions Classification (NIC)* (4th ed.) by J. M. Dochterman & G. M. Bulechek (2004), St. Louis, MO: Mosby; and *Nursing Outcomes Classification (NOC)* (3rd ed.) by S. Moorhead, M. Johnson, and M. Maas (2004), St. Louis, MO: Mosby.

NURSING RESEARCH   Evidence-Based Practice for the Client with Venous Leg Ulcers

Chronic leg ulcers due to venous insufficiency are a challenge to treat and heal. Oxygen is necessary for tissue repair and to prevent infection; however, peripheral perfusion to deliver oxygen to the tissues is impaired in clients with chronic venous insufficiency. Using measurements of transcutaneous tissue oxygen ($TcPO_2$), a group of nurse researchers evaluated the effects of four different positions and supplemental oxygen on a small group of subjects with venous ulcers (Wipke-Tevis et al., 2001). Not surprisingly, these researchers found lower extremity resting $TcPO_2$ levels in clients with venous ulcers than in healthy adults. Changes in position resulted in minimal $TcPO_2$ changes in tissue surrounding the ulcer. When supplemental oxygen was given, $TcPO_2$ levels were higher in the supine position than with the legs elevated, sitting, or standing. These results suggest that control of peripheral circulation and tissue oxygenation may be impaired in clients with venous ulcers.

IMPLICATIONS FOR NURSING
The results of this study support advising clients with chronic venous ulcers to stay off their feet and rest in bed as much as possible to promote healing of venous ulcers. Remove compression stockings and devices while the client is in bed to promote perfusion of subcutaneous tissues and of the region surrounding the ulcer itself. Discuss the effects of position on peripheral tissue perfusion with clients, and encourage frequent rest periods during the day. Consider discussing the option of supplemental oxygen therapy for a client with delayed ulcer healing with the primary care provider.

CRITICAL THINKING IN CLIENT CARE
1. What is the usual response of blood vessels to changing positions from supine or sitting to standing? How does this compare with the results found here?
2. What is required for tissue healing? What measures can the nurse take to promote tissue healing in a client with impaired peripheral tissue perfusion?
3. How do the measures used to treat arterial and venous ulcers compare? Explain the rationale for differing treatment measures.

Pathophysiology

Varicose veins are classified as primary (with no involvement of deep veins) or secondary (caused by the obstruction of deep veins). In both cases, long-standing increased venous pressure stretches the vessel wall. This sustained stretching impairs the ability of the venous valves to close, causing them to become incompetent.

The erect position produces a twofold negative effect on the veins. When standing, the leg veins resemble vertical columns and must withstand the full force of venous blood pressure. Prolonged standing, the force of gravity, lack of leg exercise, and incompetent venous valves all weaken the muscle-pumping mechanism, reducing venous blood return to the heart. As standing continues, the amount of blood pooled in the veins increases, further stretching the vessel wall. The venous valves become increasingly incompetent.

Manifestations

Although varicose veins may be asymptomatic, most cause manifestations such as severe aching leg pain, leg fatigue, leg heaviness, itching, or feelings of heat in the legs. The degree of valvular incompetence does not seem to correlate well with the extent of symptoms. The menstrual cycle tends to worsen symptoms, suggesting a possible correlation with hormonal factors in women. Assessment reveals obvious dilated, tortuous veins beneath the skin of the upper and lower leg. If varicose veins are long standing, the skin above the ankles may be thin and discolored, with a brown pigmentation. See the Manifestations box below.

Complications

Complications of varicose veins include venous insufficiency and stasis ulcers. Chronic stasis dermatitis may also develop. Superficial venous thrombosis may develop in varicose veins, especially during and after pregnancy, following surgery, and in clients on estrogen therapy (oral contraceptives or hormone replacement therapy).

NURSING CARE OF THE OLDER ADULT
Chronic Venous Stasis

Disorders of venous stasis are common after the fifth decade of life. Aging affects vessels and tissues, increasing the risk for venous insufficiency and varicose veins. In addition, mobility frequently declines with aging, reducing the effect of the muscle pump in promoting venous return.

Regular exercise, walking in particular, is an important part of the treatment plan. Safety when walking is an important issue for older clients. Assess the client's mobility and stability during ambulation. If appropriate, suggest using a walker and quad-cane as needed. Assist older clients holding jobs that require prolonged standing to identify strategies to minimize standing and incorporate periods of activity into their work.

Following surgery or during treatment for stasis ulcers, older clients may need additional assistance with home care and maintenance. Initiate referral to social services as needed to arrange for home nursing care, meals, assistance with ADLs, and home maintenance services as indicated. In some instances, temporary placement in an extended care facility is necessary until the client and family can assume care.

MANIFESTATIONS   of Varicose Veins

- Severe, aching pain in the leg
- Leg fatigue, heaviness
- Itching of the affected leg (stasis dermatitis)
- Feelings of warmth in the leg
- Visibly dilated veins
- Thin, discolored skin above the ankles
- Stasis ulcers

INTERDISCIPLINARY CARE

Varicose veins usually can be managed using conservative measures, although surgery may be required if symptoms are severe, when complications develop, or for cosmetic reasons.

Diagnosis

While varicose veins often are diagnosed by the history and physical examination, diagnostic tests may be ordered.

- *Doppler ultrasonography* or *duplex Doppler ultrasound* may be performed to identify specific locations of incompetent valves. This test is particularly useful before surgery to identify valves that allow reflux of blood from the femoral, popliteal, or peripheral deep veins into the superficial veins (Tierney et al., 2005).
- *Trendelenburg test* may be performed to determine the underlying cause of superficial venous insufficiency. The leg is elevated, then an elastic tourniquet is placed around the distal thigh. The varicosities then are observed as the client stands. When valves of the deep veins are incompetent, the veins remain flat on standing; they rapidly distend when the superficial venous valves are the underlying cause.

Treatments

Although there is no real cure, conservative measures are the core of treatment for most clients with uncomplicated varicose veins. These measures often relieve symptoms and prevent complications by improving venous circulation and relieving pressure on venous tissues. Properly fitted graduated compression stockings are commonly prescribed. They compress the veins, propelling blood back to the heart. Compression stockings augment the muscle pumping action of the legs. When worn during times of prolonged standing and in combination with frequent leg elevation, compression stockings often prevent progression of the condition and development of complications.

Regular, daily walking also is important. Prolonged sitting and standing are discouraged, although elevating the legs for specified periods during the day is beneficial. Leg elevation promotes venous return, prevents venous stasis, and decreases leg heaviness and fatigue.

Compression Sclerotherapy

In compression sclerotherapy, a sclerosing solution is injected into the varicose vein and a compression bandage is applied for a period of time. This obliterates the vein. Venous blood is rerouted through healthy vessels whose valves are not compromised. Compression sclerotherapy may be used to treat small, symptomatic varicosities. It may be the primary treatment, or it may be used in conjunction with varicose vein surgery. While compression sclerotherapy may be done for cosmetic reasons, complications such as phlebitis, tissue necrosis, or infection may occur and need to be considered prior to the procedures.

Surgery

Surgical treatment of varicose veins generally is reserved for clients who are very symptomatic, experience recurrent superficial venous thrombosis, and/or develop stasis ulcers. The objective of surgery is to remove the diseased veins. It may be considered for cosmetic reasons.

Surgery usually involves extensive ligation and stripping of the greater and lesser saphenous veins (Kasper et al., 2005). The evening before surgery, the surgeon marks all incompetent superficial and perforating varicose veins with a permanent ink marker. Under either regional or general anesthesia, the greater saphenous vein is removed and the connected smaller tributaries that have not naturally clotted off are tied off. Multiple small incisions may be made over the varicosities, allowing removal of the affected segments of the vein. Incompetent tributaries that communicate with larger vessels also are ligated. For clients with less extensive disease or clients seeking cosmetic improvement, surgery may involve only the removal of the lesser saphenous vein through an incision in the popliteal fossa.

Postoperative care includes applying pressure bandages for a minimum of 6 weeks, elevating the extremities to minimize postoperative edema, and gradually increasing amounts of ambulation. Sitting and standing are prohibited during the initial recovery period, and are gradually reintroduced as deemed appropriate by the surgeon.

NURSING CARE

Health Promotion

Health promotion activities to reduce the incidence of varicose veins include teaching all clients, particularly young women, the benefits of regular exercise continued over the lifetime. Discuss the effect of prolonged sitting or standing on the legs, and encourage the client whose occupation involves these activities to periodically get up and move or to sit with the legs elevated. Encourage all clients to maintain normal weight for their height.

Assessment

Focused assessment of the client with varicose veins includes the following:

- *Health history:* Complaints of leg pain, aching, heaviness, or fatigue; ankle swelling; history of venous thrombosis.
- *Physical examination:* Visible, dilated, tortuous superficial veins in lower extremities.

Nursing Diagnoses and Interventions

In planning and providing nursing care for clients with varicose veins, emphasis is placed on the importance of health teaching to manage the symptoms of varicose veins, particularly because there is no cure for the disease. Nursing care for clients who have undergone surgical treatment for varicose veins focuses on assessing and promoting wound healing and preventing infection. Nursing diagnoses may include those related to pain, impaired tissue perfusion and skin integrity, and a risk for impaired neurovascular function.

Chronic Pain

Varicose veins can lead to pooling of venous blood in the lower extremities. Venous congestion can cause a dull ache or feeling of pressure in the legs, particularly after prolonged standing. As venous pressure rises, arterial circulation and delivery of oxygen and nutrients to tissues is impaired. Tissue ischemia contributes to the pain. The pain associated with varicose veins tends to be chronic, developing and progressing gradually over a long period of time.

- Assess pain, including its intensity, duration, and aggravating and relieving factors. *Pain assessment allows collaborative planning with the client to identify appropriate interventions.*
- Inquire about current measures being used by the client to manage pain and its effects. Ask about the effectiveness of current management strategies and the desire to change. *Chronic pain management ultimately falls to the client. Strategies to address the pain must meet the client's needs.*

> **PRACTICE ALERT**
> Suggest keeping a diary of pain intensity, timing, precipitating events, and effectiveness of relief measures. Systematic tracking of pain is an important measure in improving its management.

- Teach and reinforce nonpharmacologic pain management strategies such as progressive relaxation, imagery, deep breathing, distraction, and meditation. *The effectiveness of such strategies is well documented. Nonpharmacologic measures provide a variety of options for controlling pain while maintaining independence. These measures also can reduce reliance on analgesics.*
- Collaborate with the client to establish a pain control plan. *Collaborative planning for pain management increases the client's sense of control and reduces powerlessness. This, in turn, enhances the ability to cope with pain and its effects.*
- Regularly evaluate the effectiveness of planned interventions and pain management strategies. *Regular evaluation allows modification of the care plan as needed, as well as providing a measure of disease progression. Increasing or poorly controlled pain may necessitate additional collaborative interventions to manage the disorder.*

Ineffective Tissue Perfusion: Peripheral

Varicose veins and venous stasis impair delivery of nutrients and oxygen to peripheral tissues as elevated venous pressures interfere with blood flow through the capillary beds. Improving venous blood flow reduces venous pressures and promotes arterial flow to peripheral tissues.

- Assess peripheral pulses, capillary refill, skin color and temperature, and extent of edema. *Assessment of arterial flow and tissue perfusion provides baseline and continuing data for evaluating the effectiveness of interventions.*
- Teach application and use of properly fitted elastic graduated compression stockings. *Elastic compression stockings compress the veins, promoting venous return from the lower extremities. During ambulation, the stockings enhance the blood-pumping action of the muscles. Because elastic stockings inhibit blood flow through small superficial ves-*

sels, they should be removed at least once each day for at least 30 minutes.

> **PRACTICE ALERT**
> Instruct to maintain a program of regular exercise, such as walking for 20 to 30 minutes several times a day. Exercise stimulates circulation and promotes blood flow through the vascular system. When ambulation is restricted, active ROM exercises help maintain muscle tone, joint mobility, and venous return.

- Advise to elevate the legs for 15 to 20 minutes several times a day and to sleep with the legs elevated above the level of the heart. *Elevating the legs promotes venous return, reducing tissue congestion and improving arterial circulation. Improved venous return also increases the cardiac output and renal perfusion, promoting elimination of excess fluid and decreasing peripheral edema.*

Risk for Impaired Skin Integrity

Ineffective venous valve function impairs venous return and increases venous pressures. These increased pressures oppose arterial blood flow and the delivery of oxygen and nutrients to the cells. As a result, tissues are vulnerable to any additional insult, and may break down.

- Assess lower extremity color, temperature, moisture, and for evidence of pressure or breakdown on admission and at each visit. *Initial and continuing assessment allows timely detection of early signs of skin and tissue breakdown. This, in turn, allows early institution of measures to prevent further tissue damage and promote healing.*
- Teach foot and skin care measures such as daily cleansing with nondrying soap, gentle drying, and lotions to prevent skin dryness and cracking. *Cleansing removes potentially harmful microorganisms and stimulates circulation. Care is taken to keep the skin moist and supple, promoting its function as the first line of defense against infection.*
- Discuss the importance of adequate nutrition and fluid intake. *Adequate nutrients are necessary to maintain tissue integrity and promote healing. A diet high in protein, carbohydrates, and vitamins and minerals promotes growth and maintenance of skin cells, provides energy, and helps prevent skin breakdown. Adequate hydration helps maintain the moisture and turgor of skin, reducing the risk of drying and breakdown.*

Risk for Peripheral Neurovascular Dysfunction

Severe varicose veins can lead to chronic venous insufficiency, impaired arterial circulation, and ultimately, disrupted sensation in the affected extremity. Impaired neurologic function increases the client's risk for injury and infection of the extremity, because minor trauma may go unnoticed.

- Assess circulation, sensation, and movement of the lower extremities. *Disrupted circulation and venous congestion may interfere with sensory and motor function of the affected extremity. The potential for nerve and muscle involvement is especially high in clients with venous stasis ulcers.*

- Teach measures to protect the extremities from injury, such as always wearing shoes or firm slippers, cotton socks to absorb moisture, and testing the temperature of bath water with a thermometer or the upper extremities before stepping in. *Sensation in the lower extremities may be affected by poor circulation, necessitating additional measures to protect the legs and feet from injury.*

Community-Based Care

Most clients with varicose veins provide self-care at home. Include the following topics when preparing the client and family for home care:

- Leg elevation and exercise program
- Application and use of graduated elastic compression stockings
- Foot and leg care (see Box 35–4)
- Measures to avoid injury and skin breakdown
- Symptoms or potential complications to report to the physician.

Provide information about suppliers for elastic stockings and any other required supplies. If venous stasis ulcers have developed, consider referral to home health services for regular assessment of healing and additional teaching.

DISORDERS OF THE LYMPHATIC SYSTEM

The lymphatic system, which includes the lymphatic vessels and the lymph nodes, is a unique part of the circulatory system. The lymphatic system returns plasma and plasma proteins filtered out of the capillaries from interstitial tissues to the bloodstream. This fluid is called *lymph*. The lymphatic system consists of closed capillaries leading to larger lymphatic venules and lymphatic veins. These vessels contain smooth muscle and one-way valves that help move fluid toward the heart. Lymphatic vessels share the same sheath as arteries and veins; arterial pulsations and skeletal muscle contractions compress the lymphatic vessels to assist in maintaining lymph flow. As lymph moves through the lymphatic system, it is filtered through thousands of bean-shaped lymph nodes clustered along the vessels. Within these nodes, phagocytes remove foreign material from the lymph, preventing it from entering the bloodstream.

THE CLIENT WITH LYMPHADENOPATHY

Lymphadenopathy, enlarged lymph nodes, may be localized or generalized. Localized lymphadenopathy usually results from an inflammatory process (e.g., streptococcal pharyngitis or an infected wound). The node enlarges as lymphocytes and monocytes proliferate within the node to destroy infectious material. Palpable lymph nodes often develop in response to minor trauma or a localized infection. Generalized lymphadenopathy usually is associated with malignancy or disease. Malignant cells or other abnormal cells invade the node, causing it to enlarge.

Lymphangitis, inflammation of the lymph vessels draining an infected area of the body, is characterized by a red streak along the inflamed vessels, pain, heat, and swelling. Fever and chills also may be present. Local lymph nodes are swollen and tender.

Treatment for lymphadenopathy and lymphangitis focuses on identifying and treating the underlying condition. Elevating the body part and applying heat to inflamed lymphatic vessels help reduce swelling and promote blood flow to the affected area.

THE CLIENT WITH LYMPHEDEMA

Lymphedema may be a primary or a secondary disorder, resulting from inflammation, obstruction, or removal of lymphatic vessels. It is characterized by extremity edema due to accumulation of lymph. *Primary lymphedema* is uncommon, affecting about 1 in 10,000 people. It affects females more frequently than males, and may be associated with a genetic disorder such as Turner syndrome or Klinefelter syndrome. See the accompanying Genetic Considerations box.

Secondary lymphedema is an acquired condition, resulting from damage, obstruction, or removal of lymphatic vessels. The most common worldwide cause of secondary lymphedema is *filariasis,* infestation of the lymphatic vessels by filaria, a nematode worm. Other important causes of secondary lymphedema include recurrent episodes of bacterial lymphangitis, obstruction of lymph vessels by tumors, and surgical or radiation treatment for breast cancer (Kasper et al., 2005).

GENETIC CONSIDERATIONS
Primary Lymphedema

- Primary lymphedema develops as a result of agenesis, hypoplasia, or obstruction of lymphatic vessels.
- *Congenital lymphedema* appears shortly after birth; two other forms of lymphedema develop later, one at the time of puberty (*lymphedema praecox*), the other usually after age 35 (*lymphedema tarda*).
- Congenital lymphedema and lymphedema praecox may be inherited as an autosomal dominant trait with variable penetrance.
- Lymphedema also may be inherited (although less commonly) as an autosomal or sex-linked recessive disorder (Kasper et al., 2005).

Pathophysiology and Manifestations

Obstruction of lymph drainage prevents fluid and protein molecules from interstitial tissues from returning to the circulation. The protein molecules increase the osmotic pressure in interstitial tissues, drawing in additional fluid that causes edema in the soft tissues. One or both extremities may be affected.

The edema begins distally, progressing up the limb to involve the entire extremity. Initial edema is soft and pitting; with chronic congestion, subcutaneous tissues become fibrotic, causing thick, rough skin and a woody texture of the limb (*brawny edema*). In contrast, the edema associated with venous disorders is softer, and the skin often is hyperpigmented with evidence of stasis dermatitis. Lymphedema generally is painless, although the limb may feel heavy.

INTERDISCIPLINARY CARE

Interdisciplinary care for the client with lymphedema focuses on relieving edema and preventing or treating infection. The disorder may be difficult to treat effectively, and can lead to progressive disability due to the weight and awkwardness of the affected extremity.

Diagnosis

Abdominal or pelvic ultrasound and CT scans are used to detect obstructing lesions. MRI can show edema and identify lymph nodes and enlarged lymphatic vessels. More invasive procedures such as lymphangiography and radioactive isotope studies may occasionally be necessary to identify the lymphatic defect causing lymphedema.

- *Lymphangiography* uses injected contrast media to illustrate lymphatic vessels on x-rays. Organic dyes are used to identify a distal lymphatic vessel, and then a contrast medium is injected into the vessel for visualization of the lymphatic system of the limb. In primary lymphedema, lymph vessels are absent or hypoplastic (underdeveloped). In secondary lymphedema, lymph channels often are dilated; it may be possible to determine the level of obstruction (Kasper et al., 2005).
- *Lymphoscintigraphy* involves injecting a radioactively tagged substance into distal subcutaneous tissues of the extremity, then mapping its flow through the lymphatic system. The pattern of lymph fluid distribution and transport is abnormal in clients with lymphedema.

Treatments

Meticulous skin and foot care is vital to prevent infection in the affected extremity. Shoes should always be worn to reduce the risk of injury. Careful cleansing and use of emollient lotions are recommended to prevent drying of the skin. Exercise is encouraged, as are frequent periods of leg elevation. The foot of the bed is raised by 15 to 20 degrees at night to promote lymph flow. Elastic graduated compression stockings may be ordered for use during the day. In some cases, an intermittent pneumatic compression device to reduce edema may be prescribed for home use.

Antibiotics are given to prevent and treat infection, which can be recurrent and difficult to eradicate. Diuretic therapy may be used intermittently, particularly when primary lymphedema is exacerbated by the menstrual cycle or seasonal variability (Tierney et al., 2005).

Clients who do not respond to conservative treatment measures or who experience recurrent episodes of cellulitis and lymphangitis may require surgical treatment. Microvascular techniques may be used to create anastomoses between obstructed lymphatic vessels and adjacent veins, providing channels to redirect lymph into the venous system. Successful surgery may improve both extremity function and its cosmetic appearance (Tierney et al., 2005).

NURSING CARE

Nursing care for clients with lymphatic disorders focuses on reducing edema, preventing tissue damage related to the edema, and promoting effective coping with the effect of the disorder on body image and function.

Nursing Diagnoses and Interventions

Nursing diagnoses for the client with lymphedema may include *Impaired Tissue Integrity, Excess Fluid Volume,* and *Disturbed Body Image.*

Impaired Tissue Integrity

Obstructed lymphatic flow leads to fluid congestion of the interstitial spaces of subcutaneous tissue. The resulting edema compresses and damages tissues of the affected extremity. Subcutaneous tissues become fibrotic, reducing their protective functions of shock absorption and insulation. In addition, obstructed lymphatic flow reduces the effectiveness of lymph nodes in filtering and removing foreign material and pathogens from the body. This increases the risk for local tissue infection such as *cellulitis*, a diffuse bacterial infection of the skin. Cellulitis increases the risk for skin and tissue breakdown and, if not effectively treated, can lead to sepsis.

> **PRACTICE ALERT**
> Frequently inspect the skin of the affected extremity, documenting condition with each assessment. Promptly report areas of pallor, redness, or apparent inflammation. Breaks in the skin surface allow microbial invasion, and increase the risk for infection. Prompt identification and treatment of any lesions is vital to prevent further tissue breakdown and infection.

- Apply well-fitting elastic graduated compression stockings or intermittent pneumatic pressure devices as ordered. *Elastic stockings and/or pneumatic pressure devices oppose the movement of fluid out of capillaries and improve its reabsorption into vascular spaces for transportation back to the heart.*

> **PRACTICE ALERT**
> Remove elastic stockings and intermittent pressure devices every 8 hours or at each home visit to inspect the underlying skin for evidence of redness, irritation, dryness, or breakdown. Elastic graduated compression stockings, antiembolic stockings, and pneumatic compression devices compress small vessels nourishing the skin and subcutaneous tissue. Periodic removal not only allows inspection of the underlying skin, but also allows restoration of blood flow to these small vessels and the tissues.

- Instruct to elevate the extremities while seated and during sleep. *Elevation of the extremities diminishes venous congestion, promotes venous return, facilitates arterial circulation and tissue perfusion, and helps reduce the accumulation of excess fluids in interstitial spaces of the affected extremity.*

PRACTICE ALERT
Use preventive skin care devices as indicated. Collected fluid in the affected extremity increases its weight and interferes with regular movement. The increased weight places greater pressure on surfaces of the limb that come in contact with furniture. Protective devices such as egg-crate foam, sheepskin, pillows, or padding help prevent tissue compression, promoting circulation and reducing the risk of skin and tissue breakdown.

- Keep skin clean and dry, especially in interdigital spaces. Teach skin and foot care to the client and family. *Clean, dry skin provides the first line of defense against infection. Significant limb edema can interfere with reaching the distal extremity and cleaning interdigital spaces. The dark, moist spaces between the toes are an excellent environment for bacterial growth. Teaching fosters self-care and independence, as well as preparing the client and family to manage this often chronic condition.*
- Discuss the importance of adhering to the therapeutic regimen. *Lymphedema generally is a chronic condition; effective management requires active client participation in planning and implementing care to reduce edema and maintain tissue integrity.*

Excess Fluid Volume
In lymphedema, obstruction, destruction, or congenital malformation of lymphatic vessels interferes with the normal circulation of lymphatic fluid. As a result, lymph collects in the subcutaneous tissues of the affected extremity, causing excess fluid volume of that extremity. Some clients may benefit from intermittent diuretic therapy and dietary sodium restriction.

PRACTICE ALERT
Monitor intake and output and/or weight (daily or weekly). Use consistent scales, timing, and clothing for accurate weight measurements. Intake and output records and short-term changes in weight reflect fluid balance. Measures of fluid balance permit evaluation of the effectiveness of interventions such as restricted sodium intake and diuretic therapy.

- Discuss the rationale for restricted sodium intake if ordered. Teach ways to maintain the recommended sodium restriction, and assist to choose foods that are low in sodium. *Sodium causes retention of extracellular water; restricting dietary sodium may help prevent additional fluid accumulation in interstitial spaces.*
- During acute periods, assess the affected extremity daily for increased edema; measure girth of the extremity using consistent technique. *The size of the affected extremity provides a measure of the effectiveness of ordered interventions and progression of the disorder.*

Disturbed Body Image
The disproportionate size of an extremity or extremities due to lymphedema can profoundly affect body image. During early stages of the disease, conservative measures may effectively reduce the edema and size of the affected limb. However, as the disease progresses, conservative measures may become less effective, leading to more permanent disfigurement. Mobility may be impaired, and the client may develop an increasingly negative self-perception.

- Encourage discussions about usual coping patterns and perception of self. *Knowledge of existing coping patterns and behaviors helps the nurse assess the client's ability to cope with the current situation. This knowledge is then used to reinforce effective coping mechanisms and help develop more effective coping strategies. This exchange also allows the client to voice feelings related to actual or perceived changes in body image.*
- Accept the client's perception of self and of the impact of the changes in appearance. *Nonjudgmental acceptance of the client's view of self and of the effects of changes in appearance builds trust and promotes rapport. A trusting relationship promotes the client's ability to take an active role in managing the disorder, participate in healthcare decisions, and adhere to the plan of care. Nonjudgmental listening also promotes mutual respect and demonstrates caring and compassion.*
- Encourage active participation in self-care. Assist with identifying alternative self-care strategies when the extent of edema interferes with performing some aspects of self-care such as trimming toenails or washing feet. *The client initially may have difficulty viewing or touching the affected body part. Gentle encouragement and support from the nurse helps the client assume self-care and accept the affected body part. Brainstorming to identify alternative care strategies promotes the client's independence even when total self-care is not feasible.*

Community-Based Care
When preparing the client with chronic lymphedema and family to manage the disorder, include the following teaching topics:

- Recommended program of exercise and elevation of the extremity
- Foot and skin care
- Use of elastic graduated compression stockings and/or intermittent pressure devices
- Importance of wearing elastic stockings during the majority of waking hours, removing them once during the daytime and while sleeping
- Measures to prevent infection in the affected extremity, such as wearing gloves while gardening
- Signs and symptoms to report to the healthcare provider (e.g., manifestations of tissue breakdown or infection, increasing edema, or evidence of compromised circulation)
- Use and precautions associated with any prescribed medications
- Sodium-restricted diet if ordered.

Provide information about contacts for questions, and make referrals as needed. Evaluate the need for home health, home maintenance assistance, and other services such as physical or occupational therapy.

MediaLink Care Plan Activity: Lymphedema

EXPLORE MediaLink

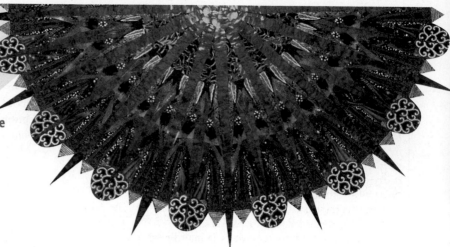

Prentice Hall Nursing MediaLink DVD-ROM
Audio Glossary
NCLEX-RN® Review

COMPANION WEBSITE www.prenhall.com/lemone
Audio Glossary
NCLEX-RN® Review
Care Plan Activity: Lymphedema
Case Study: Abdominal Aortic Aneurysm
MediaLink Application
  Calcium Channel Overdose
  Peripheral Vascular Disease
Links to Resources

CHAPTER HIGHLIGHTS

- Essential hypertension, blood pressure of 140/90 or higher with no clearly identified cause, rarely causes symptoms but is a major risk factor for coronary heart disease, heart failure, stroke, and renal insufficiency.

- Prehypertension, a newly identified category, is an average blood pressure of 120–139/80–89. Clients with prehypertension are advised to make lifestyle changes indicated for hypertension (weight loss, exercise, dietary changes, limited alcohol intake, and stress reduction), but generally are not treated with medications unless other risk factors such as diabetes or kidney disease are present.

- Systolic hypertension, an elevated systolic blood pressure without elevation of the diastolic pressure, is common in older adults and contributes to complications such as coronary heart disease and stroke.

- Medications to treat hypertension include diuretics, alpha- and beta-adrenergic blockers, ACE inhibitors and angiotensin II blockers, calcium channel blockers, and vasodilators. A combination of two or more drugs often is required for effective blood pressure control.

- Aneurysms, abnormal dilation of a blood vessel, commonly affect the aorta and the iliac arteries, particularly in older men. A slowly expanding abdominal aortic aneurysm that does not produce symptoms or impair flow through the renal arteries may not be

repaired, particularly in an older client. Percutaneously inserted endovascular splints provide an alternative to surgery for abdominal aortic aneurysms.

- Peripheral vascular disease, obstruction or occlusion of peripheral arteries by atherosclerotic plaque, is common and a leading cause of disability and amputation.

- Smoking cessation and regular daily exercise are key components of treatment for peripheral vascular disorders such as atherosclerosis, thromboangiitis obliterans, and Raynaud's disease.

- Venous thrombosis, particularly of the deep veins of the legs and pelvis, develops as a result of venous stasis, blood vessel damage, and increased coagulability of the blood. The developing clot may fragment or break loose, becoming an embolus that typically lodges in the pulmonary circulation (pulmonary embolus). Chronic venous insufficiency and venous stasis may develop as a result of deep venous thrombosis.

- Prophylactic anticoagulation and mobilization of the client are the primary preventive measures for venous thrombosis. Monitoring coagulation studies and assessing for evidence of bleeding (overt or covert) are important nursing measures for the client on anticoagulant therapy.

- Lymphadenopathy (enlarged lymph nodes), lymphangitis (inflammation of the lymph vessels), and lymphedema are the most common disorders affecting the lymph system.

TEST YOURSELF NCLEX-RN® REVIEW

1 A potential blood donor whose blood pressure is found to average 180/106 on two different readings tells the nurse, "I don't understand how it could be so high—I feel just fine." The appropriate response by the nurse is:
  1. "This is probably just a false reading due to 'white coat syndrome.' Don't worry about it."
  2. "It is unusual that you are not having some symptoms such as severe headaches and nosebleeds."
  3. "High blood pressure often has few or no symptoms; that's why it is called the 'silent killer.'"
  4. "You probably should have your blood pressure rechecked in 3 months or so and then follow up with your primary care provider if it is still high."

2 The nurse teaching a client about the DASH diet determines that additional teaching is necessary when the client states:
  1. "I'm glad I can still eat as much pasta as usual; I was afraid I would have to give up my weekly lasagna."
  2. "It will be a challenge to incorporate all those servings of fruits and vegetables into my diet."
  3. "Having a handful of nuts when the pre-dinner 'munchies' hit is a good idea."
  4. "I will enjoy having frozen yogurt as my bedtime snack on occasion."

3 The nurse teaching a client about his new prescription for Diovan HCT, a combination angiotensin II receptor blocker and thiazide diuretic, includes which of the following in his instructions? (Select all that apply.)

1. Use a potassium-based salt substitute to prevent hypokalemia while taking this drug.
2. Use caution when rising from bed or a chair to prevent dizziness.
3. Take the drug at bedtime to reduce the risk of falling due to light-headedness.
4. Report a persistent disruptive cough to your physician.
5. You may stop taking this drug once your blood pressure is within the normal range for 2 months.

4 A client is complaining of new-onset calf and foot pain. The nurse notes that the leg below the knee is cool and pale, and that dorsalis pedis and posterior tibial pulses are absent. The priority nursing intervention is to:

1. notify the physician.
2. place a cradle over the leg to prevent pressure from bedding.
3. position the leg flat, supported in anatomic position.
4. prepare to initiate heparin therapy.

5 An 86-year-old client with a newly diagnosed abdominal aortic aneurysm wonders if he will need surgery to repair the aneurysm, even though he feels fine. The nurse's response is based on the knowledge that:

1. the risk of surgical repair is lower than the risk that the aneurysm will rupture.
2. opening the abdomen for the surgical procedure greatly increases the risk of rupture.
3. surgery is indicated for type A aneurysms.
4. a percutaneously inserted endovascular stent may be considered because of his age.

6 An expected assessment finding in a client with peripheral atherosclerosis would be:

1. pallor of the legs and feet when dependent.
2. increased hair growth on the affected extremity.
3. higher blood pressure readings in the affected extremity.
4. impaired sensation in the affected extremity.

7 All of the following are appropriate home care measures for the client with peripheral vascular disease. Place them in order of priority.

1. foot and leg care
2. smoking cessation
3. daily inspection of feet and legs
4. regular daily exercise
5. weight loss strategies

8 The nurse evaluates her teaching of a client admitted with deep venous thrombosis as effective when the client states:

1. "I'll use a hard-backed, upright chair when sitting instead of my recliner."
2. "I'll get my blood drawn as scheduled and notify the doctor if I have any unusual bleeding or bruising."
3. "I understand why I am not allowed to exercise for the next 6 weeks and will take it easy."
4. "I'll have my wife buy a low-cholesterol cookbook and we'll make an appointment with the dietician to learn about a low-fat, low-cholesterol diet."

9 A client with visible varicose veins tells the nurse that she wants to have surgery to remove them, because "my legs ache every evening and they are really ugly!" The most appropriate response would be:

1. "Often measures such as elevating your legs and elastic stockings can relieve the discomfort associated with varicose veins."
2. "Surgery will have a good cosmetic effect, but will not relieve the discomfort associated with varicose veins."
3. "All varicose veins should be surgically removed to restore adequate blood flow to your legs and prevent gangrene."
4. "Surgery is never indicated unless the varicose veins are interfering with circulation. Have you tried cosmetic measures to cover them up?"

10 Which of the following nursing interventions is of highest priority for the client with lymphedema?

1. Elevate affected extremities at night.
2. Assist to don elastic compression stockings during the day.
3. Carefully dry and apply emollient lotion to affected extremities after bathing.
4. Reinforce the importance of taking prescribed diuretics.

See Test Yourself answers in Appendix C.

BIBLIOGRAPHY

American Heart Association. (2005). *Heart disease and stroke statistics—2005 update.* Dallas, TX: Author.

Aortic aneurysms: Synthetic graft prevents ruptures. (2005). *Nursing, 35*(6), 34.

Applying antiembolism stockings isn't just pulling on socks. (2004). *Nursing, 34*(8), 48–49.

Bartley, M. K. (2006). Preventing venous thromboembolism. *Nursing, 36*(1), Critical Care 64cc1, 64cc3–64cc4.

Beese-Bjurstrom, S. (2004). Hidden danger: Aortic aneurysms & dissections. *Nursing, 34*(2), 36–42.

Bonner, L. (2004). Clinical. The preventions and treatment of deep vein thrombosis. *Nursing Times, 100*(29), 38–42.

Canadian Hypertension Society. (2005). Management of hypertension. *Canadian Nurse, 101*(5), 25.

Chant, T. (2004). Clinical update: Peripheral vascular disease. *Primary Health Care, 14*(8), 29–34.

Copstead, L. C., & Banasik, J. L. (2005). *Pathophysiology* (3rd ed.). St. Louis, MO: Elsevier/Saunders.

Crowther, M., & McCourt, K. (2004). Get the edge on deep vein thrombosis: Head off progression of this deadly condition by knowing when to assess and what to look for during patient screening. *Nursing Management, 35*(1), 21–30.

_____. (2005). Venous thromboembolism: A guide to prevention and treatment. *Nurse Practitioner, 30*(8), 26–29, 32–34, 39–45.

Dee, R. (2003). Issues in geriatrics. Getting a leg up on varicose veins. *Clinical Advisor, 6*(1), 65–67.

Deglin, J. H., & Vallerand, A. H. (2003). *Davis's drug guide for nurses* (8th ed.). Philadelphia: F. A. Davis.

Dochterman, J., & Bulechek, G. (2004). *Nursing interventions classification (NIC)* (4th ed.). St. Louis, MO: Mosby.

Dunn, D. (2005). Preventing perioperative complications in special populations. *Nursing, 35*(11), 36–45.

Elton, G. (2004). Review: Elastic compression stockings prevent post-thrombotic syndrome in patients with deep venous thrombosis. *Evidence-Based Nursing, 7*(3), 86.

Fontaine, K. L. (2005). *Healing practices: Alternative therapies for nursing* (2nd ed.). Upper Saddle River, NJ: Prentice Hall Health.

Foxton, J. (2004). Actions to identify and reduce the risk of atherothrombosis in susceptible patients. *Professional Nurse, 19*(11), 30–33.

Gendreau-Webb, R. (2005). Is it a kidney stone . . . or abdominal aortic aneurysm? *Nursing Made Incredibly Easy, 3*(1), 44–47, 49.

Glover, A. J. (2005). How to detect and defend against DVT. *Nursing, 35*(10), Hospital Nursing 32hn1–32hn2, 32hn4.

Goldhaber, S. Z., McRae, S. J., & Wang, J. (2005, April 1). How to use low-molecular-weight heparin to prevent DVT. *Patient Care for the Nurse Practitioner.*

Gould, S. D., & Spandorfer, J. M. (2005, May 1). Unilateral leg swelling: Clues to cause and ways to treat. *Patient Care for the Nurse Practitioner.*

Graham, J. (2005). Heel pressure ulcers and ankle brachial pressure index. *Nursing Times, 101*(4), 47–48.

Jones, L. E. B. (2005). Endovascular stent grafting of thoracic aortic aneurysms: Technological advancements provide an alternative to traditional surgical repair. *Journal of Cardiovascular Nursing, 20*(6), 376–384.

Kasper, D. L., Braunwald, E., Fauci, A. S., Hauser, S. L., Longo, D. L., & Jameson, J. L. (Eds.). (2005). *Harrison's principles of internal medicine* (16th ed.). New York: McGraw-Hill.

King, M. J., & DiFalco, E. G. (2004). Addressing the pain. Lymphedema: Skin and wound care in an aging population. *Ostomy/Wound Management, 50*(5), 10–12.

Klein, D. G. (2005). Thoracic aortic aneurysms. *Journal of Cardiovascular Nursing, 20*(4), 245–250.

Lehne, R. A. (2004). *Pharmacology for nursing care* (5th ed). St. Louis: Saunders.

McCaffrey, R., Ruknui, P., Hatthakit, U., & Kasetsomboon, P. (2005). The effects of yoga on hypertensive persons in Thailand. *Holistic Nursing Practice, 19*(4), 173–180.

McCance, K. L., & Huether, S. E. (2006). *Pathophysiology: The biologic basis for disease in adults and children* (5th ed.). St. Louis, MO: Mosby.

Miller, E. R., III, & Jehn, M. L. (2004). New high blood pressure guidelines create new at-risk classification: Changes in blood pressure classification by JNC 7. *Journal of Cardiovascular Nursing, 19*(6), 367–373.

Moll, S., & Severson, M. A. (2004). Deep vein thrombosis: The hidden threat. *Care Management* (Suppl), 5–47.

Moore, J. (2005). Hypertension: Catching the silent killer. *Nurse Practitioner, 30*(10), 16–18, 23–24, 26–27+.

Moorhead, S., Johnson, M., & Maas, M. (2004). *Nursing outcomes classification (NOC)* (3rd ed.). St. Louis, MO: Mosby

Morris, C. M. (2005). Comorbidities increase hypertension dangers. *Clinical Advisor for Nurse Practitioners, 8*(3), 46–48.

Nadeau, C., & Varrone, J. (2003). Treat DVT with low molecular weight heparin. *Nurse Practitioner: American Journal of Primary Health Care, 28*(10), 22–23, 26, 29–31.

NANDA International. (2005). *NANDA nursing diagnoses: Definitions & classification 2005–2006.* Philadelphia: Author.

National Heart, Lung, and Blood Institute. (2003). *Facts about the DASH eating plan* (NIH Publication No. 03-4082). Retrieved from http://nhlbi.hih.gov

_____. (2004a). *Morbidity & mortality: 2004 chart book of cardiovascular, lung, and blood diseases.* Bethesda, MD: National Institutes of Health.

_____. (2004b). *The seventh report of the Joint National Committee on prevention, detection, evaluation, and treatment of high blood pressure.* Bethesda, MD: National High Blood Pressure Education Program, National Institutes of Health.

_____. (2005). NHLBI study: High blood pressure not well controlled among older men and women. *NIH News.* Retrieved from http://www.nhlbi.nih.gov/new/press/05-07-26.htm

Porth, C. M. (2005). *Pathophysiology: Concepts of altered health states* (7th ed.). Philadelphia: Lippincott.

Rice, K. L. (2005). How to measure ankle/brachial index. *Nursing, 35*(1), 56–57.

Rothrock, J. C. (2003). *Alexander's care of the patient in surgery* (12th ed.). St. Louis, MO: Mosby.

Ruff, D. (2005). Conservative management of varicose veins. *Nursing Times, 101*(4), 51–52, 54.

Skulski, C. (2004). Endovascular stent insertion for abdominal aortic aneurysm: A nursing perspective. *Canadian Operating Room Nursing Journal, 22*(3), 6, 9–10, 12.

Spencer, J. W., & Jacobs, J. J. (2003). *Complementary and alternative medicine: An evidence-based approach* (2nd ed.). St. Louis, MO: Mosby.

Spratto, G. R., & Woods, A. L. (2003). *2003 edition PDR® nurse's drug handbook™.* Clifton Park, NY: Delmar Learning.

Then, K. L., & Ranking, J. A. (2004). Hypertension: A review for clinicians. *Nursing Clinics of North America, 39*(4), 793–814.

Tierney, L. M., McPhee, S. J., & Papadakis, M. A. (2005). *Current medical diagnosis & treatment* (44th ed.). New York: McGraw-Hill.

Townsend, E., Griffiths, G., Rucker, M., Winter, R., & Lewis, M. (2005). Clinical. Setting up a screening service for abdominal aortic aneurysm. *Nursing Times, 101*(5), 36–38.

U.S. Preventive Services Task Force. (2004). Screening for high blood pressure: Recommendations and rationale. *American Journal of Nursing, 104*(11), 82–85, 87.

_____. (2005). Screening for abdominal aortic aneurysm: Recommendation statement. *The American Journal for Nurse Practitioners, 9*(5), 55–60.

Van Blerk, D. (2004). Evaluating an intermittent compression system for thromboembolism prophylaxis. *Professional Nurse, 20*(4), 48–49.

Way, L. W., & Doherty, G. M. (2003). *Current surgical diagnosis & treatment* (11th ed.). New York: McGraw-Hill

Widmar, B. (2005). When cure is care: Diagnosis and management of pulmonary arterial hypertension. *Journal of the American Academy of Nurse Practitioners, 17*(3), 104–112.

Wilkinson, J. M. (2005). *Nursing diagnosis handbook* (8th ed.). Upper Saddle River, NJ: Prentice Hall.

Wipke-Tevis, D. D., Stotts, N. A., Williams, D. A., Froelicher, E. S., & Hunt, T. K. (2001). Tissue oxygenation, perfusion, and position in patients with venous leg ulcers. *Nursing Research, 50*(1), 24–32.

Wong, J., & Wong, S. (2005). Evidence-based care for the elderly with isolated systolic hypertension. *Nursing & Health Sciences, 7*(1), 67–75.

Woods, A. (2004). Loosening the grip of hypertension. *Nursing, 34*(12), 36–45.

Woods, S. L., Froelicher, E. S., Motzer, S. A., & Bridges, E. (2004). *Cardiac nursing* (5th ed.). Philadelphia: Lippincott.

Wung, S., & Aouizerat, B. E. (2004). Newly mapped gene for thoracic aortic aneurysm and dissection. *Journal of Cardiovascular Nursing, 19*(6), 409–416.

Yang, J. C. (2005). Prevention and treatment of deep vein thrombosis and pulmonary embolism in critically ill patients. *Critical Care Nursing Quarterly, 28*(1), 72–79.

Yucha, C. B., Tsai, P. S., Calderon, K. S., & Tian, L. (2005). Biofeedback-assisted relaxation training for essential hypertension: Who is most likely to benefit? *Journal of Cardiovascular Nursing, 20*(3), 198–205.

UNIT 10 BUILDING CLINICAL COMPETENCE
Responses to Altered Peripheral Tissue Perfusion

FUNCTIONAL HEALTH PATTERN: Activity-Exercise

■ Think about clients with altered activity-exercise patterns and hematologic or peripheral vascular disorders for whom you have cared during your clinical experiences, and how the disease/disorder affected their activities.

- ■ What were the clients' major medical diagnoses (e.g., hypertension, anemia, leukemia, aneurysm, peripheral vascular disease, chronic venous insufficiency)?
- ■ What kinds of manifestations did each of these clients have? How were these manifestations similar or different among clients with different health conditions?
- ■ How did the clients' patterns of activity and exercise contribute to their health problems? Conversely, how did the clients' health status interfere with their daily activities and ability to exercise? Did the clients exercise regularly? Were the clients' symptoms affected by exercise, temperature changes, or changes in position? Did you observe changes in skin color, condition or temperature, hair distribution, or sensation? What other chronic medical conditions were present? What was your clients' history of alcohol or tobacco use?

■ The Activity-Exercise Pattern describes patterns of activity, exercise, leisure, and recreation. Disorders that affect the blood or vascular system can lead to insufficient physiologic energy for activities, disrupting the activity-exercise pattern.
   Blood transports oxygen, nutrients, hormones, and metabolic wastes; is vital to immune function; maintains hemostasis and contributes to homeostasis. Changes in the amount or composition of blood affect its function and ability to meet cellular metabolic demands, leading to manifestations such as:

- ■ Fatigue (low RBC or hgb levels ► reduced oxygen-carrying capacity ► tissue hypoxia ► decreased cellular energy production ► weakness, fatigue, shortness of breath with activity)
- ■ Frequent infections (impaired WBC production or increased WBC destruction ► impaired immune surveillance ► increased incidence of infections)
- ■ Bruising, petechiae, bleeding tendency (impaired bone marrow function ► decreased platelet production ► impaired ability to form stable clots ► bleeding into tissues and external)

■ With each heartbeat, blood moves through a system of vessels that transport oxygenated blood to organs and tissues and return deoxygenated blood to the heart and lungs. The lymphatic system filters and returns excess tissue fluid (lymph) to the bloodstream.
   Disorders of peripheral blood and lymphatic flow include constriction, obstruction, inflammation, and spasm. Arterial obstruction leads to tissue ischemia and insufficient oxygen to meet metabolic needs. Obstruction of a vein or lymph vessel increases pressure behind the obstruction, pushing fluid into interstitial spaces (edema), and interfering with oxygen delivery to the tissues. Manifestations often associated with peripheral vascular disorders include:

- ■ Intermittent claudication and impaired sensation (arterial occlusion ► decreased blood flow ► tissue ischemia ► pain, neuron damage ► paresthesias, impaired sensation)
- ■ Edema (venous or lymphatic vessel obstruction ► increased fluid pressure in capillary beds ► imbalance between capillary fluid loss and resorption ► increased interstitial fluid)

■ Priority nursing diagnoses within the Activity-Exercise Pattern that may be appropriate for clients with hematologic or peripheral vascular disorders include:

- ■ *Ineffective Peripheral Tissue Perfusion* as evidenced by changes in skin color and temperature, lack of hair growth, skin irritations or ulcers
- ■ *Activity Intolerance* as evidenced by weakness, fatigue, vital sign changes with activity
- ■ *Fatigue* as evidenced by difficulty completing usual daily activities, frequent desire to rest
- ■ *Impaired Home Maintenance* as evidenced by inability to maintain family roles
- ■ *Risk for Peripheral Neurovascular Dysfunction* as evidenced by changes in color, temperature, sensation of extremities.

■ Two nursing diagnoses from other functional health patterns often are of high priority for the client with altered hemotologic or peripheral tissue perfusion:

- ■ *Impaired Tissue Integrity* (Nutritional-Metabolic)
- ■ *Effective Therapeutic Regimen Management* (Health Perception-Health Management)

CLINICAL SCENARIO

You have been assigned to work with the following four clients for the 0700 shift on a cardiac medical-surgical unit. Significant data obtained during report are as follows:

■ Theresa Cartwright is a 34-year-old female admitted for anticoagulant therapy after developing a deep venous thrombosis after a fall down the steps and hitting her calf. She was started on heparin yesterday and needs blood drawn for an activated partial thromboplastin time (aPTT) to determine her morning dose of heparin.

■ Bessie Gregg is a 56-year-old with a 10-year history of alcoholism. She was admitted 2 days ago with pallor, shortness of breath, heart palpitations, weakness, and fatigue. She is agitated and requesting to be discharged.

■ Scott Jacoby is a 25-year-old with Down syndrome. He was admitted yesterday with an upper respiratory infection. On assessment he was pale, T 101°F, P 100, R 30 with dyspnea on exertion, BP of 118/86, and multiple bruises and petechiae on his arms and legs. He is scheduled for a bone marrow examination this morning.

■ Robert Tucker is a 65-year-old admitted 3 hours ago with moderate pain in the midabdominal region. On admission, a pulsating mass was felt in the midabdomen and a bruit was found over the same area. He is now complaining of severe pain in the midabdominal area.

Questions

In what order would you visit these clients after report?

1. _____
2. _____
3. _____
4. _____

2 What top two priority nursing diagnoses would you choose for each of the clients presented above? Can you explain, if asked, the rationale for your choices?

	Priority Nursing Diagnosis #1	Priority Nursing Diagnosis #2
Theresa Cartwright		
Bessie Gregg		
Scott Jacoby		
Robert Tucker		

3 Mrs. Cartwright needs further teaching regarding anticoagulant therapy when she makes which statement?
1. "The heparin will be continued for four to five days for the Coumadin to reach a good effect."
2. "I need to continue to have blood drawn to watch my drug levels as long as I am taking these drugs."
3. "I cannot continue to take birth control pills while I am taking these drugs."
4. "I need to take the medication at the same time every day for the drug to be effective."

4 The nurse explains to Mrs. Gregg that she needs a diet high in folic acid to treat her manifestations. Mrs. Gregg understands this diet when she picks which meal plan?
1. chili with kidney beans, roll, and milk
2. pork roast with baked potato and lemonade
3. spaghetti with meat sauce and iced tea
4. chicken and dumplings with coffee

5 Which is the most important for the client with leukemia to report?
1. constipation and straining with bowel movements
2. fever and burning on urination
3. weight loss and decreased appetite
4. dyspnea and shortness of breath with exercising

6 Which nursing interventions should reduce the risk of rupture of an aneurysm?
1. Administer anticoagulant therapy medications.
2. Instruct patient to hold the breath while moving.
3. Maintain the patient on bed rest with the legs flat.
4. Place the patient in a room near the nurse's station.

7 Which discharge instructions does the nurse teach the hypertensive client? (Select all that apply.)
1. Maintain normal body weight.
2. Eat a diet rich in fruits and vegetables.
3. Reduce potassium intake.
4. Limit alcohol to no more than 20 oz. of beer or 6 oz. of wine per day.
5. Engage in aerobic exercise for 1 hour three times a week.
6. Stop smoking.

8 Which nursing diagnosis has the highest priority for the client with varicose veins?
1. *Body Image Disturbance*
2. *Impaired Tissue Perfusion*
3. *Activity Intolerance*
4. *Risk for Infection*

9 With a history of Raynaud's disease, which is a priority teaching instruction for the client?
1. Enter a smoking cessation program.
2. Reduce dietary fats and carbohydrates.
3. Wear gloves and socks in cold weather.
4. Begin an exercise program.

10 A prescription for the calcium channel blocker diltiazem (Cardizem) is ordered for the client with hypertension. What will the nurse instruct the client regarding administration of the medication?
1. Limit fluids to decrease the development of peripheral edema.
2. Notify the physician for a pulse of less than 60 beats per minute.
3. Increase fiber in the diet because diarrhea may be a side effect.
4. Report tachycardia and an increase in blood pressure.

11 When the client is placed on warfarin (Coumadin) therapy, which laboratory studies would you expect to draw? (Select all that apply.)
1. activated partial thromboplastin time (aPTT)
2. international normalized ratio (INR)
3. partial thromboplastin time (PTT)
4. complete blood cell count (CBC)
5. white blood cell count (WBC)
6. prothrombin time (PT)

12 A client with history of hemophilia fell and cut his leg while hiking in the woods. Which intervention should the client do until help arrives?
1. Apply a tourniquet above the cut.
2. Splint the leg to prevent movement.
3. Apply pressure to the femoral artery.
4. Apply gentle pressure over the cut.

CASE STUDY

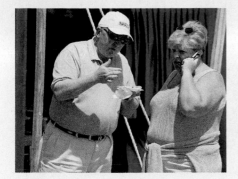

Grace Schmidt is a 49-year-old female who works as a teaching assistant at an elementary school. She comes to the medical clinic complaining of a throbbing headache and dizziness. Her height and weight are 5'6" and 245 pounds. Upon assessment her vital signs are P 100, R 16, BP lying is 180/115, sitting is 170/110, and standing is 165/105. Her skin is cool and dry. Her capillary refill is 4 seconds. She denies smoking, drinks an occasional glass of wine, and does not participate in a regular exercise program. She states that her job can be stressful at times. Nutrition assessment indicates a diet high in fats and sodium. She denies any family history of hypertension or heart disease. She is married and has a daughter and son who live in the same town. A medical diagnosis of hypertension is determined.

Based on Mrs. Schmidt's assessment, blood pressure readings, and weight, the priority nursing diagnosis of *Ineffective Health Maintenance* is identified for planning nursing care.

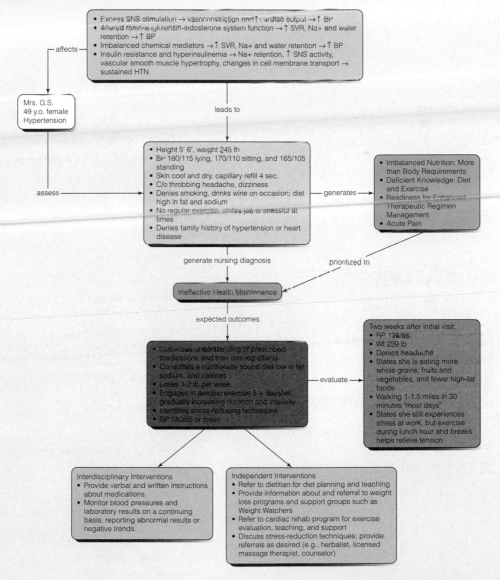

Mrs. G.S.
49 y.o. female
Hypertension

affects

- Excess SNS stimulation → vasoconstriction and ↑ cardiac output → ↑ BP
- Altered renin-angiotensin-aldosterone system function → ↑ SVR, Na+ and water retention → ↑ BP
- Imbalanced chemical mediators → ↑ SVR, Na+ and water retention → ↑ BP
- Insulin resistance and hyperinsulinemia → Na+ retention, ↑ SNS activity, vascular smooth muscle hypertrophy, changes in cell membrane transport → sustained HTN

leads to

assess

- Height 5' 6", weight 245 lb
- BP 180/115 lying, 170/110 sitting, and 165/105 standing
- Skin cool and dry, capillary refill 4 sec.
- C/o throbbing headache, dizziness
- Denies smoking, drinks wine on occasion; diet high in fat and sodium
- No regular exercise, states job is stressful at times
- Denies family history of hypertension or heart disease

generates

- Imbalanced Nutrition: More than Body Requirements
- Deficient Knowledge: Diet and Exercise
- Readiness for Enhanced Therapeutic Regimen Management
- Acute Pain

generate nursing diagnosis

prioritized to

Ineffective Health Maintenance

expected outcomes

- Verbalizes understanding of prescribed medications and their desired effects
- Consumes a nutritionally sound diet low in fat, sodium, and calories
- Loses 1-2 lb per week
- Engages in aerobic exercise 5 + days/wk, gradually increasing duration and intensity
- Identifies stress-reducing techniques
- BP 140/85 or lower

evaluate

Two weeks after initial visit:
- BP 136/86
- Wt 239 lb
- Denies headache
- States she is eating more whole grains, fruits and vegetables, and fewer high-fat foods
- Walking 1-1.5 miles in 30 minutes "most days"
- States she still experiences stress at work, but exercise during lunch hour and breaks helps relieve tension

Interdisciplinary Interventions
- Provide verbal and written instructions about medications.
- Monitor blood pressures and laboratory results on a continuing basis, reporting abnormal results or negative trends.

Independent Interventions
- Refer to dietitian for diet planning and teaching
- Provide information about and referral to weight loss programs and support groups such as Weight Watchers
- Refer to cardiac rehab program for exercise evaluation, teaching, and support
- Discuss stress-reduction techniques; provide referrals as desired (e.g., herbalist, licensed massage therapist, counselor)

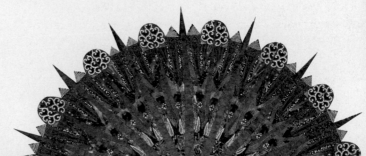

UNIT
11

Responses to Altered Respiratory Function

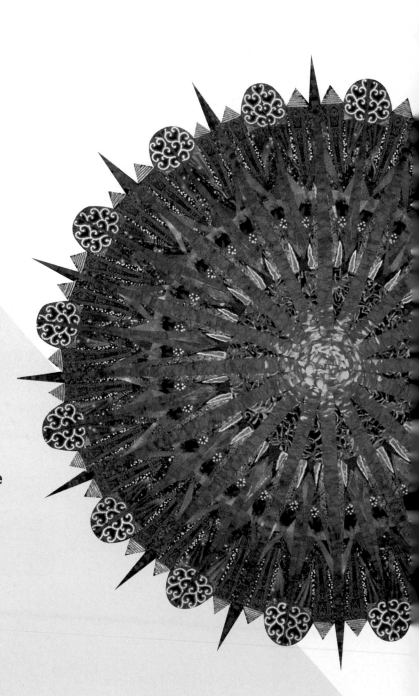

CHAPTER 36
Assessing Clients with Respiratory Disorders

CHAPTER 37
Nursing Care of Clients with Upper Respiratory Disorders

CHAPTER 38
Nursing Care of Clients with Ventilation Disorders

CHAPTER 39
Nursing Care of Clients with Gas Exchange Disorders

CHAPTER 36 Assessing Clients with Respiratory Disorders

LEARNING OUTCOMES

- Describe the anatomy, physiology, and functions of the respiratory system.
- Explain the mechanics of ventilation.
- Compare and contrast factors affecting respiration.

- Identify specific topics for consideration during a health history interview of the client with health problems involving the respiratory system.
- Describe normal variations in assessment findings for the older adult.
- Identify manifestations of impairment of the respiratory system.

CLINICAL COMPETENCIES

- Conduct and document a health history for clients having or at risk for alterations in the respiratory system.
- Conduct and document a physical assessment of respiratory structures and functions.

- Monitor the results of diagnostic tests and report abnormal findings.

EQUIPMENT NEEDED

- Tongue blade
- Penlight
- Nasal speculum

- Metric ruler
- Marking pen
- Stethoscope with diaphragm

MEDIALINK

Resources for this chapter can be found on the Prentice Hall Nursing MediaLink DVD-ROM accompanying this textbook, and on the Companion Website at
http://www.prenhall.com/lemone

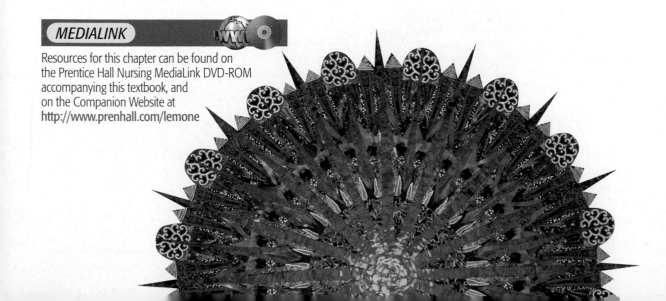

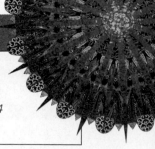

KEY TERMS

apnea, *1223*	**friction rub**, *1226*	**tachypnea**, *1223*
atelectasis, *1223*	**lung compliance**, *1216*	**tidal volume (TV)**, *1214*
bradypnea, *1223*	**oxyhemoglobin**, *1216*	**vital capacity (VC)**, *1214*
crackles, *1226*	**surfactant**, *1216*	**wheezes**, *1226*

The respiratory system provides the cells of the body with oxygen and eliminates carbon dioxide, formed as a waste product of cellular metabolism. The events in this process, called respiration, are:

■ *Pulmonary ventilation:* Air is moved into and out of the lungs.

■ *External respiration:* Exchange of oxygen and carbon dioxide occurs between the alveoli and the blood.

■ *Gas transport:* Oxygen and carbon dioxide are transported to and from the lungs and the cells of the body via the blood.

■ *Internal respiration:* Exchange of oxygen and carbon dioxide is made between the blood and the cells.

ANATOMY, PHYSIOLOGY, AND FUNCTIONS OF THE RESPIRATORY SYSTEM

The respiratory system functions as a whole, but is divided into the upper respiratory system and the lower respiratory system for discussion of respiratory disorders in the following chapters.

The Upper Respiratory System

The upper respiratory system serves as a passageway for air moving into the lungs and carbon dioxide moving out to the external environment (Figure 36–1 ■). As air moves through these structures, it is cleaned, humidified, and warmed.

The Nose

The nose is the external opening of the respiratory system. The external nose is given structure by the nasal, frontal, and maxillary bones as well as plates of hyaline cartilage. The nostrils (also called the external nares) are two cavities within the nose, separated by the nasal septum. These cavities open into the nasal portion of the pharynx through the internal nares. The nasal cavities just behind the nasal openings are lined with skin that contains hair follicles, sweat glands, and sebaceous glands. The nasal hairs filter the air as it enters the nares. The rest of the cavity is lined with mucous membranes that contain olfactory neurons and goblet cells that secrete thick mucus. The mucus not only traps dust and bacteria but also contains lysozyme, an enzyme that destroys bacteria as they enter the nose. As mucus and debris accumulate, mucosal ciliated cells move it toward the pharynx, where it is swallowed. The mucosa is highly vascular, warming air that moves across its surface.

Three structures project outward from the lateral wall of each nasal cavity: the superior, middle, and inferior turbinates. The turbinates cause air entering the nose to become turbulent

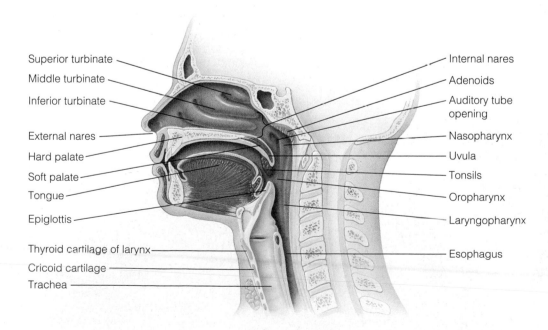

Figure 36–1 ■ The upper respiratory system.

and also increase the surface area of mucosa exposed to the air. As air moves through this area, heavier particles of debris drop out and are trapped in the mucosa of the turbinates.

The Sinuses

The nasal cavity is surrounded by paranasal sinuses (Figure 36–2 ■), located in the frontal, sphenoid, ethmoid, and maxillary bones. Sinuses lighten the skull, assist in speech, and produce mucus that drains into the nasal cavities to help trap debris.

The Pharynx

The pharynx, a funnel-shaped passageway about 5 inches (13 cm) long, extends from the base of the skull to the level of the C6 vertebra. The pharynx serves as a passageway for both air and food. It is divided into three regions: the nasopharynx, the oropharynx, and the laryngopharynx.

The nasopharynx serves only as a passageway for air. Located beneath the sphenoid bone and above the level of the soft palate, the nasopharynx is continuous with the nasal cavities. This segment is lined with ciliated epithelium, which continues to move debris from the nasal cavities to the pharynx. Masses of lymphoid tissue (the tonsils and adenoids) are located in the mucosa high in the posterior wall; these tissues trap and destroy infectious agents entering with the air. The auditory (eustachian) tubes also open into the nasopharynx, connecting it with the middle ear.

The oropharynx lies behind the oral cavity and extends from the soft palate to the level of the hyoid bone. It serves as a passageway for both air and food. An upward rise of the soft palate prevents food from entering the nasopharynx during swallowing. The oropharynx is lined with stratified squamous epithelium that protects it from the friction of food and damage from the chemicals found in food and fluids.

The laryngopharynx extends from the hyoid bone to the larynx. It is also lined with stratified squamous epithelium, and serves as a passageway for both food and air. Air does not move into the lungs while food is being swallowed and moved into the esophagus.

The Larynx

The larynx is about 2 inches (5 cm) long. It opens superiorly at the laryngopharynx and is continuous inferiorly with the trachea. The larynx provides an airway and routes air and food into the proper passageway. As long as air is moving through the larynx, its inlet is open; however, the inlet closes during swallowing. The larynx also contains the vocal cords, necessary for voice production.

The larynx is framed by cartilages, connected by ligaments and membranes. The thyroid cartilage is formed by the fusion of two cartilages; the fusion point is visible as the Adam's apple. The cricoid cartilage lies below the thyroid cartilage; other pairs of cartilages form the walls of the larynx. The epiglottis, also a cartilage, normally projects upward to the base of the tongue; however, during swallowing, the larynx moves upward and the epiglottis tips to cover the opening to the larynx. If anything other than air enters the larynx, a cough reflex expels the foreign substance before it can enter the lungs. This protective reflex does not work if the person is unconscious.

The Trachea

The trachea begins at the inferior larynx and descends anteriorly to the esophagus to enter the mediastinum, where it divides to become the right and left primary bronchi of the lungs. The trachea is about 4 to 5 inches (12 to 15 cm) long and 1 inch (2.5 cm) in diameter. It contains 16 to 20 C-shaped rings of cartilage joined by connective tissue. The mucosa lining the trachea consists of pseudostratified ciliated columnar epithelium containing seromucous glands that produce thick mucus. Dust and debris in the inspired air are trapped in this mucus, moved toward the throat by the cilia, and then either swallowed or coughed out through the mouth.

The Lower Respiratory System

The lower respiratory system includes the lungs and the bronchi (Figure 36–3 ■ and Figure 36–4 ■).

The Lungs

The center of the thoracic cavity is filled by the mediastinum, which contains the heart, great blood vessels, bronchi, trachea, and esophagus. The mediastinum is flanked on either side by the lungs (see Figure 36–3). Each lung is suspended in its own pleural cavity, with the anterior, lateral, and posterior lung surfaces lying close to the ribs. The hilus, on the mediastinal surface of each lung, is

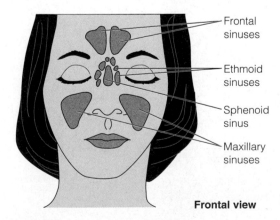

Frontal view

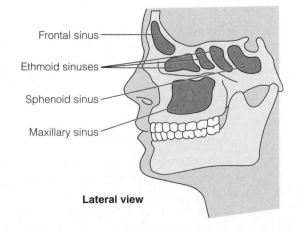

Lateral view

Figure 36–2 ■ Sinuses, frontal and lateral views.

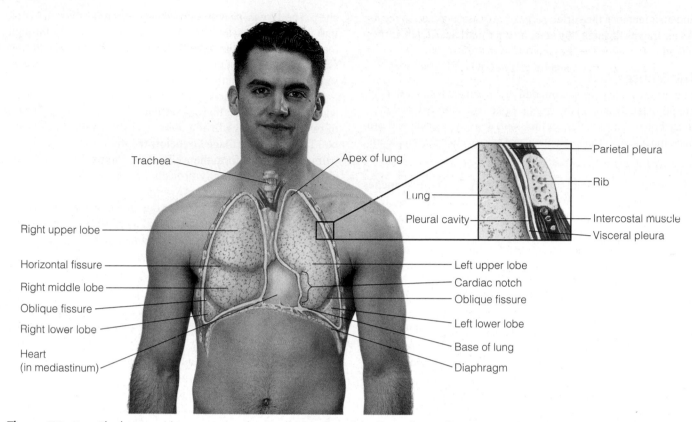

Figure 36–3 ■ The lower respiratory system, showing the location of the lungs, the mediastinum, and layers of visceral and parietal pleura.

where blood vessels of the pulmonary and circulatory systems enter and exit the lungs. The primary bronchus also enters in this area. The apex of each lung lies just below the clavicle, whereas the base of each lung rests on the diaphragm. The lungs are elastic connective tissue, called stroma, and are soft and spongy.

The two lungs differ in size and shape. The left lung is smaller and has two lobes, whereas the right lung has three lobes. Each of the lung lobes contains a different number of bronchopulmonary segments, separated by connective tissue.

There are 8 segments in the two lobes of the left lung and 10 segments in the three lobes of the right lung.

The vascular system of the lungs consists of the pulmonary arteries, which deliver blood to the lungs for oxygenation, and the pulmonary veins, which deliver oxygenated blood to the heart. Within the lungs, the pulmonary arteries branch into a pulmonary capillary network that surrounds the alveoli. Lung tissue receives its blood supply from the bronchial arteries and drains by the bronchial and pulmonary veins.

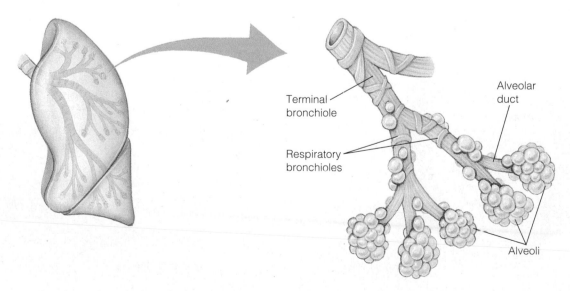

Figure 36–4 ■ Respiratory bronchi, bronchioles, alveolar ducts, and alveoli.

The Pleura

The pleura is a double-layered membrane that covers the lungs and the inside of the thoracic cavities (see Figure 36–3). The parietal pleura lines the thoracic wall and mediastinum. It is continuous with the visceral pleura, which covers the external lung surfaces. The pleura produces pleural fluid, a lubricating, serous fluid that allows the lungs to move easily over the thoracic wall during breathing. The pleura's two layers also cling tightly together and hold the lungs to the thoracic wall. The structure of the pleura creates a slightly negative pressure in the pleural space (which is actually a potential rather than an actual space), necessary for lung function.

The Bronchi and Alveoli

The trachea divides into right and left primary bronchi; in comparison to the left primary bronchus, the right primary bronchus is shorter, wider, and situated more vertically (making aspiration of foreign bodies into the right primary bronchus more likely). The point where the trachea divides is innervated with sensory neurons; activities such as tracheal suctioning may induce coughing and bronchospasm from stimulation of these neurons. These main bronchi subdivide into the secondary (lobar) bronchi, with the right middle lobe bronchus being smaller in diameter and length, and sometimes it bends sharply near its bifurcation. The secondary bronchi then branch into the tertiary (segmental) bronchi, and then into smaller and smaller bronchioles, ending in the terminal bronchioles, which are extremely small (see Figure 36–4). These branching passageways collectively are called the bronchial or respiratory tree. From the terminal bronchioles, air moves into air sacs (called respiratory bronchioles), which further branch into alveolar ducts that lead to alveolar sacs and then to the tiny alveoli. During inspiration, air enters the lungs through the primary bronchus and then moves through the increasingly smaller passageways of the lungs to the alveoli, where oxygen and carbon dioxide exchange occurs in the process of external respiration. During expiration, the carbon dioxide is expelled.

Alveoli cluster around the alveolar sacs, which open into a common chamber called the atrium. The adult lung has approximately 300 million alveoli, providing an enormous surface for gas exchange (Porth, 2005). Alveoli have extremely thin walls of a single layer of squamous epithelial cells over a very thin basement membrane. The external surface of the alveoli are covered with pulmonary capillaries. The alveolar and capillary walls form the respiratory membrane. Gas exchange across the respiratory membrane occurs by simple diffusion. The alveolar walls also contain cells that secrete a surfactant-containing fluid, necessary for maintaining a moist surface and reducing the surface tension of the alveolar fluid to help prevent collapse of the lungs.

The Rib Cage and Intercostal Muscles

The lungs are protected by the bones of the rib cage and the intercostal muscles. There are 12 pairs of ribs, which all articulate with the thoracic vertebrae (Figure 36–5 ■). Anteriorly, the first 7 ribs articulate with the body of the sternum. The 8th, 9th, and 10th ribs articulate with the cartilage immediately above the ribs. The 11th and 12th ribs are called floating ribs, because they are unattached.

The sternum has three parts: the manubrium, the body, and the xiphoid process. The junction between the manubrium and the body of the sternum is called the manubriosternal junction or the angle of Louis. The depression above the manubrium is called the suprasternal notch.

The spaces between the ribs are called the intercostal spaces. Each intercostal space is named for the rib immediately above it (e.g., the space between the third and fourth ribs is designated as the third intercostal space). The intercostal muscles between the ribs, along with the diaphragm, are called the inspiratory muscles.

FACTORS AFFECTING VENTILATION AND RESPIRATION

Many factors affect ventilation and respiration. Those discussed here include changes in volume and capacity; air pressures; oxygen, carbon dioxide, and hydrogen ion concentrations in the blood; airway resistance, lung compliance, and elasticity; and alveolar surface tension.

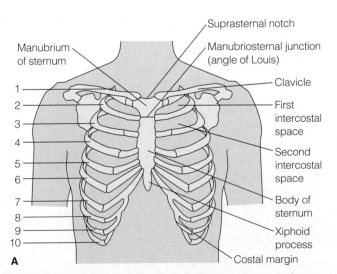

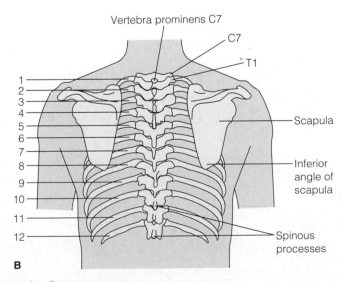

Figure 36–5 ■ *A,* Anterior rib cage, showing intercostal spaces. *B,* Posterior rib cage.

Respiratory Volume and Capacity

Respiratory volume and capacity are affected by gender, age, weight, and health status.

- **Tidal volume (TV)** is the amount of air (approximately 500 mL) moved in and out of the lungs with each normal, quiet breath.
- *Inspiratory reserve volume (IRV)* is the amount of air (approximately 2100 to 3100 mL) that can be inhaled forcibly over the tidal volume.
- *Expiratory reserve volume (ERV)* is the approximately 1000 mL of air that can be forced out over the tidal volume.
- The *residual volume* is the volume of air (approximately 1100 mL) that remains in the lungs after a forced expiration.

- **Vital capacity (VC)** refers to the sum of TV + IRV + ERV and is approximately 4500 mL in the healthy client.
- About 150 mL of air never reaches the alveoli (the amount remaining in the passageways) and is called anatomic dead space volume.

Pulmonary function tests measure these and other respiratory volumes and capacities, and are described and illustrated in Box 36–1.

Air Pressures

Pulmonary ventilation depends on volume changes within the thoracic cavity. A change in the volume of air in the thoracic

---

BOX 36–1 Pulmonary Function Tests

Pulmonary function tests (PFTs) are performed in a pulmonary function laboratory. After preparing the client, a nose clip is applied and the unsedated client breathes into a spirometer or body plethysmograph, a device for measuring and recording lung volume in liters versus time in seconds. The client is instructed how to breathe for specific tests: for example, to inhale as deeply as possible and then exhale to the maximal extent possible. Using measured lung volumes, respiratory capacities are calculated to assess pulmonary status. The specific values determined by PFT and illustrated in the figure include the following.

- *Total lung capacity (TLC)* is the total volume of the lungs at their maximum inflation. Four values are used to calculate TLC.
  - a. *Total volume (TV)*, the volume inhaled and exhaled with normal quiet breathing (also called tidal volume)
  - b. *Inspiratory reserve volume (IRV)*, the maximum amount that can be inhaled over and above a normal inspiration
  - c. *Expiratory reserve volume (ERV)*, the maximum amount that can be exhaled following a normal exhalation.
  - d. *Residual volume (RV)*, the amount of air remaining in the lungs after maximal exhalation.
- *Vital capacity (VC)* is the total amount of air that can be exhaled after a maximal inspiration. It is calculated by adding together the IRV, TV, and the ERV.

- *Inspiratory capacity* is the total amount of air that can be inhaled following a normal quiet exhalation. It is calculated by adding the TV and IRV.
- *Functional residual capacity (FRC)* is the volume of air left in the lungs after a normal exhalation. The ERV and RV are added to determine the FRC.
- *Forced expiratory volume (FEV$_1$)* is the amount of air that can be exhaled in 1 second.
- *Forced vital capacity (FVC)* is the amount of air that can be exhaled forcefully and rapidly after maximum air intake.
- *Minute volume (MV)* is the total amount or volume of air breathed in 1 minute.

In older clients, residual capacity is increased, and vital capacity is decreased. These age-related changes result from the following:

- Calcification of the costal cartilage and weakening of the intercostal muscles, which reduce movement of the chest wall
- Vertebral osteoporosis, which decreases spinal flexibility and increases the degree of kyphosis, further increasing the anterior-posterior diameter of the chest
- Diaphragmatic flattening and loss of elasticity.

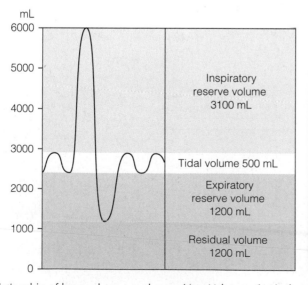
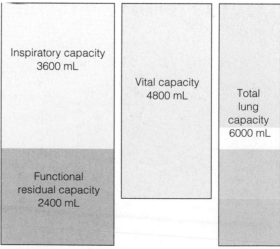

The relationship of lung volumes and capacities. Volumes (mL) shown are for an average adult male.

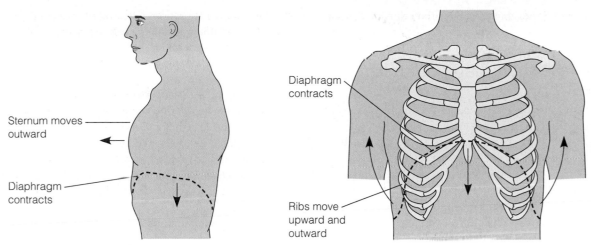

Figure 36–6 ■ Respiratory inspiration: lateral and anterior views. Note the volume expansion of the thorax as the diaphragm flattens.

cavity leads to a change in the air pressure within the cavity. Because gases always flow along their pressure gradients, a change in pressure results in gases flowing into or out of the lungs to equalize the pressure.

The pressures normally present in the thoracic cavity are the intrapulmonary pressure and the intrapleural pressure. The intrapulmonary pressure, within the alveoli of the lungs, rises and falls constantly as a result of the acts of ventilation (inhalation and exhalation). The intrapleural pressure, within the pleural space, also rises and falls with the acts of ventilation, but it is always less than (or negative to) the intrapulmonary pressure. Intrapulmonary and intrapleural pressures are necessary not only to expand and contract the lungs, but also to prevent their collapse.

Pulmonary ventilation has two phases: inspiration, during which air flows into the lungs; and expiration, during which gases flow out of the lungs. The two phases make up a single breath, and normally occur from 12 to 20 times each minute. A single inspiration lasts for about 1 to 1.5 seconds, whereas an expiration lasts for about 2 to 3 seconds.

During inspiration, the diaphragm contracts and flattens out to increase the vertical diameter of the thoracic cavity (Figure 36–6 ■). The external intercostal muscles contract, elevating the rib cage and moving the sternum forward to expand the lateral and anteroposterior diameter of the thoracic cavity, decreasing intrapleural pressure. The lungs stretch and the intrapulmonary volume increases, decreasing intrapulmonary pressure slightly below atmospheric pressure. Air rushes into the lungs as a result of this pressure gradient until the intrapulmonary and atmospheric pressures equalize.

Expiration is primarily a passive process that occurs as a result of the elasticity of the lungs (Figure 36–7 ■). The inspiratory muscles relax, the diaphragm rises, the ribs descend, and the lungs recoil. Both the thoracic and intrapulmonary pressures increase, compressing the alveoli. The intrapulmonary pressure rises to a level greater than atmospheric pressure, and gases flow out of the lungs.

Oxygen, Carbon Dioxide, and Hydrogen Ion Concentrations

The rate and depth of respirations are controlled by respiratory centers in the medulla oblongata and pons of the brain and by chemoreceptors located in the medulla and in the carotid and aortic bodies. The centers and chemoreceptors respond to changes in the concentration of oxygen, carbon dioxide, and hydrogen ions

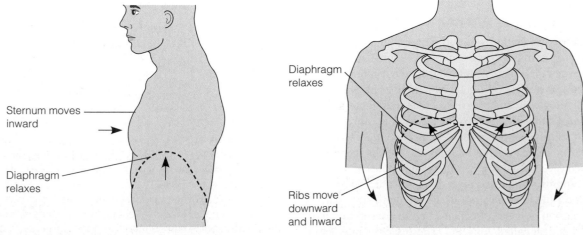

Figure 36–7 ■ Respiratory expiration: lateral and anterior views.

in arterial blood. For example, when carbon dioxide concentration increases or the pH decreases, the respiratory rate increases. This process is further described in Chapter 10 ∞.

Airway Resistance, Lung Compliance, and Elasticity

Respiratory passageway resistance, lung compliance, and lung elasticity also affect respiration.

- Respiratory passageway resistance is created by the friction encountered as gases move along the respiratory passageways, by constriction of the passageways (especially the larger bronchioles), by accumulations of mucus or infectious material, and by tumors. As resistance increases, gas flow decreases.
- **Lung compliance** is the distensibility of the lungs. It depends on the elasticity of the lung tissue and the flexibility of the rib cage. Compliance is decreased by factors that decrease the elasticity of the lungs, block the respiratory passageways, or interfere with movement of the rib cage.
- Lung elasticity is essential for lung distention during inspiration and lung recoil during expiration. Decreased elasticity from disease such as emphysema impairs respiration.

Alveolar Surface Tension

A liquid film of mostly water covers the alveolar walls. At any gas–liquid boundary, the molecules of liquid are more strongly attracted to each other than to gas molecules. This produces a state of tension, called surface tension, that draws the liquid molecules even more closely together. The water content of the alveolar film compacts the alveoli and aids in the lungs' recoil during expiration. In fact, if the alveolar film were pure water, the alveoli would collapse between breaths.

   Surfactant, a lipoprotein produced by the alveolar cells, interferes with this adhesiveness of the water molecules, reducing surface tension, and helping expand the lungs. With insufficient surfactant, the surface tension forces can become great enough to collapse the alveoli between breaths, requiring tremendous energy to reinflate the lungs for inspiration.

BLOOD GASES

Gases are transported by the blood to provide cells with oxygen and to remove carbon dioxide produced during cellular activities.

Oxygen Transport and Unloading

Oxygen is carried in the blood either bound to hemoglobin or dissolved in the plasma. Oxygen is not very soluble in water, so almost all oxygen that enters the blood from the respiratory system is carried to the cells of the body by hemoglobin. This combination of hemoglobin and oxygen is called **oxyhemoglobin**.

   Each hemoglobin molecule is made of four polypeptide chains, with each chain bound to an iron-containing heme group. The iron groups are the binding sites for oxygen; each hemoglobin molecule can bind with four molecules of oxygen.

   Oxygen binding is rapid and reversible. It is affected by temperature, blood pH, partial pressure of oxygen (P_{O_2}), partial pressure of carbon dioxide (P_{CO_2}), and serum concentration of an organic chemical called 2,3-DPG. These factors interact to ensure adequate delivery of oxygen to the cells.

The relative saturation of hemoglobin depends on the P_{O_2} of the blood, as illustrated in the oxygen-hemoglobin dissociation curve (Figure 36–8 ■).

- Under normal conditions, the hemoglobin in arterial blood is 97.4% saturated with oxygen. Hemoglobin is almost fully saturated at a P_{O_2} of 70 mmHg. As arterial blood flows through the capillaries, oxygen is unloaded, so that the oxygen saturation of hemoglobin in venous blood is 75%.
- The affinity of oxygen and hemoglobin decreases as the temperature of body tissues increases above normal. As a result, less oxygen binds with hemoglobin, and oxygen unloading is enhanced. Conversely, as the body is chilled, oxygen unloading is inhibited.
- The oxygen-hemoglobin bond is weakened by increased hydrogen ion concentrations. As blood becomes more acidotic, oxygen unloading to the tissues is enhanced. The same process occurs when the partial pressure of carbon dioxide increases because this decreases the pH.
- The organic chemical 2,3-DPG is formed in red blood cells and enhances the release of oxygen from hemoglobin by binding to it during times of increased metabolism (as when body temperature increases). This binding alters the structure of hemoglobin to facilitate oxygen unloading.

Carbon Dioxide Transport

Active cells produce about 200 mL of carbon dioxide each minute; this amount is exactly the same as that excreted by the lungs each minute. Excretion of carbon dioxide from the body requires transport by the blood from the cells to the lungs. Carbon dioxide is transported in three forms: dissolved in plasma, bound to hemoglobin, and as bicarbonate ions in the plasma (the largest amount is in this form).

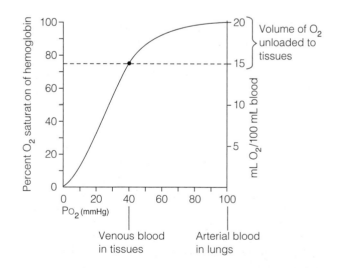

Figure 36–8 ■ Oxygen-hemoglobin dissociation curve. The percent O_2 saturation of hemoglobin and total blood oxygen volume are shown for different oxygen partial pressures (P_{O_2}). Arterial blood in the lungs is almost completely saturated. During one pass through the body, about 25% of hemoglobin-bound oxygen is unloaded to the tissues. Thus, venous blood is still about 75% saturated with oxygen. The steep portion of the curve shows that hemoglobin readily off-loads or on-loads oxygen at P_{O_2} levels below about 50 mmHg.

The amount of carbon dioxide transported in the blood is strongly influenced by the oxygenation of the blood. When the P_{O_2} decreases, with a corresponding decrease in oxygen saturation, increased amounts of carbon dioxide can be carried in the blood. Carbon dioxide entering the systemic circulation from the cells causes more oxygen to dissociate from hemoglobin, in turn allowing more carbon dioxide to combine with hemoglobin and more bicarbonate ions to be generated. This situation is reversed in the pulmonary circulation, where the uptake of oxygen facilitates the release of carbon dioxide.

ASSESSING RESPIRATORY FUNCTION

Function of the respiratory system is assessed by findings from diagnostic tests, a health assessment interview to collect subjective data, and a physical assessment to collect objective data. Sample documentation of an assessment of the respiratory system is included in the box on this page.

Diagnostic Tests

The results of diagnostic tests of respiratory function are used to support the diagnosis of a specific disease, to provide information to identify or modify the appropriate medications or therapy used to treat the disease, and to help nurses monitor the

> **SAMPLE DOCUMENTATION**
> **Assessment of the Lungs**
>
> *57-year-old male, history of smoking 2 packs cigarettes/day for 37 years; continues to smoke despite previous discussions. Works as a dry-wall installer. No family history of cancer or TB. States he has trouble breathing, especially at night. Often sleeps on a recliner "to breathe better." Complains of a cough, but denies sputum production. Diagnosed 3 years ago with emphysema. Color of face is dusky red. Fingernails pink. Respirations 30, unlabored, regular (R varies from 26 to 32 on visits to the clinic). Thoracic assessment = intercostal bulging, barrel chest, diminished lung sounds bilaterally in lower lobes. Crackles present in upper lobes, not cleared by coughing. Discussed possible use of low-flow nasal oxygen at night to help with breathing; will check with primary provider.*

client's responses to treatment and nursing care interventions. Diagnostic tests to assess the structures and functions of the respiratory system are described in the Diagnostic Tests table below and summarized in the bulleted list that follows. More information is included in the discussion of specific disorders in Chapters 37, 38, and 39 ∞.

DIAGNOSTIC TESTS of the Respiratory System

NAME OF TEST Sputum Studies

- Culture and sensitivity
- Acid-fast smear and culture
- Cytology

PURPOSE AND DESCRIPTION Culture and sensitivity of a single sputum specimen is done to diagnose bacterial infections, identify the most effective antibiotic, and evaluate treatment.

Sputum is examined for presence of acid-fast bacillus, specifically tuberculosis. A series of three early morning sputum specimens is used.

Sputum is examined for presence of abnormal (malignant) cells. A single sputum specimen is collected in a special container of fixative solution.

RELATED NURSING CARE See Procedure 36–1 on page 1220 for obtaining a sputum specimen. Sputum specimens may also be obtained during bronchoscopy (described later) if the client is unable to provide a specimen.

NAME OF TEST Arterial blood gases (ABGs)

PURPOSE AND DESCRIPTION This test of arterial blood is done to assess alterations in acid–base balance caused by a respiratory disorder, a metabolic disorder, or both. A pH of less than 7.35 indicates acidosis and a pH of more than 7.45 indicates alkalosis (see Chapter 10 ∞). To determine a respiratory cause, assess the Pa_{CO_2}: If pH is decreased and Pa_{CO_2} is increased, respiratory acidosis is indicated.

Normal values:
pH: 7.35–7.45
Pa_{CO_2}: 35–45 mmHg

Pa_{O_2}: 75–100 mmHg
HCO_3: 24–28 mEq/L
BE: ± 2 mEq/L

RELATED NURSING CARE Arterial blood is collected in a heparinized needle and syringe. Sample is placed on an icebag and taken immediately to the lab. If client is receiving oxygen, indicate on lab slip. Apply pressure to puncture site for 2–5 minutes, or longer if needed. Do not collect blood from the same arm used for an IV infusion.

NAME OF TEST Pulse oximetry

PURPOSE AND DESCRIPTION This noninvasive test is used to evaluate or monitor oxygen saturation of the blood. A device that uses infrared light is attached to an extremity (most commonly the finger, but can also be used on the toe, earlobe, or nose) and light is passed through the tissues or reflected off bony structures.

Normal value: 90%–100%

RELATED NURSING CARE Assess for factors that may alter findings, including faulty placement, movement, dark skin color, and acrylic nails.

(continued)

PROCEDURE 36–1 OBTAINING A SPUTUM SPECIMEN

GATHER SUPPLIES

- Sterile sputum container, specimen cup, or mucous trap
- Mouth care supplies
- Sterile suction kit, if necessary
- Gloves

BEFORE THE PROCEDURE

If the sputum specimen is to establish the initial diagnosis, obtain the specimen before starting oxygen and/or antibiotic therapy. Antibiotics reduce the bacterial count, making it difficult to identify the infecting organism. Oxygen therapy dries mucous membranes, making it more difficult to obtain a specimen. Unless otherwise instructed, obtain the specimen early in the morning, just after awakening. Respiratory secretions tend to pool during sleep; it is easier to obtain a specimen before normal coughing and daily activity has cleared them.

Provide for privacy, and explain the procedure. Emphasize the importance of coughing deeply to obtain sputum from the lower respiratory tract, avoiding expectoration of saliva. Increasing fluid intake prior to obtaining the specimen can help liquefy secretions, making them easier to expectorate.

DURING THE PROCEDURE

1. Use standard precautions.
2. Provide for mouth care prior to obtaining the specimen to reduce contamination by oral flora.
3. Instruct to cough deeply several times, expectorating mucus into the container.
4. Close the container securely.
5. Label the container with name and other identifying data, time and date, and any special conditions, such as antibiotic or oxygen therapy. Enclose specimen container in a clean plastic bag, and take to the laboratory or refrigerate as ordered to preserve the specimen.
6. To obtain a specimen by suctioning:
   - Provide mouth care.
   - Obtain a sterile mucous trap. Using aseptic technique, attach the trap to the suction apparatus between the suction catheter and tubing.
   - Preoxygenate for suctioning as needed.
   - Perform tracheal suctioning using aseptic technique via either the nasotracheal route, endotracheal tube, or tracheostomy. Lubricate the catheter with sterile normal saline. Apply no suction as the catheter is being inserted into the trachea; apply suction for no longer than 10 seconds while withdrawing the catheter.
   - Detach the mucous trap; close and label. Clear the suction catheter and tubing with normal saline after removing the mucus trap. Dispose of equipment appropriately.
7. A sputum specimen also may be obtained during bronchoscopy procedure.

AFTER THE PROCEDURE

Provide mouth care as needed. Teach the importance of completing all ordered antibiotic prescriptions to ensure complete eradication of microorganisms. Document the time and date that the specimen was obtained; and note color, consistency, and odor of sputum.

GENETIC CONSIDERATIONS
Respiratory Disorders

- Deficiency of alpha$_1$-antitrypsin (a protein that protects the body from damage by its immune cells) is caused by a mutation of a gene located on chromosome 14. Deficiency of this protein leaves the lung susceptible to emphysema.
- Asthma, a disease that affects more than 5% of the population, is an inheritable disease with a number of responsible genes. (There are also other causes of asthma.)
- Cystic fibrosis is the most common fatal genetic disease in the United States today. All gene defects result in defective transport of chloride and sodium by epithelial cells. As a result, the amount of sodium chloride is increased in body secretions. Thick mucus is produced that clogs the lungs, leads to infection, and blocks pancreatic enzymes from reaching the intestines to digest food.
- A familial history of lung cancer increases the risk of developing lung cancer, and small-cell lung cancer has a definite genetic component. In addition, researchers have found that lung cancer patients who never smoked are more likely than smokers to have one of two genetic mutations linked to the disease.

Health Assessment Interview

A health assessment interview to determine problems with respiratory structure and function may be conducted during a health screening, may focus on a chief complaint (such as shortness of breath), or may be part of a total health assessment. If the client has a problem with respiratory function, analyze its onset, characteristics, course, severity, precipitating and relieving factors, and any associated symptoms, noting the timing and circumstances. For example, ask the client:

- Describe the problems you are having with your breathing. Is your breathing more difficult if you lie flat? Is it painful to breathe in or out?
- When did you first notice that your cough was becoming a problem? Do you cough up mucus? What color is the mucus?
- Have you had nosebleeds in the past?

During the interview, carefully observe the client for difficulty in breathing, pausing to breathe in the middle of a sentence, hoarseness, changes in voice quality, and cough. Ask about present health status, medical history, family health history, and risk factors for illness. These areas of the client's health status include information about the nose, throat, and lungs.

To determine present health status, ask about pain in the nose, throat, or chest. Information about cough includes what type of cough, when it occurs, and how it is relieved. The client should describe any sputum associated with the cough. Is the client experiencing any dyspnea (difficult or labored breathing)? How is the dyspnea associated with activity levels and time of day? Is the client having chest pain? How is this related to activity and time of day? Note the severity, type, and location of the pain. Explore problems with swallowing, smelling, or taste. Also ask about nosebleeds and nasal or sinus stuffiness or pain, and about current medication use, aerosols or inhalants, and oxygen use.

Document past medical history by asking questions about a history of allergies, asthma, bronchitis, emphysema, pneumonia, tuberculosis, or congestive heart failure. Other questions include a history of surgery or trauma to the respiratory structures and a history of other chronic illnesses such as cancer, kidney disease, and heart disease. If the client has a health problem involving the respiratory system, ask about medications used to relieve nasal congestion, cough, dyspnea, or chest pain. Document a family history of allergies, tuberculosis, emphysema, and cancer.

The client's personal lifestyle, environment, and occupation may provide clues to risk factors for actual or potential health problems. Question the client about a history of smoking and/or exposure to environmental chemicals (including smog), dust, vapors, animals, coal dust, asbestos, fumes, or pollens. Other risk factors include a sedentary lifestyle and obesity. Also ask the client about use of alcohol and substances that are injected (such as heroin) or inhaled (such as cocaine or marijuana).

Interview questions categorized by functional health patterns follow.

FUNCTIONAL HEALTH PATTERN INTERVIEW: Respiratory System

Functional Health Pattern	Interview Questions and Leading Statements
Health Perception–Health Management	■ Describe any respiratory problems (such as allergies, asthma, bronchitis, frequent cold, pneumonia, tuberculosis, emphysema), injuries or surgery of the nose, throat, or lungs you have had.
	■ If you had such problems, how were they treated (for example, medications, surgery, breathing treatments, oxygen, environmental control of allergens, other)?
	■ Do you use oxygen for your respiratory problem? If so, how and when do you use it and at what flow rate?
	■ Do you now or have you ever smoked tobacco? If so, what type, how long, and how much? If you no longer smoke, when did you quit?
	■ Do you notice more respiratory problems at certain seasons of the year? Explain.
	■ Do you do anything to decrease environmental irritants in your home or at work? Describe if so.
	■ When was your last chest x-ray and TB skin test? What were the results of those tests?
	■ Do you have annual flu shots? Have you had a pneumonia shot (if over age 65)?
	■ Do certain foods, pollens, dust, or animals seem to increase your difficulty breathing? Explain.
	■ Do you work or do hobbies in an area where you are exposed to paints, glues, dust, pollen, fumes, or chemicals that might irritate your respiratory system? If so, describe.
Nutritional–Metabolic	■ Describe your usual 24-hour intake of food and fluids.
	■ Has your appetite been affected by your respiratory problem? Is it difficult for you to eat because of your breathing problems? Explain.
	■ Has there been a recent change in your weight? Explain.
Elimination	■ Has having this health problem made it more difficult for you to have a bowel movement?
	■ For women: Have you had difficulty controlling your urine when you cough?
Activity–Exercise	■ Describe your usual activities in a 24-hour period.
	■ What type of exercise do you usually do? Has this changed, and if so, how?
	■ Has your ability to care for yourself changed with this respiratory problem? Explain.
	■ Has your energy level decreased since you have had this problem with breathing? If so, how has it affected your daily life?
	■ How many flights of stairs can you climb before you become short of breath?
	■ Do certain activities make you very tired? Explain.
	■ Are your activities interrupted by frequent coughing? Explain.
	■ Do you cough up phlegm or sputum? If so, describe its amount, color, odor, and the presence of blood.
Sleep–Rest	■ Does having this problem interfere with your ability to rest and sleep? Explain.
	■ How many pillows do you use at night to breathe more easily? Has this changed?
	■ Do you ever wake up coughing?

(continued)

FUNCTIONAL HEALTH PATTERN INTERVIEW: Respiratory System (continued)

Cognitive–Perceptual	■ Do you have any pain in your sinuses, nose, chest, with breathing? If so, using a scale from 0 to 10, with 10 being the most severe pain, how would your rate that pain? Describe where and when you have the pain, how often you have it, what makes it worse, and what you do to relieve it. ■ Are there times when you feel anxious, restless, apprehensive, confused, or faint? Describe what you do if you have these feelings. ■ Do you know how to use the medications, inhalers, or oxygen prescribed for your respiratory problem?
Self-Perception–Self-Concept	■ How does having this condition make you feel about yourself?
Role–Relationships	■ How has having this condition affected your relationships with others? ■ Has having this condition interfered with your ability to work? Explain. ■ Is there a history of lung disease in your family? Explain.
Sexuality–Reproductive	■ Has this condition interfered with your usual sexual activity?
Coping–Stress-Tolerance	■ Has having this condition created stress for you? If so, does your breathing seem to be more difficult when you are stressed? ■ Have you experienced any kind of stress that makes the condition worse? Explain. ■ Describe what you do when you feel stressed.
Value–Belief	■ Describe how specific relationships or activities help you cope with this problem. ■ Describe specific cultural beliefs or practices that affect how you care for and feel about this problem. ■ Are there any specific treatments (such as being on a machine that breathes for you) that you would not use to treat this problem?

Physical Assessment

Physical assessment of the respiratory system may be performed either as part of a total assessment, or alone for a client with known or suspected problems. The techniques used to assess the respiratory system are inspection, palpation, percussion, and auscultation. In addition, note the client's level of consciousness, restlessness, and anxiety level, and assess the color of the lips and nail beds. Normal age-related findings for the older adult are summarized in Table 36–1.

The room should be warm and well lighted. Ask the client to remove all clothing above the waist; give women a gown to wear during the examination. Conduct the examination with the client in the sitting position. Prior to the examination, collect all necessary equipment and explain the techniques to the client to decrease anxiety.

TABLE 36–1 Age-Related Changes in the Respiratory System

AGE-RELATED CHANGE	SIGNIFICANCE
■ ↓ elastic recoil of lungs during expiration because of less elastic collagen and elastin. ■ Loss of skeletal muscle strength in the thorax and diaphragm. ■ Alveoli are less elastic, more fibrotic, and have fewer functional capillaries. ■ Cough is less effective. ■ Po_2 reduces as much as 15% by age 80.	The older adult often has an increased anterior-posterior chest diameter, with kyphosis and barrel chest. There is a reduction in vital capacity and an increase in residual volume, with decreased effectiveness in coughing up phlegm or sputum. All of these changes greatly increase the risk of respiratory infections (such as pneumonia), especially if the person becomes immobile. They also mean that respiratory infections are more difficult to treat.

RESPIRATORY ASSESSMENTS

Technique/Normal/Findings	Abnormal Findings

Nasal Assessment

Inspect the nose for changes in size, shape, or color. *The nose should be midline in the face, of the same color as the face, and the nares should be symmetric.*	■ The nose may be asymmetrical as a result of previous surgery or trauma. ■ The skin around the nostrils may be red and swollen in allergies or upper respiratory infections.

Technique/Normal/Findings	Abnormal Findings
Inspect the nasal cavity. Use an otoscope with a broad, short speculum. Gently insert the speculum into each of the nares and assess the condition of the mucous membranes and the turbinates. *The septum should be midline with pink mucosa and without drainage.*	■ The septum may be deviated. ■ Perforation of the septum may occur with chronic cocaine abuse. ■ Red mucosa indicates infection. ■ Purulent drainage indicates nasal or sinus infection. ■ Allergies may be indicated by watery nasal drainage, pale turbinates, and polyps on the turbinates.
Assess ability to smell (cranial nerve I, olfactory). Ask the client to breathe through one nostril while pressing the other one closed. Ask the client to close his or her eyes. Place a substance with an aromatic odor under the client's nose (use ground coffee or alcohol) and ask the client to identify the odor. Test each nostril separately. *This test is usually done only if the client has problems with the sense of smell, but the client should be able to distinguish different odors.*	■ Changes in the ability to smell may be the result of damage to the olfactory nerve or to chronic inflammation of the nose. ■ Zinc deficiency may cause a loss of the sense of smell.

Sinus Assessment

Technique/Normal/Findings	Abnormal Findings
Palpate the frontal and maxillary sinuses. *The sinuses should not be tender to palpation.*	■ Frontal and maxillary sinuses are tender to palpation with allergies or sinus infections.

Thoracic Assessment

Technique/Normal/Findings	Abnormal Findings
Assess respiratory rate. *The normal respiratory rate is 12 to 20 breaths per minute.*	■ **Tachypnea** (rapid respiratory rate) is seen in **atelectasis** (collapse of lung tissue following obstruction of the bronchus or bronchioles), pneumonia, asthma, pleural effusion, pneumothorax, congestive heart failure, anxiety, and in response to pain. ■ Damage to the brainstem from a stroke or head injury may result in either tachypnea or **bradypnea** (low respiratory rate). ■ Bradypnea is seen with some circulatory disorders, lung disorders, and as a side effect of some medications. ■ **Apnea**, cessation of breathing lasting from a few seconds to a few minutes, may occur following a stroke or head trauma, as a side effect of some medications, or following airway obstruction.
Inspect the anteroposterior diameter of the chest. The anteroposterior diameter of the chest should be less than the transverse diameter. *Normal ratio is 1:2.*	■ The anteroposterior diameter is equal to the transverse diameter in barrel chest, which typically occurs with emphysema.
Inspect for intercostal retraction or bulging. *There should be no retraction or bulging.*	■ Retraction of intercostal spaces may be seen in asthma. ■ Bulging of intercostal spaces may be seen in pneumothorax.

Technique/Normal/Findings	Abnormal Findings

Inspect and palpate for chest expansion. Place your hands with the fingers spread apart palm down on the client's posterolateral chest. Gently press the skin between your thumbs (Figure 36–10 ■). Ask the client to breathe deeply. As the client inhales, watch your hands for symmetry of movement. *Chest expansion should be bilaterally symmetric, with the examiner's hands moving 5 to 10 cm apart.*

- Thoracic expansion is decreased on the affected side in atelectasis, pneumonia, pneumothorax, and pleural effusion.
- Bilateral chest expansion is decreased in emphysema.

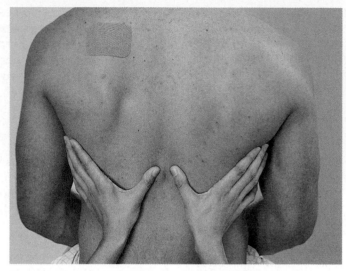

Figure 36–10 ■ Palpating for chest expansion.

Gently palpate the location and position of the trachea. *The trachea should be midline.*

- The trachea shifts to the unaffected side in pleural effusion and pneumothorax and shifts to the affected side in atelectasis.

Palpate for tactile fremitus. Ask the client to say "ninety-nine" as you palpate at three different levels for a vibratory sensation called tactile fremitus, which occurs as sound waves from the larynx travel through patent bronchi and lungs to the chest wall. *Fremitus is symmetric and easily palpated in the upper regions of the lungs.*

- Tactile fremitus is decreased in atelectasis, emphysema, asthma, pleural effusion, and pneumothorax. It is increased in pneumonia if the bronchus is patent.

Percuss the lungs for dullness over shoulder apices and over anterior, posterior, and lateral intercostal spaces (Figure 36–11 ■). *The normal percussion tone over normal lung tissue is resonance.*

- Dullness is heard in clients with atelectasis, lobar pneumonia, and pleural effusion.
- Hyperresonance is heard in those with chronic asthma, emphysema, and pneumothorax.

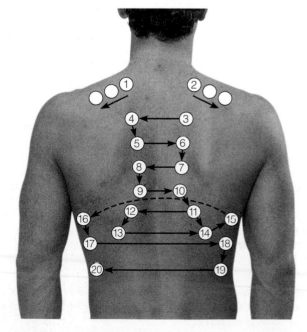

Figure 36–11 ■ Sequence for lung percussion.

Technique/Normal/Findings	Abnormal Findings
Percuss the posterior chest for diaphragmatic excursion. Systematic percussion of the posterior chest from a level of lung resonance to the level of diaphragmatic dullness reveals *diaphragmatic excursion, a measurement of the level of the diaphragm.* First percuss downward over the posterior thorax while the client exhales fully and holds the breath. Mark the spot at which the sound changes from resonant to dull. Then ask the client to inhale and hold the breath while you percuss downward again to note the descent of the diaphragm. Again mark the spot where the sound changes. *Measure the difference in diaphragmatic excursion which normally varies from about 3 to 5 cm (Figure 36–12 ■).*	■ Diaphragmatic excursion is decreased in emphysema, ascites, on the affected side in pleural effusion, and in pneumothorax. ■ A high level of dullness or a lack of excursion may indicate atelectasis or pleural effusion.

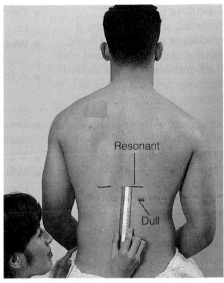

Figure 36–12 ■ Measuring diaphragmatic excursion.

Breath Sound Assessment

Auscultate the lungs for breath sounds with the diaphragm of the stethoscope by having the client take slow deep breaths through the mouth. Listen over anterior, posterior, and lateral intercostal spaces (Figure 36–13 ■). *The three different types of normal breath sounds are vesicular, bronchovesicular, and bronchial (Table 36–2).*

■ Bronchial breath sounds (expiration > inspiration) and bronchovesicular breath sounds (inspiration = expiration) are heard over lungs filled with fluid or solid tissue.
■ Breath sounds are decreased or diminished over atelectasis, emphysema, asthma, pleural effusion, and pneumothorax.
■ Breath sounds are increased over lobar pneumonia.
■ Breath sounds are absent over collapsed lung, surgical removal of lung, pleural effusion, and primary bronchus obstruction.

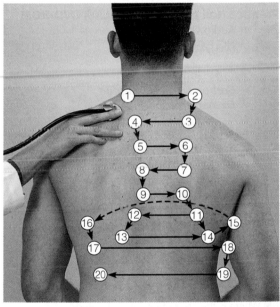

Figure 36–13 ■ Sequence for lung auscultation.

TABLE 36–2 Normal Breath Sounds

TYPE OF BREATH SOUND	CHARACTERISTICS
Vesicular	■ Soft, low-pitched, gentle sounds ■ Heard over all areas of the lungs except the major bronchi ■ Have a 3:1 ratio for inspiration and expiration, with inspiration lasting longer than expiration
Bronchovesicular	■ Medium pitch and intensity of sounds ■ Have a 1:1 ratio, with inspiration and expiration being equal in duration ■ Heard anteriorly over the primary bronchus on each side of the sternum, and posteriorly between the scapulae
Bronchial	■ Loud, high-pitched sounds ■ Gap between inspiration and expiration ■ Have a 2:3 ratio for inspiration and expiration, with expiration longer than inspiration ■ Heard over the manubrium

CHAPTER 37

Nursing Care of Clients with Upper Respiratory Disorders

LEARNING OUTCOMES

- Relate anatomy and physiology of the upper respiratory tract to commonly occurring disorders and risk factors for these disorders.

- Describe the pathophysiology of common upper respiratory tract disorders, relating their manifestations to the pathophysiologic process.

- Discuss nursing implications for medications and other interdisciplinary care measures to treat upper respiratory disorders.

- Describe surgical procedures used to treat upper respiratory disorders and their implications for client care and recovery.

- Identify health promotion activities related to reducing the incidence of upper respiratory disorders, describing the appropriate population and setting for implementing identified measures.

- Discuss treatment options for oral and laryngeal cancers with their implications for the client's body image and functional health.

CLINICAL COMPETENCIES

- Assess functional health status of clients with upper respiratory disorders, using data to identify and prioritize holistic nursing care needs.

- Use nursing research and evidence-based practice to plan and implement nursing care for clients with upper respiratory disorders.

- Provide safe and effective nursing care for clients having surgery involving the upper respiratory system and/or with a tracheostomy.

- Safely and knowledgeably administer medications and prescribed treatments for clients with disorders of the upper respiratory tract.

- Provide appropriate teaching for the client and family affected by upper respiratory tract disorders.

- Evaluate the effectiveness of care, reassessing and modifying the plan of care as needed to achieve desired client outcomes.

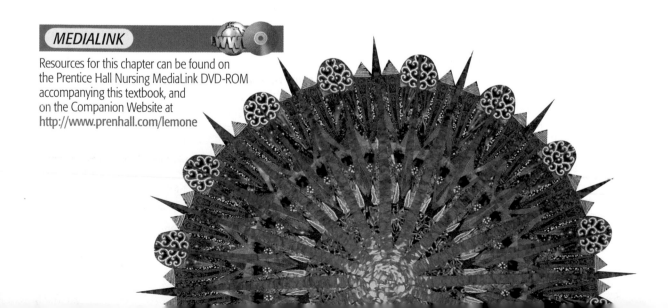

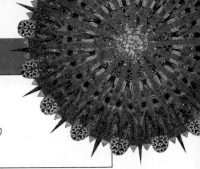

Upper respiratory disorders may affect the nose, paranasal sinuses, tonsils, adenoids, larynx, and pharynx. Upper respiratory disorders may be minor, such as the common cold. However, a patent upper airway is necessary for effective breathing. Acute and even life-threatening problems develop when upper airway patency is affected (e.g., by laryngeal edema). Upper respiratory disorders can affect breathing, communication, and body image. When breathing is compromised because of swelling, bleeding, or accumulation of secretions, fear and anxiety develop.

Nursing care focuses on maintaining the airway, managing pain and symptoms, promoting effective communication, and providing psychologic support for the client and family. Prior to proceeding with this chapter, review the anatomy and physiology, diagnostic tests, and assessment of the upper respiratory system in Chapter 36 ∞ as needed.

INFECTIOUS OR INFLAMMATORY DISORDERS

Constant exposure of the upper respiratory tract to the environment makes it vulnerable to a variety of infectious and inflammatory conditions. Although most upper respiratory infections and inflammations are minor, complications may result. In the frail older adult, the risk of serious problems following an upper respiratory infection can be significant.

Rhinitis, inflammation of the nasal cavities, is the most common upper respiratory disorder. Rhinitis may be either acute or chronic. *Acute viral rhinitis*, or the common cold, is discussed below. Chronic rhinitis includes allergic, vasomotor, and atrophic rhinitis. *Allergic rhinitis,* or hay fever, results from a sensitivity reaction to allergens such as plant pollens. It tends to occur seasonally. The etiology of *vasomotor rhinitis* is unknown. Although its manifestations are similar to those of allergic rhinitis, it is not linked to allergens. *Atrophic rhinitis* is characterized by changes in the mucous membrane of the nasal cavities.

THE CLIENT WITH VIRAL UPPER RESPIRATORY INFECTION

Viral upper respiratory infections (URIs or the common cold) are the most common respiratory tract infections and are among the most common human diseases. URIs are highly contagious and are prevalent in schools and work environments. The incidence of acute URI peaks during September and late January, coinciding with the opening of schools, as well as toward the end of April. Most adults experience two to four colds each year (Porth, 2005).

FAST FACTS

- Rhinoviruses are the most common cause of viral URIs.
- Colds due to rhinovirus are more common in early fall and late spring.
- More than 100 different serotypes of rhinovirus have been identified.
- Parainfluenza viruses, respiratory syncytial viruses (RSV), coronaviruses, and adenoviruses also can cause URIs.
- Colds due to RSV, coronavirus, and adenovirus peak in winter and spring (Porth, 2005).

Pathophysiology

More than 200 strains of virus cause URI, including rhinoviruses, adenoviruses, parainfluenza viruses, coronaviruses, and respiratory syncytial virus (see the section that follows for more information about RSV). Occasionally, more than one virus may be present. Viruses causing acute URIs spread by aerosolized droplet nuclei during sneezing or coughing or by direct contact. The virus usually spreads when the hands and fingers pick it up from contaminated surfaces and carry it to the eyes and mucous membranes of the susceptible host. Infected clients are highly contagious, shedding virus for a few days prior to and after the appearance of symptoms. Although immunity is produced to the individual virus strain, the number of viruses causing URI ensures that most people continue to experience colds throughout their lifetimes.

Viscous mucous secretions in the upper respiratory tract trap invading organisms, preventing contamination of more vulnerable areas. Cells of the upper respiratory tract are infected when the virus attaches to receptors on the cell. Local immunologic defenses, such as secretory IgA antibodies in respiratory secretions, then attempt to inactivate the antigen, producing a local inflammatory response. The mucous membranes of the nasal passages swell and become hyperemic and engorged. Mucus-secreting glands become hyperactive. These responses to the virus produce the typical manifestations of viral URI.

Manifestations and Complications

Acute viral upper respiratory infection often presents as the common cold. Nasal mucous membranes appear red (*erythematous*) and *boggy* (swollen). Swollen mucous membranes, local vasodilation, and secretions cause nasal congestion. Clear, watery secretions lead to **coryza**, profuse nasal discharge. Sneezing and coughing are common. Sore throat is common, and may be the initial symptom. Systemic manifestations of acute viral URI may include low-grade fever, headache, malaise, and muscle aches. Symptoms generally last for a few days up to 2 weeks. Although acute viral URI is typically mild and self-limited, its effects on the immune defenses of the upper respiratory tract can increase the risk for more serious bacterial infections, such as sinusitis or otitis media.

INTERDISCIPLINARY CARE

Because most acute viral upper respiratory infections are self-limiting, self-care is appropriate and encouraged. Medical treatment is usually required only when complications such as sinusitis or otitis media develop.

Diagnosis of acute viral URI is usually based on the history and physical examination. Diagnostic testing may be indicated if a complication such as bacterial infection is suspected. A white blood count (WBC) may be ordered to assess for leukocytosis (an elevated WBC). Cultures of purulent discharge may also be obtained.

Treatment is symptomatic. Adequate rest, maintaining fluid intake, and avoiding chilling help relieve systemic symptoms such as fever, malaise, and muscle ache. Instruct clients to cover the mouth and nose with tissue when coughing or sneezing, and to dispose of soiled tissues properly. Additionally, avoiding crowds helps prevent spread of the infection to others.

Medications

Medications may be recommended to shorten the duration of the illness and relieve symptoms. Mild decongestants or over-the-counter (OTC) antihistamines may help relieve coryza and nasal congestion. Nasal sprays such as phenylephrine (Neo-Synephrine) rapidly relieve nasal congestion, but may lead to dependence and rebound congestion if used for more than a few days at a time. Warm saltwater gargles, throat lozenges, or mild analgesics may be used for sore throat. Although no specific antiviral therapy has been shown to be effective in shortening the duration of a URI, experimental vaccines to prevent acute viral URI are in developmental stages. For the nursing implications of decongestants and common antihistamines see the box below.

MEDICATION ADMINISTRATION **Decongestants and Antihistamines**

DECONGESTANTS
Phenylephrine (Neo-Synephrine, others)
Phenylpropanolamine (Comtrex, Ornade, Triaminic, others)
Pseudoephedrine (Sudafed, Actifed, others)

Decongestants promote vasoconstriction, reducing the inflammation and edema of nasal mucosa and relieving nasal congestion. They are very effective when applied topically (by nasal spray) because of their rapid onset of action. However, the duration of effect is short, followed by vasodilation and rebound congestion. Because of their rapid effect and short duration, these preparations are habit forming. Chronic use may lead to *rhinitis medicamentosa,* a rebound phenomenon of drug-induced nasal irritation and inflammation.

Nursing Responsibilities
- Assess for contraindications, such as hypertension or chronic heart disease. These drugs stimulate the sympathetic nervous system, increasing peripheral vascular resistance, blood pressure, and heart rate.
- Evaluate medication regimen for potential interactions such as antihypertensive medications and monoamine oxidase (MAO) inhibitors.

Health Education for the Client and Family
- Do not use more than the recommended dose.
- Check with the physician before taking decongestants if you are taking any prescription medications or are being treated for high blood pressure or heart disease.
- Use nasal sprays for no more than 3 to 5 days.
- Increase fluid intake to relieve mouth dryness.
- These drugs may cause nervousness, shakiness, or difficulty sleeping. Stop the drug if these effects occur.
- In some states, drugs containing pseudoephedrine may require a prescription or be kept behind the counter to reduce its use in preparing methamphetamine.

ANTIHISTAMINES
Brompheniramine (Dimetane, others)
Chlorpheniramine (Chlor-Trimeton, others)
Clemastine (Tavist)
Dexchlorpheniramine (Dexchlor, others)
Diphenhydramine (Benadryl, others)
Triprolidine (Actidil, Myidil)

Nonsedating
Cetirizine (Zyrtec)
Fexofenadine (Allegra)
Loratadine (Claritin)

Antihistamines are widely available with and without a prescription. They are frequently combined with decongestants in over-the-counter cold and allergy preparations. Antihistamines relieve the systemic effects of histamine and dry respiratory secretions through an anticholinergic effect. Most antihistamines cause drowsiness; nonsedating forms are less likely to interfere with alertness. Diphenhydramine is used in numerous over-the-counter sleep aids as well as in cold and allergy preparations.

Nursing Responsibilities
- Before administering or recommending these drugs, assess for possible contraindications, including the following:
  - Acute asthma or lower respiratory disease that may be aggravated by drying of secretions
  - Hypersensitivity to antihistamines
  - Glaucoma (increased intraocular pressure)
  - Impaired gastrointestinal motility or obstruction
  - Prostatic hypertrophy or other urinary tract obstruction
  - Heart disease.
- For clients who must remain alert while on antihistamine therapy, recommend nonsedating forms.

Health Education for the Client and Family
- Do not drive or operate machinery while taking over-the-counter or prescription forms of antihistamines known to be sedating.
- Stop the drug and notify your doctor immediately if you develop confusion, excessive sedation, chest tightness, wheezing, bleeding, or easy bruising while taking antihistamines.
- Do not use alcohol or other CNS depressants while taking antihistamines.
- Hard candy, gum, ice chips, and liquids help relieve mouth dryness caused by antihistamines.

Complementary Therapies

Complementary therapies are appropriate for treating most acute viral URI. Herbal remedies such as echinacea and garlic may have antiviral and antibiotic effects (Fontaine, 2005). Echinacea also is thought to stimulate the immune system, improving the body's response to infection. Taken at the first sign of infection, echinacea may reduce the duration and symptoms, although clinical trials have shown no consistent benefit (National Center for Complementary and Alternative Medicine, 2005). The recommended dose of echinacea varies, depending on the part of the plant used in the preparation. It should not be used for longer than 2 weeks. It is contraindicated for use during pregnancy and lactation, and in people who have an autoimmune disease such as rheumatoid arthritis.

Dietary supplements such as vitamin C and zinc also are promoted as measures to reduce the severity and duration of URI. Again, however, no consistent benefit is demonstrated in clinical trials. Although selected studies have shown a beneficial effect of zinc gluconate lozenges to reduce the duration of an induced URI, no such benefit was found when zinc was compared with placebo to treat naturally occurring URI (National Institutes of Health, 2002).

Aromatherapy with essential oils such as basil, cedarwood, eucalyptus, frankincense, lavender, marjoram, peppermint, or rosemary can reduce congestion and promote comfort and recovery. Teach clients that these essential oils are to be used only for inhalation, not for internal consumption.

Acupuncture and acupressure have been shown to be effective in treating URI in adults, particularly when combined with use of Chinese herbs (Spencer & Jacobs, 2003). Their beneficial effect is most likely related to stimulation of the immune response by acupuncture and acupressure.

 NURSING CARE

Health Promotion

Clients can limit their incidence of acute viral URI by frequent hand washing and avoiding exposure to crowds. Maintaining good general health and stress-reducing activities support the immune system and help prevent acute viral URI. Teach the client that becoming chilled or going out in the rain do not cause colds, and that URI are more likely to occur during periods of physical or psychologic stress.

Community-Based Care

The primary nursing role in caring for clients with acute viral URI is educational. Self-care is appropriate for most clients unless the problem is recurrent or a complication occurs. Acute viral URI may interfere with work and recreational activities. Unless limited by symptoms, normal daily activities and roles usually can be maintained. Additional rest during the acute phase of illness is recommended. Additional fluid intake and a well-balanced diet help support the immune response, hastening recovery.

Include the following topics in teaching for home care:

- Using disposable tissues to cover the mouth and nose while coughing or sneezing to reduce airborne spread of the virus

- Blowing the nose with both nostrils open to prevent infected matter from being forced into the eustachian tubes
- Washing hands frequently, especially after coughing or sneezing, to limit viral transmission
- Using OTC preparations for symptomatic relief; precautions related to the sedating effects of antihistamines
- Limiting use of nasal decongestants to every 4 hours for only a few days at a time to prevent rebound effect.

THE CLIENT WITH RESPIRATORY SYNCYTIAL VIRUS

Respiratory syncytial virus (RSV) is a common virus that is the primary cause of respiratory illnesses in young children and the majority of lower respiratory disease in infants. Older children and adults also are commonly and repetitively infected by RSV, but the disease is milder, usually presenting as a common cold. However, the elderly and people who are immunocompromised may develop severe pneumonitis when exposed to RSV (Kasper et al., 2005). The disease may be fatal among people who have undergone or are preparing to undergo bone marrow transplant (Tierney et al., 2005).

RSV is transmitted in much the same way as other URI: via contaminated hands or objects and by coarse droplets spread by coughing and sneezing. The incubation period is 4 to 6 days.

In adults, the manifestations of RSV are those of other common URI, including rhinorrhea, sore throat, and cough. Headache, malaise, and low-grade fever may occur. In older adults, RSV may present as lower respiratory infection with fever or pneumonia (Kasper et al., 2005). While the illness also presents as URI in infants, it is more likely to progress to pneumonia, bronchiolitis, and tracheobronchiolitis in this population.

Treatment for adults with upper respiratory RSV is symptomatic (see the preceding section on URI). When the lower respiratory tract is involved, hydration and other measures to mobilize respiratory secretions are important. Intubation and mechanical ventilation may be necessary if hypoxia develops. Aerosolized ribavirin (Virazole, an antiviral drug) may be prescribed for older adults and immunocompromised clients with RSV pneumonia.

Nursing care is supportive. The focus of nursing care for the adult with URI manifestations of RSV is on teaching for self-care, identification of complications, and prevention of viral spread. When lower respiratory symptoms are present, nursing care is similar to that provided for clients with pneumonia (see Chapter 38 ∞).

THE CLIENT WITH INFLUENZA

Influenza, or *flu*, is a highly contagious viral respiratory disease characterized by coryza, fever, cough, and systemic symptoms such as headache and malaise. Influenza usually occurs in epidemics or pandemics, although sporadic cases do occur. Localized outbreaks of influenza usually occur about every 1 to 3 years. Global epidemics (pandemics) are less frequent, developing every 10 to 15 years until the past two decades. A recently identified strain of avian (bird) influenza has raised concerns about a potential future pandemic. This strain of influenza virus has not yet demonstrated the ability to spread between humans; however, concerns are that it will mutate to allow person-to-person spread. This viral strain has a mortality rate of greater than 50% in people who have been infected due to close association with infected birds. See Box 37–1 for more information about avian influenza.

Although influenza tends to be mild and self-limited in healthy adults, older adults and people with chronic heart or pulmonary disease have a high incidence of complications (such as pneumonia) and a higher risk for mortality related to the disease and its complications (Kasper et al., 2005).

Pathophysiology

Influenza virus is transmitted by airborne droplet and direct contact. Three major strains of the virus have been identified as influenza A virus, influenza B virus, and influenza C virus. Influenza A is responsible for most infections and the most severe outbreaks of influenza. This is primarily due to its ability to alter its surface antigens, bypassing previously developed immune defenses to the virus. New strains of influenza virus are named according to the strain, geographic origin, and year the strain was identified (e.g., A/Taiwan/89). Surface antigens of the specific virus may be used to further differentiate influenza A viruses. Outbreaks of influenza B virus are generally less extensive and less severe than those caused by

influenza A virus. Illness associated with influenza C virus is mild and often goes unrecognized.

FAST FACTS

- Type A influenza viruses are found in birds, pigs, whales, and humans.
- Type A influenza is believed to have caused three pandemics, in 1918, 1957, and 1968.
- Type B influenza viruses are commonly found among humans, and often are responsible for influenza outbreaks but not pandemics.
- Type C influenza viruses, found in humans, pigs, and dogs, typically cause mild respiratory infections (National Institute of Allergy and Infectious Diseases, 2006).

The incubation period for influenza is short, only 18 to 72 hours. The virus infects the respiratory epithelium. It rapidly replicates in infected cells and is released to infect neighboring cells. Inflammation leads to necrosis and shedding of serous and ciliated cells of the respiratory tract. This allows extracellular fluid to escape, producing rhinorrhea. With recovery, serous cells are replaced more rapidly than ciliated cells, leading to continued cough and coryza. Systemic manifestations of influenza likely are caused by release of inflammatory mediators such as tumor necrosis factor alpha, interleukin alpha, and interleukin 6 (Kasper et al., 2005). The humoral and cell-mediated immune responses

BOX 37–1 Focus on Avian Influenza

Influenza viruses are common in nature, found in wild birds such as ducks and shore birds. Although these birds carry the virus, they usually are not harmed by it. Movement of the virus into domesticated flocks of ducks and chickens can not only devastate populations of these birds, but can also spread the virus to other domestic animals such as pigs.

Avian influenza is caused by a type A influenza virus identified as H5N1. Type A influenza viruses are subclassified by two proteins found on the surface of the virus, hemagglutinin (HA) and neuraminidase (NA). HA allows the virus to attach to a cell and initiate an infection, whereas NA allows the virus to exit the host cell after replicating. Currently, there are only three known subtypes of influenza A circulating among humans (H1N1, H1N2, and H3N2). The H5N1 virus, which is particularly virulent and spread by migratory birds, raises fears of a potential human pandemic should it evolve to become transmissible from human to human. Influenza viruses are very changeable, undergoing small, continuous changes as well as occasional large and abrupt changes. *Antigenic drift* is the term for small changes that occur continuously as a virus makes copies of itself. These changes help the virus elude the immune system, and necessitate the production of new vaccines every year. Sudden, dramatic changes occur when two different strains of influenza virus (for example, avian influenza and human influenza) infect the same cell and exchange genetic material. These changes, called *antigenic shift*, create a new subtype of the virus to which people have little or no immunity.

As of March 2006, the World Health Organization (WHO) reported a cumulative total of 186 confirmed human cases of avian

influenza A, with the majority of these cases occurring in Viet Nam. Among these confirmed cases, more than half of the people infected died (105 deaths) (WHO, 2006). It is important to note that the cases being reported probably represent the most seriously ill people and milder infections may not be reflected in reported numbers. Most reported cases of avian influenza A have occurred in previously healthy children and young adults.

Symptoms of avian influenza include typical flulike manifestations such as fever, cough, sore throat, and myalgias. In addition, affected people may develop eye infections, pneumonia, and respiratory distress, including acute respiratory distress syndrome (ARDS; see Chapter 39 ∞ for more information about ARDS and its manifestations).

No vaccine to protect against H5N1 virus has yet been developed for commercial use. Measures are being taken, however, to develop pre-pandemic vaccines based on current strains of H5N1 influenza virus, to increase the capacity for vaccine production in the United States, and to research new types of vaccines. Some currently available antiviral medications may effectively treat avian influenza; however, the virus implicated in deaths in southeast Asia was found to be resistant to amantadine and rimantadine, two commonly used drugs to treat influenza (General information, 2006).

A severe pandemic of avian influenza could disrupt all aspects of life, not only causing severe illness and death, but also overwhelming the healthcare system, impacting social services, and causing significant economic loss. Advance preparations such as those currently being undertaken by the WHO and the United States and other countries can reduce the impact of a pandemic.

are activated by influenza infection, and are supplemented by other local and systemic responses (such as interferons).

Manifestations

Infection with influenza virus produces one of three syndromes: uncomplicated nasopharyngeal inflammation, viral upper respiratory infection followed by bacterial infection, or viral pneumonia. The onset is rapid; profound malaise may develop in a matter of minutes.

Manifestations of influenza include abrupt onset of chills and fever, malaise, muscle aches, and headache. Respiratory manifestations include dry, nonproductive cough, sore throat, substernal burning, and coryza (see the box below). Acute symptoms subside within 2 to 3 days, although fever may last as long as a week. The cough may be severe and productive. Along with fatigue and weakness, the cough can persist for days or several weeks.

Complications

The respiratory epithelial necrosis caused by influenza increases the risk for secondary bacterial infections. Sinusitis and otitis media are frequent complications of influenza. Tracheobronchitis, inflammation of the trachea and bronchi, may develop. Although trachcobronchitis is not a serious health risk, its manifestations may persist for up to 3 weeks.

Influenza is clearly linked to an increased risk for pneumonia, particularly in older adults. Changes in respiratory function associated with aging, including decreased effectiveness of cough and increased residual lung volume, pose little risk in the healthy older adult but greatly increase the risk for pneumonia associated with influenza. Primary influenza viral pneumonia, while uncommon, is a serious complication that may be fatal. It typically develops within 48 hours of the onset of influenza, often in clients with preexisting heart valve or pulmonary disease. Influenza pneumonia progresses rapidly and can cause hypoxemia and death within a few days. Bacterial pneumonia is more likely to occur in older at-risk adults but also may affect otherwise healthy adults. It usually presents as a relapse of influenza, with a productive cough and evidence of pneumonia on the chest x-ray. See Chapter 38 ∞ for more information about pneumonia.

Other respiratory complications of influenza include exacerbation of chronic obstructive pulmonary disease (COPD),

chronic bronchitis, or asthma. Sinusitis (discussed later in this chapter) also may develop.

Reye's syndrome is a rare but potentially fatal complication of influenza. Although it is more likely to affect children, it also has been identified in older adults. It is most often associated with influenza B virus. Reye's syndrome develops within 2 to 3 weeks after the onset of influenza. It has a 30% mortality rate. Hepatic failure and encephalopathy develop rapidly in clients with Reye's syndrome.

While uncommon, other potential complications of influenza include myositis (inflammation of skeletal muscles), myocarditis (inflammation of the heart muscle), and central nervous system (CNS) disorders such as encephalitis and Guillain-Barré syndrome.

INTERDISCIPLINARY CARE

Preventing community outbreaks and protecting vulnerable populations (e.g., older adults and people with chronic diseases) are the primary focus for interdisciplinary care related to influenza. Medical treatment of influenza focuses on establishing the diagnosis, providing symptomatic relief, and preventing complications.

Prevention

Preventing influenza by immunizing at-risk populations is an important aspect of care. Immunization with polyvalent (containing antigens of several viral strains) influenza virus vaccine is about 85% effective in preventing influenza infection for several months to a year (Tierney et al., 2005). Annual immunization is recommended for at-risk clients, including people over the age of 65, residents of nursing homes, adults and children with chronic cardiopulmonary disorders (e.g., asthma) or chronic metabolic diseases such as diabetes, and healthcare workers who have frequent contact with high-risk clients. Additionally, family members of at-risk clients should be vaccinated to reduce the client's risk of exposure. The vaccine is given in the fall, prior to the annual winter outbreak. Live attenuated vaccine, administered by intranasal spray, is available for healthy people under age 50.

Diagnosis

The diagnosis of influenza is based on history, clinical findings, and knowledge of an influenza outbreak in the community. A chest x-ray and WBC count may be done to rule out complications such as pneumonia. The WBC count is commonly decreased in influenza; bacterial infections usually cause increased WBCs.

Medications

Yearly immunization with influenza vaccine is the single most important measure to prevent or minimize symptoms of influenza. Although the vaccine is readily available and inexpensive, only about 30% of at-risk clients are vaccinated each year. Many may fear a reaction from the vaccine, although the vaccines are highly purified and reactions are rare. About 5% of people experience mild symptoms of low-grade fever, malaise, or myalgia for up to 24 hours after vaccination. Because the vaccine is produced in eggs, it should not be given to people who are allergic to

---

MANIFESTATIONS of Influenza

RESPIRATORY MANIFESTATIONS
- Coryza
- Cough, initially dry becoming productive
- Substernal burning
- Sore throat

SYSTEMIC MANIFESTATIONS
- Fever and chills
- Malaise
- Muscle aches
- Fatigue

egg protein. Serious adverse reactions to influenza vaccine are rare. Guillain-Barré syndrome, an acute neurologic disorder characterized by muscle weakness and distal sensory loss, has been associated with certain batches of vaccine.

Amantadine (Symmetrel) or rimantadine (Flumadine) may be used for prophylaxis in unvaccinated people who are exposed to the virus. If the drug is given before or within 48 hours of exposure, it inhibits viral shedding and prevents or decreases the symptoms of influenza. If possible, unvaccinated people should receive the vaccine along with the antiviral drug. The drug is continued for several weeks or for the duration of the influenza outbreak. Some strains of type A influenza virus have been found to be resistant to amantadine and rimantadine, potentially limiting their effectiveness in preventing or treating an influenza outbreak.

Amantadine, rimantadine, and the antiviral drugs zanamivir (Relenza), oseltamivir (Tamiflu), and ribavirin (Virazole) also may be used to reduce the duration and severity of flu symptoms. Both zanamivir and ribavirin are administered by inhalation; the other drugs are given orally. Zanamivir can precipitate bronchospasm in clients with a history of asthma or COPD, so it is not recommended for use in these clients (Food and Drug Administration, 2000). See Chapter 12 ∞ for nursing implications for antiviral drugs.

Over-the-counter analgesics such as aspirin, acetaminophen, or nonsteroidal anti-inflammatory drugs (NSAIDs) provide symptomatic relief of fever and muscle ache. Antitussives may decrease cough, promoting rest. Antibiotics are not indicated unless secondary bacterial infection occurs.

 # NURSING CARE

Health Promotion

Stress the importance of yearly influenza vaccination for clients in high-risk groups and their families. Teach about spread of the disease, including measures to reduce the risk of contracting influenza, such as avoiding crowds and people who are ill.

Assessment

Unless there is a known outbreak of influenza in the community, it can be difficult to differentiate the manifestations of influenza from those of other URI.

- *Health History:* Known exposure to virus; current symptoms, their onset and duration; presence of dyspnea, chest pain, productive cough, facial pain or pressure in sinus areas; current medications, history of influenza vaccine; chronic diseases such as heart disease, COPD, or diabetes; known medication allergies.
- *Physical Examination:* General appearance; vital signs including temperature; skin color; lung sounds; abdominal exam.
- *Diagnostic Tests:* WBC, throat and sputum cultures, and chest x-ray for evidence of bacterial infection or pneumonia.

Nursing Diagnoses and Interventions

Although the symptoms of influenza are distressing, most people with the illness provide self-care and do not contact a healthcare provider. Recommendations to rest in bed during the acute phase of the illness and limit activities until recovery are appropriate for influenza.

Severe disease or complications of influenza may necessitate hospitalization for respiratory support and management. For these clients, nursing care focuses on maintaining airway clearance, breathing patterns, and adequate rest.

Ineffective Breathing Pattern

Muscle aches, malaise, and elevated temperature may increase the respiratory rate and alter the depth of respirations, decreasing effective alveolar ventilation. Shallow respirations also increase the risk of *atelectasis* (lack of ventilation in an area of lung).

> **PRACTICE ALERT**
> Monitor respiratory rate and pattern. Tachypnea and/or rapid, shallow respirations may impair effective alveolar ventilation and gas exchange.

- Pace activities to provide for periods of rest. *Tachypnea increases the work of breathing, causing fatigue; fatigue, in turn, can further impair ventilation and reduce the effectiveness of coughing.*
- Elevate the head of the bed. *The upright position improves lung excursion and reduces the work of breathing by lowering the diaphragm, moving abdominal contents downward, creating less resistance to diaphragmatic excursion, and slightly decreasing venous return.*

Ineffective Airway Clearance

Swelling and congestion of mucous membranes, extracellular fluid exudate, and impaired ciliary action due to cell damage increase the risk of impaired airway clearance in influenza. The older adult is at particular risk because of normally reduced ciliary activity and increased lung compliance.

> **PRACTICE ALERT**
> Monitor the effectiveness of cough and ability to remove airway secretions. Fatigue and general malaise may impair the ability to cough effectively and mobilize secretions.

- Maintain adequate hydration. Assess mucous membranes and skin turgor for evidence of dehydration. *Fever and decreased oral fluid intake may lead to dehydration and increased viscosity of secretions. Thick, viscous secretions are more difficult to expectorate.*
- Increase the humidity of inspired air with a bedside humidifier. *Increasing the water content of inhaled air helps loosen thick secretions and soothe mucous membranes.*
- Teach effective cough techniques. Administer analgesics as ordered. *The huff cough is effective to maintain open airways and it spares energy. (See Box 39–5 for client teaching of this technique.) Relieving muscle ache increases the ability to cough effectively.*

Disturbed Sleep Pattern

Airway congestion, malaise, muscle aches, and persistent cough may interfere with the ability to rest, increasing fatigue and prolonging recovery.

- Assess sleep patterns using subjective and objective information. *The client may appear to be sleeping but not achieving normal sleep patterns because of influenza symptoms. Both subjective and objective data are important to accurately assess sleep.*
- Provide antipyretic and analgesic medications at or shortly before bedtime. *These drugs promote comfort by reducing fever and relieving muscle aches.*

PRACTICE ALERT

If necessary, request a cough suppressant for nighttime use. Cough suppressants are not recommended during the day because coughing promotes airway clearance. They may, however, be necessary at night to allow rest.

Risk for Infection

Infection control measures are recommended to prevent person-to-person transmission of influenza and control influenza outbreaks in healthcare facilities.

- Use standard precautions and encourage all staff and visitors to frequently wash hands. *Hand washing is a primary infection control measure for infections transmitted via respiratory secretions.*
- Instruct clients and visitors to control respiratory secretions by using tissues, and to maintain a distance of at least 3 feet from others when coughing or sneezing. Provide masks for clients and visitors who are unable to control secretions. *Limiting the spread of aerosolized secretions by covering the nose and mouth and maintaining distance from other people can reduce the spread of the disease to vulnerable populations.*
- Use droplet precautions for clients with suspected or confirmed influenza: private room, masks for caregivers and visitors, and a mask for the client when transporting within the facility. *These measures limit the spread of respiratory secretions.*

Using NANDA, NIC, and NOC

Chart 37–1 illustrates linkages between NANDA nursing diagnoses, nursing interventions, and nursing outcomes for the client with influenza.

Community-Based Care

Encourage appropriate self-care for clients with influenza. Discuss the following topics related to home care:

- Increase rest during the acute, febrile phase of the illness.
- Maintain a liberal fluid intake even if anorexic.
- Appropriately use OTC medications for symptom relief.
- Employ hygiene measures such as using disposable tissues and frequent hand washing to reduce spread of the disease.
- Know manifestations of potential complications of influenza to report to the primary care provider.

THE CLIENT WITH SINUSITIS

Sinusitis is inflammation of the mucous membranes of one or more of the sinuses (see Figure 36–2). Sinusitis is a common condition that usually follows an upper respiratory infection

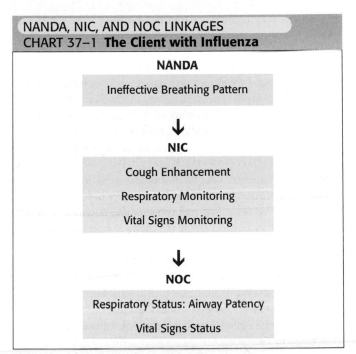

NANDA, NIC, AND NOC LINKAGES
CHART 37–1 The Client with Influenza

NANDA

Ineffective Breathing Pattern

↓

NIC

Cough Enhancement

Respiratory Monitoring

Vital Signs Monitoring

↓

NOC

Respiratory Status: Airway Patency

Vital Signs Status

Data from NANDA's Nursing Diagnoses: Definitions & Classification 2005–2006 by NANDA International (2005), Philadelphia; Nursing Interventions Classification (NIC) (4th ed.) by J. M. Dochterman & G. M. Bulechek (2004), St. Louis, MO: Mosby; and Nursing Outcomes Classification (NOC) (3rd ed.) by S. Moorhead, M. Johnson, and M. Maas (2004), St. Louis, MO: Mosby.

such as acute viral upper respiratory infection or influenza. Common causative organisms include streptococci, *S. pneumoniae, Haemophilus influenzae,* and staphylococci. The risk of sinusitis is higher when the immune system is suppressed by immunosuppressive drugs or HIV infection. Sinusitis is common and difficult to treat in people who have AIDS.

Physiology Review

The sinuses (or *paranasal sinuses*) are air-filled cavities in the facial bones that open into the turbinates of the nasal cavity. They are lined with ciliated mucous membranes that help move fluid and microorganisms out of the sinuses into the nasal cavity. The sinuses normally are sterile. Air within the sinuses has a lower oxygen content than inspired air.

Pathophysiology

Sinusitis develops when nasal mucous membranes swell or other disorders obstruct sinus openings, impairing drainage. Mucous secretions collect in the sinus cavity, serving as a medium for bacterial growth. The nasal and sinus mucous membranes are continuous; therefore, bacteria generally spread to the sinuses via the opening into the nasal turbinates. The inflammatory response provoked by bacterial invasion draws serum and leukocytes to the area to combat the infection, increasing swelling and pressure.

Any process that impairs drainage from the sinuses may precipitate sinusitis. These include nasal polyps, deviated septum, rhinitis, tooth abscess, or swimming or diving trauma. In hospitalized clients, sinusitis may develop following prolonged nasotracheal intubation. Usually more than one sinus is infected. The frontal and maxillary sinuses are usually involved in adults.

Sinusitis may be acute or chronic. Chronic sinusitis results when acute sinusitis is untreated or inadequately treated. With continued infection, bacteria can become isolated, producing chronic inflammation. Over time, mucous membranes become thickened. Fungal infections may cause chronic infections, especially in immunosuppressed clients. Other factors that may contribute to chronic sinusitis are smoking, a history of allergy, and habitual use of nasal sprays or inhalants.

Manifestations and Complications

The client with acute sinusitis often looks sick. Manifestations of sinusitis include pain and tenderness across the infected sinuses, headache, fever, and malaise. The pain usually increases with leaning forward. When the maxillary sinuses are involved, pain and pressure are felt over the cheek. The pain may be referred to the upper teeth. Frontal sinusitis causes pain and tenderness across the lower forehead. Infection of the ethmoid sinus produces retro-orbital pain and pain over the high lateral aspect of the nose. Sphenoid sinusitis, the rarest form, may cause pain in the occiput, vertex, or middle of the head. Symptoms often worsen for 3 to 4 hours after awakening and then become less severe in the afternoon and evening as secretions drain. The intensity and location of headache pain may change as sinuses drain. In acute sinusitis, the pain is usually constant and severe. In chronic sinusitis, the pain is described as dull and may be constant or intermittent.

Other symptoms include nasal congestion, purulent nasal discharge, and bad breath. The nasal mucous membrane is red and swollen. Purulent drainage may be noted at the opening to the middle turbinate. This may be the only sign of chronic sinusitis. Swallowed secretions irritate and inflame the throat, and may cause nausea or vomiting.

Complications develop when the infection spreads to surrounding structures (Box 37–2). These include periorbital abscess or cellulitis, cavernous sinus thrombosis, meningitis, brain abscess, or sepsis. Eustachian tube edema may lead to hearing loss.

INTERDISCIPLINARY CARE

Treatment of sinusitis focuses on restoring drainage of obstructed sinuses, controlling infection, relieving pain, and preventing complications.

BOX 37–2 Potential Complications of Sinusitis

Local Complications
- Orbital cellulitis
- Subperiosteal abscess
- Orbital abscess
- Cavernous sinus thrombosis
- Mucocele
- Osteomyelitis

Intracranial Complications
- Meningitis
- Epidural abscess
- Subdural abscess
- Brain abscess
- Venous sinus thrombosis

Diagnosis

The diagnosis of acute sinusitis usually can be made using the history and physical exam. Diagnostic studies such as CT scan or sinus x-rays generally are done only when sinusitis is persistent, chronic, or recurrent. See Chapter 36 ∞ for more information about diagnostic studies and their nursing implications.

- *Sinus x-rays* are evaluated. Sinuses are normally translucent because they are filled with air; affected sinuses appear cloudy or opaque. A visible air-fluid level or thickening of the sinus mucosa may be seen in infected sinuses.
- *CT scan* is a more sensitive indicator of acute and chronic sinusitis and often is performed without preceding x-rays.
- *Magnetic resonance imaging (MRI)* may be ordered if malignancy of the sinus is suspected.

Medications

Antibiotic therapy directed at the usual organisms causing sinusitis typically is prescribed. Amoxicillin (possibly combined with clavulanate [Augmentin]), trimethoprim-sulfamethoxazole (Bactrim, Septra), cefuroxime (Ceftin), cefaclor (Ceclor), ciprofloxacin (Cipro), or clarithromycin (Biaxin) are commonly used antibiotics for sinusitis. Antibiotic therapy is continued for 10 to 14 days; occasionally a longer course is prescribed to prevent relapse. If the sinusitis does not respond to treatment with oral antibiotics, hospitalization and intravenous antibiotic therapy may be required. See Chapter 12 ∞ for nursing care related to antibiotic therapy.

Oral or topical (in the form of nasal sprays) decongestants such as pseudoephedrine or phenylephrine are also prescribed to reduce mucosal edema and promote sinus drainage. Antihistamines may decrease nasal congestion and facilitate sinus drainage, but they also tend to increase the viscosity of secretions and hinder drainage. For this reason, they may not be as effective as decongestants. Saline nose drops or sprays promote sinus drainage, as does inhalation of warm steam.

PRACTICE ALERT
To administer topical drugs, the client's head is tilted backward and to the side on which the drops are to be instilled. The client may need to remain in position for 5 minutes to allow the drops to reach the posterior nares.

Systemic mucolytic agents such as guaifenesin may be useful to liquefy secretions, promoting sinus drainage. Aerobic exercise also promotes mucous flow and may be recommended.

Surgery

Clients who do not respond to pharmacologic measures and who experience persistent facial pain, headache, or nasal congestion may require *endoscopic sinus surgery*. Detailed evaluation of the sinuses by CT scan is done prior to surgery. Under local or general anesthesia, a fiberoptic nasal endoscope is inserted to visualize the sinus opening. If obstruction is present, it can be removed, restoring patency and drainage. This surgery is most effective for local disease, recurrent acute sinusitis, and for removing anatomic obstructions (Way & Doherty,

2003). Clients who have endoscopic sinus surgery usually do not require nasal packing postoperatively. Instead, frequent nasal cleaning and irrigation with normal saline are performed. The client is instructed to sneeze with the mouth open and avoid blowing the nose, lifting, or straining for a week following surgery.

Antral irrigation can be done in the physician's office under local anesthesia. A 16-gauge needle is inserted under the inferior turbinate of the nose into the maxillary sinus on the affected side. Saline solution is instilled to irrigate the area and wash out the sinus of purulent exudate. The client is seated with the head forward and mouth open to allow drainage of the solution through the nose and mouth. A culture of the exudate may be obtained to determine appropriate antibiotic therapy.

The *Caldwell-Luc procedure* may be necessary if endoscopic sinus surgery is unsuccessful. It is performed under local or general anesthesia. An incision is made under the upper lip into the maxillary sinus, and diseased mucous membrane and periosteum are removed. An opening between the maxillary sinus and lateral nasal wall, a "nasal antral window," is created to increase aeration of the sinus and promote drainage into the nasal cavity. The area is packed with gauze for 24 to 48 hours postoperatively. The gauze packing obstructs nasal breathing while it is in place. As the maxillary sinus heals, exposed bone is covered by mucosa. The upper lip and teeth may be numb for several months after the procedure because of nerve trauma. Chewing may be impaired on the affected side. Only liquids are given for the first 24 hours, followed by a soft diet. The client is instructed to avoid wearing dentures and the Valsalva maneuver (no blowing the nose, coughing, or straining at stool) for about 2 weeks after the packing has been removed to prevent bleeding.

In *external sphenoethmoidectomy,* an incision along the side of the nose from the middle of the eyebrow is used to open and remove diseased tissue from the sphenoid or ethmoid sinuses (Figure 37–1 ■). Nasal polyps may also be removed using this approach. Nasal packing is inserted, and an eye pressure patch is applied to decrease periorbital edema. Care is similar to that following the Caldwell-Luc procedure.

Complementary Therapies

Complementary therapies may help relieve symptoms of sinusitis and promote comfort. Aromatherapy using herbs such as

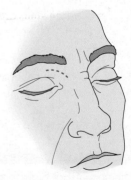

Figure 37–1 ■ Incision to access ethmoid and frontal sinuses. Resulting scar is nearly invisible in folds of the eye.

basil, marjoram, or eucalyptus in a vaporizer or on a handkerchief, herbal teas made from goldenseal, yarrow, or coltsfoot, hot or cold compresses or steam inhalation, and acupressure may be employed (Fontaine, 2005).

NURSING CARE

Health Promotion

Measures to prevent sinusitis are those that promote nasal drainage: encouraging liberal fluid intake, judicious use of nasal decongestants as needed, and treating any obstructive process. Encourage clients with URI to blow their nose with both nares open. Advise clients that use of saline nasal sprays can help maintain patency of the opening to the sinuses, promoting drainage and reducing the risk of obstruction and infection.

Assessment

Focused assessment of the client with suspected sinusitis includes the following:

- *Health History:* Complaints of frontal or periorbital headache, cheek, teeth, or ear pain; timing of pain and changes in intensity over course of the day; nasal discharge or postnasal drip; other symptoms; previous sinus problems; current medications, known medication allergies.
- *Physical Examination:* General appearance; vital signs including temperature; inspect nasal and pharyngeal mucous membranes; percuss sinuses for tenderness.
- *Diagnostic Tests:* WBC and differential, cultures of sinus drainage, sinus x-rays or other imaging studies.

Nursing Diagnoses and Interventions

The client with sinusitis is often acutely uncomfortable. Obstructed and congested sinuses cause pain and pressure that increase with position changes and leaning forward. Treatment usually is community based, making education the key nursing role. When the client is hospitalized for intravenous antibiotic therapy or sinus surgery, *Pain* and *Imbalanced Nutrition* are priority nursing diagnoses.

Pain

Although sinus surgery is relatively minor, both the incision and postoperative swelling can cause discomfort. Nasal packing, if used, contributes to the discomfort.

- Assess pain using a standardized pain scale. Administer analgesics as ordered. *Relief of pain promotes a feeling of well-being and enhances recovery.*
- Apply ice packs to the nose. *Cold compresses reduce swelling, control bleeding, and provide local analgesia.*
- Elevate the head of the bed to Fowler's or high-Fowler's position for 24 to 48 hours after surgery. *Elevating the operative site minimizes tissue swelling and promotes comfort.*

Imbalanced Nutrition: Less than Body Requirements

Postoperatively, the sense of smell, an appetite stimulus, is diminished by nasal packing. Mouth discomfort from the incision and numbness of the upper teeth also may impact appetite and eating.

- Provide clear liquid diet progressing to soft foods as tolerated. High-calorie dietary supplements may be used. *A progressive diet is used to assess the ability to swallow without choking and allay fears. Foods high in calories and nutritional value provide for metabolic and healing requirements.*
- Monitor intake, output, and weight. *This information allows assessment of overall fluid balance and the adequacy of dietary intake.*
- Elevate the head of the bed during meals. *The upright position facilitates swallowing and minimizes risk of aspiration.*

Community-Based Care

Teaching for clients with sinusitis and their families focuses on following through with appropriate treatment and promoting comfort. Discuss the following topics when preparing for home care:

- The importance of completing the entire course of prescribed antibiotics to achieve cure and prevent the development of antibiotic-resistant bacteria. Assist in developing a schedule that helps ensure all doses are taken.
- Measures to prevent superinfections (such as vaginitis or oral thrush) during the prolonged course of treatment (e.g., consume 8 oz of yogurt containing live bacterial cultures daily while on antibiotics).
- Use of systemic or topical decongestants to promote sinus drainage.
- Maintaining a liberal fluid intake to reduce the viscosity of mucous drainage.
- Use of a humidifier or steam inhalation to promote sinus drainage.
- Sleeping with the head of the bed elevated to a 45-degree angle and on the unaffected side to promote drainage of affected sinuses.
- Application of a warm, moist pack to the area of pain and tenderness to promote comfort.
- Notify the physician if symptoms do not improve with treatment or if signs of a complication develop, such as increased pain, and redness and swelling on the side of the nose or around the eyes.
- Postoperative instructions to prevent bleeding, such as avoiding blowing the nose for 7 to 10 days and avoiding strenuous activity such as heavy lifting for about 2 weeks.
- Use of saline nasal sprays postoperatively to keep the nasal mucosa moist.

THE CLIENT WITH PHARYNGITIS OR TONSILLITIS

Pharyngitis, acute inflammation of the pharynx, is one of the most commonly identified clinical problems. Although it is usually viral in origin, pharyngitis may also be caused by bacterial infection. *Group A beta-hemolytic streptococcus* (strep throat) is the most common cause of bacterial pharyngitis. Other bacteria that may cause pharyngitis include *Neisseria gonorrhoeae,* a gram-negative diplococcus that is sexually transmitted, *Mycoplasma,* and *Chlamydia trachomatis.*

Tonsillitis is acute inflammation of the palatine tonsils. Although it is sometimes viral in origin, tonsillitis is usually due to streptococcal infection. The incidence of streptococcal infections is greatest between late fall and spring, especially in cold climates. Viral tonsillitis may occur in epidemics in people living in crowded conditions, such as military recruits.

Pathophysiology and Manifestations

Pharyngitis and tonsillitis are contagious and spread by droplet nuclei. Incubation varies from a few hours to several days, depending on the organism. Viral infections are communicable for 2 to 3 days. Symptoms usually resolve within 3 to 10 days after onset.

Viral pharyngitis may be attributed to the same viruses causing the common cold: rhinovirus, coronavirus, or parainfluenza virus. Pharyngitis caused by adenovirus, influenza virus, or Epstein-Barr virus (associated with infectious mononucleosis) may be particularly severe.

Acute pharyngitis causes pain and fever. The pain may vary from a scratchy sore throat to one so painful that swallowing is difficult. Streptococcal pharyngitis is usually marked by an abrupt onset, with fever of 101°F (38.3°C) or higher, severe sore throat with dysphagia, malaise, and often arthralgias and myalgias. Anterior lymph nodes are often enlarged and tender. Exudate (pus) may be seen on the pharynx and tonsils (Figure 37–2 ■). In contrast, the onset of viral pharyngitis is often gradual, with manifestations of low-grade fever, sore throat, mild hoarseness, headache, and rhinorrhea. The pharyngeal membranes appear mildly red with vascular congestion. Infectious mononucleosis, caused by the Epstein-Barr virus, often presents as acute pharyngitis, with visible patches of exudate on the pharynx or tonsils (Kasper et al., 2005). The cervical lymph nodes are enlarged and tender as well. See the accompanying box for the manifestations of pharyngitis and tonsillitis.

In tonsillitis, the tonsils appear bright red and edematous. White exudate is present on the tonsils; pressing on a tonsil may produce purulent drainage. The uvula may also be reddened and swollen. Cervical lymph nodes are usually tender and enlarged.

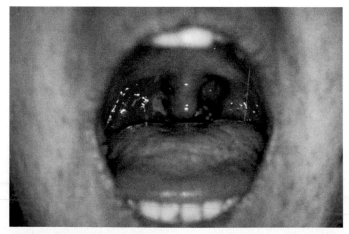

Figure 37–2 ■ The appearance of the oral pharynx and tonsils in acute pharyngitis and tonsillitis.

Source: Biophoto Associates, Photo Researchers, Inc.

MANIFESTATIONS of Pharyngitis and Tonsillitis

LOCAL
- Sore throat
- Possible dysphagia and otalgia
- Tender, swollen anterior cervical lymph nodes
- Hoarse voice
- Red, swollen pharyngeal mucous membranes and/or tonsils
- Possible visible exudate on pharyngeal membranes and/or tonsils

GENERAL
- Fever
- General malaise
- Arthralgia, myalgia

The client with tonsillitis complains of a sore throat, difficulty swallowing, general malaise, fever, and otalgia (pain referred to the ear). Manifestations are often more severe in adolescents and adults than in children. Infection may extend via the eustachian tubes to cause acute otitis media. This may lead to further damage such as spontaneous rupture of the eardrums and mastoiditis. See Chapter 48 ∞ for more information about otitis media.

Complications

Although bacterial pharyngitis may be mild and indistinguishable from viral pharyngitis by its signs and symptoms, it can lead to significant complications such as abscess, scarlet fever, toxic shock syndrome, rheumatic fever, or acute poststreptococcal glomerulonephritis.

Peritonsillar abscess, or *quinsy,* is a potential complication of tonsillitis. It usually results from group A beta-hemolytic streptococcus infection extending from the tonsils to the surrounding tissue. The abscess causes pus formation behind the tonsil with marked swelling and asymmetric deviation of the uvula. The degree of swelling may make it difficult to swallow anything other than liquids. The client may exhibit thickening of the voice, drooling, and a tonic contraction of the muscles of mastication, called trismus.

Rare (1% to 3%) but serious complications of streptococcal pharyngitis and tonsillitis include acute glomerulonephritis and rheumatic fever, abnormal immune responses to the infection. Acute glomerulonephritis generally presents with sudden onset of hematuria, proteinuria, and less commonly, hypertension and edema within 7 to 10 days after the acute infection. Rheumatic fever typically presents 3 to 5 weeks after acute infection with fever, painful or swollen joints, rash, and heart murmur. Other complications of bacterial infection include sinusitis, otitis media, mastoiditis, and cervical adenitis.

INTERDISCIPLINARY CARE

Both viral and bacterial pharyngitis are usually self-limited diseases. However, because of the risk for serious complications associated with streptococcal sore throat, an effort is usu-

ally made to establish an accurate diagnosis and treat bacterial pharyngitis.
- *Throat swab* is obtained and examined for streptococcus antigen using the latex agglutination (LA) antigen test or enzyme immunoassay (ELISA) testing. These tests allow rapid identification of the antigen (in as little as 10 minutes for the LA test) but are not highly sensitive. When the test is positive, treatment for strep throat is initiated. If the test is negative, the swab is cultured to ensure that streptococcus organisms are not present. Even throat cultures are not always accurate, with approximately 10% false negative and 20% false positive results. See Chapter 36 ∞ for nursing care related to obtaining a throat swab.
- *Complete blood count (CBC)* may be done on severely ill clients or to rule out other causes of pharyngitis. The WBC count is usually normal or low in viral infections and elevated in bacterial infections.

Antipyretics and mild analgesics such as aspirin or acetaminophen provide symptomatic relief for throat pain and associated myalgias. Penicillin is the drug of choice for group A streptococci. Erythromycin, amoxicillin, or cefuroxime (Ceftin, Kefurox) may be used if the client is allergic to penicillin. Antibiotic therapy is continued for at least 10 days. The client is no longer contagious after 24 hours of antibiotic therapy.

A peritonsillar abscess is drained by needle aspiration or by incision and drainage. The area is first sprayed with a topical anesthetic such as Cetacaine and then injected with a local anesthetic. The sitting position is preferred for the procedure, because it enables expectoration of blood and pus. (See the accompanying Nursing Care Plan for nursing care of the client with a peritonsillar abscess.) Tonsillectomy is done either immediately or 6 weeks after incision and drainage of peritonsillar abscess.

Tonsillectomy (surgical removal of the tonsils) is indicated for recurrent or chronic infections that have not responded to antibiotic therapy, hypertrophy of the tonsils with risk of airway obstruction, peritonsillar abscess, repeated attacks of purulent otitis media, and tonsil malignancy. Adenoid tissue usually is removed at the same time. Bleeding is the most significant postoperative complication of tonsillectomy, and may develop up to 2 weeks following the surgery.

NURSING CARE

Because of the risk of significant complications associated with streptococcal pharyngitis, encourage all clients with symptoms that persist for several days or that include fever, lymphadenopathy, and myalgias to seek evaluation and treatment.

Home care is appropriate for acute uncomplicated pharyngitis. Treatment focuses on adequate rest and relief of symptoms. A liquid or soft diet is useful when swallowing is difficult. Increased fluid intake is encouraged, especially when febrile. Warm saline gargles, moist inhalations, and application of an ice collar are soothing to the sore throat.

Following tonsillectomy, ensure a patent airway by placing the client in semi-Fowler's position with the head turned to the side to allow secretions to drain from the mouth and pharynx.

NURSING CARE PLAN   A Client with Peritonsillar Abscess

Monica Wunderman, age 27, was recently treated for tonsillitis caused by infection by group A streptococcus. She presents to the emergency department 10 days later appearing acutely ill. She states that her throat is so sore that she has difficulty swallowing even liquids. Barbara Ironhorse, the ED nurse, completes an assessment of Ms. Wunderman.

ASSESSMENT
Findings include T 102°F (38.8°C). An acutely swollen and reddened area of the soft palate is noted in her mouth, half occluding the orifice from the mouth into the pharynx. Yellow exudate is present. CBC reveals an elevated WBC of 16,000/mm³. A diagnosis of peritonsillar abscess is made. Needle aspiration of the abscess is performed.

DIAGNOSES
- *Acute Pain* related to swelling
- *Risk for Ineffective Airway Clearance* related to pain and swelling
- *Deficient Fluid Volume* related to fever and difficulty in swallowing fluids

EXPECTED OUTCOMES
- Have minimal or no pain.
- Maintain a patent airway as demonstrated by normal respiratory rate and rhythm.
- Maintain optimal fluid intake as evidenced by consumption of fluids and semiliquid foods, moist mucous membranes, normal skin turgor, and normal temperature.

PLANNING AND IMPLEMENTATION
- Teach that ice-cold fluids may be easier to swallow than hot or room temperature beverages and may provide a local analgesic effect.
- Advise to avoid citrus juices, hot or spicy foods, and rough-textured foods for 1 week.
- Teach pain management strategies such as applying an ice collar as desired and gargling with warm saline or mouthwash solution every 1 to 2 hours for the first 24 to 48 hours after aspiration of the abscess.
- Instruct to take medications as prescribed.

EVALUATION
When Ms. Ironhorse contacts Ms. Wunderman by telephone 2 days after her visit to the emergency department, she reports complete relief of symptoms. She is afebrile, taking fluids without difficulty, and has had no difficulty breathing. She has not experienced any pain.

CRITICAL THINKING IN THE NURSING PROCESS
1. Describe common symptoms of infectious or inflammatory diseases of the upper airway and discuss methods of symptom relief.
2. Describe common pharmacologic interventions for these disorders.
3. What themes of nursing diagnoses emerge for clients with these types of disorders?
   See Evaluating Your Response in Appendix C.

Keep the airway in place until the gag and swallowing reflexes have returned. Apply an ice collar to reduce swelling and pain. Notify the surgeon immediately if excessive bleeding or hemorrhage occurs. If there is no bleeding, allow water and cracked ice as desired. Warm saline mouthwashes are helpful in managing thick oral secretions following tonsillectomy. A liquid or semiliquid diet is recommended for several days.

Community-Based Care
Discuss the following topics when preparing the client for home care:
- The importance of completing the full 10 days of antibiotic therapy if prescribed
- Using warm saline gargles or throat lozenges for symptomatic relief
- Signs and symptoms of possible complications of streptococcal infection such as glomerulonephritis or rheumatic fever
- Monitoring temperature in the morning and evening until well to ensure that the infection has not spread to deeper tissues
- Proper use and disposal of tissues and frequent hand washing to prevent spreading the infection to others.

For the client who has had a peritonsillar abscess drainage or tonsillectomy, provide the following instructions:
- Postoperative mouth and throat care
- Avoiding use of aspirin for 2 weeks to reduce the risk of postoperative bleeding

- Manifestations of bleeding to report to the physician (delayed hemorrhage may occur for up to 1 week postsurgery).

THE CLIENT WITH A LARYNGEAL INFECTION
The larynx, located between the upper airways and the lungs, protects the lower respiratory tract from inhaled substances other than air, and allows speech. The larynx includes the epiglottis, which covers the larynx during swallowing, and the glottis, or vocal cords. Either portion of the larynx may become inflamed.

Epiglottitis
Epiglottitis, inflammation of the epiglottis, is an uncommon disorder that presents as a medical emergency. *H. influenzae* infection is the most common cause of epiglottitis. Epiglottitis is a rapidly progressive cellulitis that begins between the base of the tongue and the epiglottis. The epiglottis itself becomes swollen and inflamed; swelling of adjacent tissues pushes the epiglottis posteriorly. This swelling and edema threaten the airway. Adults usually present with a 1- to 2-day history of sore throat, *odynophagia* (painful swallowing), dyspnea, and possibly drooling and stridor.

Using a tongue blade to view the oropharynx is avoided; this may precipitate laryngospasm and airway obstruction. The epiglottis is visualized using a flexible fiberoptic laryngoscope to establish the diagnosis. The epiglottis appears red, swollen, and edematous. Nasotracheal intubation may be required to ensure airway patency. The client is admitted to a critical care unit and intravenous antibiotic therapy is initiated. Ceftriaxone (Rocephin), cefuroxime (Ceftin), or ampicillin/sulbactam (Unasyn) may be prescribed. If allergic to penicillin, a combination of clindamycin (Cleocin) and either trimethoprim-sulfamethoxazole (TMP-SMZ) or ciprofloxacin (Cipro) may be used. Dexamethasone, a systemic corticosteroid, is also given to suppress the inflammatory response and rapidly reduce swelling of the epiglottis.

Nursing care for the client with acute epiglottitis focuses on monitoring and maintaining airway patency. Monitor oxygen saturation continuously. Observe closely for signs of airway obstruction, including nasal flaring, restlessness, stridor, use of accessory muscles, and decreased oxygen saturation measurements. If the client is not intubated, supplies for emergency intubation should be kept in the unit. Epiglottitis is frightening for both the client and the nurse. Maintaining a calm, reassuring manner is an essential nursing role.

Laryngitis

Laryngitis, inflammation of the larynx, is a common disorder that may occur alone or in conjunction with other upper respiratory infections. It is commonly associated with a viral URI such as influenza. It may also occur with bronchitis, pneumonia, or other respiratory infections. Excessive use of the voice, sudden changes in temperature or exposure to dust, irritating fumes, smoke, or other pollutants can also cause acute or chronic laryngitis. It is more common in the winter and in colder climates.

In laryngitis, the mucous membrane lining the larynx becomes inflamed; the vocal cords also may become edematous. The primary symptom of laryngitis is a change in the voice. Hoarseness or *aphonia*, complete loss of the voice, may occur. The throat is often sore and scratchy, and a dry, harsh cough may be present.

There is no specific treatment for viral laryngitis. Any identified precipitating factors such as overuse of the voice and exposure to irritants should be eliminated. Voice rest is advised, as is abstinence from tobacco and alcohol, which are chemical irritants. Treatment may also include inhaling steam or spraying the throat with antiseptic solutions. Identifying and eliminating irritants are helpful to prevent future attacks.

Impaired verbal communication is the priority nursing problem for clients with laryngitis. The meaning of messages is conveyed not only by the words used, but also by the tone and loudness of voice. Instruct to rest the voice as much as possible. Encourage speaking in short sentences or using alternate methods of communication, such as writing. Resting the voice hastens recovery and decreases throat discomfort. Advise to use soothing throat lozenges, sprays, or other comfort measures such as gargling with a warm antiseptic solution. Help identify potential irritants, such as fumes, chemicals, or cold temperature, to prevent future bouts of laryngitis.

THE CLIENT WITH DIPHTHERIA

Diphtheria is an acute, contagious disease caused by *Corynebacterium diphtheriae,* a small aerobic pathogen. This disease, which primarily affects adults, is uncommon in the United States. Waning immunity due to lack of periodic booster immunizations is the primary risk factor for diphtheria in the United States.

The disease is spread through droplet nuclei and by contamination of articles such as eating utensils. Asymptomatic carriers can be a factor in spreading this infection. People who have recovered from diphtheria can harbor bacteria in their throats for up to 4 weeks. Diphtheria is easily spread in areas where sanitation is poor, living conditions are crowded, and access to health care is limited. Immunization is readily available, and infants and children are usually immunized against diphtheria, pertussis, and tetanus concurrently.

Pathophysiology and Manifestations

C. diphtheriae infects the mucous membranes of the respiratory tract and can invade skin lesions. The tonsils and pharynx are common sites of infection. Toxins released by the organism inflame mucosal surfaces of the pharynx. Exudate from inflamed tissues forms a thick, grayish, rubbery pseudomembrane over the posterior pharynx and sometimes into the trachea. This pseudomembrane adheres to inflamed, eroded surfaces and interferes with eating, drinking, and breathing. The airway may be obstructed, necessitating tracheostomy to maintain respirations. The toxins damage the heart and CNS and may cause myocarditis and paralysis of cranial or peripheral nerves.

Clients with diphtheria develop fever, malaise, sore throat, and malodorous breath. In severe cases, the neck may be warm and swollen because of lymphadenopathy. Isolated patches of gray or white exudate grow and extend to form a gray membrane that becomes progressively thicker. Dislodging the membrane often causes bleeding. Symptoms of airway obstruction, such as stridor and cyanosis, can develop quickly.

INTERDISCIPLINARY CARE

Collaborative care goals for diphtheria are to prevent its transmission, treat the infection, neutralize toxins, and provide respiratory support. The diagnosis is confirmed by a throat culture. Gram-stain or immunofluorescent antibody stains may also be used.

Strict isolation procedures are instituted, and all contacts are screened and immunized. Booster shots are given to people who were immunized 5 or more years previously. Unimmunized contacts are treated with immunization and antibiotics.

Diphtheria antitoxin is given to neutralize free toxin and prevent further toxin production. Diphtheria antitoxin is produced in horses; a skin test for sensitivity to horse serum should precede immunization. Anaphylaxis is a risk during antitoxin therapy; epinephrine must be readily available. Antibiotics such as penicillin or erythromycin are administered to eliminate the organism.

NURSING CARE

Clients with diphtheria require intensive nursing care. The client is placed on bed rest and monitored closely for airway obstruction is relieved or more definitive care can be given. Endotracheal intubation may be attempted. If intubation is unsuccessful, an immediate cricothyrotomy or tracheotomy must be performed to open the airway.

CT scan is used to identify laryngeal fractures; however, emergency treatment may be required prior to diagnosis to ensure airway patency and preserve life. Soft-tissue injuries may be managed conservatively with bedside humidifier, intravenous fluids, antibiotics, and corticosteroids to reduce edema. More severe injuries require endotracheal intubation or immediate tracheostomy. Nursing care related to caring for the client with a tracheostomy is presented later in this chapter. See Chapter 39 ∞ for more information about endotracheal intubation and nursing care for the intubated client.

 ## NURSING CARE

PRACTICE ALERT
The priority of nursing care in laryngeal obstruction or trauma is restoring a patent airway to prevent cerebral anoxia and death. Laryngeal obstruction and trauma are medical emergencies requiring immediate intervention.

Closely monitor clients at risk for laryngeal obstruction (e.g., following neck trauma, newly extubated clients, and people receiving medications with a high risk of anaphylaxis, such as intravenous antibiotics or radiologic dyes) for manifestations of obstruction, including dyspnea, nasal flaring, tachypnea, anxiety, wheezing, and stridor. Suction the airway as needed; small aspirated foreign bodies might possibly be removed by suctioning. If obstruction is complete, initiate a cardiopulmonary arrest procedure and perform the Heimlich maneuver until the obstruction is relieved or the emergency response team arrives. Prepare to assist with emergency intubation or tracheotomy as needed. Provide emotional support, reassurance, and teaching for the client and family to reduce anxiety.

Community-Based Care
Health promotion and teaching for home care focus on preventing laryngeal obstruction and early intervention techniques. Everyone should be aware of the risk factors for adult aspiration. Caution clients who wear dentures to take small bites, chewing each bite carefully before swallowing. Discuss the relationship between excess alcohol intake and food aspiration. Participate in promoting training of the general public in CPR and the Heimlich maneuver. The more people who are adequately trained in emergency procedures, the more likely it is that emergency procedures will be initiated in a timely manner. Clients with a known risk for anaphylaxis, such as people with a previous anaphylactic response and those allergic to bee venom, should wear a Medic-Alert tag and carry a bee-sting kit to allow early intervention to prevent severe laryngeal edema and spasm.

THE CLIENT WITH OBSTRUCTIVE SLEEP APNEA

Sleep apnea, intermittent absence of airflow through the mouth and nose during sleep, is a serious and potentially life-threatening disorder. It affects at least 2% of middle-aged women and 4% of middle-aged men. Sleep apnea is a leading cause of excessive daytime sleepiness, and may contribute to other problems such as poor work performance and motor vehicle crashes (Kasper et al., 2005; McCance & Huether, 2006). Recent studies have linked sleep apnea with an increased risk for hypertension, ischemic heart disease, and exacerbation of heart failure.

Types of sleep apnea include obstructive and central. In *obstructive sleep apnea,* the more common type, the respiratory drive remains intact, but airflow ceases due to occlusion of the oropharyngeal airway. *Central sleep apnea* is a rare neurologic disorder that involves transient impairment of the neurologic drive to respiratory muscles.

Risk Factors

In addition to male gender, risk factors for obstructive sleep apnea include increasing age and obesity. Large neck circumference (>17 inches in men and >16 inches in women) also is a known risk factor for obstructive sleep apnea (Porth, 2005). Use of alcohol and other CNS depressants may contribute to sleep apnea.

Pathophysiology

During sleep, skeletal muscle tone decreases (except the diaphragm). The most significant decrease occurs during rapid eye movement (REM) sleep (Porth, 2005). Loss of normal pharyngeal muscle tone permits the pharynx to collapse during inspiration as pressure within the airways becomes negative in relation to atmospheric pressure. The tongue is also pulled against the posterior pharyngeal wall by gravity during sleep, causing further obstruction. Obesity or skeletal or soft-tissue changes that decrease inspiratory tone, such as a relatively large tongue in a relatively small oropharynx, contribute to the problem. Airflow obstruction causes the oxygen saturation, Po_2, and pH to fall, and the Pco_2 to rise. This progressive asphyxia causes brief arousal from sleep, which restores airway patency and airflow. Sleep can be severely fragmented because these episodes may occur hundreds of times each night.

Manifestations

Narrowed upper airways produce loud snoring during sleep, often years before obstructive sleep apnea occurs. Excessive daytime sleepiness, headache, irritability, and restless sleep also are common manifestations. See the box on the next page.

Complications

Recurrent episodes of apnea and arousal during sleep have secondary physiologic effects. Sleep fragmentation and loss of slow-wave sleep are thought to contribute to neurologic and behavior problems such as excessive daytime sleepiness, impaired intellect, memory loss, and personality changes. Recurrent nocturnal asphyxia and negative intrathoracic pressure due to airway

---

MANIFESTATIONS of Obstructive Sleep Apnea

- Loud, cyclic snoring
- Periods of apnea lasting 15 to 120 seconds during sleep
- Gasping or choking during sleep
- Restlessness, thrashing during sleep
- Daytime fatigue and sleepiness
- Morning headache
- Personality changes, depression
- Intellectual impairment
- Impotence
- Hypertension

---

obstruction increase the workload of the heart. People with coronary heart disease may develop myocardial ischemia and angina. Dysrhythmias such as significant bradycardia and dangerous tachydysrhythmias may develop. Left ventricular function may be impaired and heart failure may occur. Systemic blood pressure remains high during sleep and may contribute to systemic hypertension that affects more than 50% of people with obstructive sleep apnea (Kasper et al., 2005). Pulmonary hypertension also may develop. Sudden cardiac death is believed to be a potential fatal complication of obstructive sleep apnea.

Obstructive sleep apnea is a common condition in people who are morbidly obese. When these clients undergo gastric bypass surgery to treat their obesity, sleep apnea places them at significant risk for postoperative respiratory complications. Not only does the obesity interfere with chest movement and ventilation, it increases metabolic demands and carbon monoxide production. Anesthetic and analgesics used during surgery and in the postoperative period can lead to hypoxemia due to muscle relaxation and depression of the respiratory drive (Deutzer, 2005).

INTERDISCIPLINARY CARE

The goal of care for obstructive sleep apnea is to restore airflow and prevent the adverse effects of the disorder. Sustained weight loss may cure obstructive sleep apnea.

Diagnosis

The diagnosis of obstructive sleep apnea is based on *polysomnography,* an overnight sleep study. Several variables are recorded during the study, including:

- Electroencephalogram and measurements of ocular activity and muscle tone
- Recordings of ventilatory activity and airflow
- Continuous arterial oxygen saturation readings
- Heart rate.

Transcutaneous arterial P_{CO_2} readings also may be monitored during the study. Because sleep studies are time consuming and expensive, overnight monitoring of oxygen saturation by pulse oximetry may be used to confirm the diagnosis of sleep apnea when symptoms indicate a high probability of the disorder (Kasper et al., 2005). Nursing implications for pulmonary function studies and pulse oximetry are presented in

Chapter 36 ∞. See Chapter 43 ∞ for more information about electroencephalography.

Treatments

Mild to moderate obstructive sleep apnea may be treated by weight reduction, alcohol abstinence, improving nasal patency, and avoiding the supine position for sleep. Although weight reduction often cures the disorder, maintaining optimal weight is difficult. Oral appliances designed to keep the mandible and tongue forward also may be prescribed.

Nasal continuous positive airway pressure (CPAP) is the treatment of choice for obstructive sleep apnea. Positive pressure generated by an air compressor and administered through a tight-fitting nasal mask (Figure 37–5 ■) splints the pharyngeal airway, preventing collapse and obstruction. With proper training, this device is well tolerated by the client. Nasal airways can become dry and irritated with CPAP, so an in-line humidifier or a room humidifier is recommended. A newer device, the BiPAP ventilator, delivers higher pressures during inhalation and lower pressures during expiration, providing less resistance to exhaling.

Surgery

Tonsillectomy and adenoidectomy may relieve upper airway obstruction in some clients. Excision of obstructive tissue from the soft palate, uvula, and posterior lateral pharyngeal wall may be accomplished by *uvulopalatopharyngoplasty (UPPP).* Although only about 50% of these surgeries are successful in treating sleep apnea, UPPP is useful in selected cases. In severe cases, tracheostomy may also be performed to bypass the area of obstruction.

NURSING CARE

Obstructive sleep apnea usually is treated in the home. Nursing care focuses on teaching the client and family about equipment use and strategies to decrease contributing factors such as obesity and alcohol intake. The following nursing diagnoses are appropriate for clients with sleep apnea:

- *Disturbed Sleep Pattern* related to repeated apneic episodes
- *Fatigue* related to interrupted sleep patterns

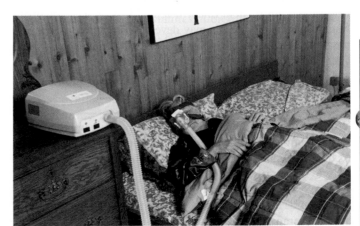

Figure 37–5 ■ A client using a nasal mask and CPAP to treat sleep apnea.
Source: Custom Medical Stock Photo, Inc.

MEDIALINK Case Study: Sleep Apnea

- If desired, arrange a visit by a rehabilitated laryngectomy client who has mastered an alternative form of verbal communication and has a positive attitude about rehabilitation. *Many clients and their families find that they are better able to communicate their fears with someone who has gone through the same experience they are facing.*

See the accompanying nursing research box for more information about assistive devices for use in the early postoperative period.

Impaired Swallowing

Disruption of laryngeal structures by the tumor itself or due to radiation or surgery can impair the swallowing mechanism. Additionally, even when a total laryngectomy has been performed and a connection between the oropharynx and trachea no longer exists, swallowing may cause fear of choking.

- Maintain intravenous fluids and enteral feedings or parenteral nutrition until adequate food and fluids can be ingested orally. *It is important to maintain nutritional and fluid balance until normal eating can be resumed.*
- Postoperatively, initiate oral intake with soft foods, not liquids. *Soft foods are easier to handle and swallow initially. As recovery progresses, thickened liquids can be swallowed and, eventually, a normal diet can be resumed.*
- Following total laryngectomy, reassure that choking is not possible, because there is no connection between the esophagus and trachea. *Clients often fear that swallowing will result in choking and they will be unable to cough effectively.*
- Instruct to initiate a swallow by placing a small amount of food on the back of the tongue, flex the head forward, and then think "swallow." *Swallowing is no longer an automatic function and needs to be relearned.*

PRACTICE ALERT
Provide for privacy during initial attempts at eating. Eating in the presence of others may cause embarrassment until confidence in eating is regained. Privacy also reduces distractions, allowing concentration on swallowing.

Imbalanced Nutrition: Less than Body Requirements

Large laryngeal tumors often place pressure on the esophagus and may cause dysphagia (difficulty swallowing) or odynophagia (painful swallowing). In either case, difficulty eating may ultimately impair nutrition. Additionally, cancer often produces a hypermetabolic state, increasing calorie requirements. If surgery is performed, difficulty swallowing and a fear of aspiration in the early postoperative period also interfere with eating. Enteral or parenteral feedings are usually needed initially to meet nutritional status. After a total laryngectomy, the senses of taste and smell are disrupted. Although the sense of taste may be partially recovered, clients may complain that eating no longer is pleasurable.

- Assess nutritional status using height and weight charts, reported weight loss, and anthropometric measurements such as skin folds. *Thorough assessment of nutritional status is important in planning to meet current and anticipated calorie needs.*

PRACTICE ALERT
Monitor food and fluid intake and urinary output. Pain or fatigue, rather than a sensation of fullness, may prompt the decision to stop eating, resulting in inadequate intake.

- Evaluate current and preferred eating habits and foods, as well as understanding of nutrition. *This evaluation provides additional information about nutrition as well as a basis for future planning.*

NURSING RESEARCH | **Evidence-Based Practice: The Client Undergoing Laryngectomy**

Communication methods and content among clients who had undergone surgery for head or neck cancer were evaluated in this pilot study of the use of electronic speech-generating devices (SGDs) (Happ et al., 2005). The researchers also looked at the quality (ease and client satisfaction) of communications among study participants, as well as barriers to SGD use and the effect of client factors such as age and illness severity on communications. All study participants were alert and able to write legibly; the majority had at least some experience using a computer.

Although 60% of study participants were found to be able to use SGDs with minimal assistance and instruction, the devices were used in only 17% of observed communications; writing and nonverbal communications were used the majority of the time. Barriers to use of the devices included placement of the device out of the client's reach, mechanical malfunctions, and impatience of caregivers with the time required for typed communications. Clients expressed frustration with the lack of a standard keyboard and with the impersonality of the computerized voice. Overall, the devices were found to be useful as one of several methods of communication used by the client.

IMPLICATIONS FOR NURSING
Speech-generating devices can facilitate communication for selected clients, particularly when the content of the message is complex. Training of clients, caregivers, and family members is necessary for effective use of these devices, however. Preoperatively, clients scheduled for laryngectomy should be instructed in communication methods to use after surgery, including use of gestures, written messages (including predeveloped messages, such as "I am in pain"), and use of any assistive communication devices.

CRITICAL THINKING IN CLIENT CARE
1. In this study, SGDs often were found out of the client's reach. What planning should the nurse do to help ensure that assistive communication devices are accessible to the client?
2. Clients in this study were literate and many had at least some experience using computers. Do you think results of the study would differ if the study population had less education, was illiterate, or had minimal English language proficiency? Why or why not?
3. Develop a teaching plan for a preoperative laryngectomy client using the nursing diagnosis *Deficient Knowledge: Postoperative Communication Strategies.*

PRACTICE ALERT
Weigh daily. Daily weight is an accurate measure of both fluid balance and nutritional status.

- Refer to a dietitian for further evaluation, planning, and education. *A professional can identify nutritional needs and help plan a diet that will meet them.*
- Encourage experimentation with foods of different textures and temperatures. *Very cold foods or foods of a soft texture may be easier to swallow.*
- Encourage frequent, small meals rather than three large meals per day. *Frequent, small quantities of food improve overall intake when dysphagia, odynophagia, or fatigue interfere with nutrition.*
- Recommend liquid supplements such as Ensure when calorie needs are not being met. Provide information about where to obtain nutritional supplements. *Liquid dietary supplements provide balanced nutrition as well as additional calories and are an effective way of increasing intake. They are available without prescription in major supermarkets.*
- Provide mouth care before meals and supplemental feedings. Provide a topical anesthetic such as viscous lidocaine before eating for stomatitis or esophagitis related to radiation or chemotherapy. *The tumor or its treatment may cause bad breath or a foul taste in the mouth, which suppresses appetite. Inflamed mucosa may make eating uncomfortable. A topical anesthetic may relieve this discomfort and thus promote food intake.*
- Provide an antiemetic 30 minutes before eating as needed to relieve nausea. *Nausea interferes with food intake. An antiemetic can relieve nausea and make eating possible.*
- Suggest enteral (tube) feedings via nasogastric or gastrostomy tube if the client is unable to consume enough food to maintain weight and nutritional status. *Both cancer and surgery increase calorie needs. Supplemental enteral feedings may be necessary to prevent catabolism and to promote healing and recovery.*

PRACTICE ALERT
Following laryngectomy, place in semi-Fowler's or Fowler's position. Elevating the head of the bed facilitates swallowing of oral secretions and helps prevent regurgitation of tube feedings.

- Instruct to perform mouth rinses before initiating feeding postoperatively. *Rinsing helps clean the mouth and also provides practice in using tongue and cheek muscles to control fluid in the mouth.*
- Refer to a physical or speech therapist for swallowing rehabilitation following laryngectomy. *Because surgery changes the relationship of the trachea, esophagus, and oropharynx, swallowing needs to be relearned before eating.*
- Reinforce swallowing instructions. *Reinforcement promotes learning.*

Anticipatory Grieving

The client with laryngeal cancer faces not only the diagnosis of cancer, which is often perceived as a death sentence, but also the prospect of mutilating surgery. If laryngectomy is necessary, the client grieves the loss of both a body part and an important function, speech, a vital aspect of social interaction and often necessary for one's career. It also enables people to express their needs when they cannot meet them alone. The loss of speech, therefore, is a major loss. In addition, the tracheal stoma changes the manner in which the client breathes. If radical neck dissection is required, loss of neck musculature and function also alters body image and self-concept.

- Provide opportunities for expressing feelings of grief, anger, or fear about the diagnosis of cancer, the impending surgery, and the anticipated loss of speech. *The client with laryngeal cancer needs the opportunity (and may need permission) to grieve anticipated losses. A cancer diagnosis may precipitate grieving for unfulfilled plans and expectations, even though a cure may be anticipated. Laryngectomy causes a major change in body image, with loss of a vital body part and creation of a stoma. The client also grieves the loss of speech. This loss can have a significant impact on occupation and social interaction.*

PRACTICE ALERT
Provide a calm, supportive environment with adequate privacy and emotional support for the client and family members as they work through the grieving process. It is important for the client and family to know that their feelings of loss are real and accepted by caregivers.

- Help the client and family discuss the potential impact of the loss on family structure and function. *Discussion helps family members understand each other's feelings and support one another.*
- Refer for psychologic or spiritual counseling as appropriate. *Counseling and spiritual guidance can help the client and family deal with the diagnosis and proposed treatment, and help prevent a sense of defeat and hopelessness.*
- Help identify additional resources, such as coping strategies that have been successfully used in the past to deal with crises. *This exercise helps the client and family identify strengths they can use to deal with the present situation.*

Using NANDA, NIC, and NOC

Chart 37–3 shows links between NANDA nursing diagnoses, NIC, and NOC for the client with laryngeal cancer.

Community-Based Care

Teaching for the client with a benign laryngeal tumor emphasizes management of contributing factors. Stress the importance of not yelling or screaming. Refer clients, particularly singers, to a speech therapist for voice training. Emphasize the need to keep the voice within its normal range to reduce vocal cord stress. Encourage smoking cessation, particularly if the client is also a singer. Discuss the relationship of industrial pollutants to laryngeal tumors and help explore ways of reducing pollutant exposure.

Teaching the client and family about laryngeal cancer, treatment options, and home care related to those treatments is an important nursing responsibility. Include the following topics when teaching:

- Clarification of treatment options, including risks and benefits.
- Importance of early intervention to reduce the risk of local spread and metastasis.

Pneumocystis Pneumonia

People with acquired immune deficiency syndrome (AIDS) and others with significant immunocompromise are at risk for developing an opportunistic pneumonia caused by *Pneumocystis*, a common parasite found worldwide. Immunity to *Pneumocystis* is nearly universal, except in immunocompromised people. Opportunistic infection may develop in people treated with immunosuppressive or cytotoxic drugs for cancer or organ transplant and in people with genetic or acquired immunodeficiency. People with AIDS account for most cases (60%) of *Pneumocystis* pneumonia (PCP) (Copstead & Banasik, 2005).

Infection with *Pneumocystis* produces patchy involvement throughout the lungs, causing affected alveoli to thicken, become edematous, and fill with foamy, protein-rich fluid. Gas exchange is severely impaired as the disease progresses.

PCP has an abrupt onset with fever, tachypnea and shortness of breath, and a dry, nonproductive cough. Respiratory distress can be significant, with intercostal retractions and cyanosis.

Table 38–3 compares the manifestations of infectious pneumonias.

Aspiration Pneumonia

Aspiration of gastric contents into the lungs results in a chemical and bacterial pneumonia known as *aspiration pneumonia*. Major risk factors for aspiration pneumonia include emergency surgery or obstetric procedures, depressed cough and gag reflexes, and impaired swallowing. Older surgical clients are at significant risk. Enteral nutrition by either nasogastric or gastric tube also increases the risk for aspiration pneumonia. Vomiting is not always apparent; silent regurgitation of gastric contents may occur when the level of consciousness is decreased. Measures to reduce the risk for aspiration pneumonia include minimizing the use of preoperative medications, promoting anesthetic elimination from the body, and preventing nausea and gastric distention.

The low pH of gastric contents causes a severe inflammatory response when aspirated into the respiratory tract. Pul-monary edema and respiratory failure may result. Common complications of aspiration pneumonia include abscesses, bronchiectasis (chronic dilation of the bronchi and bronchioles), and gangrene of pulmonary tissue.

INTERDISCIPLINARY CARE

Prevention is a key component in managing pneumonia. Identifying vulnerable populations and instituting preventive strategies are measures to reduce the mortality and morbidity associated with pneumonia. With early identification of the infecting organism, appropriate treatment, and support of respiratory function, most clients recover uneventfully. However, pneumonia remains a serious disease with significant mortality, especially in aged and debilitated populations.

Diagnosis

The history and physical examination, along with diagnostic testing, are used to establish the diagnosis, determine the extent of lung involvement, and identify the causative organism. See Chapter 36 ∞ for more information about the following tests and their nursing implications:

- *Chest x-ray* is obtained to determine the extent and pattern of lung involvement. Fluid, infiltrates, consolidated lung tissue, and atelectasis (areas of alveolar collapse) appear as densities on the film. The *CT scan* provides a more detailed image of pulmonary tissue and may be used when the chest x-ray is not diagnostic.

- *Sputum Gram stain* rapidly identifies the infecting organisms as gram-positive or gram-negative bacteria. Antibiotic therapy can then be directed at the predominant type of organism until culture and sensitivity results are obtained.

- *Sputum culture and sensitivity* is ordered to identify the infecting organism and determine the most effective antibiotic therapy. When obtaining sputum for culture, it is important to obtain secretions from the lower respiratory tract, not the mouth and nasal passages. See Procedure 36–1 on page 1220.

TABLE 38–3 Manifestations of Infectious Pneumonias

TYPE	ONSET	RESPIRATORY MANIFESTATIONS	SYSTEMIC MANIFESTATIONS
Pneumococcal or lobar pneumonia	Abrupt	Cough productive of purulent or rust-colored sputum; pleuritic or aching chest pain; decreased breath sounds and crackles over affected area; possible dyspnea and cyanosis	Chills and fever
Bronchopneumonia	Gradual	Cough, scattered crackles; minimal dyspnea and respiratory distress	Low-grade fever
Legionnaires' disease	Gradual	Dry cough; dyspnea	Chills and fever; general malaise; headache; confusion; anorexia and diarrhea; myalgias and arthralgias
Primary atypical pneumonia	Gradual	Dry, hacking, nonproductive cough	Fever, headache, myalgias, and arthralgias predominate
Viral pneumonia	Sudden or gradual	Dry cough	Flulike symptoms
Pneumocystis pneumonia	Abrupt	Dry cough; tachypnea and shortness of breath; significant respiratory distress	Fever

- *Complete blood count (CBC) with white blood cell (WBC) differential* shows an elevated WBC (11,000/mm^3 or higher) with increased circulating immature leukocytes (a left shift) in response to the infectious process. White blood cell changes are minimal in viral and other pneumonias.
- *Serology testing*, blood tests to detect antibodies to respiratory pathogens, may be used to identify the infecting organism when blood and sputum cultures are negative.
- *Pulse oximetry*, a noninvasive method of measuring arterial oxygen saturation, is ordered to continuously monitor gas exchange. The Sao_2 normally is 95% or higher. An Sao_2 of less than 95% may indicate impaired alveolar gas exchange.
- *Arterial blood gases (ABGs)* may be ordered to evaluate gas exchange. Respiratory secretions or pleuritic pain can interfere with alveolar ventilation. Alveolar inflammation can interfere with gas exchange across the alveolar-capillary membrane, especially if exudate or consolidation is present. An arterial oxygen tension (Pao_2) of less than 75 to 80 mmHg indicates impaired gas exchange or alveolar ventilation. See Chapters 10 and 36 ∞ for more information about gas transport, ABGs, and normal or expected values.
- *Fiberoptic bronchoscopy* may be done to obtain a sputum specimen or remove secretions from the bronchial tree (Figure 36–9). Nursing responsibilities related to bronchoscopy are summarized in the Diagnostic Tests box in Chapter 36 ∞.

Immunization

Vaccines offer some degree of protection against the most common bacterial and viral pneumonias.

Pneumococcal vaccine, made of antigens from 23 types of pneumococcus, usually imparts lifetime immunity with a single dose. The vaccine is recommended for people who have a high risk of adverse outcome from bacterial pneumonias; people over age 65; those with chronic cardiac or respiratory conditions, diabetes mellitus, alcoholism, or other chronic diseases; and immunocompromised people. A one-time revaccination is recommended for selected populations, including people over age 65 who were immunized more than 5 years previously and before age 65, people with chronic renal failure or immunosuppressive conditions (e.g., malignancy), and people receiving chemotherapy with selected agents (CDC, 2005).

Influenza vaccine is also recommended for high-risk populations. The predominant strain of influenza virus varies from year to year. A new vaccine formulation is prepared yearly, incorporating antigens of the influenza strains predicted to be the most prevalent for the upcoming flu season (typically the winter months). Vulnerable populations for whom yearly vaccine is recommended include those listed above as well as healthcare workers and residents of long-term care facilities. The vaccine contains egg protein, and is not recommended for people who have a severe allergy to eggs or who have previously experienced a severe hypersensitivity response to the vaccine.

Medications

Medications used to treat pneumonia may include antibiotics to eradicate the infection and bronchodilators to reduce bronchospasm and improve ventilation.

Initial antibiotic therapy is based on the results of sputum Gram stain and the pattern of lung involvement shown on a chest x-ray. Considerations such as the presence of cardiovascular disease or residence in a long-term care facility also are considered in the initial antibiotic choice. Typically, a broad-spectrum antibiotic such as a macrolide (e.g., clarithromycin, azithromycin, or erythromycin), a penicillin or a second- or third-generation cephalosporin, or a fluoroquinolone (e.g,. ciprofloxacin) is ordered until the results of sputum culture and sensitivity tests are available. Table 38–4 lists commonly prescribed antibiotics for selected pneumonias; nursing implications for selected antibiotics are summarized in Chapter 12 ∞.

When an inflammatory response to the infection causes bronchospasm and constriction, bronchodilators may be ordered to improve ventilation and reduce hypoxia. Bronchodilators generally belong to one of two major groups: the

TABLE 38–4 Antibiotic Therapy for Selected Pneumonias

CAUSATIVE ORGANISM	ANTIBIOTIC OF CHOICE	ALTERNATIVE ANTIBIOTICS
Streptococcus pneumoniae	Penicillin G; amoxicillin	Erythromycin, cephalosporins, doxycycline, fluoroquinolone, clindamycin, vancomycin, trimethoprim-sulfamethoxazole (TMP-SMZ), linezolid
Haemophilus influenzae	Second- or third-generation cephalosporins, doxycycline, azithromycin, TMP-SMZ	Fluoroquinolones, clarithromycin
Staphylococcus aureus	Penicillinase-resistant penicillin (e.g., nafcillin); vancomycin for methicillin-resistant organisms	Cephalosporins, vancomycin, clindamycin; ciprofloxacin, fluoroquinolones, TMP-SMZ
Mycoplasma pneumoniae	Erythromycin, doxycycline	Clarithromycin, azithromycin, fluoroquinolone
Klebsiella pneumoniae	Third-generation cephalosporin (with aminoglycoside if severe); metronidazole	Aztreonam, imipenem-cilastatin, fluoroquinolone
Legionella pneumophila	Macrolide + rifampin; fluoroquinolone	TMP-SMZ, doxycycline + rifampin
Pneumocystis	TMP-SMZ, pentamidine + prednisone	Dapsone + trimethoprim, clindamycin + primaquine, trimetrexate + folinic acid
Chlamydia pneumoniae	Doxycycline	Macrolide, fluoroquinolone

sympathomimetic drugs, such as albuterol sulfate (Proventil) and metaproterenol (Alupent); or the methylxanthines, such as theophylline and aminophylline. Use of these drugs and related nursing implications are discussed in detail in the section on asthma in Chapter 39 ∞.

An agent to "break up" mucus or reduce its viscosity may be prescribed. Acetylcysteine (Mucomyst), potassium iodide, and guaifenesin (a common ingredient in expectorant cough syrups) help to liquefy mucus, making it easier to expectorate. For many clients, however, increasing fluid intake is an effective means of liquefying mucus.

Treatments

When mucous secretions are thick and viscous, increasing fluid intake to 2500 to 3000 mL per day helps liquefy secretions, making them easier to cough up and expectorate. If the client is unable to maintain an adequate oral intake, intravenous fluids and nutrition may be required.

Incentive spirometry may be used to promote deep breathing, coughing, and clearance of respiratory secretions. Endotracheal suctioning may be required if the cough is ineffective. This invasive technique is discussed in Chapter 39 ∞ in the section describing nursing care for the client with acute respiratory failure. On occasion, bronchoscopy is used to perform pulmonary toilet and remove secretions.

OXYGEN THERAPY Oxygen therapy may be indicated for the client who is tachypneic or hypoxemic.

Inflammation of the alveolar-capillary membrane interferes with diffusion of gases across the membrane. Diffusion is affected by several other factors, including the partial pressure of gases on each side of the membrane. Increasing the percentage of inspired oxygen above that of room air (21%) increases the partial pressure of oxygen in the alveoli and enhances its diffusion into the capillaries. Supplemental oxygen therefore improves oxygenation of the blood and tissues in clients with pneumonia.

Depending on the degree of hypoxia, oxygen may be administered by either a low-flow or high-flow system. Low-flow systems include the nasal cannula, simple face mask, partial rebreathing mask, and nonrebreathing mask (Figure 38–3 ■). A nasal cannula can deliver 24% to 45% oxygen concentrations with flow rates of 2 to 6 L/min. The nasal cannula is comfortable and does not interfere with eating or talking. A simple face mask delivers 40% to 60% oxygen concentrations with flow rates of 5 to 8 L/min. Up to 100% oxygen can be delivered by the nonrebreather mask, the highest concentration possible without mechanical ventilation. When the amount of oxygen delivered must be precisely regulated, a high-flow system such as a Venturi mask is used (Figure 38–4 ■). The Venturi mask regulates the ratio of oxygen to room air, allowing precise regulation of the oxygen percentage delivered, from 24% to 50%. Severe hypoxia may necessitate intubation and mechanical ventilation. Endotracheal intubation and methods of mechanical ventilation are discussed in Chapter 39 ∞.

CHEST PHYSIOTHERAPY Chest physiotherapy, including percussion, vibration, and postural drainage, may be prescribed to reduce lung consolidation and prevent atelectasis.

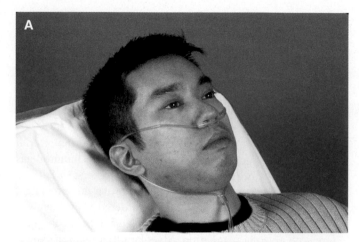

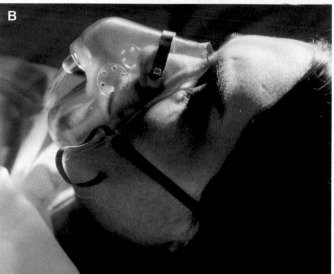

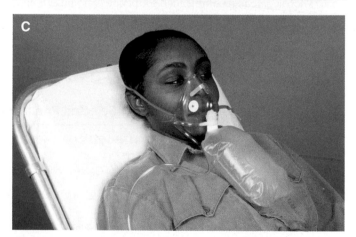

Figure 38–3 ■ Low-flow oxygen delivery devices: A, nasal cannula; B, simple face mask; C, nonrebreather mask.

Source: A, C, Michal Heron, Pearson Education/PH College; *B,* Tony McConnell, Photo Researchers, Inc.

Percussion is performed by rhythmically striking or clapping the chest wall with cupped hands (Figure 38–5A ■), using rapid wrist flexion and extension. Cupping traps air between the palm and the client's skin, setting up vibrations through the chest wall that loosen respiratory secretions. The trapped air also provides a cushion, preventing injury. When per-

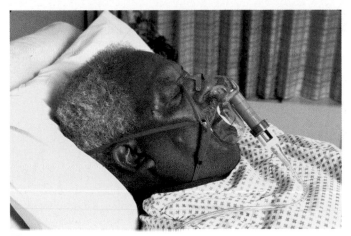

Figure 38–4 ■ Venturi mask, a high-flow oxygen delivery system.
Source: Michal Heron, Pearson Education/PH College

formed correctly, percussion produces a hollow, popping sound. Percussion may also be done using a mechanical percussion cup. The breasts, sternum, spinal column, and kidney regions are avoided during percussion.

Vibration facilitates secretion movement into larger airways. It usually is combined with percussion, although it may be used when percussion is contraindicated or poorly tolerated. Vibration is performed by repeatedly tensing the arm and hand muscles while maintaining firm but gentle pressure over the affected area with the flat of the hand (Figure 38–5B).

Percussion and vibration are done in conjunction with *postural drainage*, which uses gravity to facilitate removal of secretions from a particular lung segment. The client is positioned with the segment to be drained superior to or above the trachea or mainstem bronchus. Drainage of all lung segments requires a variety of positions (Figure 38–6 ■); rarely do all segments require drainage. Bronchodilators or nebulizer treatments are administered as ordered prior to postural drainage. It is best to perform postural drainage before meals to avoid nausea and vomiting.

Complementary Therapies

Although complementary therapies do not replace conventional treatment for pneumonia, they often promote comfort and speed recovery. The herb echinacea is widely used to stimulate immune function and treat URIs. Because viral URIs often precede pneumonia, echinacea may be helpful in preventing pneumonia. Recent research, however, shows mixed results for the effectiveness of echinacea in reducing the duration and severity of URI (National Center for Complementary and Alternative Medicine [NCCAM], 2005). Goldenseal, which often is sold in combination with echinacea, is used to treat bacterial, fungal, and protozoal infections of the mucous membranes of the respiratory tract.

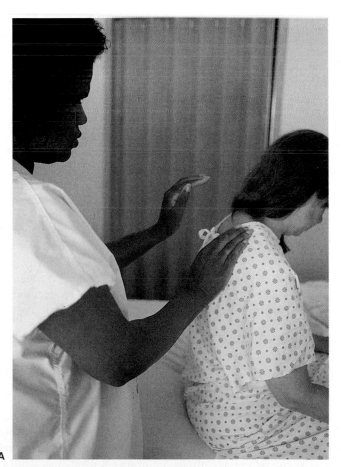

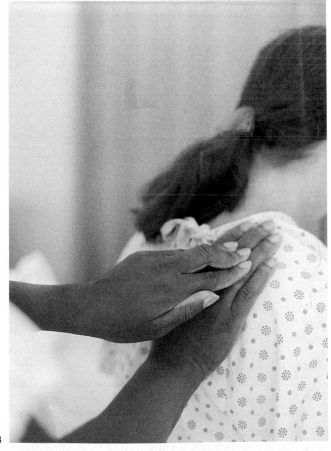

Figure 38–5 ■ *A,* Percussing (clapping) the upper posterior chest. Notice the cupped position of the nurse's hands. *B,* Vibrating the upper posterior chest.

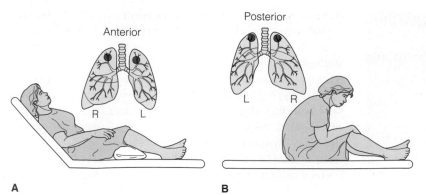

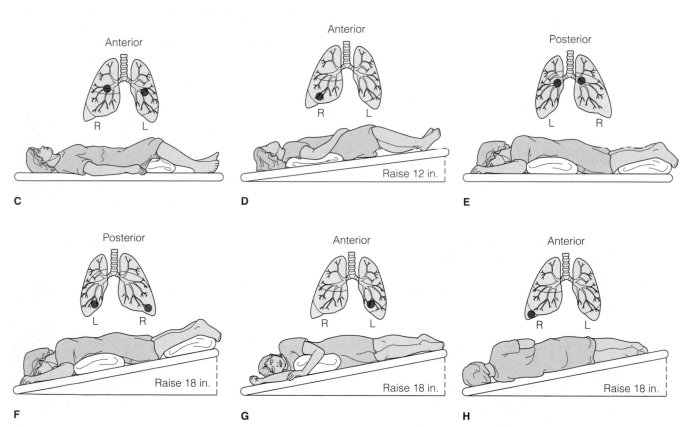

Figure 38–6 ■ Positions for postural drainage. *A,* Left and right anterior apical. *B,* Left and right posterior apical. *C,* Left and right anterior upper. *D,* Right middle lobe. *E,* Superior lower lobes. *F,* Left and right lower posterior. *G,* Left lower lateral. *H,* Right lower lateral.

Ma huang contains the active ingredient ephedra, which has been used to relieve bronchospasm and ease breathing. The primary active ingredient in ephedra is epinephrine, a cardiac and CNS stimulant. Because of the dangers associated with its use, sale of herbal products containing ephedra has been banned (NCCAM, 2004). Advise clients inquiring about the use of Chinese herbal remedies to reduce pneumonia symptoms to inquire if any recommended product contains ma huang or ephedra, and to avoid such products.

NURSING CARE

Health Promotion

Health promotion activities focus on pneumonia prevention. Make clients in high-risk groups aware of the benefits of immunizations against influenza and pneumococcal pneumonia. A single dose of pneumococcus vaccine usually produces im-

munity to most strains of pneumococcal pneumonia, although repeat doses may be needed for older adults and people who are immunosuppressed. (Pneumococcus vaccine is contraindicated for people receiving immunosuppressive therapy.) Annual influenza vaccine helps prevent pneumonia, because pneumonia often occurs as a sequela to influenza.

PRACTICE ALERT
Inquire about allergic responses to eggs or previous influenza vaccinations prior to administering influenza vaccine. A significant hypersensitivity response may occur in clients who are allergic to egg protein.

Additional measures to screen for and detect pneumonia in older adults are appropriate. Frequent pulmonary assessment and aggressive interventions help prevent problems. Restoring and maintaining mobility improves ventilation and helps mobilize secretions. Promoting adequate fluid intake is necessary because fluid helps liquefy secretions, making them easier to expectorate.

Assessment

Focused assessment of the client with pneumonia includes the following:

- *Health History:* Current symptoms and their duration; presence of shortness of breath or difficulty breathing, chest pain and its relationship to breathing; cough, productive or nonproductive, color, consistency of sputum; other symptoms; recent upper respiratory or other acute illness; chronic diseases such as diabetes, chronic lung disease, or heart disease; current medications; medication allergies.
- *Physical Examination:* Presentation, apparent distress; level of consciousness, vital signs including temperature; skin color, temperature; respiratory excursion, use of accessory muscles of respiration; lung sounds.
- *Diagnostic Tests:* WBC with differential, sputum Gram stain, culture and sensitivity, chest x-ray or CT scan.

Nursing Diagnoses and Interventions

Clients with lower respiratory disorders such as pneumonia may have multiple nursing care needs, depending on the severity of the illness. Alveolar ventilation and the process of alveolar respiration can be affected by inflammation and secretions. **Hypoxemia**, low levels of oxygen in the blood, and tissue hypoxia may result. Nursing care focuses on supporting optimal respiratory function and promoting rest to reduce metabolic and oxygen needs. Priority nursing diagnoses include *Ineffective Airway Clearance, Ineffective Breathing Pattern,* and *Activity Intolerance.*

Ineffective Airway Clearance

The inflammatory response to infection causes tissue edema and exudate formation. In the lungs, the inflammatory response can narrow and potentially obstruct bronchial passages and alveoli. Assessment findings supporting this nursing diagnosis include adventitious breath sounds such as crackles (rales), rhonchi, and wheezes; dyspnea and tachypnea; coughing; and indicators of hypoxia such as cyanosis, reduced SaO_2 levels, anxiety, and apprehension.

- Assess respiratory status, including vital signs, breath sounds, SaO_2, and skin color at least every 4 hours. *Early identification of respiratory compromise allows intervention before tissue hypoxia is significant.*
- Assess cough and sputum (amount, color, consistency, and possible odor). *Assessment of the cough and nature of sputum produced allows evaluation of the effectiveness of respiratory clearance and the response to therapy.*
- Monitor ABG results; report increasing hypoxemia and other abnormal results to the physician. *Blood gas changes may be an early indicator of impaired gas exchange due to airway narrowing or obstruction.*
- Place in Fowler's or high-Fowler's position. Encourage frequent position changes and ambulation as allowed. *The upright position promotes lung expansion; position changes and ambulation facilitate the movement of secretions.*

- Assist to cough, deep breathe, and use assistive devices. Provide endotracheal suctioning using aseptic technique as ordered. *Coughing, deep breathing, and suctioning help clear airways.*
- Provide a fluid intake of at least 2500 to 3000 mL per day. *A liberal fluid intake helps liquefy secretions, facilitating their clearance.*
- Work with the physician and respiratory therapist to provide pulmonary hygiene measures, such as postural drainage, percussion, and vibration. *These techniques help mobilize and clear secretions.*
- Administer prescribed medications as ordered, and monitor their effects. *If the infecting organism is resistant to the prescribed antibiotic, little improvement may be seen with treatment. Bronchodilators help maintain open airways but may have adverse effects such as anxiety and restlessness.*

Ineffective Breathing Pattern

Pleural inflammation often accompanies pneumonia, causing sharp localized pain that increases with deep breathing, coughing, and movement, which can lead to rapid and shallow breathing. Distal airways and alveoli may not expand optimally with each breath, increasing the risk for atelectasis and decreasing gas exchange. Fatigue from the increased work of breathing is an additional problem in pneumonia. This, too, can lead to decreased lung inflation and an ineffective breathing pattern.

> **PRACTICE ALERT**
> Assess respiratory rate, depth, and lung sounds at least every 4 hours. Tachypnea and diminished or adventitious breath sounds may be early indicators of respiratory compromise.

- Provide for rest periods. *Rest reduces metabolic demands, fatigue, and the work of breathing, promoting a more effective breathing pattern.*
- Assess for pleuritic discomfort. Provide analgesics as ordered. *Adequate pain relief minimizes splinting and promotes adequate ventilation.*
- Provide reassurance during periods of respiratory distress. *Hypoxia and respiratory distress produce high levels of anxiety, which tends to further increase tachypnea and fatigue and decrease ventilation.*
- Administer oxygen as ordered. *Oxygen therapy increases the alveolar oxygen concentration and facilitates its diffusion across the alveolar-capillary membrane, reducing hypoxia and anxiety.*
- Teach slow abdominal breathing. *This breathing pattern promotes lung expansion.*
- Teach use of relaxation techniques, such as visualization and meditation. *These techniques help reduce anxiety and slow the breathing pattern.*

Activity Intolerance

Impaired airway clearance and gas exchange interfere with oxygen delivery to body cells and tissues. At the same time, the infectious process and the body's response to it increase metabolic demands on the cells. The net result of this imbalance between oxygen delivery and oxygen demand is a lack of physiologic energy to maintain normal daily activities.

■ Assess activity tolerance, noting any increase in pulse, respirations, dyspnea, diaphoresis, or cyanosis. *These assessment findings may indicate limited or impaired activity tolerance.*

PRACTICE ALERT

Activity intolerance may be an early sign of cardiorespiratory compromise, particularly in the older adult or client with preexisting heart disease. New or worsening manifestations of activity intolerance should be reported to the physician.

■ Assist with self-care activities, such as bathing. *Assistance with ADLs reduces energy demands.*
■ Schedule activities, planning for rest periods. *Rest periods minimize fatigue and improve activity tolerance.*
■ Provide assistive devices, such as an overhead trapeze. *These assistive devices facilitate movement and reduce energy demands.*
■ Enlist the family's help to minimize stress and anxiety levels. *Stress and anxiety increase metabolic demands and can decrease activity tolerance.*
■ Perform active or passive range-of-motion (ROM) exercises. *Exercises help maintain muscle tone and joint mobility, and prevent contractures if bed rest is prolonged.*
■ Provide emotional support and reassurance that strength and energy will return to normal when the infectious process has resolved and the balance of oxygen supply and demand is restored. *The client may be concerned that activity intolerance will continue to be a problem after the acute infection is resolved.*

Using NANDA, NIC, and NOC

Links between NANDA nursing diagnoses, NIC, and NOC for the client with pneumonia are outlined in Chart 38–1.

Community-Based Care

Clients with pneumonia usually are treated in the community, unless their respiratory status is significantly compromised (e.g., altered mental status, tachypnea, tachycardia, hypotension, hypo- or hyperthermia, and altered blood gases) or if risk factors such as advanced age and/or coexisting heart, kidney, or liver disease are present.

Discuss the following topics when preparing the client and family for home care:

■ The importance of completing the prescribed medication regimen as ordered; potential drug side effects and their management, including manifestations that necessitate stopping the drug and notifying the physician
■ Recommendations for limiting activities and increasing rest
■ Maintaining adequate fluid intake to keep mucus thin for easier expectoration
■ Ways to maintain adequate nutritional intake, such as small, frequent, well-balanced meals
■ The importance of avoiding smoking or exposure to secondhand smoke to prevent further irritation of the lungs

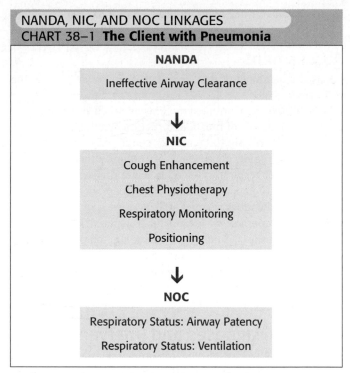

NANDA, NIC, AND NOC LINKAGES
CHART 38–1 The Client with Pneumonia

NANDA

Ineffective Airway Clearance

↓

NIC

Cough Enhancement

Chest Physiotherapy

Respiratory Monitoring

Positioning

↓

NOC

Respiratory Status: Airway Patency

Respiratory Status: Ventilation

Data from *NANDA's Nursing Diagnoses: Definitions & Classification 2005–2006* by NANDA Interational (2005), Philadelphia; *Nursing Interventions Classification (NIC)* (4th ed.) by J. M. Dochterman & G. M. Bulechek (2004), St. Louis, MO: Mosby; and *Nursing Outcomes Classification (NOC)* (3rd ed.) by S. Moorhead, M. Johnson, and M. Maas (2004), St. Louis, MO: Mosby.

■ Manifestations to report to the physician, such as increasing shortness of breath, difficulty breathing, increased fever, fatigue, headache, sleepiness, or confusion
■ The importance of keeping all follow-up appointments to ensure disease cure.

The accompanying Nursing Care Plan provides further nursing interventions for clients treated in the community.

Clients with respiratory compromise or who are elderly or debilitated may require home care assistance to remain at home. Provide referrals to home intravenous services, home health nursing services, and home maintenance services as indicated. Community services such as Meals-on-Wheels can provide support to reduce the energy demands of meal preparation.

THE CLIENT WITH SEVERE ACUTE RESPIRATORY SYNDROME

Severe acute respiratory syndrome (SARS) is a lower respiratory illness of unknown etiology first described in people in Asia in the fall of 2002. Since then, this emerging disease has been identified in clients in North America, Australia, and Europe, although the majority of identified cases are in China (including Hong Kong and Singapore) (World Health Organization, 2003). The primary population affected by SARS is previously healthy adults ages 25 to 70 years.

Pathophysiology

The infective agent responsible for SARS is a coronavirus not previously identified in humans. This virus appears to spread

NURSING CARE PLAN   A Client with Pneumonia

Mary O'Neal is a 35-year-old executive assistant and a part-time college student. On returning home from class one evening, she begins to chill. She alternates between chills and sweats all night. Staying home from work, she remains in bed most of the next day. Her fever continues, and she develops a cough and dull aching chest pain. When the cough becomes productive of rust-colored sputum the following day, she seeks medical treatment from her family doctor.

ASSESSMENT

Debby Kowalski, RN, the family practice clinic nurse, admits Mrs. O'Neal to the clinic and obtains the nursing assessment. Mrs. O'Neal denies any previous history of respiratory diseases "other than the usual colds, flu, and such." She also denies any history of smoking or medication allergies. She says her symptoms began abruptly with the onset of the chills. She describes her chest pain as a dull ache that was initially substernal but now is localized in her lower lateral right chest. The pain increases with deep breathing, coughing, and moving. Her cough is increasing in frequency and severity, and her sputum appears rusty brown. Her vital signs are BP 116/74, P 104 and regular, R 26, T 101.8°F (38.7°C). Skin warm and flushed, with no evidence of cyanosis. Respirations shallow, unlabored; respiratory excursion equal. Diminished breath sounds in bases bilaterally, crackles noted in right posterior and lateral base. Faint pleural rub heard at right midaxillary line.

A STAT CBC shows a WBC of 18,900/mm³; differential shows increased numbers of neutrophils and immature WBCs (bands). Ms. Kowalski has Mrs. O'Neal rinse with an antiseptic mouthwash and then collects a sputum specimen for culture and Gram stain prior to seeing the physician.

The physician orders a chest x-ray after examining Mrs. O'Neal. Based on her history, examination, and the chest x-ray, he makes the diagnosis of acute bacterial pneumonia, probably pneumococcal. He prescribes oral penicillin V, 500 mg every 6 hours for 10 days. He asks Mrs. O'Neal to return for a follow-up appointment in 10 days and refers her back to Ms. Kowalski for appropriate teaching.

DIAGNOSES

- *Ineffective Breathing Pattern* related to pleuritic chest pain
- *Hyperthermia* related to inflammatory process
- *Deficient Knowledge* about pneumonia and its treatment

EXPECTED OUTCOMES

- Maintain normal pulmonary function.
- Describe measures to minimize elevations in body temperature.
- Identify a schedule for taking her medication that will facilitate compliance with the regimen.
- Describe manifestations that should be reported to the physician.

PLANNING AND IMPLEMENTATION

- Assess knowledge and understanding of pneumonia and its effects.
- Assist to develop a medication schedule that coordinates with normal daily routine.
- Teach about the following:
  a. Importance of avoiding use of a cough suppressant except at night to facilitate rest
  b. Ways to increase fluid intake to reduce fever and maintain thin mucus for easy expectoration
  c. Beneficial effects of rest, especially during the acute phase of her illness
  d. Safe use of aspirin and acetaminophen to reduce fever
  e. Importance of taking all prescribed medication doses as scheduled
  f. Common side effects of penicillin V and their management
  g. Early manifestations of penicillin allergy that necessitate stopping the medication and notifying the physician
  h. Signs of complications of pneumonia or worsening pneumonia to report.

EVALUATION

The sputum culture confirms *S. pneumoniae* as the cause of Mrs. O'Neal's pneumonia. When she returns for her follow-up appointment, she reports that she began to feel better after 2 days on the penicillin and returned to work the following Monday. Her examination reveals good breath sounds throughout with no adventitious sounds. The follow-up sputum culture is free of pathogens.

CRITICAL THINKING IN THE NURSING PROCESS

1. Do any of the factors identified in the case study increase Mrs. O'Neal's risk for acute bacterial pneumonia?
2. Mrs. O'Neal's WBC differential showed increased neutrophil and band counts. Describe the reason for and effect of this change.
3. Even though Mrs. O'Neal has no history of medication allergies, anaphylactic shock remains a potential risk. Describe the sequence of events leading to anaphylactic shock, its initial symptoms, and immediate nursing interventions.
4. Had Mrs. O'Neal required hospitalization to treat her acute pneumonia, interruption of her usual activities and responsibilities could lead to anxiety. Develop a care plan for this situation, using the nursing diagnosis *Ineffective Role Performance* related to hospitalization.

See Evaluating Your Response in Appendix C.

---

primarily by contact with respiratory secretions. Other potential sources of the infection are through direct contact with an infected person or contaminated object, and exposure of the eyes or mucous membranes to respiratory secretions (CDC, 2004). Contact with contaminated water or sewage may transmit the disease, suggesting fecal–oral transmission as well (Kasper et al., 2005).

The virus infects cells of the respiratory tract, leading to surface necrosis and sloughing of pneumocytes in the alveolar spaces and formation of hyaline membranes (a fibrin and protein "film" that interferes with gas exchange within the alveoli). The alveolar damage is accompanied by inflammation of interstitial pulmonary tissues with infiltration by lymphocytes and monocytes. The virus also is found in the blood, urine, and feces.

Manifestations and Complications

The incubation period for SARS is generally 2 to 7 days, although it may be as long as 10 days in some people. Fever higher than 100.4°F (38°C) is typically the initial manifestation of the disease. The high fever may be accompanied by chills, headache, malaise, and muscle aches. After 1 to 2 days, respiratory manifestations of SARS develop, including nonproductive cough, shortness of breath, dyspnea, and possible hypoxemia. Respiratory symptoms may worsen, progressing to respiratory distress, during the second week of the illness.

Although the majority of people with SARS recover, up to 20% of affected clients require intubation and mechanical ventilation (see Chapter 39 ∞). Acute respiratory distress syndrome (ARDS) or multiorgan dysfunction (see Chapter 11 ∞) may develop. The overall mortality rate for SARS is about 11%. The disease is less severe in children than in adults (Kasper et al., 2005).

INTERDISCIPLINARY CARE

Prompt identification of SARS, infection control measures, and reporting of the disease are vital to control this potentially fatal disease. Healthcare providers and public health personnel should report cases of SARS to state and local health departments.

Diagnosis

Diagnostic testing for SARS may include the following:

- *Serology tests* (including enzyme-linked immunosorbent assay [ELISA] or immunofluorescence tests) for antibodies to the coronavirus may performed, but often are undetectable during the acute stage of the illness.
- *Reverse-transcriptase polymerase chain reaction (RT-PCR)* testing of respiratory and blood samples provides a rapid mechanism for identifying the virus, but only about 33% of early samples are positive.
- *Chest x-ray* may be normal or show interstitial infiltrates in a focal or generalized patchy pattern. In late stages of SARS, consolidation may be evident.
- *Pulse oximetry (oxygen saturation)* often shows hypoxemia in the respiratory phase of the illness.
- *CBC* often demonstrates a low lymphocyte count early in the disease. Leukopenia and thrombocytopenia may develop at the peak of the respiratory illness.
- *Creatinine phosphokinase (CPK or CK), ALT*, and *AST* levels may be markedly increased in SARS.
- *Sputum specimen* is obtained. Gram stain and culture are performed on the specimen to rule out other causes of pneumonia.
- *Blood culture* may be done to identify possible bacteremia.

Medications

At this time, no medications have been shown to be consistently effective in treating SARS. Antibiotic and/or antiviral therapy targeted at community-acquired forms of pneumonia may be administered if the diagnosis is unclear.

Infection Control

Because healthcare workers are at risk for developing SARS after caring for infected clients, infection control precautions

should be immediately instituted when SARS is suspected. Standard precautions (see Appendix A ∞) are implemented along with contact and airborne precautions. The CDC (2005) recommends hand hygiene, gown, gloves, eye protection, and an N95 respirator to prevent transmission of SARS in healthcare settings.

When clients with SARS are managed in the community, they are advised to remain home for 10 days after the fever has resolved and until respiratory symptoms are absent or minimal. Members of the household are advised to wash hands frequently or use alcohol-based hand rubs. The client is advised to cover the mouth and nose with tissue when coughing or sneezing and to wear a surgical mask during close contact with uninfected people. Sharing of utensils, towels, and bedding should be avoided. Routine cleaning (e.g., washing with soap and hot water) is adequate to disinfect objects and no special precautions are necessary for disposing of waste.

Treatments

Care of the client with SARS is supportive. Oxygen may be administered to treat hypoxemia. Intubation and mechanical ventilation may be required if respiratory failure or ARDS develops.

NURSING CARE

Nursing care of the client with SARS focuses on preventing spread of the disease to others and providing respiratory support.

Health Promotion

Use respiratory and contact infection control precautions in addition to standard precautions when caring for all clients with suspected SARS to prevent spread of the disease to healthcare workers or other clients.

Assessment

Focused assessment data for the client with suspected SARS include the following. For more complete respiratory assessment, see Chapter 36 ∞.

- *Health History:* Current symptoms, including fever, malaise, shortness of breath, and cough; onset of symptoms; recent international travel or exposure to a person known to have SARS.
- *Physical Assessment:* Vital signs including temperature; respiratory status, including respiratory rate, depth, and effort; presence of cough; adventitious lung sounds.

Nursing Diagnoses and Interventions

The client with SARS poses a risk for spread of the infection to healthcare workers and others. In addition, while many people with this disease experience only mild symptoms and recover fully and uneventfully, others develop severe respiratory distress and may require significant respiratory support. Gas exchange may be impaired, leading to significant hypoxemia. In addition to the nursing diagnoses discussed in the previous section on pneumonia, *Impaired Gas Exchange* and *Risk for Infection* are priority nursing diagnoses.

Impaired Gas Exchange

SARS causes hypoxemia of varying degrees in affected clients. Significant hypoxemia may necessitate intubation and mechanical ventilation to support cellular function until recovery occurs.

- Monitor vital signs, color, oxygen saturation, and ABGs. Assess for manifestations such as anxiety or apprehension, restlessness, confusion, lethargy, or complaints of headache. *These assessment data alert the nurse and care providers to potential hypoxemia or hypercapnia due to impaired gas exchange.*

PRACTICE ALERT
Promptly report signs of respiratory distress, including tachypnea, tachycardia, nasal flaring, use of accessory muscles, intercostal retractions, cyanosis, increasing restlessness, anxiety, or decreased level of consciousness (LOC). These may be early manifestations of respiratory failure and inability to maintain ventilatory effort.

- Promptly report worsening ABGs and oxygen saturation levels. *Close assessment of these values allows timely intervention as needed.*
- Maintain oxygen therapy and mechanical ventilation as ordered. Hyperoxygenate prior to suctioning. *Oxygen and mechanical ventilation support alveolar gas exchange. Hyperoxygenation prior to suctioning reduces the degree of hypoxemia that occurs during suctioning.*
- Place in Fowler's or high Fowler's position. *Sitting positions decrease pressure on the diaphragm and chest, improving lung ventilation and decreasing the work of breathing.*
- Minimize activities and energy expenditures by assisting with activities of daily living (ADLs), spacing procedures and activities, and allowing uninterrupted rest periods. *Rest is vital to reduce oxygen and energy demands.*

PRACTICE ALERT
Avoid sedatives and respiratory depressant drugs unless mechanically ventilated. These medications can further depress the respiratory drive, worsening respiratory failure.

- If intubation and mechanical ventilation are necessary, explain the procedure and its purpose to the client and family, providing reassurance that this *temporary* measure improves oxygenation and reduces the work of breathing. Alert that talking is not possible while the endotracheal tube is in place, and establish a means of communication. *Thorough explanation is important to relieve anxiety.*

See the section in Chapter 39 ∞ on respiratory failure for more information about caring for a client who is intubated and mechanically ventilated.

Risk for Infection

The spread of SARS is a risk both in the healthcare facility and the community in which the client resides. Respiratory and contract precautions are recommended to prevent the spread of SARS via respiratory secretions or contact with the virus.

- Place the client in a private room with airflow control that prevents air within the room from circulating into the hall-

way or other rooms. A negative flow room in which air is diluted by at least six fresh-air exchanges per hour is recommended. *A negative flow room and multiple fresh-air exchanges dilute the concentration of virus within the room and prevent its spread to adjacent areas.*

- Use standard precautions and respiratory and contact isolation techniques as recommended by the CDC, including wearing respirators, gowns, and eye protection when caring for clients with SARS. *These measures are important to prevent the spread of SARS to others.*
- Discuss the reasons for and importance of respiratory and contact isolation procedures during treatment. *Maintenance of infection control precautions during and immediately following the febrile and respiratory phases of SARS is vital to prevent its spread to healthcare workers and the community.*
- Place a mask on the client when transporting to other parts of the facility for diagnostic or treatment procedures. *Covering the client's nose and mouth during transport minimizes air contamination and the risk to visitors and personnel.*
- Inform all personnel having contact with the client of the diagnosis. *This allows personnel to take appropriate precautions.*
- Assist visitors to mask prior to entering the room. *Providing visitors with appropriate masks or respirators reduces their risk of infection.*
- Teach the client how to limit transmitting the disease to others:
  a. Always cough and expectorate into tissues.
  b. Dispose of tissues properly, placing them in a closed bag.
  c. Wear a mask if sneezing or unable to control respiratory secretions.
  d. Do not share eating utensils, towels, bedding, or other objects with others, because this disease may also be spread by contact with contaminated objects.

Teaching appropriate precautions helps prevent the spread of SARS to others while allowing as much freedom from restraints as possible.

Community-Based Care

Many clients with SARS experience only mild symptoms and are appropriately cared for in the community. Teaching about home care and infection control precautions is vital to prevent spread of this disease to the community. Include the following topics when teaching for home care:

- The disease, its origin, and how it is spread
- Manifestations of impaired respiratory status to report to the physician
- Preventing spread of the disease to others:
  - Cover the mouth and nose with tissues when coughing or sneezing. Personally dispose of tissues in a paper bag or the garbage. Wear a surgical mask during close contact with other members of the household.
  - Limit interactions outside the home; do not go to work, school, or other public areas until you have been free of fever for 10 days and your respiratory symptoms are resolving.
  - Remind all members of the household to wash hands (or use an alcohol-based hand sanitizer) frequently, particularly after direct contact with body fluids.

- Do not share eating utensils, towels, or bedding with others. These items can be cleaned with soap and hot water between uses. Clean contaminated surfaces with a household disinfectant.
- Monitoring uninfected members of the household for signs of the illness (Instruct to report fever or respiratory symptoms to the physician.)

THE CLIENT WITH LUNG ABSCESS

A **lung abscess** is a localized area of lung destruction or necrosis and pus formation. The most common cause of lung abscess is aspiration and resulting pneumonia. Risk factors, therefore, are those for aspiration: decreased LOC due to anesthesia, injury or disease of the central nervous system (CNS), seizure, excessive sedation, or alcohol abuse; swallowing disorders; dental caries; and debilitation secondary to cancer or chronic disease. Lung abscess also may occur as a complication of some types of pneumonia, including those due to *S. aureus*, *Klebsiella*, and *Legionella*.

Pathophysiology and Manifestations

A lung abscess forms after lung tissue becomes consolidated (i.e., after alveoli become filled with fluid, pus, and microorganisms). Consolidated tissue becomes necrotic. This necrotic process can spread to involve the entire bronchopulmonary segment and progress proximally until it ruptures into a bronchus. With rupture, the contents of the abscess empty into the bronchus, leaving a cavity filled with air and fluid, a process known as *cavitation*. If purulent material from the abscess is not expectorated, the infection may spread, leading to diffuse pneumonia or a syndrome similar to acute respiratory distress syndrome (discussed in Chapter 39 ∞).

Manifestations of lung abscess typically develop about 2 weeks after the precipitating event (aspiration, pneumonia, and so on). Their onset may be either acute or insidious. Early symptoms are those of pneumonia: productive cough, chills and fever, pleuritic chest pain, malaise, and anorexia. The temperature may be significantly elevated, 103°F (39.4°C) or higher. When the abscess ruptures, the client may expectorate large amounts of foul-smelling, purulent, and possibly blood-streaked sputum. Breath sounds are diminished, and crackles may be noted in the region of the abscess. A dull percussion tone is also present.

INTERDISCIPLINARY CARE

The diagnosis of lung abscess usually is based on the history and presentation. The CBC may indicate leukocytosis. Sputum culture may not show the organism involved unless rupture occurs. Chest x-ray shows a thick-walled, solitary cavity with surrounding consolidation, although differentiating lung abscess from consolidation can be difficult until cavitation occurs.

Lung abscess is treated with antibiotic therapy, usually intravenous clindamycin (Cleocin), amoxicillin-clavulanate (Augmentin), or penicillin (Tierney et al., 2005). Postural drainage may be ordered to relieve obstruction and promote drainage. In some cases, bronchoscopy is used to drain the abscess. If the pleural space becomes involved, a chest tube (*tube thoracostomy*) may be used to drain the abscess. See the section on pneumothorax later in this chapter for further discussion of chest tubes.

NURSING CARE

Although most clients with lung abscess recover fully with appropriate antibiotic treatment, rupture and drainage of the abscess into a bronchus is a frightening experience. Nursing care needs of the client relate primarily to maintaining a patent airway and adequate gas exchange. The following nursing diagnoses may be appropriate for the client with lung abscess:

- *Risk for Ineffective Airway Clearance* related to large amounts of purulent drainage in bronchi
- *Impaired Gas Exchange* related to necrotic and consolidated lung tissue
- *Hyperthermia* related to infectious process
- *Anxiety* related to copious amounts of purulent sputum.

Health education for the client and family focuses on the importance of completing the prescribed antibiotic therapy. Most lung abscesses are successfully treated with antibiotics; however, treatment may last up to 1 month or more. Emphasize the importance of completing the entire course of therapy to eliminate the infecting organisms. Teach about the medication, including its name, dose, and desired and adverse effects. Stress the need to contact the physician if symptoms do not improve or if they become worse. Infection from lung abscess can spread not only to lung and pleural tissue but systemically, causing sepsis. If postural drainage is ordered, teach the client and family how to perform this procedure. When procedures such as bronchoscopy or thoracostomy are performed to drain the abscess, provide preoperative teaching and instruction on postoperative care.

THE CLIENT WITH TUBERCULOSIS

Tuberculosis (TB) is a chronic, recurrent infectious disease that usually affects the lungs, although any organ can be affected. This disease, caused by *Mycobacterium tuberculosis*, is uncommon in the United States, especially among young adults of European descent.

M. tuberculosis is a relatively slow-growing, slender, rod-shaped, acid-fast organism with a waxy outer capsule, which increases its resistance to destruction. Although the lungs are usually infected, tuberculosis can involve other organs as well. It is transmitted by *droplet nuclei*, airborne droplets produced when an infected person coughs, sneezes, speaks, or sings. The tiny droplets can remain suspended in air for several hours. Infection may develop when a susceptible host breathes in air containing droplet nuclei and the contaminated particle eludes the normal defenses of the upper respiratory tract to reach the alveoli.

Incidence and Prevalence

The incidence of tuberculosis fell steadily until the mid-1980s, thanks to improved sanitation, surveillance, and treatment of people with active disease. The late 1980s and early 1990s saw a resurgence of the disease, attributed primarily to the HIV/AIDS epidemic, the emergence of multiple-drug-resistant (MDR) strains of TB, and social factors such as immigration, poverty, homelessness, and drug abuse. Today, the number of people affected by TB in the United States continues to decline, with a total of 14,093 cases reported in 2005, the lowest number recorded since national reporting began in 1953 (CDC, 2006b). This decline can be attributed to TB-control programs that emphasize promptly identifying new cases and initiating and completing appropriate therapy.

Worldwide, TB continues to be a significant health problem, with an estimated 2 billion people (one-third of the world's population) infected by *M. tuberculosis*. An estimated 9 million cases of TB develop annually, with the vast majority (95%) occurring in developing countries of Asia, Africa, the Middle East, and Latin America. TB accounts for an estimated 2 million deaths each year (CDC, 2006c).

Today, TB in the United States is a disease primarily affecting immigrants, those infected with HIV, and disadvantaged populations. See the Focus on Cultural Diversity box on the primary populations affected by TB. Poor urban areas are hit the hardest—areas that are also affected by the epidemics of injection drug use, homelessness, malnutrition, and poor living conditions. Overcrowded institutions also contribute to the spread of TB; transmission in hospitals, homeless shelters, drug treatment centers, prisons, and residential facilities has been documented. People with altered immune function, including older adults (see the box on page 1282) and people with AIDS are at particular risk for tuberculosis. Some strains of *M. tuberculosis* have become resistant to the primary drugs used to treat the disease (isoniazid and rifampin), with the number of MDR cases of TB increased by 13.3% between 2004 and 2005 (CDC, 2006a).

FAST FACTS

■ Worldwide, approximately 39% of identified *M. tuberculosis* strains are MDR, demonstrating resistance to at least isoniazid and rifampin.

■ Of MDR tuberculosis strains identified worldwide, 7% are extensively drug resistant (XDR). XDR tuberculosis is resistant to isoniazid and rifampin, as well as at least three of the six main classes of second-line tuberculosis drugs (CDC, 2006a).

■ The prevalence of MDR and XDR tuberculosis in the United States is lower, with 1.6% of cases reported from 1993 through 2004 identified as MDR. Of these, 4.1% were resistant to three or more classes of antituberculosis drugs, qualifying as XDR tuberculosis (CDC, 2006a).

Risk Factors

The risk for infection by *M. tuberculosis* is affected by characteristics of the infectious person, the extent of air contamination, duration of exposure, and susceptibility of the host. The number of microbes in the sputum, frequency and force of coughing, and behaviors such as covering the mouth when coughing affect the production of droplet nuclei. In a small, closed, or poorly ventilated space, droplet nuclei become more concentrated, increasing the risk of exposure. Prolonged con-

---

FOCUS ON CULTURAL DIVERSITY
Tuberculosis

■ The TB case rate for foreign-born U.S. residents is 8.7 times higher than that for people born in the United States (CDC, 2006b).

■ Asians and Pacific Islanders living in the United States have the highest case rates, nearly 20 times higher than that for whites.

■ Case rates for blacks and Hispanics in the United States are 7 to 8 times that for whites.

---

tact, such as living in the same household, increases the risk. Less-than-optimal immune function, a problem for people in lower socioeconomic groups, injection drug users, the homeless, alcoholics, and people with HIV infection, increases the susceptibility of the host.

Pathophysiology

Pulmonary Tuberculosis

Minute droplet nuclei containing one to three bacilli that elude upper airway defense systems to enter the lungs implant in an alveolus or respiratory bronchiole, usually in an upper lobe. As the bacteria multiply, they cause a local inflammatory response. The inflammatory response brings neutrophils and macrophages to the site. These phagocytic cells surround and engulf the bacilli, isolating them and preventing their spread. *M. tuberculosis* continues to slowly multiply; some enter the lymphatic system to stimulate a cellular-mediated immune response. (See Chapter 12 ∞ for a review of immune responses.) Neutrophils and macrophages isolate the bacteria but cannot destroy them. A granulomatous lesion called a *tubercle*, a sealed-off colony of bacilli, is formed. Within the tubercle, infected tissue dies, forming a cheeselike center, a process called *caseation necrosis*.

If the immune response is adequate, scar tissue develops around the tubercle, and the bacilli remain encapsulated. These lesions eventually calcify and are visible on x-ray. The client, while infected by *M. tuberculosis*, does not develop tuberculosis disease. If the immune response is inadequate to contain the bacilli, the disease of tuberculosis can develop. Occasionally, the infection can progress, leading to extensive destruction of lung tissue. In *primary tuberculosis*, granulomatous tissue may erode into a bronchus or into a blood vessel, allowing the disease to spread throughout the lung or other organs. This severe form of tuberculosis is uncommon in adults (Kasper et al., 2005).

A previously healed tuberculosis lesion may be reactivated. *Reactivation tuberculosis* occurs when the immune system is suppressed due to age, disease, or use of immunosuppressive drugs. The extent of lung disease can vary from small lesions to extensive cavitation of lung tissue. Tubercles rupture, spreading bacilli into the airways to form satellite lesions and produce tuberculosis pneumonia. Without treatment, massive lung involvement can lead to death, or a more chronic process of tubercle formation and cavitation may

NURSING CARE OF THE OLDER ADULT — Tuberculosis

The prevalence of active tuberculosis is significantly higher among older Caucasian adults in the United States than it is in young adults (Kasper et al., 2005). Of cases among older adults, approximately 90% occur due to reactivation of a dormant bacterium. Older adults are at increased risk for reactivation tuberculosis due to age-related decreases in cell-mediated immunity. Chronic illnesses, poor nutrition, gastrectomy, alcoholism, or the long-term use of steroids and immunosuppressive agents may also reactivate dormant TB lesions.

Presenting symptoms of tuberculosis in the older adult are often vague, including coughing, weight loss, anorexia, or periodic fevers. These signs and symptoms should not be dismissed as a normal part of aging.

Residents of nursing homes are at increased risk for acquiring tuberculosis because of group living. Yearly tuberculin skin testing with purified protein derivative (PPD) is often required by state health departments. If the initial test is negative, a repeat PPD in 1 to 2 weeks is recommended. This improves sensitivity to the test so that silent cases of tuberculosis are not missed. A chest x-ray and sputum culture for acid-fast bacilli are obtained if the PPD is positive.

Successful treatment for tuberculosis includes taking at least two drugs for at least 6 to 9 months to totally eradicate the organism. Older adults usually do not develop drug-resistant forms of tuberculosis, because they acquired the disease prior to emergence of drug-resistant strains.

Assessing for Home Care

Community-dwelling older adults are susceptible to tuberculosis as well as those in care facilities. The older adult with respiratory symptoms often is treated presumptively for pneumonia, without a sputum smear and Gram stain. Older adults living in the community may not have had a tuberculin test or chest x-ray for many years.

Assess risk factors for tuberculosis:

- General health and nutritional status, including intake of specific nutrients such as vitamin D (lack of vitamin D is associated with a higher risk of developing active tuberculosis)
- Presence of a chronic disease such as silicosis, diabetes, alcoholism, or HIV infection; past history of a gastrectomy
- Past history of a positive tuberculin test that now has converted to negative
- Medications such as corticosteroids or other immunosuppressive drugs.
  Assess living and social situation:
- Natural light and ventilation in the home
- Access to clean water, cooking facilities, grocery stores, and other services
- Possible exposure to infected people, for example, sharing a household with someone with active TB, crowded living facilities, homelessness, frequent participation in senior activities,

volunteer work in residential care facilities or other institutional settings
- Access to health care

Tuberculosis is typically treated in the community; hospitalization or institutionalization rarely is necessary or desirable. For the older adult being treated for active TB in the community, assess:

- Knowledge and understanding of the disease and the prescribed treatment regimen
- Mental status and ability to follow prescribed regimen and precautions to avoid exposing others to the disease
- Transportation and ability to access healthcare services on a regular basis
- Financial resources to complete treatment and follow-up care
- Need for home health or social services to ensure adequate treatment.

Health Education for the Client and Family

Teaching focuses on improving the older adult's ability to self-manage the disease and treatment. Teach about tuberculosis and how it is spread. Emphasize the importance of taking all medications as prescribed and complying with follow-up appointments and testing. Discuss the importance of:

- Using disposable tissues to contain respiratory secretions, especially during the first 2 weeks of treatment when the disease may be transmitted to others
- Avoiding exposure to crowds or people with infectious diseases
- Eating a well-balanced diet with adequate nutrients
- Getting adequate rest, sleep, and exercise to maintain good general health
- Ensuring that housemates or others having frequent contact with the client are tested and receive prophylactic treatment if indicated.

Teach about possible side effects of the prescribed medications and the importance of reporting these to healthcare providers:

- Peripheral neuropathy (numbness, tingling, or a burning sensation of the extremities) may occur with isoniazid (INH). Pyridoxine (vitamin B_6) often is prescribed to prevent this adverse effect.
- Both INH and rifampin may cause hepatitis. Avoid alcohol while taking these drugs, and report any manifestations such as nausea and anorexia, jaundice, a change in urine or stool color, or pain in the upper right quadrant.
- Rifampin may cause an orange-red coloration of saliva and urine.
- Streptomycin can affect hearing and balance; promptly report any changes, because they may be irreversible.
- Ethambutol may affect red-green color discrimination and visual acuity. Use caution when driving or walking in unfamiliar areas and promptly report any vision changes.

---

result. People with chronic disease continue to spread *M. tuberculosis* into the environment, potentially infecting others. *Pathophysiology Illustrated: Tuberculosis* on pages 1284–1285 illustrates the pathogenesis of tuberculosis.

Clients with HIV disease are at high risk for developing active tuberculosis, due to primary infection or reactivation. HIV infection suppresses cellular immunity, which is vital to limiting the replication and spread of *M. tuberculosis*.

MANIFESTATIONS AND COMPLICATIONS The initial infection causes few symptoms and typically goes unnoticed until the tuberculin test becomes positive or calcified lesions are seen on chest x-ray. Manifestations of primary progressive or reactivation tuberculosis often develop insidiously and are initially nonspecific (see the box below). Fatigue, weight loss, anorexia, low-grade afternoon fever, and night sweats are common. A dry cough develops, which later becomes productive of purulent and/or blood-tinged sputum. It is often at this stage that the client seeks medical attention.

Tuberculosis empyema and bronchopleural fistula are the most serious complications of pulmonary tuberculosis. When a tuberculosis lesion ruptures, bacilli may contaminate the pleural space. Rupture also may allow air to enter the pleural space from the lung, causing pneumothorax.

Extrapulmonary Tuberculosis

When primary disease or reactivation allows live bacilli to enter the bronchi, the disease may spread through the blood and lymph system to other organs. These distant disease metastases may produce an active lesion, or they may become dormant and reactivate at a later time. Extrapulmonary tuberculosis is especially prevalent in people with HIV disease.

MILIARY TUBERCULOSIS Miliary tuberculosis results from hematogenous spread (through the blood) of the bacilli throughout the body. Miliary tuberculosis causes chills and fever, weakness, malaise, and progressive dyspnea. Multiple lesions evenly distributed throughout the lungs are noted on x-ray. The sputum rarely contains organisms. The bone marrow is usually involved, causing anemia, thrombocytopenia, and leukocytosis. Without appropriate treatment, the prognosis is poor.

GENITOURINARY TUBERCULOSIS The kidney and genitourinary tract are common extrapulmonary sites for tuberculosis. The organism spreads to the kidney through the blood, initiating an inflammatory process similar to that which occurs in the lungs. Reactivation can occur years after the original infection.

As the lesion then enlarges and caseates, a large portion of the renal parenchyma is destroyed. The infection then can spread to the rest of the urinary tract, including the ureters and bladder. Scarring and strictures commonly result. In men, the prostate, seminal vesicles, and epididymis may be involved. In women, tuberculosis may affect the fallopian tubes and ovaries.

Manifestations of genitourinary tuberculosis develop insidiously. Symptoms of a urinary tract infection, including malaise, dysuria, hematuria, and pyuria, develop. Flank pain may be present. Men may develop manifestations of epididymitis or prostatitis: perineal, sacral, or scrotal pain and tenderness; difficulty voiding; and fever. Women may have manifestations of pelvic inflammatory disease, impaired fertility, or ectopic pregnancy.

TUBERCULOSIS MENINGITIS Tuberculosis meningitis results when tuberculosis spreads to the subarachnoid space. In the United States, this complication most often affects older adults, usually from reactivation of latent disease. Manifestations develop gradually, with listlessness, irritability, anorexia, and fever. Headache and behavior changes are common early symptoms in the older adult. As the disease progresses, the headache increases in intensity, vomiting develops, and the level of consciousness decreases. Convulsions and coma may follow. Without appropriate treatment, neurologic effects may become permanent.

SKELETAL TUBERCULOSIS Tuberculosis of the bones and joints is most likely to occur during childhood, when bone epiphyses are open and their blood supply is rich. The organisms spread via the blood to vertebrae, the ends of long bones, and joints. Immune and inflammatory processes isolate the bacilli, and the disease often becomes evident years or decades later.

Tuberculous spondylitis usually involves the thoracic vertebrae, eroding vertebral bodies and causing them to collapse. Significant kyphosis develops, and the spinal cord may be compressed. The large, weight-bearing joints (hips and knees) are most often affected by tuberculous arthritis, although other joints may be affected, particularly if they have been previously damaged. The involved joint is painful, warm, and tender.

INTERDISCIPLINARY CARE

Tuberculosis was a major public health concern earlier in this century, before the development of effective sanitation measures and drug treatment. Developing drug-resistant strains, susceptibility of people with HIV disease, and inadequate access to health care for high-risk populations contribute to the continuing significance of tuberculosis as a significant public health threat. Interdisciplinary care, therefore, focuses on the following:

- Early detection
- Accurate diagnosis
- Effective disease treatment
- Preventing tuberculosis spread to others.

Hospitalization is rarely required to treat tuberculosis. With appropriate treatment, clients become noninfective to others fairly rapidly. However, a client with active tuberculosis may be admitted for a concurrent problem or a complication of the disease. Nurses and other healthcare workers are at risk for exposure if the disease has not yet been diagnosed. When a client

---

MANIFESTATIONS of Pulmonary Tuberculosis

- Fatigue
- Weight loss
- Anorexia
- Low-grade afternoon fever and night sweats
- Cough: initially dry, later productive of purulent and/or blood-tinged sputum

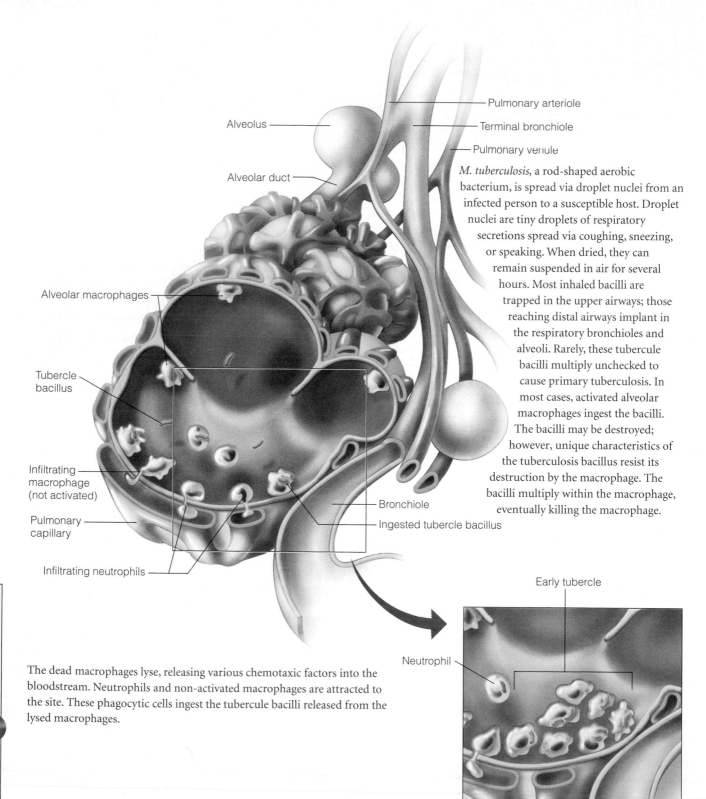

Pulmonary arteriole

Alveolus

Terminal bronchiole

Pulmonary venule

Alveolar duct

M. tuberculosis, a rod-shaped aerobic bacterium, is spread via droplet nuclei from an infected person to a susceptible host. Droplet nuclei are tiny droplets of respiratory secretions spread via coughing, sneezing, or speaking. When dried, they can remain suspended in air for several hours. Most inhaled bacilli are trapped in the upper airways; those reaching distal airways implant in the respiratory bronchioles and alveoli. Rarely, these tubercle bacilli multiply unchecked to cause primary tuberculosis. In most cases, activated alveolar macrophages ingest the bacilli. The bacilli may be destroyed; however, unique characteristics of the tuberculosis bacillus resist its destruction by the macrophage. The bacilli multiply within the macrophage, eventually killing the macrophage.

Alveolar macrophages

Tubercle bacillus

Infiltrating macrophage (not activated)

Pulmonary capillary

Bronchiole

Ingested tubercle bacillus

Infiltrating neutrophils

Early tubercle

Neutrophil

The dead macrophages lyse, releasing various chemotaxic factors into the bloodstream. Neutrophils and non-activated macrophages are attracted to the site. These phagocytic cells ingest the tubercule bacilli released from the lysed macrophages.

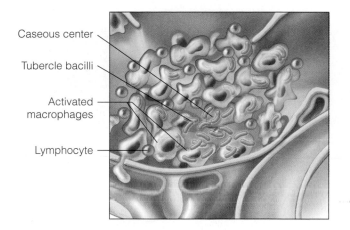

Caseous center

Tubercle bacilli

Activated
macrophages

Lymphocyte

After several weeks, a delayed hypersensitivity response to bacterial antigens destroys many of the macrophages. Concurrently, a cell-mediated immune response activates additional macrophages, which ingest and destroy the bacilli. The lysed macrophages and bacilli are surrounded by a mass of live, activated macrophages and lymphocytes. Scar (granulomatous) tissue forms, encapsulating the primary lesion. Most lesions calcify and are visible on x-ray. These lesions may remain dormant for a year or more (in some cases, many years) before being reactivated to produce secondary or reactivation tuberculosis.

When the immune and macrophage-activating responses are weakened by age or disease (e.g., HIV disease), the tuberculosis bacilli continue to multiply within the lesion. The caseous material at the center of the lesion liquefies, and the lesion grows.

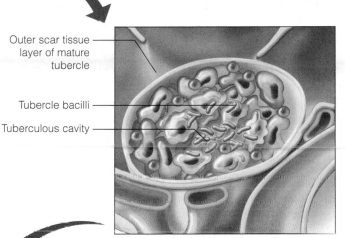

Outer scar tissue
layer of mature
tubercle

Tubercle bacilli

Tuberculous cavity

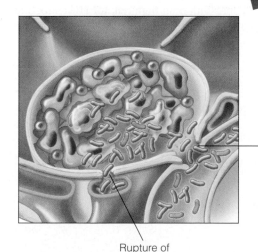

Rupture of
bronchiole wall

Rupture of
capillary wall

The enlarging lesion damages surrounding bronchial walls and blood vessels. Granulomatous tissue surrounding the lesion can erode into a bronchus, forming an air-filling cavity. Within this cavity, the bacilli multiply, spreading into the airways and the environment via infected sputum. Bacilli multiply, spreading into the airways and the environment via infected sputum. Bacilli also spread via the blood and within macrophages to regional lymph nodes, and from there to many organs and tissues. Resulting extrapulmonary lesions evolve in the same sequence as pulmonary lesions.

with tuberculosis is institutionalized, maintain respiratory isolation to minimize the risk of infection to other clients and to the healthcare workers.

Noncompliance with prescribed treatment is a major problem in treating active tuberculosis: The client can continue transmitting the disease to others, and drug-resistant strains of bacteria can develop when treatment is incomplete. Tuberculosis must be reported to local and state public health departments; contacts are identified and examined. People who share living or work environments with the client are tested and receive prophylactic treatment. Continuing contact with clients who have active TB is vital to ensure effective cure.

Screening

The tuberculin test is used to screen for tuberculosis infection. A cellular, or delayed hypersensitivity, response to *M. tuberculosis* develops within 3 to 10 weeks after the infection. Injecting a small amount of *purified protein derivative (PPD)* of tuberculin any time thereafter activates this response, attracting macrophages to the area and causing a pronounced local inflammatory response. The amount of induration surrounding the injection site is used to determine infection (see Table 38–5 and Figure 38–7 ■). It is important to remember that a positive response indicates that infection and a cellular (T-cell) response have developed; however, it does not mean that active disease is present or that the client is infectious to others.

Several methods are currently available for tuberculin testing:

■ *Intradermal PPD (Mantoux) test:* 0.1 mL of PPD (5 tuberculin units, or TU) is injected intradermally into the dorsal aspect of the forearm. This test is read within 48 to 72 hours (the peak reaction period) and recorded as the diameter of induration (raised area, not erythema) in millimeters.
■ *Multiple-puncture (tine) test:* A multiple-puncture device is used to introduce tuberculin into the skin. This test is less accurate than other testing methods. A vesicular reaction is considered positive; any other reaction must be confirmed using a Mantoux test.

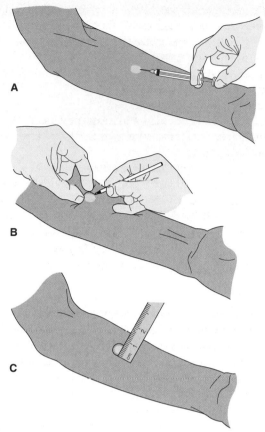

Figure 38–7 ■ *A,* Intradermal injection for tuberculin testing. *B,* The injection causes a local inflammatory response (wheal). *C,* Measurement of induration following tuberculin testing.

Although it is impractical and unnecessary to screen the entire population, the CDC recommend screening people in the following risk groups:

■ People with or at high risk for HIV infection
■ Close contacts of people who have or are suspected of having infectious TB

TABLE 38–5 Interpreting Tuberculin Test Results

AREA OF INDURATION	SIGNIFICANCE
Less than 5 mm	Negative response; does not rule out infection.
5 to 9 mm	Positive for people who: ■ Are in close contact with a client with infective TB. ■ Have an abnormal chest x-ray. ■ Have HIV infection or are immunocompromised. ■ Have an organ transplant. Negative for all others.
10 to 15 mm	Positive for people who have other risk factors: ■ Birth in a high-incidence country. ■ African American, Hispanic, Asian American in poverty areas. ■ Injection drug use. ■ Residence in a long-term care facility, correctional institution, residential care setting, homeless shelter. ■ Medical risk factors (e.g., malnutrition, diabetes, others).
Greater than 15 mm	Positive for all people.

- People with medical risk factors, such as silicosis, chronic malabsorption, end-stage renal failure, diabetes mellitus, immunosuppression, and hematologic and other malignancies
- People born in countries with a high prevalence of TB
- Medically underserved low-income populations, including racial and ethnic minorities
- Alcoholics and injection drug users
- Residents and staff of long-term residential facilities, such as long-term care facilities, correctional institutions, and mental health facilities.

False-negative responses are common in people who are immunosuppressed. A two-step procedure may be necessary to elicit a positive response. If the first test elicits a negative response, a second PPD test is given 1 week later. If the second test also is negative, the client either is free of infection or is *anergic* (unable to react to common antigens). This two-step procedure is recommended for long-term care residents and workers.

Diagnosis

A positive tuberculin test alone does not indicate active disease. Sputum tests for the bacillus and chest x-rays are routinely used to diagnose and evaluate active disease. A series of three consecutive early morning sputum specimens is typically examined for bacilli (see Procedure 36–1). Use special procedures or personal protective devices when obtaining sputum specimens. If possible, collect specimens in a room equipped with airflow control devices, ultraviolet light, or both. Alternatively, have the client step outside to collect the specimen. Wear a mask capable of filtering droplet nuclei when collecting sputum specimens. Aerosol therapy, percussion, and postural drainage may help the client produce sputum. Occasionally, endotracheal suctioning, bronchoscopy, or gastric lavage may be necessary to obtain a specimen. See the Diagnostic Tests box in Chapter 36 ∞ for nursing care related to bronchoscopy.

- *Sputum smear* is microscopically examined for *acid-fast bacilli*. *M. tuberculosis* resists decolorizing chemicals after staining. This property is called *acid fast*. The acid-fast smear provides a rapid indicator of the tubercle bacillus.
- *Sputum culture* positive for *M. tuberculosis* provides the definitive diagnosis. However, *M. tuberculosis* is slow growing, requiring 4 to 8 weeks before it can be detected using traditional culture techniques. Automated radiometric culture systems (such as Bactec) allow detection of *M. tuberculosis* in several days.
- Once the organism is detected, *sensitivity testing* is performed to identify appropriate drug therapy.
- *Polymerase chain reaction (PCR)* permits rapid detection of DNA from *M. tuberculosis*.
- *Chest x-ray* is ordered to diagnose and evaluate TB. Typical findings in pulmonary TB include dense lesions in the apical and posterior segments of the upper lobe and possible cavity formation.

Prior to initiating antituberculosis drug therapy, several additional diagnostic tests may be done to establish baseline data for monitoring potential adverse effects of the drugs.

- *Liver function tests* are obtained prior to treatment with isoniazid (INH) because this drug is hepatotoxic.

- A thorough *vision examination* is done prior to treatment with ethambutol, a commonly used antituberculosis medication. Optic neuritis is a potential adverse effect of this drug. Periodic eye examinations are scheduled during the course of therapy.
- *Audiometric testing* is performed before streptomycin therapy is initiated. Ototoxicity is a significant adverse effect of streptomycin and other aminoglycoside antibiotics. Hearing also is evaluated periodically during the course of therapy to detect any hearing loss.

Medications

Chemotherapeutic medications are used both to prevent and treat tuberculosis infection. Goals of the pharmacologic treatment of TB are to:

- Make the disease noncommunicable to others.
- Reduce symptoms of the disease.
- Effect a cure in the shortest possible time.

Prophylactic treatment is used to prevent active tuberculosis. Clients with a recent skin test conversion from negative to positive are often started on prophylactic therapy, especially when other risk factors are present. Prophylactic therapy also is used for people in close household contact with a person whose sputum is positive for bacilli. Single-drug therapy is effective for prophylactic treatment, whereas treatment of active disease always involves two or more chemotherapeutic medications. For adults, INH, 300 mg per day for a period of 6 to 12 months, is commonly used to prevent active TB.

When INH prophylaxis is contraindicated, bacilli Calmette-Guérin (BCG) vaccine may be prescribed. This vaccine is widely used in developing countries. BCG is made from an attenuated strain of *M. bovis*, a closely related bacillus that causes tuberculosis in cattle. In the United States, BCG vaccine is recommended only for infants, children, and healthcare workers with a negative tuberculin test who are repeatedly exposed to untreated or ineffectively treated people with active disease. After vaccination with BCG, a positive reaction to tuberculin testing is common. Periodic chest x-rays may be required for screening purposes.

The tuberculosis bacillus mutates readily to drug-resistant forms when only one anti-infective agent is used. Active disease is always treated with concurrent use of at least two antibacterial medications to which the organism is sensitive. The primary antituberculosis drugs can prevent development of resistance because all act by different mechanisms. However, the organism is protected within the tubercle, and 6 or more months of treatment is necessary to eradicate it.

Newly diagnosed tuberculosis is typically treated with an initial regimen of four oral antitubercular drugs, isoniazid, rifampin, and pyrazinamide, and ethambutol daily (or several times per week on a decreasing schedule of frequency) for the first 2 months of treatment. This initial regimen is followed by at least 4 additional months of therapy with isoniazid and rifampin, given daily, twice per week, or weekly. In the presence of HIV infection, treatment is continued for at least 9 months. The most common antituberculosis drugs are outlined in Table 38–6; their nursing implications are outlined in the Medication Administration box on pages 1288–1289.

TABLE 38–6 Antituberculosis Medications

DRUG AND DOSAGE	ADVERSE EFFECTS	NURSING IMPLICATIONS
Isoniazid (INH), oral: 300 mg daily or 900 mg one, two, or three times weekly	Peripheral neuropathy Hepatitis	Administer pyridoxine (vitamin B$_6$) concurrently. Monitor liver function studies (AST and ALT); avoid other hepatotoxins.
Rifampin (RMP), oral: 600 mg daily or two or three times weekly	Hepatitis Flulike syndrome; fever	As for INH. Do not miss or skip doses; flulike syndrome and fever occur when drug is resumed.
	Colors body fluids—including sweat, urine, saliva, tears, and cerebrospinal fluid (CSF)—orange-red	Contact lenses may become discolored and should not be worn.
Pyrazinamide (PZA), oral: 1 to 2 g daily; or 2 to 4 g twice weekly	Hyperuricemia Hepatotoxicity	Monitor uric acid levels. Monitor AST and ALT; avoid other hepatotoxins.
Ethambutol (EMB), oral: 800 mg to 1600 mg daily; or 2 to 4 g twice weekly	Optic neuritis	Monitor red-green color discrimination and visual acuity.
Streptomycin (SM), intramuscular: 15 mg/kg, up to 1 g daily; or 25 to 30 mg/kg twice weekly	Ototoxicity, vertigo Nephrotoxicity	Have periodic audiometric examinations conducted. Monitor renal function studies, including BUN and serum creatinine.

If a drug-resistant strain is suspected, therapy is tailored to the resistance. In some cases, four or more anti-infective drugs may be used.

Antitubercular medications have many adverse and toxic effects. Close monitoring during therapy is necessary. Most have some degree of, or risk for, hepatotoxicity. For this reason, clients should avoid using alcohol and other drugs (such as acetaminophen) or chemicals that can damage the liver. Baseline liver and renal function studies are done prior to initiating therapy. Audiometric testing also may be done before treatment is started, because several commonly used medications can affect hearing. Regular visits to a healthcare provider are necessary to evaluate regularly for adverse effects. Although none of these drugs have been proved to be teratogenic, potential adverse effects on the fetus are weighed against the benefit to the mother before they are prescribed during pregnancy.

Compliance with the prescribed regimen also is evaluated during follow-up visits. The urine can be examined for color changes characteristic of rifampin and tested for metabolites of INH. When compliance is a problem, medications are administered under direct supervision. Twice-weekly therapy is more cost effective in this instance, with a public health nurse watching the client take and swallow the prescribed medication.

MEDICATION ADMINISTRATION Antituberculosis Drugs

ISONIAZID (INH, LANIAZID, NYDRAZID)
Isoniazid is the drug of choice for tuberculosis prophylaxis and a first-line drug for treating active disease. It is effective against both intracellular and extracellular organisms. Isoniazid is used alone as a prophylactic medication and in combination with rifampin, ethambutol, or both. A fixed-dose combination form with 150 mg of INH and 300 mg of rifampin (Rifamate) is available as well.

Nursing Responsibilities
- Administer on an empty stomach 1 hour before or 2 hours after meals for maximal effect if tolerated; may be given with meals to reduce gastrointestinal effects.
- Monitor for adverse effects:
  a. Numbness and tingling of the extremities (most likely to occur in malnourished, alcoholic, or diabetic clients)
  b. Hepatotoxicity, as evidenced by abnormal liver function studies and scleral jaundice
  c. Hypersensitivity reactions, such as rash, drug fever, or evidence of anemia, bruising, bleeding, or infection related to agranulocytosis.

- Isoniazid interferes with the metabolism of diazepam (Valium), phenytoin (Dilantin), and carbamazepine. Doses of these drugs may need to be reduced to prevent toxicity.

Health Education for the Client and Family
- Take the medication as prescribed for the entire treatment period to prevent incomplete eradication of the bacteria and development of resistant strains.
- Take the medication on an empty stomach. If nausea and vomiting occur, take with meals.
- If anorexia, nausea, vomiting, and jaundice (yellowing of the skin and the whites of the eyes) develop, notify your doctor immediately.
- Take pyridoxine as prescribed to prevent peripheral neuropathy.
- Avoid alcohol and other agents that may be harmful to the liver.
- Notify your doctor if you develop signs of an allergic reaction, such as rash, fever, easy bruising, bleeding gums, or fatigue.

MEDICATION ADMINISTRATION Antituberculosis Drugs (continued)

- Use measures to prevent pregnancy while taking INH; this drug may be harmful to the developing fetus.

RIFAMPIN (RIFADIN, RIMACTANE)

Rifampin is commonly used in combination with INH and other antitubercular drugs. It is relatively low in toxicity, although it can cause hepatitis, a flulike immune response, and, rarely, renal failure. Rifampin stimulates the microsomal enzymes of the liver, increasing the rate of metabolism of many drugs and decreasing their effectiveness.

Nursing Responsibilities

- Administer on an empty stomach.
- Monitor CBC, liver function studies, and renal function studies for evidence of toxicity.
- Rifampin reduces the effect of oral contraceptives, quinidine, corticosteroids, warfarin, methadone, digoxin, and hypoglycemics. Monitor for the effectiveness of these drugs.

Health Education for the Client and Family

- Rifampin causes body fluids, including sweat, urine, saliva, and tears, to turn red-orange. This is not harmful. Avoid wearing soft contact lenses because they may be permanently stained.
- Aspirin may interfere with rifampin absorption and should not be taken concurrently.
- Fever, flulike symptoms, excessive fatigue, sore throat, or unusual bleeding may indicate an adverse reaction to the drug and should be reported to your doctor.

PYRAZINAMIDE (TEBRAZID)

Pyrazinamide typically is given with INH and rifampin for the first 2 months of tuberculosis treatment. Concurrent use of pyrazinamide allows a shorter course of therapy. As with many of the antitubercular agents, pyrazinamide is toxic to the liver. Its other principal adverse effect is hyperuricemia. Gout, however, rarely develops.

Nursing Responsibilities

- Administer with meals to reduce gastrointestinal side effects.
- Monitor liver function studies and serum uric acid levels. Notify the physician if changes are noted.

Health Education for the Client and Family

- Notify your doctor if you develop loss of appetite, nausea, vomiting, jaundice, or symptoms of gout (a painful, red, hot, swollen joint, often the great toe or elbow).
- While taking this drug, avoid using alcohol or other substances that may be harmful to the liver.

ETHAMBUTOL (MYAMBUTOL)

Ethambutol is added to the initial treatment regimen or substituted for INH when an INH-resistant strain of TB is suspected. Ethambutol is a bacteriostatic drug that reduces the development of resistance to the bactericidal first-line agents. Its principal toxic effect is optic neuritis; fortunately, this is reversible. Early signs of optic neuritis include decreased visual acuity and loss of red-green discrimination. This drug may be safe for use in pregnancy.

Nursing Responsibilities

- Record a baseline visual examination prior to therapy. Schedule periodic eye exams during the course of treatment.
- Administer with meals to reduce gastrointestinal side effects.
- Monitor liver and renal function studies and neurologic status while taking this drug. Notify the physician of abnormal findings or significant changes.

Health Education for the Client and Family

- Monitor vision daily by reading newspapers and looking at the same blue object (using usual corrective lenses, if appropriate). Notify your doctor if changes in vision or color perception occur.

STREPTOMYCIN

An aminoglycoside antibiotic, streptomycin is highly effective in treating most mycobacterial infection. Resistance may develop if it is used alone. There are two primary drawbacks to streptomycin: (1) It must be administered parenterally because it is not absorbed in the gastrointestinal tract, and (2) it has toxic effects on the kidneys and ears.

Nursing Responsibilities

- Administer by deep intramuscular injection into a large muscle mass, rotating sites to minimize tissue trauma.
- Monitor urine output, weight, and renal function studies (including BUN and serum creatinine) to detect early signs of nephrotoxicity. Report significant changes to the physician.
- Maintain fluid intake at 2000 to 3000 mL per day to minimize the concentration of drug in the kidney tubules.
- Assess hearing and balance frequently. Have audiometric testing performed as indicated.

Health Education for the Client and Family

- Maintain a daily fluid intake of at least 2.5 to 3 quarts.
- Weigh yourself on the same scale at least twice a week; report any significant weight gain to your doctor.
- Notify your doctor if hearing acuity decreases, ringing or buzzing sensations in the ear develop, or dizziness occurs.

Repeat sputum specimens and chest x-rays are used to evaluate the effectiveness of therapy. In most cases, sputum cultures for *M. tuberculosis* are negative within 2 months of therapy; virtually all clients have negative sputum cultures within 3 months. If cultures remain positive at 3 months and beyond, treatment failure and drug resistance are suspected. In this case, cultures of the organism are tested for susceptibility to antitubercular agents, and two or three previously unused drugs are added to the treatment regimen (Kasper et al., 2005).

With adherence to prescribed treatment, virtually all clients should have negative sputum cultures for *M. tuberculosis*

within 3 months. The relapse rate for current treatment regimens is less than 5%. The principal cause of treatment failure is noncompliance (Tierney et al., 2005).

NURSING CARE

Health Promotion

Tuberculosis today presents a greater threat to public health than it does to individuals. Nurses play a key role in maintaining public health. Education and tuberculosis screening are major nursing strategies to prevent TB. See the accompanying Nursing Research box regarding tuberculosis screening for a homeless population.

Public health teaching includes increasing awareness of tuberculosis as a reemerging threat. Teach clients in all settings how to reduce the spread of TB by covering their mouths when coughing or sneezing and disposing of sputum appropriately. The benefit of screening programs to identify infected (though not necessarily infective) people also needs to be included in public health education.

The best tuberculosis prevention is early diagnosis of infections and appropriate treatment to achieve cure. BCG vaccine is recommended for infants born in countries where tuberculosis is prevalent, but is not widely used in the United States. It may be administered to healthcare workers in settings where the risk of infection with MDR strains of *M. tuberculosis* is high despite rigorous infection control measures (Kasper et al., 2005).

The primary preventive strategy used in the United States is treating people with latent tuberculosis infection demonstrated by a positive tuberculin test. A 9- to 10-month course of treatment with isoniazid reduces the risk of active TB by 90% or more (Kasper et al., 2005). Isoniazid also is prescribed prophylactically for people with HIV infection who have been exposed to TB.

ASSESSMENT

Focused assessment for the client with suspected TB includes the following:

- *Health history:* Complaints of fatigue, weight loss, night sweats, difficulty breathing, cough (productive or nonproductive), bloody sputum, or chest pain; known exposure to TB; most recent tuberculin test and results; living circumstances; alcohol and other recreational drug use.
- *Physical examination:* Vital signs including temperature; general appearance; respiratory rate and lung sounds.
- *Diagnostic tests:* Tuberculin test results, presence of acid-fast bacilli in sputum, chest x-ray.

Nursing Diagnoses and Interventions

Nursing care related to tuberculosis focuses primarily on infection control and compliance with prescribed treatment. See the accompanying Nursing Care Plan on the next page.

Deficient Knowledge

Adequate knowledge and information are necessary to manage the disease and prevent its transmission to others. The client needs to understand reasons for prolonged drug therapy and the importance of complying with treatment and follow-up. Antituberculosis drugs are relatively toxic. The client needs to know how to minimize toxicity.

- Assess knowledge about the disease process; identify misperceptions and emotional reactions. *Teaching based on previous learning enhances understanding and retention of information.*
- Assess ability and interest in learning, developmental level, and obstacles to learning. *Assessment allows presentation of information in a manner tailored to the learning needs and style of the client, promoting learning.*

NURSING RESEARCH   Evidence-Based Practice: Clients with Risk for Tuberculosis

Homeless people and those living in homeless shelters have several identified risk factors for TB: high incidence of drug and alcohol abuse, lowered immune status, and crowded living conditions. Access to and participation in TB screening, however, often is problematic. Swigart and Kolb (2004) identified factors contributing to homeless persons' decisions to participate in free TB screening. Contrary to the beliefs of many healthcare providers, many homeless people chose to participate in the screening out of a desire to maintain good health and a recognition that homelessness and shelter life increased their risk of developing TB. The desire to maintain good health was particularly noted as a reason among those participants in early recovery from drug or alcohol addiction. Other major factors cited for participating included a history of lung problems, a desire to identify possible problems related to smoking, and encouragement by shelter personnel. Fear of the results and a desire "not to be bothered" had negative effects on participation. Women with children were least likely to participate in screening in this study, citing fear of being identified as ill that could result in loss of child custody.

IMPLICATIONS FOR NURSING

Outreach to homeless populations for health services, while difficult, has personal and public health benefits. The homeless often lack access to preventive and health promotion services, instead interacting with healthcare providers only intermittently when urgent care is needed. This study suggests, however, that a portion of this population desires to maintain good health and is receptive when screening and health promotion services are accessible. Shelter personnel were instrumental in getting many of the study participants to the screening. Recruiting the support of these workers can improve resident participation. Regularly scheduling a nurse in a shelter can allow trust to develop and can also improve participation in health promotion activities. This may be a particularly important strategy in shelters for women with children—bringing services to the residents to reduce the fear of being perceived as unable to care for dependent children.

CRITICAL THINKING IN CLIENT CARE

1. What factors contribute to the perception of many healthcare providers that homeless people and shelter residents do not care about maintaining good health?
2. The participants in this study were screened for their ability to understand English and to read or hear and comprehend the interview and process. How might the healthcare team need to alter its approach to reach homeless people who have mental illnesses that affect thinking and cognition?
3. Design a TB screening program using a multidisciplinary team to reach a specific population. Identify members of the team and discuss your rationale for their inclusion on the team.

NURSING CARE PLAN   A Client with Tuberculosis

Harry Facée, age 53, arrives at a metropolitan public health clinic complaining of aching chest pain that has lasted for the past few days. He says that his sputum also is bloody. He is afraid he might have lung cancer, so he came in to see a doctor.

ASSESSMENT

Raj Kamil, RN, the public health nurse at the clinic, obtains an admission history and physical examination of Mr. Facée. Mr. Kamil notes that Mr. Facée is a homeless person who has lived on the streets and in various shelters for the past "10 years or so." He usually prefers to sleep outdoors, taking refuge in shelters only during very cold or very wet weather. He has a small disability income, but usually scrounges for food or eats with other homeless people at soup kitchens. Mr. Facée states that he has had a cough for a long time, which has become worse recently. It is now productive, especially in the mornings. He also admits that he has recently been waking up drenched with sweat in the middle of the night and is more tired than usual.

Although Mr. Facée's clothes are tattered, he is fairly clean. He answers questions appropriately and intelligently. Mr. Kamil does not detect any odor of alcohol on his breath. He is very thin, almost emaciated. Mr. Facée's vital signs are BP 152/86, P 92, R 20, and T 100.2°F (37.8°C).

Suspecting tuberculosis, Mr. Kamil obtains a sputum specimen for Gram stain and culture, administers a tuberculin test, and sends Mr. Facée for a chest x-ray before he sees the clinic physician. Although the chest x-ray is inconclusive, the Gram stain is positive for acid-fast bacilli. The diagnosis of probable active pulmonary tuberculosis is made. The physician prescribes isoniazid, 300 mg orally; rifampin, 600 mg orally; and pyrazinamide, 1500 mg orally daily for 2 months, to be followed by twice weekly isoniazid 900 mg orally and rifampin 600 mg orally. The physician also orders weekly sputum cultures for the first month.

DIAGNOSES

- *Ineffective Health Maintenance* related to homelessness
- *Risk for Noncompliance with Prescribed Treatment* related to lack of understanding and resources
- *Imbalanced Nutrition: Less than Body Requirements* related to increased metabolic needs associated with infection
- *Risk for Disturbed Sensory Perception: Kinesthetic* related to effects of isoniazid therapy

EXPECTED OUTCOMES

- Keep all follow-up appointments as scheduled.
- Verbalize an understanding of his disease and its treatment.
- Follow the prescribed plan of care.
- Demonstrate measures to prevent spread of the organism to others.
- Gain 1 to 2 lb of weight per week.
- Promptly report symptoms of peripheral neuropathy, including numbness, tingling, or burning sensations.

PLANNING AND IMPLEMENTATION

- Teach about tuberculosis, and provide a client education pamphlet about the disease.
- Instruct about the prescribed medications, potential adverse effects, and the importance of completing the entire prescribed regimen.
- Emphasize the importance of continued follow-up.
- Teach and demonstrate sputum and droplet control measures.
- Escort to the local incentive shelter program for directly observed medical therapy and meals.
- Identify verbally and in writing manifestations to report to the physician.

EVALUATION

Mr. Kamil successfully enrolls Mr. Facée in the local incentive shelter program. In this program, a healthcare worker administers Mr. Facée's medications daily, watching him swallow them. He is assigned a small individual room and can eat three daily meals at the shelter. He still prefers to sleep outside when the weather permits, but he complies with the requirement for supervised medication administration because he "likes the food there." Always a clean person, Mr. Facée is able to demonstrate appropriate sputum control measures and practices them faithfully. The sputum culture done after 2 months of treatment is negative for tubercle bacilli, and his chest x-ray indicates no disease progression.

CRITICAL THINKING IN THE NURSING PROCESS

1. Many homeless people have schizophrenia or other mental diseases. How would you adapt the care plan for a homeless schizophrenic client with active tuberculosis?
2. Mr. Kamil was fortunate in having access to an incentive shelter with healthcare workers to supervise medication compliance. Identify available resources in your area for homeless clients infected with tuberculosis.
3. Develop a care plan for the nursing diagnosis *Ineffective Airway Clearance* related to mucopurulent sputum and weak cough.

See Evaluating Your Response in Appendix C.

- Identify support systems, and include significant others in teaching. *A knowledgeable significant other provides reinforcement of learning, confirmation of understanding, and encouragement for the client. Including significant others also reduces the risk of inadvertent sabotage of the treatment plan.*
- Establish a relationship of mutual trust with the client and significant others. *An atmosphere of trust increases receptiveness to teaching and learning.*
- Develop mutually acceptable learning goals with the client and significant other. *Working together to identify learning*

needs and establish goals increases the client's "ownership" and interest in the process.

- Select appropriate teaching strategies, using learning aids such as literature and visual materials that are appropriate for age, level of education, and intellect. *Teaching tailored to the client is more effective and results in better learning.*
- Teach about tuberculosis and the prescribed treatment, including:
  a. Nature of the disease and its spread
  b. Purpose of treatment and follow-up procedures

c. Measures to prevent spreading the disease to others
d. Importance of maintaining good general health by eating a well-balanced, high-protein, high-carbohydrate diet; balancing exercise with rest; and avoiding crowds and people with upper respiratory infections
e. Names, doses, purposes, and adverse effects of prescribed medications
f. Importance of avoiding alcohol and other substances that may damage the liver while taking chemotherapeutic drugs
g. Fluid intake needs of 2.5 to 3.0 quarts of fluid per day
h. Manifestations to report to the physician: chest pain, hemoptysis, difficulty breathing; anorexia, nausea, or vomiting; yellow tint to skin or sclera; sudden weight gain, swollen feet, ankles, legs, or hands; hearing loss, tinnitus, or vertigo; change in vision or difficulty discriminating colors.

Tuberculosis is a chronic disease requiring lengthy treatment with antitubercular medications. A good understanding of the disease, its treatment, and potential adverse effects of therapy prepares the client to manage care.

■ Document teaching and level of understanding. Reinforce teaching and learning as needed. *Teaching is not complete until the client can demonstrate learning of the information.*

Ineffective Therapeutic Regimen Management

The populations at highest risk for developing active tuberculosis—the homeless and members of lower socioeconomic groups—are also at high risk for being unable to manage its complex treatment regimen. Three or more costly medications that may have unpleasant or even dangerous side effects are prescribed. Frequent medical follow-up is required. Infectious diseases such as TB carry a stigma that may lead to denial of the disease or its seriousness. Alcoholics and IV drug users need to withdraw from their addiction to be successful in treating the disease. The client with HIV infection faces a potentially fatal disease and costly treatment that may well override concerns about tuberculosis management.

■ Assess self-care abilities and support systems. *Assessment is used to help determine the client's ability to follow the prescribed regimen.*

■ Assess knowledge and understanding of the disease, its complications, treatment, and risks to others. Provide additional teaching and reinforcement as indicated. *Lack of understanding is a barrier to compliance with and management of the treatment regimen.*

■ Work collaboratively to identify barriers or obstacles to managing the prescribed treatment. *Working collaboratively with the client and other members of the healthcare team provides insight for overcoming identified barriers to effective treatment.*

■ Assist the client, significant others (if available), and healthcare team members to develop a plan for managing the prescribed regimen. *Including the client in developing a plan to manage care increases the sense of control and ownership and helps ensure that personal, cultural, and lifestyle factors are considered. This increases the likelihood of compliance.*

■ Provide verbal and written instructions that are clear and appropriate for level of literacy, knowledge, and understanding. *Clearly written directions provide support and reinforcement for the client.*

■ Provide active intervention for homeless people, including shelter placement or other housing and ongoing follow-up by easily accessed healthcare providers (clinics and public health workers in the neighborhood that do not present transportation or access problems, either real or perceived). *Simple referral will not ensure compliance, especially among disenfranchised populations. Active intervention is needed to help ensure treatment compliance.*

■ Refer clients who are unlikely to comply with the treatment regimen to the public health department for management and follow-up. *Because tuberculosis presents a significant public health risk, public health follow-up is essential. In some cases, it is necessary for nurses to administer medications, observing the client swallow all pills.*

Risk for Infection

The spread of tuberculosis is a risk in any facility housing many people. It is especially high in residential care facilities for older clients and for people with AIDS. The increasing incidence of TB among homeless people and members of lower socioeconomic groups increases the risk in hospitals, emergency departments, and public and urgent care clinics. Respiratory precautions are necessary to prevent the spread of TB via microscopic airborne droplets to other clients and to healthcare workers.

■ Place the client in a private room with airflow control that prevents air within the room from circulating into the hallway or other rooms. A negative flow room in which air is diluted by at least six fresh-air exchanges per hour is recommended. *A negative flow room and multiple fresh-air exchanges dilute the concentration of droplet nuclei within the room and prevent their spread to adjacent areas.*

■ Use standard precautions and tuberculosis isolation techniques as recommended by the CDC, including wearing masks and gowns when caring for clients who do not reliably cover the mouth when coughing. *These measures are important to prevent the spread of tuberculosis to others.*

PRACTICE ALERT

Use personal protective devices to reduce the risk of transmission during client care. The Occupational Safety and Health Administration (OSHA) requires use of a HEPA-filtered respirator for protection against occupational exposure to tuberculosis. Surgical masks are ineffective to filter droplet nuclei, necessitating the use of protective devices capable of filtering bacteria and particles smaller than 1 micron.

■ Discuss the reasons for and importance of respiratory isolation procedures during initial hospitalization. When treatment is provided as an outpatient, instruct to avoid crowds and close physical contact and maintain ventilation in living facilities, particularly during the first 3 weeks of treatment. *These measures help protect others during initial treatment, when sputum is still likely to contain significant numbers of bacilli.*

■ Place a mask on the client when transporting to other parts of the facility for diagnostic or treatment procedures. *Covering the client's nose and mouth during transport minimizes air contamination and the risk to visitors and personnel.*

■ Inform all personnel having contact with the client of the diagnosis. *This allows personnel to take appropriate precautions.*

■ Assist visitors to mask prior to entering the room. *Providing visitors with appropriate masks or respirators reduces their risk of infection.*

■ Teach the client how to limit transmitting the disease to others:
  a. Always cough and expectorate into tissues.
  b. Dispose of tissues properly, placing them in a closed bag.
  c. Wear a mask if you are sneezing or unable to control respiratory secretions.
  d. The disease is not spread by touching inanimate objects, so no special precautions are required for eating utensils, clothing, books, or other objects used.

Teaching appropriate precautions helps prevent the spread of tuberculosis to others while allowing as much freedom from restraints as possible.

■ Teach how to collect sputum specimens. If necessary, have the client step outside to collect a sputum specimen. *This minimizes the risk of exposure to healthcare personnel and provides for rapid dilution of any droplet nuclei produced and their exposure to ultraviolet light (which kills the bacteria).*

■ Teach the importance of complying with the prescribed treatment for the entire course of therapy. *Completion of the entire treatment regimen is important to reduce the risk of relapse and creation of drug-resistant organisms.*

Using NANDA, NIC, and NOC

Linkages between NANDA nursing diagnoses, nursing interventions, and nursing outcomes for the client with tuberculosis are illustrated in Chart 38–2.

Community-Based Care

Most clients with TB are managed in community settings; few require institutionalization. In addition to the teaching topics and strategies identified above, discuss the following topics when preparing the client and significant others for home care:

■ Importance of screening close contacts for infection and possibly prophylactic treatment

■ Effect, dose, and timing for all medications, and potential side effects and their management

■ Importance of long-term therapy in eradicating the disease

■ Principles of good nutrition, dietary guidelines for a client with TB, and other measures to help maintain good health, such as balancing rest with exercise

■ Signs and symptoms of complications to report to the physician or healthcare provider.

Provide referrals as appropriate:

■ Smoking cessation clinics or support groups

■ Alcohol treatment facilities, Alcoholics Anonymous, other treatment programs or support groups

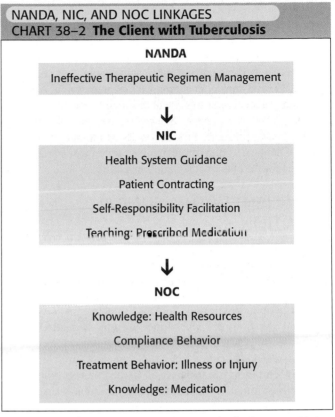

NANDA, NIC, AND NOC LINKAGES
CHART 38–2 The Client with Tuberculosis

NANDA

Ineffective Therapeutic Regimen Management

↓

NIC

Health System Guidance

Patient Contracting

Self-Responsibility Facilitation

Teaching: Prescribed Medication

↓

NOC

Knowledge: Health Resources

Compliance Behavior

Treatment Behavior: Illness or Injury

Knowledge: Medication

Data from *NANDA's Nursing Diagnoses: Definitions & Classification 2005–2006* by NANDA International (2005), Philadelphia; *Nursing Interventions Classification (NIC)* (4th ed.) by J. M. Dochterman & G. M. Bulechek (2004), St. Louis, MO: Mosby; and *Nursing Outcomes Classification (NOC) (3rd ed.)* by S. Moorhead, M. Johnson, and M. Maas (2004), St. Louis, MO: Mosby.

■ Drug treatment facilities, Narcotics Anonymous, other outpatient or inpatient treatment programs or support groups

■ Low-cost community clinics and incentive programs for people with TB

■ Counseling, support groups, and other community resources that provide additional assistance and support.

THE CLIENT WITH INHALATION ANTHRAX

Inhalation anthrax is a relatively new potential threat in the United States. This disease rarely affects humans in nature, even though both wild and domestic animals can be infected. However, *Bacillus anthracis*, the spore-forming rod responsible for causing anthrax, has been identified as an agent likely to be used as a biologic weapon. Anthrax spores can be aerosolized so they remain suspended in the air, allowing them to be inhaled into the lungs. Person-to-person transmission does not occur.

Inhalation anthrax causes initial flulike symptoms, including malaise, dry cough, and fever. This is followed by an abrupt onset of severe dyspnea, stridor, and cyanosis. Lymph nodes in the mediastinum and thorax become inflamed and enlarged. Septic shock and/or meningitis may develop. Untreated, death results from hemorrhagic thoracic lymphadenitis and hemorrhagic mediastinitis with resultant hypotension and hypoxemia (Kasper et al., 2005).

Blood cultures and chest x-ray are used to diagnose inhalation anthrax. However, because death can quickly result from the disease, people who are known or suspected to have been exposed to anthrax spores often are treated prophylactically. Ciprofloxacin (Cipro) is used to both prevent and treat inhalation anthrax. Doxycycline (Vibramycin) is an alternative to ciprofloxacin. Although an anthrax vaccine exists, its use at this time is considered experimental (Persell et al., 2002). See the section on bioterrorism in Chapter 7 ∞ for more information about anthrax and the section in Chapter 39 ∞ on respiratory failure for nursing care measures for the client with inhalation anthrax.

THE CLIENT WITH A FUNGAL INFECTION

Fungal spores are endemic, present in the air everyone breathes. Normal respiratory defense mechanisms allow few of these spores to reach the lungs. If they reach the lungs, pulmonary macrophages and neutrophils efficiently remove them in most people. When they do cause infection, it is typically mild and self-limiting. Most fungi are opportunistic, able to cause infection only in people who are immunocompromised. For this reason, clients with AIDS, renal failure, leukemia, burns, or chronic diseases, as well as people receiving corticosteroids or immunosuppressants, are particularly susceptible to fungal diseases.

Many fungal lung diseases have a geographic distribution pattern. Histoplasmosis and blastomycosis are more common in the southeastern, mid-Atlantic, and central states. California, Arizona, and western Texas are the primary sites for coccidioidomycosis, also known as San Joaquin valley fever (Kasper et al., 2005).

The course and manifestations of fungal lung diseases resemble those of tuberculosis. Lung lesions are slow to develop, and symptoms are mild. The fungus can disseminate from the lung to other organs.

Pathophysiology

Histoplasmosis

Histoplasmosis, an infectious disease caused by *Histoplasma capsulatum*, is the most common fungal lung infection in the United States. The organism is found in the soil and is linked to exposure to bird droppings and bats. Infection occurs when the spores are inhaled and reach the alveoli. Most infections develop into *latent asymptomatic disease*, much like tuberculosis, or *primary acute histoplasmosis*, a mild, self-limiting influenza-like illness. Initial chest x-rays are nonspecific; later ones show areas of calcification. *Chronic progressive disease*, usually seen in older adults, typically is limited to the lung but may involve any organ. Progressive lung changes and cavitation occur, with increasing dyspnea and eventual disabling pulmonary disease.

Regional lymph vessels spread the organism from the lungs to other parts of the body, much like the process that occurs in tuberculosis. In the healthy host, normal immune responses inactivate and remove the organism. In the immunocompromised host, however, macrophages remove the fungi but are unable to destroy them, resulting in *disseminated histoplasmosis*. This type of histoplasmosis is often fatal. Manifestations of fever, dyspnea, cough, weight loss, and muscle wasting are usual. Ulcerations of the mouth and oropharynx may be present, and the liver and spleen are enlarged.

Coccidioidomycosis

Coccidioidomycosis is an infectious disease caused by the fungus *Coccidioides immitis*. This mold grows in the soil of the arid Southwest, Mexico, and Central and South America. When inhaled, the fungus typically causes an acute, self-limiting pulmonary infection that often is asymptomatic and goes unrecognized. If manifestations do occur, they resemble those of influenza, with malaise, fever, body aches, and cough. Pleuritic pain, skin rash, and arthritis of the knees and ankles also may develop. Disseminated disease, which may affect the lymph nodes, meninges, spleen, liver, kidney, skin, and adrenal glands, is rare in immunocompetent people. When it does occur, the mortality rate is high. Meningitis is the usual cause of death.

Blastomycosis

The fungus *Blastomyces dermatitidis* causes the infectious disease blastomycosis. It occurs primarily in the south central and midwestern regions of the United States and in Canada. Men are affected more frequently than women. The lungs are the primary site for the disease, although it may spread to involve the skin, bones, genitourinary system, and, rarely, the CNS. Pulmonary symptoms include fever, dyspnea, pleuritic chest pain, and cough, which may become productive of bloody or purulent sputum. If untreated, the disseminated disease is slowly progressive and ultimately fatal.

Aspergillosis

Aspergillus spores are common in the environment, but rarely cause disease except in the immunocompromised. When they do cause infection, *Aspergillus* species invade blood vessels and produce hyphae that branch at acute angles, frequently causing venous or arterial thrombosis. In the lungs, aspergillosis can cause an acute, diffuse, self-limited pneumonitis. The manifestations of pulmonary aspergillosis include dyspnea, nonproductive cough, pleuritic chest pain, chills, and fever. If the organism invades a pulmonary blood vessel, hemoptysis or massive pulmonary hemorrhage can occur. In clients with underlying lung disease, balls of *Aspergillus* hyphae may form within cysts or cavities, usually in the upper lobes of the lung. When this occurs, symptoms often are milder and more insidious in onset, with fever, weight loss, night sweats, and cough (Kasper et al., 2005).

INTERDISCIPLINARY CARE

Most fungal lung infections can be diagnosed by microscopic examination of a sputum specimen for the fungus. (See Chapter 36 ∞ for nursing responsibilities related to collecting a sputum specimen.) Blood cultures also may be done, as well as cultures of cerebrospinal fluid if indicated. Chest x-ray may show typical changes in lung tissue or widening of the mediastinum, depending on the infecting organism.

Acute pulmonary histoplasmosis and acute pulmonary coccidioidomycosis usually resolve without treatment, although antifungal drugs may be given to shorten the disease course.

Oral itraconazole (Sporanox), a broad-spectrum antifungal agent, is commonly prescribed to treat histoplasmosis. Other fungal lung diseases and clients who are immunocompromised are often treated with intravenous amphotericin B. Surgery (lobectomy) may be indicated for clients with severe hemoptysis associated with aspergillosis.

NURSING CARE

Clients with fungal lung infections have different nursing care needs, depending on the disease and their immune status. For most clients, nursing care focuses on education. People living in high-prevalence areas or who have specific risk factors such as exposure to bird droppings (for example, by cleaning chicken coops, pigeon lofts, or barns where birds roost), decomposed vegetation, rotting wood, or stored grain need to be aware of the risk, common symptoms, and measures to reduce the risk. Clients with latent histoplasmosis may need education to maintain good general health to prevent reactivation. Teach clients receiving antifungal drugs about the specific drug, its intended and adverse effects, the duration of therapy, and symptoms to report to the physician. Include teaching about any specific precautions such as drug or food interactions. Itraconazole interacts with many medications; verify the safety of concurrent usage with all other prescribed drugs. Its use is contraindicated during pregnancy and lactation; emphasize the importance of effective birth control and of notifying the physician immediately if pregnancy occurs. Amphotericin B is a toxic drug. Administer the initial intravenous dose slowly after premedicating with an antihistamine and antiemetic as ordered to manage its adverse effects. Monitor carefully during infusion and therapy for changes in vital signs, hydration, nutrition, weight, or urine output.

DISORDERS OF THE PLEURA

The *pleura* is a thin membrane with two layers: the visceral pleura, which overlies the lung surface, and the parietal pleura, which lines the inner chest wall. Between the layers of pleura is a potential space, the *pleural cavity*, which contains a thin layer of serous fluid. As the thoracic cavity expands during inspiration, the pressure in this space becomes negative in relation to atmospheric and alveolar pressure. The expansible lung is drawn out, and air rushes into the alveoli. When the pleura is inflamed or affected by disease or injury, air or fluid can collect in the pleural cavity, restricting lung expansion, air movement, and ventilation.

THE CLIENT WITH PLEURITIS

Pleuritis (*pleurisy*), inflammation of the pleura, irritates sensory fibers of the parietal pleura, causing characteristic pain. Pleural inflammation usually occurs secondarily to another process, such as a viral respiratory illness, pneumonia, or rib injury.

The onset of pleuritis is typically abrupt. The pain is unilateral and well localized; it is usually sharp or stabbing in nature. Pain may be referred to the neck or the shoulder. Deep breathing, coughing, and movement aggravate the pain. Respirations are rapid and shallow, and chest wall movement is limited on the affected side. Breath sounds are diminished, and a pleural friction rub may be heard over the site.

The diagnosis of pleuritis is based on its manifestations. Chest x-ray and ECG may be ordered to rule out other causes of chest pain. Treatment for pleuritis is symptomatic. Analgesics and nonsteroidal anti-inflammatory drugs (NSAIDs), indomethacin (Indocin) in particular, help relieve the pain. Codeine may be ordered, both to relieve pain and to suppress the cough.

Nursing care for the client with pleuritis is directed toward promoting comfort, including administration of NSAIDs and analgesics. Positioning and splinting the chest while coughing also are helpful. Although wrapping the chest with 6-inch-wide elastic bandages may help relieve pain, this may excessively restrict chest motion, increasing the risk of impaired airway clearance.

Teach the client and family that pleuritis is generally self-limited and of short duration. Discuss symptoms to report to the physician: increased fever, productive cough, difficulty breathing, or shortness of breath. Provide information about prescription and nonprescription NSAIDs and analgesics, including the drug ordered, how to use it, and its desired and possible adverse effects.

THE CLIENT WITH A PLEURAL EFFUSION

The pleural space normally contains only about 10 to 20 mL of serous fluid. **Pleural effusion** is collection of excess fluid in the pleural space. Pleural effusions result from either systemic or local disease. Systemic disorders that may lead to pleural effusion include heart failure, liver or renal disease, and connective tissue disorders, such as rheumatoid arthritis and systemic lupus erythematosus (SLE). Pneumonia, atelectasis, tuberculosis, lung cancer, and trauma are local conditions that may cause pleural effusion.

Pathophysiology and Manifestations

Excess pleural fluid may be either *transudate*, formed when capillary pressure is high or plasma proteins are low, or *exudate*, the result of increased capillary permeability. Heart failure is the most common precipitating factor in transudate formation; it also may accompany renal failure, nephrosis, liver failure, and malignancy. Exudate, a protein-rich fluid, is seen with inflammatory processes such as infections, systemic inflammation (e.g. rheumatoid arthritis or SLE), pulmonary infarction (leading to tissue necrosis and an inflammatory response), and malignancy (Porth, 2005). Other pleural fluid collections include *empyema*, pus in the pleural cavity; *hemothorax*, the presence of blood in the cavity; *hemorrhagic pleural effusion*, a mixture of blood and pleural fluid; and *chylothorax*, a collection of lymph in the pleural space. In adults, chylothorax may result from thoracic surgery or placement of a central catheter in one of the great veins (Porth, 2005).

A large pleural effusion compresses adjacent lung tissue. This causes the characteristic manifestation of dyspnea. Pain may develop, although with inflammatory processes pleuritic pain often is relieved by formation of an effusion, as the fluid reduces friction between inflamed visceral and parietal pleura. Breath sounds are diminished or absent, and a dull percussion tone is heard over the affected area. Chest wall movement may be limited.

INTERDISCIPLINARY CARE

Chest x-ray often provides the first evidence of a pleural effusion. Because fluid typically collects in dependent regions, it is seen at the base of the affected lung on an upright chest x-ray, and along the lateral wall when the client is positioned on the affected side. CT scans and ultrasonography also are used to localize and differentiate pleural effusions.

Thoracentesis

If the cause of pleural effusion is not apparent, a thoracentesis is done. **Thoracentesis** is an invasive procedure in which fluid (or occasionally air) is removed from the pleural space with a needle. Aspirated fluid is analyzed for appearance, cell counts, protein and glucose content, the presence of enzymes such as LDH and amylase, abnormal cells, and culture.

When pleural effusion is significant and interferes with respirations, thoracentesis is the treatment of choice to remove the fluid (Figure 38–8 ■). Thoracentesis may be performed at the bedside, in a procedure room, or in an outpatient setting. Local anesthesia is used, and the procedure requires less than 30 minutes to complete. Percussion, auscultation, radiography, or ultrasonography are used to locate the effusion and needle insertion site. The amount of fluid removed is limited to 1200 to 1500 mL at one time to reduce the risk of cardiovascular collapse from rapid removal of too much fluid. Pneumothorax is a possible complication of thoracentesis if the visceral pleura is punctured or a closed drainage system is not maintained during the proce-dure. Nursing care for the client undergoing a thoracentesis is outlined in the box on the next page.

Treatments

Because pleural effusion usually occurs secondarily to another disease or disorder, medical management also focuses on treating the underlying condition to prevent further fluid accumulation. An empyema may require repeated drainage, as well as high doses of parenteral antibiotics. Occasionally, thoracotomy and surgical excision may be necessary. See the box on page 1313 for nursing care of the client undergoing thoracic surgery. Recurrent pleural effusions, often due to cancer, may be prevented by instilling an irritant, such as doxycycline bleomycin, or talc, into the pleural space to cause adhesion of the parietal and visceral pleura (*pleurodesis*). Water-seal chest tube drainage is often employed for hemothorax.

NURSING CARE

Nursing care for the client with a pleural effusion is directed toward supporting respiratory function and assisting with procedures to evacuate collected fluid. With a large pleural effusion and partial lung collapse, impaired gas exchange and activity intolerance are high-priority nursing problems. Risk for impaired gas exchange is also a priority problem during the initial period following thoracentesis.

Teaching for home care focuses on symptoms of recurrent effusion or complications following a thoracentesis to report to the physician: increasing dyspnea or shortness of breath, cough, and hemoptysis. Pleuritic pain may be an early sign of effusion and also should be reported. Further teaching about an underlying condition also may be necessary; for example, the client with heart failure may need teaching about a salt-restricted diet.

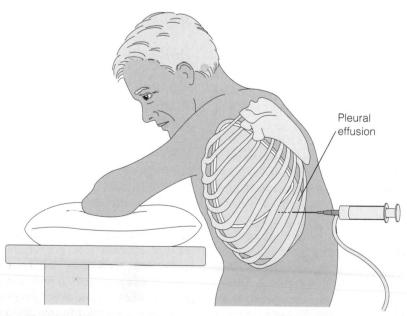

Figure 38–8 ■ Thoracentesis. With the client seated, a needle is inserted between the ribs into the pleural space to withdraw accumulated fluid.

NURSING CARE OF THE CLIENT HAVING A   Thoracentesis

BEFORE THE PROCEDURE

- Verify a signed informed consent for the procedure. *This invasive procedure requires informed consent.*
- Assess knowledge and understanding of the procedure and its purpose; provide additional information as needed. *An informed client will be less apprehensive and more able to cooperate during the thoracentesis.*
- Preprocedure fasting or sedation is not required. *Only local anesthesia is used in this procedure, and the gag and cough reflexes remain intact.*
- Administer a cough suppressant if indicated. *Movement and coughing during the procedure may cause inadvertent damage to the lung or pleura.*
- Obtain a thoracentesis tray, sterile gloves, injectable lidocaine, povidone-iodine, dressing supplies, and an extra overbed table or Mayo stand. *These supplies are used by the physician performing the procedure.*
- Position the client upright, leaning forward with arms and head supported on an anchored overbed table. *This position spreads the ribs, enlarging the intercostal space for needle insertion.*
- Inform the client that although local anesthesia prevents pain as the needle is inserted, a sensation of pressure may be felt. *A pressure sensation occurs as the needle punctures the parietal pleura to enter the pleural space.*

AFTER THE PROCEDURE

- Monitor pulse, color, oxygen saturation, and other signs during thoracentesis. *These are indicators of physiologic tolerance of the procedure.*
- Apply a dressing over the puncture site, and position on the unaffected side for 1 hour. *This allows the pleural puncture to heal.*
- Label obtained specimen with name, date, source, and diagnosis; send specimen to the laboratory for analysis. *Fluid obtained during thoracentesis may be examined for abnormal cells, bacteria, and other substances to determine the cause of the pleural effusion.*
- During the first several hours after thoracentesis, frequently assess and document vital signs; oxygen saturation; respiratory status, including respiratory excursion, lung sounds, cough, or hemoptysis; and puncture site for bleeding or crepitus. *Frequent assessment is important to detect possible complications of thoracentesis, such as pneumothorax.*
- Obtain a chest x-ray. *Chest x-ray is ordered to detect possible pneumothorax.*
- Normal activities generally can be resumed after 1 hour if no evidence of pneumothorax or other complication is present. *The puncture wound of thoracentesis heals rapidly.*

THE CLIENT WITH PNEUMOTHORAX

Accumulation of air in the pleural space is called **pneumothorax**. Pneumothorax can occur spontaneously, without apparent cause, as a complication of preexisting lung disease, as a result of blunt or penetrating trauma to the chest, or from an iatrogenic cause (e.g., following thoracentesis).

Pathophysiology

Pressure in the pleural space is normally negative in relation to atmospheric pressure. This negative pressure is vital to the process of breathing. Contraction of the diaphragm and the intercostal muscles enlarges the thoracic space. Negative intrapleural pressure draws the lung outward, increasing its volume so air rushes in to fill the expanded lung space.

When either the visceral or parietal pleura is breached, air enters the pleural space, equalizing this pressure. Lung expansion is impaired, and the natural recoil tendency of the lung causes it to collapse to a greater or lesser extent, depending on the size and rapidity of air accumulation. Table 38–7 illustrates the classifications of pneumothorax.

Spontaneous Pneumothorax

Spontaneous pneumothorax develops when an air-filled bleb, or blister, on the lung surface ruptures. Rupture allows air from the airways to enter the pleural space. Air accumulates until pressures are equalized or until collapse of the involved lung section seals the leak. Spontaneous pneumothorax may be either *primary* (*simple*) or *secondary* (*complicated*).

Primary pneumothorax affects previously healthy people, usually tall, slender men between ages 16 and 24 (Way & Doherty, 2003). The cause of primary pneumothorax is unknown. Risk factors include smoking and familial factors. Air-filled blebs tend to form in the apices of the lungs. This is considered to be a benign condition, although recurrences are common. Certain activities also increase the risk of spontaneous pneumothorax, such as high-altitude flying and rapid decompression during scuba diving.

Secondary pneumothorax, generally caused by overdistention and rupture of an alveolus, is more serious and potentially life threatening. It develops in clients with underlying lung disease, usually COPD. Middle-age and older adults are primarily affected. Secondary pneumothorax also may be associated with asthma, cystic fibrosis, pulmonary fibrosis, tuberculosis, acute respiratory distress syndrome (ARDS), and other lung diseases. Rarely, a form of secondary pneumothorax called *catamenial pneumothorax* can develop in affected women within 24 to 48 hours of the onset of menstrual flow.

MANIFESTATIONS The manifestations of spontaneous pneumothorax depend on the size of pneumothorax, extent of lung collapse, and any underlying lung disease. Typically, pleuritic chest pain and shortness of breath begin abruptly, often while at rest. The respiratory and heart rates increase as gas exchange is affected. Chest wall movement may be asymmetrical, with less movement on the affected side than the unaffected side. The affected side is hyperresonant to percussion, and breath sounds may be diminished or absent. Hypoxemia may develop, although normal mechanisms that shunt

TABLE 38–7 Types of Pneumothorax

TYPE	PATHOPHYSIOLOGY	MANIFESTATIONS
A. Spontaneous 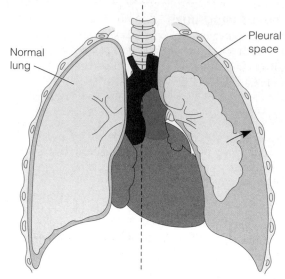	Rupture of a bleb on the lung surface allows air to enter pleural space from airways. ■ *Primary pneumothorax* affects previously healthy people. ■ *Secondary pneumothorax* affects people with preexisting lung disease (e.g., COPD).	■ Abrupt onset ■ Pleuritic chest pain ■ Dyspnea, shortness of breath ■ Tachypnea, tachycardia ■ Unequal lung excursion ■ Decreased breath sounds and hyperresonant percussion tone on affected side
B. Traumatic 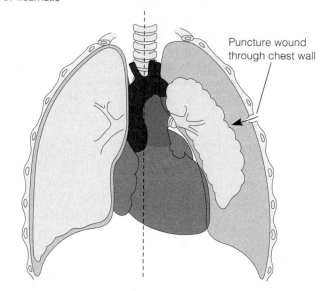	Trauma to the chest wall or pleura disrupts the pleural membrane. ■ *Open* occurs with penetrating chest trauma that allows air from the environment to enter the pleural space. ■ *Closed* occurs with blunt trauma that allows air from the lung to enter the pleural space. ■ *Iatrogenic* involves laceration of visceral pleura during a procedure such as thoracentesis or central-line insertion.	■ Pain ■ Dyspnea ■ Tachypnea, tachycardia ■ Decreased respiratory excursion ■ Absent breath sounds in affected area ■ Air movement through an open wound
C. Tension 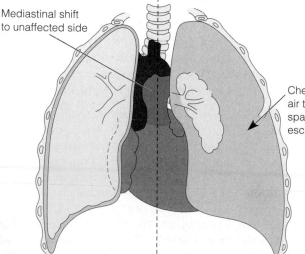	Air enters pleural space through chest wall or from airways but is unable to escape, resulting in rapid accumulation. Lung on affected side collapses. As intrapleural pressure increases, heart, great vessels, trachea, and esophagus shift toward the unaffected side.	■ Hypotension, shock ■ Distended neck veins ■ Severe dyspnea ■ Tachypnea, tachycardia ■ Decreased respiratory excursion ■ Absent breath sounds on affected side ■ Tracheal deviation toward unaffected side

Labels within illustrations:

A. Spontaneous — Normal lung; Pleural space

B. Traumatic — Puncture wound through chest wall

C. Tension — Mediastinal shift to unaffected side; Chest wound allows air to enter pleural space but prevents escape.

blood flow to the unaffected lung often maintain normal oxygen saturation levels. Hypoxemia is more pronounced in secondary pneumothorax.

Traumatic Pneumothorax

Blunt or penetrating trauma of the chest wall and pleura can cause pneumothorax. Blunt trauma, for example, due to a motor vehicle crash, fall, or during cardiopulmonary resuscitation (CPR), can lead to a *closed pneumothorax*. Fractured ribs penetrating the pleura are the leading cause of pneumothorax due to blunt trauma (Yamamoto et al., 2005). Fracture of the trachea and a ruptured bronchus or esophagus also may result from blunt trauma, leading to closed pneumothorax.

Open pneumothorax (*sucking chest wound*) results from penetrating chest trauma such as a stab wound, gunshot wound, or impalement injury. With open pneumothorax, air moves freely between the pleural space and the atmosphere through the wound. Pressure on the affected side equalizes with the atmosphere, and the lung collapses rapidly. The result is significant hypoventilation.

Iatrogenic pneumothorax may result from puncture or laceration of the visceral pleura during central-line placement, thoracentesis, or lung biopsy. During bronchoscopy, bronchi or lung tissue can be disrupted. Alveoli can become overdistended and rupture during anesthesia, resuscitation procedures, or mechanical ventilation.

MANIFESTATIONS With traumatic pneumothorax, manifestations of pain and dyspnea may be masked or missed due to other injuries. Tachypnea and tachycardia may be attributed to the primary injury. Focused assessment for evidence of pneumothorax is vital. Chest wall movement on the affected side is diminished, and breath sounds are absent. If a penetrating wound is present, air may be heard and felt moving through it with respiratory efforts. Hemothorax frequently accompanies traumatic pneumothorax. The manifestations of iatrogenic pneumothorax are similar to those of spontaneous pneumothorax.

Tension Pneumothorax

Tension pneumothorax develops when injury to the chest wall or lungs allows air to enter the pleural space but prevents it from escaping. Pressure within the pleural space becomes positive in relation to atmospheric pressure as air rapidly accumulates with each breath. The lung on the affected side collapses, and pressure on the mediastinum shifts thoracic organs to the unaffected side of the chest, placing pressure on the opposite lung as well. Ventilation is severely compromised, and venous return to the heart is impaired. Tension pneumothorax is a medical emergency requiring immediate intervention to preserve respiration and cardiac output.

MANIFESTATIONS In addition to manifestations of pneumothorax, hypotension and distended neck veins are evident as venous return and cardiac output are affected. The trachea is displaced toward the unaffected side as a result of the mediastinal shift. Signs of shock may be present. See Chapter 11 ∞ for the manifestations and treatment of shock.

INTERDISCIPLINARY CARE

Treatment for pneumothorax depends on the severity of the problem. A small simple pneumothorax may require no treatment other than monitoring with serial x-rays. Air is absorbed from the pleural space, allowing most small pneumothoraces to resolve spontaneously. A large pneumothorax with significant symptoms usually requires treatment with *thoracostomy*, or the placement of chest tubes. Surgical intervention may be necessary to prevent recurrent spontaneous pneumothorax.

Diagnosis

Oxygen saturation measurements are obtained to evaluate the effect of pneumothorax on gas exchange. ABGs may be obtained to further assess gas exchange.

The chest x-ray is an effective diagnostic tool for pneumothorax. In tension pneumothorax, air is evident on the affected side, and mediastinal structures are shifted toward the opposite or unaffected side.

Treatments

CHEST TUBES The treatment of choice for significant pneumothorax is placement of a closed-chest catheter to allow the lung to reexpand. When a tube is placed in the pleural cavity to remove air or fluid, it must be sealed to prevent air from also entering the tube and, in essence, creating an open pneumothorax. Chest tubes are sealed with a Heimlich (one-way) valve (Figure 38–9 ■) or connected to a closed drainage system with a one-way valve or "water seal." The valve or water seal prevents air from entering the chest cavity during inspiration and allows air to escape during expiration. Applying a low level of suction to the system helps to reestablish negative pressure in the pleural space, allowing the lung to reexpand.

A number of closed-drainage chest tube systems are available. Most are self-contained disposable systems (Figure 38–10 ■). Drainage from the chest tube is collected in the collection chamber. This chamber is sealed with a one-way valve or connected to a water seal chamber, which is in turn connected to the suction control regulator or chamber. Nursing care of the client with chest tubes is discussed in the box on page 1300.

A large-bore needle or plastic intravenous catheter may be inserted through the chest wall as emergency treatment of a tension pneumothorax. This allows air to escape from the affected side, relieving pressure on mediastinal structures and the opposite lung.

PLEURODESIS Although controversial, *pleurodesis*, or creation of adhesions between the parietal and visceral pleura, may be used to prevent recurrent pneumothorax. This procedure involves instilling a chemical agent such as doxycycline into the

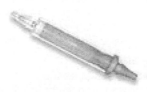

Figure 38–9 ■ The Heimlich one-way valve allows air to escape from the pleural space, helping to reestablish negative pressure and allowing the lung to reexpand.

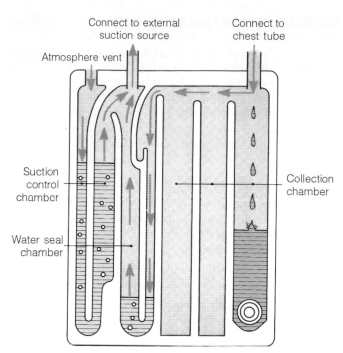

Connect to external suction source

Connect to chest tube

Atmosphere vent

Suction control chamber

Water seal chamber

Collection chamber

Figure 38–10 ■ A water seal chest drainage system with wet suction control.

pleural space. The subsequent inflammatory response creates scar tissue and adhesions between the pleural layers. This procedure reduces the recurrence rate to as low as 2% but can make subsequent surgery more difficult (Way & Doherty, 2003).

Surgery

The risk for recurrence of spontaneous pneumothorax increases with each attack. Clients at high risk for recurrent pneumothorax may have surgery to reduce the risk of future ruptures. A thoracotomy is done to excise or oversew blebs (usually at the apices of the lungs). The overlying pleura is then roughened or irritated to induce scarring and adhesion to the surface of the lung. In some cases, the parietal pleura may be partially excised. These procedures can be done using video-assisted thoracoscopic surgery (VATS), a minimally invasive surgical technique (Way & Doherty, 2003).

NURSING CARE

Health Promotion

Health promotion activities to prevent spontaneous and traumatic pneumothorax primarily involve health teaching. Initiate

---

NURSING CARE OF THE CLIENT WITH Chest Tubes

BEFORE THE PROCEDURE

- Ensure a signed informed consent for chest tube insertion. *This invasive procedure requires informed consent.*
- Provide additional information as indicated. Explain that local anesthesia will be used but that pressure may be felt as the trocar is inserted. Reassure that breathing will be easier once the chest tube is in place and the lung reexpands. *The client may be extremely dyspneic and anxious and may need reassurance that this invasive procedure will provide relief.*
- Gather all needed supplies, including thoracostomy tray, injectable lidocaine, sterile gloves, chest tube drainage system, sterile water (if required), and a large sterile catheter-tipped syringe to use as a funnel for filling water seal and suction chambers as needed. *These supplies are used during the insertion procedure to establish a water seal drainage system.*
- Position as indicated for the procedure. *Either an upright position (as for thoracentesis) or side-lying position may be used, depending on the site of the pneumothorax.*
- Assist with chest tube insertion as needed. The procedure may be performed in a procedure room, in the surgical suite, or at the bedside. *Although chest tube insertion is a relatively simple procedure, nursing assistance is necessary to support the client and rapidly establish a closed drainage system.*

AFTER THE PROCEDURE

- Assess respiratory status at least every 4 hours. *Frequent assessment is necessary to monitor respiratory status and the effect of the chest tube.*
- Maintain a closed system. Tape all connections, and secure the chest tube to the chest wall. *These measures are important*

to prevent inadvertent tube removal or disruption of system integrity.
- Keep the collection apparatus below the level of the chest. *Pleural fluid drains into the collection apparatus by gravity flow.*
- Check tubes frequently for kinks or loops. *These could interfere with drainage.*
- Check the water seal or negative pressure indicator frequently. The water level should fluctuate with respiratory effort. Periodic air bubbles in the water seal chamber or air leak meter are normal and indicate that trapped air is being removed from the chest. *Frequent assessment of the system is important to ensure appropriate functioning.*
- Measure drainage every 8 hours, marking the level on the drainage chamber. Report drainage that is cloudy, in excess of 70 mL per hour, or red, warm, and free flowing. *Red, free-flowing drainage indicates hemorrhage; cloudiness may indicate an infection. Emptying the drainage would disrupt integrity of the closed system.*
- In systems using water to regulate suction, periodically assess water level in the suction control chamber, adding water as necessary. *Adequate water in the suction control chamber prevents excess suction from being placed on delicate pleural tissue.*
- Assist with frequent position changes and sitting and ambulation as allowed. *Chest tubes should not prevent performance of allowed activities. Care is needed to prevent inadvertent disconnection or removal of the tubes.*
- When the chest tube is removed, immediately apply a sterile occlusive petroleum jelly dressing. *An occlusive dressing prevents air from reentering the pleural space through the chest wound.*

and participate in programs to prevent smoking among children and teenagers. Teach safe behaviors such as always wearing a seat beat in an automobile, driving safely, and using precautions to prevent falls when working or recreating in high places.

Assessment

The client with pneumothorax may be in acute respiratory distress, necessitating rapid and focused assessment.

- *Health History:* Current symptoms and their duration; precipitating factors or activities if known; previous episodes of pneumothorax; smoking history; chronic pulmonary diseases such as COPD.
- *Physical Assessment:* General appearance and degree of apparent respiratory distress; evidence of chest trauma; vital signs, oxygen saturation, skin color, LOC, respiratory excursion, percussion tone, and breath sounds anterior and posterior chest; neck vein inspection, position of trachea; peripheral pulses.
- *Diagnostic Tests:* Chest x-ray, ABGs.

Nursing Diagnoses and Interventions

Maintaining or restoring adequate alveolar ventilation and gas exchange is of highest priority for the client with a pneumothorax. Chest tubes may interfere with physical mobility, contributing to a high risk for injury.

Impaired Gas Exchange

Loss of negative pressure in the pleural cavity and the resulting collapse of lung tissue can cause poor chest expansion and loss of alveolar ventilation. As the pneumothorax is removed or reabsorbed, ventilation and gas exchange improve.

- Assess and document vital signs and respiratory status, including rate, depth, lung sounds, and oxygen saturation at least every 4 hours. *Frequent assessment is important to monitor the adequacy of respirations and lung expansion.*

PRACTICE ALERT
Evaluate chest wall movement, position of the trachea, and neck veins frequently. Early identification of tension pneumothorax and appropriate interventions are vital to preserve cardiorespiratory function.

- Place in Fowler's or high-Fowler's position. *This position facilitates lung expansion.*
- Administer oxygen as ordered. *Supplemental oxygen is given to improve oxygenation of the blood and tissues.*

PRACTICE ALERT
Provide emotional support, particularly in early stages and during chest tube insertion. Dyspnea and hypoxemia can cause extreme anxiety and apprehension, impairing the ability to cooperate with procedures.

- Assess chest tube, system function, and drainage at least every 2 hours. *The system must remain patent and intact to function effectively.*
- Provide for rest. *Adequate rest is important to conserve energy and reduce oxygen demand.*

Risk for Injury

Pain and the presence of chest tubes can reduce the perceived ability to ambulate and provide self-care. Moderate activity is encouraged unless respiratory function is significantly impaired. Caution is taken to maintain integrity of the chest tube system. If the tube is inadvertently pulled out or system integrity is disrupted, the pneumothorax may increase or infection may develop.

PRACTICE ALERT
Avoid placing tension on chest tubes during positioning, ambulation, and care activities. The chest tubes are minimally secured to the chest wall and can be dislodged if tension is placed on them.

- Secure a loop of drainage tubing to the sheet or gown. *Looping the drainage tubing prevents direct pressure on the chest tube itself.*
- When turning to the affected side, ensure that neither the chest tube nor drainage tubing is kinked or occluded under the client. *This maintains patency of the system.*
- Teach the client how to ambulate with the drainage system, keeping the system lower than the chest. In most cases, suction can be discontinued during ambulation. *Ambulation facilitates lung ventilation and expansion. Drainage systems are portable to allow ambulation while chest tubes are in place. Keeping the drainage system lower than the chest promotes drainage and prevents reflux.*
- Observe insertion site for redness, swelling, pain, or drainage. Report any signs of infection, including fever, to the physician. *Interruption of skin integrity by chest tube insertion increases the risk for infection.*
- If a connection comes loose, reconnect it as soon as possible. *A closed, sealed system is vital to prevent air from entering the pleural space and an open pneumothorax.*

PRACTICE ALERT
Seal the wound of an open pneumothorax or a wound from inadvertent tube removal as soon as possible with a sterile occlusive dressing, such as gauze impregnated with petroleum jelly. If a sterile dressing is not available, other occlusive material such as foil or plastic wrap can be used. Tape the dressing on three sides only. An occlusive dressing taped on three sides prevents the development of a tension pneumothorax by inhibiting air from entering the wound during inhalation but allowing it to escape during exhalation.

Community-Based Care

Clients who have experienced spontaneous pneumothorax need education about their future risk. After a single episode of spontaneous pneumothorax, the risk of recurrence is 40% to 50%. This risk increases with subsequent episodes (Way & Doherty, 2003). Stress the importance of quitting smoking to reduce the risk. Other activities that can precipitate recurrent episodes include mountain climbing or those involving exposure to high altitudes, flying in unpressurized aircraft, and

carbon dioxide, ABGs, and pulmonary artery pressures as ordered and indicated. Report changes to the physician. Maintain oxygen flow rates as ordered. Provide frequent mouth care to reduce the discomfort of dry mucous membranes and prevent tissue breakdown. Work with respiratory therapy to maintain effective oxygen delivery with mechanical ventilation. Administer sedation as required. Maintain fluid restriction if ordered.

Ineffective Tissue Perfusion: Cerebral

Impaired cerebral tissue perfusion is a priority problem, especially with near-drowning. Hypoxia and possible hypervolemia can lead to cerebral edema and increased intracranial pressure (IICP), further impairing blood flow. Monitor vital signs and neurologic status frequently. A change in level of consciousness or behavior is typically the earliest sign of IICP. Changes noted on an intracranial pressure monitor also provide early evidence of IICP. Increasing systolic blood pressure and pulse pressure and slowed heart rate are late signs. Other manifestations may include pupillary changes and decreasing muscle strength. Report changes promptly to the physician. Elevate the head of the bed and keep the head in neutral position to promote drainage

from the cranial vault. Maintain effective ventilation and oxygenation; hypercapnia and hypoxemia increase cerebral edema. Administer sedation, osmotic diuretics, or corticosteroids as ordered to reduce cerebral edema. Maintain fluid restriction. Space activities and promote rest to reduce metabolic demands.

Community-Based Care

Teach clients who do not require hospitalization for inhalation injury about symptoms that may indicate a complication and should be reported to the physician: increasing dyspnea, cough productive of purulent or pink frothy mucus, confusion, or other changes. Manifestations of respiratory damage may not be apparent for 24 to 48 hours following the injury.

Significant hypoxia due to near-drowning or carbon monoxide poisoning may cause permanent neurologic effects. Work with the family to develop communication techniques and identify remaining strengths. Help the family identify future care needs and means for meeting them, such as home health, personal care aides, or long-term care facilities. Provide social services and support group referrals.

LUNG CANCER

THE CLIENT WITH LUNG CANCER

Lung cancer is the leading cause of cancer deaths among all racial groups in the United States, accounting for 31% of all cancer deaths in men and 27% of all cancer deaths in women. In 2005, more than 168,000 people died from lung cancer in the United States; an estimated 184,800 new cases were diagnosed in that same year (American Cancer Society [ACS], 2005). It is a major health problem with a grim prognosis: Most people with lung cancer die within 1 year of the initial diagnosis.

Incidence and Risk Factors

The incidence of lung cancer varies from state to state and among nations. It increases with age, occurring most commonly in clients over age 50. Family clusters of lung cancer suggest a genetic predisposition; however, exposure to tobacco smoke may be necessary for expression of the trait. Cigarette smoke, which contains 43 known chemical carcinogens and cancer promoters, is clearly the most significant cause of lung cancer (ACS, 2005). More than 80% of lung cancer cases are related to smoking, and the disease is 10 times more common in smokers than nonsmokers. There is a dose–response relationship between smoking and lung cancer; the more the person smokes and the longer the person smokes, the greater the risk. Even former smokers who have abstained for a number of years have a higher risk of developing lung cancer than nonsmokers. Exposure to ionizing radiation and inhaled irritants, asbestos in particular, is also recognized as a risk factor for lung cancer (Porth, 2005). Exposure to radon, a radioactive gas, also is identified as a lung cancer risk factor (ACS, 2005). Radon forms as radium, an element present in the earth's crust, disintegrates. Radon tends to accumulate in closed spaces where air circulation is poor, such as caves, mines, and energy-efficient houses.

FAST FACTS

- In the United States, the incidence of lung cancer is second to prostate cancer in men and breast cancer in women.
- Lung cancer is, however, the leading cause of cancer deaths in the United States, responsible for 31% of cancer deaths in men and 27% of cancer deaths in women.
- Tobacco use and exposure to cigarette smoke are the leading risk factors for lung cancer.

Pathophysiology

Lung cancer develops as damaged bronchial epithelial cells mutate over time to become neoplastic. The genetic abnormality commonly seen is on chromosome 3, with loss of genetic material. Alterations of tumor suppressor genes also are seen in some types of lung cancer.

The vast majority of primary lung lesions are *bronchogenic carcinoma,* tumors of the airway epithelium. These tumors are further differentiated by cell type: small-cell carcinoma, adenocarcinoma, squamous cell carcinoma, and large-cell carcinoma. For clinical purposes, the latter three cell types frequently are classified together as non–small-cell carcinomas. *Small-cell carcinomas,* which account for approximately 25% of lung cancers, grow rapidly and spread early. These tumors have paraneoplastic properties; that is, they produce manifestations at sites that are not directly affected by the tumor. Small-cell lung carcinomas can synthesize bioactive products and hormones such as adrenocorticotropic hormones (ACTH), antidiuretic hormone (ADH), a parathormone-like hormone, and gastrin-releasing peptide. *Non–small-cell carcinoma* accounts for about 75% of lung cancers. Each cell type differs in its incidence, presentation, and manner of spread. Table 38–8 outlines the incidence and unique characteristics of each cell type.

TABLE 38–8 Comparison of Lung Cancer Cell Types

	CELL TYPE AND PREVALENCE	PRESENTATION AND ASSOCIATED MANIFESTATIONS	SPREAD
	Small-cell (oat cell) carcinoma: 20% to 25% of all lung cancers	Central lesion with hilar mass common, early mediastinal involvement, no cavitation; SIADH, Cushing's syndrome, thrombophlebitis	Aggressive tumor; more than 40% of clients have distant metastasis at time of presentation
	Adenocarcinoma: 20% to 40% of all lung cancers	Peripheral mass involving bronchi; few local symptoms; hypertrophic pulmonary osteoarthropathy	Early metastasis to CNS, skeleton, and adrenal glands
	Squamous cell carcinoma: 30% to 32% of all lung cancers	Central lesion located in large bronchi; client presents with cough, dyspnea, atelectasis, and wheezing; hypercalcemia common	Spreads by local invasion
	Large-cell carcinoma: 10% to 15% of all lung cancers	Usually, peripheral lesion that is larger than that associated with adenocarcinoma and tends to cavitate; gynecomastia, thrombophlebitis	Early metastasis

Bronchogenic cancer, regardless of cell type, tends to be aggressive, locally invasive, and have widespread metastatic lesions. Tumors begin as mucosal lesions that grow to form masses that obstruct the bronchi or invade adjacent lung tissue. All types frequently spread via the lymph system to nodes and other organs such as the brain, bones, and liver.

Manifestations

The manifestations of lung cancer are related to the location and spread of the tumor. Clients may present with symptoms related to the primary tumor, manifestations of metastatic disease, or with systemic symptoms. Initial symptoms often are attributed to smoking or chronic bronchitis. Chronic cough is common, as is hemoptysis. Wheezing and shortness of breath occur as a result of airway obstruction. Dull, aching chest pain occurs as the tumor spreads to the mediastinum; pleuritic pain occurs when the pleura is invaded. Hoarseness and/or dysphagia indicates pressure of the tumor on the trachea or esophagus.

Systemic and paraneoplastic manifestations of lung cancer include weight loss, anorexia, fatigue, and weakness; bone pain, tenderness, and swelling; clubbing of the fingers and toes; and various endocrine, neuromuscular, cardiovascular, and hematologic symptoms. The *Multisystem Effects of Lung Cancer* are illustrated on the next page.

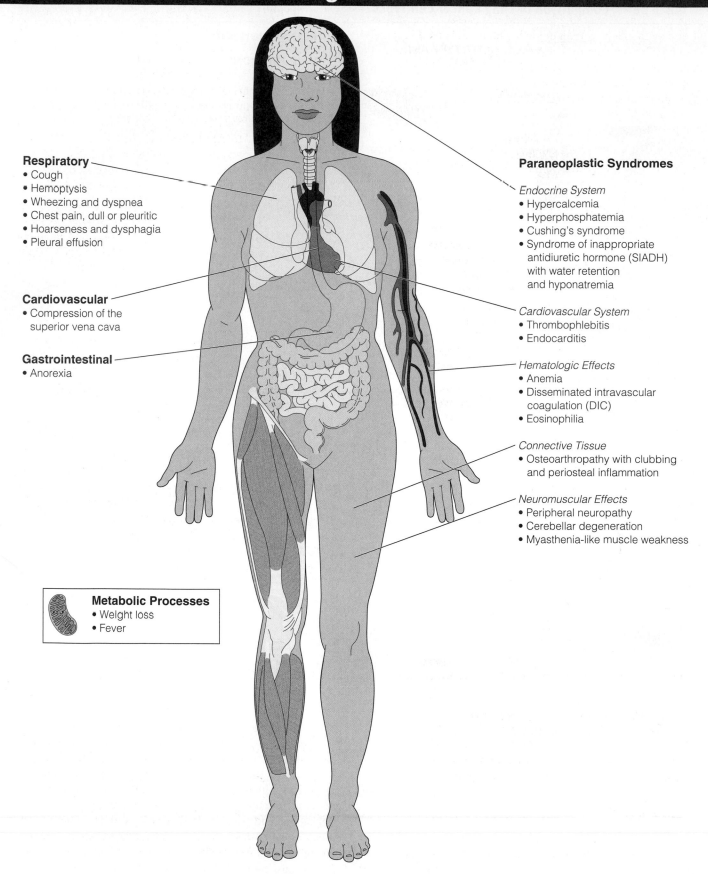

Respiratory
- Cough
- Hemoptysis
- Wheezing and dyspnea
- Chest pain, dull or pleuritic
- Hoarseness and dysphagia
- Pleural effusion

Cardiovascular
- Compression of the superior vena cava

Gastrointestinal
- Anorexia

Metabolic Processes
- Weight loss
- Fever

Paraneoplastic Syndromes

Endocrine System
- Hypercalcemia
- Hyperphosphatemia
- Cushing's syndrome
- Syndrome of inappropriate antidiuretic hormone (SIADH) with water retention and hyponatremia

Cardiovascular System
- Thrombophlebitis
- Endocarditis

Hematologic Effects
- Anemia
- Disseminated intravascular coagulation (DIC)
- Eosinophilia

Connective Tissue
- Osteoarthropathy with clubbing and periosteal inflammation

Neuromuscular Effects
- Peripheral neuropathy
- Cerebellar degeneration
- Myasthenia-like muscle weakness

Confusion, impaired gait and balance, headache, and personality changes may indicate brain metastasis. Bone metastases cause bone pain, pathologic fractures, and possible spinal cord compression, as well as thrombocytopenia and anemia if bone marrow is invaded. When the liver is affected, symptoms of liver dysfunction and biliary obstruction—including jaundice, anorexia, and upper right quadrant pain—are evident.

Complications and Course

Superior vena cava syndrome, partial or complete obstruction of the superior vena cava, is a potential complication of lung cancer, particularly when the tumor involves the superior mediastinum or the mediastinal lymph nodes. Obstructed venous flow from the head and neck produces the symptoms of superior vena cava syndrome (edema of the neck and face, headache, dizziness, vision disturbances, and syncope) and may develop acutely or more gradually. Veins of the upper chest and neck are dilated; flushing occurs, followed by cyanosis. Cerebral edema may affect the level of consciousness; laryngeal edema may impair respirations.

Paraneoplastic syndromes commonly associated with lung cancer include syndrome of inappropriate ADH secretion (SIADH) with fluid retention, hyponatremia, and edema, Cushing's syndrome (see Chapter 19 ∞) related to abnormal ACTH production, and hypercalcemia. Lung tumors also may produce procoagulation factors, increasing the risk for venous thrombosis, pulmonary embolism, and thrombotic endocarditis. In lung cancer, neuromuscular symptoms such as muscle weakness and wasting of the limbs may be the first indication of the disease (Porth, 2005).

At the time of diagnosis, cancer of the lung typically is well advanced, with distant metastasis present in 55% of clients and regional lymph node involvement in another 25%. The prognosis is generally poor: The overall 5-year survival rate is only 15% (ACS, 2005).

INTERDISCIPLINARY CARE

Because lung cancer typically is advanced when diagnosed and the prognosis generally is poor, prevention of the disease must be a primary goal for all healthcare providers. With 80% of lung cancer related to cigarette smoking, reducing tobacco use can have a significant impact on the death rate from lung cancer—a far greater impact than advances in treatment.

Establishing an accurate diagnosis is the first step in treating lung cancer. Treatment decisions are based on the tumor location, type of cancer cell, staging of the tumor, and the client's ability to tolerate treatment. Lung cancer is staged by the tumor size, location, degree of invasion of the primary tumor, and the presence of metastatic disease. Lung cancer staging is summarized in Table 38–9. Surgery is the treatment of choice for most forms of lung cancer.

Diagnosis

- *Chest x-ray* usually provides the first evidence of lung cancer. It is particularly reliable as a diagnostic tool when compared with previous chest x-ray. In high-risk populations, the chest x-ray may be used as a screening tool for lung cancer.
- *Sputum specimen* is sent for *cytologic examination* to establish the diagnosis of lung cancer. The sputum sample is collected on arising in the morning. If malignant cells are found in the sputum, more expensive and invasive examinations may be unnecessary. However, a sputum sample negative for malignant cells does not rule out lung cancer; it may simply indicate that the tumor is not shedding cells into mucous secretions.

TABLE 38–9 Lung Cancer Staging

	PRIMARY TUMOR (T STAGE)	REGIONAL LYMPH NODES (N)	DISTANT METASTASIS (M)
Stage 0	T_0—No evidence of primary tumor T_X—Malignant cells in bronchopulmonary secretions, but no tumor visualized		M_X—Presence of distant metastasis cannot be assessed
Stage I	T_1S—Carcinoma *in situ*	N_0—No regional lymph node metastasis	M_0—No distant metastasis
Stage II	T_1—Tumor that is 3 cm in diameter or less, with no evidence of invasion T_2—Tumor that is greater than 3 cm in diameter, or invades visceral pleura, or has associated atelectasis or pneumonitis	N_1—Metastasis or direct extension to peribronchial or ipsilateral hilar nodes	
Stage III	T_3—Tumor with direct extension into an adjacent structure, or any tumor with associated pleural effusion or atelectasis or pneumonitis of entire lung	N_2—Metastasis to ipsilateral mediastinal or subcarinal nodes	
Stage IV	T_4—Tumor that invades mediastinum or involves the heart, great vessels, trachea, esophagus, vertebral body, or carina; presence of malignant pleural effusion	N_3—Metastasis to contralateral mediastinal, scalene, or supraclavicular nodes	M_1—Distant metastasis present

- *Bronchoscopy* is frequently done to visualize and obtain tissue for biopsy from the tumor. When a tumor mass or suspicious tissue is identified visually, a cable-activated instrument is used to obtain a biopsy specimen. If the tumor cannot be seen, the airways may be flushed with a saline solution (bronchial washing) to obtain cells for cytologic examination. Nursing care of the client undergoing a bronchoscopy is included in the Diagnostic Tests box in Chapter 36 ∞.
- *CT scan* is used to evaluate and localize tumors, particularly tumors in the lung parenchyma and pleura. It also is done prior to needle biopsy to localize the tumor. CT scanning can also detect distant tumor metastasis and evaluate tumor response to treatment.
- Cells or tissue for *cytologic examination and biopsy* may be obtained by aspirating fluid from a pleural effusion, percutaneous needle biopsy, and lymph node biopsy. These procedures may be done in an outpatient or a surgical setting.
- *CBC, liver function studies,* and *serum electrolytes* including calcium are obtained to evaluate for evidence of metastatic disease or paraneoplastic syndromes.
- *Tuberculin test (PPD)* is performed to rule out tuberculosis as the cause of symptoms and abnormalities seen on chest x-ray.
- *Pulmonary function tests (PFTs)* and *ABGs* may be performed prior to the initiation of treatment if the client has manifestations of respiratory insufficiency (e.g., dyspnea, activity intolerance, low oxygen saturation levels).

See Chapter 36 ∞ for nursing care related to commonly used diagnostic tests for lung cancer.

Medications

Combination chemotherapy (often combined with radiation therapy and/or surgery) is the treatment of choice for small-cell lung cancer because of its rapid growth, dissemination, and sensitivity to cytotoxic drugs. Used in combination, chemotherapeutic drugs allow tumor cells to be attacked at different parts of the cell cycle and in different ways, increasing the effectiveness of therapy. Fifty percent of clients with tumors at early stages achieve complete tumor remission with combination chemotherapy. When a complete tumor response is achieved in the first few cycles of chemotherapy, the chances for long-term survival are much greater.

Combination chemotherapy is used also as an adjunct to surgery or radiation therapy for other types of lung cancer. It may be used to reduce the size of advanced local tumors prior to surgery, and to lengthen survival when distant metastases are present. See Chapter 14 ∞ for further discussion of chemotherapy.

Bronchodilators may be prescribed to reduce airway obstruction. Analgesics and pain management strategies are vital when the cancer is advanced. See Chapter 9 ∞ for more information about postoperative and cancer pain management.

Surgery

Surgery offers the only real chance for a cure in non–small-cell lung cancer. Unfortunately, most tumors are inoperable or only partially resectable at the time of diagnosis. The 5-year survival rate following curative surgery in clients with resectable tumors is about 30%, with most clients succumbing to metastatic disease within 5 years (Kasper et al., 2005). The type of surgery performed depends on the location and size of the tumor, as well as the client's pulmonary and general health. The goal of surgery is to remove all involved tissue while preserving as much functional lung as possible. Table 38–10 outlines various surgical procedures used to treat lung cancer. Nursing care for the client having lung surgery is outlined in the box on page 1313.

Radiation Therapy

Radiation therapy is used alone or in combination with surgery or chemotherapy for lung cancer. The treatment goal may be either cure or symptom relief (palliative). Prior to surgery, radiation therapy is used to "debulk" tumors. When cancer has spread by direct extension to other thoracic structures and surgery is not feasible, radiation therapy may be the treatment of choice. It also may be used to relieve manifestations such as cough, hemoptysis, pain due to bone metastasis, and dyspnea from bronchial obstruction. Complications of lung cancer, such as superior vena cava syndrome, may be treated with radiation.

TABLE 38–10 Types of Surgery for Lung Cancer

PROCEDURE	DESCRIPTION	USED FOR
Laser bronchoscopy	Bronchoscopy-guided laser used to resect tumor	Tumors localized in a main bronchus
Mediastinoscopy	Visualization of the mediastinum using an endoscope passed through a suprasternal incision	Evaluation and biopsy of a mediastinal tumor and lymph nodes
Thoracotomy	Incision into the chest wall	Access the lung and thoracic cavity for surgery
Wedge resection	Removal of a small section (wedge) of peripheral lung tissue	Small, peripheral lung tumors
Segmental resection	Removal of an individual bronchovascular segment of a lobe	Peripheral lung tumor with no evidence of extension to the chest wall or metastasis
Sleeve resection (bronchoplastic reconstruction)	Resection of a section of a major bronchus with reconstruction of remaining normal bronchus	Small lesion of a major bronchus
Lobectomy	Removal of a single lung lobe	Tumors confined to a single lobe
Pneumonectomy	Removal of an entire lung	Tumor widespread throughout the lung, involving the main bronchus, or fixed to the hilum

NURSING CARE OF THE CLIENT HAVING Lung Surgery

PREOPERATIVE CARE

- Provide routine preoperative nursing care as outlined in Chapter 4 ∞.
- Note any history of smoking, respiratory and cardiac diseases, and other chronic conditions in the nursing history. *These factors may affect the response to surgery and the risk for postoperative complications.*
- Provide emotional and psychologic support for the client and family. *In addition to facing surgery, the client may be adjusting to a new diagnosis of cancer and the possibility that surgical intervention will be only partially successful.*
- Instruct about postoperative procedures, including respiratory therapy, breathing exercises, and coughing techniques. Allow practice time. *Learning will be easier in the preoperative period, when pain and analgesia are not affecting mental function.*
- If the client will return from surgery with an endotracheal tube and mechanical ventilation, establish a means of communication using hand or eye signals or a magic slate. *Establishing a means of communication prior to surgery reduces postoperative anxiety at being unable to speak.*
- If the client will return to the ICU, introduce the client and family to the unit and any machines, such as ventilators and monitors, that will be used. *The knowledge that this is an expected part of surgical recovery reduces the client's and family's postoperative anxiety.*

POSTOPERATIVE CARE

- Assess and provide routine postoperative care as outlined in Chapter 4 ∞.
- Assess for adequate pain control, and provide analgesics as needed. *Incisional pain commonly causes altered breathing patterns in the client who has undergone lung surgery.*
- Frequently assess respiratory status, including color, oxygen saturation, respiratory rate and depth, chest expansion, lung sounds, percussion tone, and ABGs. *Maintaining adequate ventilation and gas exchange postoperatively is vital to reduce mortality and morbidity. Gas exchange may be impaired*

by complications of lung surgery, including pneumothorax, atelectasis, bronchospasm, pulmonary embolus, bronchopleural fistula, and ARDS.

- Assist with effective coughing techniques, postural drainage, and incentive spirometry. Perform endotracheal suctioning as needed while intubated. *Surgical manipulation and anesthesia can increase the mucous production, leading to airway obstruction. Aggressive pulmonary hygiene is important to prevent this complication.*
- Monitor and maintain effective mechanical ventilation. *This is vital to ensure adequate ventilation and gas exchange in the early postoperative period.*
- Maintain patent chest tubes and a closed drainage system. Monitor chest tube output every hour initially, then every 2 to 4 or 8 hours as indicated. Notify the physician if chest tube output exceeds 70 mL per hour and/or is bright red, warm, and free flowing. *Maintaining a patent, intact chest drainage system is vital to reestablish negative pressure within the chest cavity and reexpansion of the lungs. Increased amounts of warm, free-flowing blood indicate intrathoracic hemorrhage that may necessitate surgical intervention.*
- Assess for signs of infection involving the incision or chest tube site(s). Use strict aseptic technique in caring for incisions and invasive monitoring devices. *The postoperative client is at risk for incisional infections, empyema in the chest cavity, and pneumonia.*
- Assist with turning and to ambulate as soon as possible. *Early mobility is important to prevent possible complications, such as pneumonia or pulmonary embolus.*
- Assess and maintain nutritional status. Initiate enteral or parenteral nutrition early if intubation and mechanical ventilation will be required for an extended period. Provide frequent small feedings once extubated. *Maintaining nutritional status promotes wound healing and prevents negative nitrogen balance. Giving frequent small feedings reduces the fatigue associated with eating.*

Radiation therapy may be delivered by external beam to the primary tumor site or by intraluminal radiation, or brachytherapy. Radiation therapy and related nursing care are discussed further in Chapter 14 ∞. Specific nursing measures for the client undergoing radiation therapy for lung cancer are outlined in the Nursing Care box on page 1314.

Complementary Therapies

Research indicates that a significant number of clients diagnosed with lung cancer use complementary and alternative medicine (CAM). In one study of clients with lung cancer in eight European nations, 23.6% used CAM therapies (Molassiotis et al., 2006). The CAM remedies used included herbal medicines, medicinal teas, homeopathy, animal extracts, and spiritual therapies. While these therapies may be safe when used alone, the potential for interactions with conventional medical treatment must be considered. Inquire of clients about their use of complementary and alternative therapies, and inform members of the healthcare team when present.

 NURSING CARE

Health Promotion

The incidence of lung cancer is decreasing as the use of tobacco products declines. Teach people of all ages, particularly children and teenagers, about the link between cigarette smoking and lung cancer. Not smoking and avoiding exposure to secondhand smoke is the primary preventive measure for lung cancer. In addition, explain the risk of lung cancer to clients with occupational risk factors, exposure to asbestos products in particular.

Assessment

Nursing assessment related to lung cancer focuses on identifying risk factors for the disease, early manifestations of lung cancer, and respiratory function in the client undergoing treatment.

- *Health History:* Current symptoms, including chronic cough, shortness of breath, blood-tinged sputum; systemic

NURSING CARE OF THE CLIENT RECEIVING Radiation Therapy

Although radiation therapy is well controlled and specifically directed toward the tumor cells, some normal cells are also damaged in the process of treatment. Nursing care and client teaching help the client cope with uncomfortable side effects associated with radiation therapy.

Nursing Responsibilities
- Monitor for potential complications:
  a. Radiation pneumonitis—dyspnea on exertion, dry cough, fever
  b. Pericarditis—chest pain, pericardial friction rub; muffled heart sounds, paradoxical pulse, ECG abnormalities (Notify the physician if symptoms develop.)
  c. Esophagitis—pain, sore throat, difficulty swallowing.
- Encourage adequate fluid intake to liquefy respiratory secretions.
- Provide local analgesics and local anesthetics such as viscous lidocaine as ordered to relieve dysphagia and sore throat.
- Offer small frequent meals of soft, cool foods and liquids to maintain nutritional status.

Health Education for the Client and Family
- If dyspnea or pneumonitis develop, teach positioning, pursed-lip techniques, and relaxation exercises to facilitate breathing.
- Reassure that pneumonitis is generally a self-limiting process and should resolve when the course of radiotherapy is completed.
- Teach the manifestations of pericarditis, which may develop during treatment or up to 1 year after its completion. Chest pain or pressure, rapid heartbeat, and fever may signal pericarditis; increasing fatigue, dyspnea, and light-headedness can indicate a chronic process with pericardial effusion and possible cardiac tamponade.
- Instruct to eliminate hot, spicy, or acidic foods from the diet if esophagitis is a problem. Alcohol and tobacco should also be avoided.
- Adequate rest and nutrition are important to alleviate the symptoms of radiation fatigue, which is common in clients receiving radiation therapy for lung cancer. The fatigue is generally temporary.

---

manifestations such as recent weight loss, fatigue, anorexia, bone pain; smoking history; occupational exposure to carcinogens; chronic diseases such as COPD.
- *Physical Examination:* General appearance; skin color, evidence of clubbing; weight and height; vital signs; respiratory rate, depth, excursion; lung sounds to percussion and auscultation.
- *Diagnostic Tests:* CBC and coagulation studies, serum electrolytes and osmolality, liver and renal function studies; chest x-ray and CT scan results; ABGs and oxygen saturation levels.

Nursing Diagnoses and Interventions

The client with lung cancer is facing invasive treatments with undesirable side effects, possibly surgery, and typically a poor prognosis for long-term survival. Nursing care needs are diverse, related to respiratory status, the cancer itself and possible metastases, and the treatment plan. Priority nursing diagnoses related to respiratory function include *Ineffective Breathing Pattern* and *Activity Intolerance*. *Pain* and *Anticipatory Grieving* also are likely to be high-priority problems. See the accompanying Nursing Care Plan on page 1315.

Ineffective Breathing Pattern

Breathing pattern and ventilation may be affected by the tumor itself or by treatment of the tumor. Thoracic surgery increases the risk due to the incision and disruption of the muscles of respiration. Maintaining effective lung ventilation is particularly important postoperatively to reexpand remaining lung tissue and prevent surgical complications.

- Assess and document respiratory rate, depth, and lung sounds at least every 4 hours; evaluate more frequently in the immediate postoperative period or as indicated by condition. *Early detection of signs of respiratory compromise or adventitious lung sounds is vital for effective intervention.*

PRACTICE ALERT
Monitor oxygen saturation, exhaled carbon dioxide, and/or blood gas results, reporting changes from normal. Changes in levels of blood oxygen or exhaled CO_2 may be early indications of respiratory compromise.

- Frequently assess and document pain level (using a standard pain scale); provide analgesics as needed. *Pain and attempting to avoid chest movement to prevent additional pain can lead to rapid, shallow respirations and ineffective ventilation.*
- Elevate the head of the bed to 60 degrees. *Elevating the head of the bed reduces pressure on the diaphragm and permits optimal lung expansion.*
- Assist to turn, cough, and deep breathe and use incentive spirometry. Help splint the chest with a pillow or blanket when coughing. *These measures promote airway clearance.*
- Suction airway as needed. *Suctioning may be required to remove secretions that the client is unable to cough up and expectorate.*

PRACTICE ALERT
Maintain chest tube integrity and patency by ensuring uninterrupted gravity flow. Chest tubes help reestablish negative pressure in the thoracic cavity, allowing the lung to fully reexpand.

- Provide chest physiotherapy with percussion and postural drainage as needed or ordered. *Percussion and postural drainage help maintain airway patency and effective respirations.*
- If mechanical ventilation is instituted, work with respiratory therapy and use analgesia or sedation as needed to synchronize respirations with the ventilator. *Coordination of the*

NURSING CARE PLAN A Client with Lung Cancer

After coughing up bloody sputum one morning, James Mueller, a 68-year-old retired mill worker, sees his physician. A chest x-ray shows a suspicious density in the central portion of his right lung. Mr. Mueller is admitted to the hospital the following Monday for diagnostic tests.

ASSESSMENT

Anita Sarros, RN, admits Mr. Mueller to the oncology unit and obtains a nursing history. Mr. Mueller is married and has three grown children. He worked in a local paper mill for 35 years before retiring at age 62. He describes himself as "pretty healthy," except for a chronic smoker's cough. He started smoking as a young man in the army. He has a 50 pack-year smoking history, having smoked a pack a day for 50 years, since age 18. Mr. Mueller says he briefly quit smoking following a small heart attack 3 years ago, but started again after 4 months. On further questioning, Mr. Mueller says his cough has been productive for the past few months, especially in the morning, and that he is shorter of breath than usual with activity.

Mr. Mueller's examination data include BP 162/86, P 78 and regular, R 20, and T 98.4°F (36.9°C). Color good, skin warm and dry. Inspiratory and expiratory wheezes noted in right chest but good breath sounds throughout. No other abnormal findings are noted on examination. The physician orders early morning sputum specimens times 3 days for cytologic examination and schedules a CT scan of the chest the morning after admission.

Mr. Mueller's CBC shows mild anemia, but remaining routine laboratory tests are essentially normal. Sputum cytology is positive for small-cell bronchogenic cancer. The CT scan shows a central mass approximately 4 cm in diameter with involved mediastinal and subclavicular lymph nodes. A small mass is also noted on the lumbar spine. After conferring with his physician and an oncologist, Mr. Mueller decides to undergo a trial course of chemotherapy.

DIAGNOSES

- *Ineffective Airway Clearance* related to tumor mass
- *Risk for Imbalanced Nutrition: Less than Body Requirements* related to effects of chemotherapy
- *Risk for Compromised Family Coping* related to new diagnosis of lung cancer
- *Deficient Knowledge* about lung cancer and aids to smoking cessation

EXPECTED OUTCOMES

- Maintain a patent airway.
- Maintain current weight.
- Express feelings and concerns about the effect of cancer on the family unit.
- Participate in care.
- Contact appropriate support groups.
- Verbalize an understanding of the disease, its treatment, and prognosis.

- Develop a plan to stop smoking.

PLANNING AND IMPLEMENTATION

- Teach coughing, deep breathing, and hydration measures to facilitate airway clearance.
- Discuss symptoms to report to the physician: increased dyspnea or hemoptysis, severe stridor or wheezing, chest pain.
- Discuss measures to relieve nausea associated with chemotherapy, including premedication with a prescribed antiemetic.
- Have dietitian consult with Mr. and Mrs. Mueller to develop a diet plan for maintaining ideal weight.
- Discuss possible effects of lung cancer with Mr. and Mrs. Mueller.
- Encourage Mr. and Mrs. Mueller to call a family conference to discuss the disease with their children and grandchildren.
- Evaluate family members' knowledge and understanding of lung cancer, correcting misinformation and teaching as needed.
- Have an American Cancer Society volunteer contact the family.
- Refer to local cancer support group.
- Refer to home health department for follow-up and further teaching.
- Work with Mr. Mueller to develop a plan to stop smoking.
- Ask the physician for a prescription for nicotine patches or gum for Mr. Mueller.

EVALUATION

Mr. Mueller had his first chemotherapy treatment in the hospital and was discharged 4 days after admission. After 3 months of chemotherapy, his tumor shows little regression, and a liver scan reveals further metastasis. He and his wife decide to stop chemotherapy, a decision with which the children reluctantly agree. Mr. and Mrs. Mueller are referred to hospice services. With the help of hospice nurses and volunteers, Mr. Mueller is able to remain at home. His pain is managed initially with oral MS Contin, a sustained-release form of morphine sulfate, and later with an intravenous morphine infusion. Mr. Mueller dies at home with his family at his side 9 months after his diagnosis of lung cancer.

CRITICAL THINKING IN THE NURSING PROCESS

1. The oncologist prescribed a chemotherapy regimen of cyclophosphamide, doxorubicin, and vincristine. Describe how each of these drugs works against cancer cells, and discuss the rationale for using this combination.
2. Develop a care plan to deal with the specific side effects for the above treatment regimen.
3. Mr. Mueller had small-cell (oat cell) cancer. How would his presentation and treatment differ if the diagnosis had been non–small-cell adenocarcinoma, stage $T_2N_2M_0$?

See Evaluating Your Response in Appendix C.

---

client's respiratory effort with ventilator-delivered breaths is important for fully effective mechanical ventilation.

- Provide reassurance and emotional support. *These measures help relieve anxiety and promote an effective breathing pattern.*

Activity Intolerance

Both resectional lung surgery and inoperable lung cancer reduce the amount of functional lung tissue and surface area for gas diffusion. This can lead to activity intolerance if the oxygen supply is insufficient to meet the body's oxygen demand.

PRACTICE ALERT

Assess and document physiologic responses to activity, including pulse, respiratory rate, dyspnea, and fatigue. These assessments are good indicators of activity tolerance.

- Plan rest periods between activities and procedures. *Rest periods reduce oxygen demands and fatigue.*
- Assist the postoperative client to increase activities gradually. *Increasing activity levels gradually improves exercise tolerance.*
- Teach measures to conserve energy while performing ADLs, such as sitting while showering and dressing and wearing slip-on shoes. *These energy-conserving measures reduce oxygen demand and allow the client to remain independent as long as possible.*
- Keep frequently used objects within easy reach. *This helps conserve energy.*
- Administer oxygen as prescribed. Teach the client and family about home oxygen use if appropriate. *Supplemental oxygen can help improve activity and exercise tolerance.*
- Encourage maintenance of physical activity to tolerance. *Maintaining activity levels to the degree possible improves physical and emotional well-being.*
- Allow family members to provide assistance as needed. *This helps the client conserve energy and allows the family to retain a sense of usefulness.*

Pain

Pain is a priority problem in both the postoperative period as well as in the terminal stages of cancer. Poorly managed pain prolongs recovery from surgery. In the terminal cancer client, chronic and acute pain must be managed effectively to allow a peaceful death.

- Assess and document pain using a standardized pain scale and objective data. *Pain is a subjective experience, best evaluated by the client. Changes in vital signs, guarded movement, or unwillingness to move may indicate unreported pain.*
- Provide analgesics as needed to maintain comfort. *Postoperative recovery and restoration of function is facilitated by adequate pain management.*
- For cancer pain, maintain an around-the-clock medication schedule using narcotic, nonsteroidal anti-inflammatory drugs, and other medications as ordered. *Addiction is not a concern in terminal cancer; providing adequate pain relief that does not allow "breakthrough" pain is important.*
- Provide or assist with comfort measures, such as massage, positioning, distraction, and relaxation techniques. *These techniques promote relaxation and enhance pain relief.*
- Assist the client and family to plan and engage in activities that distract from pain such as reading, watching television, and engaging in social interactions. *Distraction helps the client focus away from the pain.*
- Spend as much time with the client as possible; allow family members to remain with the client. *Physical presence of the nurse and family provides emotional support for the client.*

Anticipatory Grieving

Because lung cancer often is advanced when diagnosed, the client faces the very real prospect of dying from the disease. Grieving for the anticipated loss of life is a normal response as the client and family begin to adapt to the diagnosis. Nursing care goals are to promote expression of feelings and thoughts about the loss, and to help the client and family initiate grief work, make decisions, and use appropriate resources and coping mechanisms to deal with the loss.

- Spend time with the client and family. *Time is necessary to develop a trusting, therapeutic relationship.*
- Answer questions honestly; do not deny the probable outcome of the disease. *Honesty reinforces reality and provides a sense of control over decisions to be made.*
- Encourage the client and family to express their feelings, fears, and concerns. *Open expression of feelings helps to promote understanding and acceptance.*
- Assist with understanding the grieving process and acceptance of feelings as normal. *Feelings of guilt, anger, or depression may cause the client to withdraw from others. Explanation of the grieving process enhances understanding and ability to cope.*
- Help identify strengths and coping measures that have been used effectively in the past. Provide positive reinforcement for effective coping behavior. *Past effective coping measures can help the client and family deal with the present situation and regain a sense of control.*
- Help the client and family make decisions regarding treatment and care. *This also is important to give them a sense of control.*
- Encourage use of other support systems, such as spiritual and social groups. Refer the client and family to support groups, social support services, and hospice care as indicated. Provide American Cancer Society literature and information as appropriate. *These support systems provide emotional support and help the client and family cope with the diagnosis.*
- Discuss advance directives (the Living Will) and power of attorney for health care with the client and family. *These documents give the client and family a sense of control over medical care provided if the client is no longer able to express his or her own wishes.*

Using NANDA, NIC, and NOC

Linkages between NANDA nursing diagnoses, nursing interventions, and nursing outcomes for the client with lung cancer are illustrated in Chart 38–3.

Community-Based Care

A primary teaching need to prepare the client and family affected by lung cancer for home care is information about the disease itself, expected prognosis, and planned treatment strategies. Provide honest information; do not promote false hope. Include the following additional topics in teaching for home care:

- Importance of quitting smoking, especially if surgery has been performed. (The client with lung cancer may have dif-

NANDA, NIC, AND NOC LINKAGES
CHART 38–3 **The Client with Lung Cancer**

NANDA

Ineffective Coping

↓

NIC

Coping Enhancement

Decision-Making Support

Support System Enhancement

NOC

Coping

Decision Making

Social Support

Data from *NANDA's Nursing Diagnoses: Definitions & Classification 2005–2006* by NANDA Interational (2005), Philadelphia; *Nursing Interventions Classification (NIC)* (4th ed.) by J. M. Dochterman & G. M. Bulechek (2004), St. Louis, MO: Mosby; and *Nursing Outcomes Classification (NOC)* (3rd ed.) by S. Moorhead, M. Johnson, and M. Maas (2004), St. Louis, MO. Mosby.

ficulty recognizing the need to stop smoking. Include information about the effects of nicotine and the tars in cigarette smoke on healing and already compromised lung tissue.)
- Planned treatments such as chemotherapy or radiation therapy, including expected effects and usual side effects of each
- Strategies to cope with noxious effects of radiation or chemotherapy
- Activities and exercises to improve strength and regain function for the postoperative client
- The need to continue coughing and deep-breathing exercises at home
- Symptoms to report to the physician: fever, increasing or continued shortness of breath, cough, increased or purulent sputum, redness, pain, swelling, or incisional drainage
- Use of prescribed medications, including desired and potential side effects and interactions with other drugs or foods
- Use of analgesics and other pain relief measures for postoperative or cancer pain
- Information about hospice services, home health, local cancer support groups for clients and caregivers, and American Cancer Society services.

Refer the client and family for home health services including nursing care, assistance with ADLs, respiratory care, and respite care as needed.

EXPLORE MEDIALINK

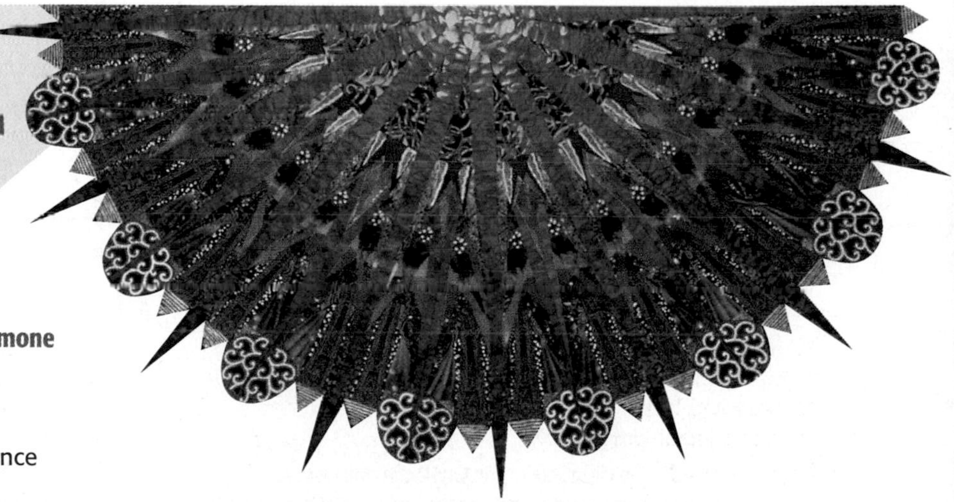

Prentice Hall Nursing MediaLink DVD-ROM
Audio Glossary
NCLEX-RN® Review

Animation
Tuberculosis

COMPANION WEBSITE www.prenhall.com/lemone
Audio Glossary
NCLEX-RN® Review
Care Plan Activity: Pneumonia
Case Study: TB Medication and Compliance
MediaLink Applications
    Health Promotion Among Vulnerable Populations
    SARS
Links to Resources

CHAPTER HIGHLIGHTS

- Pneumonia, inflammation of the respiratory bronchioles and alveoli, usually is bacterial in origin. Different organisms are usually found in hospital-acquired pneumonia than in community-acquired pneumonia. Nursing care focuses on promoting airway clearance, supporting effective gas exchange, and promoting rest.
- Infection control measures, including standard, airborne, and contact precautions, are vital to prevent the spread of viral severe acute respiratory syndrome.

- Tuberculosis affects many people worldwide; in the United States, the primary affected populations are immigrants, people with compromised immunity, and people living in crowded or unsanitary conditions.
- The tuberculin test (PPD) detects a cellular immune response to *M. tuberculosis*, indicating infection, but not necessarily active disease.
- Effective tuberculosis treatment is a public health concern, requiring therapy and compliance monitoring, contact follow-up, and assessment for adverse treatment effects.

- Fungal lung infections tend to have a geographic pattern of distribution. People with compromised immune status are more likely to be affected. Their manifestations resemble those of pneumonia or tuberculosis.
- Disorders of the pleura, such as pleural effusion and pneumothorax, can affect lung expansion, ventilation, and gas exchange when significant.
- Tension pneumothorax develops when air enters the pleural space but is unable to escape, collapsing the lung on the affected side and placing pressure on the unaffected lung and mediastinum. Ventilation, gas exchange, venous return, and cardiac output can be significantly affected.
- Trauma may affect the chest wall (rib fracture, flail chest), the surface of the lungs (pulmonary contusion), or the airways and alveoli (smoke inhalation and near-drowning). Flail chest and pulmonary contusion often occur concurrently; hemothorax also frequently develops with chest trauma. Chest trauma (chest wall or airways) can endanger effective ventilation and gas exchange.
- Lung cancer, the leading cause of cancer deaths, typically is advanced when diagnosed. Surgery, radiation therapy, and chemotherapy are used to treat lung cancer, often in combination.
- Superior vena cava syndrome (impaired venous drainage from the head and neck) and paraneoplastic syndromes (abnormal hormone production, fluid and electrolyte imbalance, and altered clotting with possible venous thrombosis and pulmonary emboli) may complicate lung cancer.

TEST YOURSELF NCLEX-RN® REVIEW

1 Admitting orders for a client with acute bacterial pneumonia include an intravenous antibiotic every 8 hours, oxygen per nasal cannula at 5 L/min, continuous pulse oximetry monitoring, bed rest with bathroom privileges and chair at bedside as desired, diet as tolerated, sputum specimen for C&S, CBC, urinalysis, and chemistry panel. Which order should the nurse carry out first?
 1. Start the oxygen per nasal cannula.
 2. Insert an intravenous catheter and start the prescribed antibiotic.
 3. Provide a dinner tray to the client.
 4. Obtain the sputum specimen.

2 When assessing a client with bacterial pneumonia, the nurse notes that the client's overall skin tone is somewhat gray and there is a bluish tinge around the client's lips. The nurse should: (Place the following in the correct order of priority.)
 1. start oxygen.
 2. assess breath sounds.
 3. notify the physician.
 4. raise the head of the bed.
 5. obtain oxygen saturation level.

3 The nurse evaluating a tuberculin test result 72 hours after it was administered notes an area of induration 9 mm in diameter. What additional information would indicate to the nurse that this is a positive result? The client
 1. resides in a long-term care facility.
 2. was born in Southeast Asia.
 3. has HIV disease.
 4. is an injection drug user.

4 The nurse teaching a client taking prophylactic daily isoniazid (INH) following tuberculin test conversion includes which of the following in the instructions?
 1. This drug turns your urine red-orange. This is harmless.
 2. Report numbness and tingling of your extremities to your doctor.
 3. You will need to have periodic eye examinations during treatment.
 4. Do not use aspirin while taking this drug because abnormal bleeding may occur.

5 Which of the following statements made by a client with a new diagnosis of lung cancer would indicate that the nurse's teaching has been effective?
 1. "Well, since I'm going to die anyway, I may as well go home, put my affairs in order, and spend the rest of my time in the easy chair."
 2. "I understand that because the cancer has already spread, I will be undergoing aggressive cancer treatment for the next several years to beat this thing."
 3. "Even though I can't undo the damage caused by cigarette smoking, I will try to quit to prevent further damage to my lungs."
 4. "Having the 'big C' is very scary; I'm just glad it is one of the more curable forms of cancer."

6 The nurse caring for a client following a lobectomy notes 100 mL of red drainage in the chest drainage container since checking it 30 minutes previously. The nurse should: (Select all that apply.)
 1. empty the chest-tube drainage system.
 2. note the finding and reevaluate drainage in 30 minutes.
 3. notify the surgeon.
 4. assess vital signs and level of consciousness.
 5. apply pressure to the chest tube insertion site.

7 The nurse caring for a client having a thoracentesis appropriately assists the client to:
 1. sit upright leaning forward during the procedure.
 2. breathe deeply as the needle is inserted.
 3. remain on quiet bed rest for 4 hours following the procedure.
 4. cough as the fluid is withdrawn.

8 The nurse teaches a client being discharged from the emergency department with a diagnosis of fractured rib to:
 1. avoid using pain medications to prevent respiratory depression.
 2. use elastic roller bandages (ACE wraps) to stabilize the chest wall and promote comfort.
 3. remain on bed rest for a week to allow the fracture to stabilize.
 4. use a small pillow to splint the area when coughing.

9 Which of the following assessment findings of a client with smoke inhalation does the nurse find of greatest concern?
 1. ash-like material in the sputum
 2. respiratory rate of 36
 3. skin and mucous membranes pink
 4. fine crackles in bilateral bases

10 Which of the following nursing diagnoses does the nurse identify as of highest priority for a client with tension pneumothorax?
 1. *Decreased Cardiac Output*
 2. *Ineffective Breathing Pattern*
 3. *Acute Pain*
 4. *Risk for Aspiration*

See Test Yourself answers in Appendix C.

BIBLIOGRAPHY

Ahrens, T., Kollef, M., Stewart, J., & Shannon, W. (2004). Effect of kinetic therapy on pulmonary complications. *American Journal of Critical Care, 13*(5), 376–383.

Ailinger, R. L., Armstrong, R., Nguyen, N., & Lasus, H. (2004). Latino immigrants' knowledge of tuberculosis. *Public Health Nursing, 21*(6), 519–523.

American Cancer Society. (2005). *Cancer facts and figures 2005.* Atlanta: Author.

American Thoracic Society, CDC, & Infectious Diseases Society of America. (2003). Treatment of tuberculosis. *MMWR Recommendations and Reports, 55*(RR11), 1–77. Retrieved from: http://cdc.gov/mmwr/preview/mmwrhtml/rr5211al.htm

Banning, M. (2005). Community acquired pneumonia: Common causes, treatment and resistance. *Nurse Prescribing, 3*(5), 195–200.

Barry, R. M. (2004). Penetrating chest wounds. *RN, 67*(5), 36, 42.

Carlisle, D. (2005). Targeted TB prevention. *Community Practitioner, 78*(11), 385–386.

Cava, M. A., Fay, K. E., Beanlands, H. J., McCay, E. A., & Wignall, R. (2005). Risk perception and compliance with quarantine during the SARS outbreak. *Journal of Nursing Scholarship, 37*(4), 343–347.

Centers for Disease Control and Prevention (CDC). (2004). Fact sheet. Basic information about SARS. Retrieved from www.cdc.gov/ncidod/sars/pdf/factsheet.pdf.

_____. (2005). Public health guidance for community-level preparedness and responses to severe acute respiratory syndrome (SARS) Version 2/3. Retrieved from www.cdc.gov/ncidod/sars/guidance/index.htm

_____. (2006a). Emergence of *Mycobacterium tuberculosis* with extensive resistance to second-line drugs—worldwide, 2000–2004. *MMWR, 55*(11), 301–305.

_____. (2006b). Trends in tuberculosis—United States, 2005. *MMWR, 55*(11), 305–308.

_____. (2006c). World TB day—March 24, 2006. *MMWR, 55*(11), 301.

Chatterjee, M. (2005). Vulnerable TB patients slipping through the net. *Nursing Times, 101*(6), 7.

Chernecky, C., Sarna, L., Waller, J. L., & Bracht, M. L. (2004). Assessing coughing and wheezing in lung cancer: A pilot study. *Oncology Nursing Forum, 31*(6), 1095–1101.

Clinical rounds: Bioterrorism. How to identify inhalation anthrax. (2004). *Nursing, 34*(10), 34–35.

Coleman, P. R. (2004). Pneumonia in the long-term care setting: Etiology, management and prevention. *Journal of Gerontological Nursing, 30*(4), 14–23, 54–55.

Copstead, L. C., & Banasik, J. L. (2005). *Pathophysiology* (3rd ed.). St. Louis, MO: Elsevier/Saunders.

Darlison, L. (2005). Respiratory care. Lung cancer: An update on current diagnostic techniques and treatment. *Nursing Times, 101*(14), 42–44, 46.

DeBoer, S., & O'Connor, A. (2004). Prehospital and emergency department burn care. *Critical Care Nursing Clinics of North America, 16*(1), 61–73.

Dent, M. (2004). Hospital-acquired pneumonia: The "gift" that keeps on taking. *Nursing, 34*(2), 48–51.

Dick, J., Lewin, S., Rose, E., Zwarenstein, M., & van der Walt, H. (2004). Changing professional practice in tuberculosis care: An educational intervention. *Journal of Advanced Nursing, 48*(5), 434–442.

Dochterman, J., & Bulechek, G. (2004). *Nursing interventions classification (NIC)* (4th ed.). St. Louis, MO: Mosby.

Dreher, H. M., Dean, J. L., Moriarty, D. M., Kaiser, R., Willard, R., O'Donnell, S., et al. (2004). What you need to know about SARS now. *Nursing, 34*(1), 58–63.

Dunn, L. (2005). Pneumonia: Classification, diagnosis and nursing management. *Nursing Standard, 19*(42), 50–54.

Fontaine, K. L. (2005). *Healing practices: Alternative therapies for nursing* (2nd ed.). Upper Saddle River, NJ: Prentice Hall Health.

Gift, A. G., Jablonski, A., Stommel, M., & Given, C. W. (2004). Symptom clusters in elderly patients with lung cancer. *Oncology Nursing Forum, 31*(2), 203–210.

Grap, M. J., Munro, C. L., Hummel, R. S. III, Elswick, R. K., McKinney, J. L., & Sessler, C. N. (2005). Effect of backrest

elevation on the development of ventilator-associated pneumonia. *American Journal of Critical Care, 14*(4), 325–333.

Hilton, P. (2004). Clinical. Evaluating the treatment options for spontaneous pneumothorax. *Nursing Times, 100*(28), 32–33.

Hoyert, D. L., Heron, M., Murphy, S. L., & Kung, H. C. (2006). Deaths: Final data for 2003. Health & Stats. Retrieved from www.cdc.gov/nchs/products/pubs/pubd/hestats/finaldeaths03

Jantarakupt, P., & Porock, D. (2005). Dyspnea management in lung cancer: Applying the evidence from chronic obstructive pulmonary disease. *Oncology Nursing Forum, 32*(4), 785–797.

Joseph, H. A., Shrestha-Kuwahara, R., Lowry, D., Lambert, L. A., Panlilio, A. L., Raucher, B. G., et al. (2004). Factors influencing health care workers' adherence to work site tuberculosis screening and treatment policies. *American Journal of Infection Control, 32*(8), 456–461.

Kasper, D. L., Braunwald, E., Fauci, A. S., Hauser, S. L., Longo, D. L., & Jameson, J. L. (Eds.). (2005). *Harrison's principles of internal medicine* (16th ed.). New York: McGraw-Hill.

Kim, S., & Crittenden, K. S. (2005). Risk factors for tuberculosis among inmates: A retrospective analysis. *Public Health Nursing, 22*(2), 108–118.

Kleinpell, R. M., & Elpern, E. H. (2004). Community-acquired pneumonia: Updates in assessment and management. *Critical Care Nursing Quarterly, 27*(3), 231–240.

Ladd, E. (2005). The use of antibiotics for viral upper respiratory tract infections: An analysis of nurse practitioner and physician prescribing practices in ambulatory care, 1997–2001. *Journal of the American Academy of Nurse Practitioners, 17*(10), 416–424.

Lakasing, E., & Tester, M. (2006). How to manage lung cancer in primary care. *Practice Nursing, 17*(1), 35–39.

Lehne, R. A. (2004). *Pharmacology for nursing care* (5th ed.). St. Louis, MO: Saunders.

Leonard, M. K., Osterhlot, D., Kourbatova, E. V., Del Rio, C., Wand, W., & Blumberg, H. M. (2005). How many sputum specimens are necessary to diagnose pulmonary tuberculosis? *American Journal of Infection Control, 33*(1), 58–61.

McCance, K. L., & Huether, S. E. (2006). *Pathophysiology: The biologic basis for disease in adults & children* (5th ed.). St. Louis, MO: Mosby.

McInnes, K., & Satian, L. (2005). Keeping SARS out: An education program for SARS screeners in one Ontario hospital. *Journal for Nurses in Staff Development, 21*(2), 73–78.

Merrel, P., & Mayo, D. (2004). Inhalation injury in the burn patient. *Critical Care Nursing Clinics of North America, 16*(1), 27–38.

Molassiotis, A., Panteli, V., Patiraki, E., Ozden, G., Platin, N., Madsen, E., et al. (2006). Complementary and alternative medicine use in lung cancer patients in eight European countries. *Complementary Therapies in Clinical Practice, 12*(1), 34–39.

Montgomery, S. S., Burke, E. M., Wissman, S. A., Feldman, D. S., & Leier, C. V. (2005). Natural course of large spontaneous pneumothorax. *Heart & Lung, 34*(5), 332–334.

Moorhead, S., Johnson, M., & Maas, M. (2004). *Nursing outcomes classification (NOC)* (3rd ed.). St. Louis, MO: Mosby.

Myrianthefs, P. M., Kalafati, M., Samara, I., & Baltopoulos, G. J. (2004). Nosocomial pneumonia. *Critical Care Nursing Quarterly, 27*(3), 241–257.

NANDA International. (2005). *Nursing diagnoses: Definitions and classification 2005–2006.* Philadelphia: Author.

National Center for Complementary and Alternative Medicine. (2004). Consumer advisory. Ephedra. Retrieved from http://www.nccam.nih.gov/health/alerts/ephedra/consumeradvisory

_____. (2005). Herbs at a glance. Echinacea. Retrieved from http://www.nccam.nih.gov/health/echinacea/

National Center for Health Statistics. (2005). *Health, United States, 2005 with Chartbook on trends in the health of Americans.* Hyattsville, MD: U.S. Government Printing Office.

Neafsey, P. J. (2005). Medication news. Ketolides: New antimicrobials for community-acquired pneumonia. *Home Healthcare Nurse, 23*(3), 141–143.

Nyamathi, A., Berg, J., Jones, T., & Leake, B. (2005). Predictors of perceived health status of tuberculosis-infected homeless. *Western Journal of Nursing Research, 27*(7), 896–914.

Porth, C. M. (2005). *Pathophysiology: Concepts of altered health states* (7th ed.). Philadelphia: Lippincott.

Pruitt, B., & Jacobs, M. (2006). Best-practice interventions: How can you prevent ventilator-associated pneumonia? *Nursing, 36*(2), 36–42.

Ross, J. L. (2005). Near drowning. *RN, 68*(7), 36, 42.

Rothrock, J. C. (2003). *Alexander's care of the patient in surgery* (12th ed.). St. Louis, MO: Mosby.

Ryan, B. (2005). Pneumothorax: Assessment and diagnostic testing. *Journal of Cardiovascular Nursing, 20*(4), 251–253.

Sarna, L., Brown, J. K., Cooley, M. E., Williams, R. D., Chernecky, C., Padilla, G., et al. (2005). Quality of life and meaning of illness in women with lung cancer. *Oncology Nursing Forum, 32*(1), E9–E19.

Schleder, B. J. (2004). Taking charge of hospital-acquired pneumonia. *The Nurse Practitioner, 29*(3), 50–53.

Spencer, J. W., & Jacobs, J. J. (2003). *Complementary and alternative medicine: An evidence-based approach* (2nd ed.). St. Louis, MO: Mosby.

Swigart, V., & Kolb, R. (2004). Homeless persons' decisions to accept or reject public health disease-detection services. *Public Health Nursing, 21*(2), 162–170.

Tierney, L. M. Jr., McPhee, S. J., & Papadakis, M. A. (Eds.). (2005). *Current medical diagnosis & treatment* (44th ed.). New York: McGraw-Hill.

Todd, B. (2005). Emerging infections. *Legionella* pneumonia: Many cases of Legionnaire disease go unreported or unrecognized. *American Journal of Nursing, 105*(11), 35–36, 38.

Tolomiczenko, G. S., Kahan, M., Ricci, M., Strathern, L., Jeney, C., Patterson, K., et al. (2005). SARS: Coping with the impact at a community hospital. *Journal of Advanced Nursing, 50*(1), 101–110.

Toth, A., Fackelmann, J., Pigott, W., & Tolomeo, O. (2004). Tuberculosis prevention and treatment: Occupational health, infection control, public health, general duty staff, visiting, parish nursing or working in a physician's office—all nursing roles are key in improving tuberculosis control. *Canadian Nurse, 100*(9), 27–30.

Tseng, H., Chen, T., & Chou, S. (2005). SARS: Key factors in crisis management. *Journal of Nursing Research, 13*(1), 58–64.

Understanding pleural effusion. (2004). *Nursing, 34*(8). 64.

Vecchiarino, P., Bohannon, R. W., Ferullo, J., & Malijanian, R. (2004). Short-term outcomes and their predictors for patients hospitalized with community-acquired pneumonia. *Heart & Lung, 33*(5), 301–307.

Way, L. W., & Doherty, G. M. (2003). *Current surgical diagnosis & treatment* (11th ed.). New York: McGraw-Hill.

Wilkinson, J. M. (2005). *Nursing diagnosis handbook* (8th ed.). Upper Saddle River, NJ: Prentice Hall.

Williams, V. G. (2006). Tuberculosis: Clinical features, diagnosis and management. *Nursing Standard, 20*(22), 49–53.

Willis, D., VanSickle, D., Van Riper, S., & Valerio, C. (2005). Pneumonia: Bringing JCAHO and CMS to the bedside. *American Journal of Nursing, 105*(3), 72A, 72C–72D.

Wing, S. (2004). Pleural effusion: Nursing care challenge in the elderly. *Geriatric Nursing, 25*(6), 348–354.

Withy, K., & Alper, B. S. (2005). Stat consult. Acute bronchitis. *Clinical Advisor for Nurse Practitioners, 8*(1), 73–74, 77.

Woods, A., & Hathaway, L. (2004). Treating community-acquired pneumonia. *Nurse Practitioner, 29*(6), 11.

World Health Organization. (2003). Cumulative number of reported probable cases of severe acute respiratory syndrome (SARS). *Communicable Disease Surveillance & Response (CSR).* Author.

Yamamoto, L., Schroeder, C., Morley, D., & Beliveau, C. (2005). Thoracic trauma: The deadly dozen. *Critical Care Nursing Quarterly, 28*(1), 22–40.

CHAPTER 39 Nursing Care of Clients with Gas Exchange Disorders

LEARNING OUTCOMES

- Relate the pathophysiology and manifestations of obstructive, pulmonary vascular, and critical respiratory disorders to their effects on ventilation and respiration (gas exchange).

- Compare and contrast the etiology, risk factors, and vulnerable populations for disorders affecting ventilation and gas exchange within the lungs.

- Describe interdisciplinary care and the nursing role in health promotion and caring for clients with disorders that affect the ability to ventilate the lungs and exchange gases with the environment.

- Discuss interdisciplinary interventions to provide airway and ventilatory support for the client with respiratory failure, and nursing responsibilities in caring for clients requiring airway and ventilatory support.

- Describe the nursing implications for medications used to promote ventilation and gas exchange.

CLINICAL COMPETENCIES

- Assess functional health status of clients with disorders affecting ventilation and gas exchange.

- Use assessed data and knowledge of the effects of the disorder and prescribed treatment to identify priority nursing diagnoses and plan care for clients with disorders affecting ventilation and gas exchange.

- Use the nursing process and evidence-based nursing research to plan and implement individualized nursing care for clients, including measures to promote ventilation and gas exchange.

- Plan and provide appropriate teaching for health promotion among vulnerable populations and to prepare clients and families for community-based care.

- Evaluate the effectiveness of nursing interventions and teaching, revising strategies and teaching plans as needed.

- Safely and knowledgeably coordinate interdisciplinary care and administer prescribed medications and treatments for clients with disorders affecting ventilation and gas exchange.

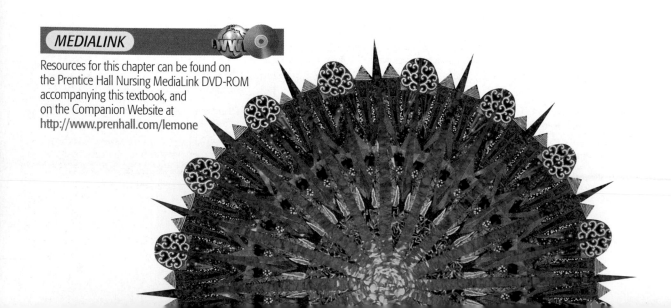

MEDIALINK

Resources for this chapter can be found on the Prentice Hall Nursing MediaLink DVD-ROM accompanying this textbook, and on the Companion Website at http://www.prenhall.com/lemone

KEY TERMS

acute respiratory distress syndrome (ARDS), *1365*
asthma, *1321*
atelectasis, *1343*
bronchiectasis, *1344*
chronic bronchitis, *1331*

chronic obstructive pulmonary disease (COPD), *1330*
cor pulmonale, *1352*
cystic fibrosis (CF), *1340*
emphysema, *1332*
pulmonary embolism, *1347*

pulmonary hypertension, *1352*
respiratory failure, *1353*
sarcoidosis, *1346*
status asthmaticus, *1323*
weaning, *1360*

Normal function of the lower respiratory system depends on several organ systems: the central nervous system, which stimulates and controls breathing; chemoreceptors in the brain, aortic arch, and carotid bodies, which monitor the pH and oxygen content of blood; the heart and circulatory system, which provide for blood supply and gas exchange; the musculoskeletal system, which provides an intact thoracic cavity capable of expanding and contracting; and the lungs and bronchial tree, which allow air movement and gas exchange. Impaired function of any of these systems affects ventilation and respiration. As a result, tissues may become *hypoxic*, with inadequate oxygen to support metabolic activity.

Although some of the disorders discussed in this chapter can affect ventilation (air movement into and out of the airways and alveoli), all can have significant effects on gas exchange. The mechanisms by which they affect gas exchange differ:

- In reactive airway disease (asthma) and obstructive disorders, air trapping reduces the amount of oxygen available to drive gas exchange.
- Interstitial lung disorders affect the ability of the lungs to expand and the work of breathing, again, reducing alveolar oxygenation and gas exchange.
- Pulmonary vascular disorders affect blood flow to the lungs or a portion of the lungs, reducing gas exchange through their effects on perfusion of the lungs.
- Respiratory failure is the ultimate consequence of impaired gas exchange; the lungs cannot adequately oxygenate the blood or eliminate carbon dioxide.

With a few exceptions, the disorders discussed in this chapter are relatively common, chronic lung diseases.

FAST FACTS

- Chronic lower respiratory diseases are the fourth leading cause of death in the United States.
- The death rate for chronic lower respiratory diseases is higher for men than women.
- Whites have a higher death rate due to chronic lower respiratory diseases than blacks, Native Americans, or Hispanics; people of Asian heritage have the lowest death rate due to chronic lower respiratory diseases.
- Adults age 45 and older have the greatest risk: Chronic lower respiratory diseases are not among the leading causes of death for adults ages 25 to 44; in the 45- to 64-year-old age grouping, however, they are the sixth leading cause of death, jumping to the fourth leading cause of death for people 65 years old and older.

Source: National Center for Health Statistics, 2005.

Disorders of other body systems, such as neurologic disorders (e.g., head injury, spinal cord trauma or disorders, amyotrophic lateral sclerosis, myasthenia gravis) also can affect gas exchange through their effects on the central or peripheral nervous systems. These disorders and their effects on the respiratory system are discussed in subsequent chapters of this text.

Aging affects pulmonary ventilation and gas exchange as well. The number of alveoli decrease, and emphysematous changes (senile emphysema) reduce the surface area for gas exchange. Alveoli become less elastic, causing increased air trapping and dead space. For most older adults who remain active, these changes have minimal effect on exercise tolerance and activities of daily living (ADLs). When combined with lung disease, however, age-related pulmonary changes increase the client's risk for developing respiratory failure.

REACTIVE AIRWAY DISORDERS

In reactive airway disorders, the airways narrow in response to a stimulus. Airway narrowing limits airflow both into and out of the alveoli. Limited airflow increases the work of breathing and the residual volume of the lungs as air is trapped behind narrowed airways. Inspired air mixes with an abnormally large volume of residual air, effectively reducing the amount of oxygen available in the alveoli. Decreased alveolar ventilation further reduces oxygen available for exchange.

THE CLIENT WITH ASTHMA

Asthma is a chronic inflammatory disorder of the airways characterized by recurrent episodes of wheezing, breathlessness, chest tightness, and coughing. Inflammation causes increased responsiveness of the airways to multiple stimuli. The widespread airflow obstruction that occurs during acute episodes usually reverses either spontaneously or with treatment. While most episodes or asthma "attacks" are relatively brief, some clients with asthma may experience longer episodes with some degree of airway impairment daily. In rare cases, an acute episode of asthma is so severe that respiratory failure and death result.

Incidence and Risk Factors

In the United States, approximately 11 million people experienced at least one asthma attack in the year 2003. After several

MediaLink

Asthma Animation

years of increase, the prevalence of asthma currently is relatively stable. Hospitalizations and deaths due to asthma have decreased in recent years, likely as a result of better disease management. Asthma is a serious disease, causing more than 4000 deaths in the United States in 2002 (American Lung Association [ALA], 2005a).

FAST FACTS

- Although asthma is more common in children than adults, 5.5% to 10% of adults are affected (National Heart, Lung, and Blood Institute [NI ILBI], 2004).
- Across races, the mortality rate associated with asthma is higher in women than in men.
- The asthma mortality rate of blacks is nearly three times that of whites and is higher than that of Hispanics and other ethnic groups.
- Deaths due to asthma are rare in children and increase with age, particularly in middle and late adulthood and old age (ALA, 2005a).

A number of risk factors can be identified for asthma, although many clients develop the disease in the absence of known risk factors. Allergies play a strong role in childhood asthma, a lesser role in adults. There is a strong genetic component to the disease, although a specific pattern of inheritance has not been identified. Multiple regions on several chromosomes appear to contribute to asthma-related factors such as airway hyperreactivity and high IgE levels (Kasper et al., 2005). Environmental factors, including air pollution and occupational exposure to industrial compounds, may contribute. Respiratory viruses such as rhinovirus and influenza can precipitate asthma attacks. Other contributory factors include exercise (particularly in cold air) and emotional stress.

Physiology Review

Airways within the lungs contain crisscrossing strips of smooth muscle that control their diameter. This muscle is innervated by the autonomic nervous system. Parasympathetic (cholinergic) stimulation leads to bronchoconstriction, or narrowing of the airways. Sympathetic stimulation through β_2-adrenergic receptors causes bronchodilation, or expansion of the airways. Slight bronchoconstriction normally predominates. However, when increased airflow is necessary (e.g., during exercise), the parasympathetic system is inhibited, and stimulation of the sympathetic system causes bronchodilation. Inflammatory mediators (such as histamine) released during an antigen–antibody response act directly on bronchial smooth muscle to produce bronchoconstriction.

Pathophysiology

In asthma, the airways are in a persistent state of inflammation. During symptom-free periods, airway inflammation in asthma is subacute or quiet. Even during these periods, however, inflammatory cells such as eosinophils, neutrophils, and lymphocytes may be found in airway tissues and edema may be present. An acute inflammatory response, during which resident inflamma-

tory cells interact with inflammatory mediators, cytokines, and additional infiltrating inflammatory cells, may be triggered by a variety of factors. Common triggers for an acute asthma attack include exposure to allergens, respiratory tract infection, exercise, inhaled irritants, and emotional upsets.

Attack Triggers

Childhood asthma (which may continue into adulthood) is most often linked to inhalation of allergens such as pollen, animal dander, or household dust. Clients with allergic asthma often have a history of other allergies. Environmental pollutants, such as tobacco smoke and irritant gases (e.g., sulfur dioxide, nitrogen dioxide, and ozone), can provoke asthma. Exposure to secondhand smoke as a child is associated with a higher risk for and increased severity of asthma. Agents found in the workplace, such as noxious fumes and gases, chemicals, and dusts, may cause occupational asthma.

Respiratory infections, viral in particular, are a common internal stimulus for an asthmatic attack. Exercise-induced asthma attacks also are common, affecting 40% to 90% of people with bronchial asthma (Porth, 2005). Loss of heat or water from the bronchial surface may contribute to exercise-induced asthma. Exercising in cold, dry air increases the risk of an asthma attack in susceptible people.

Emotional stress is a significant etiologic factor for attacks in as many as half of clients with asthma. Common pharmacologic triggers include aspirin and other nonsteroidal anti-inflammatory drugs, sulfites (which are used as preservatives in wine, beer, fresh fruits, and salad), and beta-blockers.

Responses

When a trigger such as inhalation of an allergen or irritant occurs, an *acute* or *early response* develops in the hyperreactive airways predisposed to bronchospasm. Sensitized mast cells in the bronchial mucosa release inflammatory mediators such as histamine, prostaglandins, and leukotrienes. Resident and infiltrating inflammatory cells also produce inflammatory mediators such as cytokines, bradykinin, and growth factors. These mediators stimulate parasympathetic receptors and bronchial smooth muscle to produce bronchoconstriction. They also increase capillary permeability, which allows plasma to escape and leads to mucosal edema. Mucous production is stimulated; excess mucus collects in the narrowed airways.

The attack is prolonged by the *late phase response,* which develops 4 to 12 hours after exposure to the trigger. Inflammatory cells such as basophils and eosinophils are activated, and they damage airway epithelium, produce mucosal edema, impair mucociliary clearance, and produce or prolong bronchoconstriction. The degree of hyperreactivity depends on the extent of inflammation. Together, bronchoconstriction, edema and inflammation, and mucous secretion narrow the airway. Airway resistance increases, limiting airflow and increasing the work of breathing (Figure 39–1 ■).

Limited expiratory airflow traps air distal to the spastic, narrowed airways. Trapped air mixes with inspired air in the alveoli, reducing its oxygen tension and gas exchange across the alveolar-capillary membrane. Distended alveoli compress alveolar capillaries, reducing blood flow and further affecting

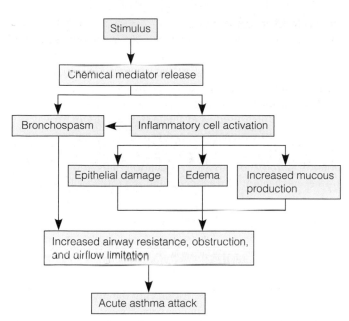

Figure 39–1 ■ The pathogenesis of an acute episode of asthma.

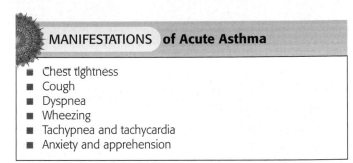

MANIFESTATIONS of Acute Asthma

- Chest tightness
- Cough
- Dyspnea
- Wheezing
- Tachypnea and tachycardia
- Anxiety and apprehension

gas exchange. As a result, hypoxemia develops. Hypoxemia and increased lung volume due to trapping stimulate the respiratory rate. Hyperventilation causes the $PaCO_2$ to fall, leading to respiratory alkalosis. (See Chapter 10 ∞ for more information about acid–base imbalances.)

To summarize, in an acute asthma attack, inflammatory mediators are released from sensitized airways followed by activation of inflammatory cells. These events lead to bronchoconstriction, airway edema, and impaired mucociliary clearance. Airway narrowing limits airflow and increases the work of breathing; trapped air mixes with inhaled air, impairing gas exchange.

Manifestations and Complications

An asthma attack is characterized by a subjective sensation of chest tightness, cough, dyspnea, and wheezing (see the Manifestations box above). The onset of symptoms may be either abrupt or insidious, and an attack may subside rapidly or persist for hours or days. A sense of chest constriction and nonproductive cough are common early manifestations of an attack. During an attack, tachycardia, tachypnea, and prolonged expiration are common. Diffuse wheezing is heard on auscultation. With more severe attacks, use of the accessory muscles of respiration, intercostal retractions, loud wheezing, and distant breath sounds may be noted. Fatigue, anxiety, apprehension, and severe dyspnea that allows speaking only one or two words between breaths may occur with persistent severe episodes. The onset of respiratory failure is marked by inaudible breath sounds with reduced wheezing and an ineffective cough. Without careful assessment, this apparent relief of symptoms can be misinterpreted as an improvement.

The frequency of attacks and severity of symptoms vary greatly from person to person. Although some people have infrequent, mild episodes, others have nearly continuous manifestations of cough, dyspnea on exertion, and wheezing with periodic severe exacerbations (Table 39–1).

Status asthmaticus is severe, prolonged asthma that does not respond to routine treatment. Without aggressive therapy, status asthmaticus can lead to respiratory failure with hypoxemia, hypercapnia, and acidosis. Endotracheal intubation, mechanical ventilation, and aggressive drug treatment may be necessary to sustain life.

(Side tab: MEDIALINK — Case Study: Acute Asthma Attack)

TABLE 39–1 Classification of Asthma Severity

CLASSIFICATION	SYMPTOM FREQUENCY	NIGHTTIME SYMPTOMS
Mild intermittent	■ No more than twice a week ■ Brief attacks (hours to days) of varied intensity ■ Asymptomatic and normal peak expiratory flow rate between attacks	No more than twice a month
Mild persistent	■ More than twice a week but less than once a day ■ Exacerbations may affect activity	More than twice a month
Moderate persistent	■ Daily symptoms ■ Daily short-acting bronchodilator use ■ Exacerbations affect activity ■ Exacerbations more than twice a week; may last for days	More than once a week
Severe persistent	■ Continual symptoms ■ Limited physical activity ■ Frequent exacerbations	Frequent

Source: Adapted from Expert Panel Report 2: Guidelines for the Diagnosis and Management of Asthma, Publication No. 97-4051 by National Education and Prevention Program, 1997, Bethesda, MD: National Institutes of Health.

In addition to acute respiratory failure, other complications associated with acute asthma include dehydration, respiratory infection, atelectasis, pneumothorax, and cor pulmonale.

Cough-Variant Asthma

Asthma is one of the three most common causes of chronic cough (the other two being postnasal drip and gastroesophageal reflux disease [GERD]) (Kasper et al., 2005; Martin, 2003). Cough can be initiated by either upper airway irritants (e.g., postnasal drip or GERD) or by inflammation or constriction of the lower airways. Most commonly, cough associated with asthma is accompanied by classic asthma symptoms such as chest constriction, dyspnea, and wheezing. Clients with *cough-variant asthma*, however, have persistent cough without wheezing or dyspnea, often delaying diagnosis. These clients do have significant airway inflammation and demonstrate the pathophysiologic features of asthma.

INTERDISCIPLINARY CARE

The diagnosis of asthma is based primarily on the history and manifestations. Treatment goals are twofold. Daily management focuses on controlling symptoms and preventing acute attacks. During an acute attack, therapy is directed toward restoring airway patency and alveolar ventilation.

Diagnosis

Diagnostic tests are used to determine the degree of airway involvement during and between acute episodes and identify causative factors such as allergens. See Chapter 36 ∞ for more information about and the nursing care related to these diagnostic tests.

- *Pulmonary function tests (PFTs)* are used to evaluate the degree of airway obstruction. Pulmonary function testing done before and after use of an aerosolized bronchodilator helps determine the reversibility of airway obstruction. The residual volume of the lungs may be increased and vital capacity decreased or normal even during periods of remission. The forced expiratory volume and peak expiratory flow rate are the most valuable pulmonary function studies to evaluate the severity of an asthma attack and the effectiveness of treatment measures. See Box 36–1.
- *Challenge* or *bronchial provocation testing* uses an inhaled substance such as methacholine or histamine with PFTs to confirm the diagnosis of asthma by detecting airway hyper-responsiveness.
- *Arterial blood gases (ABGs)* are drawn during an acute attack to evaluate oxygenation, carbon dioxide elimination, and acid–base status. ABGs initially show hypoxemia with a low PaO_2, and mild respiratory alkalosis with an elevated pH and low $PaCO_2$ due to tachypnea. Severe airflow obstruction causes significant hypoxemia and respiratory acidosis (pH less than 7.35 and $PaCO_2$ greater than 42 mmHg), indicative of respiratory failure and the need for mechanical ventilation. See Chapter 10 ∞ for more information about arterial blood gases and their interpretation.
- *Skin testing* may be done to identify specific allergens if an allergic trigger is suspected for asthma attacks.

Disease Monitoring

Peak expiratory flow rate (PEFR) is used on a day-to-day basis to evaluate the severity of bronchial hyperresponsiveness. Small, inexpensive meters to measure PEFR are available. Readings taken at varying times of day over several weeks are used to establish the client's personal best or normal PEFR. This value is then used to evaluate the severity of airway obstruction. Traffic signal colors are used for simplicity: *green* (80% to 100% of personal best) indicates asthma that is under control; *yellow* (50% to 80%) is caution, indicating a need for further medication or treatment; and *red* (50% or less) signals an immediate need for a bronchodilator and medical treatment if the level does not immediately return to the yellow range (Porth, 2005).

Preventive Measures

Asthma attacks often can be prevented by avoiding allergens and environmental triggers. Modifying the home environment by controlling dust, removing carpets, covering mattresses and pillows to reduce dust mite populations, and installing air filtering systems may be useful. Pets may need to be removed from the household. Eliminating all tobacco smoke in the home is vital. Wearing a mask that retains humidity and warm air while exercising in cold weather may help prevent attacks of exercise-induced asthma. Early treatment of respiratory infections is vital to prevent asthma exacerbations.

Medications

Medications are used to prevent and control asthma symptoms, reduce the frequency and severity of exacerbations, and reverse airway obstruction. Drugs used for long-term control of asthma are taken daily to maintain control of the disease. The primary drugs in this group are anti-inflammatory agents, long-acting bronchodilators, and leukotriene modifiers. Quick-relief medications provide prompt relief of bronchoconstriction and airflow obstruction with associated wheezing, cough, and chest tightness. Short-acting adrenergic stimulants (rapid-acting bronchodilators), anticholinergic drugs, and methylxanthines fall into this category.

A stepwise approach for managing asthma is recommended. This approach is based on the severity of disease (see Tables 39–1 and 39–2). For all clients, a short-acting inhaled β_2-agonist is recommended for quick relief of acute symptoms. Up to three treatments at 20-minute intervals or a single nebulizer treatment may be used as needed. Strategies for long-term control may need to be modified if a short-acting bronchodilator is needed more than twice a week (NHLBI, 2003).

Many of the drugs used for continued asthma management and relief of an acute attack can be administered by a metered-dose inhaler (MDI), dry powder inhaler (DPI), or nebulizer. The advantages of administering medications locally by inhalation include rapid onset and reduced systemic effects of the drugs. In an MDI, a chemical propellant is used to deliver the medication when the canister is depressed. DPI, in contrast, contain no propellant. Instead, the medication is released by inhaling rapidly through the mouthpiece. Box 39–1 outlines client teaching for use of an MDI or DPI.

TABLE 39-2 Stepwise Approach to Asthma Management for Adults

STEP/DISEASE SEVERITY	PREFERRED TREATMENT	ALTERNATE OR AS NEEDED TREATMENT
Step 1: mild intermittent	No daily medication needed	Systemic corticosteroids for severe exacerbations
Step 2: mild persistent	Low-dose inhaled corticosteroids	Cromolyn, leukotriene modifier, nedocromil, or sustained-release theophylline
Step 3: moderate persistent	Low-to-moderate dose inhaled corticosteroids *and* long-acting inhaled β_2-agonist	Increase inhaled corticosteroid dose *or* combine inhaled corticosteroid with leukotriene modifier or theophylline
Step 4: severe persistent	High-dose inhaled corticosteroid *and* long-acting inhaled β_2-agonist	Add systemic corticosteroid

Source: Adapted from *Expert Panel Report 2: Guidelines for the Diagnosis and Management of Asthma, Update on Selected Topics 2002,* Publication No. 02-5074 by National Education and Prevention Program, 2003, Bethesda, MD. National Institutes of Health.

BRONCHODILATORS Most asthmatics need bronchodilator therapy to control their symptoms. Inhalation of nebulized medication is the preferred means of administration. The primary bronchodilators used include adrenergic stimulants, methylxanthines, and anticholinergic agents. These drugs often are administered in combination with an anti-inflammatory agent.

Adrenergic stimulants (β_2-agonists) affect receptors on smooth muscle cells of the respiratory tract, causing smooth muscle relaxation and bronchodilation. Long-acting adrenergic stimulants such as inhaled salmeterol and oral sustained-release albuterol are used in conjunction with anti-inflammatory drugs to control symptoms, but are not appropriate to treat an acute episode of asthma. Inhaled short-acting beta-adrenergic agonists such as albuterol, bitolterol, pirbuterol, and terbutaline, administered by MDI or DPI, are the treatment of choice for quick relief. They act within minutes, but their duration generally is short, lasting only 4 to 6 hours. Tachycardia and muscle tremors, common side effects of adrenergic agonists, are minimal with inhalation therapy.

BOX 39-1 Client Teaching: Using a Metered-Dose Inhaler or Dry Powder Inhaler

Metered-Dose Inhaler

- Firmly insert a charged metered-dose inhaler canister into the mouthpiece unit or spacer (if used).
- Remove mouthpiece cap. Shake canister vigorously for 3 to 5 seconds.
- Exhale slowly and completely.
- Holding the canister upside down, place the mouthpiece in the mouth, closing lips around it if a spacer is being used. When no spacer is used, hold the mouthpiece directly in front of the mouth.
- Press and hold the canister down while inhaling deeply and slowly for 3 to 5 seconds (see figure).

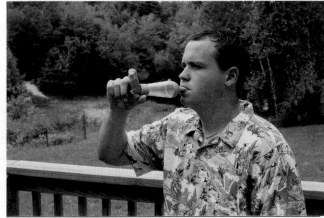

Source: Michal Heron, Pearson Education/PH College

- Hold breath for 10 seconds, release pressure on the container, remove from mouth, and exhale. Wait 20 to 30 seconds before repeating the procedure for a second puff.

- Rinse the mouth after using the inhaler to minimize systemic absorption and drying of the mucous membranes.
- Rinse the inhaler mouthpiece and spacer after use; store in a clean location.

Dry Powder Inhaler

- Keep the inhaler and medication in a clean, dry location. Do not refrigerate or store in a humid place (for example, the bathroom).
- Remove the cap and hold the inhaler upright. Inspect to be sure that the mechanism is clean and the mouthpiece is clear.
- If necessary, load the dose into the inhaler, following manufacturer's directions.
- Hold the inhaler level with the mouthpiece end facing down.
- Breathe slowly and completely. Tilt your head back slightly.
- Place the mouthpiece in your mouth with your teeth over the mouthpiece. Seal your lips around the mouthpiece. Do not block the inhaler with your tongue.
- Breathe in rapidly and deeply through your mouth over 2 to 3 seconds to activate the flow of medication.
- Remove the inhaler from your mouth and hold your breath for 10 seconds.
- Exhale slowly through pursed lips to allow the medication to enter distal airways. Never exhale into the inhaler mouthpiece to prevent clogging.
- Rinse your mouth or brush your teeth after using the inhaler to avoid a bad taste from the medication and to prevent a yeast infection (if a corticosteroid medication is being used).
- Store the inhaler in a clean, sealed plastic bag; do not wash the inhaler unless so directed by the manufacturer. The mouthpiece should be cleaned weekly using a dry cloth.

MEDIALINK

Metered-Dose Inhaler Video

Anticholinergic medications prevent bronchoconstriction by blocking parasympathetic input to bronchial smooth muscle. Ipratropium bromide, an anticholinergic drug administered by MDI, is useful when asthma symptoms are poorly controlled by adrenergic stimulants alone. Anticholinergic drugs act more slowly than adrenergic stimulants, requiring up to 60 to 90 minutes to achieve maximal effect.

Theophylline is a methylxanthine used as adjunctive treatment for asthma. It relaxes bronchial smooth muscle and may also inhibit the release of chemical mediators of the inflammatory response. Monitoring of serum theophylline levels is necessary because of wide individual variations in metabolism and elimination of the drug and its toxic effects. Serum levels of 10 to 20 mcg/mL or lower are recommended. Theophylline may be used as a long-term bronchodilator, given once or twice daily. A related drug, aminophylline, may be administered intravenously to treat an acute, severe exacerbation of the disease.

ANTI-INFLAMMATORY AGENTS Corticosteroids and two nonsteroidal anti-inflammatory agents, cromolyn sodium and nedocromil, are used to suppress airway inflammation and reduce asthma symptoms.

Corticosteroids block the late response to inhaled allergens and reduce bronchial hyperresponsiveness. The preferred route of administration is by MDI or DPI to minimize systemic absorption and reduce the adverse effects of prolonged steroid use (cushingoid effects). For a severe acute attack, corticosteroids may be given systemically to alleviate symptoms and induce remission.

Cromolyn sodium and nedocromil are used to prevent acute episodes of asthma. They reduce airway hyperreactivity and inhibit the release of mediator substances. These drugs are used for long-term control of asthma, not quick relief. They have a wide margin of safety and few side effects.

LEUKOTRIENE MODIFIERS Leukotriene modifiers, montelukast (Singulair), zafirlukast (Accolate), and zileuton (Zyflo Filmtab), are oral medications that reduce the inflammatory response in asthma. They appear to improve lung function, diminish symptoms, and reduce the need for short-acting bronchodilators. These drugs affect the metabolism and excretion of other medications such as warfarin and theophylline and may cause liver toxicity.

Nursing implications for medications used to treat asthma are outlined in the Medication Administration box on pages 1327–1328.

Complementary Therapies

A number of herbal preparations and other complementary therapies have been shown to be helpful in treating asthma. Dietary therapies, environmental medicine, and nutritional supplements are the complementary therapies most widely recommended by healthcare professionals for asthma (Spencer & Jacobs, 2003). Nutritional and dietary therapies may include elimination of certain foods or food additives (e.g., sulfite) from the diet, often in the absence of a documented food allergy or relationship between consumption and the onset of asthma symptoms. Although the evidence is inconsistent, some studies suggest that increasing intake of ascorbic acid, an antioxidant, zinc, and magnesium may help alleviate manifestations of asthma. People with mild asthma may benefit from addition of omega-3 polyunsaturated fatty acids to the diet, experiencing less severe and fewer acute attacks (Spencer & Jacobs, 2003).

Herbal preparations may include atropa belladonna (the natural form of atropine) or ephedra (also called ma huang), an herb that contains ephedrine. These herbals have effects similar to those of drugs used to treat asthma, and should not be used in combination with sympathetic stimulants or anticholinergic preparations. Because of the dangers associated with its use, sale of herbal products containing ephedra has been banned (National Center for Complementary and Alternative Medicine, 2004). Advise clients asking about the use of Chinese herbal remedies to treat asthma to inquire if any recommended product contains ma huang or ephedra, and to avoid such products. Capsaicin also may relieve acute asthma symptoms. Other herbal preparations include quercetin and grape seed extract. Refer clients interested in using natural preparations to a qualified herbalist, and emphasize the importance of talking to the physician before using these preparations along with conventional treatment.

In addition to herbals, other complementary therapies such as biofeedback, yoga, breathing techniques, acupuncture, homeopathy, and massage have been found to alleviate or help control asthma symptoms.

NURSING CARE

Nurses encounter clients with asthma both in the acute care setting during an acute exacerbation and as outpatients or in homes. The priority nursing care needs differ with each setting.

Health Promotion

Although specific measures to prevent asthma have not yet been identified, the link between parental smoking and childhood asthma is strong. Discuss this link with young people and families with children. Encourage all clients to not start smoking, and if they do smoke, to quit. Provide referrals to smoking cessation clinics, help groups, or a care provider for nicotine patches as needed to facilitate quitting. Additional evidence suggests that early exposure to certain infectious diseases and to other children and limited use of antibiotics reduces the risk for developing asthma (NHLBI, 2003).

Assessment

Assessment of the client experiencing an acute asthma attack must be very focused and timely.

- *Health History:* Current symptoms, including chest tightness, shortness of breath, dyspnea; duration of current attack; measures used to relieve symptoms and their effect; identified precipitating factors for the attack; frequency of attacks; current medications; known allergies.
- *Physical Examination:* Apparent level of distress; color; vital signs; respiratory rate and excursion, breath sounds throughout lung fields; apical pulse.
- *Diagnostic Tests:* Forced expiratory volume, peak expiratory flow rate; arterial blood gases.

MEDICATION ADMINISTRATION   Asthma

ADRENERGIC STIMULANTS
Epinephrine
Isoproterenol (Isuprel)
Metaproterenol (Alupent, Metaprel)
Terbutaline (Brethaire, Brethine)
Isoetharine (Bronkosol, Bronkometer)
Albuterol (Proventil, Ventolin)
Bitolterol (Tornalate)
Pirbuterol (Maxair)
Salmeterol (Serevent)
Formoterol (Foradil)
***Combination products:* albuterol/ipratropium**
(Combivent); salmeterol/fluticasone (Advair)

Adrenergic stimulants affect sympathetic receptors in the respiratory tract. Administered by metered-dose inhalers or dry powder inhalers, these drugs are the treatment of choice for acute bronchial asthma. Nearly all of the drugs in this class (epinephrine and isoproterenol being the exceptions) selectively activate β_2-receptors at the doses typically used to treat asthma. β_2-receptor activation results in smooth muscle relaxation and bronchodilation. Formoterol and salmeterol are highly selective to β_2-receptors, resulting in fewer adverse effects. Formoterol and salmeterol have been shown to increase the risk of serious asthma exacerbations and death, however. The U.S. Food and Drug Administration (FDA, 2005b) recommends using these drugs only when the disease cannot be adequately controlled with other medications.

Oral forms of adrenergic agonists may be used for prophylaxis but are not effective in treating an acute attack because of their slow onset. When administered orally or parenterally, their effect on sympathetic nervous system receptors can produce undesirable side effects such as nervousness, irritability, tachycardia, and cardiac dysrhythmias.

Nursing Responsibilities
- Use with caution in clients with hypertension, cardiovascular disease or dysrhythmias, hyperthyroidism, or diabetes.
- When given to a client who is hypoxemic and acidotic, these drugs may cause potentially dangerous cardiac stimulation.
- When given by MDI, wait 1 to 2 minutes between puffs to allow airways to dilate, permitting the second dose to reach distal airways.
- Observe for desired effect of reduced dyspnea and wheezing. Central nervous system stimulation (anxiety, irritability, and insomnia) and tremor are common side effects.

Health Education for the Client and Family
- Use the prescribed inhaler or nebulizer as directed.
- If you are taking a bronchodilator along with another medication by inhalation, use the bronchodilator first to open airways and enhance the effectiveness of the second medication.
- Rinse the mouth after using inhalers to reduce systemic absorption of the medication.
- Keep a log to track your bronchodilator use. If the drug becomes less effective, or if you need a higher dosage or more frequent doses than prescribed, contact your physician.
- Report palpitations, irregular pulse, and other side effects to the physician.

METHYLXANTHINES
Theophylline (Bronkotabs, Quibron, Slo-Phyllin Theolair, Theo-Dur, others)
Aminophylline (Somophyllin)

The methylxanthines are central nervous system (CNS) stimulants chemically related to caffeine. These drugs produce bronchodilation through relaxation of bronchial smooth muscle. As CNS stimulants, they produce adverse effects such as nervousness, insomnia, and tremors. When administered in large doses, convulsions may result.

Once the drugs of choice for preventing and treating asthma attacks, they are now used primarily to prevent nocturnal asthma in affected adult clients. Theophylline has a narrow margin of safety and high potential for toxicity. Because the metabolism and excretion of theophylline vary significantly from person to person—affected by such factors as age, smoking, genetic factors, alcoholism, and other chronic diseases—monitoring of serum levels is vital.

Nursing Responsibilities
- The therapeutic blood level for theophylline is 10 to 20 mcg/mL.
- Monitor for manifestations of toxicity. Anorexia, nausea, vomiting, restlessness, insomnia, cardiac dysrhythmias, and seizures are early manifestations. Other manifestations include epigastric pain, hematemesis, diarrhea, headache, irritability, muscle twitching, palpitations, tachycardia, flushing, and circulatory failure.
- Administer with meals or a full glass of water or milk to minimize gastric irritation.
- Monitor effect closely when administering concurrently with other medications such as barbiturates, anticonvulsants, thyroid hormone, beta blockers, bronchodilators, and others.
- Aminophylline is incompatible with many other intravenous drugs. Use a separate line or flush the line with normal saline before and after administering any other preparation.

Health Education for the Client and Family
- Oral methylxanthines are ineffective to treat an acute asthma attack; do not delay other treatment by using these drugs.
- Check with the physician before taking any over-the-counter medications or other prescription drugs while on theophylline.
- Do not smoke while using this drug.
- Report adverse effects to the physician.

ANTICHOLINERGICS
Atropine
Ipratropium bromide (Atrovent)
Tiotropium bromide (Spiriva)
Combination products: albuterol/ipratropium
(Combivent)

Anticholinergics are potent bronchodilators, blocking muscarinic receptors of the parasympathetic nervous system. Activation of muscarinic receptors produces smooth muscle contraction and bronchoconstriction; blockade of these receptors facilitates smooth muscle relaxation and bronchodilation. Atropine is used infrequently because of its tendency to dry secretions of the mucous membranes and other side effects. Ipratropium and tiotropium bromide are available as inhalers and have fewer side effects than atropine.

(continued)

MEDICATION ADMINISTRATION **Asthma (continued)**

Nursing Responsibilities

- Assess for possible contraindications to the drug, including hypersensitivity, glaucoma, prostatic hypertrophy, or bladder-neck obstruction.
- Assess for desired and/or adverse effects: improving or worsening symptoms; nausea, vomiting, abdominal cramping, anxiety, dizziness; headache.
- Provide ice chips, fluids, or hard candy to relieve dry mouth.

Health Education for the Client and Family

- To prevent overdose, take no more than the prescribed number of doses per day.
- If the drug becomes less effective over time, notify the physician; an adjustment in dosage may be needed.

CORTICOSTEROIDS

Beclomethasone dipropionate (Vanceril, Beclovent)
Triamcinolone acetonide (Azmacort)
Flunisolide (AeroBid)
Fluticasone propionate (Flovent)
Dexamethasone sodium phosphate (Decadron Phosphate Respihaler)
***Combination products:* salmeterol/fluticasone (Advair)**

The anti-inflammatory effect of corticosteroids helps both prevent and treat acute episodes. Corticosteroids are used to reduce the frequency and severity of asthma attacks and allow reduced dosages of other drugs. The beneficial effects of corticosteroids for asthma result from their ability to decrease the synthesis and release of inflammatory mediators (such as histamine and leukotrienes), reduce inflammatory cell activation and infiltration, and decrease airway edema. Corticosteroids also decrease mucous production in the airways and increase the number and receptivity of β_2-receptors (Lehne, 2004). The cushingoid side effects of corticosteroids, always a major concern with their use, are minimized when they are inhaled. Note that the combination product salmeterol/fluticasone is associated with an increased risk of serious asthma exacerbations and death. It is a second-line drug, recommended for use only when asthma is inadequately controlled using other preparations (FDA, 2005a).

Nursing Responsibilities

- Administer inhaler doses after bronchodilators to facilitate transit of the medication to distal airways.
- Assess for common side effects: sore throat; hoarseness; and oropharyngeal or laryngeal *Candida albicans* infection.
- Administer antifungal medications or gargles as ordered.

Health Education for the Client and Family

- Rinse the mouth after using the inhaler and maintain good oral hygiene to reduce the risk of fungal infections.
- These medications should not be used to alleviate the symptoms of an acute attack.
- Several weeks of continued therapy may be required before a beneficial effect is noticed.
- Notify the physician if you develop weight gain, fluid retention, muscle weakness, redistribution of fat, or mood changes.

MAST CELL STABILIZERS
Cromolyn sodium (Intal, NasalCrom)
Nedocromil (Tilade)

Cromolyn sodium and nedocromil inhibit inflammatory cells in the airway, blocking early and late responses to inhaled antigens. Both drugs also prevent bronchoconstriction in response to inhaling cold air. These drugs act primarily by stabilizing the cytoplasmic membrane of mast cells, preventing the cells from releasing inflammatory mediators such as histamine (Lehne, 2004). These drugs are used only for preventing asthma attacks, not to treat an acute attack. They are administered by metered-dose inhaler, and have a wide margin of safety. Clients using nedocromil may complain of an unpleasant taste.

Nursing Responsibilities

- Evaluate for potential adverse effects of wheezing and bronchoconstriction.

Health Education for the Client and Family

- Gargling or sipping water can decrease the throat irritation associated with nebulizer treatment.
- Use appropriate technique. Inhale deeply with head tipped back to open airways, hold breath, and then exhale. Repeat until all of the drug has been inhaled.
- These drugs are used only to prevent asthma attacks; they are not effective in treating an acute attack.
- Several weeks may be required before a beneficial effect is noted.

LEUKOTRIENE MODIFIERS
Montelukast (Singulair)
Zafirlukast (Accolate)
Zileuton (Zyflo)

Leukotriene modifiers interfere with the inflammatory process in the airways by suppressing the effects of leukotrienes, a group of inflammatory mediators. Leukotrienes are powerful bronchoconstrictors and vasodilators; blocking their synthesis or their receptors improves airflow, decreases symptoms, and reduces the need for short-acting bronchodilators. They are used for maintenance therapy in adults and children over the age of 12 as an alternative to inhaled corticosteroid therapy. They are not used to treat an acute attack.

Nursing Responsibilities

- Administer at least 1 hour before or 2 hours after meals.
- These drugs inhibit some liver enzymes, affecting the metabolism of warfarin and possibly terfenadine and theophylline. Monitor prothrombin times and theophylline blood levels.
- Monitor liver enzymes, because these drugs may be toxic to the liver.

Health Education for the Client and Family

- Take the drugs as prescribed on an empty stomach.
- Notify the physician if a change in color of stools or urine is noted or if jaundice develops.

Nursing Diagnoses and Interventions

An acute asthma attack causes fear as breathing becomes increasingly difficult and hypoxemia develops. Anxiety in turn tends to increase the severity and manifestations of the attack. Priority nursing care needs during an acute attack focus on improving airway clearance and reducing fear and anxiety. Teaching about prevention of future attacks and home management must be postponed until adequate ventilation is restored.

Ineffective Airway Clearance

Bronchospasm and bronchoconstriction, increased mucous secretion, and airway edema narrow the airways and impair airflow during an acute attack of asthma. Both inspiratory and expiratory volume are affected, decreasing the oxygen available at the alveolus for the process of respiration. Narrowed air passages increase the work of breathing, increasing the metabolic rate and tissue demand for oxygen.

PRACTICE ALERT
Frequently assess respiratory status (at least every 1 to 2 hours): respiratory rate and depth, chest movement or excursion, breath sounds, and peak expiratory flow rate. Respiratory status can change rapidly during an acute asthma attack and its treatment. Decreasing PEFRs indicate worsening airflow restriction. Slowed, shallow respirations with significantly diminished breath sounds and decreased wheezing may indicate exhaustion and impending respiratory failure. Immediate intervention is necessary.

- Monitor skin color and temperature and level of consciousness (LOC). *Cyanosis, cool clammy skin, and changes in LOC (agitation, lethargy, or confusion) indicate worsening hypoxia.*
- Assess ABG results and pulse oximetry readings; notify the physician of abnormal values or changes in status. *These values provide information about gas exchange and the adequacy of alveolar ventilation. A fall in oxygen saturation levels is an early indicator of impaired gas exchange.*

PRACTICE ALERT
Assess cough effort and sputum for color, consistency, and amount. Ineffective cough may also signal impending respiratory failure.

- Place in Fowler's, high-Fowler's, or orthopneic (with head and arms supported on the overbed table) position to facilitate breathing and lung expansion. *These positions reduce the work of breathing and increase lung expansion, especially of basilar areas.*
- Administer oxygen as ordered. If a mask is used, monitor closely for feelings of claustrophobia or suffocation. *Supplemental oxygen reduces hypoxemia. Although the mask is a very effective oxygen delivery system, it may increase anxiety.*
- Administer nebulizer treatments and provide humidification as ordered. *Nebulizer treatments are used to administer bronchodilators and other medications; humidity helps loosen secretions.*
- Initiate or assist with chest physiotherapy, including percussion and postural drainage. *Percussion and postural drainage facilitate the movement of secretions and airway clearance.*

- Increase fluid intake. *Increasing fluids helps keep secretions thin.*
- Provide endotracheal suctioning as needed. *Endotracheal suctioning may be necessary to remove secretions and improve ventilation if the client is unable to clear secretions by coughing.*

Ineffective Breathing Pattern

The physiologic changes in lung ventilation that occur during an acute asthma attack impair both lung expansion and emptying. Anxiety caused by hypoxia and dyspnea compounds the problem by increasing the respiratory rate. Collaborative and nursing interventions can help restore a more normal breathing pattern and adequate lung ventilation.

PRACTICE ALERT
Frequently assess respiratory rate, pattern, and breath sounds. Note manifestations of ineffective breathing, including rapid rate, shallow respirations, nasal flaring, use of accessory muscles, intercostal retractions, and diminished or absent breath sounds. Early identification of ineffective respirations allows timely initiation of interventions.

- Monitor vital signs and laboratory results. *Tachypnea, tachycardia, an elevated blood pressure, and increasing hypoxemia and hypercapnia are signs of compromised respiratory status.*
- Assist with ADLs as needed. *This conserves energy and reduces fatigue.*
- Provide rest periods between scheduled activities and treatments. *Scheduled rest is important to prevent fatigue and reduce oxygen demands.*
- Teach and assist to use techniques to control breathing pattern:
  a. Pursed-lip breathing
  b. Abdominal breathing
  c. Relaxation techniques including visualization and meditation.
  Pursed-lip breathing helps keep airways open by maintaining positive pressure, and abdominal breathing improves lung expansion. Relaxation techniques reduce anxiety and its effect on the respiratory rate.
- Administer medications, including bronchodilators and anti-inflammatory drugs, as ordered. Monitor for desired and possible adverse effects. *Medications are used to improve airway status and facilitate breathing.*

Anxiety

Acute exacerbations of asthma can produce significant anxiety. Fear of being unable to breathe and feelings of suffocation associated with acute asthma are significant. Financial or other concerns may cause the client to want to avoid hospitalization. Increasingly frequent and severe episodes may cause fear for the future. Hypoxia contributes to anxiety as well, stimulating the sympathetic nervous system and the fight-or-flight response.

- Assess level of anxiety. *Interventions for severe anxiety or panic differ from those for mild or moderate anxiety.*
- Assist to identify coping skills that have been successful in the past. *Successful coping helps the client regain control of the situation, reducing anxiety.*

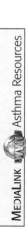

PRACTICE ALERT

Provide physical and emotional support. Remain with the client during episodes of severe anxiety; schedule time every 1 to 2 hours to be with the mildly or moderately anxious client. Answer call lights promptly. The severely anxious client may fear being alone or believe that he or she will die if someone is not on hand. Knowing that the nurse is readily available and will return regardless if help is needed reduces anxiety.

■ Listen actively to concerns; do not deny or negate the fear of dying or of being unable to breathe. *Active listening promotes trust and helps the client express concerns.*

PRACTICE ALERT

Provide clear, concise directions and explanations about procedures. Avoid presenting more information than the client is able to assimilate. Anxiety interferes with the ability to learn. Explanations may need to be repeated frequently.

■ Include the client in care planning and decisions as appropriate, without making excessive demands. *Participating in decision making increases the client's sense of control. Because high levels of anxiety interfere with the ability to make decisions, it is important to avoid placing demands on the client that may further increase the level of anxiety.*
■ Reduce excessive environmental stimuli, and maintain a calm demeanor. *This promotes rest.*
■ Allow supportive family members to remain with the client. *Significant others provide additional support and can help reduce anxiety.*
■ Assist to use relaxation techniques, such as guided imagery, muscle relaxation, and meditation. *These techniques help restore psychologic balance and reduce sympathetic stimulation and responses.*

Ineffective Therapeutic Regimen Management

Once acute asthma is under control and effective respirations have been reestablished, it is important to help the client identify contributing factors to the attack. This helps the client prevent future episodes.

■ Assess level of understanding about asthma and the prescribed treatment regimen. Provide additional information and teaching as indicated. *Assessment helps to identify and clarify misperceptions and difficulties with disease management.*
■ Discuss the client's perception of the illness and its effect on his or her lifestyle. *Open discussion can help identify conflicts between lifestyle and the treatment regimen.*

PRACTICE ALERT

Assist to identify factors that contributed to the acute episode. Identifying contributing factors increases the client's awareness of the disease and strategies to prevent future exacerbations.

■ Assist the client and significant others to identify problems or difficulties integrating the treatment regimen into their lifestyle. *Asthma and its management may necessitate lifestyle modifications to prevent acute exacerbations. This can significantly impact family members, for example, elim-*inating cigarette smoking or pets from the household, removing carpets, or daily damp-dusting to remove dust mites.
■ Assess knowledge and understanding of prescribed medications and use of over-the-counter (OTC) preparations. *This is important to determine misperceptions or possible misuse of medications.*
■ Provide verbal and written instructions. *Written instructions reinforce teaching and allow future reference.*
■ Refer to counseling, support groups, or self-help organizations. *Counseling, support groups, and self-help organizations can help the client and family adapt to living with asthma and the treatment regimen.*

Community-Based Care

Asthma is a chronic disease that is best managed by the client with assistance from medical personnel. Teaching for home care focuses on promoting the highest level of wellness and preventing and managing acute episodes and exacerbations of the disease. Topics to include in teaching are as follows:

■ Suggestions for lifestyle changes to avoid specific triggers for asthma attacks, for example:
  ■ Warm up slowly before exercising in cold weather; wear a special mask or scarf to retain air warmth and humidity while exercising.
  ■ Substitute indoor exercises during cold, dry weather.
  ■ Reduce the risk for respiratory infections (e.g., adequate rest, good nutrition, and stress management to maintain immune function, yearly influenza vaccines and immunization against pneumococcal pneumonia).
  ■ Use techniques to reduce or manage physical and psychologic stress.
■ Using PEFR meter to monitor airway status; how to manage the disease based on results
■ Using prescribed medications, including:
  ■ Name, frequency, dose, and desired effect
  ■ Potential adverse effects and their management, including effects to report to the physician
  ■ Potential interactions with other drugs (including OTC herbal preparations) or foods
  ■ If tolerance is a potential risk, how to identify it and steps to take.

Provide referrals to local or regional resources for further teaching and support as needed. Consider the need for home health services, home respiratory care services, and others as needed.

THE CLIENT WITH CHRONIC OBSTRUCTIVE PULMONARY DISEASE

Clients with chronic airflow obstruction due to chronic bronchitis and/or emphysema are said to have **chronic obstructive pulmonary disease (COPD)**.

Incidence and Risk Factors

In 2003, approximately 10.7 million Americans were affected by COPD (ALA, 2006). It is more common among whites than blacks and affects men more frequently than women. It is the fourth leading cause of death in the United States. The death rate from COPD continues to rise among black and American Indian males and among females of all ethnic groups; the death rate is stable in whites, Hispanics, and Asians. In 2002, COPD and other chronic obstructive lung diseases accounted for more than 125,500 deaths (NHLBI, 2004). In addition, COPD morbidity is significant. In people under age 65, COPD is second only to heart disease as a cause of disability, resulting in an estimated 250 million lost work-hours yearly.

FAST FACTS

- Since 2000, the number of deaths due to COPD in women has exceeded the number of men who have died due to COPD.
- Chronic bronchitis affected an estimated 8.6 million Americans in 2003.
- Women are now more than twice as likely to be diagnosed with chronic bronchitis as men.
- Approximately 3.1 million Americans have emphysema.
- While more men than women have emphysema, its prevalence is increasing in women and decreasing in men.

Source: Lung Disease Data: 2006 by the American Lung Association, 2006; retrieved from at http://www.lungusa.org.

Obstructive lung disease typically affects middle-aged and older adults. Cigarette smoking is clearly implicated as the primary cause of COPD. Even though COPD develops in a minority of smokers, smokers are 12 to 13 times more likely to die from COPD than nonsmokers (ALA, 2006). Cigarette smoke and the irritants it contains impair ciliary movement, inhibit the function of alveolar macrophages, and cause mucus-secreting glands to hypertrophy. It also produces emphysema or airway destruction and constricts smooth muscle, increasing airway resistance. Other contributing factors include air pollution, occupational exposure to noxious dusts and gases, airway infection, and familial and genetic factors (see the accompanying Genetic Considerations box).

Pathophysiology

COPD is characterized by slowly progressive obstruction of the airways. The disease is one of periodic exacerbations, often re-

GENETIC CONSIDERATIONS
Chronic Obstructive Pulmonary Disease

Severe α_1-antitrypsin (α_1AT or ATT) deficiency, present in about 1% to 2% of clients with COPD, is a proven risk factor for COPD. Normal α_1AT levels are associated with the common M allele. Two other alleles, the S allele and the Z allele, lead to reduced α_1AT levels. An estimated 25 million Americans carry a single gene associated with α_1AT deficiency and can pass that gene on to their offspring (ALA, 2006). People who inherit two Z alleles or one Z allele and one null allele have severe α_1AT deficiency. Approximately 1 in 3000 people in the United States inherit severe α_1AT deficiency (Kasper et al., 2005). An estimated 100,000 people in the United States have emphysema related to α_1AT deficiency (ALA, 2006). Although studies suggest additional genetic factors in the development of COPD, at this time none have been proven (Kasper et al., 2005).

lated to respiratory infection, with increased symptoms of dyspnea and sputum production. Unlike acute processes in which lung tissues recover, airways and lung parenchyma do not return to normal following an exacerbation; instead, they demonstrate progressive destructive changes.

Although one or the other may predominate, COPD typically includes components of both chronic bronchitis and emphysema, two distinctly different processes. Small airways disease, narrowing of small bronchioles, is also part of the COPD complex. Through different mechanisms, these processes cause airways to narrow, resistance to airflow to increase, and expiration to become slow or difficult (Figure 39–2 ■). The result is a mismatch between alveolar ventilation and blood flow or perfusion, leading to impaired gas exchange.

Chronic Bronchitis

Chronic bronchitis is a disorder of excessive bronchial mucous secretion. It is characterized by a productive cough lasting 3 or more months in 2 consecutive years (Porth, 2005). Cigarette smoke is the major factor implicated in the development of chronic bronchitis.

Inhaled irritants lead to a chronic inflammatory process with vasodilation, congestion, and edema of the bronchial mucosa. Goblet cells increase in size and number, and mucous glands enlarge. Thick, tenacious mucus is produced in increased amounts. Changes in bronchial squamous cells impair the ability to clear mucus (Kasper et al., 2005). Narrowed airways and excess secretions obstruct airflow; expiration is affected first, then inspiration. Because ciliary function is impaired, normal defense mechanisms are unable to clear the mucus and any inhaled pathogens. Recurrent infection is common in chronic bronchitis.

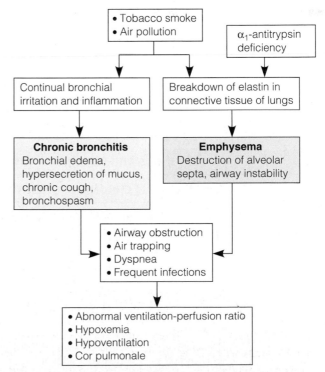

Figure 39–2 ■ The pathogenesis of chronic obstructive pulmonary disease.

An imbalance between ventilation and perfusion leads to hypoxemia, hypercapnia, and pulmonary hypertension. Pulmonary hypertension often leads to right-sided heart failure.

Emphysema

Emphysema is characterized by destruction of the walls of the alveoli, with resulting enlargement of abnormal air spaces. As in chronic bronchitis, cigarette smoking is strongly implicated as a causative factor in most cases of emphysema. Deficiency of α_1-antitrypsin, an enzyme that normally inhibits the activity of proteolytic enzymes and tissue destruction in the lungs, contributes to the development of emphysema, especially when combined with exposure to cigarette smoke.

Inflammatory cells that collect in distal airway tissues appear to lead to destruction of elastic fibers in the respiratory bronchioles and alveolar ducts. Alveolar wall destruction causes alveoli and air spaces to enlarge with loss of corresponding portions of the pulmonary capillary bed. As a result, the surface area for alveolar-capillary diffusion is reduced, affecting gas exchange. Elastic recoil is lost, reducing the volume of air that is passively expired. The loss of support tissue also affects airways, increasing the risk of expiratory collapse and further air trapping. Anatomically, either respiratory bronchioles or alveoli may be the primary tissue involved.

To summarize, COPD is a progressive, nonreversible process of airway narrowing and loss of supporting tissue. Three separate processes typically are involved:

- Chronic bronchitis with persistent airway edema, excessive mucous production, and impaired airway clearance
- Emphysema with loss of interstitial membranes and airway support tissue, resulting in airway collapse and loss of alveolar surface area for gas exchange
- Small airways disease with bronchoconstriction.

The result of these processes and their combined effects is increased work of breathing, impaired expiration with air trapping, and impaired gas exchange.

Manifestations

The clinical presentation of COPD varies from simple chronic bronchitis without disability to chronic respiratory failure and

---

BOX 39–2 Classification of COPD by Severity

Stage 0— At risk. Lung function normal, but chronic cough and sputum production are present

Stage 1—Mild COPD. Mild airflow limitation, usually with chronic cough and sputum production

Stage 2—Moderate COPD. Worsening airflow limitation, usually with progressing manifestations including dyspnea on exertion

Stage 3—Severe COPD. Further worsening of airflow limitation, increased shortness of breath, and repeated exacerbations impacting quality of life

Stage 4—Very severe COPD. Severe airflow limitation with significantly impaired quality of life and potentially life-threatening exacerbations

Source: Adapted from *Global Initiative for Chronic Obstructive Lung Disease. Pocket Guide to COPD Diagnosis, Management, and Prevention: A Guide for Health Care Professionals,* 2005, by the National Heart, Lung, and Blood Institute and the World Health Organization.

---

severe disability. Box 39–2 outlines the classifications of COPD severity. Manifestations are typically absent or minor early in the disease. When the client finally seeks care, productive cough, dyspnea, and exercise intolerance often have been present for as long as 10 years. The cough typically occurs in the mornings and often is attributed to "smoker's cough." Initially, dyspnea occurs only on extreme exertion; as the disease progresses, dyspnea becomes more severe and accompanies mild activity. Manifestations characteristic of chronic bronchitis and emphysema develop. The clinical features and manifestations of COPD are summarized in Table 39–3.

Manifestations of chronic bronchitis are a cough productive of copious amounts of thick, tenacious sputum, cyanosis, and evidence of right-sided heart failure, including distended neck veins, edema, liver engorgement, and an enlarged heart. Adventitious lung sounds, including loud rhonchi and possible wheezes, are prominent on auscultation.

Emphysema is insidious in onset. Dyspnea is the initial symptom. Initially occurring only with exertion, dyspnea may progress to become severe even at rest. Cough is minimal or absent. Air trapping and hyperinflation increase the anterior-posterior chest

---

TABLE 39–3 Clinical Features and Manifestations of COPD

	FEATURE	CHRONIC BRONCHITIS	EMPHYSEMA
History	Onset	After age 35; recurrent respiratory infections	After age 50; insidious progressive dyspnea
	Smoking	Usual	Usual
	Cough	Persistent, productive of copious mucopurulent sputum	Absent or mild with scant clear sputum, if any
Physical Examination	Appearance	Often obese; edematous and cyanotic; distended neck veins and other symptoms of right-sided heart failure	Usually thin and cachectic; barrel chest; prominent accessory muscles of respiration
	Chest	Adventitious sounds with wheezing and rhonchi; normal percussion note	Distant or diminished breath sounds; hyperresonant percussion note
Other Features	Blood gases	Hypercapnia and hypoxemia; respiratory acidosis	Normal or mild hypoxemia; normal pH
	Pulmonary function studies	Normal or decreased total lung capacity; moderately increased residual volume	Increased total lung capacity; markedly increased residual volume
	Pulmonary hypertension	May be severe	Only when advanced

diameter, causing *barrel chest*. The client often is thin, tachypneic, uses accessory muscles of respiration, and often assumes a position of sitting and leaning forward (Figure 39–3 ■). The expiratory phase of the respiratory cycle is prolonged. On auscultation, breath sounds are diminished, and the percussion tone is hyperresonant.

INTERDISCIPLINARY CARE

Although COPD can be prevented in most people, it cannot be cured. Smoking abstinence is the only certain way to prevent COPD and to slow its progression. To a certain extent, airway obstruction can be reversed and disability minimized early in the disease. Treatment generally focuses on relieving symptoms, minimizing obstruction, and slowing disability.

Diagnosis

Diagnostic tests are used to help establish the diagnosis of chronic obstructive pulmonary disease and identify the predominant component, emphysema or chronic bronchitis. These procedures also are used to assess respiratory status and monitor treatment effectiveness. See Chapter 36 ∞ for more information about these diagnostic procedures and related nursing care.

■ *Pulmonary function testing* is performed to establish the diagnosis and evaluate the extent and progress of COPD (see Box 36–1). Results are based on calculated norms for each person by age, height, sex, and weight; note these as well as all current medications on the requisition. In COPD, the total lung capacity and residual volume typically are increased. The forced expiratory volume (FEV_1) and forced vital capacity (FVC) are decreased due to narrowed airways and resistance to airflow.

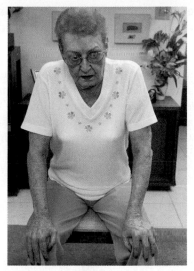

Figure 39–3 ■ Typical appearance of a client with emphysema. Note the client's anxious expression and assumption of the tripod position, leaning forward with the hands on the knees.
Courtesy of Michal Heron/Pearson Education/PH College

■ *Ventilation-perfusion scanning* may be performed to determine the extent of ventilation-perfusion mismatch—that is, the extent to which lung tissue is ventilated but not perfused (dead space), or perfused but inadequately ventilated (physiologic shunting) (Figure 39–4 ■). A radioisotope is injected or inhaled to illustrate areas of shunting and absent capillaries.

■ *Serum α_1-antitrypsin (α_1AT) levels* may be drawn to screen for deficiency, particularly in clients with a family history of obstructive airway disease, those with an early onset,

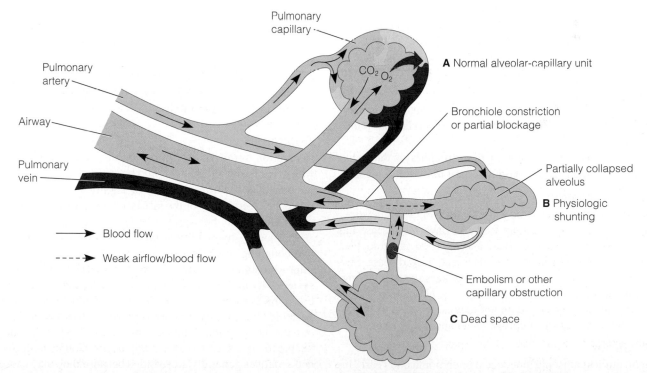

Figure 39–4 ■ Ventilation-perfusion relationships. *A,* Normal alveolar-capillary unit with an ideal match of ventilation and blood flow. Maximum gas exchange occurs between alveolus and blood. *B,* Physiologic shunting: A unit with adequate perfusion but inadequate ventilation. *C,* Dead space: A unit with adequate ventilation but inadequate perfusion. In the latter two cases, gas exchange is impaired.

women, and nonsmokers. Normal adult serum $\alpha_1 AT$ levels range from 80 to 260 mg/dL. Fasting is not required prior to this test.

■ *ABGs* are drawn to evaluate gas exchange, particularly during acute exacerbations of COPD. Clients with predominant emphysema often have mild hypoxemia and normal or low carbon dioxide tension. Respiratory alkalosis may be present due to an increased respiratory rate. Predominant chronic bronchitis and airway obstruction may cause marked hypoxemia and hypercapnia with respiratory acidosis. Oxygen saturation levels are low due to marked hypoxemia. See page 240 for steps to interpret ABGs.

PRACTICE ALERT

Hypercapnia (elevated $Paco_2$ levels) often is chronic in clients with COPD (CO_2 retainers). In these clients, administering oxygen can actually increase the $Paco_2$, leading to somnolence and acute respiratory failure. While oxygen is the drug of choice for treating clients with COPD, close monitoring is necessary during oxygen therapy.

■ *Pulse oximetry* is used to monitor oxygen saturation of the blood. Marked airway obstruction and hypoxemia often cause oxygen saturation levels of less than 95%. Pulse oximetry may be continuously monitored to assess the need for supplemental oxygen.

■ *Exhaled carbon dioxide (capnogram or $ETco_2$)* may be measured to evaluate alveolar ventilation. The normal $ETco_2$ reading is 35 to 45 mmHg; it is elevated when ventilation is inadequate, and decreased when pulmonary perfusion is impaired. $ETco_2$ monitoring can reduce the frequency of ABG determinations.

■ *Complete blood count (CBC) with white blood cell (WBC) differential* often shows increased red blood cells (RBCs) and hematocrit (erythrocytosis) as chronic hypoxia stimulates increased erythropoiesis to improve the oxygen-carrying capacity of the blood. *Polycythemia,* increased numbers of all blood cells, may be evident. Increased WBC count and a higher percentage of immature WBCs (bands) are often indicative of bacterial infection.

■ *Chest x-ray* may show flattening of the diaphragm due to hyperinflation and evidence of pulmonary infection if present.

Smoking Cessation

Smoking cessation can not only prevent COPD from developing, but also can improve lung function once the disease has been diagnosed. FEV_1 improves, and survival is prolonged, largely due to lower rates of lung cancer and heart disease. Sustained quitting is difficult; only 6% of smokers succeed in long-term abstinence from smoking (Kasper et al., 2005). Use of nicotine patches or gum and an antidepressant such as bupropion (Wellbutrin, Zyban) improve the chances of success.

Medications

Immunization against pneumococcal pneumonia and yearly influenza vaccine are recommended to reduce the risk of respiratory infections. A broad-spectrum antibiotic is prescribed if infection is suspected. Recent studies indicate that clients with

purulent sputum and increased dyspnea will likely benefit from antibiotic therapy, even if no other signs of infection are present. Prophylactic antibiotics may be ordered for clients who experience four or more disease exacerbations per year (Kasper et al., 2005).

Bronchodilators improve airflow and reduce air trapping in COPD, resulting in improved dyspnea and exercise tolerance. Bronchodilators may be given by MDI, DPI, by nebulizer, or orally. Oral administration may promote adherence, but is associated with much higher rates of adverse effects. A spacer or holding chamber may facilitate effective use of an MDI. Ipratropium bromide, an anticholinergic agent administered by MDI, is frequently prescribed. It has a longer duration of action than the short-acting β_2-adrenergic stimulant bronchodilators and few side effects. Salmeterol, a longer acting β_2-agonist, may be used in combination therapy. Oral theophylline, a methylxanthine, is a weak bronchodilator and has a narrow therapeutic range, but often is prescribed for its other effects. Theophylline stimulates the respiratory drive, strengthens diaphragmatic contractions, and improves cardiac output. As a result, dyspnea, exercise tolerance, and quality of life improve for the client with COPD. Bronchodilators are discussed in further detail in the section on asthma, and their nursing implications are outlined in the Medication Administration box on pages 1327–1328.

Corticosteroid therapy may be used when asthma is a major component of COPD. It also improves symptoms and exercise tolerance, and may reduce the severity of exacerbations and the need for hospitalization. Oral corticosteroids, such as prednisone, are used initially. If a beneficial response occurs, the amount is reduced to the lowest effective dose. Every-other-day dosing or administration by inhaler is preferred to minimize steroid side effects, such as cushingoid effects and an increased risk for osteoporosis and vertebral fractures.

$\alpha_1 AT$ replacement therapy is available for clients with emphysema due to a genetic deficiency of the enzyme. Although expensive and inconvenient ($\alpha_1 AT$ is administered weekly by intravenous infusion), it has been shown to reduce the rate of airflow decline and mortality.

Treatments

In addition to refraining from smoking, exposure to other airway irritants and allergens should be avoided. The client should remain indoors during periods of significant air pollution to prevent exacerbations of the disease. Air filtering systems or air conditioning may be useful.

Pulmonary hygiene measures, including hydration, effective coughing, percussion, and postural drainage, are used to improve clearance of airway secretions. Maintaining adequate systemic hydration is essential to keep secretions thin. Forceful coughing is often less effective than leaning forward and repeatedly "huffing," with relaxed breathing between huffs. Percussion and postural drainage may be necessary if the client is unable to clear secretions by usual means. Cough suppressants and sedatives generally are avoided because they may cause retention of secretions.

Unless disabling cardiac disease is present, a regular exercise program is beneficial for:

- Improving exercise tolerance.
- Enhancing ability to perform ADLs.
- Preventing deterioration of physical condition.

A program of regular aerobic exercise (e.g., walking for 20 minutes at least three times weekly) designed to gradually increase exercise tolerance is recommended. Activities that strengthen the muscles used for breathing and ADLs, such as swimming and golf, also are beneficial. See the Nursing Research box below.

Breathing exercises are used to slow the respiratory rate and relieve accessory muscle fatigue. Pursed-lip breathing slows the respiratory rate and helps maintain open airways during exhalation by keeping positive pressure in the airways. Abdominal breathing relieves the work of accessory muscles of respiration.

Oxygen

Long-term oxygen therapy is used for severe and progressive hypoxemia. Oxygen therapy improves exercise tolerance, mental functioning, and quality of life in advanced COPD. It also reduces the rate of hospitalization and increases length of survival. Oxygen may be used intermittently, at night, or continuously. For severely hypoxemic clients, the greatest benefit is seen with continuous oxygen. Home oxygen may be supplied as liquid oxygen, compressed gas cylinders, or oxygen concentrators.

An acute exacerbation of COPD may necessitate oxygenation and inspiratory positive-pressure assistance with a face mask or intubation and mechanical ventilation. Oxygen administered without intubation and mechanical ventilation requires caution: Administering oxygen to clients with chronic elevated carbon dioxide levels in the blood can actually increase the $PaCO_2$, leading to increased somnolence and even

respiratory failure. Close monitoring of LOC and ABGs during oxygen therapy is vital (Simmons & Simmons, 2004).

Surgery

When medical therapy is no longer effective, lung transplantation may be an option. Both single and bilateral transplants have been performed successfully, with a 2-year survival rate of 75%. Lung reduction surgery is an experimental surgical intervention for advanced diffuse emphysema and lung hyperinflation. The procedure reduces the overall volume of the lung, reshapes it, and improves elastic recoil. As a result, pulmonary function and exercise tolerance improve and dyspnea is reduced. See the box on page 1313 for nursing care of the client undergoing lung surgery. Special nursing care considerations related to lung or heart-lung transplant are summarized in Box 39–3.

Complementary Therapies

Complementary therapies may be useful to help manage symptoms of COPD. Dietary measures such as minimizing intake of dairy products and salt may help reduce mucous production and keep mucus more liquefied. Be sure to recommend measures to replace the protein and calcium in dairy products to help maintain nutritional balance.

Herbal teas made with peppermint and yarrow, coltsfoot, or comfrey may act as expectorants to help relieve chest congestion. Licorice root, which may be taken in several forms, also has expectorant and anti-inflammatory effects that may be beneficial. Licorice root can, however, cause toxicity when used for extended periods of time (Spencer & Jacobs, 2003). Refer clients to a qualified herbalist for treatment.

Acupuncture may help the client with smoking cessation, and also has been used to treat asthma and other respiratory

---

NURSING RESEARCH | **Evidence-Based Practice: Client with COPD**

The correlation between physical activity and performance of essential ADLs, quality of life, and higher level functioning is well established. This is particularly true for the elderly and people with disease-related impairment in physical abilities. Physical inactivity is both a cause and an effect of declining physical function in the elderly as well as in clients with chronic obstructive pulmonary disease.

A study by Yang and Chen (2005) looked at change processes involved in moving from inactivity to activity in clients with COPD. This study found that those who adopted more behavioral change processes (counter-conditioning, helping relationships, reinforcement management, and self-liberation) were more likely to engage in and maintain regular exercise (defined as at least 20 minutes of exercise of any intensity performed more than three times a week), usually walking. Most of these clients were aware of exercise benefits and the link between exercise and illness. Even so, 15% of study participants who achieved exercise maintenance returned to a more sedentary, inactive lifestyle.

IMPLICATIONS FOR NURSING

This study and others support a program of regular physical activity to maintain functional status and reduce symptom progression. Additionally, this study suggests the importance of providing support and tools to help the client incorporate exercise into daily

routines, rather than simply recommending an exercise program and discussing the benefits of exercise. Strategies such as regular telephone follow-ups and creation of support groups help promote self-care responsibility. Encourage COPD clients to enroll in a pulmonary rehabilitation program if one is available. If there is no organized program in the area, work with the client, family, and social support network to develop an exercise routine that can and will be maintained.

CRITICAL THINKING IN CLIENT CARE

1. Consider other populations for whom regular exercise is recommended (e.g., clients who are overweight, clients with heart failure). What strategies have been shown to improve compliance with recommendations for regular exercise in these groups? How could these strategies be adapted for clients with COPD?
2. Use the physiologic and psychologic effects of regular exercise to explain its correlation with improved symptoms in the client with COPD.
3. Consider the age of most clients with COPD. What other physical or psychosocial factors commonly limit physical activity in this population? How can you use this information in designing an appropriate exercise program?

BOX 39–3 Nursing Considerations Related to Lung Transplant

While immediate postoperative care for clients undergoing lung or heart-lung transplant is provided by specially trained interdisciplinary teams in transplant centers, increased survival following transplant means that these clients increasingly are seen in community-based settings, non-transplant hospitals, and on general nursing care units. An understanding of common post-transplant complications and care needs of the post-transplant client facilitates appropriate nursing care.

Common Post-Transplant Complications

In the early post-transplant period, the most common complications relate to the surgical procedure itself or to rejection of the transplanted organ(s).

■ *Rejection.* Acute organ rejection can occur at any time following the transplant. An acute change in FEV_1 and FVC on home spirometry often is the first indication of acute rejection. Other manifestations of rejection include fever, shortness of breath, and an elevated WBC count. Because these manifestations are similar to those of infection, the client is instructed to return to the transplant clinic or center for a transbronchial biopsy (Petty, 2003). Acute rejection is treated with increased corticosteroids and adjustment of the immunosuppressive regimen (see Chapter 13 ∞). Chronic rejection is less amenable to therapy, ultimately necessitating retransplant.

■ *Infection.* Prevention of infection is vital in lung transplant clients. Clients are encouraged to reduce their risk of infection by avoiding contact with people who have an infectious disease (e.g., URI, shingles, diseases of childhood). Prophylactic trimethoprim-sulfamethoxazole (TMP-SMZ) is administered weekly to prevent *Pneumocystis* pneumonia (see Chapter 38 ∞). Bacterial endocarditis prophylaxis also is provided as needed (see Chapter 32 ∞). The post-transplant client may not have typical manifestations of infection due to immunosuppression. Any vague symptoms with or without fever or leukocytosis are investigated. Recurrent viral infections such as CMV have been associated with chronic rejection; hence, they are aggressively treated with antiviral therapy. Treatment of other infections is targeted to the infectious organism.

Nursing Considerations for the Post-Transplant Client

Reverse isolation procedures are not necessary unless the neutrophil count is very low ($<500/mm^3$). Use good hand washing and standard precautions at all times, and aseptic technique for dressing changes, IV starts and site care, and other invasive procedures (such as urinary catheterization). Do not allow caregivers or visitors with URI to have contact with the client; a mask may be provided for short visits if contact is unavoidable. Skin surveillance and care is vital following transplant. Intact skin reduces the risk of infection; however, corticosteroid therapy increases the risk for skin tears and breakdown.

The effect of all medications on immunosuppressive therapy and the transplanted organ(s) should be carefully investigated prior to administration. Some antibiotics and other drugs can affect blood levels of immunosuppressants (Petty, 2003).

Particular attention must be paid to pulmonary hygiene. Denervation of the transplanted lung eliminates the usual cough stimuli. Regularly scheduled coughing and deep breathing, and the use of vibration, percussion, and postural drainage, are important to prevent accumulation of secretions (Petty, 2003).

---

conditions. Hypnotherapy and guided imagery are used to assist with smoking cessation. These techniques also can help the client control anxiety and breathing patterns. Refer clients to a trained professional. Nurses, physicians, psychologists, counselors, social workers and others can take professional training in hypnotherapy and guided imagery (Fontaine, 2005).

 NURSING CARE

Health Promotion

Not smoking—never starting, or quitting—is the best preventive measure for chronic obstructive pulmonary disease. Even in clients with COPD, smoking cessation improves lung function and increases survival. Educate all clients, including preschool and school-age children, about the risks of smoking. See Box 39–4.

Assessment

Focused assessment for the client with chronic obstructive pulmonary disease includes:

■ *Health History:* Current symptoms, including cough, sputum production, shortness of breath or dyspnea, activity tolerance; frequency of respiratory infections and most recent episode; previous diagnosis of emphysema, chronic bronchitis, or asthma; current medications; smoking history (in pack-years— packs per day times number of years smoked), history of exposure to secondhand smoke, occupational or other pollutants.

■ *Physical Examination:* General appearance, weight for height, mental status; vital signs including temperature; skin color and temperature; anterior-posterior:lateral chest diameter, use of accessory muscles, nasal flaring or pursed-lip breathing; respiratory excursion and diaphragmatic excursion; percussion tone; breath sounds throughout; neck veins, apical pulse and heart sounds, peripheral pulses, edema.

■ *Diagnostic Tests:* FVC and FEV_1, ABGs, hematocrit.

Nursing Diagnoses and Interventions

Clients with chronic obstructive pulmonary disease, whether hospitalized or in the community, have multiple nursing care needs. Because of the obstructive nature of the disease, airway clearance is a high priority. Nutritional deficit is common, particularly when emphysema is predominant. Because this chronic disease affects all functional health patterns, psychosocial issues are also of concern in planning nursing care. In addition to the nursing diagnoses presented here, see the Nursing Care Plan that follows.

Ineffective Airway Clearance

Both chronic bronchitis and emphysema affect the ability to maintain open airways. In chronic bronchitis, copious

BOX 39–4 Cigarette Smoking and Tobacco Use

The use of tobacco reaches back to early civilizations, when it was used in religious ceremonies and as an offering of friendship. At one time, tobacco was thought to have medicinal qualities effective against all common diseases. Widespread use of tobacco among the male population of the industrialized world began during World War I.

Tobacco is now recognized as the leading cause of preventable illness in the world. Diseases directly related to tobacco use are responsible for the deaths of more than 438,000 Americans every year. Smoking will lead to the deaths of about half of all regular cigarette smokers (ALA, 2006). In spite of this knowledge, aggressive marketing of the product continues, and its worldwide use is increasing, especially in underdeveloped countries.

The link between tobacco use and lung cancer was reported as early as 1912. In 1987, lung cancer became the leading cause of cancer-related death in the United States among both men and women.

Cigarette smoke contains over 4800 chemicals (69 of which are known to cause cancer), including nicotine (ALA, 2006). Nicotine is a highly addictive psychoactive substance that is relatively cheap and readily available. It produces euphoria, which acts as a positive reinforcer for continued use. In North American society, tobacco is more acceptable than many other dependency-producing drugs.

Tar is the particulate matter in cigarette smoke that is responsible for most of its carcinogenic and pathologic effects on the lungs. Smoke also paralyzes the cilia, reducing their ability to remove tars from contact with the respiratory epithelium. The risk for cancer and other lung diseases is dose related, affected by the age at which smoking began, the number of cigarettes smoked per day, and the number of years smoked. Smoking cessation reduces the risks associated with tobacco use. For some, such as those at risk for coronary heart disease, quitting smoking yields rapid benefits. For others, the degree of risk reduction is less immediate, but still significant.

Nurses need to do more than simply advise clients to quit smoking and talk about the risks of smoking. Nurses can take an active role in smoking cessation. Identify smoking habits, smoking-related illnesses, and previous efforts to quit. Work with the client to identify barriers and obstacles to quitting. Educate about the addictive nature of nicotine, and explain the manifestations of nicotine withdrawal (anxiety, irritability, headache, and disturbed sleep). Develop a plan with the client that specifies a target date to quit and includes ways to deal with obstacles to quitting, withdrawal symptoms, and the temptation to resume smoking. Offer self-help material at an appropriate reading level. Refer to a counselor, physician, self-help group, or smoking cessation clinic. If a relapse occurs, accept it as a normal part of rehabilitation from any addictive substance. Continue to provide support and encouragement, helping the client avoid further relapses.

Nurses can be especially effective in primary prevention of cigarette smoking and the diseases associated with it. Just as tobacco companies direct advertising at women and teens, nurses can target these populations and younger children for programs to prevent smoking. In addition, nurses need to become active in reducing minors' access to tobacco products, especially cigarettes and chewing tobacco (often the first product used by teens).

Nursing diagnoses that may be appropriate related to smoking include the following:

- *Ineffective Health Maintenance* related to tobacco use
- *Decisional Conflict* related to tobacco use
- *Ineffective Denial* related to acknowledgment of substance abuse and dependence.

amounts of thick, tenacious mucus are produced. Ciliary action is impaired, making it difficult to clear mucus from the airways. The loss of supporting tissue caused by emphysema increases the risk for airway collapse. In both cases, air is trapped distally, and less oxygen is available to the alveoli for diffusion. Normal respiratory defense mechanisms are impaired, and mucous-plugged airways provide an ideal environment for bacterial growth. Respiratory infection further impairs airway clearance and is often the cause of an acute exacerbation.

- Assess respiratory status every 1 to 2 hours or as indicated. Assess rate and pattern; cough and secretions (color, amount, consistency, and odor); and breath sounds, both normal and adventitious. *Frequent assessment is vital to monitor current status and response to treatment. Adventitious sounds should decrease with effective intervention. Diminished or absent breath sounds may indicate increasing airway obstruction and possible atelectasis.*

PRACTICE ALERT
Promptly report changes in oxygen saturation, skin color, or mental status. A drop in oxygen saturation levels, increasing cyanosis, or altered LOC indicate hypoxemia, possibly related to airway obstruction.

- Monitor ABG results. *Increasing hypoxemia, hypercapnia, and respiratory acidosis may indicate increasing airway obstruction.*
- Weigh daily, monitor intake and output, and assess mucous membranes and skin turgor. *Dehydration causes respiratory secretions to become thicker, more tenacious, and difficult to expectorate; fluid overload can further compromise respiratory status.*
- Encourage a fluid intake of at least 2000 to 2500 mL per day unless contraindicated. *Adequate fluid intake helps keep mucous secretions thin.*
- Place in Fowler's, high-Fowler's, or orthopneic position; encourage movement and activity to tolerance. *Upright positions improve ventilation and reduce the work of breathing. Activity helps mobilize secretions and prevent them from pooling.*
- Assist with coughing and deep breathing at least every 2 hours while awake. Position seated upright, leaning forward during coughing. *The upright position promotes chest expansion, increasing the effectiveness of coughing and reducing the work involved.*
- Provide tissues and a paper bag to dispose of expectorated sputum. *This important infection control measure reduces the spread of respiratory organisms to other people.*
- Refer to a respiratory therapist, and assist with or perform percussion and postural drainage as needed. *Percussion helps*

NURSING CARE PLAN   A Client with COPD

Anna Mercurio, known as "Happy" to all her friends, is an 83-year-old widow who lives with her two adult sons. During the past 15 years, Mrs. Mercurio has become increasingly short of breath while gardening and walking, two favorite activities. She also has developed a chronic cough that is particularly bad in the mornings. Ten years ago, her family physician told her that she had emphysema. She is admitted to the hospital with possible pneumonia and acute exacerbation of COPD.

ASSESSMENT

Jeff Harris, RN, admits Mrs. Mercurio to the medical unit. In the nursing history, Mr. Harris notes that she denies ever smoking, but says that her husband and two sons have been smokers "for practically their whole lives." She says she lived an active life before developing lung disease, but now her breathing and cough have progressed so that she now must rest after just a few minutes of housework or other activity. Her cough is productive of moderate to large amounts of sputum, particularly in the mornings. She developed increasing shortness of breath and sputum 2 days ago; this morning, she could not complete her morning activities without resting, so she contacted her doctor.

On physical examination, Mr. Harris notes the following: skin very warm and dry, color dusky. Pauses frequently while speaking to breathe. Respiratory rate 36, fairly shallow; coughs frequently, producing large amounts of thick, tenacious green sputum. Other vital signs: P 115 and irregular, BP 186/60, T 102.4°F (39°C). Appears very thin; weight 96 lb (43.6 kg), height 63 inches (160 cm). Anteroposterior:lateral chest diameter approximately 1:1; moderate kyphosis noted. Chest hyperresonant to percussion. Auscultation reveals distant breath sounds with scattered wheezes and rhonchi throughout lung fields. Chest x-ray shows flattening of diaphragm, slight cardiac enlargement, prominent vascular and bronchial markings, and patchy infiltrates. Initial laboratory work reveals moderate erythrocytosis, leukocytosis, and low serum albumin. Arterial blood gas results: pH 7.19; PaO_2 54 mmHg; $PaCO_2$ 59 mmHg; HCO_3^- 30 mg/dL, and O_2 saturation 88%. Admitting orders include sputum specimen for culture; intravenous penicillin G, 2 million units every 4 hours; albuterol/ipratropium (Combivent) inhaler, two puffs every 6 hours; salmeterol/fluticasone (Advair) dry powder inhaler, twice a day; bed rest with bathroom privileges; oxygen per nasal cannula at 2 L continuously; and regular diet.

DIAGNOSES

- *Ineffective Airway Clearance* related to pneumonia and COPD
- *Impaired Gas Exchange* related to acute and chronic lung disease
- *Risk for Impaired Spontaneous Ventilation* related to loss of hypoxemic respiratory drive and respiratory muscle fatigue
- *Impaired Home Maintenance* related to activity intolerance

EXPECTED OUTCOMES

- Expectorate secretions effectively.
- Return to level of pulmonary function prior to acute exacerbation.
- Demonstrate improved ABG and oxygen saturation values.
- Maintain spontaneous respirations without excess fatigue.
- Verbalize willingness to allow sons or a housekeeper to assist with daily household tasks.

PLANNING AND IMPLEMENTATION

- Assess respiratory status and LOC every 1 to 2 hours until stable, then at least every 4 hours.
- Closely monitor response to oxygen therapy, including skin color, oxygen saturation, sputum consistency, and respiratory drive.
- Increase fluid intake to at least 2500 mL per day and provide bedside humidifier.
- Elevate head of bed to at least 30 degrees at all times.
- Teach "huff" coughing technique.
- Administer medications as ordered, providing ipratropium inhaler before beclomethasone inhaler. Provide mouth care after inhalers.
- Contact respiratory therapy for percussion and postural drainage following inhaler treatments.
- Provide for uninterrupted rest periods following treatments and procedures.
- Meet with Mrs. Mercurio and her sons to develop a postdischarge care plan.
- Refer to home health department for nursing follow-up.
- Refer to social services for possible assistance with home maintenance.

EVALUATION

After the first day in the hospital, Mrs. Mercurio's condition begins to improve slowly. On discharge 6 days later, she is able to provide self-care with less fatigue and dyspnea. She is using oxygen at night only, admitting that it is just for security. Although a few scattered wheezes and rhonchi are still present in her lungs, Mrs. Mercurio's sputum is thinner, white, and easily expectorated. She will continue taking oral penicillin V for an additional 10 days at home. She will also continue using the Advair and Combivent inhalers as prescribed at home. Although Mrs. Mercurio's sons admit they will probably never be able to quit smoking, they have agreed to smoke only in the garage or outside. A home health nurse will initially evaluate Mrs. Mercurio's progress three times weekly. Arrangements have been made for a housekeeper to come twice a week for cleaning and laundry. Mrs. Mercurio is glad to be returning home and grateful for the arrangements that have been made.

CRITICAL THINKING IN THE NURSING PROCESS

1. Mrs. Mercurio has never been a smoker but had long-term exposure to secondhand smoke. How does secondhand smoke contribute to lung diseases in adults and children?
2. Mr. Harris's nursing care plan included the nursing diagnosis *Risk for Impaired Spontaneous Ventilation* related to loss of hypoxemic respiratory drive and respiratory muscle fatigue. Identify the normal physiologic events that stimulate breathing, and describe how these differ for the client with chronic hypoxemia and hypercapnia.
3. The client with an acute exacerbation of COPD is at risk for respiratory failure. What changes in Mrs. Mercurio's assessment findings could indicate this complication?
4. Develop a nursing care plan for Mrs. Mercurio for the nursing diagnosis *Deficient Diversional Activities* related to inability to continue preferred activities.

See Evaluating Your Response in Appendix C.

loosen secretions in airways; postural drainage facilitates movement of these secretions out of the respiratory tract.

PRACTICE ALERT
Provide endotracheal, oral, or nasopharyngeal suctioning as necessary. Suctioning may be necessary to stimulate cough and help clear secretions.

- Provide rest periods between treatments and procedures. *The client with COPD fatigues easily; adequate rest is important to conserve energy and reduce fatigue.*
- Administer expectorant and bronchodilator medications as ordered. Correlate timing with respiratory treatments. *Using expectorants and bronchodilators prior to coughing, percussion, and postural drainage increases their effectiveness in clearing airways.*
- Provide supplemental oxygen as ordered. *Supplemental oxygen helps maintain adequate blood and tissue oxygenation.*

PRACTICE ALERT
Prepare for intubation and mechanical ventilation if respiratory status deteriorates (increasing hypoxemia and hypercapnia, decreased LOC, cyanosis, or worsening airway obstruction). Respiratory failure is a possible complication of an acute exacerbation of COPD and requires immediate intervention to preserve life.

Imbalanced Nutrition: Less than Body Requirements

With advanced COPD, minimal activity, including eating, can cause fatigue and dyspnea. The client may be unable to consume a full meal without resting. At the same time, the increased work of breathing increases metabolic demands, and more calories are required. The client may appear cachectic (thin and wasted). Poor nutritional status further impairs immune function and increases the risk of a complicating infection.

- Assess nutritional status, including diet history, weight for height (use reference tables of desired weights), and anthropometric (skinfold) measurements. *It is important to differentiate nutritional status from body type rather than assume a nutritional impairment.*
- Observe and document food intake, including types, amounts, and caloric intake. *This information can provide direction for supplementation, if needed.*
- Monitor laboratory values, including serum albumin and electrolyte levels. *These values provide information about the adequacy of nutritional intake, including protein.*
- Consult with a dietitian to plan meals and nutritional supplements that meet caloric needs. *More concentrated sources of high-energy foods may be required to maintain caloric intake without excess fatigue. A diet high in proteins and fats without excess carbohydrates is recommended to minimize carbon dioxide production during metabolism (carbohydrates are metabolized to form CO_2 and water).*
- Provide frequent, small feedings with between-meal supplements. *Frequent, small meals help maintain intake and reduce fatigue associated with eating.*

- Place seated or in high-Fowler's position for meals. *An upright position promotes lung expansion and reduces dyspnea.*
- Assist to choose preferred foods from the menu; encourage family members to bring food from home if allowed. *Providing preferred foods encourages eating.*
- Keep snacks at the bedside. *Snacks provide additional caloric intake.*
- Provide mouth care prior to meals. *This helps enhance the appetite.*
- If unable to maintain oral intake, consult with the physician about enteral or parenteral feedings. *Maintenance of caloric and nutrient intake is vital to prevent catabolism.*

Compromised Family Coping

Chronic illness affects the entire family structure. Roles and relationships change; additional demands are placed on the family. Family members may blame the client for causing the illness or have distorted perceptions about it, even denying its existence. They may refuse to assist or participate in care. The client may develop an attitude of helplessness or dependence or may demonstrate anger, hostility, or aggression.

- Assess interactions between client and family. *Assessment helps identify desired and potential destructive behaviors.*
- Assess the effect of the illness on the family. *Assessment of family interactions, roles, and relationships assists in planning appropriate interventions.*
- Help the client and family identify strengths for coping with the situation. *Identifying personal and family strengths helps the family regain a sense of control.*
- Provide information and teaching about COPD. *Education helps the family gain an understanding of the client's condition and needs.*
- Encourage expression of feelings. Avoid judging feelings expressed or family members as "good" or "bad," "right" or "wrong." *It is important that the nurse remain objective to maintain the therapeutic relationship.*
- Help family members recognize behaviors and attitudes that may hinder effective treatment, such as continuing to smoke in the house. *Family members may be unaware of the effect of their behavior on the client's ability to change habits and cope with a disabling disease.*
- Encourage family members to participate in care. *This helps develop skills for use at home.*
- Initiate a care conference involving the client, family, and healthcare team members from a variety of disciplines. *A wide range of perspectives and areas of expertise aids in problem solving and facilitates communication.*
- If dysfunctional family relationships interfere with measures to enhance coping, advocate for the client, reaffirming his or her right to make decisions. *Dysfunctional family relationships are not likely to change simply because of illness. The nurse can better meet the client's needs by accepting his or her limitations in dealing with family members.*
- Refer the client and family to support groups and pulmonary rehabilitation programs, as available. *Support groups and structured rehabilitation programs enhance coping abilities.*

- Arrange a social services consultation. *This can help the client and family identify care and support service needs.*
- Refer community agencies or services such as home health, homemaker services, or Meals-on-Wheels as appropriate. *Agencies or community services can provide additional support beyond the family's means or capability.*

Decisional Conflict: Smoking

Smoking is more than a habit; it is an addiction. The client who must quit is facing a significant loss, not only of nicotine but also of a lifestyle. Although the client may fully comprehend the consequences of continuing to smoke, the decision to give up a part of his or her life is not easy. This fear may be expressed in such concerns as "I'll gain weight" or "What will I do with my hands?" In addition to providing practical information, a plan, and assistance with nicotine withdrawal, the nurse must support the client's decision-making process to comply with an order to stop smoking.

- Assess knowledge and understanding of the choices involved and possible consequences of each. *The decision to quit smoking ultimately belongs to the client. He or she needs a full understanding of the consequences of quitting or continuing to smoke.*
- Acknowledge concerns, values, and beliefs; listen nonjudgmentally. *The nurse needs to avoid imposing his or her values and beliefs about smoking on the client.*
- Spend time with the client, encouraging expression of feelings. *This demonstrates acceptance of the client and his or her right to make the decision.*
- Help plan a course of action for quitting smoking and adapt it as necessary. *When the client develops the plan, he or she has more ownership in it and interest in making it work.*
- Demonstrate respect for decisions and the right to choose. *Respect supports self-esteem and the ability to cope.*
- Provide referral to a counselor or other professional as needed. *Counselors or other people trained to assist with smoking cessation can help with decision making.*

Using NANDA, NIC, and NOC

Chart 39–1 shows links between NANDA nursing diagnoses, NIC, and NOC for the client with COPD.

Community-Based Care

As with any chronic disease, the client and family will have primary responsibility for disease management. Teaching is vital to promote optimal health and slow disease progression. Teaching for home care focuses on effective coughing and breathing techniques (Box 39–5), preventing exacerbations, and managing prescribed therapies.

THE CLIENT WITH CYSTIC FIBROSIS

Cystic fibrosis (CF) is an autosomal recessive disorder that affects epithelial cells of the respiratory, gastrointestinal, and reproductive tracts and leads to abnormal exocrine gland secretions (see the accompanying box). Although it can affect many organ systems, CF is particularly damaging to the lungs, leading to COPD

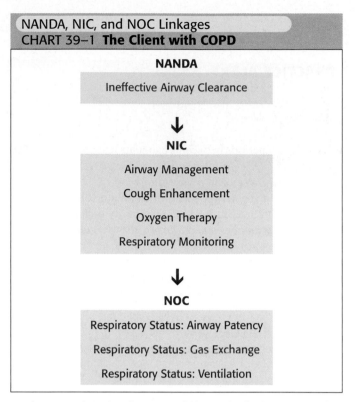

NANDA, NIC, and NOC Linkages
CHART 39–1 The Client with COPD

NANDA

Ineffective Airway Clearance

↓

NIC

Airway Management

Cough Enhancement

Oxygen Therapy

Respiratory Monitoring

↓

NOC

Respiratory Status: Airway Patency

Respiratory Status: Gas Exchange

Respiratory Status: Ventilation

Data from *NANDA's Nursing Diagnoses: Definitions & Classification 2005–2006* by NANDA International (2005), Philadelphia; *Nursing Interventions Classification (NIC)* (4th ed.) by J. M. Dochterman & G. M. Bulechek (2004), St. Louis, MO: Mosby; and *Nursing Outcomes Classification (NOC)* (3rd ed.) by S. Moorhead, M. Johnson, and M. Maas (2004), St. Louis, MO: Mosby.

in childhood and early adulthood. Respiratory manifestations of CF are the usual cause of morbidity and death from this disease. The gastrointestinal tract also is affected significantly; exocrine pancreatic insufficiency is characteristic of CF. Abnormally high sweat electrolytes also occur in CF.

Incidence and Prevalence

CF is the most common lethal genetic disease in Caucasian Americans, affecting about 1 in 2500 live births. It is less common in African Americans and rare in Asians. About 5% of

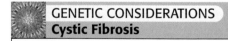

GENETIC CONSIDERATIONS
Cystic Fibrosis

The gene responsible for cystic fibrosis is at a single locus on the long arm of chromosome 7. This gene codes for a protein known as the *cystic fibrosis transmembrane conductance regulator* (CFTR). More than 1000 mutations of this gene have been identified. The most common mutation, identified as $\triangle$F508, accounts for about 66% of cystic fibrosis (Aronson & Marquis, 2004). Cystic fibrosis is an autosomal recessive disorder: It is not transmitted as a sex-linked trait, and the normal gene is dominant. People with one abnormal gene do not have the disorder but can transmit this abnormal gene to their offspring. When a child inherits an abnormal gene from both parents, the disorder is seen. Genetic screening of family members of a CF client can detect 70% to 75% of carriers of the CF gene. Screening for the CF gene is not recommended for the general population.

BOX 39–5 Client Teaching: Effective Coughing and Breathing Techniques

Pursed-lip and diaphragmatic breathing techniques help minimize air trapping and fatigue. Pursed lip breathing helps maintain open airways by maintaining positive pressures longer during exhalation. Teach the client to:

1. Inhale through the nose with the mouth closed.
2. Exhale slowly through pursed lips, as though whistling or blowing out a candle, making exhalation twice as long as inhalation.

Diaphragmatic or abdominal breathing helps conserve energy by using the larger and more efficient muscles of respiration. Teach the client to:

1. Place one hand on the abdomen, the other on the chest.
2. Inhale, concentrating on pushing the abdominal hand outward while the chest hand remains still
3. Exhale slowly, while the abdominal hand moves inward and the chest hand remains still.

Repeat these exercises as often as necessary until the techniques become incorporated into normal breathing.

Several different coughing techniques may be useful. For controlled cough technique, teach the client to:

1. Following prescribed bronchodilator treatment, inhale deeply, and hold breath briefly.
2. Cough twice, the first time to loosen mucus, the second to expel secretions.
3. Inhale by sniffing to prevent mucus from moving back into deep airways.
4. Rest. Avoid prolonged coughing to prevent fatigue and hypoxemia.

For huff coughing, teach the client to:

1. Inhale deeply while leaning forward.
2. Exhale sharply with a "huff" sound, to help keep airways open while mobilizing secretions.

In addition, include the following topics when teaching for home care:

- Maintaining adequate fluid intake, at least 2.0 to 2.5 quarts of fluid daily
- Avoiding respiratory irritants, including cigarette smoke, both primary and secondary, other smoke sources, dust, aerosol sprays, air pollution, and very cold dry air
- Preventing exposure to infection, especially upper respiratory infections
- Importance of pneumococcal vaccine and annual influenza immunization
- Prescribed exercise program, maintaining ADLs, and balancing rest and exercise
- Maintaining nutrient intake (e.g., eating small frequent meals and using nutritional supplements to provide adequate calories)
- Ways of reducing sodium intake if prescribed
- Identifying early signs of an infection or exacerbation and the importance of seeking medical attention for the following: fever, increased sputum production, purulent (green or yellow) sputum, upper respiratory infection, increased shortness of breath or difficulty breathing, decreased activity tolerance or appetite, increased need for oxygen
- Prescribed medications, including purpose, proper use, and expected effects
- Avoiding use of OTC medications unless approved by the physician
- Other prescribed therapies, such as use of home oxygen, percussion, postural drainage, and nebulizer treatments
- Use, cleaning, and maintenance of any required special equipment
- Importance of wearing an identification band and carrying a list of medications at all times in case of an emergency.

Provide referrals to home care services such as home health, assistance with ADLs as needed, home maintenance services, respiratory therapy and home oxygen services, and other agencies such as Meals-on-Wheels and senior services as indicated.

Caucasians in the United States carry the CF trait. Although the manifestations of CF usually develop in childhood, about 7% of clients with CF are diagnosed as adults. Adults now make up just over one-third of the CF population in the United States, with about 13% surviving into their 30s (Kasper et al., 2005).

Pathophysiology

The CFTR protein is involved in membrane transport of chloride and sodium in cells lining the ducts of exocrine glands (sweat glands, pancreas, liver, and reproductive systems). The genetic abnormality of CF leads to a lack or abnormality of this protein, with resulting abnormal electrolyte transport across epithelial cell membranes. Defective chloride transport causes more water and sodium reabsorption than normal. Secretions in affected organs become thick and viscous, obstructing glands and ducts. This obstruction causes dilation of secretory glands and damage to exocrine tissue. The hallmark pathophysiologic effects of CF include:

- Excess mucous production in the respiratory tract with impaired ability to clear secretions and progressive COPD
- Pancreatic enzyme deficiency and impaired digestion

- Abnormal elevation of sodium and chloride concentrations in sweat.

In the lungs, viscous mucus plugs small airways and impairs mucociliary clearance, leading to atelectasis, infection, bronchiectasis, and dilation of distal airways. Lower respiratory infections with *Staphylococcus aureus* and *Pseudomonas* are common (Porth, 2005). Acute and chronic damage to lung parenchyma causes tissue loss and extensive scarring and fibrosis. The upper lobes are involved to a greater extent than the lower lobes. Severe airway obstruction and chronic hypoxemia lead to pulmonary hypertension, right ventricular hypertrophy, and eventual cor pulmonale. Death usually results from a combination of cardiovascular changes and respiratory failure.

Pancreatic insufficiency is a frequent component of CF. It can range from slight pancreatic dysfunction to complete absence of function due to obstruction of pancreatic ducts with thick mucus and degenerative and fibrotic changes. Pancreatic insufficiency and impaired enzyme secretion lead to impaired digestion and absorption of proteins, carbohydrates, and fats.

About 8% of clients with CF develop diabetes mellitus (Porth, 2005). Liver failure is another potential complication of the disease (McCance & Huether, 2006). Because the genetic defect also affects cells of the reproductive tract, males with CF usually are sterile. Although females may have difficulty conceiving, pregnancies usually are carried to term (Kasper et al., 2005).

Manifestations

Manifestations of CF in a young adult include a history of chronic lung disease. Recurrent pneumonia, exercise intolerance, and chronic cough are typical. Other pulmonary manifestations include *clubbing* of the fingers and toes (Figure 39–5), increased anteroposterior chest diameter (barrel chest), hyperresonant percussion tone, and basilar crackles on auscultation. Distended neck veins, ascites, and peripheral edema accompany right-sided heart failure. Abdominal pain and *steatorrhea* (excess fat in the stools, causing frequent, bulky, foul-smelling stool) commonly result from associated pancreatic insufficiency. Growth and development are often retarded, resulting in small stature.

INTERDISCIPLINARY CARE

The treatment plan for cystic fibrosis is multidisciplinary, with the goals of preventing or treating respiratory complications and maintaining adequate nutrition. Psychosocial care is vital, as is genetic and occupational counseling.

Diagnosis

Although evidence of lung disease and pancreatic insufficiency suggests CF, analysis of Cl^- concentration in sweat is used to confirm the diagnosis. In CF, the Cl^- concentration is >70 mEq/L. Pilocarpine (a parasympathomimetic agent) and a small electric current are used to increase sweat production on the forearm. Absorbent paper or gauze is used to collect the sweat for analysis.

ABGs and oxygen saturation levels show hypoxemia. Pulmonary function studies reveal reduced airflow, reduced forced vital capacity (see Box 36–1 on page 1214), and reduced total lung capacity. Alveolar-capillary diffusion also is typically reduced.

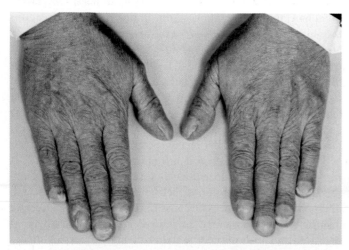

Figure 39–5 ■ Clubbing of fingers caused by chronic hypoxemia.
Source: John Radcliffe Hospital/Science Photo Library/Photo Researchers, Inc.

Medications

Immunization against respiratory infections is vital to promote optimal health. Yearly influenza vaccine is recommended, along with measles and pertussis boosters as needed.

Bronchodilator inhalers may be used to control airway constriction. Acute pulmonary infections are treated with appropriate antibiotic therapy as determined by sputum culture and sensitivity tests. A prolonged treatment course or multiple antibiotics may be required to eradicate pulmonary infections. Antibiotics may be administered by several routes, including inhalation, to achieve the desired concentration in large airways (Aronson & Marquis, 2004). Dornase alfa, recombinant human DNase, breaks down the excess DNA in the sputum of clients with CF, decreasing its viscosity and making it easier to clear. Dornase alfa, administered by aerosol, reduces the frequency of hospitalizations and the need for antibiotics for some clients.

Treatments

Chest physiotherapy with percussion and postural drainage is used to promote airway clearance. Newer airway clearance techniques include the use of the "huff" cough technique with specified breathing cycles or patterns. In one technique, a valved mask or mouthpiece is used to maintain positive expiratory pressure (PEP) for approximately 20 breaths, followed by three to five "huff" coughs. This cycle is repeated for a total of 20 minutes. The autogenic drainage technique, a form of biofeedback, involves controlled breathing at specific lung volumes and patterns to facilitate the movement of mucus into larger airways, where it can be cleared with the "huff" cough. A flutter valve device, which looks like a fat pipe, contains a steel ball within an inner cone. The weight of the ball provides intermittent PEP, which vibrates airway walls to loosen secretions.

Oxygen therapy may be required for hypoxemia. A liberal fluid intake helps reduce the viscosity of mucous secretions. A diet high in protein, fat, and calories may be necessary to maintain weight. Vitamins and minerals are supplemented to counteract excess losses in the sweat and stools. Enteral or parenteral nutrition may be required during acute exacerbations of the disease.

Surgery

Lung transplantation currently offers the only definitive treatment for CF. Lung transplantation lengthens life span and improves quality of life. Single-lung, double-lung, and heart-lung transplants have been successfully completed. Because the donor lungs do not have the CF gene, they do not develop the pathophysiologic changes of CF. Although the other defects characteristic of CF remain, these can be managed with pharmacologic therapy.

NURSING CARE

Nursing care for the client with cystic fibrosis is much the same as that for any chronic obstructive lung disease. Promoting airway clearance is the priority of nursing care. The genetic component of the disease and the client's age are important considerations. Adults with CF are just entering their productive years and face a life span that is likely to be shortened significantly. Females who do conceive face the prospect of transmitting the defective gene to their offspring.

Nursing Diagnoses and Interventions

Ineffective Airway Clearance

Bronchial hygiene measures, including vibration, percussion, and postural drainage, are the mainstay of treatment for clients with CF.

- Assess respiratory status, including vital signs, breath sounds, SaO_2, and skin color, at least every 4 hours. *Early identification of respiratory compromise allows intervention before tissue hypoxia is significant.*
- Assess cough and sputum (amount, color, consistency, and possible odor). *Assessment of the cough and nature of sputum produced allows evaluation of the effectiveness of respiratory clearance and the response to therapy.*
- Monitor ABG results; report increasing hypoxemia and other abnormal results to the physician. *Blood gas changes may be an early indicator of impaired gas exchange due to airway obstruction.*
- Place in Fowler's or high-Fowler's position. Encourage frequent position changes and ambulation as allowed. *The upright position promotes lung expansion; position changes and ambulation facilitate the movement of secretions.*
- Assist to cough, deep breathe, and use assistive devices. Provide endotracheal suctioning using aseptic technique as ordered. *Coughing, deep breathing, and suctioning help clear airways.*
- Provide a fluid intake of at least 2500 to 3000 mL per day. *A liberal fluid intake helps liquefy secretions, facilitating their clearance.*
- Work with the physician and respiratory therapist to provide pulmonary hygiene measures, such as postural drainage, percussion, and vibration. *These techniques help mobilize and clear secretions.*
- Administer prescribed medications as ordered, and monitor their effects. *If the infecting organism is resistant to the prescribed antibiotic, little improvement may be seen with treatment. Bronchodilators help maintain open airways but may have adverse effects such as anxiety and restlessness.*

Anticipatory Grieving

The client with CF and family members face the knowledge that life span is likely to be short: The median survival for males is over 32 years; for females it is 29 years (Kasper et al., 2005).

- Spend time with the client and family. *Time is necessary to develop a trusting, therapeutic relationship.*
- Answer questions honestly; do not deny the probable outcome of the disease. *Honesty reinforces reality and provides a sense of control over decisions to be made.*
- Encourage the client and family to express their feelings, fears, and concerns. *Open expression of feelings helps to promote understanding and acceptance.*
- Assist with understanding the grieving process and acceptance of feelings as normal. *Feelings of guilt, anger, or depression may cause the client to withdraw from others.*

Explanation of the grieving process enhances understanding and ability to cope.

- Help the client and family make decisions regarding treatment and care. *This also is important to give them a sense of control.*
- Encourage use of other support systems, such as spiritual and social groups. Refer the client and family to support groups, social support services, and hospice care as indicated. *These support systems provide emotional support and help the client and family cope with the diagnosis.*
- Discuss advance directives (the living will) and power of attorney for health care with the client and family. *These documents give the client and family a sense of control over medical care provided if the client is no longer able to express his or her own wishes.*

Community-Based Care

Education of the client and family affected by cystic fibrosis is essential to maintaining optimal health. The adult whose disease was diagnosed in infancy or childhood has grown up with the disease and often has a much greater knowledge level than many caregivers. However, when the initial diagnosis is made as an adolescent or young adult, teaching needs are significant. Include the following topics when teaching for home care:

- Respiratory care techniques, including percussion, postural drainage, and controlled cough techniques
- Specific breathing and coughing exercises and procedures
- The importance of avoiding respiratory irritants, such as cigarette smoke, air pollution, and occupational dusts and gases
- Measures to prevent respiratory infection, such as maintaining immunizations and optimal general health, and avoiding exposure to large crowds and infected people.

Refer to a dietitian for planning and teaching to maintain adequate nutrition and minimize gastrointestinal symptoms. Referral to community agencies and support groups is also helpful.

Discuss the genetic transmission of cystic fibrosis and refer for counseling and possible genetic testing. Help the client and family sort through the impact of the disease on future pregnancies and generations. Remember that the possibility of CF may present an ethical dilemma regarding future pregnancies. Provide support as needed.

THE CLIENT WITH ATELECTASIS

Atelectasis is not a disease but a condition associated with many respiratory disorders. It is a state of partial or total lung collapse and airlessness. It may be acute or chronic. The most common cause of atelectasis is obstruction of the bronchus ventilating a segment of lung tissue. The affected segment may be small or an entire lobe. Other causes include compression of the lung by pneumothorax, pleural effusion, or tumor; or loss of pulmonary surfactant and inability to maintain open alveoli.

The manifestations of atelectasis depend on its size. Diminished breath sounds over the affected area may be the only sign of a small atelectasis. If a large lung segment is affected, manifestations may include tachycardia, tachypnea, dyspnea, cyanosis, and

Either acute or subacute illness can occur. Acute illness occurs 4 to 8 hours after exposure and is heralded by sudden onset of malaise, chills and fever, dyspnea, cough, and nausea. The subacute syndrome is characterized by an insidious onset of chronic cough, progressive dyspnea, anorexia, and weight loss. Diffuse fibrosis occurs after repeated exposure to the organic material, leading to respiratory insufficiency.

INTERDISCIPLINARY CARE

Prevention is a key strategy for all occupational lung diseases. Containing dust and wearing personal protective devices that limit the amount of inhaled particles are essential for people who work in industries with known risks.

Chest x-ray, pulmonary function studies, bronchoscopy, and possibly lung biopsy are used to establish the diagnosis of pneumoconioses. Characteristic patterns are seen for each disorder on x-ray. Pulmonary function testing shows restrictive impairment of lung ventilation, with reduced vital capacity and reduced total lung capacity. The diffusing capacity of the lungs is also decreased. Blood gas analysis reveals hypoxemia, especially with exercise. Bronchoscopy may be performed to obtain tissue for biopsy. Specialized lung scans may be used to determine the extent of fibrosis.

Eliminating further exposure to the offending agent is an important part of disease management. There is no specific therapy. Anti-inflammatory drugs, such as corticosteroids, may reduce the inflammatory response and slow the progression of the disease. Preventing exposure to other damaging substances such as cigarette smoke and pollution is vital. Pneumococcal vaccine and annual influenza immunizations are recommended to reduce the risk of lower respiratory infections. Other care is supportive, similar to that for COPD.

NURSING CARE

Health Promotion

Teaching about the dangers of occupational lung diseases and ways to reduce their risk needs to begin early, before the disease develops. Nurses in industrial and public health settings can begin by recognizing potential dangers and teaching workers about measures to reduce dust in their work area and the use of personal protective devices such as masks. Nurses working with affected families have an excellent opportunity to begin educating children about the risks associated with the occupation.

Nursing Diagnoses and Interventions

Nursing care for clients with occupational lung diseases is similar to that for clients with COPD. Activity intolerance is a high-priority problem for many clients. Severe dyspnea can significantly interfere with ADLs. Nursing measures to reduce energy expenditures and provide for rest are essential. Caregiver role strain, either actual or potential, must be considered when the client with severe disability is being cared for at home.

Both client and family coping may be compromised. Many of these diseases develop after 20 to 30 years of exposure to the hazardous material. Clients who entered the industry following

high school may develop evidence of disease in their 40s and face the possibility of changing their occupation or developing significant disability. The resulting role strain affects all members of the family.

Other nursing diagnoses to consider for the client with an occupational lung disease follow:

- *Ineffective Breathing Pattern* related to restrictive lung disease
- *Anticipatory Grieving* related to potential loss of employment and income
- *Low Self-Esteem: Situational* related to change of occupation.

Community-Based Care

The affected client and family need teaching in preparation for home care, including:

- Prevention of further lung damage, for example, avoiding cigarette smoke and heavy air pollution
- Recommendations for pneumococcal and annual influenza immunizations; yearly tuberculin testing for clients with silicosis
- Pulmonary hygiene measures, such as liberal fluid intake, coughing, and deep-breathing exercises
- Use and care of oxygen therapy equipment if required
- Use and effects of any prescribed or recommended OTC medications.

THE CLIENT WITH SARCOIDOSIS

Sarcoidosis is a chronic, multisystem disease characterized by an exaggerated cellular immune response in involved tissues. This abnormal immune response leads to granuloma formation in the lungs, lymph nodes, liver, eyes, skin, and other organs. Its cause is unknown. Sarcoidosis primarily affects young adults between the ages of 20 and 40. In the United States, the incidence is highest in African Americans. Women are affected at a slightly higher rate than men (Kasper et al., 2005).

In sarcoidosis, multiple granulomas form; these lesions may resolve spontaneously or proceed to fibrosis. The lungs are affected in about 90% of clients with sarcoidosis. Sarcoidosis has a low mortality rate—less than 3%—but a relatively high rate (approximately 10%) of serious disability from ocular, respiratory, or other organ damage. Pulmonary hemorrhage and cardiac and respiratory failure from pulmonary fibrosis are the leading causes of death from sarcoidosis.

The manifestations of sarcoidosis vary, depending on the organ system affected. It may be asymptomatic, diagnosed by characteristic findings on routine chest x-ray. Symptoms may be insidious, with anorexia, fatigue, weight loss, fever, dyspnea, arthralgias, and myalgias. Skin lesions, uveitis, lymphadenopathy, hepatomegaly, or other manifestations may also develop.

Leukopenia, eosinophilia, and an elevated erythrocyte sedimentation rate (ESR) typically are noted in sarcoidosis. The chest x-ray helps to determine the extent of pulmonary involvement. Biopsy of a granulomatous lesion may be required to confirm the diagnosis. Pulmonary function tests reveal decreased compliance and impaired diffusing capacity.

Sarcoidosis often resolves spontaneously; therefore, treatment is indicated only when symptoms are severe or disabling.

Corticosteroid therapy is prescribed to suppress the inflammatory process when indicated. Relapse frequently occurs when corticosteroids are discontinued. Other anti-inflammatory or immune-modifier medications may also be used, including chloroquine, indomethacin, azathioprine, and methotrexate.

Nursing care for clients with sarcoidosis is directed by involved organ systems and related manifestations. Respiratory care is supportive and includes avoiding respiratory irritants and maintaining adequate ventilation. Refer for smoking cessation assistance as needed.

Teach clients with limited symptoms about the disease and symptoms to report to a healthcare provider, including shortness of breath, tearing and eye inflammation, chest pain or irregular pulse, skin lesions, and swollen and painful joints. If corticosteroid therapy is prescribed, teach the importance of taking the drug as prescribed and not stopping it abruptly. Include information about managing the side effects of corticosteroids by limiting sodium and increasing potassium in the diet, taking the medication with food or milk to minimize gastric irritation, and identifying early signs of infection.

PULMONARY VASCULAR DISORDERS

The cardiovascular and respiratory systems are closely interrelated. As blood flows through the capillary network of the pulmonary vascular system, oxygen diffuses into it, and carbon dioxide diffuses out. An effective match of alveolar ventilation and capillary perfusion is essential to maintain this process and, ultimately, tissue oxygenation and function of all organ systems. Both vascular and alveolar changes can alter gas exchange. Arteriosclerotic changes in pulmonary vasculature reduce blood flow to the alveolus. Nearly all lower respiratory system disorders potentially can affect ventilation. Many also have a secondary effect on lung perfusion, because breakdown or fibrosis of alveolar walls destroys the capillary network as well. This section focuses on primary disorders of the pulmonary vascular system.

THE CLIENT WITH PULMONARY EMBOLISM

A **pulmonary embolism** (or *thromboembolism*) is obstruction of blood flow in part of the pulmonary vascular system by an embolus. Thromboemboli, or blood clots, that develop in the venous system (deep venous thrombosis or DVT) or right side of the heart are the most frequent cause of pulmonary embolism. Other sources of emboli include tumors that have invaded venous circulation, fat or bone marrow entering the circulation due to fracture or other trauma, amniotic fluid released into the circulation during childbirth, and intravenous injection of air or other foreign substances.

Pulmonary embolism is a medical emergency. Fifty percent of deaths from pulmonary embolism occur within the first 2 hours following embolization. In many cases, DVT has not been recognized or treated; often embolization also goes undetected. Prevention is the most effective treatment strategy for pulmonary embolism.

Incidence and Risk Factors

Pulmonary embolism causes an estimated 200,000 deaths annually, making it the third leading cause of death in hospitalized clients (Tierney et al., 2005). Although many substances can become emboli, thrombus arising from the deep veins of the legs is the leading cause of pulmonary embolism. *Deep venous thrombosis* develops in approximately 5 million people per year in the United States. The risk factors for pulmonary embolus are those for DVT: stasis of venous blood flow, vessel wall damage, and altered blood coagulation.

Prolonged immobility; trauma, including hip and femur fractures; surgery (orthopedic, pelvic, and gynecologic surgery in particular); myocardial infarction and heart failure; obesity; and advanced age are risk factors for DVT. Women who use oral contraceptives or estrogen therapy are at risk, as are women during pregnancy and childbirth. See Chapter 35 ∞ for more information about DVT.

Physiology Review

The right heart receives deoxygenated blood from the systemic venous circulation. The entire output of the right ventricle enters the pulmonary circulation via the pulmonary artery. This artery branches into successively smaller arteries, arterioles, and capillaries of the pulmonary vascular system. Each alveolus of the lungs is surrounded by a meshwork of capillaries. Oxygen and carbon dioxide readily diffuse across the alveolar-capillary membrane, driven by a concentration gradient. The partial pressure of oxygen in the alveolus is greater than in the capillary; therefore, it diffuses into the blood. Carbon dioxide diffuses from the capillaries into the alveoli, driven by the higher pressure of dissolved carbon dioxide in venous blood.

A match between blood flow through the pulmonary vascular system (perfusion) and lung ventilation is necessary for effective *respiration* (gas exchange) (see Figure 39–4). Local factors regulate ventilation and perfusion to maintain this match. A low alveolar P_{O_2} constricts alveolar capillaries, directing blood flow to better ventilated areas of the lung. High alveolar P_{CO_2} levels cause local bronchodilation, increasing airflow and eliminating excess carbon dioxide.

Pathophysiology

Thrombi affecting only the deep veins of the calf rarely embolize to the pulmonary circulation. However, thrombi often propagate proximally to the popliteal and ileofemoral veins. From there, they may break loose to become an embolus. As vessels of the venous system become progressively larger, the embolus moves freely until it enters the pulmonary arterial system with its progressively smaller vessels leading to the pulmonary capillary beds (Figure 39–6 ■).

The impact of a pulmonary embolus depends on the extent to which pulmonary blood flow is obstructed, the size of the embolus, its nature, and secondary effects of the obstruction. The effects can range widely:

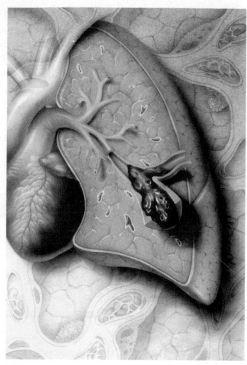

Figure 39–6 ■ A thromboembolism lodged in a pulmonary vessel.
Source: Steve Oh, M. S., Phototake NYC

- Occlusion of a large pulmonary artery with sudden death. Gas exchange is significantly reduced or prevented, and cardiac output falls dramatically as blood fails to move through the pulmonary vascular system and return to the left heart.
- Lung tissue infarction due to occlusion of a significant portion of pulmonary blood flow. Fewer than 10% of pulmonary emboli result in pulmonary infarction.
- Obstruction of a small segment of the pulmonary circulation with no permanent lung injury.
- Chronic or recurrent, possibly multiple, small emboli with recurring symptoms.

Obstruction of pulmonary blood flow by an embolus affects both perfusion and ventilation. Neurohumoral reflexes triggered by obstruction cause vasoconstriction, increasing pulmonary vascular resistance. In severe cases, this can lead to pulmonary hypertension and right ventricular heart failure. Systemically, hypotension and a drop in cardiac output may develop. Bronchoconstriction occurs in the affected area of lung. Dead space (areas of the lung that are ventilated but not perfused) increases. Alveolar surfactant decreases, increasing the risk for atelectasis.

If infarction does not occur, the fibrinolytic system (see Chapter 33 ∞) ultimately dissolves the clot, and pulmonary function returns to normal. Infarcted tissue becomes scarred and fibrotic.

Fat emboli are the most common nonthrombotic pulmonary emboli. A fat embolism usually occurs after fracture of long bone (typically the femur) releases bone marrow fat into the circulation. Adipose tissue or liver trauma may also lead to fat emboli.

Manifestations

The manifestations of pulmonary embolism depend on its size and location. Small emboli may be asymptomatic. Manifestations usually develop abruptly, over a period of minutes. The most common symptoms are dyspnea and pleuritic chest pain. Anxiety, a sense of impending doom, and cough are also common. See the box below. Diaphoresis and hemoptysis may develop. Massive pulmonary embolus can cause syncope and cyanosis. On examination, tachycardia and tachypnea are noted. Crackles may be heard on auscultation of the chest, and a cardiac gallop (S_3 and possibly S_4) may be noted. A low-grade fever may develop. It is difficult to differentiate pulmonary embolism from myocardial infarction or pneumonia by manifestations.

Characteristic manifestations of fat emboli include sudden onset of cardiopulmonary and neurologic symptoms: dyspnea, tachypnea, tachycardia, confusion, delirium, and decreased LOC. Petechiae often develop on the chest and arms.

INTERDISCIPLINARY CARE

Because deep venous thrombosis may not be identified until pulmonary embolism occurs, prevention is the primary goal in treating pulmonary embolism.

Early ambulation of medical and surgical clients is an effective means of preventing venous stasis and reducing the incidence of pulmonary embolism. External pneumatic compression of the legs is also effective for clients undergoing neurosurgery, urologic surgery, or major surgery of the hip or knee, or when anticoagulant therapy is contraindicated. Other preventive measures include elevating the legs and active and passive leg exercises.

When pulmonary embolism occurs, treatment is supportive. Oxygen therapy is initiated, and analgesics may be ordered to relieve severe pleuritic pain and anxiety. Pulmonary artery and wedge pressures are monitored with a balloon (Swan-Ganz) catheter. Cardiac outputs also may be assessed. Cardiac rhythm is monitored to detect dysrhythmias.

MANIFESTATIONS of Pulmonary Embolism

Common
- Dyspnea and shortness of breath
- Chest pain
- Anxiety and apprehension
- Cough
- Tachycardia and tachypnea
- Crackles (rales)
- Low-grade fever

Less Common
- Diaphoresis
- Hemoptysis
- Syncope
- Cyanosis
- S_3 and/or S_4 gallop

Diagnosis

The studies performed to identify DVT differ from those used to diagnose a pulmonary embolism. See Chapter 35 ∞ for diagnostic studies for venous thrombosis.

- *Plasma D-dimer levels* are highly specific to the presence of a thrombus. D-Dimer is a fragment of fibrin formed during lysis of a blood clot; elevated blood levels indicate thrombus formation and lysis (e.g., DVT and pulmonary embolism).
- *Chest CT with contrast* is the principal test used to diagnose pulmonary embolism. Chest CT effectively shows large, central PE; newer generation scanners also can detect peripheral emboli.
- *Lung scans,* including perfusion and ventilation scans, may be used. In a perfusion lung scan, radiotagged albumin is injected intravenously and distributed in the lungs by the pulmonary blood flow. The lungs are then scanned for distribution of the isotope. An area of lung in which the isotope is undetectable is suggestive of occluded blood flow and pulmonary embolism. For a ventilation scan, a radiotagged gas is inhaled and the lungs are scanned for gas distribution. Combined perfusion and ventilation scans allow identification of areas of the lungs that are ventilated but not perfused, a characteristic of pulmonary embolism.
- *Pulmonary angiography* is the definitive test for pulmonary embolism when other, less invasive tests are inconclusive. It is possible to detect very small emboli with angiography. A contrast medium injected into the pulmonary arteries illustrates the pulmonary vascular system on x-ray.
- *Chest x-ray* often shows pulmonary infiltration and occasionally pleural effusion.
- *Electrocardiogram (ECG)* is ordered to rule out acute myocardial infarction as the cause of symptoms. ECG findings commonly associated with pulmonary embolism include tachycardia and nonspecific T-wave changes.
- *ABGs* usually show hypoxemia (PaO_2 less than 80 mmHg) and often respiratory alkalosis (pH > 7.45, $PaCO_2$ < 38 mmHg) due to tachypnea and hyperventilation.
- *$ETCO_2$* may be measured to evaluate alveolar perfusion. The normal $ETCO_2$ reading is 35 to 45 mmHg; it is decreased when pulmonary perfusion is impaired.
- *Coagulation studies* are ordered to monitor the response to therapy. The *activated partial thromboplastin time (aPTT or PTT)* is used to assess the intrinsic clotting pathway and the response to heparin therapy. Desired levels with anticoagulant therapy are 1.5 to 2 times the control value. The risk of recurrent thromboembolism is high at lower levels; the risk of bleeding increases at higher levels. The *International Normalized Ratio (INR)* is used to assess the extrinsic clotting system and oral anticoagulation with warfarin (Coumadin). The goal of anticoagulant therapy is to achieve a therapeutic range of 2.0 to 3.0.

Medications

Anticoagulant therapy is the standard treatment to prevent pulmonary emboli. It is often instituted in high-risk clients who have no evidence of pulmonary embolism, to prevent possible devastating effects. In the client with DVT or a pulmonary embolus, anticoagulants are administered to prevent further clotting and embolization. See Chapter 35 ∞ for more information about anticoagulant therapy to prevent and treat DVT. See the Medication Administration box on pages 1189–1190 for the nursing implications for anticoagulant therapy.

For pulmonary embolus, heparin therapy is initiated with an intravenous bolus of 5000 to 10,000 units of heparin, followed by continuous infusion at the rate of 1000 to 1500 units per hour. The aPTT or PTT is monitored frequently until stabilized. Heparin therapy is typically continued for about 5 days or until oral anticoagulant therapy has become fully effective.

Oral anticoagulant therapy with warfarin sodium (Coumadin) is initiated at the same time as heparin. Warfarin alters the synthesis of vitamin K–dependent clotting factors and requires 5 to 7 days to be fully effective. Anticoagulant therapy is continued for 2 to 3 months when few risk factors for thromboemboli exist; long-term therapy is used when chronic disorders that increase the risk of thromboemboli are present.

Bleeding is a risk associated with anticoagulant therapy. Although major hemorrhage is uncommon, it occurs in approximately 5% of clients receiving intravenous heparin. Cardiac, hepatic, and renal disease increase the risk of significant bleeding, as does age over 60 years. Protamine, a protein that combines with heparin to inactivate it, is used to stop its anticoagulant effect if major bleeding occurs. Vitamin K is given to treat bleeding associated with Coumadin therapy.

Fibrinolytic therapy may be used to treat massive pulmonary embolus and hypotension. Streptokinase, urokinase, or tissue plasminogen activator (tPA) are used to *lyse* (disintegrate) the embolus, restore pulmonary blood flow, and reduce pulmonary artery and right heart pressures. Although fibrinolytic therapy may not reduce mortality associated with pulmonary embolus, it may reduce the incidence of pulmonary hypertension, which develops 3 to 5 years after an embolism. Fibrinolysis significantly increases the risk of bleeding, particularly cerebral bleeding. Contraindications to fibrinolysis include intracranial disease, recent stroke, active bleeding or a bleeding disorder, pregnancy, severe hypertension, and recent surgery or trauma. Because of the increased risk of hemorrhage, invasive procedures are avoided after fibrinolysis. See Chapter 31 ∞ for further discussion of fibrinolytic therapy and its nursing implications.

Surgery

When anticoagulant therapy fails to prevent recurrent emboli or is contraindicated, an umbrella-like filter may be inserted into the inferior vena cava to trap large emboli while allowing continued blood flow (see Figure 35–11). The filter usually is inserted percutaneously, via either the femoral or jugular vein.

 NURSING CARE

Health Promotion

Nurses are key in preventing pulmonary embolism. Encouraging clients to ambulate after surgery or illness, applying compression stockings or pneumatic compression devices, teaching and encouraging leg exercises, discouraging the use of pillows under the knees—all of these measures help prevent DVT and subsequent pulmonary emboli.

Teach clients to reduce the risks associated with long periods of immobility, stopping every 1 to 2 hours during long automobile trips for a brief stretch and walk, getting up every hour or so and doing leg exercises while seated during long flights, and avoiding crossing the legs to prevent venous stasis and pooling. Regular exercise such as walking also reduces the risk of DVT. Instruct clients who stand for long periods to use well-fitted elastic stockings, being careful to avoid hose that bind around the knee or thigh.

Assessment

Because pulmonary embolus can be a medical emergency, assessment may be very focused. In other instances, when emboli are small and not life threatening, a more extensive nursing assessment may be done.

- *Health History:* Chest pain, shortness of breath, other symptoms, including onset, severity, precipitating factors; history of recent surgery, venous thrombosis, or other risk factor such as childbirth or malignancy; current medications.
- *Physical Examination:* Level of consciousness, presence of respirations and pulse; color, skin temperature and moisture; vital signs including apical pulse and temperature; breath sounds and heart sounds; oxygen saturation level; neck vein distention, peripheral edema.
- *Diagnostic Tests:* Plasma D-dimer levels, coagulation studies; chest x-ray and other imaging studies; oxygen saturation and ABGs; ECG.

Nursing Diagnoses and Interventions

A large pulmonary embolus can cause a significant mismatch between pulmonary ventilation and circulation. Impaired gas exchange is a priority problem and focus for interventions. Cardiac output may be significantly affected by obstructed pulmonary blood flow. Fibrinolytic and anticoagulant therapy affect the clotting process, increasing the risk for bleeding. Anxiety accompanies pulmonary embolism almost universally.

Impaired Gas Exchange

Pulmonary embolism results in areas of the lung that are ventilated but not perfused; they receive no capillary blood flow. If the embolus is large and a major segment of the lung is unperfused, gas exchange is significantly affected. Nursing interventions are directed toward compensating for impaired gas exchange.

- Frequently assess respiratory status, including rate, depth, effort, lung sounds, and oxygen saturation. *Impaired ventilation will further compromise gas exchange and worsen hypoxemia. Oxygen saturation can be monitored continuously and noninvasively to evaluate gas exchange.*

PRACTICE ALERT
Monitor and record LOC, mental status, and skin color. Hypoxemia often causes confusion and agitation; hypercapnia may reduce LOC. Cyanosis indicates significant hypoxemia.

- Place in Fowler's or high-Fowler's position, with the lower extremities dependent. *This position facilitates maximal lung expansion and reduces venous return to the right side of the heart, lowering pressures in the pulmonary vascular system.*

PRACTICE ALERT
Start oxygen per nasal cannula or mask. Obtain a physician's order if one has not been written. Supplemental oxygen increases alveolar and arterial oxygenation. Oxygen is a drug and must be prescribed by the physician. It may, however, be initiated by the nurse in an emergency to prevent tissue hypoxia.

- Monitor ABG results, reporting abnormal findings as indicated. *ABGs are used to assess gas exchange and tissue oxygenation. An arterial line may be inserted for monitoring arterial pressure and arterial blood sampling.*
- Maintain bed rest. *Bed rest reduces metabolic demands and tissue needs for oxygen.*

Decreased Cardiac Output

The impact of a large pulmonary embolus on hemodynamic status can be significant. Pressures in the pulmonary vascular system and right heart increase; blood return to the left heart and cardiac output may significantly decrease. Nursing interventions focus on preserving an adequate blood pressure and organ function until cardiopulmonary status stabilizes. A central line for hemodynamic monitoring may be instituted. (See Chapter 32 ∞ for nursing care related to hemodynamic monitoring.)

PRACTICE ALERT
Assess and record vital signs and cardiopulmonary status every 15 to 30 minutes initially, then every 2 to 4 hours as condition stabilizes. Frequent assessment facilitates timely interventions to maintain cardiovascular status and preserve organ function.

- Auscultate heart sounds every 2 to 4 hours, reporting any abnormalities. *Sounds such as an S_3 or S_4 gallop may indicate cardiac compromise.*

PRACTICE ALERT
Record intake and output hourly. Decreased urinary output often is an early indicator of decreased cardiac output. Maintaining renal perfusion is vital to preserve renal function and prevent acute renal failure.

- Assess skin color and temperature. *These assessments monitor tissue perfusion.*
- Monitor cardiac rhythm. *A drop in cardiac output and other hemodynamic alterations resulting from pulmonary embolism can precipitate dysrhythmias. Dysrhythmias, in turn, can further impair cardiac output.*
- Administer vasopressors and other medications as ordered. Carefully monitor the response to prescribed medications. *Drugs may be prescribed to maintain adequate arterial pressure and tissue perfusion. Potent drugs such as vasopressors require careful monitoring for desired and adverse effects.*

- Monitor pulmonary artery pressures, neck vein distention, and peripheral edema. Report findings as indicated. *Right-sided heart failure is a potential complication of pulmonary embolism because of increased pulmonary artery pressures.*
- Maintain intravenous and arterial access sites as well as central lines. *The client may be in unstable and critical condition, potentially needing immediate interventions to maintain life.*

PRACTICE ALERT
Provide frequent skin care. Impaired tissue perfusion and oxygenation increase the risk of skin and tissue breakdown.

- Instruct to report chest pain or other symptoms. *Decreased cardiac output and an increased workload due to pulmonary hypertension may cause anginal pain.*

Ineffective Protection

Fibrinolytics and anticoagulant therapy impair normal clotting mechanisms, increasing the risk for bleeding and hemorrhage. This risk is particularly acute during the first 24 to 48 hours following fibrinolytic drug administration.

- Assess frequently for overt and covert signs of bleeding: bleeding gums; hematuria; obvious or occult blood in stool or vomitus; incisional bleeding, bleeding or bruising of injection sites or with minor trauma; joint pain or immobility; abdominal or flank pain. *Careful monitoring is necessary to identify early signs of abnormal bleeding and prevent potential hemorrhage.*

PRACTICE ALERT
Promptly report changes in neurologic status. Although cerebral bleeding is not evident externally, changes in LOC and other neurologic signs suggest it and should be reported immediately.

- Report coagulation study results outside the desired range for anticoagulant therapy. *Levels less than the target range may indicate an increased risk for further clot development and pulmonary emboli; levels above the target range indicate an increased risk for bleeding.*
- Keep protamine sulfate available for heparin therapy and vitamin K available for warfarin (Coumadin) therapy. *Bleeding or hemorrhage due to excess anticoagulant may require antidote administration to rapidly reverse anticoagulant effects.*
- Assess medication regimen for possible drug interactions that could potentiate or inhibit anticoagulant effects. *Drug interactions can increase the risk for hemorrhage or further embolus formation.*
- Avoid invasive procedures, injections, and venous punctures when possible, particularly during and following fibrinolytic therapy. *Invasive procedures increase the risk of tissue trauma and bleeding.*
- Maintain firm pressure on injection and venipuncture sites. Maintain pressure for 30 minutes following arterial puncture. *Firm pressure reduces the risk for bleeding into the tissues.*

PRACTICE ALERT
Use an infusion device to administer heparin infusion. Using an infusion pump or device helps prevent administration of excess medication.

- Maintain adequate fluid intake. Administer stool softeners as ordered. *These measures help prevent constipation and straining, which may precipitate bleeding of hemorrhoids.*

Anxiety

Pulmonary embolism is a physiologic and psychologic threat to safety and integrity. It is a major physiologic stressor, eliciting a strong neuroendocrine stress response. The feeling of suffocation and inability to catch one's breath that accompanies a pulmonary embolus is also a strong psychologic stressor. Fear, anxiety, and apprehension are common responses.

- Assess anxiety level. *Appropriate interventions are determined by the level of anxiety.*

PRACTICE ALERT
Provide reassurance and emotional support, listening to fears. Do not negate the fear of dying, but reassure that treatment usually restores effective respiratory function. The fear of death is very real and must not be discounted; however, it is important to provide reassurance to alleviate excess anxiety.

- Remain with the client as much as possible. *The presence of a caring nurse helps reduce fear.*
- Explain procedures and treatments, using short, simple sentences. *Providing clearly understood, simple instructions reduces fear of the unknown.*
- Reduce environmental stimuli, and use a calm, reassuring manner. *These measures help reduce anxiety (for both the nurse and the client).*
- Allow supportive family members to remain with the client as much as possible. *Calm, supportive family members provide further reassurance.*
- Administer morphine sulfate as ordered. *Morphine is given to reduce pain and anxiety.*

Using NANDA, NIC, and NOC

Linkages between NANDA nursing diagnoses, nursing interventions, and nursing outcomes for the client experiencing a pulmonary embolism are illustrated in Chart 39–2.

Community-Based Care

Discuss the following topics when preparing the client with pulmonary embolism and family members for home care:

- Use of prescribed anticoagulant, including drug interactions, scheduled laboratory testing, and manifestations of bleeding to report to the primary care provider
- Using a soft toothbrush and electric razor to reduce the risk of bleeding
- Avoiding aspirin (unless prescribed) and other OTC medications unless approved by the physician
- Importance of wearing a Medic-Alert tag for anticoagulant use

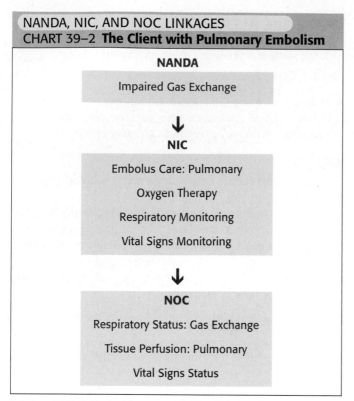

NANDA, NIC, AND NOC LINKAGES
CHART 39–2 The Client with Pulmonary Embolism

NANDA

Impaired Gas Exchange

↓

NIC

Embolus Care: Pulmonary

Oxygen Therapy

Respiratory Monitoring

Vital Signs Monitoring

↓

NOC

Respiratory Status: Gas Exchange

Tissue Perfusion: Pulmonary

Vital Signs Status

Data from *NANDA's Nursing Diagnoses: Definitions & Classification 2005–2006* by NANDA International (2005), Philadelphia; *Nursing Interventions Classification (NIC)* (4th ed.) by J. Dochterman & G. M. Bulechek (2004), St. Louis, MO: Mosby; and *Nursing Outcomes Classification (NOC)* (3rd ed.) by S. Moorhead, M. Johnson, and M. Maas (2004), St. Louis, MO: Mosby.

- Health promotion measures to reduce the risk of recurrent pulmonary embolism
- Symptoms of recurrent pulmonary embolism, such as sudden chest pain, shortness of breath, and possibly bloody sputum.

THE CLIENT WITH PULMONARY HYPERTENSION

The pulmonary vascular system is normally a high-flow, low-pressure, low-resistance system that can accommodate large increases in blood flow when necessary (e.g., during exercise). The normal mean arterial pressure in the pulmonary system is 12 to 15 mmHg (25 to 28 systolic/8 diastolic). **Pulmonary hypertension** is abnormal elevation of the pulmonary arterial pressure.

Pathophysiology

Pulmonary hypertension can develop as a primary disorder, but usually occurs secondarily to another condition. In both instances, changes in the pulmonary artery lead to abnormal growth and remodeling of pulmonary vessels. Smooth muscle cells and fibroblasts proliferate, leading to abnormal vasoconstriction and fibrosis of pulmonary vessels. Once initiated, pulmonary vascular changes are progressive and nonreversible. Vasoconstrictive substances such as endothelin 1 and thromboxane A_2 are produced in excess, while the production of va-

sodilating substances such as nitric oxide is reduced. This further contributes to vasoconstriction and increased pulmonary artery pressures. Thromboxane A_2 also stimulates platelet aggregation, promoting clot formation in pulmonary vessels. Inflammation may contribute to progression of the disease. Vasoconstriction and increased pressures in the pulmonary system increase the workload of the right ventricle, ultimately leading to right ventricular failure (Sims, 2003; Steinbis, 2004).

Primary Pulmonary Hypertension

Primary pulmonary hypertension is an uncommon disorder without identified cause. It occurs in both familial and sporadic patterns. In the familial form, a gene transmitted in an autosomal dominant pattern affects a protein receptor in the walls of pulmonary arteries, leading to abnormal vessel growth and remodeling (Sims, 2003; Steinbis, 2004). Primary pulmonary hypertension affects primarily women in their 30s or 40s.

FAST FACTS
- An estimated 300 new cases of primary pulmonary hypertension are diagnosed annually.
- Median survival after being diagnosed with primary pulmonary hypertension is 3 years (ALA, 2006).

Secondary Pulmonary Hypertension

Secondary pulmonary hypertension is more common than primary. HIV infection and collagen diseases such as scleroderma and lupus may lead to secondary pulmonary hypertension. However, its usual cause is reduced size of the pulmonary vascular bed, which may be due to vasoconstriction or widespread vessel destruction or obstruction. Hypoxemia is a potent pulmonary vasoconstrictor and a common initiating factor in pulmonary hypertension. Chronic lung diseases, sleep apnea, and hypoventilation due to obesity or neuromuscular disease can lead to hypoxemia. Alveolar wall destruction associated with emphysema leads to loss of pulmonary capillaries. Large or multiple pulmonary emboli may cause significant vessel obstruction. Other factors such as left ventricular failure or mitral stenosis also can lead to elevated pulmonary pressures. Once initiated, pulmonary hypertension becomes self-sustaining, as pulmonary vessels undergo changes that further narrow the pulmonary bed.

Manifestations

The manifestations of pulmonary hypertension are progressive dyspnea, fatigue, angina, and syncope with exertion. In secondary pulmonary hypertension, the signs and symptoms often are masked by those of the underlying disease. Dull, retrosternal chest pain may occur in addition to the manifestations of the primary disease. Primary pulmonary hypertension is a progressive disorder that generally causes a steady decline to death within 3 to 4 years.

Complications

Cor pulmonale is a condition of right ventricular hypertrophy and failure resulting from long-standing pulmonary hypertension. Chronic obstructive pulmonary disease is the most common cause of cor pulmonale.

The manifestations of cor pulmonale are those of the underlying pulmonary disorder and right-sided heart failure. Chronic productive cough, progressive dyspnea, and wheezing are common. With right-sided heart failure, peripheral edema and distended neck veins are seen. Skin is warm, moist, and both ruddy and cyanotic because of increased numbers of RBCs and hypoxemia.

INTERDISCIPLINARY CARE

The CBC commonly shows *polycythemia*, increased numbers of red blood cells. ABGs and oxygen saturation measurements reveal hypoxemia. The chest x-ray shows right heart enlargement and dilation of central pulmonary arteries. Typical ECG changes are those of right ventricular hypertrophy. An echocardiogram may be done to identify cardiac changes occurring either as a cause or result of pulmonary hypertension. Doppler ultrasonography is a noninvasive means of estimating pulmonary artery pressure, but cardiac catheterization may be required for definitive diagnosis. See Chapter 30 ∞ for nursing care of the client undergoing cardiac catheterization.

Treatment for pulmonary hypertension focuses on slowing the course of the disease, preventing thrombus formation, and reducing pulmonary vasoconstriction. Oxygen is administered to reduce hypoxemia and improve activity tolerance. If polycythemia is present, phlebotomy is performed to reduce the viscosity of the blood.

The calcium channel blockers nifedipine (Procardia) or diltiazem (Cardizem) may be given to reduce pulmonary vascular resistance and improve cardiac output. Short-acting direct vasodilators such as intravenous epoprostenol (Flolan) or treprostinol (Remodulin) or oral bosentan (Tracleer) may be used for clients who do not respond to calcium channel blockers. An oral anticoagulant (Coumadin) is given to prevent clotting (Steinbis, 2004).

Bilateral lung or heart-lung transplant is the most effective long-term treatment for primary pulmonary hypertension.

When cor pulmonale is present, salt and water restrictions as well as diuretic therapy are added to the above regimen to manage the right-sided heart failure.

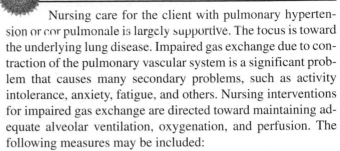

NURSING CARE

Nursing care for the client with pulmonary hypertension or cor pulmonale is largely supportive. The focus is toward the underlying lung disease. Impaired gas exchange due to contraction of the pulmonary vascular system is a significant problem that causes many secondary problems, such as activity intolerance, anxiety, fatigue, and others. Nursing interventions for impaired gas exchange are directed toward maintaining adequate alveolar ventilation, oxygenation, and perfusion. The following measures may be included:

- Monitoring breath sounds, respiratory rate, skin color, and use of accessory muscles
- Positioning for optimal lung expansion
- Coughing, deep breathing, and chest physiotherapy
- Administering prescribed vasodilators.

It is important to assess fatigue and dyspnea with activities and to plan frequent rest periods. Assist with self-care as needed to conserve energy.

With primary pulmonary hypertension, *Anticipatory Grieving* and *Hopelessness* are additional potential nursing diagnoses. When cor pulmonale is present, *Decreased Cardiac Output*, *Excess Fluid Volume*, and *Ineffective Individual Coping* must be considered.

Community-Based Care

Most care for these chronic conditions is provided in the home and community settings. Teaching is directed both at the underlying lung disease, if present, and the resulting hypertensive process. Refer to the section on COPD for teaching related to this disease, the most frequent underlying cause of cor pulmonale. In addition, provide teaching about the following topics for the client and family:

- Disease process, its management, and the prognosis
- Manifestations or changes in condition to report to the physician, such as a change in activity tolerance, increased edema, and signs of respiratory infection or exacerbation
- Importance of planned rest periods between activities and measures to conserve energy, such as using a shower chair
- Importance of not smoking due to its irritant and vasoconstrictive effects
- Prescribed medications, including their use and effects.

RESPIRATORY FAILURE

Many of the conditions discussed in this chapter and in Chapter 38, from pneumonia to acute respiratory distress syndrome, can lead to respiratory failure. In **respiratory failure**, the lungs are unable to oxygenate the blood and remove carbon dioxide adequately to meet the body's needs, even at rest.

THE CLIENT WITH ACUTE RESPIRATORY FAILURE

Respiratory failure is not a disease but a consequence of severe respiratory dysfunction. It is often defined by ABG values. An arterial oxygen level (PaO_2) of less than 50 to 60 mmHg and an arterial carbon dioxide level ($PaCO_2$) of greater than 50 mmHg are generally accepted as indicators of respiratory failure. However, clients with advanced COPD may be alert and functional with blood gas values that would indicate respiratory failure in someone whose respiratory function was previously normal. In clients with COPD, respiratory failure is indicated by an acute drop in blood oxygen levels along with increased carbon dioxide levels.

Respiratory failure can result from inadequate alveolar ventilation (hypoventilation), impaired gas exchange, or a

TABLE 39–5 Selected Causes of Respiratory Failure

TYPE OF DYSFUNCTION	EXAMPLES
Impaired Ventilation	
■ Airway obstruction	Laryngospasm, foreign body aspiration, airway edema
■ Respiratory disease	Asthma, COPD
■ Neurologic causes	Spinal cord injury, poliomyelitis, Guillain-Barré syndrome, drug overdose, stroke
■ Chest wall injury	Flail chest, pneumothorax
Impaired Diffusion	
■ Alveolar disorders	Pneumonia, pneumonitis, COPD
■ Pulmonary edema	Heart failure, ARDS, near-drowning
Ventilation-perfusion mismatch	Pulmonary embolism

significant ventilation-perfusion mismatch. COPD is the most common cause of respiratory failure. Other lung diseases, chest injury, inhalation trauma, neuromuscular disorders, and cardiac conditions can also lead to respiratory failure. Selected causes of acute respiratory failure are identified in Table 39–5.

Pathophysiology

Respiratory failure may be characterized by primary hypoxemia or a combination of hypoxemia and hypercapnia (Figure 39–7 ■). In hypoxemic respiratory failure, PaO_2 is significantly reduced, whereas $PaCO_2$ remains normal or is low due to stimulation of the respiratory center and tachypnea. Impaired diffusion across the alveolar-capillary membrane, and a ventilation-perfusion mismatch can cause a drop in arterial oxygen levels that is more rapid than the rise in carbon dioxide. Metabolic acidosis results from tissue hypoxia. The increased work of breathing can eventually lead to respiratory muscle fatigue and hypoventilation.

Hypoventilation, or reduced movement of air into and out of the lung, causes carbon dioxide retention. With significant hy-poventilation, the carbon dioxide level in the blood rises rapidly, leading to respiratory acidosis. Hypoxemia develops more slowly, and responds readily to administration of oxygen unless gas exchange also is impaired.

In summary, hypoxemia without a corresponding rise in carbon dioxide levels indicates a failure of oxygenation; hypoxemia with hypercapnia is the result of lung hypoventilation.

Manifestations and Course

The manifestations of respiratory failure are caused by hypoxemia and hypercapnia, as well as the underlying disease process. Hypoxemia causes dyspnea and neurologic symptoms such as restlessness, apprehension, impaired judgment, and motor impairment. Tachycardia and hypertension develop as the cardiac output increases in an effort to bring more oxygen to the tissues. Cyanosis is present. As hypoxemia progresses, dysrhythmias, hypotension, and decreased cardiac output may develop.

Increased carbon dioxide levels depress CNS function and cause vasodilation. Dyspnea and headache are early signs. Other manifestations include peripheral and conjunctival va-

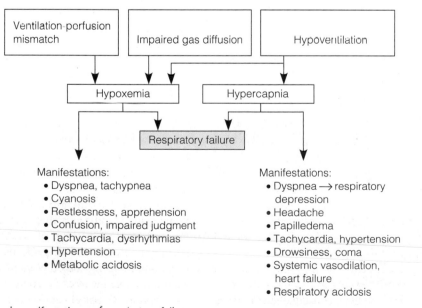

Figure 39–7 ■ Causes and manifestations of respiratory failure.

sodilation, papilledema, neuromuscular irritability, and decreased LOC. As hypercapnia worsens, the respiratory center may be depressed, reducing dyspnea and slowing respirations. Increased carbon dioxide and hydrogen ion concentrations no longer stimulate the respiratory center; hypoxemia provides the primary active breathing stimulus. Administering oxygen without ventilatory support may further reduce the drive to breathe, leading to respiratory arrest.

The prognosis for acute respiratory failure varies, depending on the underlying disease process. Respiratory failure resulting from uncomplicated drug overdose generally resolves quickly without long-term effects. When respiratory failure results from underlying lung disease, the course may be prolonged and the outcome less favorable.

FAST FACTS

Among adults requiring mechanical ventilation for acute respiratory failure:

- An estimated 62% survive to be weaned from the ventilator
- Only 43% survive to be discharged from the hospital
- About 30% remain alive at 1 year after discharge (Tierney et al., 2005).

INTERDISCIPLINARY CARE

Treatment of respiratory failure focuses on correcting the underlying cause or disease, supporting ventilation, and correcting hypoxemia and hypercapnia. Care related to disorders that can precipitate respiratory failure is discussed in the sections specific to each disorder.

Diagnosis

Exhaled carbon dioxide and ABGs are used to diagnose and monitor treatment of respiratory failure.

- $ETCO_2$ is used to evaluate alveolar ventilation. The normal $ETCO_2$ is 35 to 45 mmHg; it is elevated when ventilation is inadequate, and decreased when pulmonary perfusion is impaired.
- *ABGs* also are used to evaluate alveolar ventilation and gas exchange. With hypoxemic respiratory failure, the $PaCO_2$ may be normal, 38 to 42 mmHg, or even low due to tachypnea. A pH of less than 7.35 and low bicarbonate levels indicate metabolic acidosis, typical of hypoxemic respiratory failure.

In respiratory failure due to hypoventilation, the $PaCO_2$ is elevated, usually greater than 50 mmHg. The pH is low due to respiratory acidosis. Acidosis develops rapidly in hypoxemia and hypercapnia because of increased acid production (metabolic) and decreased acid elimination (respiratory).

Medications

Drugs used in treating respiratory failure depend on the underlying cause of the failure and the need for intubation and mechanical ventilation.

Beta-adrenergic (sympathomimetic) or anticholinergic medications may be administered by inhalation to promote bronchodilation. If mechanical ventilation is required, the drugs may be given by nebulizer attached to the ventilator. Methylxanthine

bronchodilators (theophylline derivatives) may be given intravenously. See the box on pages 1327–1328 and the asthma section of this chapter for more information about bronchodilators and their nursing implications. Corticosteroids, administered by inhalation or intravenously, may be ordered to reduce airway edema. Antibiotics are given to treat any underlying infection.

Sedation and analgesia often are required during mechanical ventilation to decrease pain and anxiety. Benzodiazepines such as diazepam (Valium), lorazepam (Ativan), or midazolam (Versed) may be used for sedation and to inhibit the respiratory drive. Intravenous morphine or fentanyl provides analgesia and also inhibits the respiratory drive, allowing more effective mechanical ventilation. Occasionally, the client's respiratory drive competes with the ventilator despite sedation, decreasing its effectiveness and increasing the work of breathing. A neuromuscular blocking agent may be necessary to induce paralysis and suppress the ability to breathe. Nursing implications of neuromuscular blockers are described in the Medication Administration box on page 1356.

Oxygen Therapy

Oxygen is administered to reverse hypoxemia in acute respiratory failure. In general, the goal is to achieve an oxygen saturation of 90% or greater without oxygen toxicity. A PaO_2 of about 60 mmHg usually is adequate to meet the oxygen needs of body tissues. Higher levels do not significantly increase oxygen saturation and may lead to hypoventilation in clients with chronic hypercapnia. As little as 1 to 3 L of oxygen per nasal cannula or 28% oxygen per Venturi mask may correct hypoxemia in advanced COPD. Oxygen concentrations of 40% to 60% may be required when diffusion is impaired (e.g., in pneumonia or ARDS). High concentrations are used only for short periods to avoid oxygen toxicity. Both the oxygen concentration and duration of therapy contribute to oxygen toxicity. Continued high oxygen concentrations impair the synthesis of surfactant, reducing lung compliance (ease of inflation). ARDS or absorption atelectasis may develop.

When respiratory failure is caused by hypoventilation or usual oxygen delivery systems do not correct hypoxemia, a tight-fitting mask to maintain *continuous positive airway pressure* (CPAP) may be used. CPAP increases lung volume, opening previously closed alveoli, improving ventilation of underventilated alveoli, and improving ventilation-perfusion relationships.

Airway Management

If the upper airway is obstructed or positive-pressure mechanical ventilation is necessary to correct hypoxemia and hypercapnia, an endotracheal tube that extends from the mouth or nose into the trachea is inserted (Figure 39–8 ■). To maintain positive-pressure ventilation, the tube is cuffed with an air-filled or foam sac just above the end of the tube. When the cuff is inflated, it obstructs the upper airway, preventing air from escaping back into the nose or mouth. Excess pressure of the cuff can cause tissue ischemia and necrosis of the trachea. To minimize this risk, high-volume, low-pressure ("floppy") cuffs are used. Tubes with low-pressure cuffs may be left in place for 3 to 4 weeks.

MEDICATION ADMINISTRATION **Neuromuscular Blockers**

NONDEPOLARIZING NEUROMUSCULAR BLOCKERS
Rocuronium (Zemuron)
Pancuronium bromide (Pavulon)
Atracurium besylate (Tracrium)
Cisatracurium (Nimbex)

Nondepolarizing neuromuscular blockers competitively block the action of acetylcholine (ACh) at skeletal muscle receptors, preventing muscle depolarization and contraction. Complete muscle paralysis is achieved within minutes. Facial muscles are affected first, followed by muscles of the limbs, neck, and trunk. The muscles of respiration (the diaphragm and intercostal muscles) are least sensitive to the effects of neuromuscular blockers and are paralyzed last. When the drug is discontinued or an antagonist is given, muscles recover in reverse order; respiratory function is recovered first.

Nursing Responsibilities
- Prior to administering, assess endotracheal tube placement and ensure effective mechanical ventilator function. The risk of hypoxemia and organ damage is significant if respiratory muscles are paralyzed without adequate ventilatory support in place.
- Administer the drug by slow intravenous injection and/or intravenous infusion as prescribed.

- Keep an acetylcholinesterase (AChE) inhibitor such as neostigmine (Prostigmin) available at the bedside to rapidly reverse neuromuscular effects if needed.
- Administer morphine sulfate, diazepam (Valium), or other antianxiety agent or sedative as ordered. Neuromuscular blockers provide no sedation or pain relief; muscle paralysis produces extreme anxiety.
- Instill artificial tears every 2 to 4 hours.
- Suction oral cavity as needed to remove saliva.
- *Never* turn off ventilator alarms when administering neuromuscular blockers. Should the tubing become disconnected or plugged, the client is unable to breathe independently or call for help.
- Treat the client as though awake and alert. Although unable to respond, mental function is unaffected.

Health Education for the Client and Family
- Reassure that the ability to move and communicate will return when the drug is discontinued.
- Teach the family about the effects of the drug and the reason for its use. Explain that the client can hear and understand what is going on.

A tracheostomy may be performed if long-term ventilatory support is required. Although a tracheostomy is more comfortable and easier to secure in place, complications such as cuff necrosis and increased risk of infection are associated with tracheostomy as well as endotracheal intubation. Table 39–6 compares the advantages, disadvantages, and possible complications of endotracheal tubes and tracheostomy.

When the client is able to maintain effective respirations and ventilatory support is no longer required, the endotracheal tube is removed (*extubation*). Gag, cough, and swallow reflexes must be intact to prevent aspiration. After oxygenation and suctioning, the cuff is deflated and the tube removed. Humidified oxygen is provided immediately following removal. Close observation for respiratory distress is vital following extubation. Inspiratory stridor within the first 24 hours indicates laryngeal edema, which may necessitate reintubation. Sore throat and a hoarse voice are common after extubation. Oral intake is reinitiated slowly, with careful assessment of swallowing.

Mechanical Ventilation

Mechanical ventilation is indicated when alveolar ventilation is inadequate to maintain blood oxygen and carbon dioxide levels. Specific indications for mechanical ventilation include:
- Apnea or acute ventilatory failure
- Hypoxemia unresponsive to oxygen therapy alone
- Increased work of breathing with progressive client fatigue.

The most common indicator for ventilation support is respiratory muscle fatigue or its potential (Fenstermacher & Hong, 2004). Drug overdose, neural disorders, chest wall injury, and airway problems such as severe asthma or COPD can lead to acute ventilatory failure. Disorders that affect alveolar-capillary diffusion, such as pulmonary contusion, pneumonia, and ARDS, may necessitate mechanical ventilation to attain adequate oxygenation. Positive-pressure ventilation increases lung volume, helps redistribute fluid from the alveolar to the interstitial space, and helps reduce the oxygen demand caused by increased work of breathing.

TYPES OF VENTILATORS Two broad general classifications of mechanical ventilators are available. Negative-pressure ventilators create negative (subatmospheric) pressure externally to draw the chest outward and air into the lungs, mimicking spontaneous breathing. The iron lung, cuirass ventilator, and PulmoWrap are examples of negative-pressure ventilators. Negative-pressure ventilators primarily are used by clients with neuromuscular disorders (e.g., post-polio syndrome, amyotrophic lateral sclerosis) that interfere with the ability to maintain adequate ventilation. They also may be used by clients who primarily require ventilator support during sleep.

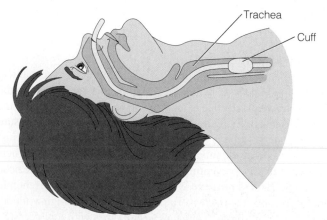

Trachea

Cuff

Figure 39–8 ■ Nasal endotracheal (nasotracheal) intubation.

TABLE 39–6 A Comparison of Endotracheal Tubes and Tracheostomy

	ADVANTAGES	DISADVANTAGES	POTENTIAL COMPLICATIONS
Oral endotracheal tube	■ More easily inserted ■ Larger tube can be used, facilitating work of breathing, suctioning	■ More difficult to secure ■ Can be obstructed by biting ■ Communication and mouth care more difficult ■ Increased risk of lower respiratory infection	■ Obstruction or displacement ■ Pressure necrosis of lip ■ Tracheoesophageal fistula
Nasal endotracheal tube	■ More easily secured and stabilized ■ Well tolerated by client ■ Facilitate communication and oral hygiene	■ Necessitates smaller tube, which may impede removal of secretions ■ Increased risk of lower respiratory infection	■ Obstruction or displacement ■ Pressure necrosis of nares ■ Obstruction of sinus drainage, possible sinusitis ■ Tracheoesophageal fistula
Tracheostomy	■ Easily secured and stabilized ■ Enable swallowing, speech, and oral hygiene ■ Avoid upper airway complications	■ Require surgical incision ■ Increased risk of lower respiratory infection	■ Hemorrhage due to incision or vessel erosion by tube ■ Wound infection ■ Subcutaneous emphysema ■ Tracheoesophageal fistula ■ Tracheal infarction and stenosis

Positive-pressure ventilators are used more often than negative-pressure ones, especially in treating acute respiratory failure (Figure 39–9 ■). These ventilators push air into the lungs, rather than drawing it in like negative-pressure ventilators. Either invasive ventilation using an endotracheal tube or tracheostomy or noninvasive positive-pressure ventilation may be used. Increasingly, noninvasive techniques, which use a nasal or face mask, nasal plugs, or an oral mouthpiece, are being used (Fenstermacher & Hong, 2004).

Noninvasive ventilation (NIV) provides ventilator support using a tight-fitting face mask, thus avoiding intubation. Its primary use is to support clients with obstructive sleep apnea, neu-

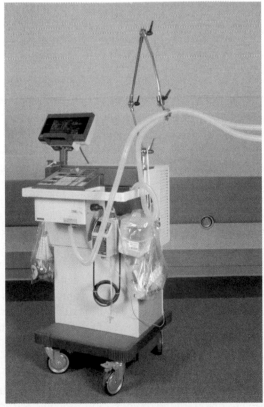

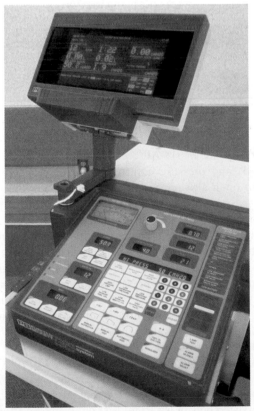

A
B

Figure 39–9 ■ *A*, Positive-pressure ventilator and *B*, the control panel used to set the mode, rate, limits, and percentage of oxygen delivered.

romuscular disease, or impending respiratory failure (e.g., advanced COPD). NIV also may be used for clients in respiratory failure who refuse intubation. The degree of success varies, primarily limited by client intolerance due to the physical and psychologic discomfort of wearing a mask when dyspneic (Kasper et al., 2005). NIV tends to be more successful in clients without significant underlying lung disease (e.g., respiratory failure related to neuromuscular disease).

Several variables are used to trigger, cycle, and limit airflow with positive-pressure ventilators. The *trigger* prompts the ventilator to deliver a breath. The client's inspiratory effort triggers *ventilator-assisted breaths. Ventilator-controlled breaths* usually are triggered by a preset time interval (e.g., a breath is delivered every 5 seconds for a rate of 12 breaths per minute). The ventilator *cycle,* or duration of inspiration, can be limited by volume, pressure, flow, or time. *Volume-cycled ventilators* deliver air until a preset volume is delivered. *Pressure-cycled ventilators* cycle off when a preset pressure is achieved within the airways. *Flow-cycled ventilators* are cycled by a preset inspiratory flow rate, and *time-cycled ventilators* deliver air for a set time interval. Airflow delivered by the ventilator also can be limited by factors such as airway pressure (e.g., a volume-cycled ventilator can be set to immediately stop inspiratory flow if airway pressure exceeds a preset value).

MODES OF VENTILATION A number of different *modes* or patterns of ventilation may be used with positive-pressure ventilators. The mode determines whether a breath is initiated by the client or the ventilator and the pattern of airway support provided by the ventilator. CPAP, bilevel airway pressure support, assist-control mode ventilation, synchronized intermittent mandatory ventilation, positive end-expiratory pressure, pressure support ventilation, and pressure-control ventilation are common modes of ventilation in use today (Table 39–7).

Continuous positive airway pressure applies positive pressure to the airways of a spontaneously breathing client. CPAP may be used with either endotracheal intubation or a tight-fitting face mask. All breathing is spontaneous (client triggered) and pressure controlled. CPAP is used to help maintain open airways and alveoli, decreasing the work of breathing. *Bilevel ventilators* (BiPAP) provide inspiratory positive airway pressure as well as airway support during expiration. Bilevel ventilation is primarily used at night with a tight-fitting mask (nasal, facial, or oral). Three modes of ventilation can be used with BiPAP: spontaneous breathing (S); timed mode (T), in which pressure-supported breaths are delivered at a predetermined rate; and spontaneous/timed (S/T), in which the ventilator switches to timed mode if spontaneous breathing falls below a preset rate (International Ventilator Users Network, 2006).

Assist-control mode ventilation (ACMV or AC) is frequently used to initiate mechanical ventilation and when the client is at risk for respiratory arrest (e.g., overdose or head injury). Assisted breaths are triggered by inspiratory effort; however, if the respiratory rate falls below a preset number (e.g., 14 per minute), ventilator-controlled breaths are delivered. All breaths, assisted and controlled, are delivered at a specific tidal volume or pressure and inspiratory flow rate.

Synchronized intermittent mandatory ventilation (SIMV) allows the client to breathe spontaneously, without ventilator assistance, between delivered ventilator breaths. Mandatory or ventilator-controlled breaths are delivered at a preset rate, volume, and/or pressure, coordinated with the client's inspiratory efforts. This mode of ventilation is used to support ventilation, to exercise respiratory muscles between ventilator-assisted breaths, and during the weaning process (Kasper et al., 2005).

Positive end-expiratory pressure (PEEP) requires intubation and can be applied to any of the previously described ventilator modes. With PEEP, a positive pressure is maintained in the airways during exhalation and between breaths. Keeping alveoli open between breaths improves ventilation-perfusion relationships and diffusion across the alveolar-capillary membrane. This reduces hypoxemia and allows use of lower percentages of inspired oxygen. PEEP is particularly useful for treating ARDS.

In *pressure support ventilation* (PSV), ventilator-assisted breaths are delivered when the client initiates an inspiratory effort. The cycle is flow limited; inspiration is terminated when inspiratory airflow falls below a preset rate. This mode decreases the work of breathing. It can be used in combination with SIMV when the respiratory drive is depressed. Ventilator support can be gradually withdrawn during weaning.

Pressure-control ventilation (PCV), in contrast, controls pressure within the airways to reduce the risk of airway trauma (e.g., following thoracic surgery). Ventilation is time triggered and time cycled, but pressure is limited. The ventilator maintains a preset airway pressure throughout inspiration. Because all breaths are controlled by the ventilator, heavy sedation may be required to prevent competition between inspiratory effort and ventilator control.

VENTILATOR SETTINGS In addition to choosing the mode of ventilation, other parameters are set to meet individual client needs when positive-pressure ventilation is used (Table 39–8).

For most adult clients, the rate is initially set between 12 and 15 breaths per minute. With ACMV or SIMV, the client's respiratory rate often is higher than the ventilator setting due to spontaneous breathing. Exhaled carbon dioxide (ET_{CO_2}) or the Pa_{CO_2} may be used to determine the rate. A Pa_{CO_2} of less than 38 mmHg indicates hyperventilation and respiratory alkalosis; the set rate is reduced. A Pa_{CO_2} above 42 mmHg or an ET_{CO_2} greater than 45 mmHg indicates hypoventilation and a need to increase the rate.

The tidal volume setting controls the amount of gas delivered with each ventilator breath. The normal adult tidal volume at rest is about 7 mL/kg of body weight, or 400 to 550 mL. The tidal volume delivered by mechanical ventilation is slightly higher (500 to 750 mL) to compensate for tubing dead space. Higher tidal volumes can cause lung tissue trauma.

The percentage of oxygen delivered with ventilator breaths is adjusted to maintain the oxygen saturation and Pa_{O_2} within acceptable ranges. Because prolonged delivery of high oxygen concentrations increases the risk of oxygen toxicity and

TABLE 39-7 Modes of Positive-Pressure Ventilator Operation

MODE	DESCRIPTION	PATTERN
Spontaneous breathing	Client has full control of rate, tidal volume, pressures.	
Assist-control mode ventilation (ACMV)	Client can trigger ventilator to deliver breaths at preset volume or pressure and inspiratory flow rate; breaths will be delivered at preset rate if client does not initiate.	
Synchronized intermittent mandatory ventilation (SIMV)	Mandatory breaths delivered by ventilator are synchronized with client's inspiratory effort.	
Continuous positive airway pressure (CPAP)	Positive pressure is maintained in airways; all breaths are spontaneous.	
Positive end-expiratory pressure (PEEP)	Used in conjunction with other ventilator modes; positive airway pressure is maintained throughout respiratory cycle.	
Pressure support ventilation (PSV)	Pressurized inspiratory flow supports the client's inspiratory effort, decreasing the work of breathing.	

TABLE 39–8 Ventilator Settings

PARAMETER	DESCRIPTION
Rate (*f*)	Number of ventilator-delivered breaths per minute: usually 12 to 15 in adults using ACMV; may be lower in SIMV
Tidal volume (V_t)	Amount of gas delivered with each ventilator breath: usually 8 to 10 mL/kg of body weight
Oxygen concentration (FIO_2)	Percentage of oxygen delivered with ventilator breaths; can be set between 21% (room air) and 100%
I:E ratio	Duration of inspiration to expiration: usually 1:2 to 1:1.5
Flow rate	Speed at which air is delivered
Sensitivity	Effort required by client to initiate a ventilator-assisted breath
Pressure limit	Maximal pressure within airways that will terminate a ventilator breath

pulmonary fibrosis, the FIO_2 is set at the lowest possible level for adequate tissue oxygenation. For most clients, the goal is to maintain an oxygen saturation level of greater than 90%. Lower oxygen saturation levels may be appropriate for clients with long-standing COPD.

COMPLICATIONS Although endotracheal intubation and mechanical ventilation can be lifesaving in respiratory failure, they are not without risk. Improper endotracheal tube placement or advancement of the tube into a mainstem bronchus can result in ventilation of one lung only. The inflated lung becomes overdistended and traumatized, and the uninflated lung develops atelectasis. In noninvasive ventilation, associated complications include gastric dilation, aspiration, facial skin necrosis, drying of the eyes and mucous membranes, stress, and claustrophobia (Fenstermacher & Hong, 2004).

Nosocomial Pneumonia Infection is a significant risk associated with intubation and mechanical ventilation. Normal upper respiratory tract defense mechanisms are bypassed, with loss of air humidification and trapping of pathogens. Oral secretions and gastric contents can enter the respiratory tree through the open epiglottis. Frequent, meticulous oral hygiene is vital in preventing ventilator-associated pneumonia. Often the cough reflex is inhibited or impaired by the underlying disease process and the continued presence of the endotracheal tube. Even when strict asepsis is used for suctioning and other respiratory procedures, the lower airways are contaminated within 24 hours of intubation (Urden et al., 2006). Secretions often become thick and tenacious, increasing the risk of atelectasis.

Barotrauma *Barotrauma* (also called *volutrauma*) is lung injury due to alveolar overdistention. Both the volume of delivered gas and the pressures under which it is delivered can contribute to barotraumas. As a result, overdistended alveoli rupture, allowing air to escape into the pulmonary interstitial spaces and the mediastinum, pleural space, and other tissues. Subcutaneous emphysema, pneumothorax, and pneumomediastinum are possible results of barotrauma. *Subcutaneous emphysema,* or air in the subcutaneous tissue, causes tissue swelling of the chest, neck, and face. A "crackling" or air-bubble-popping sensation is felt on palpation of subcutaneous emphysema. Swelling may be massive. Once the cause is corrected, the air is gradually reabsorbed.

Pneumothorax is identified by signs of unequal chest expansion, a sudden loss or significant decrease in breath sounds on the affected side, and a hyperresonant percussion tone. Rapid chest tube insertion is necessary to prevent tension pneumothorax and cardiovascular compromise. *Pneumomediastinum* is the presence of air in the mediastinum, the space between the lungs that contains the heart, great vessels, trachea, and esophagus. Air in the mediastinal space can interfere with the function of all of these organs and lead to such complications as pneumopericardium (air in the pericardial sac). Pneumomediastinum may have few manifestations, but the chest x-ray shows widening of the mediastinal space.

Cardiovascular Effects Positive-pressure ventilation increases intrathoracic pressure, which can interfere with venous return to the heart and ventricular filling. As a result, cardiac output falls. Use of PEEP increases the effects of mechanical ventilation on cardiac output. The decreased cardiac output can affect liver and kidney function secondarily.

Gastrointestinal Effects Gastrointestinal complications are commonly associated with prolonged mechanical ventilation. Stress ulcers (erosive gastritis) may develop, leading to painless gastrointestinal hemorrhage. Histamine H_2-receptor blockers or sucralfate are often used to prevent stress ulcers. Air leaks around the endotracheal tube can cause gastric distention; a nasogastric tube often is inserted to prevent vomiting. Sedation and other medications used during mechanical ventilation can slow intestinal motility, leading to constipation.

WEANING The process of removing ventilator support and reestablishing spontaneous, independent respirations is called **weaning**. Weaning begins only after the underlying process causing respiratory failure has been corrected or stabilized. The process and time required for weaning depend on factors such as preexisting lung condition, duration of mechanical ventilation, and the client's general condition, both physical and psychologic. In all cases, the vital signs, respiratory rate, extent of dyspnea, blood gases, and clinical status are used to evaluate weaning and its progress.

Following a brief period of mechanical ventilation, T-piece or CPAP may be used for weaning. In T-piece weaning, the ventilator is removed for brief periods during which oxygen is delivered using a T-piece (Figure 39–10 ■). The duration of periods off the ventilator is gradually increased until the client can

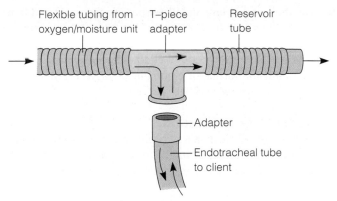

Figure 39–10 ■ A T-piece, or "blow-by" unit, for weaning from mechanical ventilation.

maintain adequate independent respirations for several hours. Vital signs, oxygen saturation, ET_{CO_2}, and Pa_{O_2} are carefully monitored during the process. The client is placed back on the ventilator at previous settings if signs of respiratory distress develop. When mechanical ventilation is no longer needed, the endotracheal tube is removed. CPAP weaning follows a similar process, with trials of spontaneous breathing supported by the ventilator in CPAP mode.

SIMV and PSV are used for weaning when the duration of mechanical ventilation has been longer and reconditioning of respiratory muscles is needed. When SIMV is used, the number of mandatory ventilator-assisted breaths is gradually decreased as ABGs, ET_{CO_2}, and the respiratory rate are monitored. When the client is able to tolerate SIMV at 4 breaths per minute without rest periods of greater ventilatory support, CPAP or T-piece weaning is attempted prior to extubation (Kasper et al., 2005).

Weaning is the primary use for pressure-support ventilation. Initially, PSV is set slightly below peak inspiratory pressures required during volume-cycled ventilation. Pressure support levels are gradually decreased, often in a cyclic pattern of periods of minimal support alternating with higher support to recondition respiratory muscles. When the PSV level is just enough to overcome endotracheal tube resistance, support is discontinued and the client is extubated (Kasper et al., 2005).

Terminal Weaning When an illness is terminal or irreversible with a poor prognosis, terminal weaning may be requested by the client or family. *Terminal weaning* is the gradual withdrawal of mechanical ventilation when survival without assisted ventilation is not expected. Unlike weaning when recovery is expected, which usually occurs in an intensive care unit, the client is moved to a quiet medical-surgical or hospice room or even home prior to initiating terminal weaning. Family members are encouraged to remain with the client throughout the process. If possible, decisions about sedation and analgesia prior to and during weaning are made with the client, as are decisions about hydration and nutritional support following weaning. Ventilator support is gradually withdrawn using the same modes described earlier (SIMV, PSV). Analgesia and sedation are given to promote comfort during weaning.

Nutrition and Fluids

Attention also must be paid to fluid and electrolyte status and adequate nutrition. Mechanical ventilation promotes sodium and water retention due to its effects on cardiac output. Renal perfusion is decreased, stimulating the renin–angiotensin–aldosterone system to retain sodium and water. A Swan-Ganz catheter is often inserted to monitor pulmonary artery pressures and cardiac output. An arterial line allows repeated blood gas analysis and continuous arterial pressure monitoring. Serum electrolytes are drawn frequently, and intake, output, and daily weight are carefully monitored.

Enteral or parenteral nutrition are provided during mechanical ventilation, because the endotracheal tube prohibits eating. A nasogastric, gastrostomy, or jejunostomy feeding tube is placed for enteral nutrition. A jejunostomy tube may be used to reduce the risk of regurgitation and aspiration.

 NURSING CARE

Health Promotion

Education is a primary strategy to prevent respiratory failure. Teach all clients and the public about the risks of smoking, water safety, the value of a working smoke detector, and measures to prevent smoke inhalation in a fire. Discuss the importance of pneumococcal vaccine and annual influenza immunizations for people who are at high risk, including those over age 65 and people with chronic diseases. Teach clients with spinal cord injury or neuromuscular disease to use effective breathing and coughing techniques to maintain airway patency. Work with clients addicted to narcotic drugs to attain and maintain drug-free status. Teach clients with COPD about measures to reduce their risk of respiratory infection and symptoms to report to the physician.

Assessment

Focused assessment data related to respiratory failure include the following:

■ *Health History:* Current manifestations, their duration, and identified precipitating factors (may need to be obtained from family members if mental status is affected); history of previous episodes; chronic diseases such as COPD, occupational lung disease; current medications.

■ *Physical Examination:* LOC, mental status; vital signs; color and oxygen saturation; respiratory assessment including rate and depth, use of accessory muscles, respiratory excursion, auscultation; cardiovascular assessment including heart rate and sounds, neck vein distention, peripheral pulses, evidence of clubbing.

■ *Diagnostic Tests:* ABGs, chest x-ray, pulmonary artery pressure and wedge pressure readings, cardiac output.

Nursing Diagnoses and Interventions

Clients in respiratory failure are often unstable and critically ill. They require both intensive medical care and intensive nursing care. Priority nursing needs relate to maintaining ventilation and a patent airway. Perhaps less obvious, but no less critical, nursing care needs relate to preventing injury and managing anxiety.

Impaired Spontaneous Ventilation

In acute respiratory failure, fatigue from the work of breathing may impair the ability to maintain adequate ventilation. This is a concern both prior to initiation of mechanical ventilation and during the weaning process.

- Assess and document respiratory rate, vital signs, and oxygen saturation every 15 to 30 minutes. *Close monitoring is vital to detect early signs of increasing respiratory distress and inability to sustain adequate breathing.*

PRACTICE ALERT
Promptly report signs of respiratory distress, including tachypnea, tachycardia, nasal flaring, use of accessory muscles, intercostal retractions, cyanosis, increasing restlessness, anxiety, or decreased LOC. These may be early manifestations of respiratory failure and inability to maintain ventilatory effort.

- Promptly report worsening ABGs and oxygen saturation levels. *Close assessment of these values allows timely intervention as needed.*
- Administer oxygen as ordered, monitoring response. Observe closely for respiratory depression, especially in the client with COPD. *Oxygen administration reduces the hypoxemic respiratory drive. Chronically high $PaCO_2$ levels depress the respiratory center; hypoxemia may provide the only respiratory drive.*
- Place in Fowler's or high-Fowler's position. *Sitting positions decrease pressure on the diaphragm and chest, improving lung ventilation and decreasing the work of breathing.*
- Minimize activities and energy expenditures by assisting with ADLs, spacing procedures and activities, and by allowing uninterrupted rest periods. *Rest is vital to reduce oxygen and energy demands.*

PRACTICE ALERT
Avoid sedatives and respiratory depressant drugs unless mechanically ventilated. These medications can further depress the respiratory drive, worsening respiratory failure.

- Prepare for endotracheal intubation and mechanical ventilation:
  a. Obtain an intubation tray with a selection of sterile endotracheal tubes and laryngoscope with a variety of adult blades.
  b. Check laryngoscope lamp; replace battery pack or bulb as needed.
  c. Set up for endotracheal suction, bringing continuous suction head, container, tubing, sterile catheter and glove kits, and sterile normal saline to the bedside.
  d. Notify respiratory therapy to set up the ventilator.
  e. Notify radiology that a portable chest x-ray will be needed on completion of intubation to verify correct placement of the endotracheal tube.
  Intubation and mechanical ventilation may be required to maintain ventilation and gas exchange.

- Explain the procedure and its purpose to the client and family, providing reassurance that this is a temporary measure to reduce the work of breathing and allow rest. Alert that talking is not possible while the endotracheal tube is in place, and establish a means of communication. *Thorough explanation is important to relieve anxiety.*

Ineffective Airway Clearance

Ineffective airway clearance may either cause respiratory failure or occur as a result of interventions. Impaired ventilation frequently leads to acute respiratory failure, particularly in clients with COPD or asthma. Chest trauma also can impair airway patency as a result of pulmonary contusion and ineffective cough. Although intubation and mechanical ventilation can be lifesaving measures, they also increase the risk of respiratory infection and ineffective secretion management.

PRACTICE ALERT
Frequently assess respiratory rate, chest movement, lung sounds, oxygen saturation, $ETCO_2$, and ABGs. Intubation and mechanical ventilation do not ensure adequate oxygenation and ventilation. Displacement of the endotracheal tube or obstruction by respiratory secretions impairs ventilation.

- Suction as needed to maintain a patent airway. Indicators for suctioning include crackles and rhonchi on auscultation, frequent coughing or setting off of the high-pressure alarm, and increasing restlessness or anxiety. Procedure 39–1 outlines endotracheal suctioning. *Although clients with a tracheostomy can usually cough up secretions, the length and diameter of endotracheal tubes makes this extremely difficult. Even with humidification, secretions often become thick and tenacious, further inhibiting their removal.*
- Obtain sputum for culture if it appears purulent or is odorous. *Culture is necessary to identify pathogens and guide antibiotic therapy.*
- Perform percussion, vibration, and postural drainage as ordered. *These techniques help loosen secretions and move them into larger airways for removal by coughing or suctioning.*

PRACTICE ALERT
Evaluate endotracheal tube cuff pressure by measurement (should have no more than 20 to 25 mmHg of pressure) or by auscultating the suprasternal notch for a hissing sound at the end of inspiration. The minimum effective cuff pressure to maintain alveolar ventilation is used to reduce the risk of tracheal ischemia and necrosis.

- Firmly secure endotracheal or tracheostomy tube. Provide adequate slack on ventilator tubing to prevent tension on the tube when turning, positioning, or transferring to chair or stretcher. If necessary, loosely restrain hands. *These measures are important to ensure proper airway placement and prevent its inadvertent removal.*
- Assess fluid balance and maintain adequate hydration. *Adequate hydration helps liquefy secretions.*

PROCEDURE 39–1 ENDOTRACHEAL SUCTIONING

GATHER SUPPLIES

- Suction unit with connecting tubing and connector at the bedside
- If an in-line suction catheter is not present
  a. Sterile suction catheter (size 12 to 16 Fr) and glove-kit or suction catheter and sleeve
  b. Sterile normal saline
- Personal protective devices as indicated: goggles, mask, gown

BEFORE THE PROCEDURE

Explain the procedure and why it is being done. Tell the client that although suctioning is not painful, it is uncomfortable. While suction is being applied, breathing is difficult but these periods last only 10 seconds. Stress that suctioning allows removal of secretions and stimulates coughing, which helps clear secretions from smaller airways. Establish a means of communicating; for example, tell the client to raise a finger or rapidly blink if unable to tolerate suctioning.

DURING THE PROCEDURE

1. Use standard precautions.
2. Prepare the suction unit by turning it on and regulating it to no more than −80 to −120 mmHg.
3. Open sterile saline bottle, leaving the cap loosely in place.

With an In-Line Catheter

- Wearing exam gloves, attach the catheter to suction tubing.
- Adjust the oxygen (FIo_2) to 100%; allow three breaths.
- Manipulating the catheter through the plastic shield (to maintain its sterility), insert the catheter without applying suction until resistance is met; apply suction while slowly withdrawing the catheter with a twirling motion (see figure).
- Suction for no longer than 10 seconds (count the seconds or watch the clock—the time passes more quickly than you think), then allow to rest for three to five breaths. Repeat the procedure as needed for a total of no more than three times.
- Remove suction tubing from the catheter, clear the tubing, turn off suction, and remove and discard gloves.

With a Separate Catheter-and-Glove Kit

- Open suction catheter/glove kit. Remove saline cup, and fill with sterile normal saline.
- Put on sterile gloves, and attach catheter to suction tubing, keeping dominant hand sterile; lubricate catheter tip with sterile saline.
- Use the nondominant hand to adjust oxygen (FIo_2) to 100%; allow three breaths.
- Using the nondominant hand, disconnect ventilator tubing from the endotracheal tube. Manipulating the suction catheter with the dominant (sterile) hand and the suction control valve with the nondominant (nonsterile) hand, insert the catheter, without applying suction until resistance is met. Then, apply suction while slowly withdrawing the catheter, using a twirling motion.

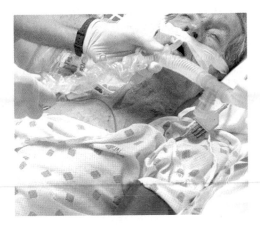

- Suction for no longer than 10 seconds. Reconnect the ventilator, and allow to rest for three to five breaths; clear suction tubing with sterile saline.
- Repeat the preceding two steps as needed for a total of three times.
- Reconnect ventilator tubing to the endotracheal tube.
- Clear suction tubing, turn off suction, and remove the catheter, discarding it with the gloves.

4. Provide three additional breaths at 100% oxygen, then readjust to the previous ordered level.
5. Note color, quantity, consistency, and odor of sputum.
6. Assess lung sounds and tolerance of the procedure.
7. Wash hands.

AFTER THE PROCEDURE

Document assessment before and after suctioning, along with the character of the sputum and the client's tolerance of the procedure. Report changes in sputum character, such as purulence or an odor that may indicate infection.

Risk for Injury

Many factors increase the risk for injury in acute respiratory failure. Hypoxemia and hypercapnia affect the level of consciousness and may impair mental status. Endotracheal intubation and mechanical ventilation carry risks of tracheal damage and trauma to the lungs. Neuromuscular blockade, if used, presents a significant risk for injury as the client is unable to breathe spontaneously, communicate, and move.

- Assess frequently, noting the following:
  a. LOC, orientation, and awareness
  b. Condition of mucosa of mouth and nose

c. Respiratory: lung sounds, chest excursion, and ventilator pressures

d. Cardiovascular: vital signs, skin color, capillary refill, and peripheral pulses

e. Gastrointestinal: bowel sounds; test gastric secretions and feces for occult blood

f. Genitourinary: urine output, daily weight

g. Skin and extremities

Complications associated with respiratory failure and mechanical ventilation can affect many body systems. Frequent assessment allows early detection and intervention.

PRACTICE ALERT

Do not bypass or turn off any ventilator alarms. The intubated client is unable to communicate verbally and cannot call for help. If neuromuscular blockers are used, the client is also unable to breathe without ventilator support.

- Report condition changes such as increasing air leak around the cuff and decreased breath sounds or chest movement. *These may be manifestations of a complication of intubation and ventilation, such as tracheal necrosis, displacement of the endotracheal tube into the right mainstem bronchus, pneumothorax, or atelectasis.*
- Turn and reposition frequently, taking care to stabilize endotracheal tube during movement. *Repositioning helps maintain tissue perfusion and prevent skin and tissue breakdown.*
- Keep skin and linens clean, dry, and wrinkle-free. Protect pressure areas with padding, egg-crate, or heel and elbow protectors. *The client may not be able to perceive and report pain, and move voluntarily to reduce pressure, necessitating excellent skin care.*
- Perform passive range-of-motion exercises every 4 to 8 hours. *These exercises maintain joint flexibility and help prevent contractures associated with long-term immobility.*

- Keep side rails up and use soft restraints as needed. *These safety measures are important to prevent falls, inadvertent disconnection of the ventilator, or dislodging of the endotracheal tube.*
- Administer histamine H_2-blockers and sucralfate as ordered. *Stress gastritis and possible gastrointestinal hemorrhage are common, preventable complications of mechanical ventilation.*

Anxiety

Critical illness creates anxiety for any client. In acute respiratory failure, this anxiety is compounded by the presence of an endotracheal tube or tracheostomy, mechanical ventilator, numerous monitors and equipment, and, potentially, neuromuscular blockade and paralysis of voluntary muscles. Fear of continued dependence on the mechanical ventilator and inability to return to a normal life may compound this anxiety.

PRACTICE ALERT

Frequently monitor anxiety level. High levels of anxiety increase oxygen use and often interfere with the ability to work with the respirator. This can increase hypoxemia and further increase anxiety; intervention is necessary to break this cycle.

See the accompanying Nursing Research box for information about assessing and managing pain in clients who are intubated.

- Remain with the client as much as possible. *The frequent and continuing presence of a caregiver provides reassurance that help is readily available.*
- Explain all monitors, procedures, unusual sounds, and machinery. *Understanding of the environment and various sounds and alarms reduces anxiety.*
- Provide a simple means of communication, such as a slate, picture board, or alphabet board. If neuromuscular blockade is used, use methods such as looking to the right for "yes" and left for "no." Reassure that endotracheal tube removal re-

---

NURSING RESEARCH   Evidence-Based Practice for the Client Who Is Intubated

Clients who are intubated cannot communicate verbally. Subjective experiences, then, such as pain may not be recognized and effectively treated in these clients. This retrospective study by Gélinas and colleagues (2004) used a standardized instrument to look at the assessment and management of pain as documented in the records of 52 clients undergoing mechanical ventilation. A total of 183 pain episodes were analyzed. In the majority of episodes, observable indicators of pain (such as restlessness, changes in vital signs, muscle tension) were recorded. Subjective reports were recorded only 29% of the time. Following intervention, pain was reassessed only about 60% of the time, usually using objective data and rarely (8%) using subjective information. The study concluded that documentation of pain and its management was incomplete or inadequate for intubated clients.

IMPLICATIONS FOR NURSING

Pain is now considered as the fifth vital sign, necessitating frequent assessment and monitoring. Unrelieved pain is known to reduce healing and prolong recovery. Observable indicators of

pain are not always present; some clients deal with pain by attempting to relax muscles and doze. When neuromuscular blockers or other anesthetic agents are administered to clients who are intubated and mechanically ventilated, objective pain indicators are lost in addition to the ability to subjectively report pain. However, it is important to remember that nursing practice standards dictate that pain level be assessed regularly and both before and following interventions to reduce or relieve pain.

CRITICAL THINKING IN CLIENT CARE

1. What tools are available to assist the nurse in evaluating the client's subjective perception of pain?
2. How can the nurse adapt these tools to use for a client under neuromuscular blockade (consciousness intact but unable to move voluntary muscles)?
3. What factors might contribute to pain in the client who is intubated and mechanically ventilated?
4. Identify five nonpharmacologic measures the nurse could implement to reduce or relieve pain in intubated and ventilated clients.

stores the ability to speak. *The inability to speak and call out for help is frightening for the client. Providing an alternate means of communication helps reduce anxiety.*

■ Encourage frequent family visits, especially if the time of visitations is being limited. Encourage family participation in care. *Family visits help reduce anxiety and feelings of abandonment. Allowing family members to participate in care helps reduce their anxiety as well.*

■ Explain to the family that the client can hear and understand. Emphasize the importance of talking to the client, not over or about the client. *The family may not understand that the client may be mentally alert although unable to respond. Talking to the client about everyday things reduces the client's sense of isolation and fear.*

■ Provide distraction with radio or television if allowed. *Distraction helps reduce the focus on machines and unusual sounds of monitors and alarms.*

■ Attend to physical needs promptly and completely. *This provides reassurance that needs will be met even though the client is unable to ask for assistance.*

■ Reassure that intubation and mechanical ventilation is a temporary measure to allow the lungs to rest and heal. Reinforce that the client will be able to breathe independently again. *The client may fear continued dependence on mechanical ventilation.*

PRACTICE ALERT
Provide sedation and antianxiety medications as needed, especially when neuromuscular blockade is used. Although neuromuscular blockade paralyzes voluntary muscles, the level of consciousness is unimpaired.

Using NANDA, NIC, and NOC

Linkages between NANDA nursing diagnoses, nursing interventions, and nursing outcomes for the client with respiratory failure are illustrated in Chart 39–3.

Community-Based Care

Prior to hospital discharge, teach the client and family about the following topics:

■ Factors that precipitated respiratory failure and measures to prevent it in the future (e.g., the impact of respiratory irritants on compromised lungs)

■ Measures to prevent future episodes such as remaining indoors with an air filter or air conditioning when pollution levels are high, obtaining influenza and pneumonia immunizations, and avoiding exposure to cigarette smoke

■ Effective coughing and pulmonary hygiene measures such as percussion, vibration, and postural drainage.

Acute respiratory failure resulting from an acute insult such as pneumonia or near-drowning often resolves with few long-term sequelae. When respiratory failure results from an underlying disease such as COPD, the prognosis is less optimistic. Clients with end-stage COPD may have repeated episodes of respiratory failure, with a gradual loss of respiratory function and reserve. These clients may choose terminal weaning rather

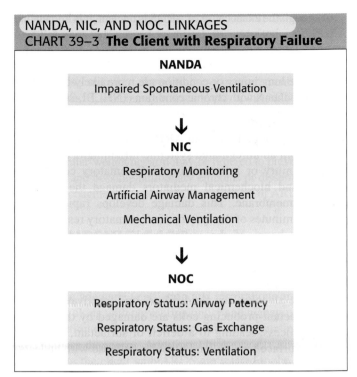

NANDA, NIC, AND NOC LINKAGES
CHART 39–3 The Client with Respiratory Failure

NANDA

Impaired Spontaneous Ventilation

↓

NIC

Respiratory Monitoring

Artificial Airway Management

Mechanical Ventilation

↓

NOC

Respiratory Status: Airway Patency

Respiratory Status: Gas Exchange

Respiratory Status: Ventilation

Data from *NANDA's Nursing Diagnoses: Definitions & Classification 2005–2006* by NANDA International (2005), Philadelphia; *Nursing Interventions Classification (NIC)* (4th ed.) by J. M. Dochterman & G. M. Bulechek (2004), St. Louis, MO: Mosby; and *Nursing Outcomes Classification (NOC)* (3rd ed.) by S. Moorhead, M. Johnson, and M. Maas (2004), St. Louis, MO. Mosby.

than a future of increasing disability. Discuss what to expect during the terminal weaning process with the client and family. Discuss use of sedation prior to and during the weaning process. Explain that medications are used to reduce respiratory distress and dyspnea during weaning. Assure the client and family that nursing support is continuously available during the weaning process and that family and other supporters such as clergy are allowed to remain with the client.

THE CLIENT WITH ACUTE RESPIRATORY DISTRESS SYNDROME

Acute respiratory distress syndrome (ARDS) is characterized by noncardiac pulmonary edema and progressive refractory hypoxemia. First identified in 1967, ARDS has been known by various names, such as shock lung and adult hyaline membrane disease. It is widely recognized as a severe form of acute respiratory failure. The mortality rate associated with acute respiratory distress syndrome, while declining, remains around 30% to 40% (ALA, 2006).

FAST FACTS
■ Approximately 150,000 Americans are affected by ARDS annually (NHLBI, 2006).
■ Most clients recover near-normal lung function within 6 months of developing ARDS.
■ Mortality associated with ARDS often is due to multiple-organ system dysfunction related to ineffective tissue oxygenation (ALA, 2006).

Acute Respiratory Distress Syndrome

Acute respiratory distress syndrome (ARDS) is a severe form of acute respiratory failure that occurs in response to pulmonary or systemic insults. ARDS is characterized by noncardiogenic pulmonary edema caused by inflammator damage to alveolar and capillary walls. Many disorders ma precipitate ARDS, although sepsis is the most common.

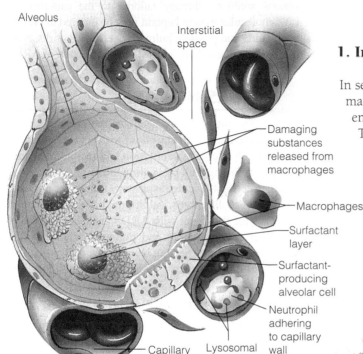

1. Initiation of ARDS

In sepsis-induced ARDS, bacterial toxins cause macrophages and neutrophils to adhere to endothelial surfaces of the alveoli and capillaries. The macrophages release oxidants, inflammatory mediators, enzymes, and peptides that damage the capillary and alveolar walls. In response, neutrophils release lysosomal enzymes causing further damage.

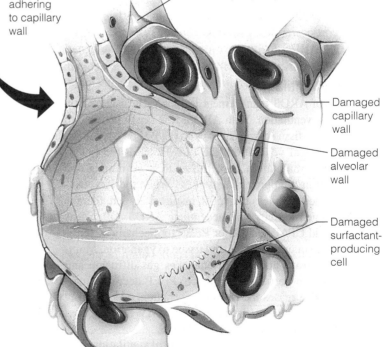

2. Onset of Pulmonary Edema

The damaged capillary and alveolar walls become more permeable, allowing plasma, proteins, and erythrocytes to enter the interstitial space. As interstitial edema increases, pressure in the interstitial space rises and fluid leaks into alveoli. Plasma proteins accumulating in the interstitial space lower the osmotic gradient between the capillary and interstitial compartment. As a result, the balance is disrupted between the osmotic force that pulls fluid from the interstitial space into the capillaries and the normal hydrostatic pressure that pushes fluid out of the capillaries. This imbalance causes even more fluid to enter alveoli.

4. End-Stage ARDS

Fibrin and cell debris from necrotic cells combine to form hyaline membranes, which line the interior of the alveoli and further reduce alveolar compliance and gas exchange. Because CO_2 cannot diffuse across hyaline membranes, $PaCO_2$ levels now begin to rise while PaO_2 levels continue to fall. Rising $PaCO_2$ levels can lead to respiratory acidosis. Without respiratory support, respiratory failure will develop.
Even with aggressive treatment, almost 50% of clients with ARDS die.

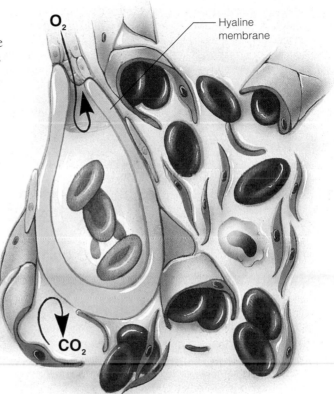

3. Alveolar Collapse

Protein-rich fluid accumulates in the alveoli, inactivating surfactant and damaging type II alveolar cells that produce surfactant. (Surfactant is important in maintaining alveolar compliance—the ability of tissue to stretch or distend.) As active surfactant is lost, the alveoli stiffen and collapse, leading to atelectasis, which increases breathing effort.

Decreased alveolar compliance, atelectasis, and fluid-filled alveoli interfere with gas exchange across the alveolar-capillary membrane. Blood oxygen (PaO_2) levels fall. Because carbon dioxide diffuses more readily than oxygen, however, blood carbon dioxide ($PaCO_2$) levels also fall initially as tachypnea causes more CO_2 to be expired.

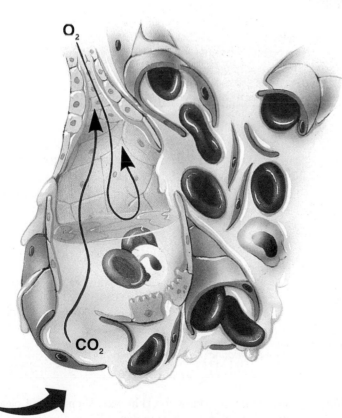

NURSING CARE PLAN   A Client with ARDS

Peggy Adamson is a 36-year-old single woman admitted to the hospital following a near-drowning in a local lake. On admission to the emergency department, Ms. Adamson is alert and oriented, having been rescued and resuscitated within 2 minutes of the accident. Rescuers report that she seemed to have aspirated "a lot" of water as she was water-skiing when the accident occurred. She is admitted to the intensive care unit for observation. Oxygen is started per nasal cannula at 6 L/min, intravenous fluids are administered to correct electrolyte imbalances, and 40 mg of furosemide (Lasix) is given intravenously for hypervolemia.

ASSESSMENT

Nadia Mucha cares for Ms. Adamson the evening of the day after her admission. Throughout her stay, Ms. Adamson has remained alert and oriented with stable vital signs. Her respiratory rate has been 20 to 24 per minute, with scattered crackles, oxygen saturations of around 94%, and a PaO_2 of 75 to 80 mmHg on 6 L/min of oxygen. Her pulse has been 96 to 100 and regular. On her initial assessment, Ms. Mucha notes that Ms. Adamson seems apprehensive and anxious. Although her blood pressure is 116/74, unchanged from previous levels, her heart rate is up to 106 and respiratory rate is 28 per minute. Her lungs have scattered crackles but good breath sounds throughout, unchanged from previous assessments. Ms. Adamson's oxygen saturation has dropped to 84%, so Ms. Mucha orders ABGs and increases the oxygen to 8 L/min. ABG results show PaO_2, 65 mmHg; respiratory alkalosis, pH, 7.48; and $PaCO_2$, 32 mmHg.

Ms. Mucha orders a portable chest x-ray and notifies the physician of the ABG results and the change in Ms. Adamson's status. The physician orders a nonrebreather mask at 8 L/min and repeat ABGs in 1 hour. The chest x-ray reveals scattered infiltrates and a normal heart size.

Ms. Adamson's oxygen saturation continues to fall, and subsequent blood gases show a PaO_2 of 55 mmHg. The attending physician diagnoses probable ARDS and orders nasotracheal intubation and mechanical ventilation.

DIAGNOSES

- *Ineffective Breathing Pattern* related to anxiety
- *Impaired Gas Exchange* related to effects of near-drowning
- *Anxiety* related to hypoxemia
- *Risk for Decreased Cardiac Output* related to mechanical ventilation
- *Risk for Injury* related to endotracheal intubation

EXPECTED OUTCOMES

- Breathe effectively with the mechanical ventilator.
- Demonstrate improved oxygen saturation, $ETCO_2$, and ABG values.
- Express fears related to intubation and mechanical ventilation.
- Demonstrate reduced anxiety levels (relaxed facial expression, ability to rest).
- Maintain adequate cardiac output and tissue perfusion.
- Tolerate endotracheal intubation and mechanical ventilation without evidence of infection or barotrauma.

PLANNING AND IMPLEMENTATION

- Obtain all necessary supplies and notify respiratory therapy and radiology in preparation for intubation and mechanical ventilation.
- Explain the purpose and procedure of intubation.
- Provide an opportunity to express fears related to intubation and mechanical ventilation; answer questions and provide reassurance.
- Discuss communication strategies while intubated; obtain a magic slate.
- Administer analgesics and/or sedatives as ordered.
- Monitor oxygen saturation and $ETCO_2$ levels every 30 to 60 minutes initially after instituting mechanical ventilation; report changes to the physician.
- Obtain ABGs as ordered or indicated; monitor and report results.
- Suction via endotracheal tube as needed to maintain clear airways.
- Allow periods of uninterrupted rest.
- Monitor vital signs every 1 to 2 hours.
- Assess skin color, capillary refill, and the presence of edema every 4 hours.
- Monitor urine output hourly; report output of less than 30 mL per hour.
- Assess lung sounds and chest excursion every 1 to 2 hours.

EVALUATION

Ms. Adamson is intubated and placed on a volume-cycled ventilator at 50% FIO_2 and a tidal volume of 700 mL in the assist-control mode at 16 breaths per minute. She has difficulty working with the ventilator initially, so a fentanyl drip is ordered to reduce her anxiety. Ms. Adamson's oxygen saturation, $ETCO_2$, and ABG results do not begin to improve until 5 mmHg of PEEP is added to ventilator settings. After 3 days of mechanical ventilation with PEEP and aggressive fluid and diuretic therapy, Ms. Adamson begins to improve. She is placed on SIMV, and over the course of another 3 days she is gradually weaned off the ventilator to a face mask with CPAP. She eventually recovers fully, with minimal apparent long-term effects.

CRITICAL THINKING IN THE NURSING PROCESS

1. Endotracheal intubation and mechanical ventilation were effective in supporting Ms. Adamson's respiratory status as she recovered from ARDS. Discuss a possible sequence of events had it not been possible to wean her from the ventilator.
2. How might the presentation and management of an acute episode of respiratory failure due to ARDS differ from respiratory failure related to COPD?
3. What measures can nurses take to prevent the development of ARDS?
4. Develop a nursing care plan for Ms. Adamson for the nursing diagnosis *Powerlessness* related to endotracheal intubation and mechanical ventilation.

See Evaluating Your Response in Appendix C.

- Assess heart and lung sounds frequently. *Increasing crackles or abnormal heart sounds may indicate heart failure.*
- Weigh daily at the same time. *Accurate daily weights are the best indicator of fluid volume status.*

- Frequently provide good skin care, keeping skin clean and dry and protecting pressure points. *Tissue hypoxia increases the risk of skin breakdown, which in turn increases the risk of infection and sepsis.*

- Maintain intravenous fluids as ordered. *Intravenous fluids are given to maintain vascular volume and prevent dehydration.*
- Administer analgesics, sedatives, and neuromuscular blockers as needed. *These medications may be prescribed to decrease cardiac workload.*

Dysfunctional Ventilatory Weaning Response

The client with dysfunctional ventilatory weaning response has difficulty adjusting to reduced mechanical ventilator support, prolonging the weaning process. Airway congestion, inadequate rest or nutrition, pain, anxiety, and a nonsupportive environment are factors that can contribute to difficulty weaning. With ARDS, the pathologic processes of the disease and its effects on gas exchange may be responsible for a prolonged or ineffective weaning process.

Assessment findings indicative of dysfunctional weaning include:

- Dyspnea, apprehension, or agitation
- Decreasing oxygen saturation level
- Cyanosis or pallor, diaphoresis
- Increased blood pressure, pulse, and respiratory rate
- Diminished or adventitious breath sounds, use of accessory muscles
- Decreased LOC
- Deteriorating ABG values
- Shallow, gasping breaths or paradoxic abdominal breathing.

Nursing interventions for dysfunctional weaning include the following:

- Assess vital signs every 15 to 30 minutes following changes in ventilator settings and during T-piece trials. *Vital signs, heart and respiratory rates in particular, can provide early signs of hypoxemia and poor tolerance of the weaning process.*

PRACTICE ALERT

Frequently monitor oxygen saturation, ETco$_2$, and ABGs following changes in ventilator settings. These values are used to assess the adequacy of ventilation and gas exchange during the weaning process.

- Place in Fowler's or high-Fowler's position. *Fowler's position facilitates lung expansion and reduces the work of breathing.*
- Fully explain all weaning procedures, along with expected changes in breathing. *Adequate explanations help reduce anxiety and improve the ability to cooperate.*
- Remain with the client during initial periods following changes of ventilator settings or T-piece trials. *This provides reassurance and allows close monitoring of the response.*
- Limit procedures and activities during weaning periods. *Reducing energy expenditures and cardiac work facilitates the weaning process.*
- Provide diversion, such as television or radio. *Diversion helps distract the focus from breathing.*
- Begin weaning procedures in the morning, when the client is well rested and alert; weaning may be discontinued overnight to provide rest. *The work of breathing increases during the weaning process; adequate rest is important.*
- When SIMV is used for weaning, decrease the SIMV rate by increments of two breaths per minute. *Slow reduction of ven-*

tilator support allows respiratory muscle reconditioning and gradual resumption of the work of breathing.

- Avoid administering drugs that may depress respirations during the weaning process (except as ordered at night to facilitate rest when ventilator support is provided). *Sedatives or analgesics that depress respirations can impair the weaning process.*

PRACTICE ALERT

Frequently assess respiratory status following weaning and extubation. Keep an intubation kit readily available following extubation; be prepared for emergency reintubation. Laryngeal spasm or laryngeal edema may develop following extubation, necessitating reintubation to maintain respirations.

- Keep oxygen at the bedside following weaning and extubation. *Supplemental oxygen may be necessary to maintain adequate blood and tissue oxygenation.*
- Provide pulmonary hygiene with percussion and postural drainage. *Maintaining patent airways and adequate alveolar ventilation is vital during the weaning process.*

Using NANDA, NIC, and NOC

Linkages between NANDA nursing diagnoses, nursing interventions, and nursing outcomes for the client with ARDS are illustrated in Chart 39–4.

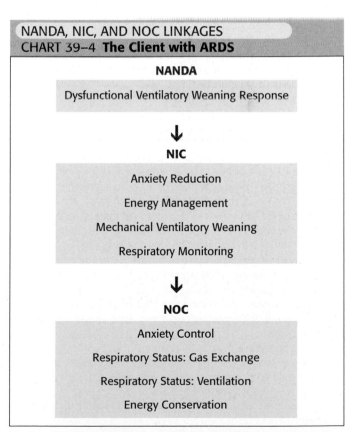

NANDA, NIC, AND NOC LINKAGES
CHART 39–4 The Client with ARDS

NANDA

Dysfunctional Ventilatory Weaning Response

↓

NIC

Anxiety Reduction

Energy Management

Mechanical Ventilatory Weaning

Respiratory Monitoring

↓

NOC

Anxiety Control

Respiratory Status: Gas Exchange

Respiratory Status: Ventilation

Energy Conservation

Data from *NANDA's Nursing Diagnoses: Definitions & Classification 2005–2006* by NANDA International (2005), Philadelphia; *Nursing Interventions Classification (NIC)* (4th ed.) by J. M. Dochterman & G. M. Bulechek (2004), St. Louis, MO: Mosby; and *Nursing Outcomes Classification (NOC)* (3rd ed.) by S. Moorhead, M. Johnson, and M. Maas (2004), St. Louis, MO: Mosby.

Community-Based Care

When preparing the client who has recovered from ARDS and the family for home care, discuss the following topics:

- ARDS did not result from something they did or did not do, but developed as a consequence of serious illness. Provide factual information about ARDS.
- Maximal respiratory function following ARDS is usually achieved within 6 months; respiratory function may remain significantly impaired. This may necessitate changes in occupation, lifestyle, and family roles.

- Avoiding smoking and exposure to secondhand smoke and environmental pollutants is vital to prevent further lung damage.
- Obtain immunization for pneumococcal pneumonia and annual influenza immunizations to prevent further episodes of serious respiratory disease.

Provide referrals to home health and respiratory care services as indicated, as well as for occupational therapy and counseling as needed.

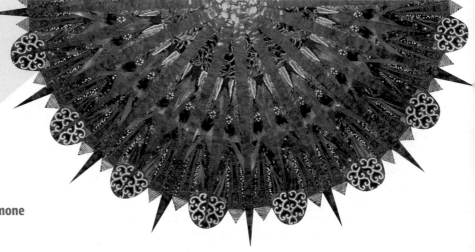

EXPLORE MediaLink

Prentice Hall Nursing MediaLink DVD-ROM
  Audio Glossary
  NCLEX-RN® Review

Animation/Video
  ARDS
  Asthma
  Metered-Dose Inhalers
  Using a Nebulizer

COMPANION WEBSITE www.prenhall.com/lemone
  Audio Glossary
  NCLEX-RN® Review
  Care Plan Activity: Acute Asthma Attack
  Case Study: Acute Asthma Attack
  Exercise: Compare and Contrast
  MediaLink Application: Respiratory Disorders
  Links to Resources

CHAPTER HIGHLIGHTS

- Obstructive disorders of the lower respiratory system, including asthma, COPD, and cystic fibrosis, impair airflow into and out of the lungs, often affecting the outflow of air to a greater extent than inflow. As a result, air trapped in the alveoli increases the residual volume of the lungs and reduces functional residual capacity. Alveolar ventilation is reduced as well. The net result is less available oxygen in the alveoli and impaired gas exchange.

- In many instances, acute episodes of asthma can be avoided through the use of inhaled steroids to reduce airway inflammation, inhaled long-acting bronchodilators, and frequent self-monitoring of expiratory flow rate. Nursing care focuses on teaching for self-management, and providing care during acute episodes of airway constriction.

- Chronic obstructive pulmonary disease (COPD) is a long-term process of progressive lung dysfunction. COPD involves two different disease processes: chronic bronchitis, characterized by airway edema and excessive mucous production, and emphysema, characterized by destruction of supporting tissue with enlargement of respiratory bronchioles and alveolar spaces and loss of surface area for gas exchange.

- Smoking and exposure to tobacco smoke is the single greatest risk factor for COPD. A small percentage of cases result from an inherited deficiency of α_1-antitripsin, an enzyme that inhibits lung

tissue destruction. Although smoking cessation does not reverse COPD, it does slow the progress of the disease.

- Cystic fibrosis, inherited as an autosomal recessive disorder, causes thick, viscous secretions in affected organs, primarily the lungs, pancreas, sweat glands, and reproductive tract. In the lungs, small airway clearance is impaired, leading to atelectasis, bronchiectasis, infection, and dilation of distal airways with air trapping and impaired gas exchange. Chest physiotherapy and early treatment of respiratory infections are key components of disease management. Ultimately, lung or heart-lung transplant may be required.

- Occupational lung diseases, pneumoconiosis and hypersensitivity pneumonitis, damage interstitial tissues of the lungs, leading to fibrosis and scarring that causes the lungs to become stiff and noncompliant. Lung volumes decrease, the work of breathing increases, and gas diffusion is impaired. Most occupational lung diseases are progressive and nonreversible. Interdisciplinary care is similar to that provided for clients with COPD.

- Pulmonary vascular disorders affect blood flow through the pulmonary vascular system and gas exchange. Pulmonary embolism, obstruction of pulmonary blood flow, is a potentially critical condition usually resulting from deep venous thrombosis. Sudden onset of chest pain and dyspnea with changes in hemodynamic status are possible manifestations of pulmonary embolism. Prevention through early ambulation, lower extremity exercises, and sequential compression devices is the most effective treatment for pulmonary embolism.

- In primary and secondary forms of pulmonary hypertension, constriction of pulmonary vessels and remodeling of the pulmonary vascular bed increase pressure in the pulmonary system and right heart, ultimately leading to right-sided heart failure (cor pulmonale). Treatment focuses on slowing disease progression through oxygen therapy, administration of vasodilators and anticoagulants, and supporting client function.

- Hypoventilation, impaired gas exchange, and significant ventilation-perfusion mismatch (e.g., pulmonary embolism) can lead to respiratory failure. Hypoventilation leads to hypoxemia and hypercapnia, whereas in impaired gas exchange or ventilation-perfusion mismatch, hypoxemia predominates.

- The manifestations of respiratory failure relate directly to the effects of hypoxemia (dyspnea, restlessness, apprehension, impaired judgment, motor impairment, tachycardia, hyper- or hypotension, and cyanosis) and hypercapnia (dyspnea, headache, peripheral and conjunctival vasodilation, papilledema, neuromuscular irritability, and decreased LOC).

- Respiratory support often is required, using positive-pressure ventilators. Variables of mechanical ventilation include the mode or cycle of ventilation, the flow rate and amount, pressures delivered, and the oxygen concentration. Either invasive or noninvasive techniques may be used.

- Complications of mechanical ventilation include lung and mucous membrane trauma and infection, reduced cardiac output, gastric dilation, impaired communication, and stress.

- ARDS is noncardiac pulmonary edema caused by a diffuse inflammatory response with increased pulmonary capillary permeability leading to interstitial and alveolar edema and impaired gas exchange. As the process continues, lung compliance decreases, increasing the work of breathing, and atelectasis and consolidation of lung tissue develop. Respiratory failure with refractory hypoxemia result.

- Mechanical ventilation and measures to support physiologic function are the primary treatments for ARDS. The mortality rate, however, remains high at about 50%.

TEST YOURSELF NCLEX-RN® REVIEW

1. All of the following nursing diagnoses are appropriate for a client with an acute asthma attack. Which is of highest priority?
   1. *Anxiety* related to difficulty breathing
   2. *Ineffective Airway Clearance* related to bronchoconstriction and increased mucous production
   3. *Ineffective Breathing Pattern* related to anxiety
   4. *Ineffective Health Maintenance* related of lack of knowledge about attack triggers and appropriate use of medications

2. The nurse caring for a client with asthma notices that the client's respirations have slowed and he is no longer coughing. Breath sounds are diminished throughout his lung fields and absent in the bases. The nurse should:
   1. notify the physician.
   2. allow the client to rest undisturbed.
   3. obtain a chest x-ray.
   4. ask family members to leave.

3. When teaching use of a metered-dose inhaler (MDI), the nurse instructs her client to:
   1. take quick shallow breaths in rapid succession while holding the canister down.
   2. use the inhaler containing the anti-inflammatory drug first, then the bronchodilator.
   3. use the anti-inflammatory drug as needed to treat acute episodes of wheezing.
   4. rinse the mouth after using the inhaler to reduce systemic absorption of the drug.

4. Which of the following would be an expected assessment finding in a client admitted with chronic obstructive airway disease?
   1. AP chest diameter equal to or greater than lateral chest diameter
   2. mental confusion and lethargy
   3. 3+ pitting edema of ankles and lower legs
   4. oxygen saturation readings of 85% or less

5. An appropriate goal for a client admitted with an acute exacerbation of COPD would be:
   1. will verbalize self-care measures to regain lost lung function.
   2. arterial blood gases will be within normal limits by discharge.
   3. will maintain SaO_2 of 90% or higher.
   4. will identify strategies to help reduce number of cigarettes smoked per day.

6. Which of the following statements best represents a nurse's understanding of use of supplemental oxygen in clients with COPD?
   1. Because oxygen is flammable, the client should not smoke.
   2. Oxygen is used only at night for clients with COPD.
   3. Oxygen is never used for clients with COPD because they may become dependent on it.
   4. The client needs to be closely monitored for signs of respiratory depression.

7. The home care nurse working with a client who has cystic fibrosis specifically directs the home care aide to report which of the following? (Select all that apply.)
   1. thick, tenacious milky white sputum
   2. fever
   3. bulky, fatty stools
   4. difficulty clearing mucous secretions
   5. increasing shortness of breath and fatigue

8. A client in skeletal traction suddenly develops right-sided chest pain and shortness of breath. The nurse should:
   1. check for Homans' sign.
   2. start oxygen per nasal cannula.
   3. administer the prescribed analgesic.
   4. elevate the head of the bed to 45 degrees.

9. The nurse caring for a client with COPD recognizes which of the following as an early sign of possible respiratory failure?
   1. restlessness and tachypnea
   2. deep coma
   3. hypotension and tachycardia
   4. decreased urine output

10 The nurse caring for a client undergoing mechanical ventilation for acute respiratory failure plans and implements which of the following measures to help maintain effective alveolar ventilation?

1. Keeps the client in supine position.
2. Increases the tidal volume on the ventilator.
3. Maintains ordered oxygen concentration.
4. Performs endotracheal suctioning as indicated.

See Test Yourself answers in Appendix C.

BIBLIOGRAPHY

American Lung Association (ALA). (2005a). *Asthma in adults fact sheet.* Retrieved from http://www.lungusa.org

_____. (2005b). *Chronic obstructive pulmonary disease (COPD) fact sheet.* Retrieved from http://www.lungusa.org

_____. (2005c). Trends in asthma morbidity and mortality. American Lung Association Epidemiology & Statistic Unit, Research and Program Services. Retrieved from http://www.lungusa.org

_____. (2006). *Lung disease data: 2006.* Retrieved from http://www.lungusa.org

Aronson, B. S., & Marquis, M. (2004). Care of the adult patient with cystic fibrosis. *Medsurg Nursing, 13*(3), 143–154.

Barnett, M. (2006). COPD: The role of the nurse. *Journal of Community Nursing, 20*(2), 18–20, 22.

Belza, B., Steele, B. G., Hunziker, J., Lakshminaryan, S., Holt, L., & Buchner, D. M. (2001). Correlates of physical activity in chronic obstructive pulmonary disease. *Nursing Research, 50*(4), 195–202.

Berkowitz, D. S., & Coyne, N. G. (2003). Understanding primary pulmonary hypertension. *Critical Care Nursing Quarterly, 26*(1), 28–34.

Bialous, S. A., & Sarna, L. (2004). Sparing a few minutes for tobacco cessation. *American Journal of Nursing, 104*(12), 54–62.

Boyle, A. H., & Locke, D. L. (2004). Update on chronic obstructive pulmonary disease. *Medsurg Nursing, 13*(1), 42–48.

Burns, S. M. (2004). The science of weaning: When and how? *Critical Care Nursing Clinics of North America, 16*(3), 379–386.

_____. (2005). Mechanical ventilation of patients with acute respiratory distress syndrome and patients requiring weaning: The evidence guiding practice. *Critical Care Nurse, 25*(4), 14–16, 18, 20–24.

Capriotti, T. (2005). Changes in inhaler devices for asthma and COPD. *Medsurg Nursing, 14*(3), 185–194.

Cardin, T., & Marinelli, A. (2004). Pulmonary embolism. *Critical Care Nursing Quarterly, 27*(4), 310–324.

Carlson, B. W., & Mascarella, J. J. (2003). Living with illness. Changes in sleep patterns in COPD. *American Journal of Nursing, 104*(12), 71–72, 74.

Caroci, A. D. S., & Lareau, S. C. (2005). Descriptors of dyspnea by patients with chronic obstructive pulmonary disease versus congestive heart failure. *Heart & Lung, 33*(2), 102–110.

Charlebois, D. (2005). Early recognition of pulmonary embolism: The key to lowering mortality. *Journal of Cardiovascular Nursing, 20*(4), 254–259.

Cheever, K. H. (2005). An overview of pulmonary arterial hypertension: Risks, pathogenesis, clinical manifestations, and management. *Journal of Cardiovascular Nursing, 20*(2), 108–118.

Copstead, L. C., & Banasik, J. L. (2005). *Pathophysiology* (3rd ed.). St. Louis, MO: Elsevier/Saunders.

Covey, M. K., & Larson, J. L. (2004). Beats & breaths. Exercise and COPD. *American Journal of Nursing, 104*(5), 40–43.

DeJong, S. R., & Veltman, R. H. (2004). The effectiveness of a CNS-led community-based COPD screening and intervention program. *Clinical Nurse Specialist, 18*(2), 72–79.

Dochterman, J., & Bulechek, G. (2004). *Nursing interventions classification (NIC)* (4th ed.). St. Louis, MO: Mosby.

Esmond, G., Butler, M., & McCormack, A. M. (2006). Comparison of hospital and home intravenous antibiotic therapy in adults with cystic fibrosis. *Journal of Clinical Nursing, 15*(1), 52–60.

Farquhar, S. L., & Fantasia, L. (2005). Pulmonary anatomy and physiology and the effects of COPD. *Home Healthcare Nurse, 23*(3), 167–176.

Fenstermacher, D., & Hong, D. (2004). Mechanical ventilation: What have we learned? *Critical Care Nursing Quarterly, 27*(3), 256–294.

Fontaine, K. L. (2005). *Healing practices: Alternative therapies for nursing* (2nd ed.). Upper Saddle River, NJ: Prentice Hall Health.

Frazier, S. C. (2005). Implications of the GOLD report for chronic obstructive lung disease for the home care clinician. *Home Healthcare Nurse, 23*(3), 109–116.

Gélinas, C., Fortier, M., Viens, C., Fillion, L., & Puntillo, K. (2004). Pain assessment and management in critically ill intubated patients: A retrospective study. *American Journal of Critical Care, 13*(2), 126–135.

Gronkiewicz, C., & Borkgren-Okonek, M. (2004). Acute exacerbation of COPD: Nursing application of evidence-based guidelines. *Critical Care Nursing Quarterly, 27*(4), 336–352.

Grossman, S., & Grossman, L. C. (2005). Pulmonary care. Pathophysiology of cystic fibrosis: Implications for critical care nurses. *Critical Care Nurse, 25*(4), 46–51.

Higgins, P. A. (1998). Patient perception of fatigue while undergoing long-term mechanical ventilation: Incidence and associated factors. *Heart & Lung, 27*(3), 177–183.

Hoyert, D. L., Heron, M., Murphy, S. L., & Kung, H. C. (2006). Deaths: Final data for 2003. Health E-Stats. Retrieved from http://www.cdc.gov/nchs/products/pubs/pubd/hestats/finaldeaths03/finaldeaths03.htm

International Ventilator Users Network (IVUN). (2006). *Home ventilator guide.* Post-Polio Health International (PHI). Retrieved from http://www.post-polio.org/IVUN/HomeVentGuide05S.pdf

Jacobs, M. (2005). Ease the stress of managing ARDS. *Nursing Made Incredibly Easy! 3*(1), 6–15, 17–18.

Kane, C., & Galanes, S. (2004). Adult respiratory distress syndrome. *Critical Care Nursing Quarterly, 27*(4), 325–335.

Kapella, M. C., Larson, J. L., Patel, M. K., Covey, M. K., & Berry, J. K. (2006). Subjective fatigue, influencing variables, and consequences in chronic obstructive pulmonary disease. *Nursing Research, 55*(1) 10–17.

Kasper, D. L., Braunwald, E., Fauci, A. S., Hauser, S. L., Longo, D. L., & Jameson, J. L. (Eds.). (2005). *Harrison's principles of internal medicine* (16th ed.). New York: McGraw-Hill.

Khan, N. U. A., & Novahed, A. (2005). Pulmonary embolism and cardiac enzymes. *Heart & Lung, 34*(2), 142–146.

Koschel, M. J. (2004). Emergency. Pulmonary embolism. *American Journal of Nursing, 104*(6), 46–50.

Lehne, R. A. (2004). *Pharmacology for nursing care* (5th ed.). Philadelphia: Saunders.

Lenaghan, N. A. (2000). The nurse's role in smoking cessation. *Medsurg Nursing, 9*(6), 298–302.

Lindgren, V. A., & Ames, N. J. (2005). Caring for patients on mechanical ventilation: What research indicates is best practice. *American Journal of Nursing, 105*(5), 50–61.

Markou, N. K., Myrianthefs, P. M., & Baltopoulos, G. J. (2004). Respiratory failure: An overview. *Critical Care Nursing Quarterly, 27*(4), 353–379.

Martin, R. J. (2003). Cough-variant asthma. Retrieved from http://www.medscape.com/viewarticle/465233.

McCance, K. L., & Huether, S. E. (2006). *Pathophysiology: The biologic basis for disease in adults and children* (5th ed.). St. Louis, MO: Mosby.

Meek, P. M. (2005). Patients with acute exacerbations of COPD saw anxiety as a sign, rather than cause, of breathlessness. *Evidence-Based Nursing, 8*(2), 61.

Moorhead, S., Johnson, M., & Maas, M. (2004). *Nursing outcomes classification (NOC)* (3rd ed.). St. Louis, MO: Mosby.

Mukherjee, R., & Burge, P. S. (2006). Occupational asthma. *Practice Nursing, 17*(2), 77–80.

National Center for Complementary and Alternative Medicine. (2004). Consumer advisory. Ephedra. Retrieved from http://www.nccam.nih.gov/health/alerts/ephedra/consumeradvisory.

National Center for Health Statistics. (2005). *Health, United States, 2005 with Chartbook on trends in the health of Americans.* Hyattsville, MD: U.S. Government Printing Office.

National Heart, Lung, and Blood Institute. (2006). ARDS. Retrieved from: www.nhlbi.nih.gov/health/dci/Diseases/Ards.

_____. (2003). *Expert panel report: Guidelines for the diagnosis and management of asthma. Update on selected topics 2002.* (NIH Publication No. 02-5074). Bethesda, MD: Author.

_____. (2004). *Morbidity & mortality: 2004 chart book of cardiovascular, lung, and blood diseases.* Bethesda, MD: Author.

_____. (2005). *Global initiative for chronic obstructive lung disease. Pocket guide to COPD diagnoses, management, and prevention.* Bethesda, MD: Author.

NANDA International. (2005). *Nursing diagnoses: Definitions and classification 2005–2006.* Philadelphia: Author.

O'Leary-Kelley, C. M., Puntillo, K. A., Barr, J., Stotts, N., & Douglas, M. K. (2005). Nutritional adequacy in patients receiving mechanical ventilation who are fed enterally. *American Journal of Critical Care, 14*(3), 222–231.

O'Neill, P. (2004). Hospital nursing. Nutrition series: Nutrition for a patient with COPD can be complicated. *Nursing, 34*(12), 32hn6, 32hn8.

Petty, M. (2003). Lung and heart-lung transplantation: Implications for nursing care when hospitalized outside the transplant center. *Medsurg Nursing, 12*(4), 250–259.

Porth, C. M. (2005). *Pathophysiology: Concepts of altered health states* (7th ed.). Philadelphia: Lippincott.

Roman, M. (2005). Clinical "how to." Tracheostomy tubes. *Medsurg Nursing, 14*(2), 143–144.

Simmons, P., & Simmons, M. (2004). Informed nursing practice: The administration of oxygen to patients with COPD. *Medsurg Nursing, 13*(2), 82–85.

Sims, J. M. (2003). What's new in pulmonary artery hypertension. *Dimensions of Critical Care Nursing, 22*(4), 167–170.

Smyth, M. (2005a). Acute respiratory failure, part 1. Failure in oxygenation. *American Journal of Nursing, 105*(5), Critical Care Extra, 72GG–72JJ, 72MM, 7200.

_____. (2005b). Acute respiratory failure, part 2. Failure of ventilation: Exploring the other cause of acute respiratory failure. *American Journal of Nursing, 105*(6), Critical Care Extra 72AA–72DD.

Spencer, J. W., & Jacobs, J. J. (2003). *Complementary and alternative medicine: An evidence-based approach* (2nd ed.). St. Louis, MO: Mosby.

Steinbis, S. (2004). What you should know about pulmonary hypertension. *The Nurse Practitioner, 29*(4), 8–10, 13–15, 19.

Theander, K., & Unosson, M. (2004). Fatigue in patients with chronic obstructive pulmonary disease. *Journal of Advanced Nursing, 45*(2), 172–177.

Tierney, L. M., McPhee, S. J., & Papadakis, M. A. (2005). *Current medical diagnosis & treatment* (44th ed.). New York: Lange Medical Books/McGraw-Hill.

Urden, L. D., Stacy, K. M., & Sough, M. E. (2006). *Thelan's critical care nursing* (5th ed.). St. Louis: Mosby.

U.S. Food and Drug Administration (FDA). (2005a). *Alert for healthcare professionals. Fluticasone propionate; salmeterol xinafoate (marketed as Advair Diskus).* Retrieved from http://www.fda.gov/cder/drug/InfoSheets/HCP/fluticasonelHCP.htm.

U.S. Food and Drug Administration. (2005b). *Alert for healthcare professionals. Formoterol fumarate (marketed as Foradil).* Retrieved from http://www.fda.gov/cder/drug/InfoSheets/HCP/formoterolHCP.htm.

Wilkinson, J. M. (2005). *Nursing diagnosis handbook with NIC interventions and NOC outcomes* (8th ed.). Upper Saddle River, NJ: Prentice Hall Health.

Winters, A. C. (2004). Management of acute severe asthma. *Critical Care Nursing Clinics of North America, 16*(3), 285–291.

Yang, J. C. (2005). Prevention and treatment of deep vein thrombosis and pulmonary embolism in critically ill patients. *Critical Care Nursing Quarterly, 28*(1), 72–79.

Yang, P. S., & Chen, C. H. (2005). Exercise stage and processes of change in patients with chronic obstructive pulmonary disease. *Journal of Nursing Research, 13*(2), 97–104.

UNIT 11 BUILDING CLINICAL COMPETENCE
Responses to Altered Respiratory Function

FUNCTIONAL HEALTH PATTERN: Activity-Exercise

■ Think about clients with respiratory disorders and altered patterns of activity and exercise for whom you have cared in your clinical experiences.

- What were the clients' major medical diagnoses affecting the respiratory system (e.g., upper respiratory infection, laryngeal cancer, pneumonia, tuberculosis, asthma, pleural effusion, pneumothorax, chronic obstructive pulmonary disease, respiratory failure)?
- What manifestations did each of these clients have? Were these manifestations similar or different?
- How did the clients' health status interfere with their activity and exercise? Was their breathing difficult or painful? Did the clients experience shortness of breath with activity or at rest? How many pillows did they use to sleep? Did your clients have a dry or productive cough? What color, odor, and consistency was the sputum? Did they smoke? Had they been exposed to environmental smoke or pollution? Did your clients have a history of respiratory disorders? Were they taking any medications or using oxygen? Had they had a chest x-ray and a tuberculosis skin test?

■ The Activity-Exercise Pattern describes the client's usual patterns of exercise and activity. Disorders that affect physiologic energy production affect the Activity-Exercise Health Pattern. The respiratory system provides oxygen to support cellular metabolism and eliminates carbon dioxide (a metabolic waste product) with each breath. This occurs through ventilation, the movement of air into and out of the lungs, and respiration, the exchange of oxygen and carbon dioxide between air and blood that occurs in the alveoli, respiratory bronchioles, and tissues.

The upper respiratory system cleans, humidifies, and warms air entering the lungs. Upper respiratory disorders affect breathing, communication, and body image.

Lower respiratory system disorders affect air movement (ventilation) and gas exchange across the alveolar-capillary membrane (respiration).

- Rhinorrhea (antigen [a viral pathogen or allergen] ▶ inflammation and release of chemical mediators ▶ mucosal vasodilation and release of WBCs and fluid from capillaries ▶ mucosal edema and watery discharge from the nose)
- Cough (irritants or excess secretions in respiratory tract ▶ stimulation of cough receptors in tracheobronchial wall ▶ impulses transmitted to medullary center ▶ rapid inhalation of large volume of air ▶ closure of glottis and rapid contraction of abdominal and expiratory muscles ▶ increased intrathoracic pressure ▶ sudden opening of glottis and explosive air expulsion)
- Dyspnea (discrepancy between respiratory muscle strength, stretch; bronchial smooth muscle contraction; decreased lung compliance or inspiratory capacity ▶ stimulation of receptors in lungs, thorax, or cerebral cortex ▶ dyspnea, a subjective perception of difficulty breathing)
- Cyanosis (decreased oxygen tension in alveoli ▶ decreased diffusion of oxygen into capillaries ▶ decreased blood oxygen tension ▶ increased amount of deoxygenated hemoglobin ▶ gray to blue or purple color of skin and mucous membranes)
- Wheezing (bronchoconstriction, airway inflammation or obstruction ▶ turbulent airflow through narrowed airway ▶ high- or low-pitched musical breath sounds).

■ Priority nursing diagnoses within the Activity-Exercise Pattern that may be appropriate for clients with respiratory disorders include:

- *Ineffective Breathing Pattern* as evidenced by shortness of breath, dyspnea, orthopnea, retractions, nasal flaring, altered chest excursion
- *Ineffective Airway Clearance* as evidenced by ineffective cough, diminished or abnormal breath sounds, cyanosis, restlessness
- *Impaired Gas Exchange* as evidenced by cyanosis, abnormal respiratory rate and rhythm, nasal flaring, tachycardia, diaphoresis, confusion
- *Impaired Spontaneous Ventilation* as evidenced by dyspnea, use of accessory muscles, tachycardia, apprehension.

■ Two nursing diagnoses from other functional health patterns often are of high priority for the client with altered respiratory function:

- *Disturbed Sleep Pattern* (Sleep-Rest)
- *Anxiety* (Self-Perception-Self-Concept)

CLINICAL SCENARIO

You have been assigned to work with the following clients on a respiratory unit. Significant data obtained during report are as follows:

- Jack Holt, a 65-year-old male, has bacterial pneumonia. Vital signs are T 101°F, P 94, R 30, BP 146/88. He is complaining of chest pain with breathing and has a productive cough of rusty-colored sputum. His SaO2 is 90% in room air.
- Maggie Sawyer, an 82-year-old female, is being discharged today following treatment for a deep venous thrombosis. She has congestive obstructive pulmonary disease. Suddenly she complains of difficulty breathing, chest pain, coughing, restlessness, and a feeling that she is going to die.
- James Mohr, a 25-year-old male, sustained head, neck, and chest injuries and has a tracheostomy from a motor vehicle crash. His vital signs were stable at the last assessment. He begins coughing and puts on his call light.
- Amy Campbell, a 30-year-old female, is being treated after having a severe asthma attack. Her current vital signs are T 99°F, P 64, R 26, BP 124/84. She has inspiratory and expiratory wheezing. Her O2 sat reading is 94% on 4 L O2 via nasal cannula.

Questions

1 In what order would you visit these clients after report?

1. _____
2. _____
3. _____
4. _____

2 What top two priority nursing diagnoses would you choose for each of the clients presented above? Can you explain, if asked, the rationale for your choices?

	Priority Nursing Diagnosis #1	Priority Nursing Diagnosis #2
Jack Holt		
Maggie Sawyer		
James Mohr		
Amy Campbell		

3 The older adult is prone to respiratory problems due to which age-related changes in the respiratory system? (Select all that apply.)

1. loss of skeletal muscle strength in the thorax
2. increased elastic recoil of lungs during expiration
3. alveoli that are less elastic and more fibrotic
4. decreased residual volume of lung
5. decreased effectiveness of coughing

4 Bacterial pneumonia is spread by droplets. When using standard precautions, which equipment is necessary to prevent its spread?

1. Wear a gown when bathing the client.
2. Wear a gown and gloves when touching the client.
3. Wear a mask and gloves when suctioning the client.
4. Wear a cap to keep hair from touching the client.

5 For the client receiving percussion and vibration with postural drainage for left lower lobe pneumonia, which position most facilitates removal of secretions?

1. semi-Fowler's position with arms elevated
2. right Sims' position with head in Trendelenberg
3. high-Fowler's position leaning on a bedside tray
4. left Sims' position with head flat

6 On discharge, the nurse teaches Mrs. Sawyer ways to prevent pulmonary embolism. Which instruction is appropriate?

1. Use pillows under the knees when in bed.
2. Apply knee-high elastic stockings when ambulating.
3. Exercise the legs vigorously to encourage blood flow.
4. Stop every 1 to 2 hours to stretch legs when traveling.

7 Mr. Mohr will be discharged with a tracheostomy. What should the nurse teach the client about tracheostomies?

1. The tracheostomy will not interfere with lifting when returning to work.

2. Water skiing is allowed, but swimming in a pool or lake is not allowed.
3. Showering is allowed as long as the tracheostomy is covered with a washcloth.
4. A small amount of alcohol is allowed but smoking is not allowed.

8 Amy Campbell is instructed to take her asthma medications in which order?

1. atrovent, cromolyn, and albuterol
2. albuterol, atrovent, and cromolyn
3. cromolyn, atrovent, and albuterol
4. albuterol, cromolyn, and atrovent

9 When admitted to the emergency department, which laboratory studies would you expect to obtain on a client with an inhalation injury?

1. arterial blood gases, carboxyhemoglobin levels, electrolytes
2. sputum cultures and sensitivity, serology testing, sputum Gram stain
3. methemoglobin levels, venous blood gases, white blood cell count
4. complete blood cell count, oxygen saturation, sputum specimen

10 Arterial blood gases results are ordered on a client with acute respiratory distress. The results are: pH, 7.22; PaO_2, 50 mmHg; $PaCO_2$, 58 mmHg; HCO_3^-, 29 mEq/L. How would a nurse interpret these results?

1. respiratory acidosis
2. respiratory alkalosis
3. metabolic acidosis
4. metabolic alkalosis

11 Corticosteroids are ordered to decrease the inflammatory process of asthma. Which comment indicates the client understands how to take corticosteroids?

1. "Corticosteroids have very few side effects to worry about."
2. "I understand that I cannot stop taking the medication abruptly."
3. "I can stop taking the corticosteroids as soon as I feel better."
4. "I can take an over-the-counter medication if I develop a cold."

12 Which are early manifestations of pulmonary tuberculosis?

1. tachypnea, tachycardia, activity intolerance
2. bradypnea, foul-smelling sputum, weight gain
3. blood-tinged sputum, high-grade fever, fatigue
4. low-grade fever, night sweats, dry cough

Directions: Read the clinical scenarios below and answer the questions that follow. To complete this exercise successfully, you will use not only knowledge of the content in this unit, but also principles related to setting priorities and maintaining client safety.

CASE STUDY

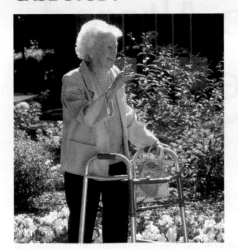

Gladys Hamer is an 83-year-old female who is seen in the emergency department with complaints of shortness of breath and fever. Her vital signs are T 102.4°F, P 115 and irregular, R 35 and shallow, BP 160/66. Her height is 63" and weight is 96 pounds. On assessment, her skin is very dry and warm. Her color is dusky. Scattered wheezes and rhonchi are heard throughout all lung fields. Her chest is hyperresonant to percussion. A pulse oximeter is applied and the O_2 sat reading is 88%. Mrs. Hamer has a past medical history of emphysema for 10 years, complaints of shortness of breath on exertion, and has a chronic cough productive of thick, grayish sputum. Her spouse passed away 5 years ago and she has lived with her two adult sons since then.

Blood is drawn for arterial blood gases and results are pH, 7.19; Pao_2, 54 mmHg, $Paco_2$, 55 mmHg; HCO_3^-, 30 mEq/L. These results indicate respiratory acidosis. Based on her current assessment, arterial blood gas results, and past medical history, a medical diagnosis of chronic obstructive pulmonary disease (COPD) is determined.

When planning nursing care for Mrs. Hamer, the nursing diagnosis of *Impaired Gas Exchange* related to acute and chronic lung disease is appropriate for implementing nursing interventions.

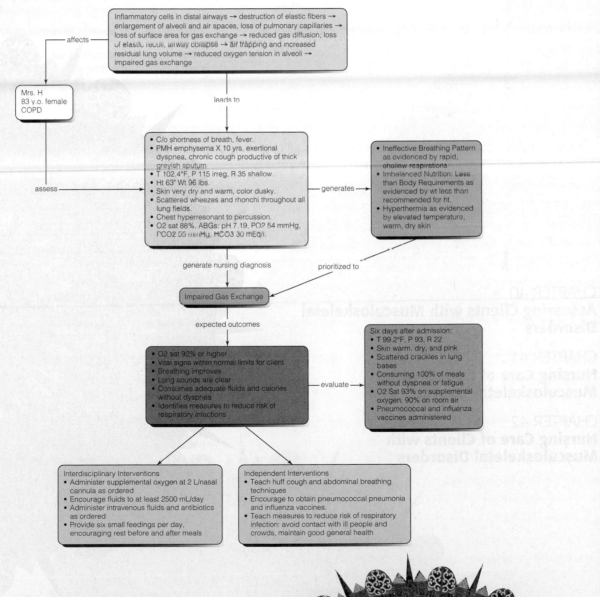

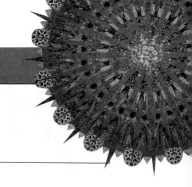

KEY TERMS

bursitis, *1394*	**kyphosis,** *1391*	**scoliosis,** *1391*
crepitation, *1392*	**lordosis,** *1391*	**synovitis,** *1394*
hematopoiesis, *1380*	**ossification,** *1381*	**tendonitis,** *1394*

The tissues and structures of the musculoskeletal system perform many functions, including support, protection, and movement. The musculoskeletal system has two subsystems: the bones and joints of the skeleton, and the skeletal muscles.

These subsystems work together to allow the body to perform both gross, simple movements such as closing a door, and fine, complex movements such as repairing a watch.

ANATOMY, PHYSIOLOGY, AND FUNCTIONS OF THE MUSCULOSKELETAL SYSTEM

The musculoskletal system is composed of bones of the skeletal system; ligaments, tendons, and muscles of the muscular system; and joints. The bones serve as the framework for the body and for the attachment of muscles, tendons, and ligaments. Innervated by the nervous system, contraction and relaxation of muscles permit movement at joints.

The Skeleton

Bones form the body's structure and provide support for soft tissues. They also protect vital organs from injury and serve to move body parts by providing points of attachment for muscles. Bones also store minerals and serve as a site for **hematopoiesis** (blood cell formation).

The human skeleton is made up of 206 bones (Figure 40–1 ■). Bones of the skeletal system are divided into the axial skeleton and the appendicular skeleton. The axial skeleton includes the bones of the skull, the ribs and sternum, and the vertebral column. The appendicular skeleton consists of all the bones of the limbs, the shoulder girdles, and the pelvic girdle.

Bone Structure

Bone cells include osteoblasts (cells that form bone), osteocytes (cells that maintain bone matrix), and osteoclasts (cells that resorb bone). Bone matrix is the extracellular element of bone tissue; it consists of collagen fibers, minerals (primarily calcium and phosphate), proteins, carbohydrates, and ground substance. Ground substance is a gelatinous material that facilitates diffusion of nutrients, wastes, and gases between the blood vessels and bone tissue. Bones are covered with periosteum, a double-layered connective tissue. The outer layer of the periosteum contains blood vessels and nerves; the inner layer is anchored to the bone.

Bones consist of a rigid connective tissue called osseous tissue, of which there are two types: Compact bone is smooth and dense; spongy bone contains spaces between meshworks of bone. Both types contain the same elements and are found in almost all bones of the body.

The basic structural unit of compact bone is the Haversian system (also called an osteon). The Haversian system consists of a central canal, called the Haversian canal; concentric layers of bone matrix, called lamellae; spaces between the lamellae, called lacunae; osteocytes within the lacunae; and small channels, called canaliculi (Figure 40–2 ■).

Spongy bone has no Haversian systems. Instead, the lamellae are arranged in concentric layers called trabeculae that branch and join to form meshworks. The spongy sections of long bones and flat bones contain tissue for hematopoiesis. In the adult, these sections, called red marrow cavities, are present in the spongy center of flat bones (especially the sternum) and in only two long bones: the humerus and the head of the femur. This red marrow is active in hematopoiesis in adults.

Bone Shapes

Bones are classified by shape (Figure 40–3 ■):

- *Long bones* are longer than they are wide. They have a midportion, or shaft, called a diaphysis and two broad ends, called epiphyses (Figure 40–4 ■). The diaphysis is compact bone and contains the marrow cavity, which is lined with endosteum. Each epiphysis is spongy bone covered by a thin layer of compact bone. Long bones include the bones of the arms, legs, fingers, and toes.

- *Short bones*, also called cuboid bones, are spongy bone covered by compact bone. They include the bones of the wrist and ankle.

- *Flat bones* are thin and flat, and most are curved. Their disklike structure consists of a layer of spongy bone between two thin layers of compact bone. Flat bones include most bones of the skull, the sternum, and the ribs.

- *Irregular bones* are of various shapes and sizes and, like flat bones, are plates of compact bone with spongy bone between. Irregular bones include the vertebrae, the scapulae, and the bones of the pelvic girdle.

Bone Remodeling in Adults

Although the bones of adults do not normally increase in length and size, constant remodeling of bones, as well as repair of damaged bone tissue, occurs throughout life. In the bone remodeling process, bone resorption and bone deposit occur at all periosteal and endosteal surfaces. Hormones and forces that

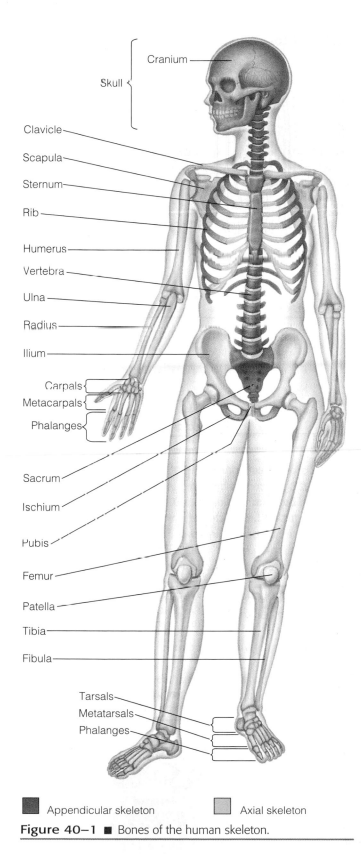

Cranium
Skull
Clavicle
Scapula
Sternum
Rib
Humerus
Vertebra
Ulna
Radius
Ilium
Carpals
Metacarpals
Phalanges
Sacrum
Ischium
Pubis
Femur
Patella
Tibia
Fibula
Tarsals
Metatarsals
Phalanges

■ Appendicular skeleton   ■ Axial skeleton

Figure 40–1 ■ Bones of the human skeleton.

put stress on the bones regulate this process, which involves a combined action of the osteocytes, osteoclasts, and osteoblasts. Bones that are in use, and are therefore subjected to stress, increase their osteoblastic activity to increase **ossification** (the development of bone). Bones that are inactive undergo increased osteoclast activity and bone resorption.

The hormonal stimulus for bone remodeling is controlled by a negative feedback mechanism that regulates blood calcium levels. This stimulus involves the interaction of parathyroid hormone (PTH) from the parathyroid glands and calcitonin from the thyroid gland. When blood levels of calcium decrease, PTH is released; PTH then stimulates osteoclast activity and bone resorption so that calcium is released from the bone matrix. As a result, blood levels of calcium rise, and the stimulus for PTH release ends. Rising blood calcium levels stimulate the secretion of calcitonin, inhibit bone resorption, and cause the deposit of calcium salts in the bone matrix. Thus, bones are necessary to regulate blood calcium levels. Calcium ions are necessary for the transmission of nerve impulses, the release of neurotransmitters, muscle contraction, blood clotting, glandular secretion, and cell division. Of the body's 1200 to 1400 g of calcium, over 99% is present as bone minerals.

Bone remodeling is also regulated by the response of bones to gravitational pull and to mechanical stress from the pull of muscles. Although the exact mechanism is not fully understood, it is known that bones that undergo increased stress are heavier and larger. This finding supports Wolff's law, which states that bone develops and remodels itself to resist the stresses placed on it.

The process of bone repair following a fracture is discussed in Chapter 41.

Muscles

The three types of muscle tissue in the body are skeletal muscle, smooth muscle, and cardiac muscle (Table 40–1). This discussion focuses on skeletal muscle, the only muscle that allows musculoskeletal function. Skeletal muscles attach to and cover the bones of the skeleton. Skeletal muscles promote body movement, help maintain posture, and produce body heat. They may be moved by conscious, voluntary control or by reflex activity. The body has approximately 600 skeletal muscles (Figure 40–5 ■).

Skeletal muscles are thick bundles of parallel multinucleated contractile cells called fibers. Each single muscle fiber is itself a bundle of smaller structures called myofibrils. The myofibrils have alternating light and dark bands that give skeletal muscle its striated (striped) appearance under an electron microscope. Myofibrils are strands of smaller repeating units called sarcomeres, which consist of thick filaments of myosin and thin filaments of actin, proteins that contribute to muscle contraction.

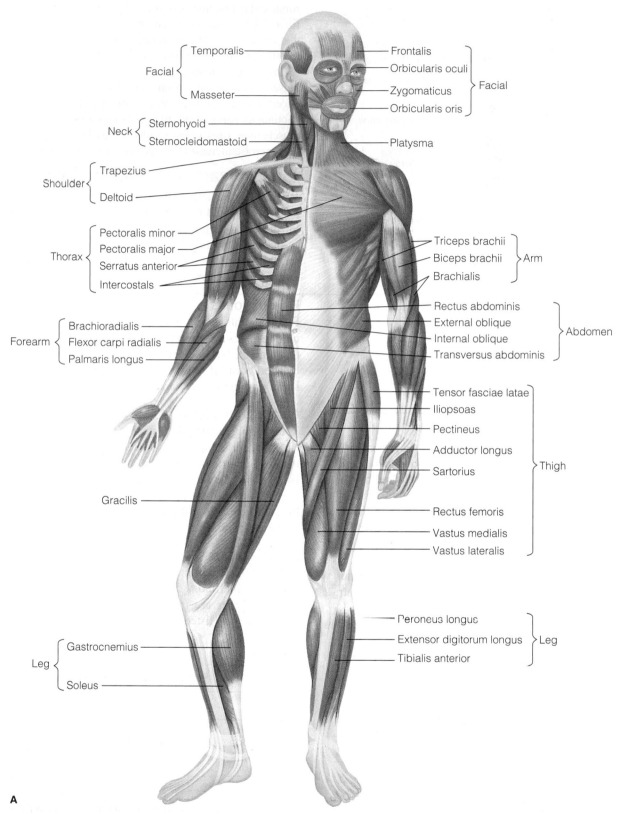

Figure 40–5 ■ *A,* Muscles of the anterior body. *B,* Muscles of the posterior body.

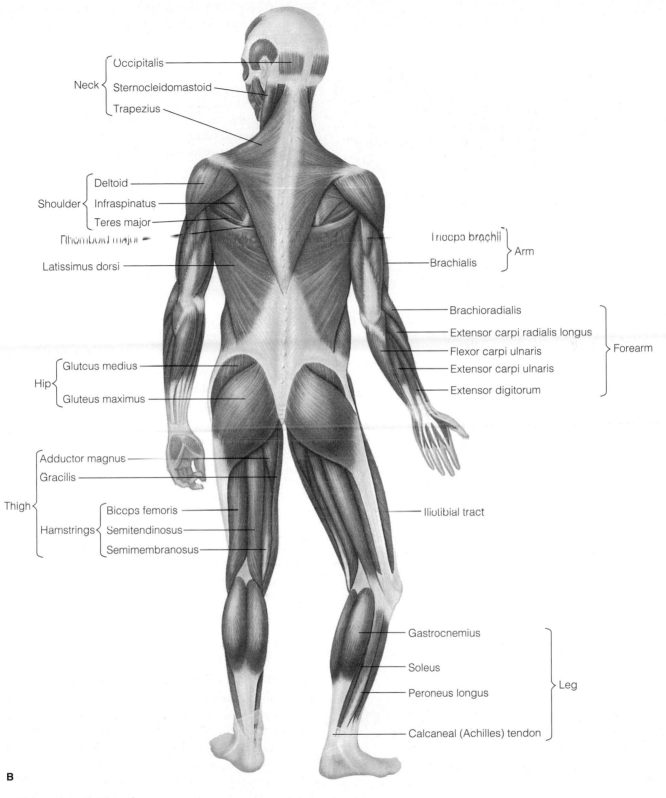

B

Figure 40–5 ■ Continued

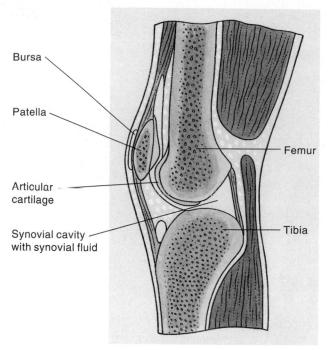

Figure 40–6 ■ Structure of a synovial joint (knee).

joints are found at all articulations of the limbs. They have several characteristics:

■ The articular surfaces are covered with articular cartilage.
■ The joint cavity is enclosed by a tough, fibrous, double-layered articular capsule; internally, the cavity is lined with a synovial membrane that covers all surfaces not covered by the articular cartilage.
■ Synovial fluid fills the free spaces of the joint capsule, enhancing the smooth movement of the articulating bones.

Bursae are small sacs of synovial fluid that cushion and protect bony areas that are at high risk for friction, such as the knee

TABLE 40–3 Movements Allowed by Synovial Joints

MOVEMENT	DESCRIPTION
Abduction	Move limb away from body midline
Adduction	Move limb toward body midline
Extension	Straighten limbs at joint
Flexion	Bend limbs at joint
Dorsiflexion	Bend ankle to bring top of foot toward shin
Plantar flexion	Straighten ankle to point toes down
Pronation	Turn forearm to place palm down
Supination	Turn forearm to place palm up
Eversion	Turn out
Inversion	Turn in
Circumduction	Move in circle
Internal rotation	Move inward on a central axis
External rotation	Move outward on a central axis
Protraction	Move forward and parallel to ground
Retraction	Move backward and parallel to ground

and the shoulder. Tendon sheaths are a form of bursae, but they are wrapped around tendons in high-friction areas.

The fibrous capsules that surround synovial joints are supported by ligaments, dense bands of connective tissue that connect bones to bones. Ligaments limit or enhance movement, provide joint stability, and enhance joint strength. Tendons are fibrous connective tissue bands that connect muscles to the periosteum of bones and enable the bones to move when skeletal muscles contract. When muscles contract, increased pressure causes the tendon to pull, push, or rotate the bone to which it is connected.

ASSESSING MUSCULOSKELETAL FUNCTION

Structures and functions of the musculoskeletal system are assessed by findings from diagnostic tests, a health assessment interview to collect subjective data, and a physical assessment to collect objective data. Sample documentation of an assessment of the musculoskeletal system is given in the accompanying box.

Diagnostic Tests

The results of diagnostic tests of musculoskeletal structure and function are used to support the diagnosis of a specific injury or disease, to provide information to identify or modify the appropriate medications or therapy used to treat the disease, and to help nurses monitor the client's responses to treatment and nursing care interventions. Diagnostic tests to assess the structures and functions of the musculoskeletal system are described in the table on the next page and summarized in the bulleted list that follows. More information is included in the discussion of specific injuries or diseases in Chapter 41 and 42 ∞.

■ Blood tests are used to monitor levels of alkaline phosphatase, calcium, uric acid, and creatine kinase, commonly increased in bone and joint diseases and muscle trauma (Table 40–4).
■ Radiologic examinations, including x-rays, CT scans, MRIs, and bone scans, are done to identify and evaluate bone density and structure in conditions such as arthritis, interverte-

---

SAMPLE DOCUMENTATION
Assessment of the Musculoskeletal System

58-year-old Hispanic male, employed as a roofer, comes to the orthopedic clinic for evaluation of chronic knee pain. Client states "The pain in my knees is worse when I get up in the morning and when I carry something heavy at work." Posture erect, gait even without obvious limp. Bones of lower extremities appear equal in size and shape bilaterally. No swelling noted, bulge test negative for fluid around knee. Crepitus heard in both knees during flexion and extension. ROM in both knees slightly decreased. No obvious decrease in muscle mass. Client states knee pain during ROM is a 3 on a 1 to 10 scale. Referred to clinic physician for further evaluation, including x-rays of both knees.

DIAGNOSTIC TESTS   of the Musculoskeletal System

NAME OF TEST Blood chemistry

PURPOSE AND DESCRIPTION See Table 40–4

RELATED NURSING CARE No special preparation is needed.

NAME OF TEST X-ray

PURPOSE AND DESCRIPTION X-rays are done to identify and evaluate bone density and structure. Injection of contrast medium with an accompanying x-ray may be done to visualize joint structures, intervertebral disks, and wounds deep in muscle.

RELATED NURSING CARE No special preparation needed for standard x-rays. If contrast medium is used, assess for allergy to shellfish, iodine, or contrast medium used in previous tests. If allergy is present, test will not be performed.

NAME OF TEST Computed tomography (CT) scan

PURPOSE AND DESCRIPTION Provides a three-dimensional picture used to evaluate musculoskeletal trauma and bony abnormalities.

RELATED NURSING CARE No special preparation is needed.

NAME OF TEST Magnetic resonance imaging (MRI)

PURPOSE AND DESCRIPTION Used in diagnosis and evaluation of avascular necrosis, osteomyelitis, tumors, disk abnormalities, and tears in ligament or cartilage. Uses radio waves and magnetic fields; gadolinium may be injected to increase visualization of bony or muscular structures.

RELATED NURSING CARE Assess for metallic implants or metal on clothing (metallic implants, such as clips on aneurysms, pacemakers, or shrapnel, will prohibit having an MRI).

NAME OF TEST Bone scan

PURPOSE AND DESCRIPTION Degree of uptake of a radioisotope (based on blood supply to bone) is measured with a Geiger counter and recorded on paper. Uptake is increased in osteomyelitis, osteoporosis, cancers of the bone, and in some fractures. Uptake is decreased in avascular necrosis.

RELATED NURSING CARE No special preparation is needed; tell client to increase oral fluids after the test to aid in excretion of the radioisotope.

NAME OF TEST Bone density (BD)
- Dual energy x-ray absorptiometry (DEXA)
- Quantitative ultrasound (QUS)
- Bone mineral density (BMD)
- Bone absorptiometry

PURPOSE AND DESCRIPTION Bone density examinations are done to evaluate bone mineral density and to evaluate degree of osteoporosis. DEXA can calculate the size and thickness of bone. Osteoporosis is diagnosed if the peak bone mass level is below >2.5 standard deviations.

Normal Value: 1 standard deviation below peak bone mass.

RELATED NURSING CARE No special preparation is needed. Assess for previous fractures, which may increase bone density.

NAME OF TEST Arthroscopy

PURPOSE AND DESCRIPTION An endoscopic examination of the interior surfaces of a joint, used to perform surgery and diagnose diseases of the patella, meniscus, and synovial and extrasynovial membranes. In addition, fluid may be drained from the joint and tissue removed for biopsy. A fiber-optic endoscope is inserted into the joint, either with local anesthesia or general anesthesia.

RELATED NURSING CARE If general anesthesia is used, client is NPO after midnight. Following the procedure, assess for bleeding and swelling, apply ice to the area if prescribed, and teach client to avoid excessive use of the joint for 2 to 3 days.

NAME OF TEST Arthrocentesis

PURPOSE AND DESCRIPTION Done to obtain synovial fluid from a joint for diagnosis (such as infections) or to remove excess fluid. A needle is inserted through the joint capsule and fluid is aspirated.

RELATED NURSING CARE
No special preparation is needed. Apply compression dressing and assess for bleeding and leakage of fluid following the procedure.

(continued)

DIAGNOSTIC TESTS of the Musculoskeletal System (continued)

NAME OF TEST Electromyogram (EMG)

PURPOSE AND DESCRIPTION Measures the electrical activity of skeletal muscles at rest and during contraction; useful in diagnosing neuromuscular diseases. Needle electrodes are inserted into skeletal muscle (as on the legs) and electrical activity can be heard, viewed on an oscilloscope, and recorded on graph paper. Normally, there is no electrical activity at rest.

RELATED NURSING CARE Tell client not to drink fluids containing caffeine or to smoke for 3 hours before the test, and not to take medications such as muscle relaxants, anticholinergics, or cholinergics.

NAME OF TEST Somatosensory evoked potential (SSEP)

PURPOSE AND DESCRIPTION Measures nerve conduction along pathways to evaluate evoked potential of muscle contractions. Used to identify dysfunction of lower motor neurons as well as muscle disease. Transcutaneous or percutaneous electrodes are applied to the skin and provide recordings.

RELATED NURSING CARE No special preparation is needed.

---

bral disk disease, musculoskeletal trauma, muscle tears, osteomyelitis, and bone tumors.

- Bone density examinations (dual energy x-ray absorptiometry [DEXA], quantitative ultrasound [QUS], and bone mineral density [BMD]) are done to evaluate bone mineral density and evaluate the degree of osteoporosis.
- An arthroscopy uses a fiber-optic endoscope to examine the joint interior, to diagnose diseases, and to perform surgery. An arthrocentesis is done to withdraw fluid from a joint by needle aspiration.
- Both electromyogram (EMG) and somatosensory evoked potential (SSEP) are tests of the electrical activity of skeletal muscle.

Regardless of the type of diagnostic test, the nurse is responsible for explaining the procedure and any special preparation needed, for assessing for medication use that may affect the outcome of the tests, for supporting the client during the examination as necessary, for documenting the procedures as appropriate, and for monitoring the results of the tests.

Genetic Considerations

When conducting a health assessment interview and a physical assessment, it is important for the nurse to consider genetic influences on health of the adult. During the health assessment interview, ask about family members with health problems affecting musculoskeletal structure or function. In addition, ask about a family history of arthritis, abnormally long bones, children with muscular dystrophy, and amyotrophic lateral sclerosis (ALS). During the physical assessment, assess for any manifestations that might indicate a genetic disorder (see the box on the next page). If data are found to indicate genetic risk factors or alterations, ask about genetic testing and refer for appropriate genetic counseling and evaluation. Chapter 8 ∞ provides further information about genetics in medical-surgical nursing.

Health Assessment Interview

A health assessment interview to determine problems with musculoskeletal structure and/or function may be conducted

TABLE 40–4 Blood Tests with Purposes Specific to the Musculoskeletal System

NAME OF TEST	PURPOSE	NORMAL VALUE
Alkaline phosphatase (ALP)	To identify bone diseases. Increased in bone cancer, Paget's disease, healing fractures, rheumatoid arthritis, osteoporosis.	42–136 unit/L ALP[1] 20–130 unit/L ALP[2] (increases slightly with aging)
Calcium (Ca)	To monitor calcium levels and detect calcium imbalances. Decreased with lack of calcium and vitamin D intake, and malabsorption from the gastrointestinal tract. Increased in bone cancer and multiple fractures.	4.5–5.5 mEq/L or 9–11 mg/dL (serum)
Phosphorus (P), phosphate (PO₄)	To assess phosphorus levels. Increased with bone tumors and healing fractures.	1.7–2.6 mEq/L or 2.5–4.5 mg/dL
Rheumatoid factor (RF)	To diagnose rheumatoid arthritis (RA) (positive for RA at >1:80) Also increased in lupus erythematosus and scleroderma.	<1:20 titer
Uric acid	To diagnose and monitor the treatment of gout. Panic level considered >12 mg/dL.	Male: 3.5–8.0 mg/dL Female: 2.8–6.8 mg/dL
Human leukocyte antigen (HLA)	To diagnose diseases such as juvenile RA or ankylosing spondylitis.	Match or no match; no normal values
Creatine kinase (CK)	To diagnose muscle trauma or disease. Increased in muscular dystrophy and traumatic injuries (specifically, CPK-MM isoenzyme)	94%–100%

GENETIC CONSIDERATIONS
Musculoskeletal Disorders

■ Myotonic dystrophy is an inherited disorder in which the muscles become weak, have a decreased ability to relax, and eventually waste away. Other parts of the body affected are mental deficiency, hair loss, and cataracts. Although rare, the disease does increase in severity with each successive generation.

■ Marfan's syndrome, an autosomal dominant disorder of connective tissue, affects the bones, lungs, eyes, heart, and blood vessels. It is characterized by abnormally long extremities, and is believed to have affected Abraham Lincoln. The aspect of the disease that is most life threatening is the effect on the cardiovascular system. The average life span of a person with Marfan's syndrome is 30 to 40 years (Porth, 2005).

■ Ellis-van Creveld syndrome is a rare genetic disorder characterized by a variety of physical alterations, including short-limb dwarfism, additional fingers or toes, malformed wrists, cardiac abnormalities, and partial tooth eruption.

■ Duchenne muscular dystrophy, an X-linked disorder, affects primarily males. It is one of the most common muscular dystrophies, and is characterized by rapid muscle degeneration early in life.

■ Amyotropic lateral sclerosis (ALS) is a neurologic disease that affects the motor neurons in the spinal cord and brain, eventually resulting in paralysis and death.

■ Other musculoskeletal diseases believed to have a genetic component include rheumatoid arthritis, osteoarthritis, gout, muscular dystrophy, ankylosing spondylitis, lupus erythematosus, and scleroderma.

during a health screening, may focus on a chief complaint (such as joint pain), or may be part of a total health assessment. Health problems affecting the neurologic system may manifest as problems with musculoskeletal function and an assessment of both systems may be necessary. (See Chapter 43 ∞ for assessment of the neurologic system.) If the client has problems with musculoskeletal structure or function, analyze its onset, characteristics, course, severity, precipitating and relieving factors, and any associated symptoms, noting the timing and circumstances. For example, ask the client:

■ Describe the pain you have had in your elbow. Does the pain increase with movement? Have you noticed any redness or swelling?

■ Did you injure your ankle before you began to experience difficulty walking?

■ Is your pain worse in the morning, or does it get worse throughout the day?

The primary manifestations of altered function of the musculoskeletal system are pain and limited mobility. Specific descriptors of the pain, its location, and its nature are important. Other significant information includes associated manifestations, such as fever, fatigue, changes in weight, rash, and/or swelling. Also collect information about the client's lifestyle: type of employment, ability to carry out activities of daily living (ADLs) and provide self-care, exercise or participation in sports, use of alcohol or drugs, and nutrition. Explore past injuries and measures to self-treat pain (such as over-the-counter [OTC] medications, prescribed medications, application of heat or cold, splinting, wrapping, or rest).

Interview questions categorized by functional health patterns are listed in the Functional Health Pattern Interview table on page 1390.

Physical Assessment

Physical assessment of the musculoskeletal system may be performed either as part of a total assessment, or alone for a client with known or suspected problems. The techniques used to assess the musculoskeletal system are inspection, palpation, and measurement of muscle mass and range of motion (ROM). The client should be comfortably dressed in clothing that lets you see the movement of all joints clearly. The client may be standing, sitting, or lying down; the sequence of the examination should be such that the client does not have frequent position changes. An assessment of the older adult, the client in pain, or the client who is weak may take extra time. Normal age-related findings for the older adult are summarized in Table 40–5.

TABLE 40–5 Age-Related Changes in the Musculoskeletal System

AGE-RELATED CHANGE	SIGNIFICANCE
Bones and Joints: ■ ↓ bone mass and minerals. ■ ↓ calcium reabsorption, a slow resorption of the interior of long bones, and slower production of new bone on the outside surface of bones. ■ Vertebrae shorten and intervertebral disks thin, and kyphosis often occurs. ■ Cartilage on bone surfaces in joints deteriorates and bone spurs may occur.	Decreased bone mass as well as decreased calcium absorption contributes to bones that are often thinner and weaker, with an increased risk of fractures with trauma. As the spinal column shortens, height decreases. Loss of joint cartilage and formation of bone spurs makes movement more painful and may even limit mobility.
Muscles ■ Muscle fibers atrophy and fibrous tissue slowly replaces muscle tissue. ■ ↓ muscle mass and strength. ■ ↓ muscle movements, especially in the arms and legs. ■ Range of motion decreases. ■ Tendons shrink and harden. ■ Muscle cramping is common.	Regular exercise is very important in decreasing the loss associated with aging in terms of maintaining muscle mass, strength, and agility.

Technique/Normal Findings	Abnormal Findings

Joint Assessment

Inspect the joints for deformity, swelling, and redness. *There should be no visible deformity, swelling, or redness of joints.*

- Diseases of the joints may be manifested by such deformities as tissue loss, tissue overgrowth, contractures, or irreversible shortenings of muscles and tendons.
- Edema in a joint may cause obvious bulging.
- Redness, swelling, and pain are evidence of an inflammation or infection in the joint.

Palpate the joints for tenderness, warmth, crepitation, consistency, and muscle mass. *Joints should be nontender and consistent bilaterally, and without visible or palpable excess warmth, crepitation, or masses.*

- Inflammation and injury cause joint pain.
- Arthritis, bursitis, tendonitis, and osteomyelitis (infection of a bone) result in painful, hot joints.
- **Crepitation** (a grating sound) is present in a joint when the articulating surfaces have lost their cartilage, such as in arthritis.

Range-of-Motion Assessment

Assess joint ROM by asking the client to perform activities specific to each joint, as follows: *All bilateral joints should move through full range of motion.*
Temporomandibular joint: "Open your mouth wide, and then close your mouth." (As the client opens and closes the mouth, palpate the temporomandibular joints with your index and middle fingers, as shown in Figure 40–8 ■.)

- Clicking or popping noises, decreased ROM, pain, and swelling may indicate temporomandibular joint syndrome or, in rare cases, osteoarthritis.

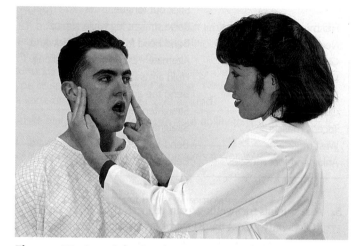

Figure 40–8 ■ Palpating the temporomandibular joints.

Cervical spine:
45-degree flexion: "Touch your chin to your chest."
55-degree extension: "Look at the ceiling."
40-degree lateral bending: "Try to touch your right ear to your right shoulder." Repeat with the left side.
70-degree rotation: "Try to touch your chin to each shoulder."

- Neck pain and limited extension with lateral bending are seen with herniated cervical disks and in cervical spondylosis.
- An immobile neck with head and neck thrust forward is seen with ankylosing spondylitis.

Lumbar spine:
75- to 90-degree flexion: "Touch your toes with your fingers" (Figure 40–9A ■).
30-degree extension: "Bend backward slowly."
35-degree lateral bending: "Bend right and left" (Figure 40–9B).
30-degree rotation: "Twist your shoulders right and left" (Figure 40–9C).

- Decreased movement or pain with movement may indicate an abnormal spinal curvature, arthritis, herniated disk, or spasm of paravertebral muscles.

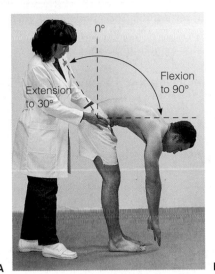
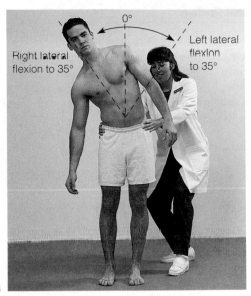
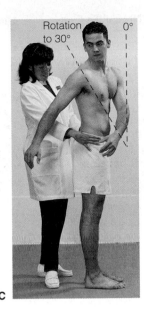

Figure 40-9 ■ *A,* Forward flexion of spine. *B,* Lateral flexion of spine. *C,* Rotation of spine.

Technique/Normal Findings	Abnormal Findings
Fingers: Flexion: "Make a fist." Extension: "Open your hand." Abduction: "Spread your fingers." Adduction: "Close your fingers."	■ Flexion and extension of fingers are decreased in arthritis. ■ Heberden's nodes and Bouchard's nodes are hard, nontender nodules on the dorsolateral parts of the distal and proximal interphalangeal joints, respectively. They are common in osteoarthritis. ■ Stiff, painful, swollen finger joints are seen in acute rheumatoid arthritis. ■ Boutonnière and swan-neck deformities are seen in chronic rheumatoid arthritis. ■ Swollen finger joints with a white chalky discharge may be seen in chronic gout.
Wrists: 90-degree flexion: "Bend wrist down." 70-degree extension: "Bend wrist up." 55-degree ulnar deviation: "Bend wrist toward little finger." 20-degree radial deviation: "Bend wrist toward thumb."	■ Bilateral chronic swelling in the wrist is seen in arthritis.
Elbows 160-degree flexion: "Touch your hands to your shoulders." 180-degree extension: "Straighten your elbows." 90-degree supination: "Bend your elbows 90 degrees, and turn hands palm up." 90-degree pronation: "Bend your elbows 90 degrees, and turn fists down."	■ Swollen, tender, inflamed elbows are apparent in gouty arthritis and rheumatoid arthritis. ■ Pain and tenderness at the lateral epicondyle occur in tennis elbow.

Technique/Normal Findings	Abnormal Findings
Shoulders: 180-degree flexion: "Hold your arms straight up and out." 50-degree hyperextension: "Put your straight arm behind your back." 90-degree internal rotation: "Put your forearm behind your lower back." 180-degree abduction: "Raise your straight arm up and out to your side." 50-degree adduction: "Put your straight arm across your chest."	■ Pain and tenderness over the biceps tendon occurs with **tendonitis** (inflammation of a tendon). ■ The arm cannot be abducted fully when the supraspinatus tendon of the shoulder is ruptured. ■ Pain and limited abduction is also seen with **bursitis** (inflammation of a bursa) and calcium deposits in this area.
Toes: 90-degree flexion: "Walk on your toes."	■ The great toe is excessively abducted in hallux valgus. ■ The joint above the great toe is swollen, inflamed, and painful in gouty arthritis. ■ There is hyperextension of the metatarsophalangeal joint and flexion of the proximal interphalangeal joint with hammer toes.
Ankles: 20-degree dorsiflexion: "Point your foot to the ceiling." 45-degree plantar flexion: "Point your foot to the floor." 30-degree inversion: "Walk on the outside of your feet." 20-degree eversion: "Walk on the inside of your feet."	■ Contractures of the Achilles tendon may occur in clients with rheumatoid arthritis or following prolonged bed rest.
Knees: 130-degree flexion: "Do a deep knee bend." 180-degree extension: "Sit down and hold your legs straight out in front of you."	■ Swelling over the suprapatellar pouch is seen with inflammation and fluid in the articular capsule of the knee. **Synovitis** is inflammation of the synovial membrane lining the articular capsule of a joint. It is common with knee trauma. ■ Swelling over the patella is seen in bursitis.
Hips: (The client is lying down.) 120-degree flexion: "Bring bent knee up to your chest." 30-degree hyperextension: "Lie on the abdomen, and lift up one leg at a time." 45-degree abduction: "Hold your leg straight, and move it out to the side." 40-degree internal rotation: "Bend your knee, and swing it toward your other leg." 45-degree external rotation: "Bend your knee, and swing it out to the side."	■ Movement of the hip is limited and/or painful in arthritis.

Technique/Normal Findings	Abnormal Findings

Special Assessments

Perform Phalen's test. Ask the client to hold the wrist in acute flexion for 60 seconds (Figure 40–10 ■). *There should be no tingling, numbness, or pain.*

- Numbness and burning in the fingers during Phalen's test may indicate carpal tunnel syndrome.

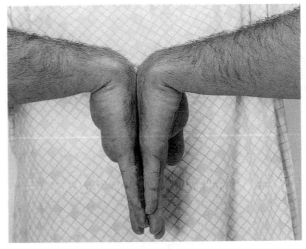

Figure 40–10 ■ Phalen's test.

Check for small amounts of fluid on the knee by conducting the bulge test. Milk upward on the medial side of the knee, and then tap the lateral side of the patella (Figure 40–11 ■). *No bulge of fluid should appear on the medial side of the knee.*

- A fluid bulge indicates increased fluid in the knee joint rather than soft tissue swelling.

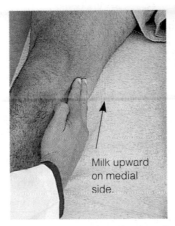 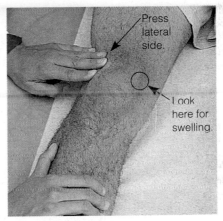

Milk upward on medial side.

Press lateral side.

Look here for swelling.

Figure 40–11 ■ Checking for the bulge sign.

Check for larger amounts of fluid by conducting the ballottement test, to detect large amounts of fluid in the knee. Apply downward pressure on the knee with one hand while pushing the patella backward against the femur with the other hand (Figure 40–12 ■). *There should be no movement of the patella. The patella should rest firmly over the femur.*

- Increased fluid will cause a tapping sound as the patella displaces the fluid and hits the femur.

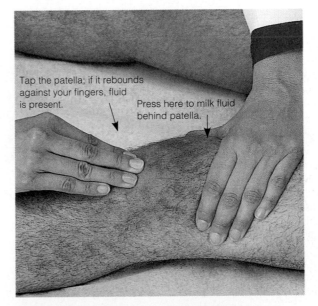

Tap the patella; if it rebounds against your fingers, fluid is present.

Press here to milk fluid behind patella.

Figure 40–12 ■ Checking for ballottement.

Technique/Normal Findings	Abnormal Findings

Perform McMurray's test. While reclining, ask the client to turn the flexed knee toward the center of the body. Stabilize the knee with one hand, and apply pressure on the lower leg with the other hand (Figure 40–13 ■). *There should be no pain or clicking.*

- Pain, locking (inability to fully extend the knee), or a popping sound may indicate an injury to a meniscus, a disk of cartilaginous tissue in the knee.

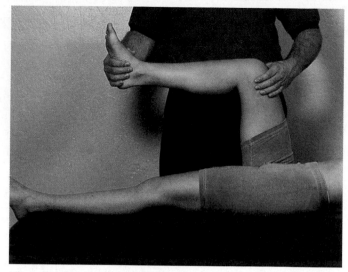

Figure 40–13 ■ McMurray's test.

Perform the Thomas test. Ask the client to lie down and extend one leg while bringing the knee of the opposite leg to the chest (Figure 40–14 ■). *The extended leg should not rise off the table.*

- A hip flexion contracture will cause the extended leg to rise off the table.

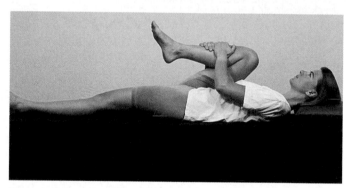

Figure 40–14 ■ Thomas test for hip contracture.

EXPLORE MediaLink

Prentice Hall Nursing MediaLink DVD-ROM
Audio Glossary
NCLEX–RN® Review

Animation
Joint Movement

COMPANION WEBSITE www.prenhall.com/lemone
Audio Glossary
NCLEX–RN® Review
Care Plan Activity: Musculoskeletal Disorders
Case Study: Knee Pain
MediaLink Application: Musculoskeletal Injuries of
Health Care Providers
Links to Resources

TEST YOURSELF NCLEX-RN® REVIEW

1 Your client has an epiphyseal fracture. Based on this information, what classification of bone is involved?
1. irregular
2. flat
3. long
4. short

2 When asking a client to move an extremity away from the body midline, you are assessing:
1. abduction.
2. adduction.
3. extension.
4. flexion.

3 Your client asks you, "Why is blood being examined for uric acid?" What would be your most accurate response?
1. "A uric acid test is done to see if your gout medication is effective."
2. "A uric acid test is done to diagnose rheumatoid arthritis."
3. "Do you have a family history of muscle or bone disease?"
4. "Tell me how you got that big bruise on your hip."

4 What age woman would be most likely to have a bone density examination?
1. teenager
2. a woman in her 20s
3. a woman in her 40s
4. a woman in her 60s

5 With aging, bone mass and calcium absorption decrease. What risk is increased as a result?
1. obesity
2. weakness
3. fractures
4. deformity

6 What would you ask the client to do in order to assess facial muscle strength?
1. "Close your eyes tightly."
2. "Stick out your tongue."
3. "Bend your head forward."
4. "Open your eyes widely."

7 What term is used to document a grating sound when a joint is moved?
1. crackles
2. arthritis
3. synovitis
4. crepitation

8 While conducting the ballottement test, you note the patella rebounds against your fingers. What does this finding indicate?
1. deformity of the elbow
2. infection of the metatarsals
3. fluid in the knee joint
4. crepitus in the hip joint

9 During the physical assessment of a young adult, you note a lateral, S-shaped curve of the spine. What is the name of this condition?
1. lordosis
2. scoliosis
3. kyphosis
4. musclosis

10 What are the most common manifestations of musculoskeletal disorders?
1. pain and limited mobility
2. swelling and exaggerated reflexes
3. cyanosis and decreased pulses
4. pallor and decreased ROM

See Test Yourself answers in Appendix C.

BIBLIOGRAPHY

Abdelhafiz, A., Lowles, R., Alam, N., Adebajo, A., & Philp, I. (2003). Clinical assessment of symptomatic osteoarthritis in older people. *Age and Aging, 32*(3), 359–360.

Amella, E. (2004). Presentation of illness in older adults: If you think you know what you're looking for, think again. *American Journal of Nursing, 104*(10), 40–52.

Asrani, C. (2003). Assessment of a patient with joint pain. *National Journal of Homeopathy, 5*(4), 245–246.

Assessment of a limb in a cast. (2003). *Nursing Times, 99*(31), 27.

Bickley, L., & Szilagyi, P. (2005). *Bates' guide to physical examination and history taking* (9th ed.). Philadelphia: Lippincott.

Burrow, J., & McLarnon, N. (2004). Foot assessment: Recognizing potential problems. *Nursing & Residential Care, 6*(2), 68–71.

Cole, E. (2004). Assessment and management of the trauma patient. *Nursing Standard, 18*(41), 45–52, 54.

Della-Giustina, D., & Nolan, R. (2004). Evaluation and management of low back pain. *Emergency Medicine, 36*(7), 20–26, 27–28.

Eliopoulos, E. (2005). *Gerontological nursing* (6th ed.). Philadelphia: Lippincott Williams & Wilkins.

Fredericson, M., & Wun, C. (2003). Differential diagnosis of leg pain in the athlete. *Journal of the American Podiatric Medical Association, 93*(4), 321–324.

Jarvis, C. (2004). *Physical examination & health assessment.* St. Louis, MO: Mosby.

Kasper, C., Talbot, L., & Gaines, J. (2002). Skeletal muscle damage and recovery. *AACN Clinical Issues: Advanced Practice in Acute and Critical Care, 13*(2), 237–247.

Kee, J. (2005). *Prentice Hall handbook of laboratory & diagnostic tests with nursing implications.* Upper Saddle River, NJ: Prentice Hall.

Leclercq, C. (2003). General assessment of the upper limb. *Hand Clinics, 19*(4), 557–564.

McConnell, E. (2002). Clinical do's & don'ts. Assessing neurovascular status in a casted limb. *Nursing, 32*(9), 20.

National Institutes of Health. (2003). *Genes and disease. Muscle and bone diseases.* Retrieved from http://www.ncbi.nlm.nih.gov/books/bv.fcgi?rid=gnd.section.59

Porth, C. (2005). *Pathophysiology: Concepts of altered health states* (7th ed.). Philadelphia: Lippincott.

Schultz, J. (2004). Clinical evaluation of the shoulder. *Physical Medicine and Rehabilitation Clinics of North America, 15*(2), 351–371.

Watson, R. (2001). Assessing the musculoskeletal system in older people. *Nursing Older People, 13*(5), 29–30.

Weber, J., & Kelley, J. (2006). *Health assessment in nursing* (3rd ed.). Philadelphia: Lippincott.

Bone Healing

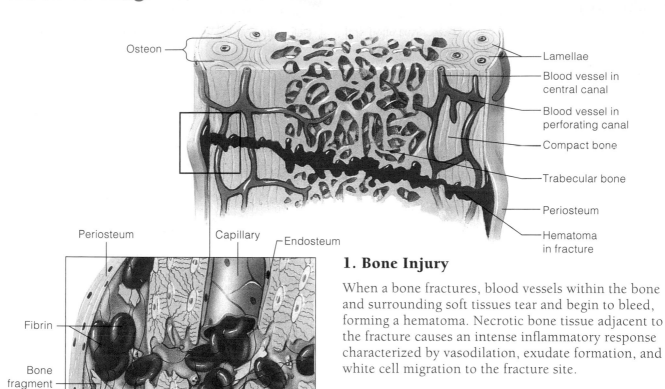

Osteon — Lamellae

Blood vessel in central canal

Blood vessel in perforating canal

Compact bone

Trabecular bone

Periosteum

Hematoma in fracture

1. Bone Injury

When a bone fractures, blood vessels within the bone and surrounding soft tissues tear and begin to bleed, forming a hematoma. Necrotic bone tissue adjacent to the fracture causes an intense inflammatory response characterized by vasodilation, exudate formation, and white cell migration to the fracture site.

Periosteum — Capillary — Endosteum

Fibrin

Bone fragment

Osteocyte

2. Fibrocartilaginous Callus Formation

Clotting factors within the hematoma form a fibrin meshwork. Within 48 hours, fibroblasts and new capillaries growing into the fracture form granulation tissue that gradually replaces the hematoma. Phagocytes begin to remove cell debris.

Osteoblasts, bone-forming cells, proliferate and migrate into the fracture site, forming a fibrocartilaginous callus. The osteoblasts build a web of collagen fibers from both sides of the fracture site that eventually unites to connect bone fragments, thus splinting the bone. Chondroblasts lay down patches of cartilage that provide a base for bone growth.

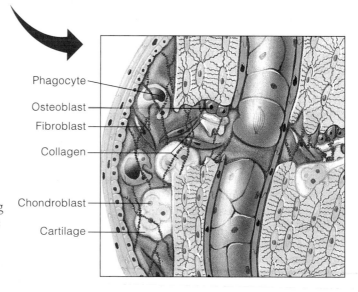

Phagocyte

Osteoblast

Fibroblast

Collagen

Chondroblast

Cartilage

4. Bone Remodeling

Osteoblasts continue to form new woven bone, which is in turn organized into the lamellar structures of compact bone. Osteoclasts resorb excess callus as it is replaced by mature bone.

    As the bone heals and is subjected to the mechanical stress of everyday use, osteoblasts and osteoclasts respond by remodeling the repair site along the lines of force. This ensures that the repaired section of bone eventually resembles the structure of the uninjured part.

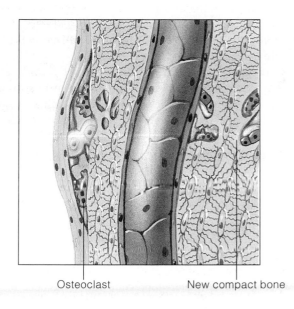

Osteoclast   New compact bone

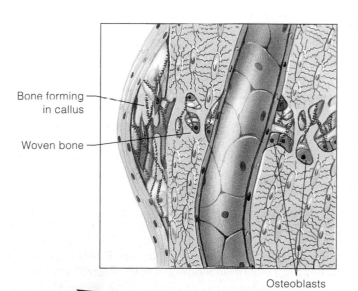

Bone forming in callus

Woven bone

Osteoblasts

3. Bony Callus Formation

Osteoblasts continue to proliferate and synthesize collagen fibers and bone matrix, which are gradually mineralized with calcium and mineral salts to form a spongy mass of woven bone. The trabeculae of woven bone bridge the fracture. Osteoclasts migrate to the repair site and begin removing excess bone in the callus. Bony callus formation usually continues for 2 to 3 months.

MEDIALINK

Bone Healing Animation

If compartment syndrome develops, interventions to alleviate pressure will be implemented; these may include removal of a tightly fitting cast. If the pressure is internal, a *fasciotomy*, a surgical intervention in which muscle fascia is cut to relieve pressure within the compartment, may be necessary. After a fasciotomy, the incision is left open, and passive ROM exercises are performed on the extremity.

Volkmann's contracture, a common complication of elbow fractures, can result from unresolved compartment syndrome. Arterial blood flow decreases, leading to ischemia, degeneration, and contracture of the muscle. Arm mobility is impaired, and the client is unable to completely extend the arm.

Fat Embolism Syndrome

Fat emboli occur when fat globules lodge in the pulmonary vascular bed or peripheral circulation. **Fat embolism syndrome (FES)** is characterized by neurologic dysfunction, pulmonary insufficiency, and a petechial rash on the chest, axilla, and upper arms. Long bone fractures and other major trauma are the principal risk factors for fat emboli; hip replacement surgery also poses a risk for FES.

When a bone is fractured, pressure within the bone marrow rises and exceeds capillary pressure; as a result, fat globules leave the bone marrow and enter the bloodstream. Another contributing factor may be the stress-induced release of catecholamine, which causes the rapid mobilization of fatty acids. Once the fat globules are released, they combine with platelets and travel to the brain, lungs, kidneys, and other organs, occluding small blood vessels and causing tissue ischemia.

Manifestations usually develop within a few hours to a week after injury. The manifestations result from the occlusion of the blood supply and the presence of fatty acids. Altered cerebral blood flow causes confusion and changes in level of consciousness. Pulmonary circulation may be disrupted, and free fatty acids damage the alveolar-capillary membrane. Pulmonary edema, impaired surfactant production, and atelectasis can result in significant respiratory insufficiency and manifestations of acute respiratory distress syndrome (see Chapter 39 ∞). Fat droplets activate the clotting cascade, causing thrombocytopenia. Petechiae (pin-sized purplish areas from bleeding under the skin) appearing on the skin, buccal membranes, and conjunctival sacs are thought to result from either microvascular clotting or the accompanying thrombocytopenia.

Early stabilization of long bone fractures is preventive for FES. Prompt identification and treatment of the syndrome are necessary to maintain adequate pulmonary function. In severe cases, the client may require intubation and mechanical ventilation to prevent hypoxemia. Fluid balance is closely monitored. Corticosteroids may be administered to decrease the inflammatory response of lung tissues, stabilize lipid membranes, and reduce bronchospasm (Porth, 2005).

Deep Venous Thrombosis

A *deep venous thrombosis (DVT)* is a blood clot that forms along the intimal lining of a large vein. Three precursors linked to DVT formation are (1) venous stasis, or decreased blood flow; (2) injury to blood vessel walls; and (3) altered blood coagulation (Table 41–2). Any or all of these precursors can cause a DVT to

TABLE 41–2 Precursors of Deep Venous Thrombosis

PRECURSOR	IMPLICATIONS FOR FRACTURES
Decreased blood flow	Common in fracture clients, who are immobilized and less active. Bed rest alone can decrease venous flow by 50%.
Injury to blood vessel wall	May occur as a direct result of the force that caused the fracture or from surgical manipulation.
Altered blood coagulation	May result from active blood loss. The body's attempt to maintain homeostasis leads to increased production of platelets and clotting factor.

form. Damage to the lining of the vein causes the platelets to aggregate or clump together, forming the thrombus. Fibrin, white blood cells (WBCs), and red blood cells (RBCs) begin to cling to the thrombus, and a tail forms. This tail or the entire thrombus may dislodge and move to the brain, lungs, or heart. Five percent of DVTs dislodge and enter the pulmonary circulation to form a pulmonary embolus. If the thrombus remains in the vein, venous insufficiency may result from scarring and valve damage.

If a DVT is present, there may be swelling, leg pain, tenderness, or cramping. Not all clients experience manifestations, however. For this reason, diagnostic tests, such as a venogram or Doppler ultrasound of lower extremities, may be required. A venogram requires intravenous administration of dye in the radiology department, whereas a Doppler ultrasound study is noninvasive and can be performed at the client's bedside. Doppler ultrasonography uses sound waves to form an image on a computer screen.

The best treatment for DVT is prevention. Early immobilization of the fracture and early ambulation of the client are imperative. The extremity should be elevated above the level of the heart. Frequent assessments of the injured extremity may lead to early recognition of DVT and prevent the formation of pulmonary embolus. Prophylactic anticoagulant administration is beneficial. Antiembolism stockings and compression boots increase venous return and prevent stasis of blood. Constrictive clothing should be avoided.

The diagnosis of DVT requires rapid intervention. The client is placed on bed rest for 5 to 7 days to prevent dislodgment of the clot. Fibrinolytic agents, which dissolve the clot, may be administered. Heparin may be administered intravenously to prevent more clots from forming. A vena cava filter may be placed to prevent the existing clot from entering the pulmonary circulation and forming a pulmonary embolus. In extreme cases in which anticoagulation therapy is contraindicated, a thrombectomy (surgical removal of the clot) may be necessary. See Chapter 35 ∞ for further discussion of DVT.

Infection

Infection is more likely to occur in an open fracture than a closed fracture, but any complication that decreases blood supply increases the risk of infection. Infection may result from contamination at the time of injury or during surgery.

Pseudomonas, Staphylococcus, or *Clostridium* organisms may invade the wound or bone. *Clostridium* infection is particularly serious because it may lead to severe gas gangrene and cellulitis, but any infection may delay healing and result in osteomyelitis, infection within the bone that can lead to tissue death and necrosis. (See Chapter 42 ∞ for a discussion of osteomyelitis.)

Delayed Union and Nonunion

Delayed union is the prolonged healing of bones beyond the usual time period. Many factors may inhibit bone healing, including poor nutrition, inadequate immobilization, prolonged reduction time, infection, necrosis, age, immunosuppression, and severe bone trauma resulting in multiple fragments. Delayed union is diagnosed by means of serial x-ray studies. It is important to note that x-ray findings may lag 1 to 2 weeks behind the healing process; for example, a client may be completely healed by week 13, but this fact may not be apparent on the x-ray until week 14.

Delayed union may lead to **nonunion**, which can cause persistent pain and movement at the fracture site. Nonunion may require surgical interventions, such as internal fixation and bone grafting. If infection is present, the bones are surgically debrided. Electrical stimulation of the fracture site may be as effective as bone grafting.

Reflex Sympathetic Dystrophy

Reflex sympathetic dystrophy may occur after musculoskeletal or nerve trauma. This term refers to a group of poorly understood post-traumatic conditions involving persistent pain, hyperesthesias, swelling, changes in skin color and texture, changes in temperature, and decreased motion. Diagnosis is made by the client's history and physical examination. X-rays may demonstrate spotty osteoporosis, and bone scans may reveal increased uptake of radionuclide. Treatment with a sympathetic nervous system blocking agent often alleviates the manifestations.

INTERDISCIPLINARY CARE

A fracture requires treatment to stabilize the fractured bone(s), maintain bone immobilization, prevent complications, and restore function. The diagnosis of a fracture is primarily based on physical assessments and x-rays.

Emergency Care

Emergency care of the client with a fracture includes immobilizing the fracture, maintaining tissue perfusion, and preventing infection. In the case of serious trauma, normal body alignment must be maintained and may involve cervical immobilization. Once the client is in a secure location, he or she is assessed for instability or deformity of the bone. If any deformity or instability is detected, the extremity is rapidly immobilized. Open wounds are covered with sterile dressings, and bleeding may be controlled with a pressure dressing. The extremities are assessed for the presence of pulses, movement, and sensation. The joint above and below the deformity is immobilized. Pulses, movement, and sensation are reevaluated after splinting.

The fracture is splinted to maintain normal anatomic alignment and prevent the fracture from dislocating. Splinting relieves pain and prevents further damage to the arteries, nerves, and bones. Splinting can be accomplished with air splints. If equipment is not available, the limb may be secured to the body. For example, an arm may be secured to the torso with a sling, or one leg may be strapped to the other leg.

Diagnosis

Diagnosis of a fracture begins with the history and initial assessment and usually is confirmed by radiographic tests. X-rays and bone scans are used to identify fractures (Figure 41–3 ■). Blood chemistry studies, complete blood count (CBC), and coagulation studies may be used to assess blood loss, renal function, muscle breakdown, and the risk of excessive bleeding or clotting. Diagnostic tests are described in Chapter 40 ∞.

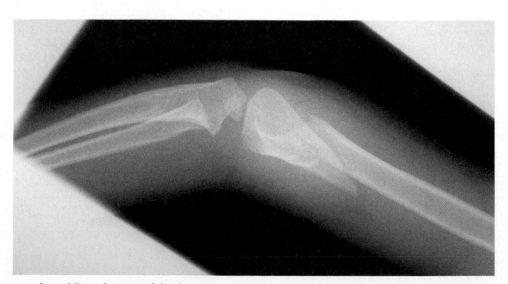

Figure 41–3 ■ X-ray of an oblique fracture of the femur.
Source: Charles Stewart and Associates.

Medications

Most clients with a fracture require pharmacologic interventions. The priority intervention focuses on relieving pain. In the case of multiple fractures or fractures of large bones, narcotics are administered initially. As healing progresses, the client begins to take oral medication for pain. Pain management for the client with a fracture is described in Box 41–3.

Stool softeners may be administered to decrease the risk of constipation secondary to narcotics and immobility. Clients who have sustained trauma are often placed on antiulcer medications or antacids. NSAIDs may be prescribed to decrease inflammation. Antibiotics may be administered prophylactically, particularly to clients with open or complex fractures. Anticoagulants may be prescribed to prevent DVT.

Treatments

Fracture treatment may involve a closed reduction and the application of a cast, or may include one or more of the following: traction, casts, surgery, and electrical bone stimulation.

TRACTION Muscle spasms usually accompany fractures and may pull bones out of alignment. Traction is the application of a straightening or pulling force to return or maintain the fractured bones in normal anatomic position. Weights are applied to maintain the necessary force (Figure 41–4 ■). Types of traction are as follows:

- In *manual traction,* the hand directly applies the pulling force.
- *Skin traction* (also called straight traction) is used to control muscle spasms and to immobilize a part of the body before surgery, with traction exerting its grabbing and pulling force through the client's skin. The most common type of skin traction is Buck's traction, in which traction tape or a foam boot is

applied to the lower portion of a client's leg and a free-hanging weight is attached to the taped or booted area (Figure 41–4A). Buck's traction is used to immobilize the leg before surgery to repair a fracture of the proximal femur. The advantage of skin traction is the relative ease of use and ability to maintain comfort. The disadvantage is that the weight required to maintain normal body alignment or fracture alignment cannot exceed the tolerance of the skin, about 6 lb per extremity. It is important to ensure that the weights remain hanging freely; they should never rest on the bed or the floor. The nurse may have to reposition the client or the weights if this occurs.

- *Balanced suspension traction* involves more than one force of pull. Several forces work in unison to raise and support the client's injured extremity off the bed and pull it in a straight line away from the body (Figure 41–4B). The advantage of this type of traction is that it increases mobility without threatening joint continuity. The disadvantage is that the increased use of multiple weights makes the client more likely to slide down in the bed.
- *Skeletal traction* is the application of a pulling force through placement of pins into the bone (Figure 41–4C). The client may receive a local, spinal, or general anesthetic, and the pins are inserted into the bone. This type of traction must be applied under sterile conditions because of the increased risk of infection. One or more pulling forces may be applied with skeletal traction. The advantage of this type of traction is that more weight can be used to maintain the proper anatomic alignment if necessary. The disadvantages include increased anxiety, increased risk of infection, and increased discomfort. The weights used for skeletal traction are not removed by the nurse. Nursing interventions for clients receiving traction are described in Box 41–4.

BOX 41–3 Pain Management in the Client with a Fracture

The client who has had musculoskeletal trauma experiences pain from many different causes:

- The interruption in the continuity of the bone itself
- Damage to ligaments and tendons
- Swelling of tissues around the trauma site
- Muscle spasms
- Tissue anoxia from swelling inside a cast, splint, or the muscle fascia sheath
- Hematoma formation
- Pressure over bony prominences from casts or splints.

The pain is often severe and may be described as sharp, aching, or burning. Carefully assess any complaint of pain; pain may be an indication of a serious complication, such as compartment syndrome, decreased tissue perfusion and neurovascular impairment, or pressure ulcers. Do not administer analgesics until the location, character, and duration of pain have been carefully assessed. After the cause of the pain has been identified, the following nursing interventions may be implemented:

1. Administer prescribed analgesics, which may include NSAIDs and narcotic analgesics. For serious fractures or following orthopedic surgery, patient-controlled analgesia (PCA) or epidural methods of providing pain relief may be used. If

medications are used on an as-needed basis, tell the client to request the medication before the pain is severe; alternatively, offer the medications at regular intervals for the first 24 to 48 hours. Reassure the client that addiction does not result from taking medications to relieve fracture or surgical pain. Most clients require only oral analgesics by the third or fourth day after orthopedic surgery.

2. Elevate the involved extremity, and apply cold (if prescribed) to help decrease swelling.

3. Monitor and drain the accumulated fluids in any drainage devices to ensure patency and to decrease the possibility of hematoma formation.

4. Encourage the client to wiggle fingers or toes on an extremity in a cast or traction to improve venous return and decrease edema.

5. Assist the client to change positions to relieve pressure and use pillows to provide support.

6. Teach the client alternative methods of pain management, such as relaxation and guided imagery.

7. Notify the physician of unrelieved pain, which may indicate a serious complication such as compartment syndrome or neurovascular impairment.

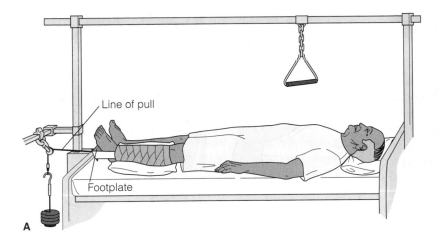

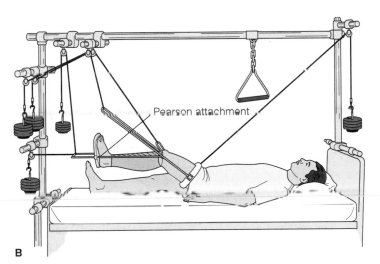

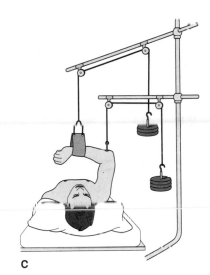

Figure 41–4 ■ Traction is the application of a pulling force to maintain bone alignment during fracture healing. Different fractures require different types of traction. *A,* Skin traction (also called straight traction) such as Buck's traction shown here, is often used for hip fractures. *B,* Balanced suspension traction is commonly used for fractures of the femur. *C,* Skeletal traction, in which the pulling force is applied directly to the bone, may be used to treat fractures of the humerus.

Labels in figure A: Line of pull; Footplate

Label in figure B: Pearson attachment

BOX 41–4 Nursing Interventions for Clients in Traction

- In skeletal traction, never remove the weights.
- In skin traction, remove weights only when intermittent skin traction has been ordered to alleviate muscle spasm.
- For traction to be successful, a countertraction is necessary. In most instances, the countertraction is the client's weight. Therefore, do not wedge the client's foot or place it flush with the footboard of the bed.
- Maintain the line of pull:
  a. Center the client on the bed.
  b. Ensure that weights hang freely and do not touch the floor.
- Ensure that nothing is lying on or obstructing the ropes. Do not allow the knots at the end of the rope to come into contact with the pulley.
- If a problem is detected, assist in repositioning. The area of the fracture must be stabilized when the client is repositioned.
- In skin traction:

a. Frequently assess skin for evidence of pressure, shearing, or pending breakdown.
b. Protect pressure sites with padding and protective dressings as indicated.
- In skeletal traction:
a. Frequent skin assessments should include pin care per policy.
b. Report signs of infection at the pin sites, such as redness, drainage, and increased tenderness.
c. The client may require more frequent analgesic administration.
- Perform neurovascular assessments frequently.
- Assess for common complications of immobility, including formation of pressure ulcers, formation of renal calculi, deep venous thrombosis, pneumonia, paralytic ileus, and loss of appetite.
- Teach the client and family about the type and purpose of the traction.

CASTS A cast is a rigid device applied to immobilize the injured bones and promote healing. The cast immobilizes the joint above and the joint below the fractured bone so that the bone will not move during healing. A fracture is first reduced manually (by hand) and a cast is then applied. Casts are applied on clients who have relatively stable fractures

The cast, which may be composed of plaster or fiberglass, is applied over a thin cushion of padding and molded to the normal contour of the body. The cast must be allowed to dry before any pressure is applied to it; simply palpating a wet cast with the fingertips will leave dents that may cause pressure ulcers. A plaster cast may require up to 48 hours to dry, whereas a fiberglass

BOX 41–5 Nursing Interventions for Clients with Internal Fixation

- Expect the client to have sutures and at least one Hemovac drain.
- Perform neurovascular assessments frequently.
- Assess the following:
  a. Wounds for drainage
  b. Hemovac for drainage of serosanguineous fluid
  c. Bowel sounds
  d. Lung sounds.

- Administer medications, such as analgesics and antibiotics, per physician's orders.
- In hip fractures, place an abductor pillow between client's legs to prevent dislocation of the hip joint.
- Arrange for physical and occupational therapy, as ordered.
- Assist with weight-bearing program, if ordered.
- Encourage early mobilization, coughing, and deep breathing, as appropriate to help prevent complications.

wire at the fracture site. The lead wire is attached to an internal or external generator, which delivers electricity through the lead wire to the cathode 24 hours a day. In noninvasive inductive stimulation, a treatment coil encircles the cast or skin directly over the fracture site. The coil is attached to an external generator that runs on batteries. The electricity goes through the skin to the fracture site. The time period for external stimulation can vary from 3 to 10 hours per day. The client may be taught to self-administer the noninvasive electrical stimulation. Electrical bone stimulation is contraindicated in the presence of infection and for upper extremities if the client has a pacemaker.

Fractures of Specific Bones or Bony Areas

Causes, manifestations, complications, treatment and selected nursing interventions are described for the following fractures: skull, face, spine, clavicle, humerus, elbow, radius/ulna, wrist/hand, ribs, pelvis, femur, hip, tibia/fibula, and ankle/foot.

Fracture of the Skull

The skull may be fractured as a result of either a fall or a direct blow. The client must be assessed for neurologic damage and any loss of consciousness (LOC) must be documented. A complete

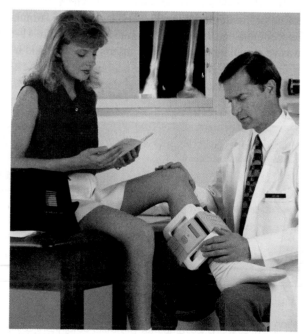

Figure 41–8 ■ External electrical bone growth stimulator.
Courtesy of Orthologic, Inc.

neurologic assessment is conducted: Pupillary reaction to light, movement and strength of all extremities, complaints of nausea and vomiting, LOC, and orientation to person, place, and time are noted. A displaced skull fracture, which is referred to as depressed, may press on the brain and cause neurologic damage. Brain injuries related to skull fractures are discussed in Chapter 44 ∞.

Fracture of the Face

Fracture of the facial bones may result from a direct blow. The client presents with hematomas, pain, edema, and bony deformity. Nondisplaced fractures are monitored to ensure the airway is not compromised. The client is observed for any neurologic deficits. Severely displaced or multiple facial fractures are treated with ORIF with wires or plates.

Nursing care focuses on maintaining the airway by helping the client clear secretions from the oropharynx. The nurse monitors the client's breathing for increased effort or tachypnea and notifies the physician immediately if these findings are noted. Pain is treated with analgesics, and body image disturbances are addressed. If the client asks to see his or her face, the nurse should plan to stay with the client and answer questions while the client looks in a mirror.

Fracture of the Spine

The spine can be injured in many ways, including sports injuries, falls, and motor vehicle crashes. The spine can be fractured in the cervical, thoracic, lumbar, or sacral area. The most severe complication of spine fracture is injury to the spinal cord (discussed in Chapter 45 ∞). A fracture to the vertebrae may cause the bones to become displaced and apply pressure on the spinal cord. This pressure on the spinal cord may result in permanent paralysis.

A nondisplaced cervical spinal fracture may be treated with a cervical collar or a halo immobilizing brace. The displaced cervical fracture is reduced by manual or skeletal traction and, eventually, application of a brace and/or surgical stabilization of the bones with plates and screws. Immobilization after a spinal fracture may last as long as 6 months.

Fracture of the Clavicle

A fracture of the clavicle commonly results from a direct blow or a fall. The most common location is midclavicular. A person with a midclavicular fracture typically assumes a protective slumping position to immobilize the arm and prevent shoulder movement. A less common fracture occurs along the distal third of the clavicle. This type of fracture may be associated with ligament damage. Injuries to the clavicle may be associated with skull or cervical fractures. The fractured bone, if displaced, may lacerate the subclavian vessels and result in hemorrhage. The fractured bone may also puncture the lung, resulting in a pneumothorax. Malunion may occur at the fracture site and result in asymmetry of the clavicles. Injury to the brachial plexus may result in numbness and decreased movement of the arm on the affected side.

A deformity may be observed or palpated along the clavicle. Treatment focuses on immobilizing the fractured bone in normal anatomic position by applying a clavicular strap, or a surgical repair may be necessary.

Fracture of the Humerus

The exact location of the fracture, the presence of displacement, and the results of the neurovascular examination determine the severity of a fracture of the humerus and the appropriate interventions. Treatment focuses on immobilizing the fractured bone in normal anatomic position. Common complications of humeral fracture include nerve and ligament damage, frozen or stiff joints, and malunion. Early interventions may prevent permanent damage.

Fractures of the proximal humerus are common in older adults. A simple nondisplaced fracture of the proximal humerus (near the humeral head) with a normal neurovascular assessment can be safely treated with immobilization. A more complicated displaced fracture of the proximal humerus with bone fragmentation requires surgical intervention. The more severe the fracture and damage to soft tissue, the more likely it is that the range of motion (ROM) of the shoulder will be impaired. Rehabilitative measures focus on increasing ROM.

The humerus may also fracture along the shaft, usually as a direct result of trauma. If the humeral shaft fracture is simple and nondisplaced, a hanging arm cast is applied. This cast maintains alignment of the fracture by using the pulling force of gravity; therefore, the client must be instructed not to rest the cast on anything to alleviate the weight. If the client is on bed rest, a hanging arm cast is not applied, because the arm would not be able to hang freely. Instead, the fracture is immobilized with external skeletal traction. This traction places the injured arm in an upright position over the face, and weights are hung off the distal portion of the humerus (see Figure 41–4C). Nursing interventions for clients with fractures of the humerus are presented in Box 41–6.

Fracture of the Elbow

The most common location of an elbow fracture is the distal humerus. Elbow fractures usually result from a fall or direct blow to the elbow. The client guards the injured extremity, holding the arm rigidly in a flexed position or an extended position. Because the radius, ulna, or humerus may be involved in the elbow fracture, all three bones must be visualized by x-ray.

Complications of an elbow fracture include nerve or artery damage and hemarthrosis, a collection of blood in the elbow joint. The most serious complication of an elbow fracture is Volkmann's contracture, which results from arterial occlusion and muscle ischemia. The client complains of forearm pain, impaired sensation, and loss of motor function. Rapid interventions are aimed at relieving pressure on the brachial artery and nerve and preventing muscle atrophy.

Nondisplaced elbow fractures are treated by immobilizing the fracture with a posterior splint or cast. The displaced frac-

---

BOX 41–6 Nursing Interventions for Clients with Fractures of the Humerus

- Perform neurovascular assessments frequently.
- Administer prescribed medications to alleviate pain.
- Encourage exercises for clients with a hanging cast:
  a. Finger exercises: Move each finger of the affected arm through complete range of motion.
  b. Pendulum shoulder exercises: Dangle the affected arm at the side, and move it forward and backward about 30 degrees in each direction.
- If client is discharged, instruct the client and family in cast care and sling application, neurovascular assessments, exercises, prescribed pain medications, and manifestations of complications.
- If client is admitted to the hospital, provide preoperative teaching.

---

ture is first reduced and then immobilized. Nursing interventions focus on alleviating pain, maintaining immobilization, and educating clients in neurovascular assessments.

Fracture of the Radius and/or Ulna

Fractures of the radius and ulna may occur as a result of either indirect injury, such as twisting or pulling on the arm, or direct injury, such as that resulting from a fall. The usual treatment of radius fractures depends on the location. The proximal radial head may be fractured from a fall on an outstretched hand. Blood commonly collects in the elbow joint and must be aspirated. If the fracture is nondisplaced, a sling is applied. If the fracture is displaced, surgical intervention is required. After surgical repair of a displaced fracture, the arm is splinted with a posterior plaster splint. The client avoids movement for the first week and then initiates movement gradually.

When both bones are broken, the fracture is usually displaced. The client complains of pain and inability to turn the palm of the hand up. A nondisplaced fracture is casted for about 6 weeks, and either a shorter cast or a brace is then applied for 6 more weeks. If the fracture is displaced, surgical intervention is performed. The physician reduces the fracture and may insert pins or screws to keep the bones in alignment. After the surgery, a cast is applied, and the client is encouraged to exercise the fingers.

Complications after a radius and/or ulnar fracture include compartment syndrome, delayed healing, and decreased wrist and finger movement. After surgery, the client also has an increased risk of infection. Nursing interventions focus on alleviating pain, maintaining immobilization, and educating clients in neurovascular assessments, the importance of elevation, and the need to inform the physician of changes in sensation or an increase in pain.

Fractures in the Wrist and Hand

Wrist fractures often result from a fall onto an outstretched hand or onto the back of the hand. A common type of wrist fracture is *Colles's fracture,* in which the distal radius fractures after a fall onto an outstretched hand. The client with a wrist fracture presents with a bony deformity, pain, numbness, weakness, and decreased ROM of the fingers. The capillary refill and sensation of the hand must be assessed.

The hand is composed of many bones. Most commonly, the metacarpals and phalanges are involved in a hand fracture. The injuring mechanism in a hand fracture varies from striking an object with a closed fist to closing a hand in a door. The client presents with complaints of pain, edema, and decreased ROM.

Comparative x-rays may be obtained to compare left and right wrists and hands. Complications of wrist and hand fractures are compartment syndrome, nerve damage, ligament damage, and delayed union. A wrist fracture is commonly treated with closed reduction, cast application, and elevation of the injured extremity. A hand fracture is splinted and elevated.

Nursing interventions focus on alleviating pain and educating the client in neurovascular assessments, the importance of elevation, and how to exercise the fingers to prevent stiffness. If the dominant hand is injured, the client will require assistance in performing activities of daily living (ADLs).

Fracture of the Ribs

Rib fractures commonly result from blunt chest trauma. The location of the fracture and involvement of underlying organs determine the severity of the injury. Fractures of the first through third ribs may result in injury to the subclavian artery or vein. Fractures of the lower ribs may result in spleen and liver injuries.

The client presents with a history of recent chest trauma. Typically, the client complains of pain along the lateral portion of the rib. Palpation of the rib reveals a bony deformity and increases pain. Deep inspiration also increases pain. The skin over the fracture site may be ecchymotic (bruised).

A complication of rib fractures is a **flail chest**, which results from the fracture of two or more adjacent ribs in two or more places and the formation of a free-floating segment that moves in the opposite direction of the rib cage. The bony instability impairs respirations. Treatment is aimed at stabilizing the flail segment and supporting respirations. Other complications of rib fractures include pneumothorax and/or hemothorax. The fractured rib may pierce the lung and injure it. The lower ribs may pierce the liver or spleen, resulting in intra-abdominal bleeding. Pneumonia may also develop from ineffective clearing of respiratory secretions.

A simple rib fracture is treated with pain medication and instructions for coughing, deep breathing, and splinting. The client is also instructed to return to the emergency room if shortness of breath develops. Nursing interventions focus on alleviating pain and teaching the client about splinting. Because deep inspiration increases pain, clients frequently avoid it. The client may be instructed to splint the injured rib with the hand or a pillow and take deep breaths and cough to decrease the chance of developing pneumonia and/or atelectasis. Incentive spirometry is encouraged.

Fracture of the Pelvis

Pelvic fractures are often caused by trauma, such as a fall or an automobile crash. The client with a pelvic fracture presents with pain in the back or hip area. A single fracture in the pelvis is treated conservatively with bed rest on a firm mattress. Log rolling increases client comfort. A pelvic fracture with two fracture sites is considered unstable and treated with surgery. An external fixator may be applied to stabilize the pelvis. In the client who is not stable for surgery, a pelvic sling may be used. The pelvic sling stabilizes the pelvis and allows the client to move in bed with less pain. Common complications include hypovolemia, spinal injury, bladder injury, urethral injury, kidney damage, and gastrointestinal trauma.

Nursing care focuses on alleviating discomfort, maintaining immobilization, and preparing the client for surgery if necessary. The nurse monitors the client for increased heart rate, decreased blood pressure, and decreasing hemoglobin levels. These findings may indicate impending hypovolemia due to bleeding into the pelvis. Any blood in the urine should be reported to the physician; this may indicate kidney, bladder, or urethral damage.

Fracture of the Shaft of the Femur

A large amount of force, such as from motor vehicle crashes, falls, or acts of violence, is required to fracture the shaft of the femur. Clients with femoral shaft fractures often have associated multiple traumas. A fracture of the femoral shaft is manifested by an edematous, deformed, painful thigh. The client is unable to move the hip or knee. Initial assessment focuses on the circulation and sensation present in the affected extremity. Pedal pulses and capillary refill in the affected extremity are compared to the unaffected extremity. Complications of a femoral shaft fracture include hypovolemia due to blood loss (which may be as great as 1.0 to 1.5 L), fat embolism, dislocation of the hip or knee, muscle atrophy, and ligament damage.

Treatment of fractures of the shaft of the femur initially includes skeletal traction to separate the bony fragments and reduce and immobilize the fracture. Depending on the location and severity of the fracture, traction may be followed by either external or internal fixation. Strength in the affected extremity is maintained through gluteal and quadricep exercises. ROM exercises for unaffected extremities are critical in preparation for ambulation. Although full weight bearing is usually restricted until x-rays demonstrate bone union, the client may be allowed to carry out non-weight-bearing activities with an assistive device.

The nurse assesses pulses in the extremity and compares them bilaterally. Sensation is evaluated by asking whether the client can feel touch and discriminate sharp from dull objects. Nursing interventions include providing pain medication, providing reassurance and decreasing anxiety, and assisting with exercises of the lower legs, feet, and toes.

Fracture of the Hip

A hip fracture refers to a fracture of the femur at the head, neck, or trochanteric regions (Figure 41–9 ■). Hip fractures are classified as intracapsular or extracapsular. *Intracapsular fractures* involve the head or neck of the femur; *extracapsular fractures* involve the trochanteric region. The majority of hip fractures involve the neck or trochanteric regions. The femoral head and neck lie within the joint capsule and are not covered in periosteum; thus, they do not have a large blood supply. Fractures at this location usually fragment, further decreasing blood supply and increasing the risk of nonunion and avascular necrosis. The trochanteric region is covered in periosteum and therefore has more blood supply than the head or neck.

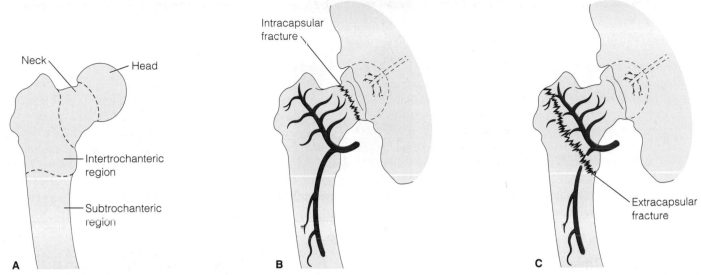

Figure 41–9 ■ Regions where hip fractures may occur: *A,* the head of the femur, the neck of the femur, and the trochanteric regions of the femur. *B,* Intracapsular fractures occur across the head or neck of the femur. *C,* Extracapsular fractures occur across the trochanteric regions. Note how both intracapsular and extracapsular fractures disrupt the blood supply to the bone.

Hip fractures result from falls and are the most common injury in the older population, requiring hospitalization of more than 300,000 older adults each year in the United States. They result in the greatest number of deaths and most serious health problems of all fractures for people 65 years or older (Centers for Disease Control and Prevention, [CDC], 2006). By the year 2040, the number of hip fractures is expected to exceed 500,000, which reflects society's increasing older population. Factors contributing to falls include problems with gait and balance, neurologic and musculoskeletal impairments, dementia, psychoactive medications, and visual impairments. Modifiable risk factors, identified through research, include lower body weakness, problems with walking and balance, and taking four or more medications or any psychoactive medications.

Hip fractures are common in older adults as a result of decreases in bone mass and the increased tendency to fall. Whether the femur breaks spontaneously and causes the fall or whether the fall causes the fracture is not always clear; regardless of the cause of the fracture, rapid interventions are required to prevent bone necrosis. Assessment findings commonly associated with a hip fracture are pain, inability to walk, and shortening and external rotation of the affected lower extremity. Rarely, the fracture dislocates posteriorly; if that occurs, the extremity may internally rotate. However, some patients with a hip fracture have only vague pain in the buttocks, knees, thighs, groin, or back and their ability to walk is unaffected. If the fracture is not visible on x-ray, a bone scan or MRI may be done to confirm the presence of the fracture.

A hip fracture may be treated with traction to decrease muscle spasms, followed by surgery; or surgery may be performed immediately or within the first 24 hours. The goal of surgery is to reduce and stabilize the fracture, thereby increasing mobility, decreasing pain, and preventing complications. Surgery usually consists of ORIF of the fracture. Fixation is accomplished by securing the femur in place with pins, screws, nails, or plates (Figure 41–10A ■). An ORIF works well for fractures in the trochanteric area. Fractures of the femoral neck frequently disrupt blood supply to the femoral head. If blood supply is disrupted, the surgeon will replace the femoral head with a prosthesis (Figure 41–10B). If the acetabulum has been damaged, the surgeon may insert a metal cup. Replacement of either the femoral head or the acetabulum with a prosthesis is called a *hemiarthroplasty*. Replacement of both the femoral head and the acetabulum is a *total hip arthroplasty (THA)*, discussed in Chapter 42 ∞.

Nursing care for a client with a hip fracture focuses on maintaining skin integrity, preventing infection, alleviating pain, maintaining circulation to the injured extremity, and increasing mobility, and is discussed in more detail in the following nursing care section.

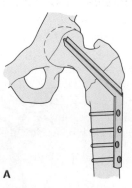
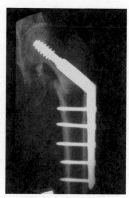
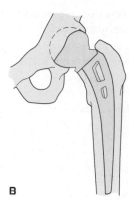

Figure 41–10 ■ Surgical fixation of hip fractures. *A,* A surgical nail or screw used to stabilize an intertrochanteric fracture. *B,* Use of a hip prosthesis (artificial hip) to replace a damaged femoral head.

Fracture of the Tibia and/or Fibula

Fractures of the lower extremities often result from a fall on a flexed foot, a direct blow, or a twisting motion. The client presents with edema, pain, bony deformity, and a hematoma at the level of injury.

Circulation and sensation are assessed to rule out common complications of the fracture, including damage to the peroneal nerve or tibial artery, compartment syndrome, hemarthroses, and ligament damage. Peroneal nerve damage may be indicated by the client's inability to point the toe on the affected side upward. Tibial artery damage may be the cause of an absent dorsalis pedis pulse on the affected side. Compartment syndrome may be present if the client develops pain on passive movement and paresthesias. An edematous knee may indicate a collection of blood in the knee joint. Ligament damage may be present if the client cannot move the knee and/or ankle.

If the fracture is closed, a closed reduction and casting are frequently performed. A long leg cast that allows for partial weight bearing is used. Partial weight bearing usually is prescribed by the physician within 10 days of the fracture. A short leg cast will be applied in 3 to 4 weeks. If the fracture is open, either external fixation or ORIF will be performed. After surgery, a cast may be applied, and weight bearing begins according to the physician's orders, usually in about 6 weeks.

Nursing care is designed to increase comfort, monitor neurovascular status, and prevent complications. The nurse instructs the client in cast care, on the use of assistive devices, how to perform neurovascular assessment, and when to follow up with the physician.

Fracture in the Ankle and Foot

The client with an ankle fracture presents with pain, limited ROM, hematoma, edema, and difficulty ambulating. Most ankle fractures are treated by closed reduction and casting. Open fractures are treated by surgical intervention and splinting.

The client with a foot fracture presents with similar symptoms; however, ROM of the ankle is not usually affected. Most foot fractures are nondisplaced and treated with closed reduction and casting. More severe displaced foot fractures may require surgery and the placement of wires to maintain reduction of the fracture.

Nursing care focuses on increasing comfort, increasing mobility, and educating the client. Analgesia is given for pain. The extremity should be elevated, and ice can be applied. The client is taught cast care, neurovascular assessment, and crutch walking.

NURSING CARE

In planning and implementing nursing care for the client with fractures, the nurse should consider the client's response to the traumatic experience. Although each client has individual needs, nursing care commonly focuses on client problems with pain, impaired physical mobility, impaired tissue perfusion, and neurovascular compromise.

Health Promotion

Trauma prevention can save lives. Many communities are educating people of all ages, from grade-schoolers to older adults, in trauma prevention. Young adults face a high risk of sustaining trauma. They need to be taught the importance of safety equipment—such as automobile seat belts, bicycle and motorized vehicle helmets, football pads, proper footwear, protective eyewear, and hard hats—in preventing or decreasing the severity of injury from trauma. Older adults should have regular screenings for osteoporosis (with a bone density test), activity levels, cognitive and affective disorders, vision impairments, and risk for falls. Older adults can reduce their risk of falling by increasing lower body strength and balance through regular physical activity, and by asking their healthcare provider or pharmacist to review their medications. Educational programs about workplace and farm safety, including information about ergonomic principles, can also help prevent musculoskeletal injuries.

Having a regular exercise program and avoiding obesity are important factors in maintaining good bone health in all adults. An adequate intake of calcium is essential to ensure proper growth, development, and maintenance of strong bones throughout life. It is important that women ensure good bone health prior to menopause, because the loss of estrogen during and after menopause decreases calcium use and increases the risk of osteoporosis. Strong bones are formed by calcium intake and weight-bearing exercise, both of which are equally important in the postmenopausal woman.

Older clients are at higher risk for musculoskeletal trauma due to falls. For these clients, home assessments must be performed and potential hazards removed. Specific teaching topics for preventing falls in older adults are outlined in the Meeting Individualized Needs box below.

Assessment

Collect the following data through the health history and physical examination (see Chapter 40 ∞).

- *Health History:* Age, history of traumatic event, history of chronic illnesses, history of prior musculoskeletal injuries, medications (ask the older adult specifically about anticoagulants and calcium supplements).
- *Physical Assessment:* Pain with movement, pulses, edema, skin color and temperature, deformity, range of motion, touch. These assessments include the 5 P's of neurovascular assessment, as follows, included in both the initial assessment and ongoing focused assessments:
- *Pain.* Assess pain in the injured extremity by asking the client to grade it on a scale of 0 to 10, with 10 as the most severe pain.
- *Pulses.* Assess distal pulses beginning with the unaffected extremity. Compare the quality of pulses in the affected extremity to those of the unaffected extremity.
- *Pallor.* Observe for pallor and skin color in the injured extremity. Paleness and coolness may indicate arterial compromise, whereas warmth and a bluish tinge may indicate venous blood pooling.
- *Paralysis/Paresis.* Assess ability to move body parts distal to the fracture site. Inability to move indicates paralysis. Loss of muscle strength (weakness) when moving is paresis. A finding of limited range of motion may lead to early recognition of problems such as nerve damage and paralysis.
- *Paresthesia.* Ask the client if any change in sensation such as burning, numbness, prickly feeling, or stinging (all these are paresthesias) has occurred.

Nursing Diagnoses and Interventions

Nursing care for clients with fractures ranges from teaching for home care treatments provided in the emergency or urgent care department (such as manual reduction and cast application) to providing interventions to maintain health and decrease the risk of complications in clients with complex or multiple fractures. Teaching is also necessary for caregivers of the older adult who is discharged home or to a long-term care or rehabilitation facility following a fractured hip. A Nursing Care Plan is included on page 1418.

Acute Pain

Pain is caused by soft tissue damage and is compounded by muscle spasms and swelling.

- Monitor vital signs. *Some analgesics decrease respiratory effort and blood pressure.*
- Ask the client to rate the pain on a scale of 0 to 10 (with 10 as the most severe pain) before and after any intervention. *This facilitates objective assessment of the effectiveness of the chosen pain relief strategy. Pain that increases in intensity or remains unrelieved with analgesics can indicate compartment syndrome.*
- For the client with a hip fracture, apply Buck's traction per physician's orders. Keep the traction weights hanging freely. *Buck's traction immobilizes the fracture and decreases pain and additional trauma.*

> **PRACTICE ALERT**
> Do not let weights lie on the bed or the floor. The weights can be removed long enough to move the client up or down in bed to ensure freely hanging weights.

- Move the client gently and slowly. *Gentle moving helps prevent the development of severe muscle spasms.*
- Elevate the injured extremity above the level of the heart. *Elevating the extremity promotes venous return and decreases edema, which decreases pain.*
- Encourage distraction or other noninvasive methods of pain relief, such as deep breathing and relaxation. *Distraction, deep breathing, and relaxation help decrease the focus on the pain and may lessen the intensity of pain.*

MEETING INDIVIDUALIZED NEEDS   Teaching Older Adults to Prevent Falls

- Begin a regular exercise program; lack of exercise leads to weakness and an increased chance of falling. Exercises that improve balance and coordination (such as t'ai chi) are the most helpful.
- Make your home safer:
  - Remove any items in your pathway, including from stairs, to avoid tripping.
  - Remove small throw rugs or use double-sided tape to keep rugs from slipping.
  - Place frequently used items within easy reach to avoid use of a step stool.
  - Install grab bars next to your toilet and in the tub or shower.
  - Use nonslip mats in the bathtub and on shower floors.

- Improve lighting, using lamp shades or frosted bulbs to reduce glare.
- Install handrails and lights in all staircases.
- Wear shoes that give good support and have thin, nonslip soles. Avoid wearing slippers and athletic shoes with deep treads.
- Ask your healthcare provider to review your medications, including prescriptions and over-the-counter medications. Some medications or a combination of medications may cause dizziness or drowsiness, leading to falls.
- Have your vision checked by an eye doctor. Your glasses may no longer have the correct prescription, or you may have developed an eye condition such as cataracts or glaucoma that limits your vision.

NURSING CARE PLAN   A Client with a Hip Fracture

Stella Carbolito is a 74-year-old Italian American with a history of osteoporosis. She is a widow and lives alone in a two-story row home. Mrs. Carbolito is retired and depends on a pension check and social security for her income. She takes pride in making all her own food from scratch.

While walking to the market one day, Mrs. Carbolito falls and fractures her left hip. She is transported by ambulance to the nearest hospital emergency department.

ASSESSMENT

During the initial assessment at the ED, abnormal findings are that Mrs. Carbolito's left leg is shorter than her right leg and is externally rotated. Distal pulses are present and bilaterally strong; both legs are warm. Mrs. Carbolito complains of severe pain but states that no numbness or burning is present. She is able to wiggle the toes on her left leg and has full movement of her right leg. Initial vital signs are as follows: T 98.0°F (36.6°C), P 100, R 18, BP 120/58. Diagnostic tests include CBC, blood chemistry, and x-ray studies of the left hip and pelvis. The CBC reveals a hemoglobin of 11.0 g/dL and a normal WBC count. Blood chemistry findings are within normal limits. The x-ray reveals a fracture of the left femoral neck. Mrs. Carbolito is admitted to the hospital with an order for 10 lb of straight leg traction. An open reduction and internal fixation (ORIF) is planned for the following day.

DIAGNOSES

- *Acute Pain* related to fractured left femoral neck and muscle spasms
- *Impaired Physical Mobility* related to bed rest and fractured left femoral neck
- *Risk for Ineffective Tissue Perfusion* related to unstable bones and swelling
- *Risk for Disturbed Sensory Perception: Tactile* related to the risk of nerve impairment

EXPECTED OUTCOMES

- Verbalize a decrease in pain.
- Verbalize the purpose of traction and surgery.
- Maintain normal neurovascular status.
- Demonstrate postoperative exercises.

PLANNING AND IMPLEMENTATION

- Assess pain on a scale of 0 to 10 before and after implementing measures to reduce pain.
- Administer narcotics per the physician's order.
- Perform neurovascular assessment every 2 to 4 hours, and document findings.
- Apply straight leg traction per physician's order.
- Encourage deep breathing and relaxation techniques.
- Teach the purpose of traction and surgery.
- Teach the purpose of and the procedure for performing isometric and flexion/extension exercises.

EVALUATION

Three days after surgery, Mrs. Carbolito is out of bed and in a chair. She verbalizes a decrease in pain. There have been no abnormal neurovascular assessments. She is able to independently perform isometric and flexion/extension exercises in both lower extremities. Discharge planning includes referrals for home care. A home health nurse will visit, and the social worker at the hospital has ordered a trapeze for her bed, an elevated toilet seat, an elevated cushion for her chair, and a walker.

CRITICAL THINKING IN THE NURSING PROCESS

1. What factors placed Mrs. Carbolito at risk for a hip fracture?
2. Mrs. Carbolito says, "I don't understand why they had to put that heavy thing on my leg before I went to surgery to get my hip fixed." What would you tell her? What preoperative factors might have decreased teaching effectiveness?
3. Describe how each of the following, if manifested by Mrs. Carbolito, would increase her risk for postoperative complications: urinary incontinence, weight more than 20% under normal for her height, chronic constipation. What nursing diagnoses and interventions would you include in her plan of care to decrease the risk?

See Evaluating Your Response in Appendix C.

- Administer pain medications as prescribed. For home care, explain the importance of taking pain medications before the pain is severe. *Analgesics alleviate pain by stimulating opiate receptor sites.*

PRACTICE ALERT
In the case of fracture in an extremity, supporting the extremity above and below the fracture can also decrease pain and muscle spasms.

Risk for Peripheral Neurovascular Dysfunction

In the client with a fracture, compartment syndrome or deep venous thrombosis can impair circulation and, in turn, tissue perfusion.

- Assess the 5 P's every 1 to 2 hours. Report abnormal findings immediately. *Unrelenting pain, pallor, diminished distal pulses, paresthesias, and paresis are strong indicators of compartment syndrome.*

PRACTICE ALERT
Pulses may remain strong, even in the presence of compartment syndrome.

- Assess nail beds for capillary refill. If nails are too thick or discolored, assess the skin around the nail. *Delayed capillary refill may indicate decreased tissue perfusion.*

PRACTICE ALERT
It may not be possible to accurately assess capillary refill in older adults who often have thickened, discolored nails. If so, test nearby skin.

- Monitor the extremity for edema and swelling. *Excessive swelling and hematoma formation can compromise circulation.*
- Assess for deep, throbbing, unrelenting pain. *Pain that is not relieved by analgesics may indicate neurovascular compromise.*

- Monitor the tightness of the cast. *Edema can cause the cast to become tight; a tight-fitting cast may lead to compartment syndrome or paralysis.*
- If cast is tight, be prepared to assist the physician with bivalving (Figure 41–11 ■). *Bivalving, the process of splitting the cast down both sides, alleviates pressure on the injured extremity.*
- If compartment syndrome is suspected, assist the physician in measuring compartment pressure. Normal compartment pressure is 10 to 20 mmHg. *Compartment pressure greater than 30 mmHg indicates compartment syndrome.*
- Elevate the injured extremity above the level of the heart. *Elevating the extremity increases venous return and decreases edema.*
- Administer anticoagulant per physician's order. *Prophylactic anticoagulation decreases the risk of clot formation.*

Risk for Infection

The client who undergoes surgical repair will have a postoperative wound. Any break in skin integrity must be monitored for infection. Wound healing in orthopedic patients is affected by the cause of the wound as well as the therapies used to repair musculoskeletal structures. It is important for nurses to understand normal wound healing processes; characteristics of musculoskeletal wounds, contamination, and drainage; and potential complications to plan for and implement appropriate interventions (Harvey, 2005).

- For clients with skeletal pins, follow established guidelines for skeletal pin site care, as outlined in the Evidenced-Based

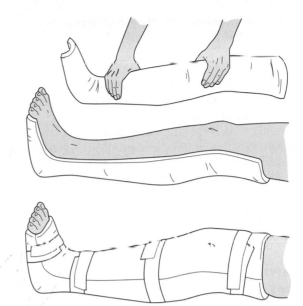

Figure 41–11 ■ Bivalving is the process of splitting the cast down both sides to alleviate pressure on or allow visualization of the extremity.

Practice box below. *Pins or wires attached to traction, casts, or external fixators stabilize a segment of bone so optimal healing can occur. However, pin infections of varying severity do occur (Holmes & Brown, 2005, pp. 1–2).*

NURSING RESEARCH   **Evidence-Based Practice for the Client with Skeletal Pins**

Clinical guidelines for specific client care interventions, such as skeletal pin care, should be based on research in order to provide the most appropriate evidence-based practice. The recommendations contained in this report from the National Association of Orthopaedic Nurses were made based on published research and are for skin care of areas surrounding the pin insertion sites. Data from the studies provided beginning guidelines, but were not conclusively useful as there were few experimental studies, and the studies were diverse in definitions and variables. However, the following recommendations were made:

- Pins located in areas with considerable soft tissue should be considered at greater risk for infection.
- After the first 48 to 72 hours (when drainage may be heavy), pin site care should be done daily or weekly for sites with mechanically stable bone–pin interfaces.
- Chlorhexidine (2 mg/mL) solution may be the most effective cleansing solution for pin site care.
- Clients and their families should be taught pin site care before discharge from the hospital. They should be required to demonstrate whatever care needs to be done and should be provided with written instructions that include signs and symptoms of infection.

IMPLICATIONS FOR NURSING
Evaluation of the literature by members of this expert panel found scanty evidence on which to base skeletal pin site interventions. The recommendations are therefore broadly stated, but do serve as a base for further research, which should examine factors such as defining pin site infection, risk for pin site infection, pin site care versus no pin site care, showering, managing crusts, skin adherence to the pins, and using dressings. The panel recommends that the guidelines should be individualized to each situation.

CRITICAL THINKING IN CLIENT CARE
1. List factors that may increase the risk for infection of skeletal pin sites. What nursing interventions may be used to reduce this risk?
2. You are caring for a client with skeletal pins for external fixation of a fracture of bones of a lower extremity. There is dried yellow drainage around the pin site. Based on clinical decision making without research to support your actions, would you remove the crusts? Why or why not?
3. You are teaching a client how to do pin care at home. Make a list of manifestations of infection the client may experience. What would you recommend if any of these manifestations occur?

Data from Holmes, S. B., & Brown, S. J. (2005). Skeletal pin site care. National Association of Orthopaedic Nurses guidelines for orthopaedic nursing. *Orthopaedic Nursing, 24*(2), 99–108.

- Monitor vital signs and lab reports of WBCs. *Increases in pulse rate, respiratory rate, temperature, and WBCs may indicate infection.*
- Use sterile technique for dressing changes. *The initial postoperative dressing will be changed by the surgeon. The nurse must change all subsequent dressings without introducing organisms into the operative site.*
- Assess the wound for size, color, and the presence of any drainage. *Redness, swelling, and purulent drainage indicate infection.*
- Administer antibiotics per physician's orders. *Prophylactic antibiotic administration inhibits bacterial reproduction and thereby helps prevent skin flora from entering the wound. In the case of "dirty wounds," such as those occurring from vehicular crashes, antibiotics are routinely administered.*

Impaired Physical Mobility

The client who has experienced a fracture requires immobilization of the fractured bone(s). Immobilization alters normal gait and mobility. The client will need to use assistive devices such as crutches, canes, slings, or walkers.

- Teach or assist client with ROM exercises of the unaffected limbs. *ROM exercises help prevent muscle atrophy and maintain strength and joint function. Flexion and extension exercises prevent the development of foot drop, wrist drop, or frozen joints.*
- Teach isometric exercises, and encourage the client to perform them every 4 hours. *Isometric exercises help prevent muscle atrophy and force synovial fluid and nutrients into the cartilage.*
- Encourage ambulation when able; provide assistance as necessary. *Ambulation maintains and improves circulation, helps prevent muscle atrophy, and helps maintain bowel function.*
- Teach and observe the client's use of assistive devices (such as canes, crutches, walkers, slings) in conjunction with the physical therapist. *Proper use of devices is necessary for safe ambulation and helps prevent the loss of joint function secondary to complications and falls.*
- Turn the client on bed rest every 2 hours. If the client is in traction, teach the client to shift his or her weight every hour. *Turning and shifting weight increase circulation and help prevent skin breakdown.*

Risk for Disturbed Sensory Perception: Tactile

The client who has sustained a fracture is at risk for nerve injury from the initial trauma, as well as from complications such as compartment syndrome.

- Assess the ability to differentiate between sharp and dull touch and the presence of paresthesias and paralysis every 1 to 2 hours. *Paresthesias develop as a result of pressure on nerves and may indicate compartment syndrome.*

PRACTICE ALERT

Paralysis is a late sign of nerve entrapment and requires that the physician be notified immediately.

- Elevate the injured extremity above the level of the heart. *Elevating the extremity decreases swelling and the risk of com-*

partment syndrome and nerve entrapment. Check the cast for fit. A tightly fitting cast can decrease blood flow to distal tissues, compress nerves, and cause compartment syndrome.

- Support the injured extremity above and below the fracture site when moving the client. *Supporting the injured extremity above and below the fracture site helps prevent displacement of bony fragments and decreases the risk of further nerve damage.*

Using NANDA, NIC and NOC

Chart 41–1 shows links between NANDA nursing diagnoses, NIC, and NOC when caring for the client with a compound fracture.

Community-Based Care

Client and family teaching focuses on individualized needs. The type of fracture and its location determine how much teaching the client and family will require. For example, a client who has a simple nondisplaced tibial fracture may need to be taught only cast care and crutch walking. An older client who has sustained a hip fracture and requires surgical intervention, by contrast, has a wider array of teaching needs, including the use of an abduction pillow, proper bending, and proper sitting. Address the following topics for home care of the client who has fractured a hip:

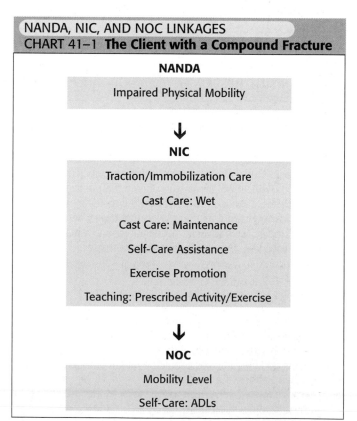

NANDA, NIC, AND NOC LINKAGES
CHART 41–1 The Client with a Compound Fracture

NANDA

Impaired Physical Mobility

↓

NIC

Traction/Immobilization Care

Cast Care: Wet

Cast Care: Maintenance

Self-Care Assistance

Exercise Promotion

Teaching: Prescribed Activity/Exercise

↓

NOC

Mobility Level

Self-Care: ADLs

Data from *NANDA's Nursing Diagnoses: Definitions & Classification 2005–2006* by NANDA International (2005), Philadelphia; *Nursing Interventions Classification (NIC)* (4th ed.) by J. M. Dochterman & G. M. Bulechek (2004), St. Louis, MO: Mosby; and *Nursing Outcomes Classification (NOC)* (3rd ed.) by S. Moorhead, M. Johnson, and M. Maas (2004), St. Louis, MO: Mosby.

- Encourage independence in ADLs:
  - Explain that the client should sit only on high chairs to prevent excess flexion of the hip; a high toilet seat can be added to a regular toilet seat.
  - Encourage the client and family to equip the shower with a rail to aid stability and prevent falls.
  - If a walker is needed, teach the client its proper use: Do not carry the walker, but lift it, advance it, and then take two steps, or use a rolling walker.
  - If a cane is needed, instruct the client to use it on the affected side.
- Stress the importance of well-balanced meals, and explain all prescribed medications.

Clients who have experienced a fracture or who have had orthopedic surgery often have a cast and require an extended period of immobilization or limited activities. Address the following topics for home care:

- Do not try to scratch under a cast with a sharp object.
- Do not get a plaster cast wet.
- Follow the physician's order for weight bearing.
- Physical therapy departments or offices often can evaluate the home environment for safety and suggest modifications as needed. Physical therapists also teach crutch walking, limited weight bearing, transferring, and other activities.
- Home care agencies can teach wound care and provide ongoing monitoring of wound healing.
- Local medical equipment and supply sources rent or sell durable equipment such as crutches, walkers, wheelchairs, overhead trapeze units, shower chairs, elevated toilet seats, grab bars, and bedside commodes. Slings or braces may be purchased through medical equipment dealers.
- Local pharmacies are good resources for dressing supplies such as antiseptic solutions or ointments, dressings, and tape.
- Fitness equipment suppliers may be able to provide rehabilitation equipment such as hand or ankle weights for strengthening exercises.

THE CLIENT WITH AN AMPUTATION

An **amputation** is the partial or total removal of an extremity. Amputation may be the result of an acute process, such as a traumatic event, or a chronic condition, such as peripheral vascular disease or diabetes mellitus. Regardless of the cause, an amputation is devastating to the client.

FAST FACTS

Amputation

- It is estimated that 350,000 people with amputations live in the United States, and that 135,000 new amputations occur each year.
- In the United States, the most common causes of lower extremity amputations are disease (70%), trauma (22%), congenital or birth defects (4%), and tumors (4%).
- Upper extremity amputation is usually due to trauma or birth defect.

Data from Moss Rehab Resource Net (2005).

The loss of all or part of an extremity has a significant physical and psychosocial effect on the client and family. Adaptation may take a long time and require much effort. Interdisciplinary health care is always important, but is especially necessary to meet the client's physical, spiritual, cultural, and emotional needs after an unexpected or planned amputation.

Causes of Amputation

Peripheral vascular disease (PVD) is the major cause of amputation of the lower extremities (see Chapter 35 ∞). Common risk factors for the development of PVD include hypertension, diabetes, smoking, and hyperlipidemia. Peripheral neuropathy also places the person with diabetes at risk for amputation. In peripheral neuropathy, loss of sensation frequently leads to unrecognized injury and infection. Untreated infection may lead to gangrene and the need for amputation. These risks are discussed in Chapter 20 ∞.

The incidence of traumatic amputations is highest among young men. Most amputations in this group result from motor vehicle crashes or accidents involving machinery at work. The client presents to the trauma center with an injury that may be life threatening; significant loss of blood and tissue may have already occurred, and shock may develop. (See Chapter 11 ∞ for a discussion of shock and trauma.) Other traumatic events that may necessitate an amputation are frostbite, burns, or electrocution.

Amputations result from or are necessitated by interruption in blood flow, either acute or chronic. In acute trauma situations, the limb is partially or completely severed, and tissue death ensues. However, replantation of fingers, small body parts, and entire limbs has been successful. In chronic disease processes, circulation is impaired, venous pooling begins, proteins leak into the interstitium, and edema develops. Edema increases the risk of injury and further decreases circulation. Stasis ulcers develop and readily become infected because impaired healing and altered immune processes allow bacteria to proliferate. The presence of progressive infection further compromises circulation and ultimately leads to gangrene (tissue death), which requires amputation.

Levels of Amputation

The level of amputation is determined by local and systemic factors. Local factors include ischemia and gangrene; system factors include cardiovascular status, renal function, and severity of diabetes mellitus. The goals are to alleviate symptoms, to maintain healthy tissue, and to increase functional outcome. When possible, the joints are preserved because they allow greater function of the extremity. Figure 41–12 ■ illustrates common sites of amputation.

Types of Amputation

Amputations may be open (*guillotine*) or closed (*flap*). Open amputations are performed when infection is present. The wound is not closed but remains open to drain. When infection is no longer present, surgery is performed to close the wound.

also be ordered to decrease the risk of peptic ulcer formation. Stool softeners may be administered to prevent constipation.

Prosthesis

The type of prosthesis selected for the client with an amputation depends on the level of the amputation as well as the client's occupation and lifestyle. Each prosthesis is based on a detailed prosthetic prescription and is custom made for the client based on the specific characteristics of the stump. Most are made of plastic and foam materials. Many factors influence the client's use of the prosthesis, including the status of the remaining limb, cognitive status, cardiovascular status, preoperative activity level, and motivation to use the prosthesis.

Clients with a lower extremity amputation are often fitted with early walking aids. Pneumatic devices that fit over the stump are used in the immediate postoperative period to allow early ambulation, decreased postoperative swelling, and improved morale. Clients may begin weight bearing as soon as 2 weeks after surgery. Clients with upper extremity amputations may be fitted for a prosthesis immediately after surgery. Rehabilitation of the client with an amputation is a team effort, involving the client, nurse, physician, physical therapist, occupational therapist, social worker, prosthetist, and vocational counselor.

NURSING CARE

Health Promotion

The goals of health promotion activities focus on preventing the progression of chronic diseases such as PVD and diabetes mellitus, and on safety. Clients with PVD from any cause need education about foot care and early recognition of decreased circulation. Education within both urban and rural populations should provide knowledge about working safely with lawn care equipment as well as farm and occupational machinery.

In addition, it is important that the public know what to do if a traumatic amputation occurs in the home, community, or workplace. The following guidelines may help preserve the amputated part until it can be surgically reattached:

- Keep the person in a prone position with the legs elevated.
- Apply firm pressure to the bleeding area, using a towel or article of clothing.
- Wrap the amputated part in a clean cloth. If possible, soak the cloth in saline (such as contact lens solution).
- Put the amputated part in a plastic bag and put the bag on ice. Do not let the amputated part come into direct contact with the ice or water.
- Send the amputated part to the emergency department with the injured person, and be sure the emergency personnel know what it is.

Assessment

Collect the following data through the health history and physical examination. Further focused assessments are described in the following nursing interventions sections.

- *Health History:* Mechanism of injury, current and past health problems, pain, occupation, ADLs, changes in sensation in

the feet, cultural and/or religious guidelines for handling the amputated part.
- *Physical Examination:* Bilateral neurovascular status of the extremities, bilateral capillary refill time, skin over the lower extremities (discoloration, edema, ulcerations, hair, gangrene).

Nursing Diagnoses and Interventions

The goals of nursing care for a person with an amputation are to relieve pain, promote healing, prevent complications, support the client and family during the process of grieving and adaptation to alterations in body image, and restore mobility. Care is individualized, and the circumstances that led to the amputation (e.g., traumatic injury or disease) also must be addressed. (See the accompanying Nursing Care Plan on page 1425.) Applying rehabilitation principles to nursing care is also important.

Acute Pain

Pain from the surgical procedure can be compounded by muscle spasms, swelling, and phantom limb pain.

- Ask the client to rate the pain on a scale of 0 to 10 (with 10 as the most severe pain) before and after any intervention. *This facilitates objective assessment of the effectiveness of the chosen pain relief strategy. Pain that increases in intensity or remains unrelieved with analgesics can indicate compartment syndrome.*
- Splint and support the injured area. *Splinting prevents additional injury by immobilizing the stump and decreasing edema while molding the stump for a good prosthetic fit.*
- Unless contraindicated, elevate the stump on a pillow for the first 24 hours after surgery. *Elevating the stump promotes venous return and decreases edema, which will decrease pain.*

> **PRACTICE ALERT**
> Elevating the stump for long periods after the immediate postoperative period increases the risk for hip contractures.

- Move and turn the client gently and slowly. *Gentle moving and turning prevents the development of severe muscle spasms.*
- Administer pain medications as prescribed. A PCA pump may be ordered by the physician. *Analgesics alleviate pain by stimulating opiate receptor sites. PCA pumps increase client control over and allow early relief of pain before it intensifies.*
- Encourage deep breathing and relaxation exercises. *These techniques increase the effectiveness of analgesics and modify the pain experience.*
- Reposition client every 2 hours; turn from side to side and onto abdomen. *Repositioning alleviates pressure from one area and distributes it throughout the body and helps prevent cramping of muscles.*

> **PRACTICE ALERT**
> Lying prone prevents hip contracture.

Risk for Infection

The client who has an amputation is at risk for wound infection. Early recognition of infection can lead to early treatment and prevent wound dehiscence.

NURSING CARE PLAN A Client with a Below-the-Knee Amputation

John Rocke is a 45-year-old divorcee with no children. He has a history of type 1 diabetes mellitus and poor control of blood glucose levels. Mr. Rocke is unemployed and currently receives unemployment compensation. He lives alone in a second-floor apartment. Mr. Rocke had developed gangrene in the foot and failed to seek prompt medical attention; as a result, a left below-the-knee amputation was necessary.

Mr. Rocke is in his second postoperative day and his vital signs are stable. The stump is splinted and has a soft dressing. The wound is approximating well without signs of infection. He has not performed ROM exercises or turning since his surgery, complaining of severe pain. When the nurse goes into the room, he yells, "Get out! I don't want anyone to see me like this." No one has visited him since his hospitalization. He is tolerating an 1800-kcal diabetic diet and is using a urinal independently. He has an order for meperidine (Demerol), 100 mg IM every 4 hours prn for pain, and cefazolin (Ancef), 1 g IV every 8 hours. He is on blood glucose coverage with regular insulin subcutaneously.

ASSESSMENT

Jane Simmons, RN, has just come on duty. She notes that the client is upset and angry. Mr. Rocke will not let anyone enter the room to give him medication or assess his vital signs.

DIAGNOSES

- *Disturbed Body Image* related to amputation of left lower leg
- *Dysfunctional Grieving* related to anger and loss of left lower leg
- *Situational Low Self-Esteem* related to appearance
- *Risk for Injury from Infection and Contractures* related to refusal of care
- *Acute Pain* related to surgery

EXPECTED OUTCOMES

- Verbalize his feelings about the amputation.
- Allow the staff to monitor his vital signs and administer medications.

- Be allowed to control his pain with a PCA pump.
- Verbalize a decrease in pain.
- Verbalize the importance of turning.
- Turn every 2 hours.

PLANNING AND IMPLEMENTATION

- Encourage verbalization of feelings.
- Actively listen to the client.
- Offer to arrange a visit with a fellow amputee.
- Ask the physician if the client can be placed on a PCA pump.
- Teach the client the importance of turning every 2 hours to prevent contractures.
- Encourage turning and lying prone
- Teach the importance of antibiotics in preventing and treating infection.

EVALUATION

One week after his surgery, Mr. Rocke is actively participating in his care. He has apologized for his behavior and has explained to Ms. Simmons that he was angry about the loss of his leg. He states, "I thought I knew what to expect but I didn't."

CRITICAL THINKING IN THE NURSING PROCESS

1. Once Mr. Rocke is ready to assist with his stump care, how would you proceed? Would you give him full responsibility for care and dressings, or would you gradually increase his participation? Why?
2. What factors in Mr. Rocke's home environment and medical history may make self-care more difficult? Do you expect Mr. Rocke to follow up on care after his discharge? Why or why not?
3. Mr. Rocke states, "Why should I exercise this leg—it was already cut off!" How would you respond? What is the purpose of exercising the stump?

See Evaluating Your Response in Appendix C.

- Assess the wound for redness, drainage, temperature, edema, and suture line approximation. *Redness is normal in the immediate postoperative period; if it persists, however, it can indicate infection. A hot area that is palpated over the incision or increased drainage may also indicate infection.*
- Take the client's temperature every 4 hours. *Increased body temperature may indicate infection.*
- Monitor WBC count. *The WBC count rises in the presence of infection.*
- Use aseptic technique to change the wound dressing. *Aseptic technique prevents the contamination of the wound with bacteria.*
- Administer antibiotics as ordered. *Antibiotics inhibit bacterial cell replication and help prevent or eradicate infection.*
- Teach the client stump-wrapping techniques. *Correctly wrapping the stump from the distal to proximal extremity increases venous return and prevents pooling of fluid, thereby reducing the chance of infection.*

Risk for Impaired Skin Integrity

Stump care is essential, not only in the postoperative healing period, but also throughout life with a prosthesis. A variety of skin problems may be caused by a prosthesis, including epidermoid cysts, abrasions, blisters, and hair follicle infections. The client must be taught stump care prior to discharge.

- Each day, preferably at night, wash the stump with soap and warm water and dry thoroughly. Inspect the stump for redness, irritation, or abrasions. *It is essential to maintain intact skin to ensure successful use of the prosthesis.*
- Massage the end of the stump, beginning 3 weeks after surgery. *Massage helps desensitize the remaining part of the limb and prevents scar tissue formation. If the skin adheres to the underlying tissue, it will tear when stressed by wearing a prosthesis.*
- Expose any open areas of skin on the remaining part of the limb for 1 hour four times a day. *Air exposure promotes healing.*

■ Change stump socks and elastic wraps each day. Wash these in mild soap and water, and allow to completely dry before using again. *Stump socks and elastic wraps must be kept clean and dry to prevent skin breakdown.*

Risk for Dysfunctional Grieving

The client who has lost an extremity is at risk for dysfunctional grieving. Denial of the need for surgery and the inability to discuss feelings compound this risk.

■ Encourage verbalization of feelings, using open-ended questions. *Asking open-ended questions allows the client to discuss feelings and communicates the listener's willingness to listen.*

■ Actively listen and maintain eye contact. *Active listening and eye contact communicate respect for what the client is expressing.*

■ Reflect on the client's feelings. *Reflection statements such as "You seem angry" allow the client to recognize feelings and perhaps develop a plan for resolution.*

■ Allow the client to have unlimited visiting hours, if possible. *Unlimited visiting hours allow increased social support.*

■ If desired by the client, provide spiritual support by encouraging activities such as visits from a spiritual leader, prayer, and meditation. *These activities often provide support during the grieving process.*

Disturbed Body Image

Although amputation is a reconstructive surgery, the client's body image will be disturbed. Risk for body image disturbance is higher in young trauma clients, in whom body image is a particularly important component of self-image.

■ Encourage verbalization of feelings. *This allows the client to communicate concerns and fears and lets the client know the nurse is willing to listen.*

■ Allow the client to wear clothing from home. *Familiar clothing provides emotional comfort and helps the client retain a sense of his or her own identity.*

■ Encourage the client to look at the stump. *Looking at and touching the stump helps the client face his or her fear of the unknown and move from denial to acceptance.*

■ Encourage the client to care for the stump. *Active participation in care increases self-esteem and independence.*

■ Offer to have a fellow amputee visit the client. *A support person who has experienced the same change gives the client the hope that he or she can regain independence.*

■ Encourage active participation in rehabilitation. *Active participation in rehabilitation increases independence and mobility.*

Impaired Physical Mobility

If time allows, the client should begin strengthening muscles preoperatively. If the amputation is the result of an emergency, exercises begin within 24 to 48 hours of surgery. The return of independent mobility boosts self-esteem and promotes adaptation to amputation.

■ Perform ROM exercises on all joints. *ROM exercises help prevent the development of joint contractures that limit mobility.*

■ Maintain postoperative stump shrinkage devices. These may be elastic bandages, shrinker socks, an elastic stockinette, or

a rigid plaster cast. *Postoperative dressings decrease edema and shape the stump for prosthetic wear.*

■ Turn and reposition the client every 2 hours. *The client with a lower extremity amputation should lie prone every 4 hours. Repositioning increases blood flow to muscles, forces synovial fluid into joints, and helps prevent contractures.*

■ Reinforce teaching by the physical therapist in crutch walking or the use of assistive devices. *These devices increase mobility by balancing the client and facilitating ambulation.*

■ Encourage active participation in physical therapy. *Physical therapy will fatigue the client in the early stage of healing. Encouragement may increase the client's participation in the physical therapy regimen and thereby increase activity tolerance.*

Using NANDA, NIC, and NOC

Chart 41–2 shows links between NANDA nursing diagnoses, NIC, and NOC when caring for the client with an amputation.

Community-Based Care

Client and family teaching includes stump care, prosthesis fitting and care, medications, assistive devices, exercises, rehabilitation, counseling, support services, and follow-up appointments. The depth of teaching depends on the cause and site of the amputation and the needs of the client. See the Meeting Individualized Needs box on the next page.

Holistic nursing care is especially important for the older client with an amputation. The normal aging process decreases

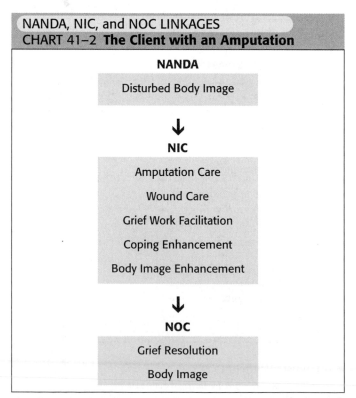

NANDA, NIC, and NOC LINKAGES
CHART 41–2 The Client with an Amputation

NANDA

Disturbed Body Image

↓

NIC

Amputation Care

Wound Care

Grief Work Facilitation

Coping Enhancement

Body Image Enhancement

↓

NOC

Grief Resolution

Body Image

Data from *NANDA's Nursing Diagnoses: Definitions & Classification 2005–2006* by NANDA International (2005), Philadelphia; *Nursing Interventions Classification (NIC)* (4th ed.) by J. M. Dochterman & G. M. Bulechek (2004), St. Louis, MO: Mosby; and *Nursing Outcomes Classification (NOC)* (3rd ed.) by S. Moorhead, M. Johnson, and M. Maas (2004), St. Louis, MO: Mosby.

MEETING INDIVIDUALIZED NEEDS   The Client with an Amputation

Amputation of a limb has significant long-term consequences for the client. The client will grieve the loss of a body part and must adjust to a new self-image. The client's ability to perform normal ADLs and to maintain his or her usual family and social roles may be significantly affected, at least initially. Depending on the client's occupation, job performance may be affected, necessitating a change of career.

The nurse may be responsible for involving multiple members of the healthcare team in the client's care and rehabilitation and coordinating their activities. Following an amputation, the client may need the services of any or all of the following:

- Social services to help with rehabilitative and financial arrangements
- Physical therapists to teach ambulation techniques, and to provide deep heat or massage
- Occupational therapists to assist the client in developing adaptive techniques to deal with the loss of a limb
- Prosthetists to develop a prosthesis for the missing limb that will meet the client's needs for ADLs and other activities
- Home health services for nursing care such as assessments and wound care
- Support group services to assist in adapting to the body image change and effects of amputation on ADLs.

ASSESSING FOR HOME CARE

Preparing the amputee for home care includes a careful assessment of the client family and support services, and the home for possible barriers to the client's safety and independence.

Assess the client's acceptance of the amputation and knowledge base about care needs, any activity restrictions or special needs, and resources for home care. Discuss home management—who is responsible for household activities such as cleaning and cooking. Inquire about arrangements that have been made for home care activities and ADLs. Evaluate the client's use of prescription and nonprescription medications, paying particular attention to possible in-

teractions and drugs that may affect the client's balance, mental alertness, or appetite. Ask about social habits, such as cigarette smoking, alcohol use, or other drug use, that may affect healing or the client's ability to provide self-care.

Assess the client's home environment for possible safety hazards or barriers to ambulation, such as:

- Scatter rugs
- Stairs between living areas of the house
- Presence of grab bars to facilitate toileting and bathing
- Access to clean water and other needs for wound care.

TEACHING FOR HOME CARE

The new amputee needs a great deal of teaching to learn to adapt to loss of a limb, whether it is an upper or lower extremity that has been lost. Because the client must be ready to learn before teaching can be effective, use therapeutic communication techniques to encourage the client to verbalize feelings about the amputation and its effects. Use active listening and teach the client ways to reduce anxiety and deal with feelings of helplessness and loss. Encourage the client to participate in care of the stump to build self-esteem and reinforce teaching. Include the following in teaching for home care:

- Teach the client to wrap the stump appropriately in preparation for fitting the prosthesis.
- Discuss positioning of the stump. Contractures are a particular problem for clients with an above-knee amputation, and can interfere with ability to effectively use a prosthesis.
- Teach the client how to perform stump exercises to maintain joint mobility and muscle tone of the affected limb.
- Encourage the client to resume physical activities as soon as possible. This improves the client's health and well-being, as well as the client's self-esteem.
- Discuss household modifications to promote independence, such as grab bars in the bathroom, faucets with single-handle controls for water flow and temperature, and handheld shower heads and shower chairs for bathing.

---

renal and liver function; hence, medications have longer half-lives. Altered circulation prolongs wound healing, and slowing of reflexes and alterations in gait may disrupt balance. A walker may be more appropriate than crutches, because older clients have less strength in the upper extremities. Safety issues, such as decreasing the risk for recurrent falls, must be addressed. The nurse should also assess the client's need for in-home assistance and make appropriate referrals to visiting nurses and home health aides.

In addition, suggest the following resources:

- The Amputee Coalition of America
- Amputee Resource Foundation of America.

THE CLIENT WITH A REPETITIVE USE INJURY

Repeatedly twisting and turning the wrist, pronating and supinating the forearm, kneeling, or raising arms over the head can result in repetitive use injuries. Clients with repetitive use injuries

pose a challenge to the healthcare team. Often these clients appear puzzled as they relate a history of manifestations that have worsened over time. They deny abrupt trauma and often worry about the ability to return to work. Repetitive use injuries are common. The number of worker's compensation claims for repetitive use injuries is steadily growing. The increase is believed to be a result of technology advances in the workplace.

Pathophysiology

Common repetitive use injuries include carpal tunnel syndrome, bursitis, and epicondylitis.

Carpal Tunnel Syndrome

The carpal tunnel is a canal through which flexor tendons and the median nerve pass from the wrist to the hand. The syndrome develops from narrowing of the tunnel and irritation of the median nerve. Carpal tunnel syndrome involves compression of the median nerve as a result of inflammation and swelling of the synovial lining of the tendon sheaths. The client complains of numbness and tingling of the thumb, index finger, and lateral ventral surface of the middle finger. The client may also complain of pain in this area that interferes with sleep and is alleviated by shaking or massaging the hand and fingers. The affected hand may become weak and the client may be unable to hold utensils or perform activities that require precision.

Carpal tunnel syndrome is one of the three most common work-related injuries. The incidence is believed to be related directly to the number of people using computers. The incidence of carpal tunnel syndrome is higher in women, especially postmenopausal women.

Bursitis

Bursitis is an inflammation of a bursa. A bursa is an enclosed sac found between muscles, tendons, and bony prominences. The bursae that commonly become inflamed are in the shoulder, hip, knee, and elbow. Constant friction between the bursa and the musculoskeletal tissue around it causes irritation, edema, and inflammation. Manifestations develop as the sac becomes engorged. The area around the sac is tender, and extension and flexion of the joint near the bursa produce pain. The inflamed bursa is hot, red, and edematous. The client guards the joint to decrease pain and may point to the area of the bursa when identifying joint tenderness.

Epicondylitis

Epicondylitis is the inflammation of the tendon at its point of origin into the bone. Epicondylitis is also referred to as *tennis elbow* or *golfer's elbow*. The exact pathophysiology of epicondylitis is unknown. Current theories attribute inflammation of the tendon to microvascular trauma. Tears, bleeding, and edema are thought to cause avascularization and calcification of the tendon. Manifestations of epicondylitis include point tenderness, pain radiating down the dorsal surface of the forearm, and a history of repetitive use.

INTERDISCIPLINARY CARE

Medical management of repetitive use disorders focuses on relieving pain and increasing mobility. Once the diagnosis is made, treatment can range from conservative measures, such as rest and pharmacologic agents, to aggressive measures such as surgery.

Diagnosis

Carpal tunnel syndrome is diagnosed by the client's history and physical examination. The history may reveal an occupation that involves areas such as computer work, jackhammer operation, mechanical work, or gymnastics. History of a radial bone fracture or rheumatoid arthritis also increases the risk of carpal tunnel syndrome. Tests specific for carpal tunnel include the Phalen test (see Chapter 40). Bursitis and epicondylitis are diagnosed by history and physical examination.

Medications

The client with a repetitive use injury usually receives NSAIDs. Narcotics also may be administered for acute flare-ups and severe pain. For the client who has epicondylitis or carpal tunnel syndrome, corticosteroids may be injected into the joint.

Treatments

Treatment of repetitive use injuries is performed first by conservative management, followed, if necessary, by surgery.

CONSERVATIVE MANAGEMENT The first steps in the care of all repetitive use injuries are to immobilize and rest the involved joint. The joint may be splinted, and ice may be applied (as described in Table 41–1) in the first 24 to 48 hours to decrease pain and inflammation. Ice application may be followed by heat application every 4 hours.

SURGERY Surgery is usually reserved for the client who does not obtain relief with conservative treatment. Surgery for carpal tunnel syndrome includes resection of the carpal ligament to enlarge the tunnel. In epicondylitis and bursitis, calcified deposits may be removed from the area surrounding the tendon or bursa.

NURSING CARE

The nursing care of a client with a repetitive use injury focuses on relieving pain, teaching about the disease process and treatment, and improving physical mobility.

Nursing Diagnoses and Interventions

Acute Pain

Swelling and nerve inflammation cause pain in the client with a repetitive use injury.

- Ask the client to rate the pain on a scale of 0 to 10 (with 10 being the most severe pain) before and after any intervention. *This facilitates objective assessment of the effectiveness of the chosen pain relief strategy.*
- Encourage the use of immobilizers. *Splinting maintains joint alignment and prevents pain due to movement of inflamed tissues.*
- Teach the client to apply ice and/or heat as prescribed. *Ice causes vasoconstriction and decreases the pooling of blood in the inflamed area. Ice may also numb the tender area. Heat decreases swelling by increasing venous return.*
- Encourage use of NSAIDs as prescribed. *NSAIDs decrease swelling by inhibiting prostaglandins.*
- Explain why treatment should not be abruptly discontinued. *Abrupt discontinuation of treatment may cause reinflammation of the injured area.*

Impaired Physical Mobility

Joint pain and swelling can impair mobility.

- Suggest interventions to alleviate pain (such as using an immobilizer and taking pain medications). *If the joint is pain free, the client will be more likely to take an active role in therapy.*
- Refer to a physical therapist for exercises. *The physical therapist can assist the client with exercise to prevent joint stiffness.*
- Suggest consultation with an occupational therapist. *Occupational therapy can help the client learn new ways to perform tasks to prevent recurring symptoms.*

Community-Based Care

Address the following topics for home care:

- Causes of and treatments for repetitive use injury.
- Rehabilitation to allow the client to return to a state of independence.
- Ways to avoid unnecessary exposure to the activities that increase risk of redeveloping the injury. Suggest evaluation of the client's work environment by an environmental risk manager who can prescribe measures to reduce the risk of repetitive use injuries. Wrist supports or an ergonomic keyboard may be useful for the client who uses a computer extensively. Appropriate desk and chair height also are important in maintaining the correct anatomic position while working.
- Information about sources for braces or other assistive devices.

EXPLORE MediaLink

Prentice Hall Nursing MediaLink DVD-ROM
  Audio Glossary
  NCLEX-RN® Review

  Animation/Video
  Bone Healing
  Crutch Instruction

COMPANION WEBSITE www.prenhall.com/lemone
  Audio Glossary
  NCLEX-RN® Review
  Care Plan Activity: Below-the-Knee Amputation
  Case Study: A Client with Fractures
  MediaLink Applications
    Compartment Syndrome
    Preventing Musculoskeletal Injuries
  Links to Resources

CHAPTER HIGHLIGHTS

- The most commonly reported musculoskeletal injuries are contusions, strains, and sprains. Immediate treatment includes RICE (rest, ice, compression, elevation) therapy.
- Dislocations may be congenital, traumatic, or pathologic. Nursing assessments include monitoring neurovascular status by assessing for increased pain, decreased or absent pulses, pale skin, inability to move a body part or extremity, and changes in sensation.
- Any of the 206 bones of the body may sustain a fracture. Fractures are closed or simple (skin is intact) or open or compound (skin integrity is interrupted); open fractures are at risk for infection. Other fracture descriptors include oblique or spiral, avulsed, comminuted, compressed, impacted, or depressed.
- Fractures heal through three phases: inflammatory, reparative, and remodeling. Healing is influenced by the age and physical condition of the client and by the type of fracture.
- Fracture complications include compartment syndrome, fat embolism syndrome, deep venous thrombosis, infection, delayed union and nonunion, and reflex sympathetic dystrophy.

- Fractures are treated with surgery, traction, and/or casts to stabilize the fractured bone, maintain bone immobilization, prevent complications, and restore function.
- Fractures of the hip are most often sustained by older adult women, and are usually the result of a fall. They are the most common injury in the older population, resulting in the greatest number of deaths and most serious health problems of all fractures for people age 65 years and older.
- Nursing care for the client with a fracture focuses on interventions for acute pain, risk for peripheral vascular dysfunction, risk for infection, impaired physical mobility, and risk for disturbed tactile sensory perception.
- An amputation is the partial or total removal of an extremity. This loss has a significant physical and psychosocial effect on the client and on the family. The most common cause for amputation of a lower extremity is peripheral vascular disease. Trauma is the most common cause for upper extremity amputation.
- Complications that may follow an amputation include infection, delayed healing, chronic stump pain, phantom pain, and

contractures. Stump care is necessary to prevent complications and to prepare the stump for a prosthesis.
- Nursing care for the client with an amputation is provided as part of the interdisciplinary team, and is focused on a return to functional health, with interventions to meet needs for acute pain,

impaired skin integrity, grieving, disturbed body image, and impaired physical mobility.
- Repetitive use injuries, especially common in the workplace, include carpal tunnel syndrome, bursitis, and epicondylitis.

TEST YOURSELF NCLEX-RN® REVIEW

1 You are teaching a young adult how to provide self-care for a sprained ankle. You explain that the reason for applying ice immediately after the injury is based on the principle that ice:
1. increases the diameter of blood vessels.
2. decreases the diameter of blood vessels.
3. is helpful in increasing white blood cells.
4. lowers the blood pressure and pulse.

2 A client with a compound, open fracture has been admitted to the emergency department and is scheduled for immediate surgery. Which of the following nursing diagnoses would be most appropriate in the immediate postoperative period?
1. *Risk for Post-Trauma Syndrome*
2. *Impaired Transfer Ability*
3. *Risk for Infection*
4. *Risk for Falls*

3 While providing care to an older woman with a cast on her left lower arm (from below the elbow to above the fingers), you perform a neurovascular assessment. Which of the following assessments indicates a possible complication?
1. slightly edematous fingers
2. warm, pink skin above the cast
3. pale, cold fingers
4. pain rating of 2 on a 1 to 10 scale

4 Which of the following minerals is essential to bone healing?
1. potassium
2. magnesium
3. sodium
4. calcium

5 You are assessing a young man with a newly applied long-leg cast. He complains of extreme pain in his leg, and his toes are cyanotic and lack sensation. What is your priority intervention?
1. Document the assessments carefully and accurately.
2. Notify the healthcare provider who applied the cast.
3. Elevate the leg on at least three pillows.
4. Apply an ice bag over the painful area.

6 Your assigned client has been diagnosed with DVT of the left lower extremity. What body system would require very careful monitoring?
1. hematologic
2. respiratory
3. digestive
4. renal

7 Although nursing diagnoses are always individualized, what is one nursing diagnosis common to all musculoskeletal injuries?
1. *Disturbed Body Image*
2. *Acute Pain*
3. *Chronic Pain*
4. *Risk for Infection*

8 At what position would you place the remaining extremity following a below-the-knee amputation during the first 24 hours after surgery?
1. elevated above the level of the heart
2. lower than the rest of the body
3. crossed over the intact extremity
4. level with the rest of the body

9 The day following a below-the-knee amputation, your client tells you that he feels as though his toes are cramping in the amputated foot. What is this experience called?
1. chronic stump pain
2. contractures
3. attention-seeking
4. phantom limb pain

10 Your husband is cutting wood with a circular saw. He suddenly screams that he has cut off his finger. What would you do with the amputated finger?
1. Don't worry about it; the important thing is to get him to the hospital.
2. Put it in a storage bag filled with warm water.
3. Tape it to his hand so the emergency personnel will know where it is.
4. Wrap it in a towel, put it in a plastic bag, and lay it on ice.

See Test Yourself answers in Appendix C.

BIBLIOGRAPHY

Altizer, L. (2003a). Forearm and humeral fractures. *Orthopaedic Nursing, 22*(4), 266–273.

_____. (2003b). Hand and wrist fractures. *Orthopaedic Nursing, 22*(3), 232–239.

_____. (2004a). Casting for immobilization. *Orthopaedic Nursing, 23*(2), 1135–1141.

_____. (2004b). Compartment syndrome. *Orthopaedic Nursing, 23*(6), 391–396.

Assessment of a limb in a cast. (2003). *Nursing Times, 99*(31), 27.

Bergland, A., & Wyller, T. (2004). Risk factors for serious fall related injury in elderly women living at home. *Injury Prevention, 10*(5), 308–313.

Bongiovanni, M., Bradley, S., & Kelley, D. (2005). Orthopedic trauma: Critical care nursing issues. *Critical Care Nursing Quarterly, 28*(1), 60–71.

Brunner, L., Eshilian-Oates, L. , & Kuo, T. (2003). Hip fractures in adults. *American Family Physician, 67*(3). Retrieved from http://www.aafp.org/afp/wooeoeow/53l7.html

Burgess, B., & Sennett, B. (2003). Traumatic shoulder instability: Nonsurgical management versus surgical intervention. *Orthopaedic Nursing, 22*(5), 345–352.

Centers for Disease Control and Prevention. (2005). Bone health. Retrieved from http://www.cdc.gov/nccdphp/dnpa/bonehealth/

Childs, S. (2003). Stimulators of bone healing: Biologic and biomechanical. *Orthopaedic Nursing, 22*(6), 421–428.

Cole, E. (2004). Assessment and management of the trauma patient. *Nursing Standard, 18*(41), 45–52, 54.

Clontz, A., Annonio, D., & Walker, L. (2004). Trauma nursing: Amputation. *RN, 67*(7), 38–44.

Davis, P. (2004). Venous thromboembolism prevention—an update. *Journal of Orthopaedic Nursing, 8*(1), 50–56.

Dochterman, J., & Bulechek, G. (2004). *Nursing interventions classification (NIC)* (4th ed.). St. Louis, MO: Mosby.

Feury, K. (2003). Injury prevention: Where are the resources? *Orthopaedic Nursing, 22*(2), 124–130.

Harris, H. (2004). Action stat. Fat embolism. *Nursing, 34*(6), 96.

Harvey, C. (2005). Wound healing. *Orthopaedic Nursing, 24*(2), 143–160.

Hip fracture. Information about a broken hip. (2004). Retrieved from http://orthopedics.about.com/cs/hipsurgery/a/brokenhip.htm

Holmes, S., & Brown, S. (2005). Skeletal pin site care. National Association of Orthopaedic Nurses guidelines for orthopaedic nursing. *Orthopaedic Nursing, 24*(2), 99–108.

Houghton, K., Peregrina, M., Gillies, D., & Herden, J. (2003). A small trial of the nursing care of patients immobilized with a Thomas splint. *Journal of Orthopaedic Nursing, 7*(4), 201–204.

Kasper, C., Talbot, L., & Gaines, J. (2002). Skeletal muscle damage and recovery. *AACN Clinical Issues: Advanced Practice in Acute and Critical Care, 13*(2), 237–241.

Kass-Wolff, J. (2004). Calcium in women: Healthy bones and much more. *Journal of Obstetrics, Gynecologic, and Neonatal Nursing, 33*(1), 21–33.

Little, D., & Alper, B. (2004). Ankle sprain. *Clinical Advisor, 7*(11), 56, 61–62.

Love, C. (2003). Carpal tunnel syndrome. *Journal of Orthopaedic Nursing, 7*(1), 33–42.

Mayo Clinic. (2006). *Dislocation; first aid.* Retrieved from http://health/first-aid-dislocation/FA0009www.mayoclinic.com

McConnel, E. (2002). Assessing neurovascular status in a casted limb. *Nursing, 32*(9), 20.

Miller, R. L. S. (2003). Reflex sympathetic dystrophy. *Orthopaedic Nursing, 22*(2), 91–101.

Moorhead, S., Johnson, M., & Maas, M. (2005). *Nursing outcomes classification (NOC)* (3rd ed.). St. Louis, Mo: Mosby.

Moss Rehab Resource Net. (2005). *Amputation fact sheet.* Retrieved from http://www.mossresourcenet.org/amputa.htm

_____. (2004). *Falls and hip fractures among older adults.* Retrieved from http://www.cdc.gov/ncipc/factsheets/falls.htm

National Center for Injury Prevention and Control. (2006). *Falls and hip fractures among older adults.* Retrieved from http://www.cdc.gov/ncipc/factsheets/falls.htm

National Institute of Arthritis and Musculoskeletal and Skin Diseases. (2004). *Questions and answers about sprains and strains.* Retrieved from http://www.niams.nih.gov/hi/topics/strain_sprain/strain_sprain.htm

NANDA International. (2005). *Nursing diagnoses: Definitions & classification 2005–2006.* Philadelphia: Author.

Porth, C. M. (2005). *Pathophysiology: Concepts of altered health states* (7th ed.). Philadelphia: Lippincott.

Proehl, J. (2004). Emergency. Accidental amputation: A frightening injury requiring quick action. *American Journal of Nursing, 104*(2), 50–53.

Reed, D. (2004). Understanding and meeting the needs of farmers with amputations. *Orthopaedic Nursing, 23*(6), 397–405.

Ruddick, S., & Scollen, C. (2003). Fracture prevention in the frail elderly. *Practice Nurse, 14*(8), 361–366.

Shannon, M., Wilson, B., & Stang, C. (2005). *Nurse's drug guide 2005.* Upper Saddle River, NJ: Prentice Hall.

Siddle, L. (2004). The challenge and management of phantom limb pain after amputation. *British Journal of Nursing, 13*(11), 664–667.

Taggart, H., Mincer, A., & Thompson, A. (2004). Caring for the orthopaedic patient who is obese. *Orthopaedic Nursing, 23*(3), 204–210.

Tierney, L., McPhee, S., & Papadakis, M. (Eds.). (2004). *Current medical diagnosis & treatment* (43rd ed.). Stamford, CT: Appleton & Lange.

Vestergaard, P., Emborg, C., Stoving, R., Hagen, C., Mosekilde, L., & Briken, K. (2003). Patients with eating disorders: A high-risk group for fractures. *Orthopaedic Nursing, 22*(5), 325–331.

Walls, M. (2002). Orthopedic trauma. *RN, 65*(7), 53–56.

Wilkinson, J. (2005). *Prentice Hall nursing diagnosis handbook with NIC interventions and NOC outcomes* (8th ed.). Upper Saddle River, NJ: Prentice Hall.

Wilson, B., Shannon, M., & Stang, C. (2005). *Prentice Hall nurse's drug guide 2005.* Upper Saddle River, NJ: Prentice Hall.

Young, T. (2004). The healing of amputation wounds. *Nursing Standard, 18*(45), 74, 76, 78.

CHAPTER 42 Nursing Care of Clients with Musculoskeletal Disorders

LEARNING OUTCOMES

- Explain the pathophysiology, manifestations, complications, interdisciplinary care, and nursing care of metabolic, degenerative, autoimmune, inflammatory, infectious, neoplastic, connective tissue, and structural musculoskeletal disorders.

- Compare and contrast the pathophysiology, manifestations, diagnosis, and treatments for osteoporosis, osteoarthritis, Paget's disease, and rheumatoid arthritis.

- Discuss the purposes, nursing implications, and health education for the client and family for medications used to treat osteoporosis, Paget's disease, gout, osteomalacia, osteoarthritis, rheumatoid arthritis, systemic lupus erythematosus, osteomyelitis, bone tumors, scleroderma, and low back pain.

- Describe the surgical procedures used to treat clients with arthritis.

CLINICAL COMPETENCIES

- Assess functional status of clients with musculoskeletal disorders, and monitor, document, and report abnormal manifestations.

- Use evidence-based research to assess clients at risk for osteoporosis and to evaluate the effectiveness of Internet use to teach older adults with rheumatoid arthritis.

- Determine priority nursing diagnoses, based on assessed data, to select and implement individualized nursing interventions for clients with musculoskeletal disorders.

- Administer topical, oral, and injectable medications used to treat musculoskeletal disorders knowledgeably and safely.

- Provide skilled care of clients having a surgical debridement for osteomyelitis and a total joint replacement.

- Integrate interdisciplinary care into care of clients with musculoskeletal disorders.

- Provide teaching appropriate for community-based self-care of musculoskeletal disorders.

- Revise plan of care as needed to provide effective interventions to promote, maintain, or restore functional health status to clients with musculoskeletal disorders.

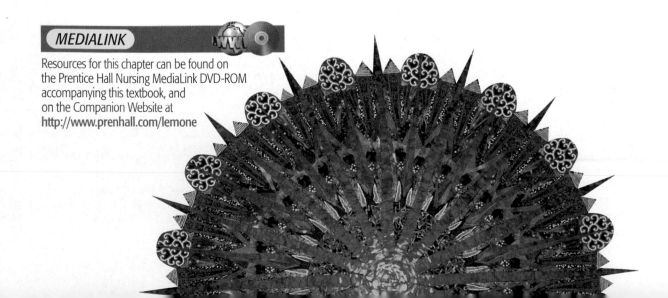

MEDIALINK

Resources for this chapter can be found on the Prentice Hall Nursing MediaLink DVD-ROM accompanying this textbook, and on the Companion Website at http://www.prenhall.com/lemone

ankylosing spondylitis (AS), *1469*
arthritis, *1433*
fibromyalgia, *1486*
gout, *1443*
Lyme disease, *1476*
muscular dystrophy (MD), *1458*
osteoarthritis (OA), *1449*
osteomalacia, *1447*

osteomyelitis, *1477*
osteoporosis, *1433*
Paget's disease, *1441*
polymyositis, *1476*
reactive arthritis (ReA), *1470*
rheumatic disorders, *1433*
rheumatoid arthritis (RA), *1459*
scleroderma, *1484*

septic arthritis, *1481*
Sjögren's syndrome, *1486*
systemic lupus
    erythematosus (SLE), *1471*
tophi, *1443*

Various metabolic, degenerative, autoimmune, inflammatory, infectious, neoplastic, connective tissue, and structural disorders may affect the musculoskeletal system. Many of these diseases have significant physical, psychosocial, and financial consequences. When these problems occur, clients experience a variety of individualized responses to their altered health status. Nursing care is directed toward meeting physiologic needs, providing education, and ensuring psychologic support for the client and family.

Arthritis refers to inflammation of the joints, while **rheumatic disorders** refer to diseases of the muscles and bones as well as the joints. These diseases affect not only the joints but also the connective tissues of the body. The various types of arthritis are discussed in this chapter in different sections, depending on the primary etiology of the disorder. Arthritis and other rheumatic disorders are widespread, affecting about 70 million people in the United States (Flynn & Johnson, 2005). Arthritic disorders are a leading cause of disability; however, their very prevalence may lead the public and healthcare professionals to treat them as normal aging processes or discount the validity of the pain and disability experienced by the person with arthritis.

There are more than 100 different types of arthritis, but the most common are osteoarthritis, rheumatoid arthritis, systemic lupus erythematosus, and gout (Moss Rehab Resource Net, 2005). The etiology of most rheumatic disorders is not clear; in many cases, the pathophysiologic processes involved are often complex and poorly understood. Many are primary disorders; others occur as secondary processes associated with another disease. The wear and tear of aging, autoimmune processes, metabolic disorders, genetic factors, and infection are also implicated as causative factors in some forms of rheumatic disease.

METABOLIC BONE DISORDERS

Metabolic bone disorders originate in the bone remodeling process, which normally involves a sequence of events of bone reabsorption and formation. In the adult, this process is primarily internal remodeling through replacement of trabecular bone. Adults replace about 25% of trabecular bone every 4 months through reabsorption of old bone by osteoclasts and formation of new bone by osteoblasts (Porth, 2005). Metabolic bone disorders may result from a variety of factors, including aging, calcium and phosphate imbalances, genetics, and changes in levels of hormones.

THE CLIENT WITH OSTEOPOROSIS

Osteoporosis, literally defined as "porous bones," is a metabolic bone disorder characterized by loss of bone mass, increased bone fragility, and an increased risk of fractures. The reduced bone mass is caused by an imbalance of the processes that influence bone growth and maintenance. Although osteoporosis may result from an endocrine disorder or malignancy, it is most often associated with aging.

The National Osteoporosis Foundation (2006) has found that osteoporosis is a health threat for an estimated 44 million Americans; 10 million people have osteoporosis and 34 million have low bone mass, increasing their risk for the disease. Although osteoporosis can occur at any age and in both men and women, 80% of those with osteoporosis are women. One in two women and one in four men over age 50 will have an osteoporosis-related fracture in his or her remaining lifetime.

Risk Factors

The risk of developing osteoporosis depends on how much bone mass is achieved between ages 25 and 35, and how much is lost later. Certain diseases, lifestyle habits, and ethnic backgrounds increase the risk of developing osteoporosis (see Focus on Cultural Diversity on page 1434). Different variables affect one's risk of osteoporosis—some can be modified and others cannot. The risk factors are summarized in Box 42–1.

BOX 42–1 Risk Factors for Osteoporosis

- A family history of osteoporosis
- Personal history of fracture after age 50
- Current low bone mass
- History of fracture in a first-degree relative
- Being female, especially Caucasian or Asian
- Being thin and/or having a small frame
- Menopause-associated low estrogen levels
- Low testosterone levels in men
- Dietary: low lifetime calcium intake, vitamin D deficiency
- Medication use: anticonvulsants, corticosteroids
- Lifestyle: inactivity, cigarette smoking, excess alcohol
- Presence of certain chronic diseases

Unmodifiable Risk Factors

Both men and women are susceptible to osteoporosis as they age, because the osteoblasts and osteoclasts undergo alterations that diminish their activity. Women have a significantly higher risk for manifestations and complications of osteoporosis because their peak bone mass is 10% to 15% less than that of men. In addition, age-related bone loss begins earlier and proceeds more rapidly in women, beginning in their 30s and accelerating before menopause. Estrogen in women and testosterone in men appear to help prevent bone loss; decreasing levels of these hormones associated with aging contribute to bone loss. Age-related bone loss in men occurs 15 to 20 years later than in women and at a slower rate.

European Americans and Asians are at a higher risk for osteoporosis than African Americans, who have greater bone density (bone mass positively correlates with the amount of skin pigmentation). Premature osteoporosis is increasing in female athletes, who have a greater incidence of eating disorders and amenorrhea. Poor nutrition and intense physical training can result in a deficient production of estrogen. Decreased estrogen, combined with a lack of calcium and vitamin D, results in a loss of bone density (Porth, 2005).

Clients who have an endocrine disorder such as hyperthyroidism, hyperparathyroidism, Cushing's syndrome, or diabetes mellitus are at high risk for osteoporosis. These disorders affect the metabolism, in turn affecting nutritional status and bone mineralization.

Modifiable Risk Factors

Modifiable risk factors include behaviors that place a person at risk for developing osteoporosis, as well as physical changes such as menopause whose contribution to osteoporosis can be modified by preventive strategies. Calcium deficiency is an important modifiable risk factor contributing to osteoporosis. Calcium is an essential mineral in the process of bone formation and other significant body functions. When there is an insufficient intake of calcium in the diet, the body compensates by removing calcium from the skeleton, weakening bone tissue. Acidosis, which may result from a high-protein diet, contributes to osteoporosis in two ways. Calcium is withdrawn from the bone as the kidneys attempt to buffer the excess acid. Acidosis also may directly stimulate osteoclast function. A high intake of diet soda with a high phosphate content also can deplete calcium stores.

With menopause and decreasing estrogen levels, bone loss accelerates in women. Estrogen promotes the activity of osteoblasts, increasing new bone formation. In addition, estrogen enhances calcium absorption and stimulates the thyroid gland to secrete calcitonin, a hormone that suppresses osteoclast activity and increases osteoblast activity.

Both cigarette smoking and excess alcohol intake are risk factors for osteoporosis. Smoking decreases the blood supply to bones. Nicotine slows the production of osteoblasts and impairs the absorption of calcium, contributing to decreased bone density. Alcohol has a direct toxic effect on osteoblast activity, suppressing bone formation during periods of alcohol intoxication. In addition, heavy alcohol use may be associated with nutritional deficiencies that contribute to osteoporosis. Interestingly, moderate alcohol consumption in postmenopausal women actually may increase bone mineral content, possibly by increasing levels of estrogen and calcitonin.

Sedentary lifestyle is another modifiable risk factor that can cause osteoporosis. Weight-bearing exercise, such as walking, influences bone metabolism in several ways. The stress of this type of exercise causes an increase in blood flow to bones, which brings growth-producing nutrients to the cells. Walking causes an increase in osteoblast growth and activity.

Prolonged use of medications that increase calcium excretion, such as aluminum-containing antacids and anticonvulsants, increase the risk of developing osteoporosis. Heparin therapy increases bone resorption, and its prolonged use is associated with osteoporosis. Antiretroviral therapy for people with AIDS or HIV infection may cause decreased bone density and osteoporosis (Porth, 2005).

Anyone who takes a glucocorticoid medication for more than 3 months is at risk for glucocorticoid-induced osteoporosis. These medications, often prescribed to control many rheumatic diseases, include prednisone (Deltasone, Orasone), prednisolone (Prelone), dexamethasone (Decadron, Hexadrol), and cortisone (Cortisone Acetate). These medications can directly affect bone cells, slowing the rate of bone formation. They also interfere with how the body uses calcium and affect levels of sex hormones, leading to bone loss. Problems that result, such as an increased possibility of fractures, can be prevented by taking a daily regimen of calcium supplements with added vitamin D and one multivitamin (American College of Rheumatology [ACR], 2004a).

Pathophysiology

Although the exact pathophysiology of osteoporosis is unclear, it is known to involve an imbalance of the activity of osteoblasts that form new bone and osteoclasts that resorb bone. Until age 35, when peak bone mass occurs, formation occurs more rapidly than does reabsorption. After peak bone mass is achieved, slightly more is lost than is gained (about 0.3% to 0.5% per year); this loss is accelerated if the diet is deficient in vitamin D and calcium. In women, bone loss increases after menopause (with loss of estrogen), then slows but does not stop at about age 60. Older women may have lost between 35% and 50% of their bone mass, older men may have lost between 20% and 35% (Mayo Clinic, 2002).

Osteoporosis affects the diaphysis (shaft of the bone) and the metaphysis (portion of the bone between the diaphysis and the epiphysis). The diameter of the bone increases, thinning the outer supporting cortex. As osteoporosis progresses, trabeculae are lost from cancellous bone (the spongy tissue of bone), and the outer cortex thins to the point that even minimal stress will fracture the bone (Porth, 2005).

Manifestations

The most common manifestations of osteoporosis are loss of height, progressive curvature of the spine, low back pain, and fractures of the forearm, spine, or hip. Osteoporosis is often called the "silent disease," because bone loss occurs without symptoms.

The loss of height occurs as vertebral bodies collapse. Acute episodes generally are painful, with radiation of the pain around the flank into the abdomen. Vertebral collapse can occur with little or no stress; minimal movements such as bending, lifting, or jumping may precipitate the pain. In some clients, vertebral collapse may occur slowly, accompanied by little discomfort. Along with loss of height, characteristic dorsal kyphosis and cervical lordosis develop, accounting for the "dowager's hump" often associated with aging. The abdomen tends to protrude and knees and hips flex as the body attempts to maintain its center of gravity (Figure 42–1 ■).

Complications

Fractures are the most common complication of osteoporosis, with the disease being responsible for more than 1.5 million fractures each year. These include 700,000 vertebral compression fractures, 300,000 hip fractures, 250,000 wrist fractures, and 300,000 fractures at other sites (National Osteoporosis Foundation, 2006). There may be no obvious manifestations of osteoporosis until fractures occur. Some fractures are spontaneous; others may result from everyday activities. While wrist and vertebral fractures have not been shown to increase disability or mortality, persistent pain and associated posture changes may restrict the client's activities or interfere with activities of daily living (ADLs).

INTERDISCIPLINARY CARE

Care of the client with osteoporosis focuses on stopping or slowing the process, alleviating the symptoms, and preventing complications. Proper nutrition and exercise are important components of the treatment program.

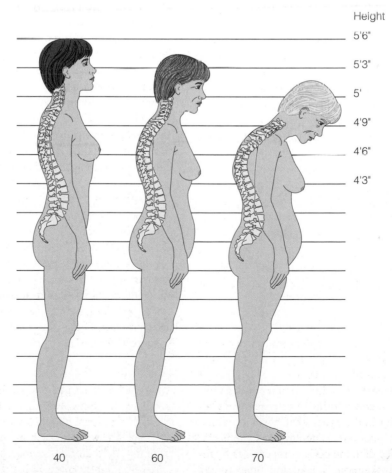

Figure 42–1 ■ Spinal changes caused by osteoporosis. As the condition progresses, height can be reduced by as much as 7 inches.

Diagnosis

The manifestations of osteoporosis can mimic those of other bone disorders, so diagnostic tests are needed to differentiate osteoporosis from other problems.

Dual-energy x-ray absorptiometry (DEXA) measures bone density in the lumbar spine or hip and is considered to be highly accurate. Ultrasound transmits painless sound waves through the heel of the foot to measure bone density. This 1-minute test is not as sensitive as DEXA, but is accurate enough for screening purposes. These tests are described in Chapter 40 ∞.

Laboratory tests include alkaline phosphatase (AST), which may be elevated following a fracture, and serum bone Gla-protein (osteocalcin), which can be used as a marker of osteoclastic activity and therefore is an indicator of the rate of bone turnover. This test is most useful to evaluate the effects of treatment, rather than as an indicator of the severity of the disease. A comparison of laboratory tests for metabolic bone diseases is outlined in Table 42–1.

Medications

Estrogen replacement therapy reduces bone loss, increases bone density in the spine and hip, and reduces the risk of fractures in postmenopausal women. It is particularly recommended for women who have undergone surgical menopause before age 50, and often is prescribed for women with other osteoporosis risk factors. Estrogen therapy alone is associated with an increased risk of endometrial cancer, so it usually is prescribed in combination with progestin (hormone replacement therapy or HRT). The choice of using HRT to prevent osteoporosis is one that must be made between the woman and her healthcare provider.

Raloxifene (Evista) is a selective estrogen receptor modulator (SERM) that appears to prevent bone loss by mimicking estrogen's beneficial effects on bone density in postmenopausal women. It does not have the risks of estrogen. Hot flashes are a common side effect, and this drug should not be taken by a woman with a history of blood clots.

Alendronate (Fosamax) and risedronate (Actonel) are from the class of drugs known as bisphosphonates. Bisphosphonates are potent inhibitors of bone resorption that may be used to prevent and treat osteoporosis. They inhibit bone breakdown, preserve bone mass, and increase bone density in the hip and vertebrae. Alendronate is especially useful for men and young adults and to prevent or treat glucocorticoid-induced osteoporosis. The nursing implications of bisphosphonates are found in the Medication Administration box on page 1437. Teriparatide (Forteo) is a synthetic parathyroid hormone, administered subcutaneously to stimulate new bone formation and mass. It is used to decrease the risk of bone fracture from osteoporosis in postmenopausal women and in men with primary or secondary hypogonadism.

Ibandronate sodium (Boniva) is the first monthly osteoporosis medication to be approved by the U.S. Food and Drug Administration (FDA). It is used for both treatment and prevention of postmenopausal osteoporosis, and reduces the number of vertebral fractures in women with osteoporosis as well as increases bone density in women who do not have the disease.

Calcitonin (Miacalcin) is a hormone that increases bone formation and decreases bone resorption. Calcitonin increases spinal bone density and reduces the risk of compression fractures; it may reduce the risk of hip fracture as well. Calcitonin usually is prescribed as a nasal spray, although it also is available in parenteral form. Because calcitonin is a protein, it can precipitate anaphylactic-type allergic responses.

Sodium fluoride stimulates osteoblast activity, increasing bone formation. When used to treat osteoporosis, bone mass of the spine increases and the risk of spinal fractures may be reduced. Fluoride therapy may, however, be associated with an increased risk of hip and other nonvertebral fractures.

Medications being investigated include vitamin D metabolites and other bisphosphonates and SERMS. See the Medication Administration Box on page 1437 for information about calcium, calcitonin, and fluoride.

TABLE 42–1 Differential Features of Osteoporosis, Osteomalacia, and Paget's Disease

DIFFERENTIATING FEATURES	OSTEOPOROSIS	OSTEOMALACIA	PAGET'S DISEASE
Pathophysiology	Resorption greater than bone formation	Inadequate mineralization of bone matrix	Excessive osteoclastic activity and formation of poor-quality bone
Calcium level (serum)	Normal	Low or normal	Normal or elevated (especially in immobilized clients)
Phosphate level (serum)	Normal	Low or normal	Normal
Parathyroid hormone level (serum)	Normal	High or normal	Normal
Alkaline phosphatase level (serum)	Normal	Elevated	Increased; not a reliable test for clients who have liver disease or are pregnant
Hydroxyproline (urine)	Not applicable	Not applicable	Increased
Radiographic findings	Osteopenia, fractures	Decreased bone density, radiolucent bands known as Looser's zones, or pseudofractures	"Punched-out" appearance of bone, increase in bone thickness, linear fractures, mosaic pattern of bone matrix

MEDICATION ADMINISTRATION   The Client with Osteoporosis

CALCIUM

Postmenopausal women, regardless of whether they take replacement estrogens, are encouraged to take calcium to prevent osteoporosis.

Nursing Responsibilities

- Help clients maintain an adequate dietary intake of calcium. The best dietary source is milk and other dairy products, including yogurt.
- Postmenopausal women who take estrogens need 1000 mg of calcium daily. Those who do not take estrogens need about 1500 mg daily to minimize osteoporosis.
- Identify alternate sources, such as skim milk and low fat yogurt, oysters, canned sardines or salmon, beans, cauliflower, and dark-green leafy vegetables.

Health Education for the Client and Family

- Take calcium carbonate in divided doses 30 to 60 minutes before meals to allow for absorption.
- Take calcium citrate with meals to minimize gastrointestinal distress.

CALCITONIN
Calcitonin-salmon injection, synthetic
Calcimar
Miacalin (injection or nasal spray)

In postmenopausal osteoporosis, calcitonin prevents further bone loss and increases bone mass if the client consumes adequate amounts of calcium and vitamin D. Calcitonin may be used in postmenopausal women who cannot or will not take estrogen.

Nursing Responsibilities

- Calcitonin is protein in nature; both the parenteral and nasal spray forms may cause an anaphylactic-type allergic response. Observe the client for 20 minutes after administration; have appropriate emergency equipment and drugs available to treat anaphylaxis.
- Alternate nostrils daily when administering calcitonin nasal spray.
- Review medical history for conditions that contraindicate use of calcitonin products: hypersensitivity to salmon calcitonin and lactation (calcitonin is secreted in breast milk and may inhibit lactation).
- Observe for side effects: nausea and vomiting, anorexia, mild transient flushing of the palms of the hands and the soles of the feet, and urinary frequency.
- Teach the client the proper technique for handling and injecting the drug at home.

Health Education for the Client and Family

- Take the medication in the evening to minimize side effects.
- Warm nasal spray to room temperature before using.
- Rhinitis (runny nose) is the most common side effect with calcitonin nasal spray. Other possible side effects include sores, itching, or other nasal symptoms. Report nosebleeds to your primary care provider.
- Nausea and vomiting may occur during initial stages of therapy; they disappear as treatment continues.
- While taking the medication, be sure to consume adequate amounts of calcium and vitamin D.

FLUORIDE

Fluoride is a mineral long recognized as essential for the normal formation of dentin and tooth enamel. Fluoride appears to decrease the solubility of bone mineral and therefore the rate of bone reabsorption. Its use in preventing and treating osteoporosis is relatively new but promising.

Nursing Responsibilities

- Monitor serum fluoride levels every 3 months.
- Have bone mineral density studies conducted at 6-month intervals to document progress of bone growth.

Health Education for the Client and Family

- Take sodium fluoride tablets after meals, and avoid milk or dairy products; these reduce gastrointestinal absorption of the medication.
- While taking fluoride, be sure to maintain an adequate calcium intake.
- Use fluoride mouth rinse immediately after brushing teeth and just before retiring at night. Do not swallow the rinse, and avoid eating or drinking for at least 30 minutes after use.
- Notify the physician if teeth become stained or mottled after repeated use of fluoride mouth rinse.

NURSING CARE

Osteoporosis is both preventable and treatable; therefore, nursing care focuses primarily on planning and implementing interventions to prevent the disease, its manifestations, and the resulting injuries. An important aspect of preventing osteoporosis is educating clients under age 35. A Nursing Care Plan for a client with osteoporosis is found on page 1438.

Health Promotion

Health promotion activities to prevent or slow osteoporosis focus on calcium intake, exercise, and health-related behaviors.

Nutrition

For clients of all ages, stress the importance of maintaining a daily calcium intake that meets National Institutes of Health (NIH) recommendations (see Chapter 10 ∞). This is particularly important for adolescent girls and young adult women who may avoid eating many high-calcium foods such as dairy products because of concerns about weight. Optimal calcium intake before ages 30 to 35 probably increases peak bone mass. Emphasize that low-fat (or nonfat) dairy products also contain calcium, although some fat in the product may enhance calcium absorption.

Milk and milk products are the best sources of calcium. The lactose in milk facilitates calcium absorption as well. Other food sources of calcium include sardines, clams, oysters, and salmon, as well as dark green, leafy vegetables such as broccoli, collard greens, bok choy, and spinach. For clients who avoid dairy products because of lactose intolerance or a vegetarian diet, suggest alternate sources.

NURSING CARE PLAN   A Client with Osteoporosis

Nancy Bauer is a 53-year-old schoolteacher. She has been married for 36 years and has two children. Mrs. Bauer is 65 inches tall. She has smoked one pack of cigarettes a day for 30 years and drinks one to two glasses of wine with dinner each evening. She does not routinely exercise. Mrs. Bauer has had symptoms of menopause for 8 years, including hot flashes in the early years and mood swings of late. She has never been on hormone replacement therapy.

Mrs. Bauer is currently seeking medical advice for continuous low back pain. The pain is not relieved with an over-the-counter analgesic, and she frequently wakes up during the night because of the pain. She is diagnosed with osteoporosis.

ASSESSMENT

The nurse practitioner notes that Mrs. Bauer's vital signs are within normal limits. She has full range of motion of all extremities and is able to stand and bend over, but she reports discomfort when returning to the upright position. Mrs. Bauer has a slightly pronounced "hump" on her upper back and is 1 inch shorter than her stated height on admission. Her muscle strength is symmetric and strong.

DIAGNOSIS

- *Acute Pain* of the lower spine related to vertebral compression
- *Deficient Knowledge* related to osteoporosis and treatment to prevent further damage
- *Imbalanced Nutrition: Less than Body Requirements* related to inadequate intake of calcium
- *Risk for Injury* related to effects of change in bone structure secondary to osteoporosis

EXPECTED OUTCOMES

- Verbalize a decrease in back pain.
- Be able to describe ways to treat her osteoporosis and prevent further complications.
- Verbalize an understanding of the current research and treatment regarding osteoporosis.
- Verbalize how stopping smoking can help prevent further progression of osteoporosis.
- Seek consultation for supplements and medications to prevent further bone loss.
- Design a program of physical activity to prevent complications of osteoporosis.
- Verbalize safety precautions to prevent fractures due to falls.

PLANNING AND IMPLEMENTATION

- Teach back strengthening exercises.
- Refer to an osteoporosis support group, if available.
- Provide realistic, yet optimistic, feedback about loss of height and bone integrity and the potential outcomes of treatment.
- Assess current knowledge base, and correct misconceptions regarding treatment of osteoporosis.
- Provide current educational literature regarding treatment of osteoporosis.
- Instruct in dietary and calcium supplements that help prevent effects of osteoporosis.
- Discuss physical exercises that help prevent complications due to osteoporosis.
- Review safety and fall precautions, and provide literature regarding how to create a safe home environment.

EVALUATION

On her return visit 6 months later, Mrs. Bauer reports that she feels much better. She is no longer irritable and does not experience mood swings, because she has been taking her prescribed hormone replacements for 6 months: She is eating products rich in calcium and taking a daily supplement of calcium with vitamin D. Mrs. Bauer has reduced her wine intake to one glass in the evening and now drinks decaffeinated coffee and tea. She also states that since she stopped smoking, she has been walking 30 to 45 minutes every day.

CRITICAL THINKING IN THE NURSING PROCESS

1. What is the rationale for stopping smoking and limiting caffeine and alcohol intake in the treatment of osteoporosis?
2. What foods would you encourage for clients at high risk for osteoporosis whose serum cholesterol and LDL/HDL ratios indicate a high risk for cardiovascular disease?
3. What physical activities would you consider beneficial in helping to prevent the effects of osteoporosis in the female client who is wheelchair bound or has limited mobility?
4. Develop a care plan for Mrs. Bauer for the nursing diagnosis *Risk for Trauma*

See Evaluating Your Response in Appendix C.

Calcium supplements are available in many forms. Most supplements (including Tums) provide calcium carbonate in the range of 200 to 600 mg per tablet. Other forms of calcium, including citrate, gluconate, and lactate, generally provide a lower amount of elemental calcium per tablet. A combination of calcium with vitamin D is recommended, particularly for older adults who may have a vitamin D deficiency that impairs their ability to absorb and use calcium.

Exercise

Teach clients the importance of physical activity and weight-bearing exercises in preventing and slowing bone loss. Suggest that clients participate in regular exercise such as walking for at least 20 minutes four or more times a week. Inform clients that swimming and pool aerobic exercises are not as beneficial for maintaining bone density because of the lack of weight-bearing activity.

Healthy Behaviors

Behaviors that help prevent osteoporosis include not smoking, avoiding excessive alcohol intake, and limiting caffeine intake to two or three cups of coffee each day.

Assessment

Collect the following data through the health history and physical examination (see Chapter 40 ∞):
- *Health History:* Age, risk factors, history of fractures, smoking history, alcohol intake, medications, usual diet, menstrual

history including menopause, usual exercise/activity level (see the Nursing Research box below), low back pain.

- *Physical Examination:* Height, spinal curves.

Nursing Diagnoses and Interventions

Nursing care of clients who have osteoporosis focuses on teaching about the disease process, helping maintain physical mobility and nutrition, and solving problems associated with pain and injury.

Health-Seeking Behaviors

At multiple points in the client's lifetime, nurses can provide vital information that will help clients use self-care strategies to reduce their risk of developing osteoporosis:

- Assess the client's health habits, including diet, exercise, smoking, and alcohol use. *The risk of developing osteoporosis in later life is affected by such things as diet, regular participation in weight-bearing exercise, and personal habits such as smoking and alcohol consumption.*
- Teach women and men of all ages the importance of maintaining an adequate calcium intake. Provide a list of calcium-rich foods, and discuss the use of calcium supplements with clients who do not consume adequate dietary calcium. *Calcium needs vary during the course of a lifetime; however, many clients never consume adequate amounts of calcium. This affects their peak bone mass and the rate of bone loss with aging. Calcium in foods is more completely absorbed than that supplied by calcium supplements.*
- Discuss the importance of maintaining a regular schedule of weight-bearing exercise, either through an exercise program or regular physical activity. *Weight-bearing exercise promotes osteoblast activity, helping maintain bone strength and integrity.*
- Refer clients to smoking-cessation programs and alcohol treatment programs as appropriate. *Smoking interferes with*

estrogen's protective effects on bones, promoting bone loss. Excess alcohol intake affects the nutritional status of the client, increasing the risk of calcium and vitamin D deficiency.

- Refer clients with significant risk factors for osteoporosis to primary care providers or clinics for bone-density evaluation. *Early identification and treatment of osteoporotic changes in bones can reduce the risk and possible long-term consequences of falls and fractures.*

Risk for Injury

Falls that would result in little or no injury in the healthy adult may cause fractures in the client with osteoporosis. Even normal movements such as twisting, bending, lifting, or rising from bed can precipitate a vertebral fracture.

- Implement safety precautions as necessary for the client who is hospitalized or in a long-term care facility. Maintain the bed in low position; use side rails if indicated to prevent the client from getting up alone; provide nighttime lighting to toilet facilities. *Most falls are preventable, particularly in hospitals and long-term care facilities.*
- Avoid using restraints (if hospitalized or a resident in a long-term care facility) if at all possible. *Restraints may actually increase the client's risk of falling and increase the risk of injury associated with a fall.*

PRACTICE ALERT

Clients may fracture osteoporotic bones when pulling against restraints.

- Teach clients who are able to participate in weight-bearing exercises to perform exercises at least three times a week for a sustained period of 30 to 40 minutes. The mechanical force of weight-bearing exercises promotes bone growth. *Bones weaken and demineralize without exercise. Walking is an*

NURSING RESEARCH   Evidence-Based Practice for the Client with Osteoporosis

Osteoporosis is a major health problem in the United States. Risk factors for osteoporosis include being white, having a small body frame, not doing weight-bearing exercises, and having a family history of osteoporosis. Nursing can do much to prevent the development of osteoporosis by assessing risk factors and teaching about diet, exercise, and lifestyle. A study by Schoen (2004) was conducted to determine the validity of items on a risk assessment screening questionnaire called the Osteoporosis Risk Assessment Tool (ORAT).

IMPLICATIONS FOR NURSING

Assessment is a critical component of the nursing process, enabling nurses to identify clients at risk for diseases, to monitor ongoing interventions, and to design teaching specific to client needs. Based on review of items contained in the ORAT, the following were retained: age, gender, body mass index, previous fractures, diagnosis of thyroid disease, use of thyroid replacement medication, estrogen replacement therapy, weight-bearing exer-

cise, family history of fractures, age at onset of menopause, use of calcium supplements, diet of calcium-rich foods, and alcohol and tobacco use. This tool is a useful means of quickly assessing clients for osteoporosis risk factors and for identifying and teaching about the prevention, diagnosis, treatment, and complications of osteoporosis.

CRITICAL THINKING IN CLIENT CARE

1. At what age do women develop maximum bone mass? (Review information in a text or on the Internet.) Based on this information, what type of teaching would be most effective?
2. Compare and contrast your teaching for a 24-year-old black woman who has a calcium-poor diet but is a nonsmoker and a thin, white 64-year-old woman who is postmenopausal and smokes.
3. While screening clients in a clinic for health risks, including osteoporosis, a man in his 70s says "Oh, I can't have bad bones . . . I'm a man!" How would you respond?

Data from Schoen, D. C. (2004). Osteoporosis. *Orthopaedic Nursing, 23*(4), 261–267.

easy, low-impact form of exercise. Swimming (including walking on the bottom of the pool) does not provide the needed weight-bearing activity.

■ Encourage older adults to use assistive devices to maintain independence in ADLs. *Walking sticks, canes, and other assistive devices encourage client independence and support activities that promote bone growth.*

■ Teach older clients about safety and fall precautions. *An assessment of the client's home for safety and fall risks may reduce the risk of fractures and, in turn, the cost of hospitalization and potential disability and/or death.*

Imbalanced Nutrition:
Less than Body Requirements

Most Americans do not maintain their recommended daily intake of calcium. Clients must therefore be made aware of the relationship between an adequate calcium intake and maintaining strong bones.

■ Teach adolescents, pregnant or lactating women, and adults through age 35 to eat foods high in calcium and to maintain a daily calcium intake of 1200 to 1500 mg. *The NIH recommends a daily calcium intake of 1200 to 1500 mg per day for adolescents and young adults, as well as for pregnant and lactating women.*

■ Encourage postmenopausal women to maintain a calcium intake of 1000 to 1500 mg daily, either through diet or a calcium supplement. *Calcium needs for postmenopausal women vary, depending on age.*

■ Teach clients taking calcium supplements the importance of taking the medication at the proper time and the side effects that may occur. *Free hydrochloric acid is needed for calcium absorption. Calcium carbonate supplement (e.g., Tums) should be taken 30 to 60 minutes before meals to allow adequate absorption. Calcium citrate supplements should be taken with meals to prevent gastrointestinal distress.*

PRACTICE ALERT
Calcium supplements should be taken in divided doses (two to three times daily) for improved distribution.

Acute Pain

Advanced stages of osteoporosis can result in pain and immobilization. Acute pain usually results from a complicating fracture, especially a compression fracture of the vertebrae.

■ Suggest anti-inflammatory pain medications for treatment of both acute and chronic phases of pain. Clients should be instructed in the amount and frequency as noted on the manufacturer's labels. *Continuous administration of ibuprofen or other nonsteroidal anti-inflammatory, drugs (NSAIDs) can be useful to provide relief from pain, but clients must be cautioned not to exceed dosage recommendations.*

PRACTICE ALERT
Teach clients on long-term anti-inflammatory medications to watch for bright red bleeding from the stomach (in vomitus) or dark black bowel movements.

■ Suggest the application of heat to relieve pain. *A heating pad may offer temporary pain relief. To avoid the "rebound effect," the heat should be removed every 20 to 30 minutes.*

Using NANDA, NIC, and NOC

Chart 42–1 shows links between NANDA nursing diagnoses, NIC, and NOC when caring for the client with osteoporosis.

Community-Based Care

The client who has osteoporosis needs education on safety and preventing falls. In addition to home safety, outdoor safety is important, too. Clients should be taught to use assistive devices for added stability, to wear rubber-soled shoes for traction, to walk on the grass when sidewalks are slippery, and to sprinkle salt or kitty litter on icy sidewalks in the winter.

Address the following topics when discussing home care:

■ Resources for medical supplies and assistive devices
■ Diet, exercise, and medications
■ Pain management
■ Maintaining good posture to help prevent stress on the spine
■ Helpful resources:
   ■ National Osteoporosis Foundation
   ■ Osteoporosis and Related Bone Diseases National Resource Center (NIH)
   ■ National Women's Health Resource Center
   ■ Older Women's League
   ■ American College of Rheumatology

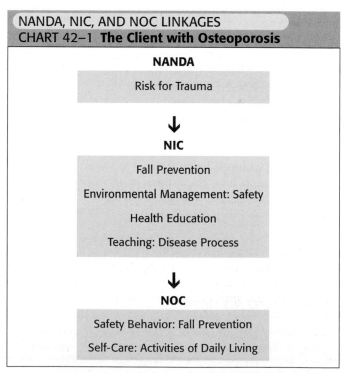

NANDA, NIC, AND NOC LINKAGES
CHART 42–1 **The Client with Osteoporosis**

NANDA

Risk for Trauma

↓

NIC

Fall Prevention

Environmental Management: Safety

Health Education

Teaching: Disease Process

↓

NOC

Safety Behavior: Fall Prevention

Self-Care: Activities of Daily Living

Data from *NANDA's Nursing Diagnoses: Definitions & Classification 2005–2006* by NANDA International (2005), Philadelphia; *Nursing Interventions Classification (NIC)* (4th ed.) by J. M. Dochterman & G. M. Bulechek (2004), St. Louis, MO: Mosby; and *Nursing Outcomes Classification (NOC)* (3rd ed.) by S. Moorhead, M. Johnson, and M. Maas (2004), St. Louis, MO: Mosby.

THE CLIENT WITH PAGET'S DISEASE

Paget's disease, also called *osteitis deformans*, is a progressive metabolic skeletal disorder that results from excessive metabolic activity in bone, with excessive bone resorption followed by excessive bone formation. This chronic remodeling results in the affected bones being larger and softer, with manifestations of bone pain, arthritis, obvious skeletal deformities, and fractures. The disorder affects bones of the axial skeleton, especially the femur, pelvis, vertebrae, and skull. The disease may affect one bone or multiple bones. The cause is unknown; however, several theories have been proposed, including hormonal imbalance, vascular disorder, neoplasm, autoimmune disorder, and inborn error of connective tissue. It is the second most common bone disease in the United States.

Paget's disease occurs in both men and women, affecting 1.5% to 8% of the population over the age of 50 in many countries. It is less common in people of Asian, Indian, and Scandinavian descent. It has a familial tendency as a result of mutations in several genes. The measles virus has been found in bone lesions, and the relevance of that finding is under investigation (Paget Foundation, 2004a).

Pathophysiology

Paget's disease progresses slowly. It usually follows a two-stage process: an excessive amount of osteoclastic bone resorption, followed by excessive osteoblastic bone formation. The initial phase presents with an abnormal increase in osteoclasts. The bones increase in size and thickness because of the acceleration in bone resorption and regeneration, resulting in a thick layer of coarse bone with a rough and pitted outer surface (Porth, 2005). Resorption of cancellous bone occurs rapidly. As new bone tissue tries to replace the loss, fibrous tissue forms in the bone marrow. The bone is at first hyperemic and soft, and bowing occurs. When this excessive bone cell activity decreases, the result is a gain in bone mass, but the newly formed bone becomes hard and brittle. This brittleness may lead to fractures.

Manifestations

Most clients with Paget's disease are asymptomatic for years, and the disease often is discovered when typical changes are seen on an incidental x-ray. Manifestations are often vague and depend on the specific area involved (see the box on this page). The most common manifestation is localized pain of the long bones, spine, pelvis, and cranium. The pain is described as a mild to moderate deep ache that is aggravated by pressure and weight bearing. It is more noticeable at night or when the client is resting. The pain usually is due to metabolic bone activity, secondary degenerative osteoarthritis, fractures, or nerve impingement. Because of the increase in blood flow to pagetic bone, flushing and warmth of the overlying skin may be apparent.

Complications

Complications of Paget's disease are as follows:
- Nerve palsy syndromes from involvement of the upper extremities

MANIFESTATIONS of Paget's Disease

MUSCULOSKELETAL EFFECTS
- Pain (in the long bones of lower extremities or joints)
- Deformity (enlargement of skull, bowing of lower extremities, and deformity of elbows and knees)
- Fractures of lower extremities
- Pathologic fractures (especially of the tibia)
- Compression fractures
- Collapse of the vertebrae, resulting in kyphosis and loss of height
- Muscle weakness

NEUROLOGIC EFFECTS
- Hearing loss
- Spinal cord injuries
- Dementia
- Pain from spinal stenosis
- Bladder and/or bowel dysfunction

CARDIOVASCULAR EFFECTS
- Congestive heart failure

METABOLIC EFFECTS
- Symptoms of hypercalcemia in immobilized clients
- Hypercalciuria and renal calculi
- Increased skin temperature over affected extremities

- Pathologic fractures from loss of bone structure
- Mental deterioration from compression of the brain when the skull is involved
- Compression of the spinal cord from affected cervical vertebrae causing quadraplegia
- Cardiovascular disease, resulting from vasodilation of the vessels in the skin and subcutaneous tissues overlying the affected bones
- Osteogenic sarcoma, seen in 5% to 10% of people with severe disease (Porth, 2005).

INTERDISCIPLINARY CARE

Care of the client with Paget's disease focuses on relieving pain, suppressing bone cell activity if necessary, and preventing or minimizing the effects of complications. Many clients with Paget's disease are asymptomatic and do not require treatment. For more severely affected clients, pharmacologic agents are usually effective. Occasionally, surgery may be required.

Diagnosis

Many of the diagnostic tests that are useful for the diagnosis of osteoporosis are equally useful for clients with Paget's disease (see Table 42–1). These include x-rays and bone scans to illustrate localized areas of demineralization in the early stages, seen as "punched-out" areas that lend a coarse, irregular appearance to the bone. In the later phase, x-rays show enlargement of the bones, tiny cracks in the long bones, and/or bowing of the weight-bearing bones. Computed tomography (CT) scans and magnetic resonance imaging (MRI) help identify possible causes of pain, including degenerative problems, spinal stenosis, or nerve root impingement. Diagnostic tests are described in Chapter 40 ∞.

Laboratory tests used in diagnosis include a serum alkaline phosphatase, which will show a steady rise as the disease progresses; the normal level (30 to 115 international units/L) may be elevated from high normal to over 3000 international units/L. A urinary collagen pyridinoline test is a sensitive indicator of the rate of bone resorption.

Medications

Clients who have mild symptoms often find relief using aspirin or NSAIDs, such as ibuprofen (Motrin) and indomethacin (Indocin). Clients who are experiencing manifestations and whose diagnostic test results are elevated are usually treated with an agent that retards bone resorption, such as calcitonin or a bisphosphonate.

Bisphosphonates such as alendronate (Fosamax), pamidronate (Aredia), and tiludronate (Skelid) are the primary treatments used for severe Paget's disease. These drugs inhibit bone resorption, possibly by attaching to the surface of the calcium/phosphate phase of bone and inhibiting osteoclast activity. They are safe and usually are well tolerated by the client. Alendronate is available as an oral preparation, and pamidronate is available for intravenous administration. Oral preparations are poorly absorbed from the GI tract, and may cause gastric or esophageal irritation. Alendronate should be given with a full glass of water on an empty stomach, at least 30 minutes before other medications or food. Pamidronate is given

as an intravenous infusion in D_5W or normal saline. It is given for 3 successive days, generally promoting a rapid response with reduced urinary excretion of hydroxyproline and pyridinium and a fall in alkaline phosphatase. Intravenous pamidronate may cause flulike symptoms, but these generally are brief. Calcium supplements also are prescribed for clients receiving bisphosphonates. After bisphosphonate treatment, clients often experience remission of symptoms for a year or more. See the Medication Administration box below for nursing implications.

Calcitonin inhibits osteoclastic resorption of bone. It also works as an analgesic for bone pain. The two derivatives of this medication are salmon (fish) and human. Salmon calcitonin (Calcimar) is generally preferred because it is inexpensive and widely available. Human calcitonin (Cibacalcin) is derived from human thyroid glands, which makes it more expensive and difficult to obtain. The parenteral form of calcitonin is used in treating Paget's disease. (Refer to the Medication Administration Box on page 1437 for nursing implications.)

Surgery

Different surgical interventions may be used to treat clients with Paget's disease, such as repairing a complete fracture through pagetic bone, realigning a knee through tibial osteotomy to decrease pain, or replacing a hip and/or knee for osteoarthritis. Because increased bleeding is a manifestation of Paget's disease, it is important to administer a potent bisphosphonate prior to surgery to decrease hypervascularity and reduce the risk of increased operative blood loss (Paget Foundation, 2004a).

MEDICATION ADMINISTRATION   The Client with Paget's Disease

BISPHOSPHONATES
Alendronate (Fosamax)   **Etidronate (Didronel)**
Pamidronate (Aredia)   **Risedronate (Actonel)**
Tiludronate (Skelid)

The bisphosphonates inhibit bone resorption, increasing the mineral density of bones and reducing the incidence of fractures. They are also used both in the prevention and treatment of osteoporosis: When used for Paget's disease, bisphosphonates slow the accelerated bone turnover associated with this disease. Bone pain is relieved, and the incidence of pathologic fractures is reduced. Cardiac and vascular manifestations of the disease also improve.

Nursing Responsibilities
- Administer alendronate with water 30 minutes before food or other medications.
- Do not give foods high in calcium, vitamins with mineral supplements, or antacids within 2 hours of administering alendronate.
- Instruct the client to avoid lying down for 30 minutes after taking the drug.
- Assess renal function studies before initiating therapy; alendronate is not recommended for use in clients with renal insufficiency.
- Dilute the prescribed dose of pamidronate in 1000 mL of D_5W or normal saline; infuse over at least 4 hours. Do not

add to calcium-containing solutions such as Ringer's or lactated Ringer's solutions.
- Monitor the IV site for signs of thrombophlebitis.
- Assess the client for signs of electrolyte imbalance or other adverse responses such as a drug fever.

Health Education for the Client and Family
- Take the medication as directed with clear water only. Consuming other beverages or food within 30 minutes of taking alendronate may interfere with its absorption and effectiveness.
- Do not lie down until after you have eaten. Alendronate can irritate the esophagus.
- Report symptoms such as new or worsening heartburn, difficulty swallowing, or painful swallowing.
- Fever with or without chills may occur while receiving intravenous pamidronate; this will subside without treatment. Flulike symptoms also may occur; these will subside within a week or so.
- Report any abnormal symptoms such as tingling around the mouth or numbness and tingling of the fingers or toes, which may indicate an imbalance of electrolytes in the blood.
- Take calcium and vitamin D supplements as instructed by your primary care provider.
- Response to these medications is gradual, and continues for months after the drug is stopped.

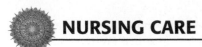 **NURSING CARE**

Nursing Diagnoses and Interventions

The nursing interventions for the client with symptomatic Paget's disease focus on pain control, prevention of injury or fractures, and education regarding the disease process and prescribed therapies.

Chronic Pain

The most common manifestation of Paget's disease is bone pain. This usually is the manifestation that prompts the client to seek health care.

- Assess the location and extent of the pain to determine the bone areas involved. *Bone pain in Paget's disease is poorly localized and is frequently described as "aching and deep."*
- Teach the client to take NSAIDs or aspirin on a regular basis as prescribed. *Pain is most noticeable at night or when the client is resting. The pain can become evident when it is aggravated by pressure and weight bearing.*
- Ensure correct placement of prescribed brace or corset. *The client may be required to wear a light brace or corset to relieve back pain and provide support when assuming an upright position. The client may need instruction in the correct application of the device and in the evaluation of pressure areas that may result from wearing the device.*
- Suggest referral for heat therapy and massage. *Heat therapy and massage can alleviate mild discomfort. Care should be taken when applying massage over areas prone to pathologic fractures.*

Impaired Physical Mobility

Clients with Paget's disease need to maintain or improve mobility so that they can perform necessary self-care activities and prevent complications of immobility.

- Provide an assistive device for use when ambulating. *During the active phase of Paget's disease, the client is prone to fractures. Bone deformities, activity intolerance, fear of falling, and pain are all factors that may make the client more prone to falls. An assistive device can provide both physical and psychologic support during ambulation, permit the client to ambulate further, and provide a device for resting during ambulation.*
- Teach good body mechanics. *The client with bone deformities should avoid activities that require lifting and twisting.*

> **PRACTICE ALERT**
> Activities as seemingly simple as lifting a heavy box may result in a fracture in the client with Paget's disease.

- Reinforce information about exercise protocols and activity regimens. *Exercise and activity protocols should be planned carefully to prevent injury and to minimize fatigue.*

Community-Based Care

A diagnosis of Paget's disease can be frightening for the client and family. It is important that they understand that this is a treatable disease, and that many manifestations of the disease will be relieved with treatment. Inform the client that remissions of the disease often last for a year or more after effective treatment. The Paget Foundation should be suggested as a resource. Discuss the following topics:

- The importance of following the prescribed treatment regimen and keeping scheduled follow-up appointments
- Because it may take several weeks to notice a response to treatment, the importance of continuing therapy during this time and after a response is obtained
- If bisphosphonates such as alendronate or pamidronate are ordered, the importance of taking supplemental calcium to prevent low blood calcium levels
- The importance of remaining active
- Safety in the home and outdoor environment to prevent falls
- The need to report to the primary care provider any sudden pain or disability, even if no trauma has occurred, because pathologic fractures are possible.

THE CLIENT WITH GOUT

Gout is a metabolic disease that occurs from an inflammatory response to the production or excretion of uric acid resulting in high levels of uric acid in the blood (hyperuricemia) and in other body fluids, including synovial fluid. The disorder is characterized by deposits of urates (insoluble precipitates) in the connective tissues of the body. Gout has an acute onset, usually at night, and often involves the first metatarsophalangeal joint (great toe). The initial acute attack is usually followed by a period of months or years without manifestations. As the disease progresses, urates are deposited in various other connective tissues. Deposits in the synovial fluids cause acute inflammation of the joint (*gouty arthritis*). Over time, urate deposits in subcutaneous tissues cause the formation of small white nodules (called **tophi**). Deposits of crystals in the kidneys can form urate kidney stones and result in kidney failure.

Gout may occur as either a primary or secondary disorder. Primary (inherited) gout is characterized by elevated serum uric acid levels resulting from either an inborn error of purine metabolism or a decrease in renal uric acid excretion due to an unknown cause. Purines are part of the structure of the nuclear compounds DNA and RNA; they also may be synthesized by the body. Impaired uric acid excretion leads to hyperuricemia in the majority of people with primary gout. In secondary gout, hyperuricemia occurs as a result of another disorder or treatment with certain medications. Disorders associated with rapid cell turnover, such as some malignancies (leukemia in particular), hemolytic anemia, and polycythemia, can increase purine metabolism. Chronic renal disease, hypertension, starvation, and diabetic ketoacidosis can interfere with uric acid excretion, as can certain drugs, including some diuretics (such as furosemide, ethacrynic acid, and chlorothiazide), pyrazinamide, cyclosporin, ethambutol, and low-dose salicylates. Alcohol ingestion appears to interfere with uric acid excretion and to accelerate its synthesis. In addition, hospitalized clients with gout are at risk for an acute attack from changes in their diet, abdominal surgery, or medications (Tierney et al., 2004).

Gout affects more than 84% of all Americans (ACR, 2005). Gout occurs more often in men, usually after age 30 years. In women, attacks of gout are rarely seen until after menopause. Obesity increases the risk of gout; about half of those with the disorder are 15% or more above their ideal weight (Flynn & Johnson, 2005).

Pathophysiology

Uric acid is the breakdown product of purine metabolism. Normally, a balance exists between its production and excretion, with approximately two-thirds of the amount produced each day excreted by the kidneys and the rest in the feces. The serum uric acid level is normally maintained between 3.4 and 7.0 mg/dL in men and 2.4 and 6.0 mg/dL in women. At levels greater than 7.0 mg/dL, the serum is saturated, and monosodium urate crystals may form. It is not known exactly how crystals of monosodium urate crystals are deposited in joints. Several mechanisms may be involved:

- Crystals tend to form in peripheral tissues of the body, where lower temperatures reduce the solubility of the uric acid.
- A decrease in extracellular fluid pH and reduced plasma protein binding of urate crystals are evident.
- Tissue trauma and a rapid change in uric acid levels may also lead to crystal deposition. A rapid increase in uric acid may occur with tissue trauma and release of cellular components.

The monosodium urate crystals may form in the synovial fluid or in the synovial membrane, cartilage, or other joint connective tissues. They may also form in the heart, earlobes, and kidneys. These crystals stimulate and continue the inflammatory process, during which neutrophils respond by ingesting the crystals. The neutrophils release their phagolysosomes, causing tissue damage, which perpetuates the inflammation.

Manifestations

The manifestations of gout are hyperuricemia, recurrent attacks of inflammation of a single joint, tophi, renal disease, and renal stones. Unless treated, the manifestations of gout appear in three stages: asymptomatic hyperuricemia, acute gouty arthritis, and tophaceous gout. See the Manifestations box on this page.

Asymptomatic Hyperuricemia

The first stage is asymptomatic hyperuricemia, with serum levels averaging 9 to 10 mg/dL. Most people with hyperuricemia do not progress to further stages of the disease.

Acute Gouty Arthritis

The second state is acute gouty arthritis. The acute attack (called a "flare"), usually affecting a single joint, occurs unexpectedly, often beginning at night. It may be triggered by trauma, alcohol ingestion, dietary excess, or a stressor such as surgery. It is often precipitated by an abrupt or sustained increase in uric acid levels. The affected joint becomes red, hot, swollen, and exquisitely painful and tender.

Approximately 50% of initial attacks of acute gouty arthritis occur in the metatarsophalangeal joint of the great toe. Other sites for acute attacks include the instep of the foot, ankles, heels, knees, wrists, fingers, and elbows. The pain, often

intense, peaks within several hours and may be accompanied by fever and an elevated white blood cell (WBC) count and sedimentation rate. The affected joints are swollen, and the skin over the joint is warm and dusky red.

Acute attacks of gouty arthritis last from several hours up to several weeks and typically subside spontaneously. There are no long-lasting sequelae, and the client enters an asymptomatic period called the intercritical period. The intercritical period may last up to 10 years; however, approximately 60% of people experience a recurrent attack within 1 year. Successive attacks tend to last longer, occur with increasing frequency, and resolve less completely than the initial attack.

Tophaceous (Chronic) Gout

Tophaceous or chronic gout occurs when hyperuricemia is not treated. The urate pool expands, and monosodium urate crystal deposits (tophi) develop in cartilage, synovial membranes, tendons, and soft tissues. They are seen most often in the helix of the ear; in tissues surrounding joints and bursae (especially around the elbows and knees); along tendons of the finger, toes, ankles, and wrists; on ulnar surfaces of the forearms; along the shins of the legs; and on other pressure points. The skin over tophi may ulcerate, exuding chalky material containing inflammatory cells and urate crystals. Tophi can also develop in the tissues of the heart and spinal epidura. Although tophi themselves are not painful, they may restrict joint movement and cause pain and deformities of the affected joints. Tophi may also compress nerves and erode and drain through the skin.

Complications

Kidney disease may occur in clients with untreated gout, particularly when hypertension is also present. Urate crystals are deposited in renal interstitial tissue. Uric acid crystals also form in the collecting tubules, renal pelvis, and ureter, forming stones. The stones can range in size from a grain of sand to a massive structure filling the spaces of the kidney. Uric acid stones can potentially obstruct urine flow and lead to acute renal failure.

MANIFESTATIONS of Gout

ACUTE GOUTY ARTHRITIS
- Usually monoarticular, affecting metatarsophalangeal joint of great toe, instep, ankle, knee, wrist, or elbow
- Acute pain
- Red, hot, swollen, and tender joint
- Fever, chills, malaise
- Elevated WBC and sedimentation rate

TOPHACEOUS (CHRONIC) GOUT
- Tophi evident on joints, bursae, tendon sheaths, pressure points, helix of ear
- Joint stiffness, limited ROM, and deformity
- Ulceration of tophi with chalky discharge

INTERDISCIPLINARY CARE

The classic presentation of acute gouty arthritis is so distinctive that the diagnosis can often be based on the client's history and physical examination. Treatment is directed toward terminating an acute attack, preventing recurrent attacks, and reversing or preventing complications resulting from crystal deposition in tissues and formation of uric acid kidney stones.

Diagnosis

Diagnostic testing is performed to establish an accurate diagnosis and direct long-term therapy. Diagnostic tests are described in Chapter 40 ∞.

Serum uric acid is nearly always elevated (usually above 7.5 mg/dL). The WBC count shows significant elevation, reaching levels as high as 20,000/mm³ during an acute attack. Eosinophil sedimentation rate (ESR or sed rate) is elevated during an acute attack from the acute inflammatory process that accompanies deposits of urate crystals in a joint. In addition, a 24-hour urine specimen is analyzed to determine uric acid production and excretion, and analysis of fluid aspirated from the acutely inflamed joint or material aspirated from a tophus shows typical needle-shaped urate crystals, providing the definitive diagnosis of gout.

Medications

Medications are used to terminate an acute attack, prevent further attacks, and reduce serum uric acid levels to prevent long-term sequelae of the disease. It is important to treat the acute attack of gouty arthritis before initiating treatment to reduce serum uric acid levels, because an abrupt decrease in serum uric acid may lead to further acute manifestations. Pharmacologic therapy is a mainstay of treatment in achieving these goals.

ACUTE ATTACK NSAIDs are the treatment of choice for an acute attack of gout. Indomethacin (Indocin) is the most frequently used NSAID for gout, although others are equally effective. Other NSAIDs that may be prescribed include ibuprofen (Motrin), naproxen (Naprosyn, Anaprox), tolmetin sodium (Tolectin), piroxicam (Feldene), and sulindac (Clinoril). Although extremely effective, NSAIDs are contraindicated for clients with active peptic ulcer disease, impaired renal function, or a history of hypersensitivity reactions to the drugs. As with other anti-inflammatory drugs, clients should be aware of possible risks and follow recommended doses carefully.

Colchicine can dramatically affect the course of an acute attack. Joint pain begins to diminish within 12 hours of the initiation of treatment and disappears within 2 days. Colchicine apparently acts by interrupting the cycle of urate crystal deposition and inflammation in an acute attack of gout. It has no anti-inflammatory effect in other forms of arthritis, and its use is limited to gout. The use of colchicine is limited by significant side effects. When administered orally, many clients develop abdominal cramping, diarrhea, nausea, or vomiting. Intravenous administration is limited by potential toxic effects including local pain, tissue damage if extravasation occurs during injection, bone marrow suppression, and disseminated intravascular coagulation (DIC). It is contraindicated for clients who have significant gastrointestinal, renal, hepatic, or cardiac disease.

Corticosteroids may also be prescribed for the client with acute gouty arthritis. If possible, the intra-articular route is preferred for monoarticular arthritis to avoid the multiple systemic effects of steroid therapy. When gout is polyarticular, corticosteroids may be administered either orally or intravenously.

Analgesics may also be prescribed during an acute episode of gouty arthritis. Either codeine or meperidine (Demerol) may be administered orally to manage the client's pain. Aspirin is avoided because it may interfere with uric acid excretion.

PROPHYLACTIC THERAPY In clients at high risk for future attacks of acute gout, prophylactic therapy with daily colchicine may be initiated. Prophylaxis is particularly useful during the first 1 to 2 years of treatment with antihyperuricemic agents. Although colchicine does not affect the serum uric acid directly, it reduces the frequency of attacks by preventing crystal deposition within the joint. The doses required to achieve this effect are small, and few side effects are associated with therapy.

Treatment to reduce serum uric acid levels is typically initiated for clients with recurring gout, tophi, or renal damage. Asymptomatic hyperuricemic clients require no treatment. Uricosuric agents are used for clients who do not eliminate uric acid adequately; allopurinol is prescribed for clients who produce excessive amounts of uric acid. Uricosuric drugs block the tubular reabsorption of uric acid, promoting its excretion and reducing serum levels. These drugs reduce the frequency of acute attacks, particularly when administered with colchicine. Probenecid (Benemid) and sulfinpyrazone (Aprazone, Anturane, Zynol) are the primary uricosuric drugs employed.

Allopurinol (Zyloprim) is a xanthine oxidase inhibitor that lowers plasma uric acid levels and facilitates the mobilization of tophi. Because of its effectiveness in lowering serum uric acid levels, it may trigger an attack of acute gout. The nursing implications for medications used to treat gout are included in the Medication Administration box on page 1446.

Complementary and Alternative Therapy

A variety of nutritional and herbal supplements may be used to help prevent gout or decrease the onset of manifestations. These include:

- Vitamin E and selenium may decrease tissue inflammation.
- Amino acids (alanine, aspartic acid, glutamic acid, and glycine) increase the ability of the kidneys to excrete uric acid.
- Dark reddish-blue berries (such as cherries and blackberries) are good sources of flavonoids, which help lower uric acid levels, decrease inflammation, and prevent or repair joint tissue damage.
- Acupuncture can provide pain relief.

Treatments

Treatments for gout, in addition to medications, include dietary management and rest.

NUTRITION Dietary purines contribute only slightly to uric acid levels in the body, and no specific diet may be recommended. If a low-purine diet is recommended, the client should be taught that

MEDICATION ADMINISTRATION The Client with Gout

COLCHICINE

Colchicine is used to terminate an acute attack of gouty arthritis and to prevent recurrent episodes of the disease. Colchicine does not alter serum uric acid levels, but appears to interrupt the cycle of urate crystal deposition and inflammatory response. It may be administered either by mouth or intravenously. Colchicine is also available as a fixed-dose combination with a uricosuric agent, probenecid (Benemid). Only plain colchicine is used to treat an acute attack of gout; combination therapy is employed to prevent further attacks.

Nursing Responsibilities

- Assess for possible contraindications to colchicines therapy, including serious gastrointestinal, renal, hepatic, or cardiac disease.
- Administer the following as ordered:
  - *Intravenous doses*: Give undiluted or diluted in up to 20 mL sterile normal saline for injection. Administer over a period of 2 to 5 minutes.
  - *Oral doses:* Give on an empty stomach to facilitate absorption.
  - Evaluate for adverse effects, including abdominal cramping, nausea, vomiting, and diarrhea, and report promptly, because these side effects may necessitate discontinuation of the drug.

Health Education for the Client and Family

- Drink 3 to 4 quarts of liquid per day.
- Report adverse responses, including gastrointestinal problems, fatigue, bleeding, easy bruising, or recurrent infections, to the physician.
- Do not drink alcohol.

URICOSURIC DRUGS
Probenecid (Benemid)
Sulfinpyrazone (Anturane)

Probenecid is a uricosuric drug that inhibits the tubular reabsorption of urate, promoting the excretion of uric acid and decreasing serum uric acid levels. Sulfinpyrazone is a uricosuric drug that potentiates the renal excretion of uric acid, reducing serum uric acid levels. It is used to prevent recurrent attacks of acute gouty arthritis and treat chronic gout.

Nursing Responsibilities

- Assess for prior hypersensitivity responses to this drug.
- Administer after meals or with milk to minimize gastric distress.
- Increase fluid intake to at least 3 L/day to prevent the formation of uric acid kidney calculi.
- Administer sodium bicarbonate or potassium citrate as ordered to maintain an alkaline urine.
- Do not administer aspirin to clients receiving probenecid because salicylates interfere with the action of the drug.
- Monitor clients receiving the following drugs concurrently with probenecid for increased or toxic effects: penicillin and related antibiotics, indomethacin, acetaminophen, naproxen, ketoprofen, meclofenamate, lorazepam, and rifampin.
- Monitor for possible adverse effects of probenecid, including headache, dizziness, hepatic necrosis, nausea and vomiting, renal colic, bone marrow depression, anaphylaxis, fever, hives, and pruritus.
- Administer sulfinpyrazone with meals or antacid to minimize gastric distress.

- Monitor clients taking sulfinpyrazone with other sulfa drugs for increased or toxic effects; monitor for hypoglycemia in clients receiving insulin or oral hypoglycemics concurrently, and monitor for bleeding or increased anticoagulant effect in clients receiving warfarin concurrently.
- Assess for contraindications to therapy with sulfinpyrazone, including active peptic ulcer disease, a history of hypersensitivity to phenylbutazone or other pyrazoles, or blood dyscrasias.

Health Education for the Client and Family

- Do not take aspirin or products containing aspirin while taking probenecid. Use acetaminophen for relief of mild pain.
- Drink at least 3 quarts of fluids per day to minimize the risk of kidney stone formation.
- Take sulfinpyrazone with meals to minimize gastric distress, and report epigastric pain, nausea, or black stools to the physician promptly

ALLOPURINOL (ZYLOPRIM)

Allopurinol acts on purine metabolism, reducing the production of uric acid and decreasing serum and urinary concentrations of uric acid. It is used for clients with manifestations of primary or secondary gout, including acute attacks, tophi, joint destruction, urinary stones, and nephropathy. It is not indicated for use in the treatment of asymptomatic hyperuricemia.

Nursing Responsibilities

- Monitor intake and output and increase fluid intake to approximately 3 L/day.
- Monitor for desired effect of decreased serum uric acid levels, and for adverse effects such as nausea, diarrhea, and rash.
- Assess BUN and creatinine levels prior to the initiation of and during treatment with allopurinol. Report signs of impaired renal function such as an elevated BUN and creatinine, decreased urine output, and dilute or frothy urine to the physician.
- Administer with meals to minimize gastric distress.
- Monitor CBC periodically because allopurinol therapy may cause bone marrow depression.
- In clients receiving warfarin concurrently, monitor prothrombin times and be alert to evidence of bleeding, because allopurinol prolongs the half-life of warfarin.
- Monitor clients receiving chlorpropamide, cyclophosphamide, hydantoin, theophylline, vidarabine, or ACE inhibitors concurrently for increased drug effects.
- Discontinue the drug and notify the physician immediately if the client develops a rash. Rash and hypersensitivity responses occur more frequently in clients receiving ampicillin, amoxicillin, or thiazide diuretics.

Health Education for the Client and Family

- Stop taking the drug and report any skin rash, painful urination, blood in the urine, eye irritation, or swelling of the lips or mouth to the physician immediately.
- Take the medication after meals to minimize gastric distress.
- Drink 3 to 4 quarts of fluid daily to maintain a urinary output greater than 2 L/day.
- Acute gouty attacks may occur during the initial stages of allopurinol therapy; continue therapy prescribed for attacks (such as colchicine) to minimize acute episodes.
- Do not take a double dose of medication if you miss a dose.

high purine foods include all meats and seafood, yeast, beans, peas, lentils, oatmeal, spinach, asparagus, cauliflower, and mushrooms. The obese client is advised to lose weight, but fasting is contraindicated for clients with gout. Alcohol intake and specific foods that tend to precipitate attacks are avoided.

A liberal fluid intake to maintain a daily urinary output of 2000 mL or more is recommended to increase urate excretion and reduce the risk of urinary stone formation. Urinary alkalinizing agents, such as sodium bicarbonate or potassium citrate, may be prescribed as well to minimize the risk of uric acid stones. It is important to monitor clients receiving these preparations carefully for signs of fluid and electrolyte or acid–base imbalances.

REST During an acute attack of gouty arthritis, bed rest is prescribed. It is continued for approximately 24 hours after the attack has subsided, because early ambulation may bring about recurrence of acute manifestations (Tierney et al., 2004). The affected joint may be elevated and hot or cold compresses may be applied for comfort.

NURSING CARE

Clients with gout provide self-care at home. Teaching focuses on self-management of pain and altered mobility.

Nursing Diagnoses and Interventions

Pain is a primary focus for nursing interventions in the client experiencing an acute attack of gout. The client's mobility is also impaired during an acute attack, both because of pain and prescribed activity limitations.

Acute Pain

The pain associated with an attack of acute gouty arthritis is intense and accompanied by exquisite tenderness of the affected joint. Measures to alleviate the pain are vital in the initial period until anti-inflammatory medications become effective and the acute inflammatory response is relieved. The following are important in teaching about pain relief:

- Position the affected joint for comfort. Elevate the joint or extremity (usually the foot) on a pillow, maintaining alignment. *Elevation and normal body alignment facilitate blood return from the affected joint, alleviating some of the edema.*
- Protect the affected joint from pressure, placing a foot cradle on the bed to keep bed covers off the foot. *A foot cradle keeps bed linens from applying pressure on the affected joint.*
- Take anti-inflammatory and antigout medications as prescribed. In the initial period, colchicine may be given hourly. *These medications reduce the acute inflammatory response, gradually relieving discomfort.*

PRACTICE ALERT
The affected joints are so painful that even the weight of a sheet can be unbearable.

- Take analgesics as prescribed. *Supplemental analgesia may be necessary in the acute period until the inflammatory response is mediated.*

- Maintain bed rest. *It is important to immobilize the affected joint and promote rest to prevent exacerbation of joint inflammation.*

Community-Based Care
Discuss the following topics with the client:
- *The disease and its manifestations.* Tell the client that initial attacks cause no permanent damage but that recurrent attacks can lead to permanent damage and joint destruction. Discuss other potential effects of continued hyperuricemia, including tophaceous deposits in subcutaneous and other connective tissues. Discuss the potential for kidney damage and kidney stones.
- *The rationale for and use of prescribed medication.* Stress the need to continue the medication until the physician discontinues it, even though the client is free of manifestations of gout. Tell the client to avoid drugs that increase uric acid blood levels: hydrochlorothiazide (HydroDIURIL), cyclosporine (Neoral, Sandimmune), furosemide (Lasix), and high dose of aspirin. Clients who need to reduce their risk of heart attacks may safely take one baby aspirin each day (Flynn & Johnson, 2005).
- The importance of a high intake of fluids each day and avoiding the use of alcohol.

THE CLIENT WITH OSTEOMALACIA

Osteomalacia, often referred to as *adult rickets,* is a metabolic bone disorder characterized by inadequate or delayed mineralization of bone matrix in mature compact and spongy bone, resulting in softening of bones. Bone mineralization requires adequate calcium and phosphate ions in extracellular fluid. When either of these ions is insufficient due to (1) inadequate calcium intake or decreased calcium absorption from the intestines because of insufficient vitamin D, or (2) increased renal losses or decreased intestinal absorption of phosphate, the bone matrix is not mineralized and cannot sustain weight bearing. Marked deformities of weight-bearing bone and pathologic fractures occur. The primary causes of osteomalacia are vitamin D deficiency and hypophosphatemia. Osteomalacia can be corrected with treatment.

Osteomalacia has been almost nonexistent in the United States because many foods are fortified with vitamin D, but its incidence is increasing among older adults, and people who adhere to strict vegetarian diets. It is a significant health problem in cultures whose diets tend to be deficient in calcium and vitamin D. Women in northern China, Japan, and northern India have a higher incidence of the disorder (Porth, 2005).

The major risk factors for vitamin D deficiency are a diet low in vitamin D, decreased endogenous production of vitamin D because of inadequate sun exposure, impaired intestinal absorption of fats (vitamin D is a fat-soluble vitamin), and disorders that interfere with the metabolism of vitamin D to its active forms. Gastrectomy and small-bowel disorders may reduce the absorptive surface of the bowel to the extent that nutrients are not completely or adequately absorbed.

Both vitamin D and calcium absorption may be affected. Hepatobiliary disorders that interfere with bile production and release, and chronic pancreatic insufficiency with inadequate pancreatic enzyme production can affect the absorption of fats and vitamin D from the bowel. Once absorbed, vitamin D is metabolized in the liver and the kidney to its active form; therefore, liver disorders such as cirrhosis and renal disorders can affect this activation. Certain drugs, such as isoniazid, rifampin, and anticonvulsants, accelerate vitamin D metabolism, resulting in less availability to the tissues. Renal excretion of vitamin D is increased in some kidney disorders such as nephrotic syndrome (Box 42–2).

Hypophosphatemia can be the result of insufficient dietary intake, excessive losses through the urine or stool, or a shift into the cells. Alcohol abuse is the most common cause of hypophosphatemia, because of related dietary deficiencies, vomiting, antacid use, and increased renal excretion of phosphate. Ingesting large amounts of nonabsorbable antacids causes increased phosphate losses in the stool. Several acquired and genetic disorders cause increased losses of phosphate in the urine.

Pathophysiology

The two main causes of osteomalacia are insufficient calcium absorption in the intestine due to a lack of calcium or resistance to the action of vitamin D and increased losses of phosphorus through the urine (Porth, 2005). In its natural form, vitamin D is obtained from certain foods and ultraviolet radiation of the sun. Vitamin D maintains adequate serum levels of calcium and phosphate for normal mineralization of the bone. Vitamin D deficiency or resistance to its action disrupts the normal mineralization of the bone, causing softening of the bone.

Vitamin D is inactive when it is absorbed from the intestine or synthesized from exposure to ultraviolet light. For vitamin D to become active, a two-step process must occur. Vitamin D (and its metabolites) is transported in the blood to the liver, where it is converted to calcidiol. Calcidiol is then transported to the kidney and transformed to an active form, calcitriol.

The active form of vitamin D is needed for optimal absorption of calcium and phosphorus from the intestine. Calcium and phosphorus are transported in the blood to the bones for normal mineralization. If there is a lack of vitamin D, calcium and phosphorus are not absorbed from the intestine, and serum calcium and phosphorus levels therefore fall. A deficiency in these minerals in turn activates the parathyroid glands, with loss of calcium and phosphorus from bone. The continued loss of calcium and phosphate in the bone disrupts bone mineralization.

Impaired bone mineralization causes abnormalities in both spongy and compact bone. The osteoid (the soft, noncalcified part of the matrix) continues to be produced but is not mineralized. This abnormal buildup of demineralized bone leads to gross deformities of the long bones, spine, pelvis, and skull, because the bone is soft and unable to bear the weight and stress of body movement.

Manifestations

The manifestations of osteomalacia include bone pain and tenderness (see the box below). As the disease progresses, fractures occur. In contrast to osteoporosis, osteomalacia is not associated with a significant occurrence of hip fractures. Instead, pathologic fractures occur in the commonly weakened areas (e.g., distal radius and proximal femur).

INTERDISCIPLINARY CARE

Osteomalacia may be difficult to differentiate from osteoporosis because the manifestations are very similar; however, once the specific cause is determined, appropriate therapy will correct the disorder.

Diagnosis

A history of inadequate dietary intake, renal failure, or some malabsorption states may suggest osteomalacia. Diagnostic

---

BOX 42–2 **Causes of Osteomalacia**

Vitamin D Deficiency
- Inadequate dietary intake
- Lack of sun exposure
- Malabsorption from intestines: gastrectomy, small-bowel disorders, gallbladder disease, chronic pancreatic insufficiency
- Renal or liver disorders
- Drug effects: isoniazid, rifampin, anticonvulsants

Phosphate Depletion
- Inadequate intake
- Impaired absorption due to chronic antacid use
- Impaired renal tubular reabsorption due to either acquired or genetic disorders

Systemic Acidosis
- Renal tubular acidosis
- Ureterosigmoidostomy
- Fanconi's syndrome

Bone Mineralization Inhibitors
- Hypophosphatasia
- Sodium fluoride or disodium etidronate (Didronel)
- Aluminum intoxication

Chronic Renal Failure

Calcium Malabsorption

MANIFESTATIONS of Osteomalacia

- Bone pain: May be vague and generalized at first, becoming more intense with activity as the disease progresses; occurs most frequently in the pelvis; long bones of the extremities, spine, and ribs.
- Difficulty changing from lying to sitting position and sitting to standing position.
- Muscle weakness: Frequently an early sign in severe cases.
- Waddling gait: May be due to pain and muscle weakness.
- Dorsal kyphosis: May occur in severe cases.
- Pathologic fractures.

tests are described in Chapter 40 ∞. Table 42–1 compares the diagnostic findings of osteomalacia with those of osteoporosis and Paget's disease. X-rays demonstrate the effects of generalized bone demineralization: trabecular bone loss, cyst formation, compression fractures, bowing and bending deformities of the long bones, and osteoid deposits, particularly in the vertebral bodies and pelvis.

Laboratory tests include serum calcium, parathyroid hormone, and alkaline phosphatase levels. Calcium may be normal or low, depending on the cause of the disease. Calcium levels may be reduced when calcium absorption is impaired or in severe vitamin D deficiency. Secondary hypoparathyroidism may shift calcium from the bone into extracellular fluid, maintaining a normal serum calcium level. Parathyroid hormone is frequently elevated as a compensatory response to hypocalcemia in renal failure or vitamin D deficiency. Alkaline phosphatase usually is elevated.

Medications

Therapeutic management of osteomalacia depends on the cause of the disease. Because the causes are so diverse, it is difficult to generalize treatment. Most clients are placed on vitamin D therapy. Calcium and phosphate supplements may be indicated. Radiologic evidence of healing often is apparent within weeks of initiating therapy.

NURSING CARE

Managing the client with osteomalacia includes assessing the client's current dietary intake of vitamin D, calcium, and phosphorus and exposure to ultraviolet light. It also includes managing client responses to bone pain and tenderness, fractures, and muscle weakness.

Teaching is important not only for the client with osteomalacia, but also for people at risk for developing the disease.

When milk and other dairy products began to be fortified with vitamin D, the incidence of childhood rickets decreased dramatically. Now many clients are unaware of the importance of vitamin D, calcium, and phosphorus to bone health.

Older adults as a group are at high risk for osteomalacia because of dietary deficiencies, age-related intestinal malabsorption, and possible physical mobility limitations that restrict their exposure to sunlight. Teach older adults about the importance of maintaining an adequate intake of milk and other dairy products that are not only rich in calcium and phosphorus, but also are fortified with vitamin D. Few other food sources provide enough vitamin D to meet recommended levels. Cod liver oil may be used as a supplement, because it contains significant amounts of vitamin D. Supplements are not recommended, however, for clients who get adequate vitamin D through dietary sources and sun exposure, because this fat-soluble vitamin may become toxic at high levels. Instruct clients who are taking supplements to report to their primary care provider symptoms such as anorexia, nausea and vomiting, frequent urination, muscle weakness, and constipation that may be indicative of hypervitaminosis D.

Teach the client with osteomalacia about safety measures to prevent falls. Discuss the importance of eliminating scatter rugs and clutter from living areas to prevent tripping. Teach the client to place a night-light in hallways and the bathroom to prevent falls associated with nighttime toileting. Suggest installing grab bars in the shower and tub and next to the toilet for safety.

Teach clients with bone pain and muscle weakness to use assistive devices such as walkers, canes, or crutches when ambulating. Provide referrals to physical therapy for teaching clients how to safely use these devices. Encourage clients to participate in a supervised exercise program such as water aerobics or t'ai chi to improve muscle strength and balance.

DEGENERATIVE DISORDERS

Degenerative disorders, especially degenerative joint disease, are the most common form of arthritis in the older adult. Both primary and secondary forms are seen in adults of all ages. Primary or idiopathic osteoarthritis, the most common type, occurs without a clear precipitating factor. Secondary osteoarthritis is associated with an identifiable cause. For instance, it may be related to trauma to a joint, inflammation, skeletal disorders such as congenital hip dysplasia, or metabolic disorders. Regardless of cause, degenerative disorders of the joints and muscles can lead to impaired mobility and chronic pain. These problems may in turn cause disability, especially in the performance of ADLs by older adults.

THE CLIENT WITH OSTEOARTHRITIS

Osteoarthritis (OA) (also labeled *degenerative joint disease*) is the most commonly occurring of all forms of arthritis, and a leading cause of pain and disability in older adults (Porth, 2005). This disease is characterized by loss of articular cartilage in articulating joints and hypertrophy of the bones at the articular margins. OA may be idiopathic (without known cause) or secondary (associated with known risk factors). OA affects more than 12% of Americans between the ages of 25 and 74 years, with about 90% of people having x-ray evidence of OA in the weight-bearing joints by age 40 (ACR, 2005; Flynn & Johnson, 2005). Men are affected more than women at an earlier age, but the rate of OA in women exceeds men by the middle adult years. The joints most affected are in the hand, wrist, neck, lower back, hip, knee, ankle, and feet. Men are more likely than women to have hip OA, whereas postmenopausal women more often have hand OA. Racial and ethnic effects on the development of OA are outlined in the box below.

FOCUS ON DIVERSITY
The Client with Osteoarthritis

- White women are more likely to have hand OA.
- Black women are more likely to have knee OA.
- Hip OA incidence is less in Chinese people.

Localized OA affects only one or two joints. Generalized OA affects three or more joints. Generalized OA may also be classified as nodal (involving the hand) or nonnodal (no hand involvement). Nodal OA may also affect the knees, hips, cervical spine, and lumbar spine. Idiopathic OA most commonly affects the terminal interphalangeal joints (*Heberden's nodes*), and less often the proximal interphalangeal joints (*Bouchard's nodes*) (Figure 42–2 ■), the joints of the thumb, the hip, the knee, the metatarsophalangeal joint of the big toe, and the cervical and lumbar spine. Secondary OA may occur in any joint from an articular injury.

Risk Factors

Idiopathic OA is associated with increasing age. It has been suggested that OA may be inherited as an autosomal recessive trait, with genetic defects causing premature destruction of the joint cartilage. The causes of secondary OA include trauma, mechanical stress, and inflammation of joint structures, joint instability, neurologic disorders, endocrine disorders, and selected medications.

Excessive weight contributes to the development of OA, especially in the hip and knee. Excess fat may have a direct metabolic effect in the development of the disease. Primary OA of the knee is almost four times more common in obese women and five times more common in obese men (Flynn & Johnson, 2005). Inactivity is another risk factor. Moderate recreational exercise has been shown to both decrease the chance of developing OA and the progression of manifestations when OA is present. People involved in strenuous, repetitive exercise (such as participating in sports) have an increased risk of developing secondary OA.

Other risk factors that are linked to OA are hormonal factors such as decreased estrogen in menopausal women, excessive growth hormone, and increased parathyroid hormone.

Pathophysiology

The cartilage that lines joints provides a smooth surface, so that the bones of the joint glide over one another without friction, and it distributes the load from one bone to the next, dissipating the mechanical stress that occurs with joint loading. This cartilage normally contains more than 70% water. More than 90% of its dry weight is collagen, which provides strength, and proteoglycans, which provide elasticity and stiffness to compression. Cartilage cells, the chondrocytes, nest in this meshwork of collagen and proteoglycans. Normal articular cartilage exudes some of its water with compression, providing lubrication for joint surfaces. This water is reabsorbed during relaxation of the joint.

In OA, proteoglycans and collagen are lost from the cartilage as a result of enzymatic degradation. The water content of the cartilage increases as the collagen matrix is destroyed. With the loss of proteoglycans and collagen fibers, the cartilage becomes yellow or brownish gray and loses its tensile strength. Surface ulcerations occur, and fissures develop in deeper layers of the cartilage. Eventually, large areas of articular cartilage are lost, and underlying bone is exposed. The bone thickens in exposed areas, reducing its ability to absorb energy in joint loading. Cysts can also develop in the bone. Cartilage-coated *osteophytes* (bony outgrowths often called "joint mice") change the anatomy of the joint. As these spurs or projections enlarge, small pieces may break off, leading to mild synovitis (inflammation of the synovial membrane).

Manifestations

The onset of OA is usually gradual and insidious, and the course slowly progressive. Pain and stiffness in one or more joints (usually weight bearing) are the first manifestations of OA. The pain is localized to the affected joints and may be described as a deep ache. It typically is aggravated by use or motion of the joint and relieved by rest, although it may become persistent as the disease progresses. Pain at night may be accompanied by paresthesias (numbness, tingling). Pain may also be referred to other parts of the body; for example, OA of the lumbosacral spine may cause severe pain along the path of the sciatic nerve. Following periods of immobility, such as sleeping all night or after a long automobile ride, involved joints may stiffen. Usually only a few minutes of activity are necessary to relieve the stiffness. Range of motion (ROM) of the joint decreases as the disease progresses, and grating or crepitus may be noted during movement. Bony overgrowth may cause joint enlargement, and flexion contractures may occur because of joint instability. In OA, enlarged joints are characteristically bony-hard and cool on palpation. Manifestations specific to affected joints are outlined in the box on the next page.

Complications

OA of the spine may involve the vertebral bodies and intervertebral disks, the diarthrodial joints, or both. *Spondylosis* is degenerative disk disease. As the intervertebral disks degenerate, disk space between the vertebrae is lost. Degenerative disk disease may be complicated by herniated disk, the protrusion of the nucleus pulposus of the disk. Herniation usually occurs in a lateral direction, potentially compressing nerve roots and causing radicular (distributed along the nerve) pain and muscle weakness. See Chapter 45 ∞ for further discussion of disk disorders.

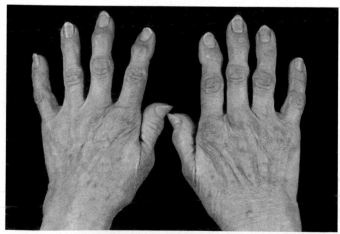

Figure 42–2 ■ Typical interphalangeal joint changes associated with osteoarthritis.

Source: L. Samsuri/Custom Medical Stock Photo.

MANIFESTATIONS of Osteoarthritis

Affected Site	Manifestations
Interphalangeal joints	■ *Heberden's nodes*—bony enlargements of distal joints; may cause pain, redness, swelling ■ *Bouchard's nodes*—bony enlargement of proximal joints
First carpometacarpal	■ Swelling, tenderness at base of thumb ■ Crepitus with movement ■ "Squared" appearance of joint
Spine	■ Localized pain and stiffness ■ Muscle spasm ■ Limited range of motion ■ Nerve root compression with radicular pain and motor weakness
Hips	■ Pain referred to inguinal area, buttock, thigh, or knee ■ Loss of internal rotation ■ Limited extension, adduction, and flexion
Knees	■ Pain and bony enlargement ■ Effusions ■ Crepitus ■ Instability and deformity with advanced disease

Disk degeneration and joint space narrowing alter the mechanics of the spinal column, promoting osteoarthritic changes in the articular processes (the facet joints) of the vertebrae. The cartilage covering the inferior and superior articular processes degenerates, causing localized pain, stiffness, muscle spasm, and limited range of motion. Osteophytes may form on articular processes, further contributing to pain and muscle spasm.

The presentation of OA in older clients is similar to that in younger adults. However, in this population, the risk of debilitation because of OA is greater, and the disease may progress faster. In addition, pain, stiffness, and limited ROM increase the risk of falls and fractures in the older adult.

INTERDISCIPLINARY CARE

At this time, no treatment is available to arrest the process of joint degeneration. Appropriate management, however, is important to relieve pain and maintain the client's function and mobility. Research is also ongoing on a new class of medications called disease-modifying osteoarthritis drugs (DMOADs) and gene therapy.

Diagnosis

The diagnosis of OA is generally based on the client's history, physical examination, and x-rays of affected joints. Diagnostic tests are described in Chapter 40 .

Characteristic changes of OA are visible in x-ray studies of affected joints. Initially, irregular joint space narrowing is seen. Progressive changes include increased density of subchondral

(under cartilage) bone, osteophyte formation at the joint periphery, and the formation of cysts in the bone. Examination of synovial fluid from involved joints can identify the type of arthritis. In addition, research of the blood level of hyaluronic acid (IIA) (a lubricating substance in cartilage and joint synovial fluid) suggests that HA may be a useful biochemical marker indicating the presence and severity of OA (National Institute of Arthritis Musculoskeletal and Skin Diseases, 2005c).

Medications

The pain of OA often can be managed through the use of analgesics such as aspirin or acetaminophen. Acetaminophen (Tylenol) is generally preferred for use in older clients because it has fewer toxic side effects. NSAIDs such as ibuprofen (Motrin), naproxen (Aleve), or ketoprofen (Orudis KT) may also be prescribed. See information with medications for rheumatoid arthritis for FDA actions concerning these drugs. These medications are discussed in more detail in Chapter 9 ∞.

Topical medications include counterirritants, salicylates, and capsaicin, sold without prescription as creams, gels, sprays, patches, or ointments to relieve pain. Counterirritants include Flexall 454 Maximum Strength Gel, ArthriCare, Bengay, and Icy Hot; salicylates include Aspercreme and Sportscreme, and capsaicin is included in Capzasin and Zostrix. The client should be taught to keep the medications away from their eyes, nose, mouth, or any open skin, and not to bandage or apply heat to the treated area. The products should be used no more than three or four times a day and discontinued immediately if severe irritation occurs.

Medications that are effective in decreasing the pain and stiffness of OA are the NSAID COX-2 inhibitors. However, because of the increased risk of adverse cardiovascular (heart attack and strokes) and gastrointestinal (bleeding) effects of most drugs in this category, several have been recalled by the FDA and the only COX-2 inhibitor being prescribed as of 2006 was celecoxib (Celebrex).

Potent anti-inflammatory medications, such as systemic corticosteroids, are seldom prescribed for clients with OA, although intra-articular corticosteroid injections may be used. With intra-articular injections, a long-acting corticosteroid medication, often mixed with a local anesthetic such as lidocaine, is injected directly into the joint space of the affected joints. Although this procedure may provide marked pain relief, it can hasten the rate of cartilage breakdown if performed more frequently than every 4 to 6 months.

Treatments

OA is initially treated conservatively, but as pain increases and joint function decreases, surgery often becomes necessary.

CONSERVATIVE TREATMENT The goals of OA treatment are to relieve pain and maintain as much normal joint function as possible. Conservative treatment may include any or all of the following:

■ ROM exercises, muscle strengthening exercises, aerobic exercises
■ Heat and ice
■ A balance between exercise and rest

- Use of a cane, crutches, or a walker
- Weight loss, if indicated
- Analgesic and anti-inflammatory medications.

VISCOSUPPLEMENTATION Viscosupplementation is a new treatment for OA of the knee. Hyaluronan, a natural component of synovial fluid, is injected directly into the knee joint. Four hyaluronan derivatives have been approved for use: Hyalgan, Supartz, Orthovisc, and Synvisc. The injection may provide pain relief and improvement in knee function for up to 1 year, but its long-term effects are unknown (Flynn & Johnson, 2005).

SURGERY Surgical procedures can provide dramatic results for clients with significant chronic pain and loss of joint function. Although elective surgical procedures are frequently avoided in the older adult, even older clients can benefit significantly if they do not have a chronic medical condition that contraindicates surgery.

Arthroscopy An *arthroscopy* is a surgical procedure in which an arthroscope (a thin tube that is lighted and has a camera in one end) is inserted into a joint. It may be done to diagnose the type of arthritis or to perform debridement by smoothing rough cartilage and flushing out the joint to remove debris. Although arthroscopic debridement and lavage of involved joints have been used, arthroscopy has not proven effective in the treatment of knee OA. It may be useful to remove large pieces of debris or repair a torn cartilage (Flynn & Johnson, 2005).

Osteotomy An *osteotomy*, an incision into or transection of the bone, may be performed to realign an affected joint, particularly when significant bony overgrowth or osteophyte formation has occurred. This procedure may also be used to shift the joint load toward areas of less severely damaged cartilage. Although osteotomy does not halt the process of OA, it may have a beneficial effect on joint function and pain, delaying the need for a joint replacement by several years.

Joint Arthroplasty A *joint arthroplasty* is the reconstruction or replacement of a joint. Arthroplasty is usually indicated when the client has severely restricted joint mobility and pain at rest. Pain is virtually eliminated, and the function of the joint is generally improved. Arthroplasty may involve partial joint replacement or reshaping of the bones of a joint. For most clients with OA, both surfaces of the affected joint are replaced with prosthetic parts in a procedure known as a *total joint replacement*. Joints that may be replaced include the hip, knee, shoulder, elbow, ankle, wrist, and joints of the fingers and toes.

In a total joint replacement, some or all of the synovium, cartilage, and bone on both sides of the joint are removed. A metallic prosthesis is inserted to replace one joint surface (generally the load-end or distal portion of a weight-bearing joint). The other joint surface is replaced by a silicone-lined ceramic or plastic prosthesis.

Most prosthetic joints are uncemented, that is, made of porous ceramic and metal components inserted so that they fit tightly into existing bone. The implant is secured by new bone growth into the prosthesis, a process that requires approximately 6 weeks. Although a longer non-weight-bearing period is necessary initially until the prosthesis is fixed in place by the

bony growth, the implant appears to have a longer useful life span than cemented prostheses. In a cemented joint replacement, methyl methacrylate (a pliable polymer that hardens to hold the prosthesis in place) is used to secure the prosthesis to existing bone. Although the client is able to resume normal activities more rapidly following a cemented joint replacement, methyl methacrylate initiates an inflammatory response, and the joint eventually loosens.

- In a *total hip replacement,* the articular surfaces of the acetabulum and femoral head are replaced. The entire head of the femur and part of the femoral neck are removed and replaced with a prosthesis (Figure 42–3 ■). The acetabulum is remodeled, and a prosthesis of high-molecular-weight polyethylene is inserted. The success rate for total hip replacement is reported to be greater than 90%. Approximately 150,000 total hip replacements are done each year in the United States; most are for treatment of OA (Boston Total Joint Association, 2004). Most hip replacements last 10 to 15 years, after which a second joint replacement, called a revision, can be performed. Potential problems associated with a total hip replacement include blood clots in leg veins, dislocation within the prosthesis, loosening of joint components from surrounding bone, and infection. If recurrent or ineffectively treated, these complications may necessitate removal of the prosthesis, resulting in severe shortening of the extremity and an unstable hip joint.
- *Total knee replacement* is performed if the client has intractable pain and x-ray films show evidence of arthritis of the knee. More than 350,000 knee replacements are performed in the United States each year (Flynn & Johnson, 2005). Several prosthetic devices involving removal of varying amounts of bone are available for knee joint replacement (Figure 42–4 ■). The femoral side of the joint is replaced with a metallic surface, and the tibial side with polyethylene. More than 80% of clients obtain significant or total relief of pain with a total knee replacement. They must, however, engage in a vigorous program of rehabili-

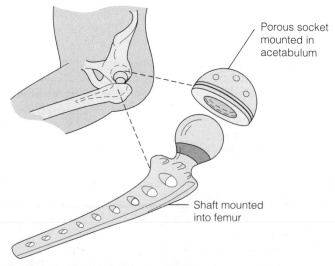

Figure 42–3 ■ Total hip prosthesis.

Porous socket mounted in acetabulum

Shaft mounted into femur

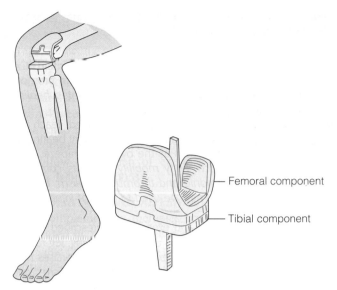

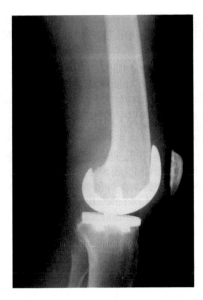

Femoral component

Tibial component

Figure 42–4 ■ Total knee replacement.

tation to achieve the best results. Joint failure is more common with knee replacement than with a total hip replacement. Loosened joint components, often on the tibial side, are the most common cause of failure. The possible complications following a total knee replacement are the same as for a total hip replacement.

■ *Total shoulder replacement* is indicated for unremitting pain and marked limitation of range of motion because of arthritic involvement of both the humeral and glenoid joint surfaces of the shoulder. The joint is immobilized in a sling or abduction splint for 2 to 3 weeks following arthroplasty. Dislocation, loosening of the prosthesis, and infection are potential problems associated with total shoulder replacement.

■ *Total elbow replacement* involves replacement of the humeral and ulnar surfaces of the elbow joint with a metal and poly-

ethylene prosthesis. Pain and disabling stiffness of the joint are indications for an elbow arthroplasty. Complications, including dislocation, fracture, tricep weakness, loosening, and infection, occur frequently.

Infection is the major complication associated with total joint replacement. Not only does infection interfere with healing and prolong recovery, but it may also necessitate removal of the prosthesis and may lead to loss of joint function. Other potential complications include circulatory impairment to the affected limb, thromboembolism, nerve damage, and dislocation of the joint.

Nursing care for the client undergoing total joint replacement is outlined in the box below. Refer to Chapter 4 ∞ for further discussion of care for the client undergoing surgery.

NURSING CARE OF THE CLIENT HAVING Total Joint Replacement

PREOPERATIVE CARE

■ Assess the client knowledge and understanding of the planned operative procedure. Provide further explanations and clarification as needed. *It is important that the client have a clear and realistic understanding of the surgical procedure and expected results. Knowledge decreases anxiety and increases the client's ability to assist with postoperative care procedures.*

■ Obtain a health history and physical assessment, including range of motion of the affected joints. *This information not only allows nurses to tailor care to the needs of the individual but also serves as a baseline for comparison of postoperative assessment data.*

■ Explain necessary postoperative activity restrictions. Teach how to use the overhead trapeze for changing positions. *The client*

who learns and practices moving techniques before surgery can use them more effectively in the postoperative period.

■ Provide or reinforce teaching of postoperative exercises specific to the joint on which surgery is to be performed. *Exercises are prescribed postoperatively to (a) strengthen muscles providing joint stability and support, (b) prevent muscle atrophy and joint contractures; and (c) prevent venous stasis and possible thromboembolism.*

■ Teach respiratory hygiene procedures such as the use of incentive spirometry, coughing, and deep breathing. *Adequate respiratory hygiene is imperative for all clients undergoing joint replacement to prevent respiratory complications associated with immobility and the effects of anesthesia. In addition, many clients undergoing total joint replacement are elderly and may have reduced mucociliary clearance.*

(continued)

THE CLIENT WITH MUSCULAR DYSTROPHY

Muscular dystrophy (MD) is a group of inherited muscle diseases that cause progressive muscle degeneration and wasting. The differences in the types of MD relate to the age at onset, the gender affected by the disorder, the muscles involved, and the rate at which the disease progresses. These factors are summarized in Table 42–2. In the majority of cases of MD, there is a positive family history.

The most common form of MD, Duchenne's muscular dystrophy, is inherited as a recessive single gene defect on the X chromosome (a sex-linked recessive disorder), and is transmitted from the mother to male children. This disorder affects males exclusively and occurs in 1 of 3500 live male births. It can be recognized early in pregnancy in about 95% of cases by genetic studies; or in late pregnancy through amniocentesis. Genetic counseling cannot be reliably used to prevent this disease because there is no way to determine if the woman carries the defective gene. The manifestations appear in early childhood, with the average life span being about 15 years after onset (Porth, 2005).

Other types of MD have an onset at any age, and a slow progression with a normal life span.

Pathophysiology

The basic defect in MD is unknown; however, three theories have been proposed. The *vascular* and *neurogenic theories* suggest that the cause is a lack of blood supply to the muscle or a disturbance in the interaction between the nerve and muscle. The *membrane theory* suggests that an alteration in the cell membranes of the muscle causes them to degenerate. Recent genetic studies have shown a deficiency in the amount of dystrophin, a muscle membrane protein, in clients with Duchenne's MD. Dystrophin plays an important role in protecting the muscle against mechanical stresses.

Manifestations

All forms of MD exhibit manifestations of muscle weakness. The specific muscles involved depend on the type of MD. As the disease progresses, the person develops difficulty with ambulation and eventually becomes wheelchair-bound and finally bed-bound. Cardiac abnormalities, endocrine abnormalities, and mental retardation may also occur.

INTERDISCIPLINARY CARE

Because there is no cure or specific treatment for MD, care focuses on preserving and promoting mobility. An interdisciplinary approach, involving many members of the healthcare team, is necessary to meet the physical and psychologic needs of these clients and their families. Diagnosis and classification of the muscular dystrophies are most often based on the manifestations and the pattern of muscle involvement. Biochemical examination, muscle biopsy, and electromyography confirm the diagnosis. Diagnostic tests are described in Chapter 40 ∞.

Tests include measuring creatine kinase (CK-MM, the isoenzyme found in skeletal muscle) which is elevated in the client with suspected MD; performing a muscle biopsy to identify fibrous connective tissue and fatty deposits that displace functional muscle fibers, and conducting an electromyogram (EMG), which will show a decrease in amplitude in MD.

NURSING CARE

Nursing care for a client with MD focuses on promoting independence and mobility and providing psychologic support for both the client and family. A holistic approach is essential in planning and implementing care.

TABLE 42–2 Types of Muscular Dystrophy

TYPE	SEX AND AGE AT ONSET	CLINICAL MANIFESTATIONS	PROGRESSION
Duchenne's	Males Ages 3 to 5	Weakness of pelvic and shoulder girdles Waddling gait Toe walking Lordosis Cardiac abnormalities Low IQ in 50% of cases	Rapid; client usually confined to wheelchair by age 15; death occurs by age 20
Myotonic	Males and females Any age	Myotonia of hand muscles Muscular weakness of arms and legs Cardiac abnormalities Endocrine abnormalities Mental retardation (common)	Slow; death usually occurs in early 50s
Becker's	Males Ages 5 to 20	Weakness of pelvic and shoulder girdles	Slow; client usually confined to wheelchair at 25 years after onset; normal life span
Facioscapulohumeral	Males and females Ages 10 to 20	Weakness of face and shoulder girdles	Slow; normal life span
Limb-girdle	Males and females Ages 20 to 40	Weakness of shoulder and pelvic girdles	Extremely variable; usually slow

Nursing Diagnoses and Interventions
Self-Care Deficit

The progressive muscle weakness that is associated with MD impairs the client's ability to perform self-care.

- Provide clients and family with supportive care during the progress of the disease. *The goal of treatment is to prolong each functional stage and delay or prevent deformity. When transition from ambulation to a wheelchair occurs, depression and grief may occur.*
- Promote independence. Encourage tasks that can be accomplished rather than letting the client struggle with tasks that may prove frustrating. *All forms of MD result in progressive muscle weakness. Management of the disease is directed toward keeping the client as functional as possible while preventing any deformities.*

Community-Based Care

Teaching the client with MD focuses on maintaining function and independence and preventing deformities. Teach prescribed exercises such as stretching and counterposturing exercises. For the client with braces, discuss skin care and ways to prevent irritation under the brace. Because the client may have weakness involving muscles of respiration, teach the client how to prevent respiratory infections, such as avoiding crowds during flu season and being immunized against pneumococcal pneumonia and influenza. Provide information about support services and organizations such as the Muscular Dystrophy Association.

AUTOIMMUNE AND INFLAMMATORY DISORDERS

Autoimmune and inflammatory disorders of the musculoskeletal system are chronic systemic rheumatic disorders, characterized by diffuse inflammatory lesions and degenerative changes in connective tissues. The disorders have similar clinical features and may affect many of the same structures and organs.

THE CLIENT WITH RHEUMATOID ARTHRITIS

Rheumatoid arthritis (RA) is a chronic systemic autoimmune disease that causes inflammation of connective tissue, primarily in the joints. Its course and severity are variable, and the range of manifestations is broad. Manifestations of RA may be minimal, with mild inflammation of only a few joints and little structural damage, or relentlessly progressive, with multiple inflamed joints and marked deformity. Most clients exhibit a pattern of symmetric involvement of multiple peripheral joints and periods of remission and exacerbation.

FAST FACTS
RA
- RA is found worldwide, affecting 1% to 2% of the total population and all races.
- RA affects 3 times as many women as men.
- The onset of RA occurs most frequently between the ages of 20 and 40 years.

The cause of RA is unknown. A combination of genetic, environmental, hormonal, and reproductive factors is thought to play a role in its development. It is speculated that infectious agents, such as bacteria, mycoplasmas, and viruses (especially Epstein-Barr virus), may play a role in initiating the autoimmune processes present in RA. Several studies have found that heavy smokers are at increased risk for developing RA. It is known that the incidence of RA has decreased during the past 40 years, supporting the theory that environmental factors may change and either promote or protect against RA (Flynn & Johnson, 2005).

The course of RA is variable and fluctuating. Remissions are most likely to occur in the first year of the disease. The rate at which joint deformities develop is not constant. Disease progression is fastest during the first 6 years, slowing thereafter. RA contributes to disability and a tendency to shorten life expectancy. About 10% of people with RA go into long-term remission within 1 year; and another 50% to 60% go into remission within 2 years (Flynn & Johnson, 2005).

RA is less common than OA, with RA affecting 1% to 2% of the population (about 2.1 million people) (Flynn & Johnson, 2005). The incidence of RA increases with age up to about 70 years. Although the onset and manifestations of RA are much the same in older and younger clients, differentiating between RA and OA in the older adult may be difficult at times. It is important to establish an accurate diagnosis, however, because the management of these disorders differs significantly. Clinical features distinguishing RA from OA are listed in Table 42–3.

For older clients, RA is managed much as it is for younger people. However, prolonged bed rest or inactivity is not prescribed for acute episodes, because it may result in irreversible immobility in the older adult. Also, medications are used with greater caution because of the increased risk of toxicity. In many cases, less emphasis is placed on preventing joint deformity and more emphasis on maintaining functional status for the older client with RA.

Pathophysiology

It is believed that long-term exposure to an unidentified antigen causes an aberrant immune response in a genetically susceptible host. As a result, normal antibodies (immunoglobulins) become autoantibodies and attack host tissues. These transformed antibodies, usually present in people with RA, are called *rheumatoid factors (RFs)*. The self-produced antibodies bind with their target antigens in blood and synovial membranes, forming immune complexes (see Chapter 13 ∞ for further information about autoimmune processes).

The damage to cartilage that occurs in RA is the result of at least three processes:

- Neutrophils, T cells, and other synovial fluid cells are activated and degrade the surface layer of the articular cartilage.
- Cytokines, especially interleukin-1 (IL-1) and tumor necrosis factor alpha (TNF-α), cause the chondrocytes to attack the cartilage.

TABLE 42–3 Comparison of the Manifestations of Rheumatoid Arthritis and Osteoarthritis

FEATURE	RHEUMATOID ARTHRITIS	OSTEOARTHRITIS
Onset	Usually insidious, may be abrupt	Insidious
Course	Generally progressive, characterized by remissions and exacerbations	Slowly progressive
Pain and stiffness	Predominant on arising, lasting >1 hour; also occurs after prolonged inactivity	Pain with activity; stiffness following periods of immobility generally relieved within minutes
Affected joints	■ Appear red, hot, swollen; "boggy" and tender to palpation; decreased ROM, weakness ■ Multiple joints affected in symmetric pattern; PIP, MCP, wrists, knees, ankles, and toes often involved	■ Affected joints may appear swollen; cool and bony hard on palpation; decreased ROM ■ One or several joints affected including hips, knees, lumbar and cervical spine, PIP and DIP, wrist, and 1st MTP joint
Systemic manifestations	Fatigue, weakness, anorexia, weight loss, fever; rheumatoid nodules; anemia	Fatigue

■ The synovium digests nearby cartilage, releasing inflammatory molecules containing IL-1 and TNF-α.

Leukocytes are attracted to the synovial membrane from the circulation, where neutrophils and macrophages ingest the immune complexes and release enzymes that degrade synovial tissue and articular cartilage. Activation of B and T lymphocytes results in increased production of rheumatoid factors and enzymes that increase and continue the inflammatory process.

The synovial membrane is damaged by the inflammatory and immune processes. It swells from infiltration of the leukocytes and thickens as cells proliferate and abnormally enlarge. The inflammation spreads and involves synovial blood vessels. Small venules are occluded, and vascular flow to the synovial tissue decreases. As blood flow decreases and metabolic needs increase (from the increased number and size of cells), hypoxia and metabolic acidosis occur. Acidosis stimulates synovial cells to release hydrolytic enzymes into surrounding tissues, starting erosion of the articular cartilage and inflammation of the supporting ligaments and tendons.

The inflammation also causes hemorrhage, coagulation, and deposits of fibrin on the synovial membrane, in the intracellular matrix, and in the synovial fluid. Fibrin develops into granulation tissue (*pannus*) over denuded areas of the synovial membrane. The formation of pannus leads to scar tissue formation that immobilizes the joint (Figure 42–5 ■).

Joint Manifestations

The onset of RA is typically insidious, although it may be acute (precipitated by a stressor such as infection, surgery, or trauma). Joint manifestations are often preceded by systemic manifestations of inflammation, including fatigue, anorexia, weight loss, and nonspecific aching and stiffness. Clients report joint swelling with associated stiffness, warmth, tenderness, and pain. The pattern of joint involvement is typically polyarticular (involving multiple joints) and symmetric. The proximal interphalangeal (PIP) and metacarpophalangeal (MCP) joints of the fingers, the wrists, the knees, the ankles, and the toes are most frequently involved, although RA can af-

fect any joint. Stiffness is most pronounced in the morning, lasting more than 1 hour. It may also occur with prolonged rest during the day and may be more severe following strenuous activity. Swollen, inflamed joints feel "boggy" or spongelike on palpation because of synovial edema. Range of motion is limited in affected joints, and weakness may be evident.

The persistent inflammation of RA causes deformities of the joint itself and supporting structures such as ligaments, tendons, and muscles. As the joint is destroyed, ligaments, tendons, and the joint capsule are weakened or destroyed. Joint cartilage and bone are also destroyed. Weakening or destruction of these supporting structures results in lack of opposition to muscle pull, causing deformity.

Characteristic changes in the hands and fingers include ulnar deviation of the fingers and subluxation at the MCP joints. Swan-neck deformity is characterized by hyperextension of the PIP joint with compensatory flexion of the distal interpha-

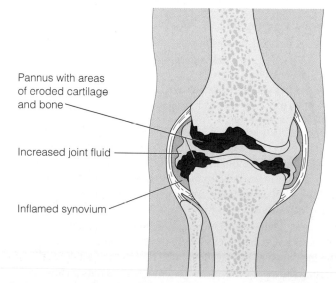

Pannus with areas of eroded cartilage and bone

Increased joint fluid

Inflamed synovium

Figure 42–5 ■ Joint inflammation and destruction in rheumatoid arthritis. Note synovial inflammation with pannus formation and the erosion of cartilage and underlying bone.

langeal (DIP) joints. A flexion deformity of the PIP joints with extension of the DIP joint is called a boutonniére deformity (Figure 42–6 ■). The ability to effect a pinch is limited by hyperextension of the interphalangeal joint and flexion of the MCP joint of the thumb.

Wrist involvement is nearly universal, leading to limited movement, deformity, and carpal tunnel syndrome. Inflammation of the elbows often causes flexion contracture.

The knees are frequently affected in RA, with visible swelling often obliterating normal contours. Instability of the knee joint along with quadriceps atrophy, contractures, and valgus (knock-knee) deformities can lead to significant disability. Ambulation may be limited by pain and deformities when the ankles and feet are involved. Typical deformities of the feet and toes include subluxation, hallux valgus (deviation of the great toe toward the other digits of the foot), lateral deviation of the toes, and cock-up toes (turned-up toes).

Spinal involvement is usually limited to the cervical vertebrae. Neck pain is common, and neurologic complications can occur.

Extra-Articular Manifestations

RA is a systemic disease with a variety of extra-articular manifestations. These are seen particularly in clients with high levels of circulating rheumatoid factor. Fatigue, weakness, anorexia, weight loss, and low-grade fever are common when the disease is active. Anemia resistant to iron therapy frequently affects clients with RA. Skeletal muscle atrophy is common, usually most apparent in the musculature around affected joints.

Rheumatoid nodules may develop, usually in subcutaneous tissue in areas subject to pressure: on the forearm, olecranon bursa, over the MCP joints, and on the toes. Rheumatoid nodules are granulomatous lesions that are firm and either movable or fixed. They may also be found in viscera, including the heart, lungs, intestinal tract, and dura.

Other possible extra-articular manifestations of RA include subcutaneous nodules, pleural effusion, vasculitis, pericarditis, and splenomegly (enlargement of the spleen). The *Multisystem Effects of RA* are illustrated on page 1462.

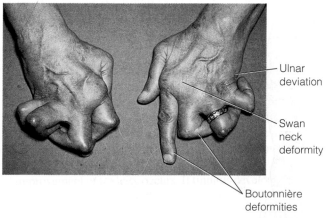

Figure 42–6 ■ Typical hand deformities associated with rheumatoid arthritis.

— Ulnar deviation

— Swan neck deformity

— Boutonnière deformities

Source: Biophoto Associates/Photo Researchers, Inc.

Increased Risk of Coronary Heart Disease

People with rheumatoid arthritis have an increased risk of developing coronary heart disease (CHD). In turn, CHD increases the risk of myocardial infarction and death; in fact, RA is associated with a shortened life expectancy (Flynn & Johnson, 2005). RA affects the heart by:

■ Direct effects on the blood vessels, with measures of C-reactive proteins (inflammatory markers) being more predictive of future cardiovascular disease than are low-density lipoprotein (LDL) levels.

■ Increased risk of having low high-density lipoprotein, high cholesterol and triglyceride levels, high blood pressure, and high levels of homocysteine—all of which increase the risk for CHD.

■ The damaging side effects that many medications, such as methotrexate and steroids, often have on coronary vessels.

INTERDISCIPLINARY CARE

The diagnosis of RA is based on the client's history, physical assessment, and diagnostic tests. Diagnostic criteria developed by the American Rheumatism Association are used as well (Box 42–3). At least four of seven criteria must be present to establish the diagnosis.

Once the diagnosis of RA has been established, the goals of therapy are to relieve pain, reduce inflammation, slow or stop joint damage, and improve well being and ability to function. No cure currently exists for RA; the goal of treatment is to relieve its manifestations. An interdisciplinary approach is used, with a balance of rest, exercise, physical therapy, and suppression of the inflammatory processes.

Because a cure is not available and traditional therapies are not always fully effective, the client with RA is vulnerable to quackery. Many nontraditional treatments, including diets, topical preparations, vaccines, hormones, plant extracts, and copper bracelets, have been put forth. These treatments are often costly, and none has been shown to be effective.

BOX 42–3 Diagnostic Criteria for Rheumatoid Arthritis

■ Morning stiffness lasting for at least 1 hour and persisting for at least 6 weeks
■ Arthritis with swelling or effusion of three or more joints persisting for at least 6 weeks
■ Arthritis of wrist, MCP, or PIP joints persisting for at least 6 weeks
■ Symmetric arthritis with simultaneous involvement of corresponding joints on both sides of the body
■ Rheumatoid nodules
■ Positive serum rheumatoid factor
■ Characteristic radiologic changes of rheumatoid arthritis noted in hands and wrists

TABLE 42–4 Examples of Nonsteroidal Anti-Inflammatory Drugs Used to Treat Rheumatoid Arthritis

DRUG	AVERAGE DOSE	COMMENTS AND PRECAUTIONS
Aspirin	600–900 mg 4 to 6 times daily	Least expensive NSAID; associated with risk of GI ulceration, bleeding, and possible hemorrhage; may cause hepatotoxicity
Diclofenac (Voltaren)	50 mg tid or qid; or 75 mg bid	Expensive; risk of hepatotoxicity
Etodolac (Lodine)	200-400 mg q6h	Expensive; may have less gastrointestinal toxicity
Fenoprofen (Nalfon)	300-600 mg tid or qid	Should not be administered to clients with impaired renal function; risk of GU effects such as dysuria, cystitis, hematuria, acute interstitial nephritis, and nephrotic syndrome
Flurbiprofen (Ansaid)	50-100 mg tid or qid, not to exceed 300 mg/day	Expensive
Ibuprofen (Motrin, Advil, others)	300 mg qid; 400-800 mg tid or qid	Available in prescription and OTC forms; less gastric distress reported than with aspirin or indomethacin; discontinue if visual disturbances develop
Indomethacin (Indocin)	25-50 mg bid or tid	A potent NSAID used for moderate to severe RA and acute episodes of chronic disease; higher incidence of adverse GI effects and CNS effects such as headache, dizziness, and depression
Ketoprofen (Orudis)	50-75 mg tid or qid	Expensive; older adults and clients with renal insufficiency require lower doses
Meclofenamate sodium (Meclomen)	100 mg bid to qid	Increased risk of adverse effects in older adults; GI effects include diarrhea and abdominal pain; anemia may develop during therapy
Nabumetone (Relafen)	1000-2000 mg per day	Most common adverse effects include diarrhea, dyspepsia, and abdominal pain
Naproxen (Aleve, Anaprox, Naprosyn)	250-500 mg bid	Available in prescription and OTC preparations
Oxaprozin (Daypro)	1200 mg daily	Expensive; risk of severe hepatotoxicity; rash may occur
Piroxicam (Feldene)	20 mg daily in a single or divided dose	Expensive; GI side effects including stomatitis, anorexia, and gastric distress may occur more frequently than with other NSAIDs
Sulindac (Clinoril)	150-200 mg bid	May be safer for use than other NSAIDs in clients with chronic renal disease; rare fatal hypersensitivity reaction with fever, liver function abnormalities, and severe skin reaction
Tolmetin (Tolectin)	200-600 mg tid	Expensive; may have higher rate of side effects including GI distress, headache, dizziness, elevated blood pressure, edema, and weight gain

etanercept (Enbrel). Leflunomide reversibly inhibits an enzyme involved in the autoimmune process, and etanercept inhibits the binding of tumor necrosis factor to receptor sites. Infliximab (Remicade) is a biologic response modifier and TNF-α receptor antagonist. Given by intravenous infusion, the drug is administered to reduce infiltration of inflammatory cells and TNF-α production. Adalimumab (Humira) is a biologic response modifier that is given to people with RA to reduce the inflammatory events of polyarthritis and slow the progression of joint damage. Given by subcutaneous injection, the drug cannot be administered if the person has an acute or chronic infection in any part of the body. Prior to initiating the drug, the person should be tested for tuberculosis.

Gold salts may be administered by mouth, but the intramuscular route is preferred because it is more effective. The mode of action of gold is unknown, but it may produce clinical remission in some clients and decrease new bony erosions. Weekly therapy is continued until significant improvement is noted unless toxic reactions occur. Clients experiencing benefit from gold therapy may be continued on monthly injections for several years. About one-third of clients on gold therapy ex-

perience toxic reactions, including dermatitis, stomatitis, bone marrow depression, and proteinuria. Mild skin reactions do not always necessitate discontinuation of therapy. CBC and urinalysis are monitored throughout treatment with gold to assess for more severe toxic responses.

Hydroxychloroquine (Plaquenil) is an antimalarial agent sometimes employed in the treatment of RA. Three to 6 months of therapy is required to achieve the desired response, and many clients do not experience significant benefit. Although hydroxychloroquine has a relatively low toxicity, it can cause pigmentary retinitis and vision loss. Clients receiving this drug require a thorough vision examination every 6 months.

Sulfasalazine, a drug regularly prescribed for chronic inflammatory bowel disease, may also be prescribed for RA. See Chapter 26 ∞ for further discussion of this drug and its nursing implications. For clients not responding to the above preparations, penicillamine may be prescribed. Although this agent may be effective in the management of RA, toxic reactions are common and can be severe, including bone marrow suppression, proteinuria, and nephrosis.

TABLE 42–5 Disease-Modifying Drugs Used to Treat Rheumatoid Arthritis

CLASS/MEDICATIONS	USUAL DOSE	ADVERSE EFFECTS	COMMENTS/NURSING RESPONSIBILITIES
Gold salts: Gold sodium thiomalate (Myochrysine) Aurothioglucose (Solganal) Auranofin (Ridaura Capsules)	Parenteral: 1st dose 10 mg; 2nd dose 25 mg, then 50 mg weekly IM Oral: 6 mg daily	■ Pruritus, dermatitis ■ Stomatitis, metallic taste ■ Renal toxicity ■ Blood dyscrasias ■ Gastrointestinal distress	■ Frequent UA and CBC ■ Monitor client after injection for flushing, fainting, dizziness, sweating, possible anaphylactic reaction
Antimalarial: Hydroxychloroquine (Plaquenil)	200-600 mg daily with meals	■ CNS reactions including irritability, nightmares, psychoses ■ Retinopathy ■ Alopecia, pruritus ■ Blood dyscrasias ■ GI disturbances	■ Should not be used during pregnancy ■ Regular ophthalmologic examination required
Sulfasalazine (Azulfidine)	2 g/day in divided doses with meals	■ Anorexia, nausea, vomiting, gastric distress ■ Decreased sperm count ■ Headache ■ Rash ■ Blood dyscrasias ■ Hypersensitivity responses including Stevens-Johnson syndrome ■ CNS, liver, and renal toxicity	■ Administer in evenly divided doses ■ Maintain high fluid intake ■ May cause yellow-orange skin or urine discoloration ■ Regular CBCs necessary
Penicillamine (Cuprimine, Depen Titratable)	125-250 mg/day initially, slowly increased to a total of 1000-1500 mg/day	■ Skin rashes ■ Fever ■ Gastrointestinal distress ■ Oral ulcers, loss of taste ■ Fever ■ Bone marrow depression with thrombocytopenia, leukopenia, anemia ■ Renal toxicity ■ May induce immune complex disorders such as Goodpasture's syndrome and myasthenia gravis	■ Regular CBC and UA necessary ■ Administer on an empty stomach ■ Discontinue during pregnancy ■ May require 2 to 3 months of therapy before benefit is seen

IMMUNOSUPPRESSIVE THERAPY Immunosuppressive or cytotoxic drugs are increasingly employed in the management of RA. Indeed, many now consider methotrexate the treatment of choice for clients with aggressive RA. Methotrexate may be used along with NSAIDs in the initial treatment plan. A weekly dose can produce a beneficial effect in as few as 2 to 4 weeks. Gastric irritation and stomatitis are the most frequent side effects associated with methotrexate, but side effects may be better controlled if folic acid is taken at the same time. Alcoholism, diabetes, obesity, advanced age, and renal disease increase the risk of toxic effects (hepatotoxicity, bone marrow suppression, interstitial pneumonitis).

Other immunosuppressive agents such as cyclosporine, azathioprine, and monoclonal antibodies have also been employed in the treatment of clients with severe, progressive, crippling disease who have failed to respond to other measures.

Treatments

The primary objectives in treating RA are to reduce pain and inflammation, preserve function, and prevent deformity.

REST AND EXERCISE A balanced program of rest and exercise is an important component in the management of clients with RA. During an acute exacerbation of the disease, the client may be hospitalized, or a short period of complete bed rest may be prescribed. For most clients, regular rest periods during the day are beneficial to reduce manifestations of the disease. Additionally, splinting of inflamed joints reduces unwanted motion and provides local joint rest. A variety of orthotic devices are available to reduce joint strain and help maintain function.

Rest must be balanced with a program of physical therapy and exercise to maintain muscle strength and joint mobility. ROM exercises are prescribed to maintain joint function and prevent contractures. Isometric exercises are used to improve muscle strength without increasing joint stress. Isotonic exercises also help improve muscle strength and preserve function. Low-impact aerobic exercises, such as swimming and walking, have been shown to benefit clients with RA without adversely affecting joint inflammation or prompting acute episodes.

PHYSICAL AND OCCUPATIONAL THERAPY Physical and occupational therapists can design and monitor individualized activity and rest programs.

HEAT AND COLD Heat and cold are used for their analgesic and muscle-relaxing effects. Moist heat is generally the most effective, and can be provided by a tub bath. Joint pain is relieved in some clients through the application of cold.

ASSISTIVE DEVICES AND SPLINTS Assistive devices, such as a cane, walker, or raised toilet seat, are most useful for clients with significant hip or knee arthritis. Splints provide joint rest and prevent contractures. Night splints for the hands and/or wrists should maintain the extremity in a position of maximum function. The best "splint" for the hip is lying prone for several hours a day on a firm bed. In general, splints should be applied for the shortest period needed, should be made of lightweight materials, and should be easily removed to perform ROM exercises once or twice a day.

NUTRITION For most clients with RA, an ordinary, well-balanced diet is recommended. Some clients may benefit from substitution of usual dietary fat with omega-3 fatty acids found in certain fish oils.

SURGERY Surgical intervention may be employed for the client with RA at a variety of disease stages. Early in the course of the disease, synovectomy (excision of synovial membrane) can provide temporary relief of inflammation, relieve pain, and slow the destructive process, helping to preserve joint function. Arthrodesis (joint fusion), may be used to stabilize joints such as cervical vertebrae, wrists, and ankles. Arthroplasty, or total joint replacement, may be necessary in cases of gross deformity and joint destruction. Total joint replacement and nursing care of clients undergoing this surgery are discussed in the preceding section on OA.

OTHER THERAPIES Several newer treatments that are not yet in widespread use may be employed in clients with progressive RA. Plasmapheresis has been used to remove circulating antibodies, moderating the autoimmune response. Total lymphoid irradiation decreases total lymphocyte levels, although serious adverse effects are associated with this treatment, and its continued efficacy has not been established.

NURSING CARE

Clients with chronic, progressive, systemic disorders such as RA have multiple nursing care needs involving many functional health patterns. Physical manifestations of the disease often result in acute and chronic pain, fatigue, impaired mobility, and difficulty performing routine tasks. The disease also has many psychosocial effects. The client has an incurable chronic disease that may lead to severe crippling. Pain and fatigue can interfere with the client's ability to perform expected roles, such as home maintenance or job responsibilities. Even though the client's hands may appear swollen or deformed, other people may not understand the systemic nature of the disease or realize the difference between RA and OA. A Nursing Care Plan for a client with RA is found on the next page.

Health Promotion

People with RA have control of their lives by becoming arthritis self-managers. They can help prevent deformities and the effects of arthritis by following prescriptions for exercise, rest, weight management, posture, and positioning. The following suggestions are outlined by the Moss Rehab Resource Net (2005):
- Never attempt an activity that cannot be stopped immediately if it proves to be beyond your power to complete it.
- Respect pain as a warning signal. When you experience pain, change your method of doing things, use equipment or tools if necessary, and take intermittent rest periods.
- Use the strongest joints available for an activity. For example, use the palm of your hand or the crook of your elbow instead of fingers for grasping while carrying.
- Avoid stress toward a position of deformity, such as when the fingers drift toward the little finger. For example, open a jar with your right hand and close a jar with your left hand.
- Avoid activities that need a tight grip, such as writing, wringing, and unscrewing.

Assessment

Collect the following data through the health history and physical examination (see Chapter 40 ∞):
- *Health History:* Pain, stiffness, fatigue, joint problems: location, duration, onset, effect on function, fever, sleep patterns, past illnesses or surgery, ability to carry out ADLs and self-care activities.
- *Physical Assessment:* Height/weight; gait; joints: symmetry, size, shape, color, appearance, temperature, range of motion, pain; skin: nodules, purpura; respiratory: cough, crackles; cardiovascular: pericardial friction rub, apical bradycardia, S_3.

Nursing Diagnoses and Interventions

Many nursing diagnoses may be appropriate for the client with RA. This section focuses on those related to its predominant manifestations and their effect on the client's life.

Chronic Pain

Pain is a constant feature of RA when the disease is active. Pain accompanies both acute inflammation and lower levels of chronic inflammation. Some clients say the pain in joints and surrounding tissue is like a deep, constant toothache. Pain can significantly affect the client's ability to provide self-care and maintain daily activities. It also contributes to the client's fatigue.
- Monitor the level of pain and duration of morning stiffness. *Pain and morning stiffness are indicators of disease activity. Increased pain may necessitate changes in the therapeutic treatment plan.*
- Encourage the client to relate pain to activity level and adjust activities accordingly. Teach the importance of joint and whole-body rest in relieving pain. *Pain is an indicator of excess stress on inflamed joints. Increasing pain indicates a need to decrease activity levels.*
- Teach the use of heat and cold applications to provide pain relief. The client may apply heat by showering or taking tub

NURSING CARE PLAN A Client with Rheumatoid Arthritis

Janice James is a 42-year-old high school science teacher who began noticing vague joint pain, fatigue, poor appetite, and general malaise, which she initially attributed to a case of the flu. However, her symptoms continued, and she reports feeling very stiff in the mornings, often taking until 10:00 or 11:00 A.M. to begin to feel "normal." She then began to notice aching in her hands and wrists, which she attributed to the quilting she loves to do in the evenings. She made an appointment with her family physician when she noticed that her knuckles and finger joints are not just achy but also swollen and hot. Noting that Mrs. James has lost 10 lb since her last visit and has mild anemia and a significantly elevated ESR, the physician refers her to the rheumatology clinic for further evaluation. Following examination, laboratory, and radiologic testing, the rheumatologist establishes a diagnosis of rheumatoid arthritis and initiates a multidisciplinary team conference to plan the management of Mrs. James's rheumatoid arthritis.

ASSESSMENT

Cathy Greenstein, RN, completes an assessment of Mrs. James. She notes that Mrs. James is well groomed and answers questions readily but appears fatigued and ill. Mrs. James relates that her job has been extremely stressful because teacher layoffs have resulted in larger class sizes and fewer teaching assistants. Despite symptoms, she continues to teach full time, but says she feels unable to keep up with all her responsibilities due to her fatigue.

Mrs. James states that she is allergic to penicillin. Her past medical history reveals only the usual childhood diseases and three uncomplicated pregnancies, resulting in the births of her children, ages 14, 11, and 9. Physical assessment findings include BP 124/78, P 82 regular, R 18, T 100.2°F (37.8°C) PO. Hands: swelling of the proximal interphalangeal (PIP) and metacarpophalangeal (MCP) joints of both hands; second and third PIP and second MCP joints on right hand are red, shiny, hot, spongy, and tender to palpation; able to extend fingers to 180 degrees but cannot make a complete fist with either hand, with flexion limited to less than 90 degrees; grip strength is weak bilaterally; wrist ROM is limited in all directions. Knees are swollen, and flexion is slightly limited; positive bulge sign in the right knee. Diagnostic findings are an ESR of 52 mm/h, a hematocrit of 30% and positive for rheumatoid factor. Few changes other than soft tissue swelling are evident on hand and wrist x-rays.

DIAGNOSES

- *Chronic Pain* related to joint inflammation
- *Impaired Home Maintenance* related to fatigue
- *Activity Intolerance* related to the effects of inflammation
- *Deficient Knowledge: Therapeutic Regimen*

EXPECTED OUTCOMES

- Verbalize effective pain management strategies:
  - Use assistive devices to minimize joint stress with ADLs:

- Verbalize a plan to reduce responsibilities for home maintenance.
- Express a willingness to plan rest breaks during the day.
- Demonstrate understanding of the prescribed therapeutic regimen and its importance for both short- and long-term benefit.

PLANNING AND IMPLEMENTATION

- Teach techniques for relieving pain and morning stiffness, including:
  - Schedule NSAIDs at equal intervals throughout the day
  - Take morning NSAID dose with milk and crackers approximately 30 minutes before rising
  - Perform ROM exercises in shower or bathtub
  - Apply local heat with paraffin dip or compress, use cold packs as needed.
  - Teach techniques to minimize joint stress while performing ADLs.
- Provide Arthritis Foundation literature and information.
- Discuss ways to delegate household tasks to other family members.
- Explore ways to incorporate 30-minute rest breaks into work schedule.
- Provide information about the disease process and its manifestations, prescribed medications with desired and adverse effects, and the importance of balancing rest and activity.

EVALUATION

The initial treatment regimen of aspirin, rest, exercise, and physical therapy succeeded in partially relieving the acute manifestations of rheumatoid arthritis in Mrs. James. However, complete remission has not been achieved. She has had difficulty scheduling rest periods at work and has had to struggle to delegate household tasks. "I don't look sick to the kids, and they seem to think housecleaning is a terrible imposition on their time. It's often easier to just do it myself than to fight about it. Besides, that way it gets done right." Mrs. James has faithfully followed the prescribed medication regimen and exercise routines, and she has kept her scheduled appointments and maintained contact with the treatment team.

CRITICAL THINKING IN THE NURSING PROCESS

1. Mrs. James is 42 years old. Would your nursing interventions differ if she were 72 years old? If so, how.
2. Rheumatoid arthritis is a chronic illness. What are the physical, emotional, and economic implications of a chronic illness that results in chronic pain and deformity?
3. Develop a nursing care plan for Mrs. James using the nursing diagnosis *Ineffective Role Performance*.
   See Evaluating Your Response in Appendix C.

baths, or using warm compresses or other local applications such as paraffin dips. For clients who find that heat increases pain and swelling during periods of acute inflammation, cold packs may be more effective. *Both heat and cold have analgesic effects and can help relieve associated muscle spasms.*

- Teach about the use of prescribed anti-inflammatory medications and the relationship of pain and inflammation. *Anti-inflammatory agents reduce chemical mediators of inflammation and swelling, relieving pain.*
- Encourage using other nonpharmacologic pain relief measures such as visualization, distraction, meditation, and progressive

relaxation techniques. *These techniques can reduce muscle tension and help the client focus away from the pain, decreasing the intensity of the pain experience.*

Fatigue

The pain and chronic inflammatory processes associated with RA lead to fatigue. Other factors contribute as well. Discomfort often disrupts the client's sleep patterns. Anemia, muscle atrophy, and poor nutrition also play a role in the development of fatigue. The client with RA may experience depression or hopelessness, with associated manifestations of fatigue.

- Encourage a balance of periods of activity with periods of rest. *Both joint and whole-body rest are important to reduce the inflammatory response.*
- Stress the importance of planned rest periods during the day. *Rest is vital during acute exacerbations of the disease but also important to maintain the client in remission.*
- Help in prioritizing activities, performing the most important ones early in the day. *Assigning priorities helps the client avoid performing relatively unimportant activities at the expense of more meaningful and important ones.*
- Encourage regular physical activity in addition to prescribed ROM exercises. *Aerobic exercise promotes a sense of well-being and restful sleep patterns.*
- Refer to counseling or support groups. *Counseling and support groups can help the client develop effective coping strategies and deal with depression and hopelessness.*

Ineffective Role Performance

Fatigue, pain, and the crippling effects of RA can interfere with the client's ability to pursue a career and fill other life roles, such as parent, spouse, or homemaker. As the client's role changes, so must the roles of other family members. This can contribute to changes in family processes, increased stress in the family, and further difficulty coping with the effects of the disease.

- Discuss the effects of the disease on the client's career and other life roles. Encourage the client to identify changes brought on by the disease. *Discussion helps the client to accept the changes and begin to identify strategies for coping with them.*
- Encourage the client and family to discuss their feelings about role changes and grieve lost roles or abilities. *Verbalization allows family members to validate and accept feelings about losses and changes, thus helping them to move into new roles.*
- Listen actively to concerns expressed by the client and family members; acknowledge the validity of concerns about the disease, prescribed treatment, and the prognosis. *Demonstrating acceptance of these feelings and concerns promotes trust and validates their reality.*

PRACTICE ALERT

Remember that grief resolution takes time and that clients may respond to loss with anger.

- Help the client and family identify strengths they can use to cope with role changes. *Identifying strengths helps the client and family to consider role changes that maintain self-esteem and dignity.*

- Encourage the client to make decisions and assume personal responsibility for disease management. *Clients who assume a personal and active role in managing their disease maintain a greater sense of self-control and self-esteem.*

Disturbed Body Image

The acute and long-term effects of RA can affect the client's body image, leading to feelings of hopelessness and powerlessness, social withdrawal, and difficulty adapting to changes. When inflammation and joint deformity occur despite compliance, the client may have difficulty accepting the need to continue therapeutic measures, particularly those that have side effects or are costly or time consuming. In addition, unproven alternative treatment strategies and quackery may become increasingly attractive to the client.

- Demonstrate a caring, accepting attitude toward the client. *This attitude helps the client accept the physical changes brought on by the disease.*
- Encourage the client to talk about the effects of the disease, both physical effects and effects on life roles. *Verbalization helps the client identify feelings and gives the nurse opportunity to validate these feelings.*
- Encourage the client to maintain self-care and usual roles to the extent possible. Discuss the use of clothing and adaptive devices that promote independence. *Independence enhances the client's self-esteem.*
- Provide positive feedback for self-care activities and adaptive strategies. *Positive reinforcement encourages the client to continue adaptive measures and maintain independence.*
- Refer to self-help groups, support groups, and other agencies that provide assistive devices and literature. *These groups and agencies can help the client develop adaptive strategies to cope with the effects of RA, enhancing the client's self-concept, body image, and independence.*

Using NANDA, NIC, and NOC

Chart 42–3 shows links between NANDA nursing diagnoses, NIC, and NOC when caring for the client with RA.

Community-Based Care

RA is typically a chronic, progressive disease. As with most diseases of this nature, involvement of the client and family in its management is vital. Education is an important nursing role in caring for clients with RA and their families. (See the Nursing Research box on page 1469). Address the following topics for home care of the client and for family members:

- Disease process and treatments, including rest and exercise
- Medications
- Management of stiffness and pain
- Energy conservation
- Use of assistive devices to maintain independence, including self-care aids such as handheld showers, long-handled brushes and shoehorns, and eating utensils with oversized or special handles
- Clothing options such as elastic waist pants without zippers, Velcro closures, zippers with large pull-tabs, and slip-on shoes
- How to apply splints and take care of skin

NANDA, NIC, AND NOC LINKAGES
CHART 42–3 The Client with Rheumatoid Arthritis

NANDA

Powerlessness

↓

NIC

Self-Esteem Enhancement

Support Group

Emotional Support

Environmental Management

Self-Care Assistance

↓

NOC

Health Beliefs: Perceived Control

Health Beliefs: Perceived Resources

Social Support

Data from *NANDA's Nursing Diagnoses: Definitions & Classification 2005–2006* by NANDA International (2005), Philadelphia; *Nursing Interventions Classification (NIC)* (4th ed.) by J. M. Dochterman & G. M. Bulechek (2004), St. Louis, MO: Mosby; and *Nursing Outcomes Classification (NOC)* (3rd ed.) by S. Moorhead, M. Johnson, and M. Maas (2004), St. Louis, MO: Mosby.

- Home and equipment modifications, such as a raised toilet seat, grab bars in the bathroom, a bath chair, or adapted counter heights for clients in a wheelchair
- Physical therapy, occupational therapy, home health and homemaker services
- Helpful resources:
  - National Institute of Arthritis and Musculoskeletal and Skin Diseases
  - American College of Rheumatology
  - Arthritis Foundation.
  - The Arthritis Society
  - American Physical Therapy Foundation
  - American Chronic Pain Association.

THE CLIENT WITH ANKYLOSING SPONDYLITIS

Ankylosing spondylitis (AS) is a chronic inflammatory arthritis that primarily affects the axial skeleton, leading to pain and progressive stiffening and fusion of the spine. The typical age of onset is between 17 and 35, with at least half a million people with AS in the United States (Spondylitis Association of America, 2006). The incidence is greater in men than women and men have more severe disease. AS is difficult to diagnose in the early stages, but may be a major cause of persistent back pain in young adults.

The cause of ankylosing spondylitis is unknown. As with the other spondyloarthropathies, there is a strong genetic component. Approximately 90% of people with ankylosing spondylitis have the HLA-B27 antigen; about 8% of the general population has this antigen (Porth, 2005).

NURSING RESEARCH | Evidence-Based Practice: Teaching the Client with Rheumatoid Arthritis

Rheumatoid arthritis (RA) is a disease that can occur at any age, but is seen most often in older adults. RA causes physical, emotional, and economic difficulties, but appropriate management can do much to reduce pain and disability, improve a sense of control, and improve quality of life. With recent advances in computer technology, the Internet has become a convenient means of providing information to people with RA. However, little is known about how many older adults use the computer to gain access to information. This study was conducted to examine the use of computers and the Internet by older adults with arthritis and to describe the characteristics of those who did use the Internet to find health information. Although one of every four older adults who participated in the study owned a computer, only slightly more than half actually used the Internet. Lack of knowledge about using the computer or about accessing the Internet were given as possible reasons.

IMPLICATIONS FOR NURSING
The Internet is a powerful method for providing health information to older adults. Although health history questions rarely contain questions about availability and use of the computer and the

Internet, it may be equally as important as asking about other components of one's dwelling. If older adults have but do not use a computer, referral to community resources that provide computer learning classes can facilitate their success in using the computer and doing online searches of the Internet for health information. In addition, prior to recommending an Internet-based health resource, nurses should review the site for content, readability, navigation features, credibility, organization, and graphic appearance.

CRITICAL THINKING IN CLIENT CARE
1. You are designing an Internet site to teach older adults about RA. What topics would you include? How would your presentation be most effective for this age group?
2. You are conducting a computer-literacy course for older adults with RA at a local library. All of them have computers, but none of them have used the Internet to find out about the disease. What sites would you recommend, and why?
3. Develop a plan to include assessment about computers on an agency's health history. What would you include to convince the agency personnel that this is important?

Data from Tak, S. H., & Hong, S. H. (2005). Use of the Internet for health information by older adults with arthritis. *Orthopaedic Nursing, 24*(2), 134–139.

Pathophysiology

Early inflammatory changes often are first noted in the sacroiliac joints. As the cartilage erodes, joint margins ossify and are replaced by scar tissue. The joints of the spine are also affected, with inflammation of the cartilaginous joints, and gradual calcification and ossification that leads to ankylosis, or joint consolidation and immobility. Other organ systems may be affected as well, including the eyes, lungs, heart, and kidneys.

Manifestations

The onset of ankylosing spondylitis is usually gradual and insidious. Clients may have persistent or intermittent bouts of low back pain. The pain is worse at night, followed by morning stiffness that is relieved by activity. Pain may radiate to the buttocks, hips, or down the legs. As the disease progresses, back motion becomes limited, the lumbar curve is lost, and the thoracic curvature is accentuated. In severe cases, the entire spine becomes fused, preventing any motion. Clients with ankylosing spondylitis may also experience peripheral arthritis, primarily affecting the hip, shoulders, and knee joints. Systemic manifestations include anorexia, weight loss, fever, and fatigue. Many clients develop uveitis (inflammation of the iris and the middle, vascular layer of the eye).

For most clients with ankylosing spondylitis, the disease is intermittent with mild to moderate acute episodes. These clients have a good prognosis with little risk of severe disability.

INTERDISCIPLINARY CARE

Diagnostic testing shows an elevated ESR during periods of active disease and typically a positive HLA-B27 antigen. The diagnosis of ankylosing spondylitis is usually confirmed with x-ray examination of the sacroiliac joints and spine. The sacroiliac joint becomes blurred and gradually obliterated. As the disease progresses, vertebrae become squared, and disk spaces narrow.

As with other forms of arthritis, the management of ankylosing spondylitis is multidimensional. Physical therapy and daily exercises are important to maintain posture and joint ROM. NSAIDs relieve pain and stiffness and allow the client to perform necessary exercises. Indomethacin (Indocin) is the NSAID most commonly used to treat ankylosing spondylitis. It may, however, have many adverse effects, including headache, nausea and vomiting, depression, and psychosis. Other drugs that may be prescribed include sulfasalazine (Azulfidine) and topical or intra-articular corticosteroids. Severe hip joint arthritis may necessitate total hip arthroplasty.

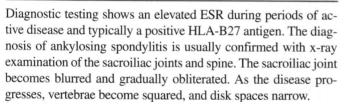 **NURSING CARE**

The primary nursing role in ankylosing spondylitis is to provide supportive care and education. To promote mobility, teach the client to take NSAIDs at regular intervals throughout the day with food, milk, or antacid. Encourage the client to maintain a fluid intake of 2500 mL or more per day. Suggest that the client perform exercises in the shower because warm, moist heat prompts mobility. Stress the importance of following the prescribed physical therapy and exercise program to maintain mobility.

Teach the client that proper positioning and posture are important. When sleeping, a bed board may be used to provide firmness, and the person should sleep in the supine position using either no pillow or only one small pillow. Other important self-care activities include losing weight if applicable, avoiding smoking, and using muscle-strengthening exercises. Suggest occupational counseling if pain and deformity are severe enough to cause work-related problems.

THE CLIENT WITH REACTIVE ARTHRITIS

Reactive arthritis (ReA) (*Reiter's syndrome*) is an acute, nonpurulent inflammatory arthritis that is believed to be a response to an exposure or infection with certain types of bacteria, including *Chlamydia* (a bacterium contracted during sexual activity) or *Salmonella, Shigella, Yersinia, or Campylobacter* (which cause dysentery from contaminated or spoiled food). This type of arthritis most often affects young men who have an inherited HLA-B27 antigen. Reactive arthritis is often found in clients with HIV infection, although the reason for the association is not clear. Reactive arthritis is typically self-limited, although it can be recurrent or progressive. About 15% to 20% of people with ReA develop a chronic arthritis or spondylitis (Spondylitis Association of America, 2006).

Manifestations

Nonbacterial urethritis is often the initial manifestation of Reiter's syndrome. In women, urethritis and cervicitis may be asymptomatic. Conjunctivitis and inflammatory arthritis follow. The arthritis is usually asymmetric, affecting large weight-bearing joints such as the knees and ankles, the sacroiliac joints, or the spine. Mouth ulcers, inflammation of the glans penis, and skin lesions may occur. The heart and aorta may also be affected.

INTERDISCIPLINARY CARE

The diagnosis of reactive arthritis is based on the client's history and presenting symptoms. Manifestations of ReA typically occur 2 to 4 weeks after the infection, and subside in 3 to 12 months. The condition has a tendency to recur. No test is specific for the disorder. Urethral or cervical cultures are obtained to rule out gonococcal infection. When *Chlamydia* is suspected, the client and sexual partner are treated with tetracycline or erythromycin. Reactive arthritis is treated symptomatically, usually with NSAIDs.

NURSING CARE

Clients with reactive arthritis usually are seen in primary care settings such as a clinic or physician's office, making the nursing role primarily one of education. Teach the client about the association of the arthritis with the precipitating infection (if identified). Stress the importance of treating the infection effectively if it is still present. Use this opportunity to provide information about sexually transmitted infections and protective measures to prevent their transmission (see Chapter 52 ∞). Discuss the usual self-limited nature of reactive arthritis, the appropriate use of prescribed NSAID preparations, and symptomatic relief measures such as application of heat and rest.

THE CLIENT WITH SYSTEMIC LUPUS ERYTHEMATOSUS

Systemic lupus erythematosus (SLE) is a chronic inflammatory connective tissue disease. It affects almost all body systems, including the musculoskeletal system. The manifestations of SLE are widely variable and are thought to result from cell and tissue damage caused by deposition of antigen–antibody complexes in connective tissues. SLE affects multiple body systems, and it can range from a mild, episodic disorder to a rapidly fatal disease process.

FAST FACTS

SLE

- Approximately 1 person in 2000 is affected by SLE (about 500,000 in the United States), with women predominating by a ratio of 9:1 over men.
- SLE usually affects women of childbearing age (when the incidence is 30 times greater than in men) but it can occur at any age.
- SLE is more common in African Americans, Hispanics, and Asians than it is in Caucasians (Porth, 2005).
- The incidence of SLE is higher in some families.

Although the exact etiology of SLE is unknown, genetic, environmental, and hormonal factors play a role in its development. Twin studies and a familial pattern of the disease point to a genetic component, as does an increased incidence of other connective tissue diseases in relatives of people with SLE. Certain human leukocyte antigen (HLA) genes are seen more frequently in people with SLE. Environmental factors such as viruses, bacterial antigens, chemicals, drugs, or ultraviolet light may play a role in activation of the pathologic mechanisms of the disease. In addition, it is felt that sex hormones may influence the development of SLE. Women with SLE have reduced levels of several active androgens that are known to inhibit antibody responses. Estrogens have been shown to enhance antibody responses and have an adverse effect in clients with SLE.

The course of SLE is mild in most clients, with periods of remission and exacerbation. The number and severity of exacerbations tend to decrease with time. In some clients, however, SLE is a virulent disease with significant organ system involvement.

Clients with active disease have an increased risk for infections, which are often opportunistic and severe. Infections such as pneumonia and septicemia are the leading cause of death in clients with SLE, followed by the effects of renal or central nervous system (CNS) involvement. See the Multisystem Effects of SLE on the next page.

Pathophysiology

The pathophysiology of SLE involves the production of a large variety of autoantibodies against normal body components such as nucleic acids, erythrocytes, coagulation proteins, lymphocytes, and platelets. Autoantibody production results from hyperreactivity of B cells (humoral response) because of disordered T-cell function (cellular immune response). The most characteristic autoantibodies in SLE are produced in response to nucleic acids, including DNA, histones, ribonucleoproteins, and other components of the cell nucleus.

SLE autoantibodies react with their corresponding antigen to form immune complexes, which are then deposited in the connective tissue of blood vessels, lymphatic vessels, and other tissues. The deposits trigger an inflammatory response leading to local tissue damage. The kidneys are a frequent site of complex deposition and damage; other tissues affected include the musculoskeletal system, brain, heart, spleen, lung, GI tract, skin, and peritoneum. The autoantibodies produced and their target tissue determine the manifestations of SLE.

A number of drugs can cause a syndrome that mimics lupus in clients with no other risk factors for the disease. Procainamide (e.g., Procan-SR, Pronestyl) and hydralazine (Apresoline, Hydralyn) are the most common drugs implicated, along with isoniazid (INH).

Renal and CNS manifestations of SLE rarely occur with drug-induced lupus, but arthritic and other systemic symptoms are common. Manifestations of drug-induced lupus usually resolve when the medication is discontinued.

Manifestations

Typical early manifestations of SLE mimic those of rheumatoid arthritis, including systemic manifestations of fever, anorexia, malaise, and weight loss, and musculoskeletal manifestations of multiple arthralgias and symmetric polyarthritis. Joint symptoms affect more than 90% of clients with SLE. Although synovitis may be present, the arthritis associated with SLE is rarely deforming.

Most people affected by SLE have skin manifestations at some point during their disease. In fact, SLE was originally described as a skin disorder and named for the characteristic red butterfly rash across the cheeks and bridge of the nose (Figure 42–7 ■).

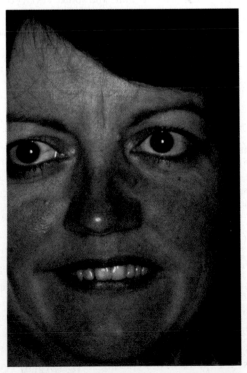

Figure 42–7 ■ The butterfly rash of systemic lupus erythematosus.

MULTISYSTEM EFFECTS of Systemic Lupus Erythematosus

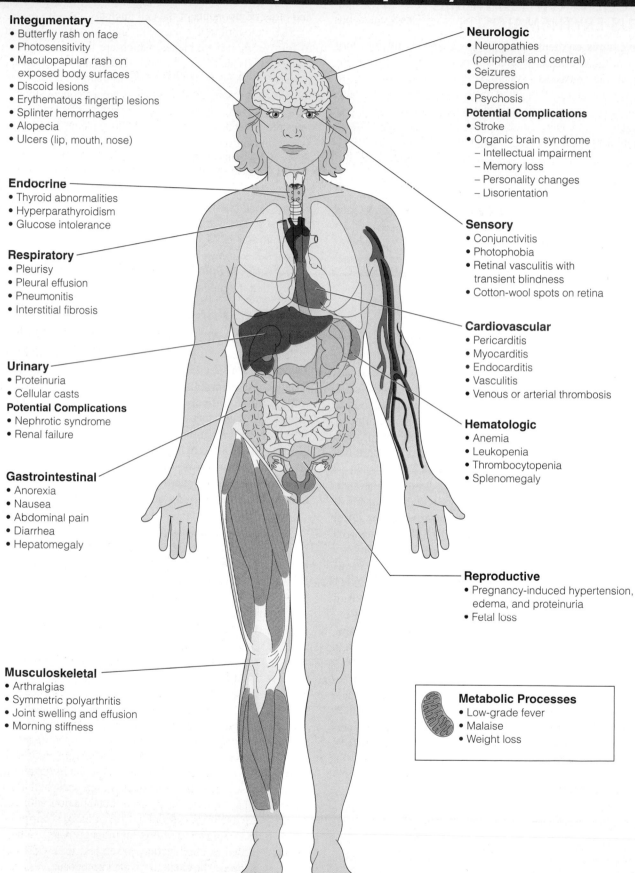

Integumentary
- Butterfly rash on face
- Photosensitivity
- Maculopapular rash on exposed body surfaces
- Discoid lesions
- Erythematous fingertip lesions
- Splinter hemorrhages
- Alopecia
- Ulcers (lip, mouth, nose)

Endocrine
- Thyroid abnormalities
- Hyperparathyroidism
- Glucose intolerance

Respiratory
- Pleurisy
- Pleural effusion
- Pneumonitis
- Interstitial fibrosis

Urinary
- Proteinuria
- Cellular casts
Potential Complications
- Nephrotic syndrome
- Renal failure

Gastrointestinal
- Anorexia
- Nausea
- Abdominal pain
- Diarrhea
- Hepatomegaly

Musculoskeletal
- Arthralgias
- Symmetric polyarthritis
- Joint swelling and effusion
- Morning stiffness

Neurologic
- Neuropathies (peripheral and central)
- Seizures
- Depression
- Psychosis
Potential Complications
- Stroke
- Organic brain syndrome
  - Intellectual impairment
  - Memory loss
  - Personality changes
  - Disorientation

Sensory
- Conjunctivitis
- Photophobia
- Retinal vasculitis with transient blindness
- Cotton-wool spots on retina

Cardiovascular
- Pericarditis
- Myocarditis
- Endocarditis
- Vasculitis
- Venous or arterial thrombosis

Hematologic
- Anemia
- Leukopenia
- Thrombocytopenia
- Splenomegaly

Reproductive
- Pregnancy-induced hypertension, edema, and proteinuria
- Fetal loss

Metabolic Processes
- Low-grade fever
- Malaise
- Weight loss

Many clients with SLE are photosensitive; a diffuse maculopapular rash on skin exposed to the sun is common. Other cutaneous manifestations include discoid lesions (raised, scaly, circular lesions with an erythematous rim), hives, erythematous fingertip lesions, and splinter hemorrhages. Alopecia is common in clients with SLE, although the hair usually grows back. Painless mucous membrane ulcerations may occur on the lips or in the mouth or nose. Common manifestations of SLE are listed in the box below.

Approximately 50% of people with SLE experience renal manifestations of the disease, including proteinuria, cellular casts, and nephrotic syndrome. Up to 10% develop renal failure as a result of the disease.

Hematologic abnormalities such as anemia, leukopenia, and thrombocytopenia are common with SLE. Cardiovascular disorders such as pericarditis, vasculitis, and Raynaud's phenomenon often occur. Less frequently, myocarditis, endocarditis, and venous or arterial thrombosis may develop. Pleurisy, pleural effusions, and lupus pneumonitis are common pulmonary manifestations of SLE.

Many clients with SLE develop transient nervous system involvement, often within the first year of the disease. Organic brain syndrome manifestations include decline in intellect, memory loss, and disorientation. Other possible neurologic manifestations include psychosis, seizures, depression, and stroke. Ocular manifestations of SLE include conjunctivitis, photophobia, and transient blindness due to retinal vasculitis.

Gastrointestinal manifestations of SLE, such as anorexia, nausea, abdominal pain, and diarrhea, may affect up to 45% of clients with the disease. The liver may be enlarged, and liver function tests may yield abnormal results.

INTERDISCIPLINARY CARE

Because of the diversity of organ system involvement and manifestations of SLE, diagnosis can be difficult. No one specific test is available to confirm the presence of this disease in all people suspected of having it. Instead, the diagnosis is based on the client's history and physical assessment, as well as laboratory studies.

As with rheumatoid arthritis, effective management of SLE requires teamwork, with active participation by both the client and members of the healthcare team. Although there is no cure for

SLE, the 10-year survival rate is greater than 70% among clients with this disease, which was once considered fatal in most cases.

Diagnosis

The multiple autoantibodies produced in SLE cause a number of abnormalities in laboratory tests. Diagnostic tests for the musculoskeletal system are described in Chapter 40 ∞.

- *Anti-DNA antibody testing* is a more specific indicator of SLE, because these antibodies are rarely found in any other disorder.
- *ESR* is typically elevated, occasionally to >100 mm/h.
- *Serum complement levels* are usually decreased as complement is consumed or "used up" by the development of antigen-antibody complexes.
- *CBC* abnormalities include moderate to severe anemia, leukopenia and lymphocytopenia, and possible thrombocytopenia.
- *Urinalysis* shows mild proteinuria, hematuria, and blood cell casts during exacerbations of the disease when the kidneys are involved. Renal function tests including *serum creatinine* and *blood urea nitrogen (BUN)* may also be ordered to evaluate the extent of renal disease.
- *Kidney biopsy* may be performed to assess the severity of renal lesions and guide therapy (see Chapter 27 ∞).

Medications

The client with mild or remittent SLE may need little or no therapy other than supportive care. Arthralgias, arthritis, fever, and fatigue can often be managed with aspirin or other NSAIDs. Aspirin is particularly beneficial for clients with SLE because its antiplatelet effects help prevent thrombosis. It may, however, cause liver toxicity and hepatitis.

Skin and arthritic manifestations of SLE may be treated with antimalarial drugs such as hydroxychloroquine (Plaquenil). Hydroxychloroquine has also been shown to be effective in reducing the frequency of acute episodes of SLE in people with mild or inactive disease. Retinal toxicity and possibly irreversible blindness are the primary concerns with this drug. For this reason, the client taking hydroxychloroquine undergoes ophthalmologic exam every 6 months.

Clients with severe and life-threatening manifestations of SLE (such as nephritis, hemolytic anemia, myocarditis, pericarditis, or CNS lupus) require corticosteroid therapy in high doses. Such clients may require 40 to 60 mg of prednisone per day initially. The dosage is tapered as rapidly as the client's disease allows, although lowering the dosage may precipitate an acute episode. Some clients with SLE require long-term corticosteroid therapy to manage symptoms and prevent major organ damage. These clients are at increased risk for corticosteroid side effects, such as cushingoid effects, weight gain, hypertension, infection, accelerated osteoporosis, and hypokalemia.

Immunosuppressive agents such as cyclophosphamide or azathioprine may be used, alone or in combination with corticosteroids, to treat clients with active SLE or lupus nephritis (see the Medication Administration box on the next page). When these agents are used in combination, lower, less toxic doses of each drug can be used. The client receiving immunosuppressive agents is at increased risk for infection, malignancy, bone marrow depression, and toxic effects specific to the drug prescribed.

MANIFESTATIONS of SLE

- Painful or swollen joints and muscle pain
- Unexplained fever
- Red rash, especially on the face
- Unusual loss of hair
- Pale, cyanotic fingers or toes
- Sensitivity to the sun
- Edema in legs and around eyes
- Ulcers in the mouth
- Enlarged glands
- Extreme fatigue

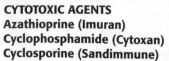

MEDICATION ADMINISTRATION — Immunosuppressive Agents for SLE

CYTOTOXIC AGENTS
Azathioprine (Imuran)
Cyclophosphamide (Cytoxan)
Cyclosporine (Sandimmune)

Certain cytotoxic or antineoplastic drugs are effective as immunosuppressive agents. They act by decreasing the proliferation of cells within the immune system and are widely used to prevent rejection following a tissue or organ transplant. They are usually administered concurrently with corticosteroid therapy, allowing lower doses of both preparations, and resulting in fewer side effects.

Nursing Responsibilities
- Monitor blood count, with particular attention to the WBC and platelet counts. Notify the physician if WBCs fall below 4000 or platelets below 75,000.
- Monitor renal and liver function studies including creatinine, BUN, creatinine clearance, and liver enzyme levels. Report any abnormal levels to the physician.
- Oral preparations should be administered with food to minimize gastrointestinal effects. Antacids may be ordered.
- Increase fluids to maintain good hydration and urinary output.
- Monitor intake and output.

- Monitor for signs of abnormal bleeding: bleeding gums, bruising, petechiae, joint pain, hematuria, and black or tarry stools.
- Use meticulous hand washing and other appropriate measures to protect the client from infection. Assess for signs of infection.
- Pulmonary fibrosis is a potential adverse effect of cyclophosphamide. Therefore, monitor the results of pulmonary function studies and be alert to clinical signs of dyspnea or cough.

Health Education for the Client and Family
- Avoid large crowds and situations where you might be exposed to infections.
- Report signs of infection such as chills, fever, sore throat, fatigue, or malaise to the physician.
- Use contraceptive measures to prevent pregnancy while you are taking these drugs because they cause birth defects.
- Avoid the use of aspirin or ibuprofen while taking these drugs. Report any signs of bleeding to the physician.
- You may stop menstruating while you are taking cyclophosphamide. The menses will resume after the drug is discontinued.
- If you are taking cyclophosphamide, be sure to report difficulty breathing or cough to the physician.

Treatments

Because of the photosensitivity associated with SLE, the client should be cautioned to avoid sun exposure. Clients should use sunscreens with a sun protection factor (SPF) rating of 15 or higher when out of doors. Topical corticosteroids may be used to treat skin lesions. Some physicians recommend avoiding the use of oral contraceptives, because estrogen can trigger an acute episode.

Clients with lupus nephritis who progress to develop end-stage renal disease are treated with dialysis (hemodialysis or peritoneal dialysis) and kidney transplantation, discussed in Chapter 29 ∞.

NURSING CARE

Nursing care for the client with mild SLE may be limited to teaching. The client with severe disease, however, has many diverse nursing needs, which vary according to the organ systems involved. Because of the close link between rheumatoid arthritis and SLE, many of the nursing diagnoses and interventions identified for the client with arthritis may be appropriate for the client with lupus. The client with lupus nephritis or end-stage renal disease has the nursing care needs outlined in the sections of Chapter 29 ∞ related to glomerulonephritis and chronic renal failure. This section focuses on the needs of the client related to the dermatologic manifestations of lupus, an increased risk for infection, and health maintenance.

Nursing Diagnoses and Interventions

The priority nursing interventions for the client with SLE are focused on problems with impaired skin integrity, ineffective protection, and impaired health maintenance.

Impaired Skin Integrity

Skin lesions are a common manifestation of SLE. A rash or discoid lesion interrupts the integrity of the skin and the first line of protection against infection, increasing the client's already high risk of infection. These lesions, which usually appear on exposed parts of the skin, can also be disfiguring and cause the client emotional distress.

- Assess knowledge of SLE and its possible effects on the skin. *Assessment allows the nurse to base teaching and information on the client's existing knowledge, improving learning and retention.*
- Discuss the relationship between sun exposure and disease activity, both dermatologic and systemic. *It is important for the client to understand that sun exposure may not only cause dermatologic manifestations but also trigger an acute episode.*
- Suggest the following strategies to limit sun exposure:
  - Avoid being out of doors during hours of greatest sun intensity (10:00 A.M. to 3:00 P.M.).
  - Use sunscreen with an SPF of 15 or higher when sun exposure cannot be avoided. Apply it 30 minutes before going out into the sun.
  - Reapply sunscreen after swimming, exercising, or bathing.
  - Wear loose clothing with long sleeves and wide-brimmed hats when out of doors.
  These strategies can help the client maintain a normal lifestyle while helping to prevent acute episodes.
- Keep skin clean and dry; apply therapeutic creams or ointments to lesions as prescribed. *These measures promote healing and reduce the risk of infection.*

Ineffective Protection

Ineffective protection can be a problem for the client with SLE, who is at increased risk for infection and multiple organ system problems because of the disease. In addition, treatment with corticosteroids or immunosuppressive agents further impairs immune responses and the ability to fight infection. The following interventions are for the client who is hospitalized.

- Wash hands before and after providing direct care. *Hand washing removes transient organisms from the skin, reducing the risk of transmission to the client.*

> ## PRACTICE ALERT
> Hands must be washed before and after providing direct care, even if gloves are worn. A decrease in this type of medical asepsis is contributing to the increasing number of hospital-acquired infections that are resistant to antibiotics.

- Use strict aseptic technique in caring for intravenous lines and indwelling urinary catheters or performing any wound care. *Aseptic technique offers protection against external and resident host microorganisms.*
- Assess frequently for infection. Monitor temperature and vital signs every 4 hours. Assess for signs of cellulitis, including tenderness, redness, swelling, and warmth. Report signs of infection to the physician promptly. *Therapy can suppress usual responses, such as elevated temperature and inflammation. The fever of infection may be mistaken for the fever commonly associated with lupus. The client receiving immunosuppressive therapy for the disease has an even higher risk for infection.*
- Monitor laboratory values, including CBC and tests of organ function; report changes to the physician. *An elevation in the WBC count with a shift to the left (increased numbers of immature leukocytes in the blood) may be an early indication of infection. Changes in liver function studies, renal function studies, myocardial enzymes, or other laboratory values may indicate organ system involvement.*
- Initiate reverse or protective isolation procedures as indicated by the client's immune status. *These procedures provide further protection from infection for the severely immunocompromised client.*
- Ensure an adequate nutrient intake, offering supplementary feedings as indicated or maintaining parenteral nutrition if necessary. *Adequate nutrition is important for healing and immune system function.*
- Teach the client the importance of good handwashing after using the bathroom and before eating. *Hand washing reduces the risk of infection with endogenous organisms.*
- Monitor for potential adverse effects of medications including thrombocytopenia and possible bleeding, fluid retention with edema and possible hypertension, loss of bone density, osteoporosis, and possible pathologic fractures, renal or hepatic toxicity, and cardiac effects, particularly in the client with fluid retention and hypervolemia. *Medications used to treat SLE have many potential adverse effects that can impair normal protective and homeostatic mechanisms.*

Impaired Health Maintenance

As with other chronic diseases, much of the responsibility for maintaining optimal health rests with the client. Disease manifestations such as fatigue, arthralgias, arthritis, and increased risk for infection can interfere with the client's ability to maintain health. Psychosocial issues can also be a significant factor in health maintenance for the client with lupus. These issues may include denial of the significance of the disease, poor coping, lack of financial and other resources, and an inadequate support system.

- Assess the ability to maintain optimal health, identifying physical and psychosocial factors that may affect health maintenance. *Before intervening to improve the client's health maintenance, the nurse must identify and understand factors affecting it.*
- Provide care and teaching in a nonjudgmental manner. *To intervene effectively, the nurse must accept the client and family as they are.*
- Encourage the client and family members to discuss the effect of the disease on their lives. *Open discussion helps the client and the nurse identify barriers to health maintenance and begin exploring alternative strategies.*
- Initiate an interdisciplinary care conference with the client and family. *In this care conference, a number of perspectives can be expressed, improving the planning of strategies for health maintenance activities.*
- Refer the client and family to counseling as needed. *Counseling may help the client and family develop the necessary coping skills to accept and deal with the disease.*
- Refer the client and family to community and social service agencies, and local support groups. *These groups and agencies are valuable resources for the client and family.*

Community-Based Care

Teaching is a critical factor in preparing clients with SLE for self-care at home. Address the following topics:

- The disease and its potential effects. Promote an optimistic outlook, stressing that the majority of clients do not require long-term corticosteroid therapy and that the disease may improve over time.
- The importance of skin care.
- The importance of avoiding exposure to infection.
- The need to follow the prescribed treatment plan, including rest and exercise, medications, and follow-up appointments. Discuss manifestations of an acute episode (often called a *flare*) and stress the importance of contacting the physician promptly if any of these manifestations occur.

> ## PRACTICE ALERT
> **Warning Signs of a Flare**
> - Increased fatigue
> - Pain, abdominal discomfort
> - Rash
> - Headache
> - Fever
> - Dizziness

- The significance of wearing a Medic-Alert tag identifying their condition and therapy such as corticosteroids or immunosuppressives.
- Family planning with the client and spouse. The use of oral contraceptives may be contraindicated for the client; if appropriate,

provide information about alternative means of birth control. Pregnancy is not contraindicated for most women with lupus. However, the pregnant client requires close monitoring because acute episodes sometimes accompany pregnancy.

- The need for preventive health care for both men and women with SLE. Women should have gynecologic and breast examinations and men should have prostate examinations each year. Both men and women should have regular screenings for cholesterol and blood pressure. Annual influenza vaccinations are important, as is pneumococcal vaccinations for older clients. If clients are taking corticosteroids or antimalarial medications, annual eye examinations should be conducted to screen for and treat any eye problems.

- Helpful resources:
  - National Institute of Arthritis and Musculoskeletal and Skin Diseases
  - Lupus Foundation of America.

THE CLIENT WITH POLYMYOSITIS

Polymyositis is a systemic connective tissue disorder characterized by inflammation of connective tissue and muscle fibers leading to muscle weakness and atrophy. When muscle fiber inflammation is accompanied by skin lesions, the disease is known as dermatomyositis. Polymyositis is an autoimmune disorder of unknown cause that affects more women than men. The onset of the disease typically occurs between the ages of 40 and 60 years, although a childhood-onset form is also seen.

The immune mechanism causing the inflammatory response in polymyositis is not clear, but autoantibodies can be identified in the majority of people with the disease. The activation of complement is thought to contribute to the inflammatory process. Inflammation leads to muscle fiber necrosis and degeneration.

Manifestations

Initial manifestations of polymyositis include muscle pain, tenderness, and weakness; rash; arthralgias; fatigue; fever; and weight loss. Skeletal muscle weakness is the predominant manifestation. Its onset may be either insidious or abrupt. Muscle weakness tends to progress over weeks to months. Muscles of the shoulder and pelvic girdles are particularly affected, making it difficult for the client to get out of chairs, climb stairs, and reach overhead. Weakness of neck flexor muscles may make it difficult to raise the head from a pillow. Affected muscles may also be tender and painful. A characteristic dusky red rash may be present on the face and upper trunk. Other manifestations include Raynaud's phenomenon, dysphagia, dyspnea, and cough (due to interstitial pneumonitis). The risk of malignancy is increased, particularly in clients with dermatomyositis.

INTERDISCIPLINARY CARE

There is no specific test to diagnose polymyositis. Autoantibodies may be identified in blood serum. Serum levels of muscle enzymes are elevated, particularly creatine kinase (CK) and aldolase levels. Biopsy of involved muscle shows patchy muscle fiber necrosis and the presence of inflammatory cells.

A combination of rest and corticosteroid therapy is prescribed for the client with polymyositis. Long-term corticosteroid therapy may be necessary to manage the disease. Immunosuppressive agents such as methotrexate, cyclophosphamide, and azathioprine may be used for clients who do not respond well to treatment with corticosteroids.

NURSING CARE

The nursing role in caring for the client with polymyositis is supportive. Measures to promote comfort are important. Muscle weakness may interfere with the client's ability to provide self-care and manage health and home. The client may have difficulty with speech because of pharyngeal muscle weakness. Provide alternate means of communication as needed, and use patience in listening. Observe closely while the client eats, because aspiration is a potential problem. Modify the client's diet as needed to maintain nutrition and safety.

Education of the client and family is an important component of care. Emphasize the need to balance periods of rest and activity. Discuss skin care to prevent dryness and infection. Teach the client about prescribed medications and their short- and long-term side effects. Provide information about safety measures while eating. Encourage family members to become trained in performance of the Heimlich maneuver and CPR. Discuss signs of respiratory infection and other possible complications of polymyositis, including renal failure and malignancy.

THE CLIENT WITH LYME DISEASE

Lyme disease is an inflammatory disorder caused by the spirochete *Borrelia burgdorferi*, which is transmitted primarily by ticks. It is the most commonly reported tick-borne illness in the United States. Geographically, Lyme disease is more prevalent in the areas where the ticks are found: in the coastal Northeast, the upper Midwest, and coastal California regions of the United States (ACR, 2004b). It has also been reported throughout Europe, Asia, and Australia. Ticks that act as vectors for Lyme disease, primarily *Ixodes dammini, I, pacificus*, and *I. scapularis* in the United States, are usually carried by mice or deer, although other animals may be infected. The most frequent time of onset is the summer months.

> **FAST FACTS**
> **Lyme Disease**
> - Lyme disease is the most common tick-transmitted disease in the United States.
> - Lyme disease occurs most often in children and young adults living in rural areas.
> - All stages of Lyme disease can be cured by antibiotics, but some people with late neurologic or arthritic involvement may not improve.

Pathophysiology

Borrelia burgdorferi enters the skin at the site of the tick bite. After an incubation period of up to 30 days, it migrates outward in the skin, forming a characteristic lesion called erythema migrans. It may also spread via lymph or blood to other skin sites, nodes, or organs. The inflammatory joint changes associated with Lyme disease closely resemble those of rheumatoid arthritis (vascular congestion, tissue infiltration by inflammatory cells, possible pannus formation, and erosion of cartilage and bone).

Manifestations

Manifestations often are seen in the skin, musculoskeletal system, and CNS. Lyme disease begins with flulike manifestations and a skin rash, followed weeks or months later by Bell's palsy or meningitis, and months to years later, by arthritis. This progression is highly individualized.

Erythema migrans is the initial manifestation of Lyme disease. This flat or slightly raised red lesion at the site of the tick bite expands over several days (up to a diameter of 50 cm), with the central area clearing as it expands. Systemic symptoms such as fatigue, malaise, fever, chills, and myalgias often accompany the initial lesion. As the disease spreads, secondary skin lesions develop, as do migratory musculoskeletal symptoms, including arthralgias, myalgias, and tendinitis. Persistent fatigue is common during this stage of the disease. Headache and stiff neck are characteristic neurologic manifestations.

Complications

With untreated infection, complications can develop months to years after the initial infection. Chronic recurrent arthritis, primarily affecting large joints (especially the knee), is common. Permanent disability may result. Other effects that may be seen weeks to months after the initial infection include meningitis, encephalitis, and neuropathies, as well as cardiac complications including myocarditis and heart block.

INTERDISCIPLINARY CARE

Both manifestations and laboratory studies are used to establish the diagnosis of Lyme disease. Culture of the organism from tissues and body fluids is difficult and slow. Antibodies to *B. burgdorferi* can be detected by either enzyme-linked immunosorbent assay (ELISA) or Western blot methods within 2 to 4 weeks of the initial skin lesion.

The early diagnosis and proper antibiotic treatment of Lyme disease are important to preventing the complications of infection. A number of antibiotics may be used to treat Lyme disease, including doxycycline (Doxy-Caps, Vibramycin), tetracycline, amoxicillin (Amoxil), cefuroxime axetil (Ceftin), or erythromycin. Therapy may be continued for up to 1 month to ensure eradication of the organism from affected tissues. The nursing implications for various classes of antibiotics are summarized in Chapter 12 ∞.

In addition to antibiotic treatment, aspirin or another NSAID may be prescribed for relief of arthritic symptoms. The affected joint may be splinted to rest the joint. When the knee is involved, weight bearing may be restricted and the use of crutches indicated.

NURSING CARE

Nursing care focuses on prevention of the disease. Many people do not protect themselves from tick bites. This protection is becoming increasingly important with a higher incidence of Lyme disease, due in part to an overpopulation of deer and the encroachment of the suburbs on once rural areas. Simple measures that can help prevent tick bites are as follows:

- Avoid tick-infested areas, especially in spring and summer, such as woods and rural areas with brush and tall weeds.
- Cover exposed skin with long-sleeved shirts and tuck pants into socks. Wearing high rubber boots may provide additional protection.
- Use insect repellents that contain DEET on clothing and exposed skin and apply permethrin to clothing prior to exposure.
- Inspect skin, especially in areas of tight-fitting clothing, after exposure.
- Remove attached ticks with fine-tipped tweezers. Grasp the tick firmly as close to the skin as possible and pull the tick's body away from the skin. If the tick's head remains in the skin, it will not cause Lyme disease (the bacteria are in the tick's midgut). Most cases occur when the tick has been feeding for at least 24 hours (Tierney et al., 2004). Clean the area with an antiseptic.

INFECTIOUS DISORDERS

Infectious disorders of bone and joints are caused by a pathogen, and are often difficult to treat. Chronic infections may result in pain, deformity, and disability.

THE CLIENT WITH OSTEOMYELITIS

Osteomyelitis is an infection of the bone. Osteomyelitis may occur as an acute, subacute, or chronic process. It occurs as a consequence of bacteremia (hematogenous osteomyelitis), invasion from a contiguous focus of infection, or skin breakdown in the presence of vascular insufficiency (Tierney et al., 2004).

Osteomyelitis can occur at any age, but adults over age 50 are more commonly affected. The older adult is at risk for osteomyelitis for several reasons. Immune function tends to decline with aging; the older adult also is more likely to have a chronic disease process that affects immune function. Circulatory status in older adults often is compromised by atherosclerotic processes, impairing blood flow to the bone. Older adults have a higher risk of pressure ulcers because of circulatory, skin, sensation, and mobility changes associated with aging. Pressure ulcers that cannot be staged and treated because of eschar formation pose a particular risk. In addition, the older adult may not demonstrate the typical signs of infection and inflammation, which allows an infectious process to become well established before it is detected.

Pathophysiology

The cause of osteomyelitis is usually bacterial; however, fungi, parasites, and viruses can also cause bone infection. *Staphylococcus aureus* is the most common infecting organism. Other organisms include *Escherichia coli, Pseudomonas, Klebsiella, Salmonella,* and *Proteus.*

NURSING CARE

The client with chronic osteomyelitis faces frequent and lengthy hospitalizations and/or treatment modalities. The prognosis is uncertain, and functional deficits and amputation are a constant concern. The ongoing expenses, loss of financial support, and role changes within the family are also client concerns.

Nursing Diagnoses and Interventions

Nursing diagnoses associated with acute osteomyelitis focus on preventing the transmission of infection and problems due to immobility. Providing comfort and client teaching are also very important.

Risk for Infection

Compromised immune status places the client with osteomyelitis at risk for superinfection. An inadequate kilocalorie intake is an additional factor that contributes to the risk.

■ Maintain strict hand washing practices. *Meticulous hand washing helps prevent the spread of infection by minimizing the entry of organisms into susceptible clients.*

> **PRACTICE ALERT**
> Careful hand washing before and after direct care is essential even if gloves are worn.

■ Administer antimicrobial therapy at specified time intervals. *Optimal blood levels of antibiotic therapy are mandatory in clients with infectious processes.*

■ Maintain the client's optimal dietary kilocalorie and protein intake. *High kilocalorie and protein intake provide the client with sufficient nutritional support for the body's needs during the stressful event of the inflammatory process.*

Hyperthermia

The infection and associated inflammatory process can cause fever in the client with osteomyelitis.

■ Monitor temperature every 4 hours and when client reports chills and/or fever. Blood cultures are frequently ordered when an acute elevation of temperature occurs. *A sudden rise in temperature in clients with either acute or chronic osteomyelitis may indicate inadequate antimicrobial management.*

■ Maintain a cool environment and provide light clothing and bedding during temperature elevation. *Proper environmental conditions and clothing enhance the evaporative process during acute temperature elevation and promote comfort.*

■ Ensure a daily fluid intake of 2000 to 3000 mL. Dehydration may result from evaporative fluid losses during acute temperature elevations. Furthermore, clients taking large doses of antibiotic therapy may experience fluid loss through excessive diarrhea as a side effect of the therapy. *Fluid replacement is necessary during this time to prevent further dehydration.*

Impaired Physical Mobility

Pain, infection, inflammation, and the use of immobilizers can all impair the mobility of the client with osteomyelitis.

■ Maintain the affected limb in functional position when immobilized. *The client may hesitate to move the involved extremity because of continuous pain; therefore, the extremity must be maintained in functional position to avoid flexion contracture.*

■ Maintain rest, and avoid subjecting the affected extremity to weight-bearing activities. *The involved extremity must be immobilized to avoid pathologic fractures caused by stress on the weakened bone.*

■ Ensure active or passive ROM exercises every 4 hours. *Flexion contracture occurs when the client remains immobile or when there is only minimal joint movement. Consult a physical therapist for plan of exercises to avoid contracture.*

Acute Pain

The client with osteomyelitis experiences pain due to swelling.

■ Use a splint or immobilizer when the client experiences acute pain from swelling. *Splinting or immobilizing the involved extremity provides support and reduces pain caused by movement.*

■ Ask the physician to order scheduled administration of narcotic and nonnarcotic analgesics on a 24-hour basis rather than as needed. *The use of 24-hour administration allows blood levels of pain-relieving medications to remain constant.*

> **PRACTICE ALERT**
> Clients are often reluctant to ask for a prn pain medication, allowing the pain to reach a level that is difficult to manage.

■ Use nonpharmacologic strategies (e.g., heat distraction, relaxation techniques) for pain management. *Pain of the muscles and joints may be controlled through nonpharmacologic interventions. Warm moist packs, warm baths, or heating pads to the involved extremity provide comfort due to vasodilation.*

■ Avoid excessive manipulation of the involved area; handle the area gently. Carefully assess the client for guarding, limping, or unwillingness to move the affected part. Communicate to other healthcare professionals the client's preferences for assistive devices and means of manipulating the involved area. *Gentle handling and minimal manipulation help reduce pain.*

Community-Based Care

Although clients may be hospitalized for acute treatment and surgery, most care is provided at home. Home health services can provide intravenous medications, if prescribed. Discuss the following topics for home care:

■ The importance of careful hand washing, especially after toileting and dressing changes.

■ The importance of taking all antibiotics as prescribed. Include information about helping prevent the yeast infections (of the mouth or vagina) often associated with prolonged antibiotic therapy by eating 8 oz of live-culture yogurt each day.

■ The need to take pain medications on a regular basis to prevent pain from becoming severe. Provide information about how to deal with side effects, such as constipation, by increasing fluid and fiber intake.

■ How to perform wound care and sources for needed equipment and supplies.

■ Rest or limited weight bearing for the affected extremity or body part. Teach how to avoid complications associated with prolonged immobilization, such as frequently shifting position, keeping skin and linens clean and dry, and doing active ROM exercises for unaffected joints.

■ The importance of maintaining good nutrition. An adequate supply of kilocalories, protein, and other nutrients is necessary for immune function and healing. Suggest frequent small meals and using nutritional supplements such as Ensure to help maintain nutritional intake.

THE CLIENT WITH SEPTIC ARTHRITIS

Septic arthritis can develop if a joint space is invaded by a pathogen. The primary risk factors for septic arthritis are persistent bacteremia (bacteria in the blood) (e.g., due to use of injectable drugs, endocarditis) and previous joint damage (e.g., due to trauma or rheumatoid arthritis). Arthroscopic surgery and total joint replacements that allow potential direct contamination of the joint are additional risk factors (Tierney et al., 2004).

Pathophysiology

The most common bacteria implicated in septic arthritis include *gonococci, S. aureus,* and streptococci. Infections by gram-negative bacteria such as *E. coli* and *Pseudomonas* are seen with increasing frequency, particularly in people who inject recreational drugs or are immunocompromised (Tierney et al., 2004).

Infection of the joint leads to inflammation with resulting synovitis and joint effusion. Abscesses may form in synovial tissues or bone underlying joint cartilage. If not treated promptly and effectively, septic arthritis can lead to destruction of the affected joint. A single joint, often the knee, is usually affected. Septic arthritis may also affect other joints such as the shoulder, wrist, hip, fingers, or elbow.

Manifestations

The onset of septic arthritis is typically abrupt, marked by pain and stiffness of the infected joint. The joint appears red and swollen, and is hot and tender to the touch. Effusion (increased fluid within the joint space) is usually present. Systemic manifestations of infection, such as chills and fever, often accompany local manifestations, although these may be muted if the client is taking anti-inflammatory medications.

INTERDISCIPLINARY CARE

Septic arthritis is a medical emergency requiring prompt treatment to preserve joint function. When it is suspected, fluid from the affected joint is aspirated and sent for Gram stain and culture. Cultures also are obtained from all likely sources of the infection, including blood, sputum, or wounds. The synovial fluid culture is always positive in nongonococcal septic arthritis but often is negative for bacteria in early gonococcal arthritis. Infected synovial fluid usually is cloudy, with a high WBC count and a low glucose level. Joint x-ray films are often normal in the initial stages, but soon show demineralization, bony erosions, and joint space narrowing.

The infected joint is treated with rest, immobilization, elevation, and systemic antibiotics. Treatment with a broad-spectrum parenteral antibiotic is initiated before the results of culture are obtained. The medication may be changed or adjusted once the organism has been identified. Antibiotic therapy is continued for at least 2 weeks after inflammatory manifestations have abated. Frequent joint aspirations may be performed to remove excess fluid and pus, and to evaluate for the continued presence of bacteria. Surgical drainage may be performed if the hip joint is involved (because of the difficulty of aspirating this joint) or when medical therapy does not rapidly eliminate bacteria from the synovial fluid. Physical therapy is implemented during the recovery period to ensure maintenance of optimal joint function.

NURSING CARE

Septic arthritis can be frightening to the client who experiences a sudden onset of joint pain and swelling and is faced with the possibility of rapid functional loss of movement. Nursing care is both supportive and educative. Clients may be hospitalized for initial treatment with intravenous antibiotics. It is important to monitor the client's response to therapy, including systemic manifestations such as fever. Position the affected joint appropriately, using pillows to elevate it as needed. Splints or traction may be used to immobilize the joint. Warm compresses may be ordered for comfort. Active ROM exercises preserve joint mobility and should be initiated as soon as the physician allows.

The client with septic arthritis needs information about the disorder, its etiology, and its treatment. Teach the client how organisms may gain entry into the joint space. Discuss the role that the use of injected drugs and sexually transmitted infections play in septic arthritis, and means to prevent infection as appropriate (e.g., using clean "works," practicing safer sex). Refer the client to a drug treatment program if necessary. Emphasize the importance of complying with all aspects of the treatment plan to prevent joint destruction and disability.

NEOPLASTIC DISORDERS

Bone tumors may be either primary (arising in the bone itself) or metastatic (seeded from a tumor elsewhere in the body). Like other tumors, bone tumors can be either benign or malignant.

THE CLIENT WITH BONE TUMORS

Benign bone tumors tend to grow slowly and do not often destroy surrounding tissues. Primary malignant tumors of the bone are rare, accounting for only about 1% of all adult cancers (Porth, 2005). Malignant tumors grow rapidly and metastasize. Virtually every malignant tumor can metastasize to bone. However, the most common metastatic bone tumors originate from primary tumors of the prostate, breast, kidney, thyroid, and lung.

Primary bone tumors arise from bone tissue itself, that is, cartilage (chondrogenic), bone (osteogenic), collagen (collagenic),

- Provide referral to physical or occupational therapy for fitting of and teaching about assistive devices for ambulating, such as a cane, crutches, or a walker. *Assistive devices can reduce the risk of falling when the client has significant weakness of an extremity or when balance has been affected by treatment of the disease.*

Acute Pain, Chronic Pain

In the client with a bone tumor, pain may be related to direct invasion of the tumor or to pathologic fractures. Clients may experience both acute and chronic pain.

- Develop strategies for controlling both acute pain (from surgery, fracture, or inflammation) and chronic pain (from progression of the disease). *Analgesics combined with nonpharmacologic methods of pain control provide optimum relief of pain. Chronic pain, when mild in nature, is best managed with NSAIDs or aspirin. Moderate pain is best managed with a combination of codeine and NSAIDs. Severe pain is best relieved with long-acting or sustained-relief narcotic analgesics.*
- Provide assistive devices (e.g., canes, walkers, crutches) when the client ambulates. *Assistive devices lessen the pain by supporting weight bearing during ambulation.*

Impaired Physical Mobility

Pain, muscle wasting, or surgical procedures can impair the physical mobility of the client with a bone tumor.

- Begin muscle strengthening and active and passive ROM exercises immediately after surgery. A continuous passive motion (CPM) machine may be used after surgical procedures to either upper or lower extremities. *Muscle strengthening exercises must be encouraged as soon as possible to prevent muscle wasting and shorten the rehabilitation period.*
- Encourage exercises that help strengthen the triceps muscles. *The triceps are the major muscles in the arms and must be strengthened to assist in use of crutches or other assistive devices.*

- For the client who has undergone an amputation of a lower extremity, encourage quadriceps and gluteal setting exercises and leg raises. *These exercises will benefit the client when the rehabilitation period begins.*

Decisional Conflict

A lack of knowledge about the diagnosis and treatment regimen can impair the client's ability to make informed decisions about the treatment plan.

- Discuss issues related to diagnosis, radiologic evaluation, biopsy, surgery, chemotherapy, radiation therapy, potential complications, alternative therapies, risks, benefits, nursing management, discharge plans, home care, and long-term treatment and follow-up. *The client requires this information in order to make informed decisions about treatment.*

Community-Based Care

The client with a primary bone tumor needs information about the disease, its potential consequences, and treatment options. Present information in a matter-of-fact manner, taking time to listen to and address the client's and family's concerns. Discuss expected effects and potential side effects of surgery, chemotherapy, and radiation therapy. Provide information about how to minimize side effects. Teach the postsurgical client about wound care, demonstrating dressing changes and stump care (if amputation has occurred). Provide the client with a list of local resources for obtaining supplies. Discuss activity and weight-bearing restrictions. Refer the client to physical therapy for teaching about ambulation and appropriate muscle-group strengthening exercises. Ensure that the client who has experienced an amputation is working with or has a referral to a prosthetic specialist. For the client with metastatic disease, discuss hospice services and support groups for clients with cancer.

CONNECTIVE TISSUE DISORDERS

Connective tissue is the most abundant and widely distributed body tissue. It not only connects body parts but also provides support; forms bones, cartilage, and the walls of blood vessels; and attaches muscles to bones. Connective tissue consists of three elements: (1) long fibers embedded in a (2) noncellular ground substance, and (3) cells specific to the class of connective tissue. Fibers made up primarily of collagen, a protein, are the most abundant in connective tissue.

Connective tissue disorders, also known as collagen diseases, are a group of immune-mediated disorders. Although they appear to have a genetic component, their cause is unknown. Because connective tissue and collagen are widely distributed in many varied tissues, these are systemic diseases with diverse manifestations.

THE CLIENT WITH SYSTEMIC SCLEROSIS (SCLERODERMA)

Systemic sclerosis, also known as **scleroderma** ("hardening of the skin"), is a chronic disease characterized by the for-

mation of excess fibrous connective tissue and diffuse fibrosis of the skin and internal organs. The cause of scleroderma is unknown, but genetic, immune, and environmental factors are thought to play a role. Although this uncommon disease is distributed worldwide, a higher incidence is noted in coal and gold miners and in people exposed to certain chemicals such as polyvinyl chloride, epoxy resins, and aromatic hydrocarbons.

FAST FACTS
Scleroderma

- Scleroderma affects approximately 300,000 people in the United States, with about one-third having the systemic form and the rest the localized form.
- Scleroderma affects women more often than men by a ratio of approximately 3:1.
- Although it can occur at any age from infants to older adults, the onset of scleroderma typically occurs between the ages of 25 and 55 years (Scleroderma Foundation, 2006).

Pathophysiology

Abnormalities in cellular immune function are believed to contribute to the development of scleroderma. Abnormal proliferation of fibrous connective tissue occurs in affected tissues, including the skin, blood vessels, lungs, kidneys, and other organs.

Scleroderma may be either localized, affecting the skin only, or generalized (systemic sclerosis), with both skin and visceral organ involvement. Localized involvement may occur as irregularly shaped patches of skin (morphea) or a line of disease on the arm, leg, or side of the face (linear scleroderma) (International Scleroderma Network, 2004). Eighty percent of people with generalized disease have limited involvement, frequently manifested by CREST syndrome, a combination of calcinosis (abnormal calcium salt deposition in the tissues), Raynaud's phenomenon, esophageal dysfunction, sclerodactyly (localized scleroderma of the fingers), and telangiectasia (dilated, superficial blood vessels). The remainder of clients with generalized systemic sclerosis have a diffuse form of the disease and a higher risk of visceral organ involvement. Infections and diseases of the cardiovascular, renal, pulmonary, and CNS are the most common causes of death in people with systemic sclerosis.

Manifestations

The initial manifestations of systemic sclerosis are usually noted in the skin, which thickens markedly. Diffuse, nonpitting swelling also is noted. As the disease progresses, the skin begins to atrophy, becoming taut, shiny, and hyperpigmented (Figure 42–9 ■). Facial skin tightening leads to loss of skin lines and a pursed-lip appearance. Skin tightness may limit mobility, particularly of the face and hands. Other skin manifestations include telangiectasias (flat, red areas caused by dilation of small blood vessels, usually noted on the face, hands, and in the mouth) and calcium deposits, usually noted around joints.

Arthralgias and Raynaud's phenomenon are common early manifestations of systemic sclerosis. Raynaud's phenomenon (intermittent attacks of small artery vasospasm) is characterized by pallor of the fingers followed by cyanosis, and then reactive hyperemia with redness. Attacks are usually triggered by cold temperatures.

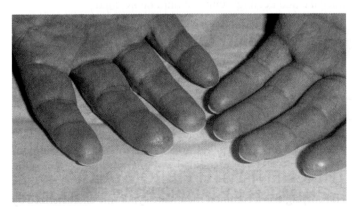

Figure 42–9 ■ Characteristic skin changes of scleroderma.

Source: Logical Images/Custom Medical Stock Photo.

The client with visceral organ involvement may have varied symptoms. Dysphagia is common, because the motility of the esophagus is affected. Pulmonary involvement can lead to exertional dyspnea due to impaired gas exchange and right sided heart failure due to pulmonary hypertension. Involvement of the heart may cause manifestations of pericarditis and dysrhythmias. Diarrhea or constipation, abdominal cramping, and malabsorption can occur when the GI tract is affected. Renal effects can lead to proteinuria, hematuria, hypertension, and renal failure.

The prognosis for localized and limited scleroderma is good; many clients have a normal life span. The course of diffuse systemic sclerosis is highly variable. This disease is usually progressive; complete remission is rare.

INTERDISCIPLINARY CARE

The manifestations of systemic sclerosis often allow diagnosis with little or no testing. No cure is currently available; treatment is symptomatic and supportive.

Diagnosis

No single diagnostic test is specific for systemic sclerosis, although a titer of 1:40 or higher for antinuclear antibody (ANA) is the most sensitive for diagnosis. Other laboratory studies that are done include an ESR, which is typically elevated from the chronic inflammatory process and a CBC, which will demonstrate anemia. A skin biopsy may be done to confirm the diagnosis.

Medications

Medications to treat systemic sclerosis are chosen based on the client's symptoms. Immunosuppressive agents and corticosteroids are of limited benefit, but may be used to slow or prevent pulmonary fibrosis and in life-threatening disease. Penicillamine may be used to treat scleroderma and pulmonary fibrosis. Calcium channel blockers such as nifedipine (Procardia) or alpha-adrenergic blockers such as prazosin (Minipress) may be prescribed for clients with Raynaud's phenomenon. When manifestations of esophagitis accompany systemic sclerosis, H₂-receptor blockers such as cimetidine (Tagamet) or ranitidine (Zantac), antacids, or omeprazole (Prilosec), which blocks all gastric secretion, may be ordered. Tetracycline or another broad-spectrum antibiotic may be prescribed to suppress intestinal flora and relieve symptoms of malabsorption. Clients with kidney disease are usually treated with angiotensin-converting enzyme (ACE) inhibitors such as captopril (Capoten) to control hypertension and preserve renal function. End-stage kidney disease is managed with dialysis and transplantation.

Physical Therapy

Physical therapy is an important part of the management of systemic sclerosis to maintain mobility of affected tissues, the hands and face in particular. Because the mouth opening, if involved, becomes increasingly smaller as the disease progresses, stretching and strengthening of facial muscles can be vital to maintaining oral food intake.

should be done 5 times and gradually increased to 10 times. Advise the client to discontinue any exercise that is painful and to seek professional advice before continuing the exercise. *Repetition of prescribed back exercises, such as the pelvic tilt, partial sit-ups, and back rolls, will strengthen the muscles that protect the spine and thus prevent back strain.*

Risk for Impaired Adjustment

The need for lifestyle changes may lead to impaired adjustment in people with back pain.

- Teach the use of appropriate body mechanics in lifting and reaching. The client should be instructed to plan the lift, keep the object being lifted close to the body, and avoid twisting when lifting. Encourage the client to obtain help when lifting. *An item is considered excessively heavy if it equals 35% of the lifter's body weight.*
- Instruct the client to modify the workplace or environment to minimize stress to the lower back. *Lumbar supports in chairs, adjustment of chair or table height, and rubber floor mats help prevent back strain or injury.*
- Encourage obese clients to lose weight. *The trunk of the body must carry excess weight when the client is obese. Obese people are farther away from the objects they lift because of their greater abdominal girth. They may also have more difficulty squatting to lift. The greater the distance between an object and the client's center of gravity, the higher the risk for straining the lower back.*

Community-Based Care

Back pain is a common problem in the United States and other industrialized countries. Nurses can have an effect on this significant problem by teaching health practices to prevent back injury to clients of all ages. Teach clients how to safely lift, bend, and turn when engaging in physical activity. Stress the importance of using large muscle groups of the legs to lift rather than bending and lifting with the smaller muscles of the back. Teach other aspects of good body mechanics, including posture, sleeping on a firm mattress, and sitting in chairs that provide good support. Discuss the positive effect of maintaining optimal body weight and good physical fitness.

THE CLIENT WITH COMMON FOOT DISORDERS

Hallux valgus, hammertoe, and Morton's neuroma are common foot disorders that cause pain or difficulty in walking. All three disorders may be caused by wearing poorly fitting or confining shoes. These disorders are more prevalent among women.

Pathophysiology

Hallux Valgus

Hallux valgus, commonly called a *bunion*, is the enlargement and lateral displacement of the first metatarsal (the great toe) (Figure 42–12 ■). Hallux valgus develops when chronic pres-

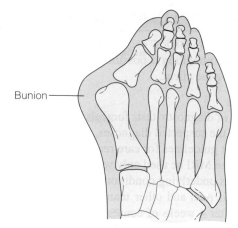

Figure 42–12 ■ Hallux valgus (bunion).

sure against the great toe causes the connective tissue in the sole of the foot to lengthen so that the stabilizing action of the great toe is gradually lost. The toe bends laterally away from the midline of the body, and the metatarsophalangeal joint (MTP) is exposed to friction during walking and becomes enlarged. As the deformity progresses, calluses form over the metatarsal head, and bursitis develops in the MTP. In severe cases, the lateral displacement of the great toe may approach 70 to 90 degrees, and the second toe may be forced upward, causing hammertoe. Although bunions may be a congenital disorder, most are caused by wearing pointed, narrow-toed shoes or high heels.

Hallux valgus is obvious on physical examination of the foot. The client may report an inability to fit into shoes. Often, the client may report joint pain or pain around calluses. In advanced or severe cases, the first metatarsal joint may have limited range of motion, particularly in dorsiflexion, and crepitus (crackling or popping) may occur during joint movement.

Hammertoe

Hammertoe (claw toe) is the dorsiflexion of the first phalanx with accompanying plantar flexion of the second and third phalanges. The condition may affect any toe, but the second toe is most commonly affected. Clients initially experience mild inflammation of the synovial membranes of the involved joints. As the deformity progresses, the dorsiflexed joint rubs against the overlying shoe, causing painful corns to develop.

Morton's Neuroma

Morton's neuroma is a tumorlike mass formed within the neurovascular bundle of the intermetatarsal spaces (Figure 42–13 ■). The neuromas usually occur in only one foot, most frequently in the third web space. Like other common foot disorders, Morton's neuroma usually is caused by wearing tight, confining shoes. The condition develops when repeated compression of the toes causes irritation and scarring of tissues surrounding the plantar digital nerve. The affected nerve becomes inflamed and swells. After repeated episodes of inflammation, the nerve fibers become fibrotic, and a neuroma forms.

Manifestations include a burning pain at the web space of the affected foot that radiates into the tips of the involved toes.

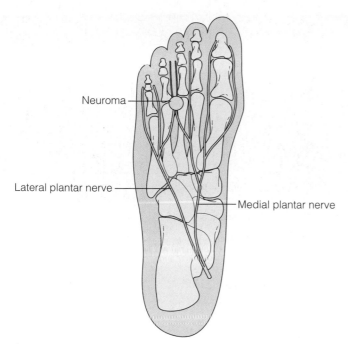

Figure 42–13 ■ Morton's neuroma.

Weight bearing usually worsens any symptoms; removing the shoe and massaging the foot often relieves the pain. The neuroma may present as a palpable mass between the affected toes. The area over the neuroma usually is tender.

INTERDISCIPLINARY CARE

Care of the client with common foot disorders such as hallux valgus, hammertoe, and Morton's neuroma focuses on relieving pain, correcting the structural deformity, and preventing reoccurrence. In most cases, all three conditions are diagnosed by inspection. X-ray films of the affected foot are taken if the need for surgery arises.

Conservative treatment for common foot disorders usually involves the use of corrective shoes. Orthotic devices that cushion and stretch the affected joints may be placed within shoes or between the client's toes. For Morton's neuroma, metatarsal pads are used to spread the client's toes and decompress the affected nerve. Analgesics may be prescribed to relieve pain and inflammation. In severe cases, corticosteroid drugs may be injected into the affected joints or surrounding tissue to relieve acute inflammation.

Surgery is reserved for clients with intractable toe deformities or pain. Hallux valgus is treated with bunionectomy; ligaments are lengthened or shortened as needed, and pins are drilled into place so the toe remains in position. Similarly, the correction of hammertoe also involves straightening the affected toe and inserting pins to retain the correction. A cast may be applied over the foot following surgery to correct toe deformities. Surgery for Morton's neuroma causes loss of sensation to a portion of the foot because removing the neuroma involves cutting out a portion of the plantar nerve.

NURSING CARE

Nursing care for clients with these foot deformities focuses on the same areas because the conservative treatment and preoperative and postoperative interventions are similar.

Nursing Diagnoses and Interventions

Pain relief, prevention of infection, and client education are important components of the nursing care of clients with foot disorders.

Chronic Pain

In the client with a foot deformity, constant pressure of footwear over the involved joint can cause pain.

■ Instruct clients to wear corrective footwear to assist in the conservative treatment of foot problems. *Pain related to foot problems can result from improper footwear that does not provide proper toe room; in addition, heels higher than 1 inch can cause constant flexion and hyperextension problems. In some instances, the client must purchase special shoes or orthotics to ensure correct fit and relief of symptoms.*

■ Suggest purchasing appropriate pads to wear over painful bunions, calluses/corns, and the ball of the foot. *Protective pads are manufactured for specific foot problems; these include bunion pads, corn pads, and metatarsal pads.*

■ Instruct clients to remove pads and inspect the skin every other day. Clients who have difficulty reaching or observing the involved foot should ask another person to do the inspection for them. *It is especially important to emphasize the need for inspection to clients who have experienced loss of sensation of the feet due to such disorders as diabetes and chronic peripheral vascular disease.*

Risk for Infection

Like all surgeries, foot surgery carries a risk of infection. This risk may be increased because of impaired peripheral circulation and exposure of the feet to the environment.

■ Teach clients proper care and cleaning of exposed pins implanted during the surgical procedure. *Pins inserted into soft tissue of the toes and bones are prone to becoming infected and can potentially result in osteomyelitis.*

■ Teach clients how to keep pins and casts dry while bathing or ambulating in inclement weather. Clients must wear a plastic bag over the cast or pins when bathing or walking in rain or snow. *When casts or pins are exposed in water, infection may result.*

Community-Based Care

For clients in all age groups, teach the importance of well-fitting footwear. Discuss the long-term effects of wearing high-heeled shoes with constricting toes with women in particular. Suggest alternatives for stylish footwear, and encourage clients to wear supportive and nonrestrictive footwear at all times. Discuss the possible effects of bunions on balance, and talk about safety measures to prevent falls and injury. Teach clients techniques to relieve pressure on affected joints.

EXPLORE MediaLink

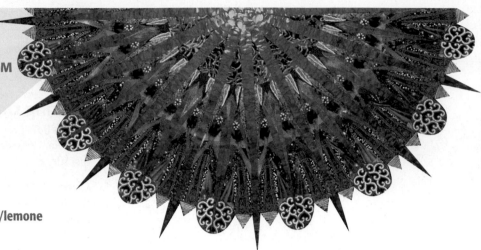

Prentice Hall Nursing MediaLink DVD-ROM
Audio Glossary
NCLEX-RN® Review

Animations
Arthritis
Carpal Tunnel
Muscular Dystrophy
Osteoporosis

COMPANION WEBSITE www.prenhall.com/lemone
Audio Glossary
NCLEX-RN® Review
Care Plan Activity: Lower Back Pain
Case Studies:
Diet and Gout
Hip Replacement
Rheumatoid Arthritis
MediaLink Applications
Compartment Syndrome
Osteoporosis Prevention
Links to Resources

CHAPTER HIGHLIGHTS

- Metabolic bone disorders begin in the bone remodeling process, and may result from aging, calcium and phosphate imbalances, genetics, and changes in hormone levels. The disorders include osteoporosis, Paget's disease, gout, and osteomalacia.

- Osteoporosis is a major health problem in the United States, with fractures being the most common complication. Health promotion activities to prevent development of the disease include a calcium-rich diet, weight-bearing exercise, and a healthy lifestyle.

- Gout is characterized by hyperuricemia and the deposit of tophi in the subcutaneous tissues. Attacks of the disease typically begin with an acutely painful inflammation of the first joint of the great toe.

- Degenerative musculoskeletal disorders include osteoarthritis (OA) and muscular dystrophy (MD). OA is the most commonly occurring of all forms of arthritis, and a leading cause of pain and disability in older adults. The disease is characterized by loss of cartilage in articulating joints and hypertrophy of bone at the articular margins. Pain and inflammation are most often conservatively managed with NSAIDs.

- If pain and disability are not controlled in clients with arthritis, total joint replacements may be performed.

- Autoimmune and inflammatory disorders of the musculoskeletal system include rheumatoid arthritis (RA), ankylosing spondylitis (AS), reactive arthritis (ReA), systemic lupus erythematosus (SLE), polymyositis, and Lyme disease.

- Although the cause of RA is unknown, it is believed to be a combination of genetic, environmental, hormonal, and reproductive factors. RA is a systemic disease, affecting one or many joints with the risk for severe contractures and deformity, and also causing fatigue, weakness, anorexia, weight loss, and fever. The primary objectives of treatment and care are to reduce pain and inflammation, preserve function, and prevent deformity.

- SLE is a chronic inflammatory connective tissue disease, affecting almost all body systems, including the musculoskeletal system. Skin lesions are a common manifestation, exhibited by a characteristic rash on the face. The client with SLE is at increased risk for infection.

- Lyme disease is caused by the spirochete *Borrelia burgdorferi*, carried and transmitted primarily by ticks. The disease can be treated effectively with antibiotics.

- Osteomyelitis and septic arthritis are infectious musculoskeletal disorders. Osteomyelitis may be the result of a bloodborne pathogen, a contiguous infection, or a complication of vascular insufficiency. Septic arthritis is a medical emergency, requiring immediate treatment to preserve joint function.

- Bone tumors may be benign or malignant, primary or metastatic. The primary manifestations of a bone tumor are pain, a mass, and impaired function. Nursing care is directed toward teaching to prevent injury and interventions to relieve pain.

- Scleroderma is a chronic disease characterized by the formation of excess connective tissue and diffuse fibrosis of the skin and internal organs. It may be either localized or generalized. Other connective musculoskeletal disorders are Sjögren's syndrome and fibromyalgia.

- Structural musculoskeletal disorders affecting the spine are manifested by scoliosis, kyphosis, and low back pain. Those commonly affecting the feet are hallux valgus, hammertoe, and Morton's neuroma.

TEST YOURSELF NCLEX-RN® REVIEW

1 Although all of the following nursing diagnoses are important when planning care for the client with osteoporosis, which is most significant in terms of long-term disability?
1. *Chronic Pain*
2. *Risk for Falls*
3. *Activity Intolerance*
4. *Acute Pain*

2 You are preparing a teaching plan for a woman with osteoarthritis. Which group of medications should you prepare to discuss?
1. opioids
2. antibiotics
3. hormones
4. NSAIDs

3 You are monitoring the laboratory reports for a client with an acute attack of gout. Which of the following measurements would you expect to be increased?
1. hematocrit
2. uric acid
3. alkaline phosphatase
4. creatinine

4 What is a potential complication of both osteoporosis and osteomalacia?
1. infection
2. blood clots
3. fractures
4. contractures

5 You are assessing a woman who has come to an orthopedic clinic complaining of knee pain. Which of the following assessments you made would indicate an increased risk for osteoarthritis?
1. being overweight by 30 pounds
2. having a history of falls
3. eating a diet high in calcium
4. walking 30 minutes each day

6 A postoperative nursing care plan for a client who has had a total knee replacement includes monitoring vital signs and laboratory results. The rationale for these interventions is to:

1. teach the client the importance of these assessments.
2. promote rapport between the client and the healthcare providers.
3. ensure adequate circulation to the involved extremity.
4. prevent the progression of infection.

7 When comparing osteoarthritis and rheumatoid arthritis, what assessment finding would be different in the client with rheumatoid arthritis?
1. Health history includes weight loss and fever.
2. Abnormal joint findings are limited to the hands.
3. Stiffness is relieved by activity.
4. Heberden's nodes are located on the finger joints

8 *Ineffective Protection* is an appropriate nursing diagnosis for the client with SLE. What would be your most important intervention for the hospitalized client?
1. Monitor laboratory findings.
2. Provide appropriate skin care.
3. Practice careful hand washing.
4. Administer prescribed medications.

9 How is the causative organism for Lyme disease spread?
1. through the bite of an infected mosquito
2. by brief contact with an infected tick
3. primarily by droplets from infected people
4. by an infected tick embedded for >24 hours

10 Of the different types of arthritis, which one is considered a medical emergency, requiring immediate diagnosis and treatment?
1. osteoarthritis
2. septic arthritis
3. reactive arthritis
4. gouty arthritis

See Test Yourself answers in Appendix C.

BIBLIOGRAPHY

Abdelhafiz, A., Lowles, R., Alam, N., Abebajo, A., & Philp, I. (2003). Clinical assessment of symptomatic osteoarthritis in older people. *Age and Aging, 32*(3), 359–360.

_____. (2005a). *FDA actions on COX-2 inhibitors & NSAIDs (Non-steroidal anti-inflammatory drugs)*. Retrieved from http://arthritis.about.com/od/arthritismedications/a/qufdaactions_p.htm

About Arthritis. (2005b). *FDA announces changes for all NSAIDSs; Bextra withdrawn from market*. Retrieved from http://arthritis.about.com/od/nsaids/a/fadaaction.htm

Altizer, L. (2004). Patient education for total hip or knee replacement. *Orthopedic Nursing, 23*(4), 383–388.

American College of Rheumatology. (2004a). *Glucocorticoid-induced osteoporosis*. Retrieved from http://www.rheumatology.org/public/factsheets/gi_osteopor_new.asp?aud=mem

_____. (2004b). *Lyme disease*. Retrieved from http://www.rheumatology.org/public/factsheets/lyme.asp?aud=mem

_____. (2005). *Background information on arthritis and rheumatology: Prevalence statistics*. Retrieved from http://www.rheumatology.org/press/index.asp?uad=mem

Arthritis Foundation. (2004). *Disease center: Osteoarthritis treatment*. Retrieved from http://www.arthritis.org/conditions/DiseaseCenter/OA/oa_treatment1.asp

Berarducci, A. (2004). Osteoporosis education: A health-promotion mandate for nurses. *Orthopaedic Nursing, 23*(2), 118–120.

Boston Total Joint Association. (2004). *Total hip replacement surgery*. Retrieved from http://www.bostontotaljoint.com/thr.html

Brown, S. (2005). Managing systemic lupus erythematosus. *Nurse 2 Nurse, 4*(11), 28–30.

Capriotti, T. (2004). The 'alphabet' of rheumatoid arthritis treatment. *Medsurg Nursing, 13*(6), 420–428.

Centers for Disease Control and Prevention. (2005). *Bone health*. Retrieved from www.cdc.gov/nccdphp/dnpa/bonehealth/

Cornell, T. (2004). Factfile. Ankylosing spondylitis: An overview. *Professional Nurse, 19*(8), 431–432.

Dochterman, J., & Bulechek, G. (2004). *Nursing interventions classification (NIC)* (4th ed.). St. Louis, MO: Mosby.

Easterbrook, L. (2003). Explaining about ... arthritis. *Working with older people, 7*(3), 7–9.

Flynn, J., & Johnson, T. (2005). *The Johns Hopkins white papers: Arthritis*. Baltimore, MD: Johns Hopkins Medicine.

Gill, J., Quisel, A., Rocca, P., & Walters, D. (2003). Diagnosis of systemic lupus erythematosus. *American Family Physician, 68*(11). Retrieved from http://www.aafp.org/afp/20031201/2179.html

Harvey, C. (2005). Wound healing. *Orthopaedic Nursing, 24*(2), 143–160.

International Scleroderma Network. (2004). *What in the world is scleroderma?* Retrieved from http://www.sclero.org

Kass-Wolff, J. (2004). Calcium in women: Healthy bones and much more. *Journal of Obstetrics, Gynecologic, and Neonatal Nursing, 33*(1), 21–33.

Kee, J. (2004). *Handbook of laboratory and diagnostic tests with nursing implications* (5th ed.). Upper Saddle River, NJ: Prentice Hall.

Lange, R., & Nies, M. (2004). Benefits of walking for obese women in the prevention of bone and joint disorders. *Orthopedic Nursing, 23*(3), 211–215.

Lucas, B. (2004). Does a pre-operative exercise programme improve mobility and function post-total knee replacement: A mini-review. *Journal of Orthopaedic Nursing, 8*(1), 25–33.

Mayo Clinic. (2002). *Osteoporosis*. Retrieved from www.mayocli8nic.com/invoke.cfm?id=DS00128

Moorhead, S., Johnson, M., & Maas, M. (2003). *Nursing outcomes classification (NOC)*. (3rd ed.). St. Louis, MO: Mosby.

Morrow, M. (2004). Duchenne muscular dystrophy–A biopsychosocial approach. *Physiotherapy, 90*, 145–150.

Moss Rehab Resource Net. (2005). *Arthritis fact sheet*. Retrieved from http://www.mossresourcenet.org/arthritis/htm

NANDA International. (2005). *Nursing diagnoses: Definitions & classification 2005–2006*. Philadelphia: Author.

National Fibromyalgia Research Association. (2004). *Fibromyalgia syndrome*. Retrieved from http://www.nfra.net/

National Institute of Arthritis and Musculoskeletal and Skin Diseases. (2003). *Systemic lupus erythematosus; lupus and quality of life*. Retrieved from http://www.niams.nih.gov/hi/topics/lupus/slehandout/

_____. (2004a). *Questions and answers about arthritis and rheumatic diseases*. Retrieved from http://www.niams.nih.gov/hi/topics/arthritis/arthrheu.htm

_____. (2004b). *Questions and answers about knee problems*. Retrieved from http://www.niams.nih.gov/hi/topics/kneeprobs/kneeqa.htm

_____. (2005a). *Fibromyalgia*. Retrieved from http://www.niams.nih.gov/hi/topics/fibromyalgia/ffibro.htm

_____. (2005b). *Hyaluronic acid shows potential as biomarker for osteoarthritis*. Retrieved from http://www.niams.nih.gov/ne/highlights/spotlight/2005/hyaluronic_acid.htm

_____. (2005c). *What is gout?* Retrieved from http://www.niams.nih.gov/hi/topics/gout/ffgout.htm

National Osteoporosis Foundation. (2006). *Fast facts*. Retrieved from http://www.nof.org/osteoporosis/diseasefacts.htm

Nivens, A. (2004). Paget's disease: A case in point. *Orthopedic Nursing, 23*(6), 355–363.

Overstreet, M. (2005). Lyme disease: The dangerous hitchhiker. *Nursing Made Incredibly Easy, 3*(3), 38–44.

Paget Foundation. (2004a). *A health professional's guide to the management of Paget's disease of the bone*. Retrieved from http://www.Paget's.org/Information/FactSheet/mgmt_of_pdisbone.html

_____. (2004b). *A nurse's guide for assessment and management of patients diagnosed with Paget's disease of bone*. New York: The Paget Foundation.

Porth, C. M. (2005). *Pathophysiology: Concepts of altered health states* (7th ed.). Philadelphia: Lippincott.

Pullen, R., Jr. (2004). Caring for a patient on Plaquenil therapy. *Nursing, 34*(6), 32hn4, 32hn16.

_____, Cannon, J., & Rushing, J. (2003). Managing organ-threatening systemic lupus erythematosus. *Medsurg Nursing, 12*(6), 368–379.

Roberts, D. (2003). Alternative therapies for arthritis treatment: Part 1. *Orthopedic Nursing, 22*(5), 335–344.

Risley, S., Thomas, M., & Bray, V. (2004). Rheumatoid arthritis, new standards of care: Nursing implications of infliximab *Journal of Orthopaedic Nursing, 8*(1), 41–49.

Schoen, D. C. (2004). Osteoporosis. *Orthopaedic Nursing, 23*(4), 261–267.

Scleroderma Foundation. (2006). *What is scleroderma?* Retrieved from http://scleroderma.org/medical/overview.shtm

Spondylitis Association of America. (2006). *Reactive arthritis/Reiter's syndrome, (ReA), Fast facts about ankylosing spondylitis (AS)*. Retrieved from http://www.spondylitis.org/about/reative.aspx

Taggart, H., Mincer, A., & Thompson, A. (2004). Caring for the orthopaedic patient who is obese. *Orthopaedic Nursing, 23*(3), 204–210.

Tak, S. H., & Hong, S. H. (2005). Use of the Internet for health information by older adults with arthritis. *Orthopaedic Nursing, 24*(2), 134–139.

Temple, J. (2004). Total hip replacement. *Nursing Standard, 19*(3), 44–51, 53.

Tierney, L., McPhee, S., & Papadakis, M. (Eds.). (2004). *Current medical diagnosis & treatment* (43rd ed.). Stamford, CT: Appleton & Lange.

Tretheway, P. (2004). Systemic lupus erythematosus. *DCCN: Dimensions of Critical Care Nursing, 23*(3), 111–115.

U. S. Food and Drug Administration (FDA). (2005). *COX-2 selective (includes Bextra, Celebrex, and Vioxx) and non-selective non-steroidal anti-inflammatory drugs (NSAIDs)*. Retrieved from http://www.fda.gov/cder/drug/infopage/COX2/

Vestergaard. P., Emborg, C., Stoving, R., Hagen, C., Mosekilde, L., & Briken, K. (2003). Patients with eating disorders: A high-risk group for fractures. *Orthopaedic Nursing, 22*(5), 325–331.

Wilkens, R. (2004). Making the most of antirheumatic drugs in older patients. *Journal of Musculoskeletal Medicine, 21*(6), 317–322.

Wilkinson, J. (2005). *Prentice Hall nursing diagnosis handbook with NIC interventions and NOC outcomes* (8th ed.). Upper Saddle River, NJ: Prentice Hall.

Wilson, B., Shannon, M., & Stang, C. (2005). *Prentice Hall nurse's drug guide 2005*. Upper Saddle River, NJ: Prentice Hall.

UNIT 12 BUILDING CLINICAL COMPETENCE
Responses to Altered Musculoskeletal Function

FUNCTIONAL HEALTH PATTERN: Activity-Exercise

■ Think about clients with altered activity-exercise patterns for whom you have cared in your clinical experiences.

- What were the clients' major medical diagnoses (e.g., sprain, joint dislocation, fracture, amputation, carpal tunnel syndrome, osteoporosis, Paget's disease, gout, osteomalacia, osteoarthritis, muscular dystrophy, rheumatoid arthritis, ankylosing spondylitis, systemic lupus erythematosus, polymyositis, Lyme disease, osteomyelitis, bone tumors, systemic sclerosis, scoliosis, low back pain, hammertoe)?
- What manifestations did each of these clients have? Were these manifestations similar or different?
- How did the clients' altered activity-exercise patterns interfere with their health status? Did pain increase with movement? Was the pain worse in the morning or did the pain increase throughout the day? Did they complain of muscle weakness or muscle cramps? Did they notice any redness or swelling of the joints? Had they ever had any muscle or bone diseases or injuries? Did they have any surgery or physical therapies for muscle or bone problems? Did they take any medications or herbal supplements for musculoskeletal disorders? Did they include foods with calcium in the diet? Did they have any family history of bone, joint, or muscle problems? Did they exercise regularly? Did they take part in strenuous activity or heavy lifting? Did they use assistive devices to move around?

■ The Activity-Exercise Pattern includes disorders that result in insufficient physiologic movement to carry out activities of daily living. Activity and exercise are affected by the ability of the musculoskeletal system to allow movement of the body and by perceived health status in two primary ways:

- Factors that result from trauma or surgery to tissues (e.g., contusion), tendons (e.g., strain, epicondylitis), ligaments (e.g., sprain), or bones (e.g., dislocation, fracture, amputation).
- Factors that result from medical disorders or deformities of joints (e.g., arthritis, gout, hammertoe), bones (e.g., osteoporosis, Paget's disease, osteomalacia, osteomyelitis, tumors, scoliosis), or muscles (e.g., muscular dystrophy, polymyositis).

■ The tissues and structures of the musculoskeletal system perform many functions, including support, protection, and movement. The bones form the body's structure and provide support for soft tissues. The bones protect vital internal organs from injury. The bones also store minerals and serve as a site for hematopoiesis (blood cell formation). The bones and joints of the skeleton and the skeletal muscles work together to allow the body to perform both gross, simple movements and fine, complex movements. Musculoskeletal disorders affect a client's perceived activity-exercise patterns, leading to manifestations such as:

- Pain (tissue damage ▶ stimulates sensory nerve endings ▶which release chemical mediators such as bradykinin and histamine ▶resulting in transmission of pain sensation to brain and nerve fibers)
- Limited mobility (disease or injury ▶causes excessive loss of movement to muscles and joints ▶resulting in reduction or restriction of range of motion to a body part)
- Edema (inflammation or infection ▶causes impaired circulation, venous pooling, and proteins leaking into the interstitium ▶resulting in edema).

■ Priority nursing diagnoses within the activity-exercise pattern that may be appropriate for clients include:

- *Risk for Disuse Syndrome* related to decreased range of motion, pain with movement, use of functional positioning splints
- *Risk for Falls* related to impaired balance, difficulty with gait, numbness of feet, decreased lower extremity strength
- *Impaired Physical Mobility* as evidenced by limited ability to perform gross/fine motor skills, uncoordinated or jerky movements, postural instability
- *Risk for Peripheral Neurovascular Dysfunction* related to musculoskeletal pain, pallor, diminished pulses, paralysis, and paresthesia.

■ Two nursing diagnoses from other functional health patterns often are of high priority for the client with altered activity-exercise patterns:

- *Impaired Skin Integrity* (Nutritional-Metabolic)
- *Risk for Disturbed Sensory Perception: Tactile (Cognitive-Perceptual)*

CLINICAL SCENARIO

You have been assigned to work with the following four clients for the 0700 shift on an orthopedic unit. Significant data obtained during report are as follows:

■ Jesse Drummond is a 70-year-old African American man with type 2 diabetes mellitus who is 3 days postoperative with bilateral below-the-knee amputations. Vital signs are T 99°F, P 88, R 24, BP 150/92. He is complaining of feeling pain in his feet.

■ Joyce Stevens is an 84-year-old who is 2 days postoperative for hip replacement surgery. Her vital signs are T 99.6°F, P 100, R 30 and shallow, BP 110/86. She is confused when spoken to. Petechiae have been noted on her arms and legs. She is complaining of difficulty breathing.

■ José Rivera, a 21-year-old, was admitted with osteomyelitis of the upper right leg. He has a history of a gunshot wound to the leg. Vital signs are T 102.6°F, P 98, R 22, BP 138/80. He is scheduled for surgical debridement of the wound this morning. He is complaining of pain and requesting pain medication.

■ Kim Wong is a 30-year-old who was admitted with manifestations of painful and swollen joints, muscle pain, pale and cyanotic fingers and toes, and edema of the legs and periorbital areas. Her vital signs are T 100.6°F, P 78, R 16, BP 108/72. She is complaining of extreme fatigue. She is to have blood drawn for complete blood count (CBC), anti-DNA antibody testing, and serum complement levels.

Questions

1 In what order would you visit these clients after report?

1. _____
2. _____
3. _____
4. _____

2 What top two priority nursing diagnoses would you choose for each of the clients presented above? Can you explain, if asked, the rationale for your choices?

	Priority Nursing Diagnosis #1	Priority Nursing Diagnosis #2
Jesse Drummond		
Joyce Stevens		
José Rivera		
Kim Wong		

3 After the amputation wound is dressed, what is the client taught to do to toughen the stump?
1. Dangle the stump for 20 minutes every hour while awake.
2. Push the stump into soft and then harder surfaces.
3. Elevate the stump on two pillows, keeping the knee straight.
4. Apply prosthesis over the compression dressing.

4 To prevent hip contractures in the client with an above-the-knee amputation, what does the nurse instruct the client to do?
1. Lie supine for short periods throughout the day.
2. Elevate the stump above the level of the heart.
3. Perform active range-of-motion exercises every 8 hours.
4. Avoid sitting in a chair for prolonged periods of time.

5 The nurse explains to the client with gout that a low-purine diet is recommended. The client understands a low-purine diet when which meal is ordered?
1. ham and asparagus casserole
2. chicken and dumplings
3. chili and spinach salad
4. shrimp and scallop pasta

6 The client's laboratory results are hematocrit of 28%, hemoglobin of 8 g/dL, WBC count of 4000/mm³, platelet count of 98,000/mL, eosinophil sedimentation rate of 100 mm/h, positive anti-DNA antibodies. What medical diagnosis is supported by these lab values?
1. systemic lupus erythmatosus
2. rheumatoid arthritis
3. ankylosing spondylitis
4. polymyositis

7 Clients who have autoimmune diseases such as systemic lupus erythematosus are at increased risk for developing what disease?
1. chronic renal failure
2. hypertension
3. liver insufficiency
4. coronary heart disease

8 A prescription for ibuprofen (Advil) is given on discharge to the client with rheumatoid arthritis. Which toxic effects of the medication does the nurse instruct the client about?
1. diarrhea, nausea, and vomiting
2. blurred vision, tinnitus, and headache
3. gastric irritation, ulceration, and bleeding
4. dizziness, dry mouth, and abdominal cramps

9 When performing a neurovascular assessment, which are included in the initial and focused assessments? (Select all that apply.)
1. pain
2. paroxysm
3. pallor
4. pulses
5. paresis
6. pallesthesia
7. paresthesia

10 Which client is at greatest risk for developing osteoporosis?
1. menopausal, Caucasian woman who smokes one pack of cigarettes a day
2. menopausal, African American woman who has diabetes and hypertension
3. premenopausal, underweight Asian woman who is allergic to dairy products
4. premenopausal, obese African American woman who has a sedentary lifestyle

11 An older adult sprained an ankle after tripping on an uneven sidewalk. Which is the MOST important intervention?
1. Use a walker when ambulating.
2. Take anti-inflammatory and pain medications to reduce ankle pain.
3. Follow a regimen of rest, ice, compression, and elevation.
4. Immobilize the ankle with an air splint.

12 Which actions by the nurse need to be followed when caring for the client with osteomyelitis?
1. Place the client in a private room and use gloves and gown with wound care and good hand washing.
2. Place the client in a semiprivate room with another infected client and use isolation precautions for both clients.
3. Place the client near the nurse's station and use standard precautions when caring for the client.
4. Place the client at the end of the hall away from other clients to prevent spread of infection and teach the client to use good hand washing.

CASE STUDY

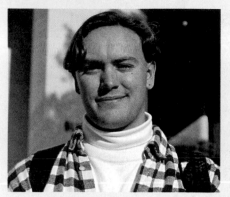

William Comfort is a 24-year-old Caucasian male admitted with a compound fracture of the left femur. He states he was riding a four-wheeler on a hill-side path and was thrown from the vehicle. He slid approximately 50 feet down the hill on his left side. His fall was stopped when his foot became tangled in some brush. On admission, his vital signs were T 99.8°F, P 100 and thready, R 24, BP 116/70. His height is 74" and weight is 198 pounds. Assessment revealed an open fracture of the left leg with bleeding and edema around the open site and severe pain on movement of the leg. Popliteal and pedal pulses are difficult to palpate. His left leg is pale and cool to touch with a capillary refill of 4 seconds. He states his leg feels numb. Multiple lacerations and abrasions are noted on his left trunk and arm. He states he does not have any medical problems and has not seen a doctor in the past 5 years. He is employed as a computer repairman. He lives in an apartment with two friends.

Blood is drawn for a baseline compete blood count (CBC) and urine is obtained for a urinalysis. An intravenous line is started in the right arm with lactated Ringer's infusing at 150 mL/h. He is given a tetanus toxoid immunization and is medicated with morphine sulfate for pain. X-rays are taken of the left leg, left arm, and abdomen. The wounds are cleansed with an antibacterial solution and antibiotic ointment is applied. He went to surgery for an open reduction of the left leg fracture and has been placed in skeletal traction to separate the bony fragments and reduce and immobilize the left leg fracture.

The pathophysiology of a femur fracture is a large amount of force applied to the shaft of the femur, resulting in breaking of the bone. An open fracture is diagnosed when the bone is broken with bone fragments protruding through the skin. Manifestations of a femur fracture are edema, and a deformed and painful thigh. The client is unable to move the hip or knee. Popliteal and pedal pulses are difficult to palpate. Capillary refill time is increased. Pallor and coolness indicate arterial compromise. Sensations to the leg may be burning, numbness, prickly feeling, or stinging. Complications of a femur fracture include hypovolemia, fat embolism, dislocation of the hip or knee, muscle atrophy, and ligament damage.

Skeletal traction is the application of a pulling force through placement of pins into the bone. Pins are inserted under sterile conditions into the bone. One or more pulling forces may be applied to maintain alignment of the femur fracture. The disadvantages of skeletal traction are increased anxiety, increased risk of infection, and increased discomfort.

When planning nursing care for Mr. Comfort, the nursing diagnosis of *Impaired Physical Mobility* related to fracture of the left femur with skeletal traction is appropriate for implementing nursing interventions.

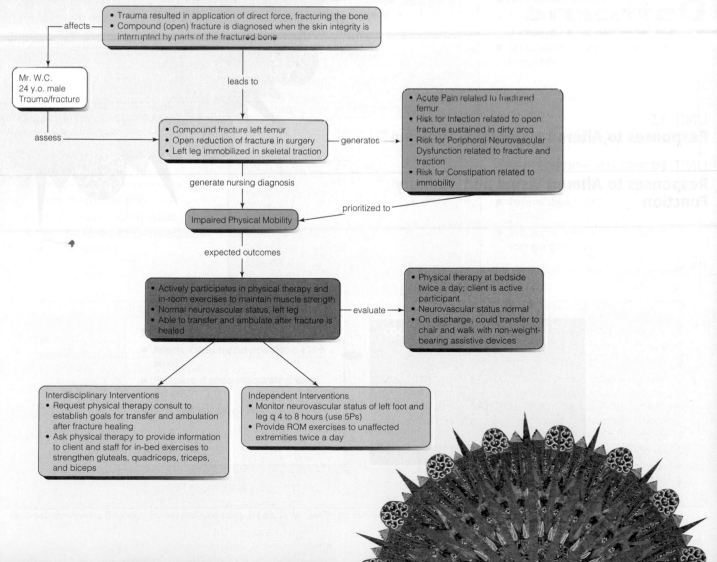

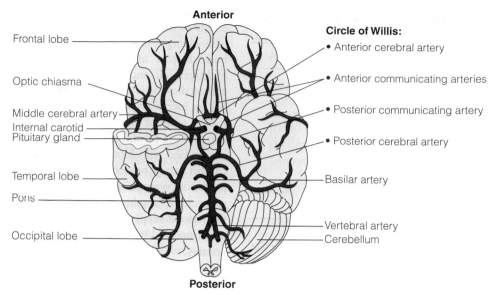

Figure 43–5 ■ Major arteries serving the brain and the circle of Willis.

The Spinal Cord

The spinal cord extends from the medulla to the level of the first lumbar vertebra (Figure 43–6 ■). It serves as a center for conducting messages to and from the brain and as a reflex center. The spinal cord is about 17 inches (42 cm) long and 0.75 inch (1.8 cm) thick. The cord is protected by the vertebrae, the meninges, and CSF. The gray matter of the cord is on the inside, and the white matter is on the outside (the reverse of the arrangement in the brain).

The spinal cord is surrounded and protected by 33 vertebrae: 7 cervical, 12 thoracic, 5 lumbar, 5 sacral, and 4 fused vertebrae, which form the coccyx. Each vertebra consists of a body and a vertebral arch formed by projections from the body. This arch encloses a space called the vertebral foramen. The vertebral foramina of all the vertebrae form the vertebral canal through which the spinal cord passes. Intervertebral foramina are spaces between the vertebrae through which spinal nerve roots pass as they exit the vertebral column.

Intervertebral disks are located between each of the movable vertebrae. Each disk is made of a thick capsule surrounding a gelatinous core called the nucleus pulposus. Ligaments that provide mobility and protection surround the vertebral column, discussed in greater detail in Chapter 45 ∞.

The roots of 31 pairs of spinal nerves, divided into the cervical, thoracic, lumbar, sacral, and coccygeal nerves, arise from the cord (see Figure 43–6). Each separates into posterior (sensory) and anterior (motor) roots. Damage to the posterior roots results in loss of sensation, whereas damage to the anterior root results in flaccid paralysis.

FUNCTIONS OF THE SPINAL CORD AND SPINAL ROOTS

Messages to and from the brain are conducted via ascending (sensory) pathways and descending (motor) pathways (Figure 43–7 ■). The major ascending tracts are the lateral and anterior spinothalamic tracts, which carry sensations for pain, temperature, and crude touch; and the posterior tracts, which carry sensations for fine touch, position, and vibra-

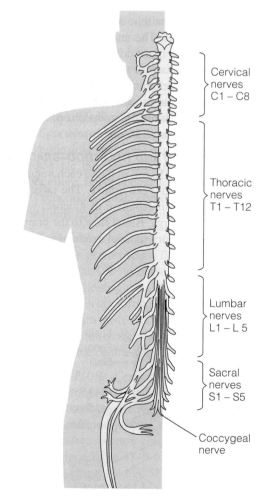

Figure 43–6 ■ Distribution of spinal nerves.

tion. The lateral and anterior corticospinal (pyramidal) tracts are descending tracts consisting of fibers that originate in the motor cortex of the brain and travel to the brainstem and then down the spinal cord. They mediate voluntary purposeful

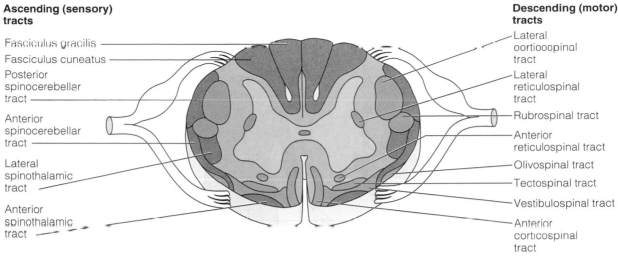

Ascending (sensory) tracts

Fasciculus gracilis
Fasciculus cuneatus
Posterior spinocerebellar tract
Anterior spinocerebellar tract
Lateral spinothalamic tract
Anterior spinothalamic tract

Descending (motor) tracts

Lateral cortioospinal tract
Lateral reticulospinal tract
Rubrospinal tract
Anterior reticulospinal tract
Olivospinal tract
Tectospinal tract
Vestibulospinal tract
Anterior corticospinal tract

Figure 43–7 ■ Ascending and descending tracts of the spinal cord.

movements and stimulate certain muscular actions while inhibiting others. They also carry fibers that inhibit muscle tone. The rubrospinal, anterior and lateral reticulospinal, and tectospinal (extrapyramidal) tracts include the pathways between the cerebral cortex, basal ganglia, brainstem, and spinal cord outside the pyramidal tract. They maintain muscle tone and gross body movements.

UPPER AND LOWER MOTOR NEURONS Upper motor neurons, such as those of the corticospinal and extrapyramidal tract, carry impulses from the cerebral cortex to the anterior gray column of the spinal cord. Damage to upper motor neurons results in increased muscle tone, decreased muscle strength, decreased coordination, and hyperactive reflexes. Lower motor neurons begin in the anterior gray column of the spinal cord and end in the muscle. Damage to lower motor neurons results in decreased muscle tone, muscle atrophy, fasciculations, and loss of reflexes.

The Peripheral Nervous System

The peripheral nervous system links the CNS with the rest of the body. It is responsible for receiving and transmitting information from and about the external environment. The PNS consists of nerves, ganglia (groups of nerve cells), and sensory receptors located outside—or peripheral to—the brain and spinal cord. The PNS is divided into a sensory (afferent) division and a motor (efferent) division. Most nerves of the PNS contain fibers for both divisions and all are classified regionally as either spinal nerves or cranial nerves.

Spinal Nerves

The 31 pairs of spinal nerves (see Figure 43–6) are named by their location:

- Cervical nerves: 8 pairs
- Thoracic nerves: 12 pairs
- Lumbar nerves: 5 pairs
- Sacral nerves: 5 pairs
- Coccygeal nerves: 1 pair

Spinal nerves exit the vertebral column through intervertebral foramina to travel to the body regions they serve. The spinal cord does not reach the end of the vertebral column; as a result, the lumbar and sacral nerve roots travel inferiorly through the vertebral canal for some distance before exiting the vertebral column through their associated intervertebral foramina. This collection of descending nerve roots is called the cauda equina.

Each spinal nerve contains both sensory and motor fibers. The sensory fibers are located in the dorsal root, and their cell bodies are located within the dorsal root ganglion. The motor fibers are located in the ventral root, and their cell bodies are located within the spinal cord. The dorsal and ventral roots merge outside the vertebral canal just past the dorsal root ganglion, forming a spinal nerve. Each spinal nerve further divides into branches called rami.

The ventral rami of the cervical, brachial, lumbar, and sacral regions form complex clusters of nerves called plexuses. The main spinal nerve plexuses innervate the skin and the underlying muscles of the arms and legs. For example, the cervical plexus innervates the diaphragm through the phrenic nerve; the brachial plexus innervates the upper extremities through the median, ulnar, and radial nerves; and the lumbar plexus innervates the anterior thigh through the femoral nerve.

An area of skin innervated by cutaneous branches of a single spinal nerve is called a dermatome. The dorsal roots of the spinal nerves carry sensations from these specific dermatomes. Dermatomes provide anatomic landmarks that are useful for locating neurologic lesions (Figure 43–8 ■).

Cranial Nerves

Twelve pairs of cranial nerves originate in the forebrain and brainstem (Figure 43–9 ■). The vagus nerve extends into the ventral body cavity, but the 11 other pairs innervate only head and neck regions. Although most are mixed nerves, three pairs (olfactory, optic, and acoustic) are solely sensory. The cranial nerves and their related functions are listed in Table 43–4.

Reflexes

A reflex is a rapid, involuntary, predictable motor response to a stimulus. Reflexes are categorized as either somatic or autonomic.

PERSISTENT VEGETATIVE STATE **Persistent vegetative state** (also called irreversible coma) is a permanent condition of complete unawareness of self and the environment and loss of all cognitive functions. Usually the result of severe brain trauma or global ischemia, this condition results from death of the cerebral hemispheres with continued function of the brainstem and cerebellum. While the homeostatic regulatory functions of the brain continue, the ability to respond meaningfully to the environment is lost. The diagnosis of persistent vegetative state requires that the condition has continued for at least 1 month (Porth, 2005).

The client has sleep–wake cycles and retains the ability to chew, swallow, and cough but cannot interact with the environment. When awake, the eyes may wander back and forth across the room, but they cannot track an object or person. In a minimally conscious state, the client is aware of the environment and can follow simple commands, manipulate objects, gesture or verbalize to indicate "yes/no" responses, and make meaningful movements (such as blinking or smiling) in response to a stimulus. With appropriate supportive care, the client may remain in this state for years.

LOCKED-IN SYNDROME **Locked-in syndrome** is distinctly different from persistent vegetative state in that the client is alert and fully aware of the environment and has intact cognitive abilities, but is unable to communicate through speech or movement because of blocked efferent pathways from the brain. Motor paralysis affects all voluntary muscles, although the upper cranial nerves (I through IV) may remain intact, allowing the client to communicate through eye movements and blinking. In essence, the client is "locked" inside a paralyzed body while remaining fully conscious of self and environment. Infarction or hemorrhage of the pons that disrupts outgoing nerve tracts but spares the RAS is the usual cause of locked-in syndrome. This condition may also result when the corticospinal tracts between the midbrain and pons are interrupted. Disorders of the lower motor neurons or muscles, such as acute polyneuritis, myasthenia gravis, or amyotrophic lateral sclerosis (ALS), may also paralyze motor responses, leading to locked-in syndrome.

BRAIN DEATH **Brain death** is the cessation and irreversibility of all brain functions, including the brainstem. Although the exact criteria for establishing brain death may vary somewhat from state to state, it is generally agreed that brain death has occurred when there is no evidence of cerebral or brainstem function for an extended period (usually 6 to 24 hours) in a client who has a normal body temperature and is not affected by a depressant drug or alcohol poisoning. Generally recognized criteria are:

- Unresponsive coma with absent motor and reflex movements
- No spontaneous respiration (apnea)
- Pupils fixed (unresponsive to light) and dilated
- Absent ocular responses to head turning and caloric stimulation (Caloric stimulation is performed by irrigating the ear with ice-cold water to test the oculovestibular reflex, a reflex controlled by the brainstem. Normally, the cold causes the eyes to first move toward the irrigated side, followed by a return to midline.)

- Flat electroencephalogram (EEG) and no cerebral blood circulation present on angiography (if performed)
- Persistence of these manifestations for 30 minutes to 1 hour and for 6 hours after onset of coma and apnea.

Apnea in the comatose client is determined by the apnea test. The ventilator is removed while maintaining oxygenation by tracheal cannula and allowing the P_{CO_2} to increase to 60 mmHg or higher. This level of carbon dioxide is high enough to stimulate respiration if the brainstem is functional. The EEG may be used to establish the absence of brain activity when brain death is suspected. A flat (isoelectric) EEG over a period of 6 to 12 hours in a client who is not hypothermic or under the influence of drugs that depress the central nervous system (CNS) is generally accepted as an indicator of brain death.

Prognosis

The prognosis for clients with altered levels of consciousness and coma varies according to the underlying cause and pathologic process. Age and general medical condition also play a role in determining outcome. Young adults may fully recover following deep coma from head injury, drug overdose, or other cause. Recovery of consciousness within 2 weeks is associated with a favorable outcome. In general, the prognosis is poor for clients who lack pupillary reaction or reflex eye movements 6 hours after the onset of coma.

INTERDISCIPLINARY CARE

Management of the client with an altered LOC or coma must begin immediately. The focus of management is to identify the underlying cause, preserve function, and prevent deterioration if possible. Airway and breathing must be maintained during the initial acute stage until the diagnosis and prognosis can be established. Intravenous fluids are used to support circulation and to correct fluid, electrolyte, and acid–base imbalances. Treatment protocols to reduce increased intracranial pressure or control seizure activity (discussed later in this chapter) may be initiated. Changes in LOC associated with craniocerebral trauma, such as hematomas, often require immediate surgical intervention.

Diagnosis

Although the client's history and physical examination findings often indicate the cause of alterations in LOC, several diagnostic tests may be useful in establishing the diagnosis. The tests used to evaluate for possible metabolic, toxic, or drug-induced disorders include both radiologic and laboratory tests.

CT and MRI scanning are done to detect neurologic damage due to hemorrhage, tumor, cyst, edema, myocardial infarction, or brain atrophy. These tests may also identify displacement of brain structures by large or expanding lesions. Radioisotope brain scan is performed to identify abnormal lesions in the brain and evaluate cerebral blood flow. Cerebral angiography allows radiographic visualization of the cerebral vascular system. This exam can identify lesions such as aneurysms, occluded vessels, or tumors, and may also be used to determine cessation of cerebral blood flow and brain death. Transcranial Doppler studies use an ultrasound velocity detector that records sound waves reflected from RBCs in blood vessels to assess cerebral blood flow. Lumbar puncture with cerebrospinal fluid (CSF) analysis is performed when infection and possible meningitis are suspected as a cause of altered LOC. EEG is used to evaluate the electrical activity of the brain. (See Chapter 43 ∞ for further information and nursing implications of neurologic tests.)

Laboratory tests are used to identify and monitor altered LOC. These may include any or all of the following:

- *Blood glucose* is measured immediately when coma is of unknown origin and hypoglycemia is suspected or possible. When the blood glucose falls to less than 40 to 50 mg/dL, cerebral function declines rapidly. The client with type 1 diabetes is at particular risk for hypoglycemia-induced coma.
- *Serum electrolytes*—sodium, potassium, bicarbonate, chloride, and calcium in particular—are measured to assess for metabolic disturbances and guide intravenous therapy. Hyponatremia, in which serum sodium levels are below 115 mEq/L (normal level: 135 to 145 mEq/L), is associated with coma and convulsions, especially if it develops rapidly.
- *Serum osmolality* is evaluated. Both hyperosmolar and hypo-osmolar states may be associated with coma. Hyperosmolality (above 320 mOsm/kg H_2O) causes cellular dehydration of brain tissue as fluid is drawn into the vascular system by osmosis. Hypo-osmolality (less than 250 mOsm/kg H_2O), by contrast, leads to cerebral edema and swelling, impairing consciousness.
- *Arterial blood gases* (ABGs) are drawn to evaluate arterial oxygen and carbon dioxide levels as well as acid–base balance. Hypoxemia is a frequent cause of altered LOC; increased levels of carbon dioxide are also toxic to the brain and can induce coma, particularly when the onset of hypercapnia is acute.
- *Liver function tests,* including bilirubin, AST, ALT, LDH, serum albumin, and serum ammonia levels, are determined to evaluate hepatic function. High ammonia levels seen in hepatic failure interfere with cerebral metabolism and neurotransmitters, affecting LOC.
- *Toxicology screening* of blood and urine is done to determine if altered LOC is the result of acute drug or alcohol toxicity. Serum alcohol levels are measured and the blood is assessed for the presence of substances such as barbiturates, carbon monoxide, or lead.

Medications

Medications are used to support homeostasis and normal function for the client with altered LOC, as well as to treat specific underlying disorders. An intravenous catheter is inserted, and fluid balance is maintained using isotonic or slightly hypertonic solutions, such as normal saline or lactated Ringer's solution. The client's response to fluid administration is monitored carefully for evidence of increased cerebral edema.

If hypoglycemia is present, 50% glucose is administered intravenously to restore cerebral metabolism rapidly. Conversely, insulin is administered to the client with hyperglycemia to reduce the blood glucose level and thus the serum osmolality. With narcotic overdose, naloxone is administered. Naloxone is a narcotic antagonist that competes for narcotic receptor sites, effectively blocking the depressant effect of the narcotic. Thiamine may be administered with glucose, particularly if the client is malnourished or known to abuse alcohol, to prevent exacerbation of Wernicke's encephalopathy, a hemorrhagic encephalopathy due to thiamine deficiency that is associated with chronic alcoholism (Tierney et al., 2005).

Any underlying fluid and electrolyte imbalance is corrected by administering medications or appropriate electrolytes. For the client who is hyponatremic and has a low serum osmolality, furosemide (Lasix) or an osmotic diuretic such as mannitol may be administered to promote water excretion. Appropriate antibiotics are administered intravenously to the client with suspected or confirmed meningitis.

Surgery

Although surgery is not indicated for most clients with altered LOC, it may be necessary if the cause of coma is an intracerebral tumor, hemorrhage, or hematoma. Surgical intervention is discussed later in this chapter, in the section on brain tumors. When there is a risk of increased intracranial pressure, the client is monitored continuously. These measures are discussed in the section on increased intracranial pressure that follows.

Other Treatments

Support of the airway and respirations is vital in the client with an altered LOC. The client who is drowsy but rousable may need little more than an oral pharyngeal airway. With more severe alterations in consciousness, the client may need endotracheal intubation to maintain airway patency, particularly if the cough and gag reflexes are absent. Mechanical ventilation is indicated when hypoventilation or apnea is present. Unless a do-not-resuscitate (DNR) order is in effect, mechanical ventilation should be initiated even if it has not been established that the disorder is reversible; without ventilatory support, cerebral anoxia develops rapidly, and brain death may ensue. ABGs are monitored frequently to determine the adequacy of ventilation. Cautious hyperventilation may be used to reduce $Paco_2$ and promote cerebral vasoconstriction to reduce cerebral edema.

Nutrition

In clients with long-term alterations in consciousness, such as vegetative state or locked-in syndrome, measures to maintain nutritional status are initiated. Enteral feedings with a gastrostomy tube are preferred if the client is unable to take enough food by mouth without aspirating. In some cases, total parenteral nutrition may be used.

NURSING CARE

Nursing care of the client with an altered LOC is planned and implemented for a variety of responses of both the client and the family of the client.

Support of the Family

Family members of a client with an altered level of consciousness are often very anxious. It is difficult for the family to deal with the client's uncertain prognosis. They may experience various conflicting emotions, such as guilt and anger. Reinforce information provided by the physician, and encourage the family to talk to the client as though he or she were able to understand. Explain that this communication may initially seem awkward, but in time it will feel appropriate. Evaluate the family's readiness to receive explanations regarding the client's treatment and care. The presence of many tubes (e.g., intravenous line, catheter, ventilator) may be overwhelming to the family. They may not perceive the seriousness of the situation if a thorough explanation is not given. Include family members in the client's care as much as they wish to be involved.

Allow significant others to stay with the client when possible. Reinforce the need for family members to care for themselves by encouraging adequate meals and rest. Offer to contact support services such as friends, neighbors, and social services that the hospital may provide. Ask family members to leave a telephone number where they can be reached, and assure them that they will be called if any significant changes occur. Encourage family members to call if they have questions or concerns.

Nursing Diagnoses and Interventions

Nursing diagnoses and interventions discussed in this section are directed toward the unconscious client and focus on problems with airway maintenance, skin integrity, contractures, and nutrition.

Ineffective Airway Clearance

Ineffective airway clearance related to loss of the cough reflex and the inability to expectorate is a major problem for the unconscious client. The cough reflex may be absent or impaired when conditions that produce coma depress the function of the medullary centers.

- Assess ability to clear secretions. Monitor breath sounds, rate and depth of respirations, dyspnea, pulse oximeter, and the presence of cyanosis. *The client's ability to clear secretions serves as the initial assessment base for developing further interventions.*
- In unconscious clients or those without an intact cough reflex, maintain an open airway by periodic suctioning, limiting the time of suctioning to 10 to 15 seconds or less. Periodic suctioning may be necessary to clear the airway of mucus, blood, or other drainage. *Suctioning for more than 15 seconds in the client with increased intracranial pressure may cause hypercapnia, which in turn vasodilates cerebral vessels, increases cerebral blood volume, and increases intracranial pressure.*

PRACTICE ALERT
If the client has a basilar skull fracture or CSF draining from the ears or nose, never suction nasally.

- Turn from side to side every 2 hours, and maintain a side-lying position with the head of the bed elevated approximately 30 degrees. Do not position the unconscious client on the back. *Turning the client from side to side facilitates respirations, prevents the tongue from obstructing the airway, and helps prevent pooling of secretions in one area of the lungs (thus decreasing the risk of pneumonia).*

- If the client has a tracheostomy, provide tracheostomy care every 4 hours and suction when secretions are present (see Chapter 37 ∞) *to maintain an open airway.*
- Monitor the results of arterial blood gas analysis and pulse oximetry. Maintain records of trends. *ABGs and pulse oximetry directly measure the oxygen content of blood and are good indicators of the lungs' ability to oxygenate the blood.*

Risk for Aspiration

The unconscious client with a depressed or absent gag and swallowing reflex is at high risk for aspiration. Drainage, mucus, or blood may obstruct the airway and interfere with oxygenation. Pooling of aspiration secretions in the lungs also increases the risk of pneumonia.

- Assess swallowing and gag reflexes every shift as appropriate to the client's level of consciousness. *Deepening levels of unconsciousness may cause a loss in swallow and gag reflexes.*
- Monitor for and report manifestations of aspiration: crackles and wheezes, dullness to percussion over an area of the lungs, dyspnea, tachypnea, and cyanosis. *Early recognition facilitates prompt intervention.*
- Provide interventions to prevent aspiration:
  - Maintain NPO status.
  - Place in the side-lying position.
  - Provide oral hygiene and suctioning as needed.
  The side-lying position allows secretions to drain from the mouth rather than into the pharynx. Oral hygiene and suctioning remove secretions that might otherwise be aspirated.

PRACTICE ALERT
Never give unconscious clients oral food and fluids because of the risk of aspiration.

Risk for Impaired Skin Integrity

The unconscious client is at risk for impaired skin integrity as a result of immobility and the inability to provide self-care. On average, healthy people change positions during sleep every 11 minutes; the unconscious client often cannot maintain the movement needed to prevent pressure on the skin, especially over bony prominences. As a result, the skin and subcutaneous tissues may become ischemic and prone to develop pressure ulcers. Perspiration and incontinence of urine and stool may exacerbate the problem. Nursing interventions are directed to maintaining the integrity not only of the skin, but also of the lips and mucous membranes.

- Assess skin every shift, especially over bony prominences, the back of the scalp, and around genitals and buttocks. *The large surface area of the skin bears weight and is in constant contact with the surface of the bed. The skin, subcutaneous tissue, and muscles, especially those tissues over bony prominences, undergo constant pressure. This impairs normal capillary blood flow, which interferes with the exchange of nutrients and waste products. Tissue ischemia and necrosis may result and lead to the development of pressure ulcers.*
- Provide proper positioning. Reposition bed-ridden clients at least every 2 hours if this is consistent with the overall treatment goals. Keep the head of the bed elevated no higher than

30 degrees unless prescribed differently. Provide special pads and mattresses that distribute weight more evenly (e.g., silicone-filled pads, egg-crate cushions, turning frames, flotation pads). Consider requesting/using a special therapeutic bed that automatically turns the client at regular intervals. Lift the client instead of dragging the client across the sheet. *When the head of the bed is elevated above 30 degrees, the client's torso tends to slide down toward the foot of the bed. Friction and perspiration cause the skin and superficial fascia to remain fixed against the bed linens while the deep fascia and skeleton slide downward. When a person is pulled rather than lifted, the skin remains fixed to the sheet while the fascia and muscles are pulled upward. These shearing forces promote tissue breakdown.*

- Provide interventions to prevent breakdown of the skin and mucous membranes:
  - Keep bed linens clean, dry, and wrinkle free.
  - Provide daily bath with mild soap.
  - Cleanse the skin after urine and fecal soiling with a mild cleansing agent.
  - Provide oral care and lubricate the lips every 2 to 4 hours.
  - Maintain accurate intake and output records.
  - Keep the cornea moist by instilling methyl cellulose solution (0.5% to 1%) and apply protective eye shields or close the eyelids with adhesive strips if the corneal reflex is absent.

Keeping linens clean, dry, and wrinkle free decreases the risk of injury from the shearing force of bed rest and protects against environmental factors that cause drying. Adequate hydration of the stratum corneum appears to protect the skin against mechanical insult. Preventing dehydration maintains circulation and decreases the concentration of urine, thereby minimizing skin irritation in people who are incontinent. Proper eye care prevents corneal abrasion and irritation.

Impaired Physical Mobility

Clients who are unconscious are unable to maintain normal musculoskeletal movement and are at high risk for contractures related to decreased movement. Because the flexor and adductor muscles are stronger than the extensors and abductors, flexor and adductor contractures develop quickly without preventive measures. Passive ROM exercises must be performed routinely to maintain muscle tone and function, to prevent additional disability, and to help restore impaired motor function.

- Maintain extremities in functional positions by providing proper support devices. Remove support devices every 4 hours for skin care and passive ROM exercises. Provide pillows for the axillary region; rolled washcloths may be placed in elevated hands; use splints to prevent plantar flexion (foot drop). *Pillows in the axillary region help prevent adduction of the shoulder. Rolled washcloths help decrease edema and flexion contracture of the fingers. Splints are useful in preventing plantar flexion.*
- Collaborate with a physical therapist to develop and implement passive range-of-motion (ROM) exercises (unless contraindicated, as for the client with increased intracranial pressure) at least four times a day, keeping the following principles in mind:

  - Place one hand above the joint being exercised. The other hand gently moves the joint through its normal range of motion.
  - Move the body part to the point of resistance, and stop.

Placing one hand above the joint provides support against gravity and prevents unwanted movement. ROM exercises help prevent contractures by stretching muscles and tendons and maintaining joint mobility.

Risk for Imbalanced Nutrition: Less than Body Requirements

The unconscious client is at risk for an alteration in nutrition related to a reduced or complete inability to eat. This is especially true for the client who is unconscious as the result of an infection or trauma, both of which increase metabolic requirements.

- Monitor nutritional status through daily weights (on bed scales) and laboratory data. For accuracy, weigh the client at the same time each day, using the same scales. Ensure that the client wears the same clothing. *Changes in laboratory data with decreased nutrition include a decrease in the levels of serum prealbumin and serum transferrin.*
- Assess the need for alternative methods of nutritional support (tube feeding or total parenteral nutrition) through collaboration with dietitian. *Clients unable to take oral food require parenteral nutrition or liquid feedings through a nasogastric, gastrostomy, or jejunostomy tube. Needs for protein, calories, zinc, and vitamin C increase during wound healing.*

THE CLIENT WITH INCREASED INTRACRANIAL PRESSURE

Increased intracranial pressure (IICP) (also labeled *intracranial hypertension*) is sustained elevated pressure (10 mmHg or higher) within the cranial cavity (Wilensky & Bloom, 2005). Transient increases in ICP occur with normal activities such as coughing, sneezing, straining, or bending forward. These transient increases are not harmful; however, sustained IICP can result in significant tissue ischemia and damage to delicate neural tissue. Cerebral edema is the most frequent cause of sustained increases in ICP. Other causes include head trauma, tumors, abscesses, stroke, inflammation, and hemorrhage.

Pathophysiology

In the adult, the rigid cranial cavity created by the skull is normally filled to capacity with three essentially noncompressible elements: the brain (80%), cerebrospinal fluid (8%), and blood (12%). A state of dynamic equilibrium exists; if the volume of any of the three components increases, the volume of the others must decrease to maintain normal pressures within the cranial cavity. This is known as the *Monro-Kellie hypothesis*. The normal intracranial pressure is 5 to 10 mmHg (measured intracranially with a pressure transducer while the client is lying with the head elevated 30 degrees) or 60 to 180 cm H_2O (measured with a water manometer while the client is lying in a lateral recumbent position).

Cerebral blood flow and perfusion are important concepts for understanding the development and effects of increased intracranial pressure. Whereas blood and CSF contribute an equal percentage to normal intracranial volume, vascular factors account for twice the amount of increase in ICP that CSF does. The brain requires a constant supply of oxygen and glucose to meet its metabolic demands; 15% to 20% of the resting cardiac output goes to the brain to meet its metabolic needs. Interruption of the cerebral blood flow leads to ischemia and disruption of the cerebral metabolism.

Pressure and chemical autoregulation are compensatory mechanisms in which cerebral arterioles change diameter to maintain cerebral blood flow when ICP increases. In pressure autoregulation, stretch receptors within small blood vessels of the brain cause smooth muscle of the arterioles to contract. Increased arterial pressure stimulates these receptors, leading to vasoconstriction; when arterial pressure is low, stimulation of these receptors decreases, causing relaxation and vasodilation. Chemical, or metabolic, autoregulation works in much the same way as pressure autoregulation. In this case, the stimulus is a buildup of metabolic by-products of cell metabolism, including lactic acid, pyruvic acid, carbonic acid, and carbon dioxide. Carbon dioxide and increased hydrogen ion concentration are potent cerebral vasodilators that may act locally or systemically to increase cerebral blood flow. Conversely, a fall in $PaCO_2$ causes cerebral vasoconstriction. Arterial oxygen tension (PaO_2) also affects cerebral blood flow, although it is a less powerful mechanism than that exerted by carbon dioxide and hydrogen ions.

IICP may result from an increase in intracranial contents from a space-occupying lesion, hydrocephalus, cerebral edema (swelling), excess cerebrospinal fluid, or intracranial hemorrhage. Displacement of some CSF to the spinal subarachnoid space and increased CSF absorption are early compensatory mechanisms. The low-pressure venous system is also compressed, and cerebral arteries constrict to reduce blood flow. Brain tissue's ability to accommodate change is relatively restricted. The relationship between the volume of the intracranial components and intracranial pressure is known as *compliance*. When the capacity to compensate for increased intracranial pressure is exceeded, increased intracranial pressure (hypertension) develops. Intracranial hypertension is a sustained state of IICP and is potentially life threatening.

Autoregulatory mechanisms have a limited ability to maintain cerebral blood flow. When autoregulation fails, cerebrovascular tone is reduced and cerebral blood flow becomes dependent on changes in blood pressure. Autoregulation may be lost either locally or globally because of several factors, including increasing intracranial pressure, local or diffuse cerebral tissue ischemia or inflammation, prolonged hypotension, and hypercapnia or hypoxia.

Manifestations

With loss of autoregulation, intracranial pressure continues to rise and cerebral perfusion falls. Cerebral tissue becomes ischemic, and manifestations of cellular hypoxia appear. The manifestations of IICP are listed in the box on this page.

Level of Consciousness

Because the neurons of the cerebral cortex are most sensitive to oxygen deficit, changes in cortical function are the earliest man-

---

MANIFESTATIONS of Increased Intracranial Pressure

- Decreased level of consciousness. *Early*: Confusion; restlessness, lethargy; disorientation, first to time, then to place and person. *Late:* Comatose with no response to painful stimuli.
- Pupillary dysfunction. Sluggish response to light progressing to fixed pupils; with a localized process, pupillary dysfunction is first noted on the ipsilateral side.
- Oculomotor dysfunction. Inability to move eye(s) upward; ptosis (drooping) of the eyelid.
- Visual abnormalities. Decreased visual acuity, blurred vision, diplopia.
- Papilledema. May be late sign.
- Motor impairment. *Early*: Hemiparesis or hemiplegia of the contralateral side. *Late:* Abnormal responses such as decorticate or decerebrate positioning; flaccidity.
- Headache. Uncommon but may occur with processes that slowly increase ICP; worse on rising in the morning and with position changes.
- Projectile vomiting without nausea.
- Cushing's response. Increased systolic blood pressure, widening pulse pressure, bradycardia.
- Respirations. Altered respiratory pattern related to level of brain dysfunction.
- Temperature. May be significantly elevated as compensatory mechanisms fail.

---

ifestations of increasing ICP (Porth, 2005). Behavior and personality changes occur; the client may become irritable and agitated. Memory and judgment are impaired, and speech pattern changes may be noted. The client's LOC decreases. As cerebral hypertension and hypoxia progress, the LOC continues to decrease in a predictable pattern to coma and unresponsiveness.

Motor Responses

Pressure on the pyramidal tract often causes weakness (hemiparesis) on the contralateral side early in IICP. As ICP continues to increase, hemiplegia and abnormal motor responses, such as decorticate or decerebrate posturing, develop (see Chapter 43 ∞ for an illustration of these postures).

Vision and Pupils

Altered vision is an early manifestation of IICP; it is caused by pressure on the visual pathways and cranial nerves. Blurred vision, decreased visual acuity, and diplopia are common. Pupillary and oculomotor responses are affected as well. Because the cause of IICP is often localized at first, pupillary changes, including gradual dilation and sluggish response to light, may initially be limited to the ipsilateral side.

Vital Signs

Ischemia of the vasomotor center in the brainstem triggers the CNS ischemic response, a late sign of IICP. Neuronal ischemia in the vasomotor center causes a marked increase in the mean arterial pressure (MAP), with a significant increase in systolic blood pressure and increased pulse pressure. The increased

MAP causes reflexive slowing of the cardiac rate. This trio of manifestations (increased MAP, increased pulse pressure, and bradycardia) is known as *Cushing's response* (or triad), and represents the brainstem's final effort to maintain cerebral perfusion (Porth, 2005). The respiratory pattern also changes, often in the predictable progression outlined earlier in Table 44–1. Although the temperature is usually normal in early stages, as ICP continues to increase, hypothalamic function is impaired and the temperature may rise dramatically.

Other Manifestations

Additional manifestations of IICP include headache, particularly on rising, that worsens with position changes. Headache is more common with slowly developing IICP and occurs because of pressure on pain-sensitive structures, such as the middle meningeal arteries, the venous sinuses, and the dura at the base of the skull. Papilledema (edema and swelling of the optic disk) may be noted on funduscopic examination. Vomiting, often projectile and occurring without warning, may develop.

Cerebral Edema

Cerebral edema is an increase in the volume of brain tissue due to abnormal accumulation of fluid. Cerebral edema is often associated with increased intracranial pressure; it may occur as a local process in the area of a tumor or injury, or it may affect the entire brain. Two types of cerebral edema have been identified and are described as follows (Porth, 2005):

- *Vasogenic edema*, an increase in the capillary permeability of cerebral vessels, occurs with impairment of the blood–brain barrier, allowing diffusion of water and protein into the interstitial spaces of the brain. A variety of pathologies, such as ischemia, hemorrhage, brain tumors and injuries, and infections (such as meningitis), may cause the increase in capillary permeability. The site of the brain injury, the level of increase in capillary permeability, and the client's systemic blood pressure influence the rate and extent of the edema's spread. Vasogenic edema is manifested by focal (localized) neurologic deficits, altered levels of consciousness, and severe intracranial hypertension.
- *Cytotoxic edema*, actual swelling of the brain cells from an increase in intracellular fluid, involves changes in the functional or structural integrity of cell membranes due to pathologies such as water intoxication (such as from the syndrome of inappropriate secretion of antidiuretic hormone [SIADH]) or severe ischemia, intracranial hypoxia, acidosis, and brain trauma. With abnormally low cerebral perfusion, oxygen and nutrients are depleted, intracranial cells switch to anaerobic metabolism, and the sodium-potassium pump in the cell walls is impaired. Sodium diffuses into the cells, pulling fluid with it. The cells swell, and intracranial pressure rises. Accumulated metabolic waste products, such as lactic acid, contribute to a rapid deterioration of cell function. Cytotoxic edema is a slowly progressive process that results in altered consciousness. The edema may be so severe that it causes cerebral infarction with brain tissue necrosis.

Cerebral edema tends to be proportional to the extent of the pathology precipitating it. Brain function is not disrupted by cerebral edema unless the edema causes an increase in ICP. When it does, a vicious cycle can ensue: Cerebral edema increases ICP, which in turn decreases cerebral blood flow. Brain tissue becomes hypoxic and ischemic, increasing toxic metabolic by-products, hydrogen ion concentration, and carbon dioxide levels in the tissue. Autoregulatory mechanisms cause vasodilation and increase cerebral blood flow, further increasing cerebral edema and intracranial pressure. Without effective intervention, the client's condition can deteriorate rapidly; intracranial pressure increases to the point where brain structures herniate.

Hydrocephalus

Hydrocephalus refers to a progressive dilatation of the ventricular system, which becomes dilated as the production of CSF exceeds its absorption (Hickey, 2003). Hydrocephalus may increase ICP when it develops acutely. It is generally classified as either noncommunicating or communicating hydrocephalus. Noncommunicating hydrocephalus occurs when CSF drainage from the ventricular system is obstructed. It may develop when a mass or tumor, inflammation or hemorrhage, or congenital malformation obstructs the ventricular system. Communicating hydrocephalus is a condition in which CSF is not effectively reabsorbed through the arachnoid villi. It may occur secondarily to subarachnoid hemorrhage or scarring from infection. In *normal pressure hydrocephalus*, seen most often in adults age 60 or older, ventricular enlargement causes cerebral tissue compression but the CSF pressure on lumbar puncture is normal. This condition may follow cerebral trauma or surgery, or the cause may not be known.

Manifestations of hydrocephalus depend on the rate of its development. They may be mild and insidious in onset, presenting as progressive cognitive dysfunctions, gait disruptions, and urinary incontinence. If the process causing hydrocephalus is an acute one, the manifestations are those of IICP.

Brain Herniation

If IICP is not treated, cerebral tissue is displaced toward a more compliant area. This can result in brain herniation, the displacement of brain tissue from its normal compartment under dural folds of the falx cerebri or through the tentorial notch or incisura of the tentorium cerebelli (Porth, 2005). Herniation of the cerebellum through the tentorium exerts pressure on the brainstem, with subsequent herniation through the foramen magnum. This is a lethal complication of IICP because it puts pressure on the vital centers of the medulla.

Brain herniation syndromes are generally categorized as supratentorial or infratentorial, depending on their location above or below the tentorium cerebelli (Figure 44–2 ■). Supratentorial herniation syndromes include cingulate herniation, central or transtentorial herniation, uncal or lateral transtentorial herniation, and infratentorial.

- *Cingulate herniation* (Figure 44–2A) occurs when the cingulate gyrus is displaced under the falx cerebri. Local blood supply and cerebral tissue are compressed, resulting in ischemia and further increases in intracranial pressure.

MRI, x-ray studies of the skull and cervical spine, EEG, or lumbar puncture for CSF if inflammation is suspected. Serum metabolic screens and hypersensitivity testing also may be performed if systemic problems are suspected.

Medications

Pharmacologic management depends on the type of headache. The goals of treatment are to reduce the frequency and severity of headaches and to limit or relieve a headache that is beginning or in progress.

The management of migraine headache includes administering medications to prevent pain (prophylactic therapy) as well as drugs to stop (or abort) a headache in progress. The client with frequent migraine headaches is a candidate for prophylactic therapy. Drugs used to reduce the frequency and severity of migraine follow:

- Methysergide maleate (Sansert) is a serotonin antagonist that competitively blocks serotonin receptors in the CNS and is also a potent vasoconstrictor.
- Propranolol hydrochloride (Inderal) is a beta-blocker that prevents dilation of vessels in the pia mater and inhibits serotonin uptake.
- Topiramate (Topamax) and valproic acid (Depakote) are CNS agents and anticonvulsants. They have been approved by the FDA for use to prevent migraines (National Headache Foundation, 2005).

When the manifestations of migraine are recognized early, several medications may be used to abort or limit the severity and duration of the headache. Ergotamine tartrate (Cafergot) is a complex drug that reduces extracranial blood flow, decreases the amplitude of cranial artery pulsation, and decreases basal artery hyperperfusion. Administered at the onset of an attack, ergotamine controls up to 70% of acute attacks. Sumatriptan (Imitrex) is available in oral, nasal spray, or subcutaneous injection forms. It binds with serotonin$_1$ receptors and is rapidly effective. Zolmitriptan (Zomig), a selective serotonin$_1$ receptor agonist, is administered orally and is effective in the treatment of acute headache. Once a migraine is in progress, a narcotic analgesic such as codeine or meperidine (Demerol) may be required. Antiemetics may be prescribed to control nausea and vomiting.

Many of the same medications used for migraine also prevent or treat cluster headache. Because the onset of cluster headaches is abrupt, abortive therapy is not possible. Medications such as ergotamine tartrate may be given in suppository form at bedtime to prevent headache during the episodic attacks. Clients may find that inhaling 100% oxygen at 7 L/min for 15 minutes at the onset of an attack relieves their headache (Tierney et al., 2005).

Nonnarcotic analgesics such as aspirin or acetaminophen may relieve tension headaches. Additionally, tranquilizers such as diazepam may reduce muscle tension.

Nursing implications for drugs commonly prescribed for headaches are described in the Medication Administration on the next page.

Alternative and Complementary Therapies

The following alternative and complementary therapies are used to relieve the pain of headaches.

- Vitamin D, elemental calcium, riboflavin (vitamin B), and magnesium
- Acupuncture
- Relaxation, guided imagery, massage
- Melatonin, 5-HTP, CoQ10
- Magnetic field therapy
- Herbal therapy
- Osteopathic manipulation

NURSING CARE

In addition to the nursing care discussed in this section, a Nursing Care Plan for a client with migraine headaches is found on page 1547.

Health Promotion

Teach clients with tension headaches relaxation techniques, such as massage and biofeedback. Counseling for chronic anxiety may also be helpful. Triggers for migraine or cluster headache should be identified and, if possible, eliminated. For example, avoiding physical and emotional stress, having regular and consistent sleep patterns, eating meals regularly, and avoiding specific foods or alcohol can be incorporated into daily life and are helpful. Specific suggestions are outlined in Box 44–2.

Assessment

Collect the following data through the health history and physical examination.

- *Health history:* History of intracerebral trauma, tumor, or infection; detailed history and description of headache characteristics; family history; triggering factors; usual diet; effects of recurring headaches on lifestyle, activities of daily living (ADLs), and role performance.
- *Physical assessment:* Skin (diaphoresis, pallor, flushing), eyes (sensitivity to light, tearing), muscle strength and movement.

Nursing Diagnoses and Interventions

The primary response of the client requiring nursing interventions is acute pain. Develop nursing interventions to help the client identify strategies for controlling the pain and discomfort of the headache.

BOX 44–2 Suggestions to Decrease Incidence of Migraine Headaches

- Wake up at the same time each morning.
- Exercise at least three times a week.
- No smoking or caffeine after 3 P.M.
- No artificial sweeteners.
- No MSG.
- Reduce or eliminate red wine, cheese, alcohol, chocolate, and caffeine.
- Try a gluten-free diet.

MEDICATION ADMINISTRATION Headaches

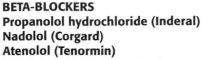

BETA-BLOCKERS
Propanolol hydrochloride (Inderal)
Nadolol (Corgard)
Atenolol (Tenormin)
Timolol maleate (Blocadren)
Beta-blockers are effective in the prophylactic treatment of headache. They act by combining with beta-adrenergic receptors to block the response to sympathetic nerve impulses, circulating catecholamines, or adrenergic drugs.

Nursing Responsibilities
- Before beginning therapy, determine pulse and blood pressure in both arms with client lying, sitting, and standing.
- Assess baseline and monitor serum glucose level, CBC, electrolytes, and liver and renal function studies.
- Note any history of diabetes or impaired renal function.
- Note the rate and quality of respirations; drugs in this category may cause dyspnea and bronchospasm.
- Administer the drug with meals to prevent gastrointestinal disturbances.
- Be alert that beta-blockers cause bradycardia and the heart rate may not rise in response to stress, such as exercise or fever. Notify the primary healthcare provider if pulse falls below 50 or if blood pressure changes significantly.
- Teach the client or family member how to take a pulse and blood pressure reading.

Health Education for the Client and Family
- Take the medication with meals to provide a coating for the gastrointestinal tract and prevent gastrointestinal disturbances.
- Return for blood work as prescribed.
- Take the last dose of the day at bedtime.
- Rise from a sitting or lying position to a standing position slowly to avoid dizziness and falls.
- Take pulse and blood pressure each day and maintain a record of readings.
- Avoid excessive intake of alcohol, coffee, tea, or cola. Consult with the healthcare provider before taking any over-the-counter medications.
- Report any cough, nasal stuffiness, or feelings of depression to the healthcare provider.

TRICYCLIC ANTIDEPRESSANTS
Imipramine hydrochloride (Tofranil)
Amitriptyline hydrochloride (Elavil)
The tricyclic antidepressants have been successful in the prophylaxis of cluster and migraine headaches. Although the exact mechanism is not known, they do prevent the reuptake of norepinephrine or serotonin, or both. They are chemically related to the phenothiazines, and as such they exhibit many of the same pharmacologic effects (e.g., anticholinergic, antiserotonin, sedative, antihistaminic, and hypotensive effects).

NURSING RESPONSIBILITIES
- Assess baseline CBC and liver function studies, heart sounds, and neurologic status before initiating prescribed therapy.

Health Education for the Client and Family
- Make position changes slowly.
- Chew sugarless gum to relieve dry mouth.
- Do not abruptly quit taking the medication.

ERGOT ALKALOID DERIVATIVES
Methysergide maleate (Sansert)
Methysergide is an ergot alkaloid derivative structurally related to LSD. It acts by stimulating smooth muscle, leading to vasoconstriction. It is thought that methysergide prevents headaches by blocking the effects of serotonin, a powerful vasodilator believed to play a role in vascular headaches. It also inhibits the release of histamine from mast cells and prevents the release of serotonin from platelets.

Nursing Responsibilities
- Note any history of renal or hepatic disease.
- Assess baseline eosinophil and neutrophil counts before beginning therapy.
- Administer the drug with meals or milk to minimize gastrointestinal irritation due to increased hydrochloric acid production.
- Assess for renal, CNS, and cardiovascular complications.
- Drug dosage should be gradually reduced over 2 to 3 weeks to prevent rebound headaches. A drug-free interval of 3 to 4 weeks is required with each 6-month course of therapy to prevent complications.
- Monitor for signs of ergotism, such as coldness or numbness of the fingers and toes, nausea, vomiting, headache, muscle pain, and weakness. Vasoconstriction may further impair peripheral circulation and increase blood pressure.

Health Education for the Client and Family
- Take the medication with meals or milk to minimize gastrointestinal upset.
- Report to the primary care provider nervousness, weakness, rashes, hair loss, or swelling of the extremities.
- Weigh daily and report any unusual weight gain to the primary care provider.
- Return to the primary care provider for a checkup at least every 6 months or as instructed. Do not take the drug on a regular basis for longer than 6 months, but do not abruptly stop taking it.
- Return for follow-up blood work as ordered.

SEROTONIN SELECTIVE AGONIST
Sumatriptan succinate (Imitrex)
Zolmitriptan (Zomig)
Rizatriptan Benzoate (Maxalt)
Binds to vascular receptors to vasoconstrict cranial blood vessels and relieve migraine headache.

Nursing Responsibilities
- Assess for history of peripheral vascular disease, renal or hepatic problems, and pregnancy.
- Evaluate relief of migraine headache, and assess for side effects of photophobia, sound sensitivity, and nausea and vomiting.

Health Education for the Client and Family
- Do not use more than two injections in a 24-hour period, and allow at least 1 hour between injections.
- Use the autoinjector to administer the medication, and follow instructions for proper method of giving the injection and disposing of the syringe.
- Report wheezing, heart palpitations, skin rash, swelling of the eyelids or face, or chest pain to the healthcare provider immediately.

CALCIUM CHANNEL BLOCKERS
Verapamil (Isoptin)
Nifedipine (Procardia)

(continued)

Help both the client and family adjust to a diagnosis of epilepsy. Address the following topics:

- The importance of wearing a Medic-Alert band or carrying a medical alert card at all times
- Avoiding alcoholic beverages and limiting coffee intake
- Taking showers versus tub baths, because of safety issues during a generalized seizure

- Factors that may trigger a seizure, such as abrupt withdrawal from medication, constipation, fatigue, excessive stress, fever, menstruation, sights and sounds such as television, flashing video, and computer screens
- Helpful resources include:
  - American Epilepsy Society
  - Epilepsy Foundation.

TRAUMATIC BRAIN INJURY

Traumatic brain injury (TBI) (also called *craniocerebral trauma*) refers to any injury of the scalp, skull (cranium or facial bones), or brain. TBI is a leading cause of death and disability in the United States. The National Head Injury Foundation defines TBI as a traumatic insult to the brain capable of causing physical, intellectual, emotional, social, and vocational changes. A TBI may be classified as a penetrating (open) head injury (e.g., resulting from a knife, bullet, or baseball bat) or a closed head injury (a blunt injury to the brain that does not result in an open skull fracture). TBI may cause problems with cognition, movement, sensation, and emotions. Even mild brain injuries, if repeated over an extended period of time, can result in cumulative neurologic and cognitive deficits.

Each year, 1.5 million Americans sustain a TBI. Of those who survive, one of every six people is unable to return to school or work when discharged from the hospital (Centers for Disease Control and Prevention [CDC], 2004b).

FAST FACTS
TBI

- Of the 1.5 million people who sustain a TBI each year, 235,000 are hospitalized and survive.
- Each year, 50,000 people die of TBI.
- Each year, 80,000 to 90,000 people experience the onset of long-term or lifelong disability associated with a TBI (CDC, 2006).

The leading causes of TBI are falls, followed by motor vehicle crashes and assaults. Elevated blood alcohol levels, not wearing motorcycle helmets, and not wearing seat belts contribute significantly to the risk of crashes and subsequent injury. Firearm use is the leading cause of death related to TBI, causing 10% of all TBI but resulting in 44% of TBI-related deaths. Nine out of 10 people with firearm-related TBI die; of those, nearly 66% are classified as suicidal in intent (CDC, 2004). Other causes of head injury include sports injuries and occupational injuries. Adults ages 15 to 44 are at the greatest risk, with the male-to-female ratio of 3-to-1 (Hickey, 2003). Other risk factors include being over the age of 75 and living in a high-crime area.

Specific damage following craniocerebral injuries is related to the mechanism of the injury (how it occurs), the nature of the injury (type), and the location of the injury (where it occurs).

Head injuries may be classified as blunt or penetrating, and can occur through several mechanisms:

- Acceleration injury is sustained when the head is struck by a moving object, such as a swinging bat.

- Deceleration injury occurs when the head hits a stationary object, such as a concrete wall.
- Acceleration-deceleration injury (also called a *coup-contrecoup* phenomenon) occurs when the head hits an object and the brain "rebounds" within the skull (Figure 44–5 ■). The brain is injured at the point of impact (the coup) and on the opposite side of the impact (the contrecoup). Two or more areas of the brain can be injured as a result of this phenomenon.
- Deformation injuries are those in which the force deforms and disrupts the integrity of the impacted body part (e.g., skull fracture).

Types of craniocerebral trauma include injuries to the skull (including fractures), injuries to the brain (including concussion and contusion), and intracranial hemorrhage (including hematomas). Brain injury can result either from the direct effects of the trauma on brain tissue or from secondary responses to trauma, such as cerebral edema, hematoma (blood clot), swelling, or increased intracranial pressure.

THE CLIENT WITH A SKULL FRACTURE

A *skull fracture* is a break in the continuity of the skull. It may occur with or without damage to the brain; however, intracranial trauma often results from skull fractures. The considerable force of impact significantly increases the risk of underlying hematoma formation. Disruption of the skull can also cause cranial nerve injury, allow bacteria to enter the cranial vault, and/or allow CSF to leak out.

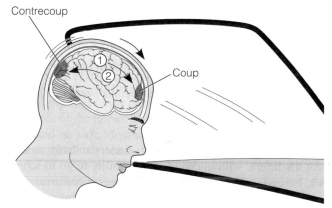

Figure 44–5 ■ Coup-contrecoup head injury. Following the initial injury (coup), the brain rebounds within the skull and sustains additional injury (contrecoup) in the opposite part of the brain.

Pathophysiology

Skull fractures are classified as open or closed. In an open fracture, the dura is torn, and in a closed fracture, the dura is not torn. Skull fractures are further classified into one of four categories: linear, comminuted, depressed, or basilar (Table 44–7).

Linear Fractures

Linear fractures are the most common, accounting for 80% of all skull fractures. They typically extend from the point of impact toward the base of the skull. Although the risk of infection or CSF leakage is minimal with this type of fracture because the dura usually remains intact, subdural or epidural hematomas (a collection of blood) frequently underlie the fracture. A hematoma (discussed later in this chapter) places pressure on underlying brain tissue, increasing both intracranial pressure and the risk of brain damage.

Comminuted and Depressed Fractures

Comminuted and depressed skull fractures increase the risk of direct damage to brain tissue from bruising (contusion) and bone fragments. However, the risk of secondary brain injury may be reduced in these fractures, because in breaking the bone, the traumatic impact energy is distributed and dissipated. If the skin overlying the fracture is lacerated or the dura is torn, the risk of infection is increased.

Basilar Fractures

Basilar skull fractures involve the base of the skull and usually are extensions of adjacent fractures, although they may occur independently. Although most basilar skull fractures are uncomplicated, they may involve the sinuses of the frontal bone or the petrous portion of the temporal bone (middle ear). If the dura is disrupted, CSF may leak through the tear. CSF leakage may include *rhinorrhea* (CSF leakage through the nose) or *otorrhea* (CSF leakage from the ear). Blood may be visible behind the tympanic membrane (hemotympanum), or ecchymosis may be noted over the mastoid process (Battle's sign). Bilateral periorbital ecchymosis ("raccoon eyes") is another possible manifestation. If CSF leakage is present, the risk of infection is high. Other complications of basilar skull fractures include injury to the internal carotid artery and compression of cranial nerve I, II, III, IV, V, VII, or VIII.

INTERDISCIPLINARY CARE

Treatment of a client with a skull fracture depends on the type and location of the fracture. Skull fracture may be only one of several head injuries.

A simple linear fracture generally requires bed rest and observation for underlying injury to brain tissue or hematoma formation. No specific treatment is required. Depressed skull fractures require surgical intervention, usually within 24 hours of the injury, to debride the wound completely and remove bone fragments, which may become embedded in brain tissue or cerebral blood vessels. If depressed deeply, the bone may be elevated. If cerebral edema is not present, a cranioplasty with insertion of acrylic bone may be performed. Basal skull fractures do not require surgery unless CSF leakage persists. Regular neurologic assessments and observation for manifestations of meningitis are required for the hospitalized client. Antibiotics may be administered prophylactically.

NURSING CARE

The client with a craniocerebral trauma may have a variety of responses and healthcare needs, depending on the location and extent of the trauma. Many of those problems with related nursing interventions are discussed in other sections of this chapter, including seizures, increased intracranial pressure, and bleeding within the brain.

Risk for Infection

The client with a skull fracture is at increased risk for infection related to access to the cranial contents through a tear in the dura. In an open, depressed fracture, the wound may be contaminated by dirt, hair, or other debris.

- Monitor for otorrhea or rhinorrhea. *Open fractures of the skull increase the possibility of leakage of CSF from the ears or nose.*
- Test drainage of clear fluid from ear and nose for glucose by using a glucose reagent strip, such as Dextrostix. *Clear drainage that tests positive for glucose indicates leakage of CSF; however, be aware that false positives may occur.*
- Observe blood-tinged fluid for "halo" sign. *CSF dries in concentric rings on gauze or tissues This sign is suggestive of CSF leakage.*
- Keep the nasopharynx and the external ear clean. Place a piece of sterile cotton in the ear, or tape a sterile cotton pad loosely under the nose; change dressings when they become wet. *Wet dressings facilitate movement of organisms.*
- Instruct client not to blow nose, cough, or inhibit sneeze; sneeze through open mouth. *Blowing the nose and coughing increase ICP. Withholding a sneeze forces bacteria backward.*
- Use aseptic technique at all times when changing head dressings or ICP monitor dressings and insertion sites. *Using aseptic technique reduces the possibility of introducing infection.*

TABLE 44–7 Types of Skull Fractures

TYPE	DESCRIPTION
Linear (simple)	Simple, clean break in skull. Occurs with low-velocity injuries.
Comminuted	Bone is crushed into small, fragmented pieces. Usually seen with high-impact injuries.
Depressed	Inward depression of bone fragments. Usually due to a powerful blow to the skull. The dura may or may not be intact. Bone fragments may penetrate into the brain tissue.
Basilar	Occurs at the base of the skull. May be linear, comminuted, or depressed.

Knowledge Deficit: Skull Fracture

The client and family need to be informed about the degree of injury that has occurred with the skull fracture. The client with a linear fracture, who may not be hospitalized, will need teaching that focuses on the need to monitor progress closely. To prevent complications, advise the client and family to go to the emergency room if the client experiences any of the following:

- Growing drowsiness or confusion
- Difficulty waking (instruct a family member to wake the client every 2 hours during the first night home)
- Vomiting (especially if projectile)
- Blurred vision
- Slurred speech
- Prolonged headache
- Blood or clear fluid leaking from the ears or nose
- Weakness in an arm or leg
- Stiff neck
- Seizure.

THE CLIENT WITH A FOCAL OR DIFFUSE TRAUMATIC BRAIN INJURY

Even when the skull and other structures overlying the brain remain intact, a blow to the head can cause significant brain injury. Closed head injuries may result in either focal or diffuse damage to the brain. They range in severity from mild to severe.

Pathophysiology

Brain injury results from both primary and secondary mechanisms. Primary injury results from the impact. A blow to the head, even with no break in the skull, can cause serious and diffuse brain injury. Injury to axons disrupts oligodendroglia, and direct mechanical disruption is caused by debris and leakage.

The immediate vascular response to the injury results in increased capillary permeability to solutes.

Secondary injury is the progression of the initial injury resulting from events that affect perfusion and oxygenation of brain cells. These events include intracranial edema, hematoma, infection, hypoxia, or ischemia. Cerebral ischemia is the most common cause of secondary brain injury (Porth, 2005). Ischemia leads to cerebral hypoxia, with consequences of increased glial permeability to sodium (cytotoxic edema), an influx of calcium with changes in electrophysiology, and release of free fatty acids and lactic acidosis.

Acute brain injury affects all body systems as well as the central nervous system. Systemic effects of acute brain injury are listed in Table 44–8.

Focal Brain Injuries

Focal brain injuries are specific, grossly observable brain lesions confined to one area of the brain. They include contusions, lacerations, and intracranial hemorrhage. The force of an impact produces contusions from direct contact with the inside of the skull that in turn may cause epidural hemorrhage and subdural and intracerebral hematomas. The mechanisms of injury are coup and/or contrecoup damage to the brain at the point of the impact and the rebound effect. The damaged brain area is surrounded by edema, contributing to IICP. Infarction and necrosis, multiple hemorrhages, and edema are found within the contused areas. The maximum effects of the injury peak in 18 to 36 hours.

Intracranial hemorrhage can result directly from the trauma (e.g., beneath a fracture) or from shearing forces on cerebral arteries and veins that occur with acceleration–deceleration. Depending on the site and rate of bleeding, manifestations may appear immediately or may not become evident for hours or even weeks. Intracranial hemorrhages and the hematomas they cause place pressure on surrounding structures, causing manifestations of an expanding focal lesion. They also cause IICP, leading to altered

TABLE 44–8 Systemic Effects of Acute Brain Injury

CAUSE	EFFECT
■ Stimulation of the sympathetic nervous system, which stimulates the adrenal cortex and medulla to increase glucocorticoid and mineralocorticoid levels	■ Increased metabolism of carbohydrates, fats, and proteins ■ Retention of sodium and water
■ Stimulation of the sympathetic nervous system, increasing the serum catecholamine levels	■ Hypertension ■ EEG changes ■ Dysrhymias (bradycardia, sinus tachycardia)
■ Altered release of ADH from the posterior pituitary ■ Neurogenic pulmonary dysfunction	■ Retention of water or diuresis and diabetes insipidus ■ Abnormal respiratory patterns ■ Reduced residual capacity with retention of CO_2, vasodilation, and increased ICP ■ Pulmonary edema
■ Stress response to trauma ■ Increased platelet, plasma fibrinogen, and thromboplastin levels	■ Hyperglycemia ■ Decreased clotting and prothrombin times ■ Vascular occlusion ■ Disseminated intravascular coagulation ■ Anemia
■ Immunosuppression ■ Decreased gastric motility and increased gastric acidity	■ Infection ■ Gastritis ■ Gastric ulcers

TABLE 44–9 Comparison of Intracranial Hematomas

TYPE/FREQUENCY	LOCATION/COMMON SITE	PRECIPITATING FACTORS	MANIFESTATIONS
Epidural Hematoma 2% to 6% of all types of head injuries	Located in the space between the skull and the dura mater Common site: the temporal bone (over the middle meningeal artery)	Skull fractures Contusion	Momentary loss of consciousness followed by a lucid period lasting from a few hours to 1 to 2 days Rapid deterioration in level of consciousness (drowsiness to confusion to coma) Seizures Headache Hemiparesis (may be ipsilateral or contralateral) Fixed dilated ipsilateral pupil Rise in blood pressure with decreases in pulse and respirations indicates a rapidly increasing hematoma
Subdural Hematoma Approximately 29% of all types of head injuries	Located in the space below the dural surface (between the dura and arachnoid and pia mater layers of meninges) Common site: may occur any place in cranium	Closed head injury Acceleration–deceleration injury Cerebral atrophy (seen in older adults) Chronic alcoholism Use of anticoagulants Contusion	Acute: ■ Headache ■ Drowsiness ■ Agitation ■ Slowed thinking ■ Confusion Subacute: ■ Same as those of acute subdural hematoma but develop more slowly Chronic: ■ Manifestations may not appear until weeks to months after injury ■ Confusion, slowed thinking, drowsiness
Intracerebral Hematoma 14% to 15% of all types of head injuries	Located directly in the brain tissue Common sites: frontal or temporal region	Gunshot wounds Depressed bone fractures Stab injury Long history of systemic hypertension Contusions	Headache Deteriorating consciousness to deep coma Hemiplegia on contralateral side Dilated pupil on the side of the clot

levels of consciousness and potential herniation syndromes. Intracranial hematomas are classified by their location as epidural, subdural, or intracerebral. Table 44–9 compares the frequency, locations, common sites, precipitating factors, and manifestations of intracranial hematomas; Figure 44–6 ■ illustrates their locations.

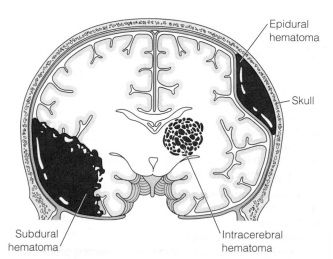

Figure 44–6 ■ Three types of hematomas: epidural hematoma, subdural hematoma, and intracerebral hematoma.

CONTUSION A *contusion* is a bruise of the surface of the brain, typically accompanied by small, diffuse venous hemorrhages. Both white and gray matter may have a bruised, discolored appearance. A decrease in pH, with accumulation of lactic acid and decreased oxygen consumption, may hinder cell function. Contusions (and other focal brain injuries) occur when the brain strikes the inner skull, often with a coup (point of impact) lesion and a contrecoup lesion on the opposite side of the brain. Contusions occur most frequently near bony prominences of the skull. Cerebral edema can follow contusion, resulting in IICP. Contusions; small, diffuse venous hemorrhages; and brain swelling are at their peak 12 to 24 hours after injury.

Manifestations of the contusion depend on the size and location of the brain injury. An initial loss of consciousness occurs; LOC may remain altered, and behavior changes such as combativeness may persist for an extended period. Full consciousness may be regained extremely slowly, and residual deficits may persist; in some clients, full LOC never really returns. Focal effects of the contusion may cause loss of reflexes, hemiparesis (muscular weakness of one-half of the body), or abnormal posturing. Manifestations of IICP may occur if cerebral edema develops. Regaining full LOC may take an extended period of time and residual deficits may persist.

TABLE 44–10 Monitoring Cerebral Oxygenation with Laboratory Values

ASSESSMENT	NORMAL RANGE OR VALUE	ABNORMAL FINDINGS
Partial pressure of oxygen in brain tissue ($Pbto_2$)	25–50 mmHg	<15 mmHg = ischemia
Intracranial pressure (ICP)	<10 mmHg	10–20 mmHg = mild to moderate increase in IICP >20 mmHg = severe increase in IICP
Mean arterial pressure (MAP)	70–110 mmHg	<60 mmHg = decreased cerebral perfusion pressure
Cerebral perfusion pressure (CPP)	70–100 mmHg	<50 mmHg = compromised cerebral blood flow
$Paco_2$	35–45 mmHg	<35 mmHg may result in cerebral vasoconstriction, further decreasing oxygenation of brain tissue
Pao_2	80–100 mmHg	If decreased, can cause tissue hypoxia and decrease oxygenation of brain tissue

Source: Data from Wilensky, E., & Bloom, S. (2005). Monitoring brain tissue oxygenation after severe brain injury. *Nursing, 35*(2), 32cc1–32cc4.

Surgery

Small subdural hematomas can frequently be reabsorbed and may be treated conservatively, with close observation and supportive care. However, the treatment of choice for epidural hematomas and large acute subdural hematomas is surgical evacuation of the clot. This can often be performed through burr holes made into the skull (Figure 44–7 ■). In an epidural hematoma, the bleeding vessel can also be ligated during this procedure, preventing further bleeding. Rebleeding may occur following evacuation of an acute subdural hematoma in older adults and clients with chronic alcoholism. A craniotomy is necessary to evacuate chronic subdural hematomas because the hematoma tends to solidify, making it difficult or impossible to remove through burr holes. Surgery is less successful in treating intracerebral hematomas because of widespread tissue damage. Supportive care to manage intracranial pressure and prevent complications is provided.

NURSING CARE

In addition to the nursing care discussed in this section, a Nursing Care Plan for a client with a subdural hematoma is found on the next page.

Health Promotion

The best way to treat any injury is to prevent it from happening. Public education must continue to stress the importance of safe driving, the dangers of driving under the influence of alcohol or drugs, and the necessity of wearing seat belts and cycle helmets. Legislation has mandated such motor vehicle changes as seat belts, child safety seats, and air bags. Other behaviors that can reduce the morbidity and mortality associated with TBI are following gun safety rules, promoting farm safety, and teaching older adults about safety (such as preventing falls) in the home.

Assessment

Collect the following data through the health history and physical examination (see Chapter 43 ∞):
- *Health history:* A history of the injury is helpful in understanding the nature of the craniocerebral trauma; knowledge about loss of consciousness assists the nurse in planning care.
- *Physical examination:* Neurologic assessment, including pupils, LOC, Glasgow Coma Scale, brainstem reflexes (cornea, cough, gag, extraocular movements), vital signs; skull and face (deformity, lacerations, bruising, bleeding); movement of extremities.

Nursing Diagnoses and Interventions

Nursing care of the client in the acute care phase initially focuses on maintaining an effective airway and breathing pattern. Nursing care is also directed toward continuous assessment and monitoring of neurologic function as well as other body systems.

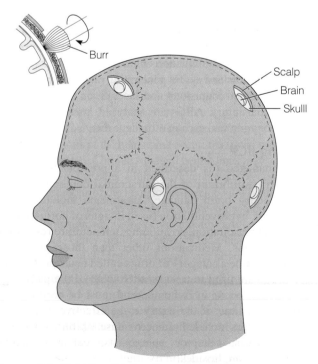

Figure 44–7 ■ Possible locations of burr holes.

NURSING CARE PLAN A Client with a Subdural Hematoma

Wong Lee is a 50-year-old tug boat mechanic who is married and has three sons. Although Mr. Lee has been through rehabilitation twice for alcoholism, he has not been able to quit drinking. His physician has explained the physical consequences and the possible interaction between alcohol and the anticoagulant Mr. Lee is taking for chronic atrial fibrillation. While attending a family reunion, during which he eats a large meal and drinks several beers, Mr. Lee joins a game of softball. Mrs. Lee is concerned that Mr. Lee has consumed too much alcohol to play ball in the heat, but Mr. Lee is adamant and states that he wants to pitch. During the end of the second inning, the batter hits a ball that strikes Mr. Lee in the head. Mr. Lee stumbles and drops to the ground, holding his head. He does not lose consciousness and gets up on his own. His sons and wife try to persuade him to go to the hospital, but Mr. Lee insists he feels fine.

Two weeks later, after an evening of consuming several mixed drinks, Mr. Lee develops a headache. He attributes the headache to a hangover, but instead of improving the next day, the headache becomes steadily worse. He becomes confused and disoriented. His wife, concerned that his drinking is increasing again, calls the physician, who admits Mr. Lee to the detoxification center at the local hospital. A CT scan is performed. The diagnosis of a subdural hematoma is made, and Mr. Lee is transferred to the neurosurgical unit.

ASSESSMENT

When Saundra Knight, the nurse on the neurosurgical unit, enters the room, she notices that Mr. Lee is sitting in bed, laughing and giddy. As she begins to talk to Mr. Lee, he states, "Don't ask me anything—I can't think. My headache is getting worse." Over the next few hours, the giddiness subsides, and Mr. Lee becomes drowsy. Ms. Knight reports a Glasgow Coma Scale score of 11. An ICP monitor is inserted and reveals increased intracranial pressure. Mr. Lee is scheduled to have burr holes and hematoma evacuation that afternoon.

DIAGNOSES

- *Risk for Ineffective Breathing Pattern* related to pressure on respiratory center by intracranial hematoma
- *Ineffective Cerebral Tissue Perfusion* related to increased intracranial pressure secondary to cerebral edema

EXPECTED OUTCOMES

- Maintain a respiratory rate and rhythm within normal limits.
- Maintain adequate cerebral perfusion, as evidenced by stable vital signs, stable neurologic status, and no decrease in level of consciousness.

PLANNING AND IMPLEMENTATION

- Perform neurologic assessment every 2 hours or as needed.
- Monitor vital signs every 2 hours or as needed.
- Explain to the family the procedure for intracranial surgery.

EVALUATION

The first day postoperatively, Mr. Lee begins breathing on his own without ventilatory support. His respiratory rate and rhythm are within normal limits, with no signs of abnormal breath sounds. The ICP monitor readings are appropriate, and Mr. Lee shows significant improvement in level of consciousness, with a Glasgow Coma Scale score of 15. Mr. Lee continues to improve and is discharged to home 5 days after surgery.

CRITICAL THINKING IN THE NURSING PROCESS

1. Describe the similarities and differences between Mr. Lee's disorder and the manifestations of other types of intracranial hematomas.
2. Mr. Lee kept trying to pull out his ICP line. You know he should not be restrained, because pulling against restraints increases restlessness and increases intracranial pressure. What would you do?
3. Write a care plan for Mr. Lee for the nursing diagnosis *Acute Confusion*.

See Evaluating Your Response in Appendix C.

MEDIALINK Care Plan Activity: Subdural Hematoma

This close monitoring provides early recognition and treatment of problems and complications, and initiation of aggressive forms of therapy that may be needed.

Many nursing diagnoses associated with traumatic brain injury correspond with those outlined previously in the sections on the client with altered LOC and IICP. Specific nursing diagnoses discussed in this section focus on problems with intracranial adaptive capacity, airway clearance, and breathing patterns.

Decreased Intracranial Adaptive Capacity

The client with a traumatic brain injury has or is at high risk for IICP. As the mechanisms that normally compensate for changes in intracranial pressure are compromised, intracranial pressure increases in disproportional response to a variety of stimuli. (See the discussion earlier in the chapter for other nursing diagnoses and interventions for the client with IICP.)

- Monitor for manifestations of IICP, including eye opening response, motor response, and verbal response. *These re-*

sponses evaluate the ability to integrate commands with conscious and involuntary movement.

- Monitor for changes in vital signs: bradycardia or tachycardia, varying breathing patterns, hypertension, and/or widening pulse pressure. Vital signs vary depending on the site of impairment. *Cushing's triad (bradycardia, increased systolic blood pressure, and increased pulse pressure) indicates brainstem ischemia leading to cerebral herniation.*
- Monitor for vomiting, headache, lethargy, restlessness, purposeless movements, and changes in mentation. *These manifestations may be early indicators of intracranial pressure changes.*
- Monitor temperature and initiate hypothermia treatment as prescribed. *Impaired hypothalamic function can interfere with temperature regulation. Hyperthermia may increase ICP.*
- Monitor fluid status: Regularly compare intake and output, review serum osmolality, and use infusion pump to administer IV fluids (if prescribed). *Osmotic diuretics, if used to treat cerebral edema, may cause hypotension and decreased cardiac output.*

The incidence of pathogenic infections of the CNS increases with the onset of AIDS. Clients who are HIV positive may have CNS infections caused by toxoplasmosis, cryptococcus, tuberculosis, herpes simplex, cytomegalovirus (CMV), or a polyoma virus (resulting in progressive multifocal leukoencephalopathy).

Pathophysiology

When pathogens enter the CNS and the meninges, an inflammatory process results. The pathology of CNS infections includes the invading pathogens, the subsequent inflammation, and the increase in intracranial pressure that may result from the inflammatory processes. Both the pathogenic damage and the IICP may result in brain damage and life-threatening complications.

Meningitis

Meningitis is an inflammation of the pia mater, the arachnoid, and the subarachnoid space. Inflammation spreads rapidly throughout the CNS because of the circulation of CSF around the brain and spinal cord. Meningitis may be acute or chronic, and it may be bacterial, viral, fungal, or parasitic in origin. Meningococcal meningitis may occur in epidemics among people who are in close contact with one another, such as military recruits and students living in dormitories. Pneumococcal meningitis, in contrast, primarily affects the very young and very old.

The organism responsible for meningitis must overcome nonspecific and specific host defense mechanisms to invade and replicate in the CSF. These defenses include the skin barrier, the blood–brain barrier, the nonspecific inflammatory response, and the immune response. Host response to the particular pathogen is responsible for the manifestations of clinical meningitis. The organisms that initiate the host response in meningitis demonstrate an affinity for the nervous system. They colonize and invade the nasopharyngeal mucosa, survive intravascularly, and penetrate the CNS if the blood–brain barrier is damaged, as can happen during surgery, the inflammatory response, or cerebral edema.

Infection of the CSF and meninges causes an inflammatory response in the pia, arachnoid, and CSF. Because the meninges and subarachnoid space are continuous around the brain, spinal cord, and optic nerves, the infection and inflammatory response are always cerebrospinal, involving both the brain and the spinal cord. Inflamed blood vessels in the area leak fluids as cell permeability increases. Purulent exudate infiltrates cranial nerve sheaths and blocks the choroid plexus and subarachnoid villi. IICP occurs as brain tissue responds to the pathogen. With an increase in ICP, cerebral perfusion decreases and cerebral autoregulation is lost.

BACTERIAL MENINGITIS The causative organisms of bacterial meningitis include *Neisseria meningitis*, meningococcus, *Streptococcus pneumoniae*, *Haemophilus influenzae*, and *Escherichia coli*. Risk factors include head trauma with a basal skull fracture, otitis media, mastoiditis, sinusitis, neurosurgery, systemic sepsis, or immunocompromise (Porth, 2005). Even when appropriate antibiotics are used, the mortality rate for adults remains at approximately 25%.

Once the pathogen enters the central nervous system, it or its toxic products (free radicals) initiate an inflammatory response in the meninges, CSF, and ventricles. Meningeal vessels become engorged, and their permeability increases. Phagocytic white blood cells migrate into the subarachnoid space, forming a purulent exudate that thickens and clouds the CSF and interferes with its flow. Rapid exudate formation causes further inflammation and edema of meningeal cells. Blood vessel engorgement, exudate formation, impaired CSF flow, and cellular edema cause the intracranial pressure to increase.

Manifestations The client with bacterial meningitis typically presents with fever and chills, headache, back and abdominal pain, and nausea and vomiting. (The older adult may not have a high fever, but may instead exhibit confusion.) Meningeal irritation causes nuchal rigidity (stiff neck) and positive Brudzinski's sign (flexion of the neck that causes the hip and knee to flex) and positive Kernig's sign (inability to extend the knee while the hip is flexed at a 90-degree angle). Photophobia is present; the client may also experience diplopia. With meningococcal meningitis, a rapidly spreading petechial rash involving the skin and mucous membranes may be noted. The client may also have IICP, manifested by decreased LOC, seizures, changes in vital signs and respiratory pattern, and papilledema. The manifestations of bacterial meningitis are listed in the box below.

Complications Complications of bacterial meningitis include arthritis, cranial nerve damage, and hydrocephalus. Cranial nerve VIII, the auditory nerve, is frequently affected, with resulting nerve deafness. Thrombophlebitis may develop in cerebral vessels, with infarction of surrounding tissues (Porth, 2005).

VIRAL MENINGITIS Acute viral meningitis, also called *aseptic meningitis*, is a less severe disease than bacterial meningitis. It can be caused by numerous viruses, such as herpes simplex, herpes zoster, Epstein-Barr virus, or cytomegalovirus (CMV). Viral meningitis most often appears after a case of mumps. Although viral infection also triggers the inflammatory response, the course of the disease is benign and of short duration. Recovery is uneventful.

Manifestations The manifestations of viral meningitis are similar to those of bacterial meningitis, although usually milder. The client may have a mild flulike illness prior to the onset of meningitis. Headache is intense and is accompanied by malaise, nausea, vomiting, and lethargy. Photophobia may be present. The

---

MANIFESTATIONS of Bacterial Meningitis

- Restlessness, agitation, and irritability
- Severe headache
- Signs of meningeal irritation:
  a. Nuchal rigidity
  b. Positive Brudzinski's sign
  c. Positive Kernig's sign
- Chills and high fever
- Confusion, altered LOC
- Photophobia (aversion to light), diplopia
- Seizures
- Signs of increased ICP (widened pulse pressure and bradycardia, respiratory irregularity, decreased LOC, headache, and vomiting)
- Petechial rash (in meningococcal meningitis)

client generally remains oriented, although possibly drowsy. Temperature is mildly elevated. Neck stiffness, positive Brudzinski's sign, and positive Kernig's sign are usually present.

Encephalitis

Encephalitis is an acute inflammation of the parenchyma of the brain or spinal cord. It is almost always caused by a virus, but it may also be caused by bacteria, fungi, and other organisms. Other less common causes include ingested lead; postvaccination encephalitis (from vaccines for measles, mumps, and rabies), and HIV (Porth, 2005). See Table 44–11 for a list of the most common causes of encephalitis.

VIRAL ENCEPHALITIS Viruses depend on living tissue for reproduction and become highly destructive when they invade brain tissue. The inflammatory response extends over the cerebral cortex, the white matter, and the meninges, with degeneration of the neurons. The pathology of encephalitis includes local necrotizing hemorrhage, which ultimately becomes generalized, with prominent edema. There is progressive degeneration of nerve cell bodies. The inflammatory response in encephalitis does not cause exudate formation as it does in meningitis. Certain viruses show a propensity for specific areas of the brain (e.g., herpes simplex virus involves frontal and temporal lobes). The virus gains access to the CNS via the bloodstream or along peripheral or cranial nerves, or it may already be present in the meninges in the client with meningitis.

The manifestations of viral encephalitis vary, depending on the organism and area of the brain affected. Usual manifestations are similar to those of meningitis, including fever, headache, seizures, stiff neck, and altered LOC. The client may be disoriented, agitated and restless, or lethargic and drowsy. As the disease progresses, the LOC deteriorates, and the client may become comatose.

ARBOVIRUS ENCEPHALITIS The arboviruses are arthropod (mosquito or tick)-borne agents that infect humans. They include many different types, including Western equine encephalitis, St. Louis encephalitis, and Rift Valley fever. Adults are most often infected with St. Louis encephalitis, with older adults affected more often. The arthropods may live in small mammals and birds, or may be carried by horses and deer. The newest arboviral encephalitis in the United States is West Nile encephalitis.

The arthropod-borne agents cause widespread degeneration of nerve cells, and edema and necrosis with or without hemorrhage occur. IICP may develop. Manifestations include fever, malaise, sore throat, nausea and vomiting, stiff neck, tremors, paralysis of extremities, exaggerated deep tendon reflexes, seizures, and altered LOC.

Brain Abscess

A brain abscess is an infection with a collection of purulent material within the brain tissue. Approximately 80% are found in the cerebrum and 20% are cerebellar.

The causes of a brain abscess include open trauma and neurosurgery; infections of the mastoid, middle ear, nasal cavity, or nasal sinuses; metastatic spread from distant foci (such as heart, lungs, skin, abscessed teeth, and dirty needles); and arising from other associated areas of infection. The immunocompromised are at increased risk for abscesses. The most common

---

TABLE 44–11 Causes of Encephalitis

CAUSE	COMMENTS
Arboviruses	Transmitted by bites from ticks and mosquitoes. Bites from ticks occur more frequently in spring. Bites from mosquitoes occur in middle to late summer. Most common types are St. Louis and Eastern and Western equine encephalitis. May destroy major parts of the lobe or hemisphere. Two-thirds of clients who develop Eastern equine encephalitis either die or develop severe residual disabilities (e.g., seizures, blindness, deafness, speech disorders, or mental retardation). The incubation is 5 to 15 days. Mortality rates associated with arboviruses are higher than those associated with enteroviruses.
Enteroviruses, such as echovirus, coxsackievirus, poliovirus, paramyxovirus (the virus that causes mumps), and varicella-zoster (the virus that causes chickenpox)	Infection occurs more frequently in summer (except infection by the mumps virus, which occurs more frequently in early winter). Some degree of protection can be afforded by immunization against measles, mumps, and poliomyelitis. Mortality rates are lower than those associated with herpes simplex type 1 virus.
Herpes simplex type 1 virus	Most common nonepidemic encephalitis in North America. Can occur any time of year and throughout the world. Has an affinity for the frontal and temporal lobes. Prognosis is grave but not hopeless: Mortality rate can be as high as 40%, and client may die within 2 weeks.
Amebic meningoencephalitis due to infection by *Naegleria* and *Acanthamoeba* protozoa	Both protozoa are found in warm freshwater. Enter the nasal mucosa of people swimming in ponds or lakes. May also be found in soil and decaying vegetation. Incidence of infection is increasing in North America.
Exogenous poisoning	May occur after ingestion of lead or arsenic or inhalation of carbon monoxide.

pathogens causing the abscess are streptococci, staphylococci, and bacteroids. Yeast and fungi may also cause brain abscess.

A brain abscess results from the presence of microorganisms in the brain tissue. If the abscess is encapsulated, it has the ability to enlarge and, therefore, behave as a space-occupying lesion within the cranium. This predisposes the client not only to the systemic effects of the inflammatory process but also to the serious consequences of increased intracranial pressure. Occasionally, the abscess does not become encapsulated; instead, it spreads through the brain tissue to the subarachnoid space and ventricular system.

Initially, the client exhibits the general symptoms associated with an acute infectious process, such as chills, fever, malaise, and anorexia. Because brain abscess generally forms after infection, the client may consider these signs to be an exacerbation of that illness. The client may experience seizures, altered LOC, and manifestations of IICP. As the abscess enlarges, specific symptoms are related to location; for example, the client with a frontal lobe abscess may have contralateral hemiparesis, expressive aphasia, focal seizures, and frontal headache.

INTERDISCIPLINARY CARE

Bacterial meningitis is a medical emergency that, if not treated immediately, can be fatal within days. Successful management depends on rapid diagnosis and aggressive treatment with antibiotics and corticosteroids to eradicate the infecting organism and support vital functions. The client may be placed in strict or respiratory isolation until the organism has been identified, depending on hospital policy. Universal precautions apply to CSF as well as blood.

Treatment for viral meningitis focuses on managing client symptoms and is supportive. Antipyretics and analgesics may provide relief. Antibiotic therapy is not indicated, and isolation precautions are not required.

Treatment of the client with a brain abscess focuses on prompt initiation of antibiotic therapy. Other manifestations are treated symptomatically, as with the client diagnosed with meningitis or encephalitis. If pharmacologic management is not effective, the abscess may be drained or, if it is encapsulated, removed.

Diagnosis

The diagnosis of meningitis is based on manifestations and diagnostic tests results. Gram stain and culture of the CSF are used to determine if a bacterial infection is present and to determine the specific infectious agent. Counterimmunoelectrophoresis (CIE) is a laboratory test that may be ordered to determine the presence of viruses or protozoa. Polymerase chain reaction techniques may be used to detect viral DNA or RNA in spinal fluid. CT scan will show an area of increased contrast surrounding a low-density core with brain abscess.

Lumbar puncture with examination of the CSF is the definitive diagnostic measure for bacterial meningitis. Data that indicate bacterial meningitis include turbid, cloudy fluid; a markedly increased white blood cell (WBC) count and protein content; and a decreased glucose content. The opening pressure on the lumbar puncture is elevated. In contrast, the client with encephalitis may have a normal CSF analysis and pressure or

may have some lymphocytes. The client with a brain abscess will have a markedly elevated pressure with elevated protein content and elevated WBC count. Glucose content is normal. (Because a lumbar puncture in the presence of a space-occupying lesion can result in brain herniation and death, a CT scan is performed first if neurologic findings support such a lesion.)

Medications

Immediate intravenous administration of a broad-spectrum antibiotic that crosses the blood–brain barrier into the subarachnoid space is instituted in cases of bacterial meningitis. Once culture reports identify the causative organism, drug therapy is continued from 7 to 21 days, using the most effective drug or drugs specific to that bacterium. The cephalosporin antibiotics are preferred. A major concern in the treatment of CNS infections is penicillin-resistant streptococci. Recommendations for treatment are for a broad-spectrum cephalosporin, such as rifampin (Rifadin), cefotaxime (Claforan), or vancomycin (Vancocin). However, as the bacteria are killed, the toxins they release increase production of inflammatory cytokines, which are potentially lethal. Steroids such as dexamethasone (Decadron) are often given with the antibiotics to suppress inflammation. The CDC recommends that the client remain on isolation for 24 hours after the start of antibiotic therapy.

Treatment for encephalitis consists of administering specific medications and preventing complications. Fungal meningitis is treated with antifungal agents, such as amphotericin-B (Amphotec), flucytosine (Ancobon), and fluconazole (Diflucan). Viral encephalitis is treated with intravenous acyclovir (Zovirax) or vidarabine (Vira-A).

Antibiotic therapy is the primary treatment for brain abscess. A combination of broad-spectrum antibiotics is used if the infecting organism is unknown.

Anticonvulsant medications such as phenytoin (Dilantin) are often prescribed to prevent or control seizure activity. Antipyretic and analgesic medications may provide symptomatic relief; however, analgesics that have a depressant effect on the CNS (such as opiates) are avoided to prevent masking of early manifestations of deteriorating LOC. The client initially may require antiemetics to control nausea and vomiting. Fluid and electrolyte status is maintained through intravenous fluid replacement until the client is able to resume oral intake.

Surgery

Surgical drainage of an encapsulated abscess may be necessary. The decision to perform surgery is based on the client's general condition, the stage of abscess development, and the site of the abscess.

NURSING CARE

Central nervous system infections are serious illnesses, with potentially life-threatening effects and complications. Nursing assessments and interventions are critical in identifying changes in the client's neurologic status and preventing complications from IICP. In addition to the nursing care described in this section, a Nursing Care Plan for a client with bacterial meningitis is found on the next page.

NURSING CARE PLAN **A Client with Bacterial Meningitis**

Monty Cook is a 22-year-old musician who plays in a local rock band. He is unmarried and lives with his parents. He is known by everyone in the community as a quiet, low-key, easygoing person and an excellent guitar player. During a performance 2 days ago, he had difficulty playing his guitar, complaining of bright stage lights blazing in his eyes. When he tried to keep his head down to prevent the lights from hurting his eyes, he noticed his neck was very stiff. After the performance, one of the newest members of the band remarked that it certainly was not their best performance. Monty responded angrily that maybe the new members of the group needed more practice. Then he stomped out and went home to bed.

He wakes at 4:00 A.M. with a severe headache, sweating, and chills; his temperature is 102°F, and he cannot bend his neck without severe pain. His mother recognizes that he is agitated and irritable, which is uncharacteristic. Frightened, she rushes him to the hospital emergency room. A lumbar puncture performed in the emergency room reveals turbid, cloudy fluid; a markedly increased WBC count; and protein with a decreased glucose content. Bacterial meningitis is the medical diagnosis. Mr. Cook is admitted to the hospital for treatment and care.

ASSESSMENT

When the nurse, Aisha Aldi, enters Mr. Cook's isolation room, she sees him thrashing about in the bed, talking incoherently, and becoming more agitated. On assessment, Ms. Aldi notes dry mucous membranes, cracked lips, and small petechiae over the upper torso and abdomen. Mr. Cook's temperature is 104°F. Kernig's sign is positive. Intravenous broad-spectrum antibiotics are prescribed and initiated. After the first 2 hours of care, Ms. Aldi notes a decrease in Mr. Cook's level of consciousness.

DIAGNOSES

- *Hyperthermia* related to infection and abnormal temperature regulation by hypothalamus
- *Disturbed Thought Processes* related to intracranial infection
- *Ineffective Protection* related to progression of illness

EXPECTED OUTCOMES

- Have a decrease in body temperature.
- Become less restless and agitated.
- Remain free of injury.

PLANNING AND IMPLEMENTATION

- Monitor vital signs every 2 hours.
- Provide sponge baths if temperature continues to rise.
- Provide a quiet, nonstimulating environment with the shades drawn.
- Provide oral care every 4 hours.
- Measure and compare intake and output every 2 hours.
- Perform neurologic assessments every 2 to 4 hours.
- Monitor for and report seizure activity and decreasing level of consciousness.
- Keep bed in low position with side rails elevated.
- Administer prescribed intravenous antibiotics.

EVALUATION

After 4 days of antibiotic therapy, Mr. Cook's temperature has returned to near normal. Ms. Aldi notes that he has begun opening his eyes and visually tracking her as she moves about the room. Mr. Cook responds to a request to squeeze Ms. Aldi's fingers and after several hours asks her what had happened. On day 5, Mr. Cook states that he feels better and his headache is gone. He ask for sips of juice and begins urinating regularly. Seven days after admission, Mr. Cook is discharged and is able to go home with his mother. He has some weakness in his legs, but otherwise has no evidence of neurologic deficits.

CRITICAL THINKING IN THE NURSING PROCESS

1. What strategies should the nurse use to decrease the environmental stimuli for Mr. Cook, and what is the rationale for doing these?
2. If you were caring for Mr. Cook in the initial phase of the illness and he became combative, what would you do?
3. Develop a plan of care for Mr. Cook for the nursing diagnosis *Acute Pain*. Consider the effect of narcotics on respiratory function in designing the plan.

See Evaluating Your Response in Appendix C.

Health Promotion

As with many other intracranial injuries and disorders, educational activities to promote health by preventing CNS infections are important nursing interventions. The following information should be provided:.

- Vaccinations for meningococcal meningitis are recommended or required for military recruits and college students (groups at increased risk for invasive meningococcal meningitis).
- Administration of prophylactic rifampin (Rifadin) is recommended for people exposed to meningococcal meningitis.
- Mosquito control with repellants, insecticides, and protective clothing.
- Destruction of the insect larvae and elimination of breeding places, such as pools of stagnant water.
- Vaccination against Japanese B encephalitis (recommended for summer travelers to rural East Asia).
- Prompt diagnosis and treatment of infections of the head, neck, and respiratory system.

Assessment

Collect the following data through the health history and physical examination (see Chapter 43 ∞). Further focused assessments are described with nursing interventions below.

- *Health history:* Risk factors (concurrent infections, other illnesses, travel), when manifestations began, severity of manifestations, current nausea and headache, seizures.
- *Physical examination:* Glasgow Coma Scale, level of consciousness, vital signs, motor function, pupillary check, cranial nerves, neck ROM, Brudzinski's sign, Kernig's sign, skin (rash, petechiae, purpura), muscle movement and strength, speech.

Nursing Diagnoses and Interventions

In planning and implementing nursing care for the client with a CNS infection, the prognosis may depend on the supportive care given. The client is often very ill, and the combination of fever, dehydration, and cerebral edema may predispose the client to

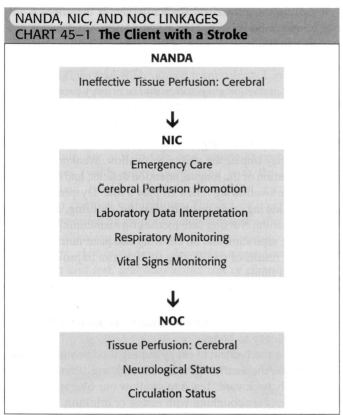

NANDA, NIC, AND NOC LINKAGES
CHART 45–1 The Client with a Stroke

NANDA

Ineffective Tissue Perfusion: Cerebral

↓

NIC

Emergency Care

Cerebral Perfusion Promotion

Laboratory Data Interpretation

Respiratory Monitoring

Vital Signs Monitoring

↓

NOC

Tissue Perfusion: Cerebral

Neurological Status

Circulation Status

Data from *NANDA's Nursing Diagnoses: Definitions & Classification 2005–2006* by NANDA International (2005), Philadelphia; *Nursing Interventions Classification (NIC)* (4th ed.) by J. M. Dochterman & G. M. Bluechek (2004), St. Louis, MO: Mosby; and *Nursing Outcomes Classification (NOC)* (3rd ed.) by S. Moorhead, M. Johnson, and M. Maas (2004), St. Louis, MO: Mosby.

and speech may continue to improve for even longer. Address the following topics in preparing the client and family for community-based care.

- Physical care, medications, physical therapy, occupational therapy, speech therapy
- Realistic expectations
- Time off for the caregiver, respite care services
- Distributors for equipment and supplies
- Home environment conducive to using equipment (e.g., a wheelchair or walker)
- Home and equipment modifications (e.g., a raised toilet seat, grab bars in the bathroom, a bath chair, a vise lid opener, a long-handled shoehorn)
- Home health services
- Community resources, such as Meals-on-Wheels, senior centers, eldercare, large-print telephone dials, stroke clubs, Life-line (emergency alerting systems through a local hospital or agency). Financial assistance may be available within the community for housekeeping and personal care assistance.
- Helpful organizational resources:
  - American Heart Association
  - National Stroke Association
  - Stroke Clubs International
  - The National Institute of Neurological Disorders and Stroke.

THE CLIENT WITH AN INTRACRANIAL ANEURYSM

An *intracranial aneurysm* is a saccular outpouching of a cerebral artery that occurs at the site of a weakness in the vessel wall. The weakness may be the result of atherosclerosis, a congenital defect, trauma to the head, aging, or hypertension. A ruptured cerebral aneurysm is the most common cause of a hemorrhagic stroke.

Incidence and Prevalence

Approximately 5 million North Americans have intracranial aneurysms; most go through life without any manifestations of bleeding. However, it is estimated that 30,000 people will have a rupture of an intracranial aneurysm each year, and two-thirds of the survivors will have serious disabilities. Intracranial aneurysms are most common in adults ages 30 to 60 (Hickey, 2003).

The exact etiology is unknown, but theories of cause include (1) a developmental defect in the vessel wall and (2) degeneration or fragility of the vessel wall due to conditions such as hypertension, atherosclerosis, connective tissue disease, or abnormal blood flow. Hypertension and cigarette smoking may be contributing factors.

Pathophysiology

Intracranial aneurysms tend to occur at the bifurcations and branches of the carotid arteries and the vertebrobasilar arteries at the circle of Willis, with most aneurysms (85%) located anteriorly. They range in size from smaller than 15 mm to larger than 50 mm. Intracranial aneurysms tend to enlarge with time, making the vessel wall thin and increasing the probability of rupture.

There are several different types of intracranial aneurysms: A *berry aneurysm* is probably the result of a congenital abnormality of the tunica media of the artery. The aneurysm usually ruptures without warning. A *saccular aneurysm* is any aneurysm with a saccular outpouching, which distends only a small portion of the vessel wall. This type of aneurysm is often caused by trauma. In a *fusiform aneurysm,* the entire circumference of a blood vessel swells to form an elongated tube. Most aneurysms of this type occur as a result of the changes of arteriosclerosis. Fusiform aneurysms act as space-occupying lesions. In a *dissecting aneurysm,* the tunica intima pulls away from the tunica media of the artery, and blood is forced between the two layers. It may result from atherosclerosis, inflammation, or trauma. *Mycotic aneurysms* are caused by emboli from infections such as bacterial endocarditis.

Intracranial aneurysms typically rupture from the dome rather than the base, forcing blood into the subarachnoid space at the base of the brain. The aneurysm may also rupture and force blood into brain tissue, the ventricles, or the subdural space. This discussion focuses on intracranial hemorrhages due to rupture of a cerebral aneurysm. See Chapter 44 ∞ for further discussion of types of intracranial bleeding and hematomas.

Manifestations

An intracranial aneurysm is usually asymptomatic until it ruptures, although very large aneurysms may cause headache and/or neurologic deficits due to pressure on adjacent intracranial structures. Small leakages of blood may occur periodically, causing headache, nausea, vomiting, and pain in the neck and back. The client may also have prodromal manifestations before the rupture occurs, such as headache, eye pain, visual deficits, and a dilated pupil.

The manifestations of a ruptured intracranial aneurysm (and subsequent subarachnoid hemorrhage) include a sudden, explosive headache; loss of consciousness; nausea and vomiting; a stiff neck and photophobia (due to meningeal irritation); cranial nerve deficits; stroke syndrome manifestations; and pituitary malfunctions (that result primarily from changes in ADH secretion).

The severity of the rupture is often inferred from the manifestations of the subarachnoid hemorrhage. The Hunt-Hess classification of subarachnoid manifestations is frequently used to classify nontraumatic subarachnoid hemorrhages. The grades of severity are:

- Grade 1: Asymptomatic, or minimal headache and slight neck rigidity
- Grade 2: Moderate to severe headache, neck rigidity, cranial nerve deficits
- Grade 3: Drowsy, lethargic, mild neurologic deficits
- Grade 4: Stuporous, moderate to severe hemiparesis, early decerebrate rigidity
- Grade 5: Deep coma, decerebrate rigidity, moribund appearance.

Fibrin and platelets seal off the bleeding point, but the escaped blood forms a clot that irritates the brain tissue. The resulting inflammatory response causes cerebral edema, and both the edema and the hemorrhage increase intracranial pressure (Hickey, 2003). Bleeding into the subarachnoid space causes meningeal irritation. Hypothalamic dysfunction and seizures are also potential complications.

Complications

The major complications of a ruptured intracranial aneurysm are rebleeding, vasospasm, and hydrocephalus.

Rebleeding

The greatest risk for rebleeding is within the first day after the initial rupture, and again in 7 to 10 days (when the initial clot breaks down). Rebleeding is manifested by a sudden severe headache, nausea and vomiting, decreasing levels of consciousness, and new neurologic deficits (Hickey, 2003). The mortality from rebleeding is as high as from the initial rupture.

Vasospasm

Cerebral vasospasm is a common but dangerous complication that occurs between 3 and 10 days after a subarachnoid hemorrhage. It is associated with a large number of deaths and disability. A cerebral vasospasm narrows the lumen of one or more cerebral vessels, causing ischemia and infarction of tissue supplied by the affected vessels. The actual cause is unknown, but it occurs in blood vessels surrounded by thick blood clots, suggesting that some substance in the clot initiates the spasm. The manifestations vary according to the degree of spasm and the area of brain affected. Regional alterations may cause focal deficits (such as hemiplegia), whereas global alterations cause loss of consciousness.

Hydrocephalus

Hydrocephalus, an abnormal accumulation of CSF within the cranial vault and dilation of the ventricles, is a potential complication of a ruptured intracranial aneurysm. Hydrocephalus is thought to be the result of obstruction of reabsorption of CSF through the arachnoid villi. The obstruction is caused by an increased protein content of the CSF because of lysis of blood in the subarachnoid space (Porth, 2005). The accumulation of cerebrospinal fluid increases intracranial pressure. Initial manifestations of hydrocephalus are typically nonspecific but commonly include decreasing levels of consciousness.

INTERDISCIPLINARY CARE

The care of the client with a ruptured intracranial aneurysm includes determining the location of the aneurysm, treating the manifestations of the hemorrhage, and preventing rebleeding and vasospasm. Interventions using radiology, angiography and a variety of procedures may be used to prevent aneurysm rupture or to stop the bleeding. Surgery is usually the treatment of choice to repair the bleeding artery.

Diagnosis

The diagnostic tests conducted to identify the site and extent of a ruptured intracranial aneurysm, as well as rebleeding, are a CT scan and bilateral carotid and vertebral cerebral angiograms. A cerebral angiogram is the gold standard for evaluating cerebral aneurysm; it can demonstrate the source of the aneurysm in about 80% to 85% of the time (Hickey, 2003). A lumbar puncture will reveal blood-tinged spinal fluid. These tests are described in Chapter 43 ∞.

Medications

Calcium channel blockers, such as nimodipine (Nimotop), are used to improve neurologic deficits due to vasospasm following subarachnoid hemorrhage from ruptured intracranial aneurysms. Administered for 21 consecutive days, it has been found to enhance collateral blood flow and reduce the incidence of ischemic deficits from arterial spasm without side effects (Hickey, 2003; Tierney et al., 2005).

Other medications that may be prescribed include anticonvulsants, such as phenytoin (Dilantin), to prevent seizures if the client has increased intracranial pressure; analgesics for headache; and stool softeners, such as docusate, to prevent constipation and straining with a bowel movement (which increases intracranial pressure and blood pressure and may cause rebleeding).

Procedures Used to Treat Aneurysm

Treatments for an intracranial aneurysm are performed either to prevent rupture or to isolate the vessel to prevent further bleeding. Clients with good neurologic status may have surgery soon after the rupture. In clients with significant neurologic deficits, surgery may be delayed until they are more stable and less at risk for vasospasm; however, the trend is toward surgery as soon as possible.

Pathophysiology

The spinal cord provides a two-way pathway for the conduction of impulses and information to and from the brain and the body, serves as a major reflex center, and (through its attached spinal nerves) is involved in the sensory and motor innervation of the entire body below the head. It consists of an outer region of white matter and an inner region of gray matter. The gray matter comprises the central canal of the cord, the posterior horns, the anterior horns, and the lateral horns. It is divided into a sensory half (dorsally) and a motor half (ventrally) and innervates somatic and visceral regions of the body. The white matter consists of tracts or pathways that convey information. The ascending (sensory) pathways carry information about proprioception, fine touch, discrimination, pain, temperature, deep pressure, and touch. The descending (motor) pathways carry information about movement. The pyramidal tracts control skilled voluntary movements (such as writing). The extrapyramidal tracts (all tracts other than the pyramidal tracts) bring about all other body movements. See Chapter 43 ∞ for further information.

When the spinal cord is injured, the primary injury causes microscopic hemorrhages in the gray matter of the cord and edema of the white matter of the cord. These initial pathologic changes are followed by the secondary injury, with mechanisms that increase the area of injury. The hemorrhages extend, eventually involving the entire gray matter. Microcirculation to the cord is impaired by edema and hemorrhage. The injured tissue releases norepinephrine, serotonin, dopamine, and histamine; these vasoactive substances cause vasospasm and further decrease microcirculation. As a result, vascular perfusion and oxygen tension of the affected area are decreased, which leads to ischemia.

When ischemia is prolonged, necrosis of both gray and white matter begins within a few hours, and within 24 hours the function of nerves passing through the injured area is lost. Although circulation returns to the white matter of the cord in about 24 hours, decreased circulation in the gray matter continues. Because edema extends the level of injury for two cord segments above and below the affected level, the extent of injury cannot be determined for up to 1 week.

Tissue repair occurs over a period of 3 to 4 weeks. Phagocytes enter the area in 36 to 48 hours after the initial injury. Neurons degenerate and are removed by microphages in the first 10 days after the injury. RBC disintegrate, and the hemorrhages are reabsorbed. Eventually the area of injury is replaced by acellular collagenous tissue, and the meninges thicken.

Forces Resulting in SCI

SCIs are the result of the application of excessive force to the spinal column. The most common cause of abnormal spinal column movements are acceleration and deceleration (forces that are applied to the body, for example, in automobile crashes and falls). *Acceleration* occurs when external force is applied in a rear-end collision; the upper torso and head are forced backward and then forward. *Deceleration* occurs in a head-on collision; the external force is applied from the front. The head and body move forward until they meet a stationary object and then are forced backward. The following forces and movements (Figure 45–5 ■) may cause a variety of spinal cord in-

juries, with the extent of injury depending on the amount and direction of motion, and the rate of application of force:

■ *Hyperflexion,* or forcible forward bending, may compress vertebral bodies and disrupt ligaments and intervertebral disks.

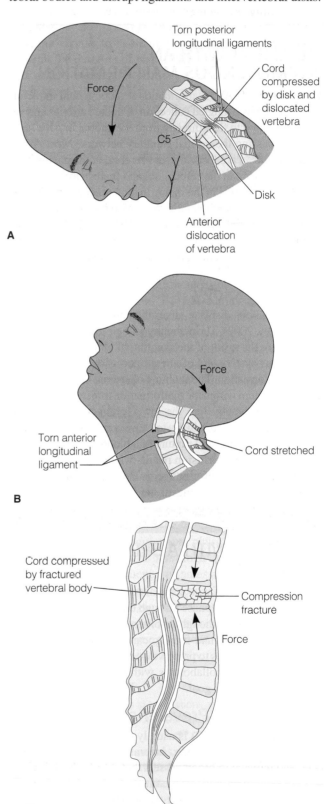

Figure 45–5 ■ Spinal cord injury mechanisms. *A,* Hyperflexion. *B,* Hyperextension. *C,* Axial loading, a form of compression.

- *Hyperextension,* or forcible backward bending, often disrupts ligaments and causes vertebral fractures. A whiplash injury is a less severe form of hyperextension, with injury to soft tissues but no vertebral or spinal cord damage.
- *Axial loading,* a form of compression, is the application of vertical force to the spinal column (for instance, by falling and landing on the feet or buttocks or by diving into shallow water).
- *Excessive rotation,* in which the head is excessively turned, may tear ligaments, fracture articular surfaces, and cause compression fractures.

The alteration of the spinal cord and soft tissues caused by these abnormal movements is called **deformation.** The spinal cord may be penetrated by bullets and other foreign objects (e.g., sharp objects used as weapons, shrapnel from explosions). Penetrating injuries may cause vertebral fractures, tear ligaments and muscles, or cut through a part or all of the spinal cord. Complete severing of the cord is rare.

Sites of Pathology

Injuries occur most often in the lumbar and cervical regions. The most frequent sites of injury of the cord are at the first, second, and fourth to sixth cervical vertebrae (C1, C2, C4 to C6); and the eleventh thoracic to second lumbar vertebrae (T11 to L2). Because the cervical spine has a wider range of movement than the rest of the spine, the cervical portion is more likely to be affected by externally applied forces. In addition, the cord fills most of the vertebral canal in the cervical and lumbar regions and thus is more easily injured. Damage to the vertebrae and ligaments causes the spinal column to become unstable, increasing the possibility of compression or stretching of the spinal cord with any further movement.

Classification of SCI

SCIs are classified according to systems, for instance (1) as complete or incomplete cord injury, (2) by cause of injury, and (3) by level of injury. In clinical practice, these classifications often overlap. In a *complete SCI* (about 45% of all injuries), the motor and sensory neural pathways are completely interrupted (transected), resulting in total loss of motor and sensory function below the level of the injury. However, "complete" does not necessarily mean the spinal cord has been severed. In an *incomplete SCI* (about 55% of all injuries), the motor and sensory pathways are only partially interrupted, with variable loss of function below the level of injury. Incomplete spinal cord injuries are further classified into syndromes as outlined in Table 45–2. Both complete and incomplete injuries can occur in paraplegia and quadriplegia (NSCIA, 2006). The alterations in function that occur as the result of a spinal cord injury vary greatly depending on the amount of tissue damage and the level of injury.

Manifestations

The spinal cord, the vertebrae, the intervertebral disks, the spinal nerves, the ligaments, and the surrounding soft tissue structures are in such close anatomic proximity that any condition or injury affecting one structure may well affect any one or all of the other structures. The conditions with the most critical effects are disorders affecting the spinal cord. Disorders and injuries of the spinal cord have the potential to affect movement, perception, sensation, sexual function, and elimination. Manifestations and complications of SCI by body system are listed in the box on the next page.

TABLE 45–2 Incomplete Spinal Cord Injury Syndromes

TYPE	CAUSE	LOCATION	DEFICITS
Central syndrome	Cord transection Hyperextension	Cervical	Spastic paralysis of the upper extremities Variable paralysis of the lower extremities Variable effects on the bowel, the bladder, and sexual function
Anterior syndrome	Damage to the anterior spinal artery Infarction of the anterior spinal artery Hyperflexion	Anterior two-thirds of the cord	Paralysis below the level of injury Loss of temperature and pain sensation below the level of injury
Posterior syndrome	Vertebral dislocation Herniated disk Compression	Nerve roots	Weakness in isolated muscle groups Tingling, pain Decreased or absent reflexes in the involved area Bowel or bladder dysfunction
Brown-Séquard syndrome	Penetrating trauma	Hemisection of the anterior and posterior cord	Paralysis below the level of injury on the ipsilateral (same) side of the body Contralateral loss of temperature and pain sensation below the level of injury Ipsilateral loss of proprioception below the level of injury
Homer's syndrome	Incomplete cord transection	Cervical sympathetic nerves	Ipsilateral ptosis of the eyelid, constricted pupil, and facial anhidrosis (inability to perspire)

MANIFESTATIONS and Complications of Spinal Cord Injury by Body System

INTEGUMENT
- Decubitus (pressure) ulcers

NEUROLOGIC
- Pain
- Areflexia
- Hypotonia
- Autonomic dysreflexia

CARDIOVASCULAR
- Spinal shock
- Paroxysmal hypertension
- Orthostatic hypotension
- Cardiac dysrhythmias
- Decreased venous return
- Hypercalcemia

RESPIRATORY
- Limited chest expansion
- Decreased cough reflex
- Decreased vital capacity

GASTROINTESTINAL
- Stress ulcers
- Paralytic ileus
- Stool impaction
- Stool incontinence

GENITOURINARY
- Urinary retention
- Urinary incontinence
- Neurogenic bladder
- Impotence
- Testicular atrophy
- Inability to ejaculate
- Decreased vaginal lubrication

MUSCULOSKELETAL
- Joint contractures
- Bone demineralization
- Osteoporosis
- Muscle spasms
- Muscle atrophy
- Pathologic fractures
- Paraplegia
- Quadriplegia

Spinal shock is the temporary loss of reflex function (called *areflexia*) below the level of injury. This response begins immediately after complete transection of the spinal cord, when connections between the brain and the spinal cord are interrupted and the cord does not function at all. The response also occurs (although in varying degrees) after partial transection as well as after spinal cord contusions, compression, and ischemia.

Normal activity of the spinal cord is dependent on constant impulses from the higher centers of the brain. When damage from an injury stops these impulses, spinal shock follows. There is loss of motor function, tendon reflexes, and autonomic function. Spinal shock may begin within 1 hour of the injury. The condition may last from a few minutes to several months (although it usually lasts from 1 to 6 weeks), and then reflex activity returns. Spinal shock ends slowly, with the gradual reappearance of reflexes, hyperreflexia (increased reflex responses), muscle spasticity, and reflex bladder emptying.

The manifestations of acute spinal shock (which vary in degree) include the following:

- Flaccid paralysis of skeletal muscles below the level of injury
- Loss of all spinal reflexes below the level of injury
- Loss of sensations of pain, touch, temperature, and pressure below the level of injury
- Absence of visceral and somatic sensations below the level of injury
- Bowel and bladder dysfunction
- Loss of the ability to perspire below the level of injury.

A person with a cervical or upper thoracic SCI may also have neurogenic shock, resulting in cardiovascular changes. These changes are due to the inability of higher centers in the brainstem to modulate reflexes. As a result, vascular beds below the level of injury dilate, and the cardiac accelerator reflex is suppressed. The client experiences hypotension and bradycardia. Other manifestations may include respiratory insufficiency due to loss of innervation of the diaphragm in C1 to C4 injuries, hypothermia, paralytic ileus, urinary retention, and oliguria.

Both bradycardia and hypotension may persist even after the spinal shock resolves. In addition to losing sympathetic control of the heart rate, the client with a high-level SCI experiences decreased peripheral resistance and loss of muscle activity. These changes result in sluggish blood flow and decreased venous return, increasing the risk for thrombophlebitis.

Complications

The complications of an SCI involve many different body systems and result often in permanent disability and loss of functional health status. The complications include but are not limited to upper and lower motor neuron deficits, paraplegia and quadriplegia, and autonomic dysreflexia. Other complications, depending on the level and severity of the injury, are ineffective respirations; altered skin integrity; increased risk of thrombosis; and alterations in bowel elimination, urinary elimination, and sexual pattern.

Upper and Lower Motor Neuron Deficits

Injuries to the spinal cord are often classified as either *upper motor neuron lesions* or *lower motor neuron lesions*. Motor neurons are functional units that carry motor impulses. The upper motor neurons (located in the cerebral cortex, thalamus, brainstem, and corticospinal and corticobulbar tracts) are responsible for voluntary movement. When these motor pathways are interrupted, the client experiences spastic paralysis and hyperreflexia and may be unable to carry out skilled movement.

Lower motor neurons (located in the anterior horn of the spinal cord, the motor nuclei of the brainstem, and the axons that reach the motor end plate of skeletal muscles) are responsible for innervation and contraction of skeletal muscles. Interruption of lower motor neurons results in muscle flaccidity and extensive muscle atrophy, with loss of both voluntary and involuntary movement. If only some of the motor neurons supplying a muscle are affected, the client experiences partial paralysis (paresis); if all motor neurons to a muscle are affected, the client experiences complete paralysis. Hyporeflexia is also present.

Paraplegia and Quadriplegia

Two common neurologic deficits resulting from an SCI are paraplegia and quadriplegia (see Figure 45–2). **Paraplegia** is paralysis of the lower portion of the body, sometimes involving the lower trunk. Paraplegia occurs when the thoracic, lumbar, and sacral portions of the spinal cord are injured, causing loss or impairment of sensory and/or motor function. **Quadriplegia**, also called *tetraplegia*, occurs when cervical segments of the cord are injured, impairing function of the arms, trunk, legs, and pelvic organs.

Autonomic Dysreflexia

Autonomic dysreflexia (also called *autonomic hyperreflexia*) is an exaggerated sympathetic response that occurs in clients with SCIs at or above the T6 level. This response, which is seen only after recovery from spinal shock, occurs as a result of a lack of control of the autonomic nervous system by higher centers. When stimuli are unable to ascend the cord, mass reflex stimulation of the sympathetic nerves below the level of the injured cord area occurs, triggering massive vasoconstriction. In response, the vagus nerve causes bradycardia and vasodilation above the level of injury. If untreated, autonomic dysreflexia can cause seizures, a stroke, or a myocardial infarction and is potentially fatal (Hickey, 2003).

Autonomic dysreflexia is triggered by stimuli that would normally cause abdominal discomfort (a full bladder is the most common cause), by stimulation of pain receptors, and by visceral contractions (Porth, 2005). Causes include fecal impaction, bladder infections or stones, intrauterine contractions, ejaculation, peritonitis, and stimulation from pressure ulcers or ingrown toenails. The most common precipitating event is a blocked urinary catheter.

The manifestations of this condition include pounding headache; bradycardia; hypertension (with readings as high as 300/160); flushed, warm skin with profuse sweating above the lesion and pale, cold, and dry skin below it; and anxiety (Porth, 2005). Dysreflexia is a neurologic emergency and requires immediate treatment.

INTERDISCIPLINARY CARE

The client with an acute SCI requires emergency assessment and care and medications; sometimes the client also requires immo-

bilization and surgery. The client is first assessed and stabilized at the scene of the accident, initially treated in the emergency room, and then admitted to the hospital intensive care unit.

Emergency Care

The danger of death from SCI is greatest when there is damage to or transection of the upper cervical region. When the injury is at the C1 to C4 level, respiratory paralysis is common, and the client who survives requires ventilator assistance to breathe. Injuries below C4 may increase the risk of respiratory failure if edema ascends the cord. It is of critical importance not to complicate the initial injury by allowing the fractured vertebrae to damage the cord further during transport to the hospital. Although at one time injuries to the high cervical cord were almost always fatal, advances in trauma care have greatly improved the survival rate.

All people who have sustained trauma to the head or spine, or who are unconscious, should be treated as though they have a spinal cord injury. Prehospital management includes rapid assessment of the ABCs (airway, breathing, circulation), immobilizing and stabilizing the head and neck, removing the person from the site of injury, stabilizing other life-threatening injuries, and rapidly transporting the person to the appropriate facility. Guidelines for emergency care are as follows:

- Avoid flexing, extending, or rotating the neck.
- Immobilize the neck, using rolled towels or blankets, or apply a cervical collar before moving the client onto a backboard.
- Secure the head by placing a belt or tape across the forehead and securing it to the stretcher.
- Maintain the client in the supine position.
- Transfer directly from the stretcher with backboard still in place to the type of bed that will be used in the hospital.

Assessment findings at the scene of the accident or in the emergency room vary according to the level of injury. The assessment findings common to the level of injury and spinal shock are outlined in Box 45–1.

The client in the emergency department with a suspected or identified SCI is also treated for respiratory problems, paralytic ileus, atonic bladder, and cardiovascular alterations. Respiratory distress in the client with a cervical-level injury is treated by placing the client on a ventilator. Oxygen is administered to the client with a thoracic-level injury. Paralytic ileus (obstruction of the intestines due to lack of peristalsis) is common in clients with a spinal cord injury and is treated by the insertion of a nasogastric tube with connection to suction. To prevent overdistention of an atonic bladder, an indwelling catheter is inserted and connected to dependent drainage. Cardiovascular status is assessed on a continuous basis by inserting invasive monitoring devices, such as a Swan-Ganz catheter, and attaching the client to a cardiac monitor; or by arterial monitoring to identify hypotension and to draw arterial blood gases (ABGs).

High-dose steroid protocol using methylprednisolone (Medrol) must be implemented within 8 hours of the injury to improve neurologic recovery. Clinical research indicates that the use of this adrenocorticosteroid is effective in preventing secondary spinal cord damage from edema and ischemia. Treatment with G_{M1} ganglioside for 3 to 4 weeks is an experimental approach that has been effective for some clients (Tierney et al., 2005).

BOX 45–1 Assessment Findings in Acute SCI

Cervical Injury
- Paralysis or weakness of extremities
- Respiratory distress manifested by changes in ABG studies, cyanosis, flaring of the nostrils, use of accessory muscles of respiration, and restlessness
- Pulse rate below 60 and systolic BP below 80
- Decreased peristalsis

Thoracic and Lumbar Injury
- Paralysis or weakness of extremities

Spinal Shock
- Loss of skin sensation
- Flaccid paralysis, areflexia
- Absent bowel sounds
- Bladder distention
- Decreasing blood pressure
- Absence of the cremasteric reflex in males (retraction of the left or right testicle in response to stimulation of the skin of, respectively, the inner left or right thigh)

- Vasopressors are used in the immediate acute care phase to treat bradycardia or hypotension due to spinal and neurogenic shock. Examples of drugs are dopamine (Intropin) to treat hypotension in neurogenic shock and dobutamine (Dobutrex) to support cardiac function. Atropine should be available at the bedside to treat bradycardia.
- Antispasmodics are used to treat spasticity in clients with spinal cord injury. Both baclofen (Lioresal) and diazepam (Valium) may be used. A discussion of nursing implications of treatment with antispasmodics is found in the Medication Administration box below.
- Analgesics such as nonsteroidal anti-inflammatory drugs (NSAIDs) and narcotics are administered to reduce pain.
- Proton pump inhibitors, such as omeprazole (Prilosec), rabeprazole (Aciphex), or pantoprazole (Protonix), are often administered to prevent stress-related gastric ulcers, a common complication in SCI.
- Unless contraindicated, anticoagulants (heparin or warfarin) may be given to prevent thrombophlebitis.
- Stool softeners may be administered as part of a bowel training program.

Diagnosis

Diagnostic tests are ordered to identify the level and extent of injury, and to detect any complications. The tests include x-ray of the spine, CT or MRI of the spine, and somatosensory evoked potential studies to locate the level of spinal cord injury by stimulating peripheral nerves and measuring response times. ABG are measured to establish a baseline or to identify problems due to respiratory insufficiency.

Medications

The pharmacologic treatment of the client with SCI is symptomatic. It is directed primarily toward decreasing edema from the injury, treating hypotension and bradycardia, and treating spasticity.

- Corticosteroids, discussed earlier in this section, may be used to decrease or control edema of the cord.

Treatments

The treatments used in the management of an SCI include surgery, stabilization, and immobilization.

SURGERY Early surgical treatment may be necessary if there is evidence of compression of the spinal cord by bone fragments or a hematoma. Surgery may also be done to stabilize and support the spine. However, many clients are treated with stabilization devices and do not require surgery. Surgeries that may be performed include a decompression laminectomy, a spinal fusion, and insertion of metal rods. Surgeries of the spine are discussed later in the chapter.

STABILIZATION AND IMMOBILIZATION As a result of one or more dislocations or fractures of the cervical vertebrae, the client with an SCI may be immobilized in some type of traction or external fixation device to stabilize the vertebral column and

MEDICATION ADMINISTRATION Antispasmodics in Spinal Cord Injury

Baclofen (Lioresal)
Chlorzoxazone (Paraflex)
Cyclobenzaprine hydrochloride (Flexeril)
Diazepam (Valium)
Orphenadrine citrate (Norflex)

These drugs depress the central nervous system and inhibit the transmission of impulses from the spinal cord to skeletal muscle. They are used to control muscle spasm and pain associated with acute or chronic musculoskeletal conditions. They are not always effective in controlling spasticity resulting from cerebral or spinal cord conditions.

NURSING RESPONSIBILITIES
- Assess the client's spasticity and involuntary movements to obtain baseline data for comparison of results of therapy.

- Do not expect therapy to have effects for 1 week.
- Administer oral medications with food to decrease gastrointestinal symptoms.

HEALTH EDUCATION FOR THE CLIENT AND FAMILY
- These drugs may cause drowsiness, diplopia, and impotence.
- Take your medications with meals to decrease gastric irritation.
- Physical improvement may take several weeks.
- Report slurred speech, drooling, or inability to carry out usual functions to the physician.
- Do not stop taking the medication without consulting your healthcare provider.

prevent any further damage (Figure 45–6 ■). Traction may also be used to stabilize the spinal column for clients who are not yet in a condition to have surgery or who have severe bleeding and edema of the injured cord. The physician applies the traction or fixation device; the nurse is responsible for assessments and interventions following the application.

Although used less frequently today, various devices provide cervical traction. For example, Gardner-Wells tongs may be used (Figure 45–7 ■). In this type of traction, the physician applies pins to the skull, approximately 1 cm above each ear, and weights are attached to the device.

The halo external fixation device is often used to provide stabilization if there is no significant involvement of the ligaments (Figure 45–8 ■). It is most often used to provide stability for fractures of the cervical and high thoracic vertebrae without cord damage. This device allows greater mobility, self-care, and participation in rehabilitation programs. The device is

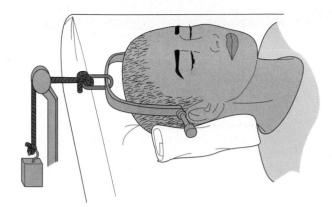

Figure 45–7 ■ Cervical traction may be applied by several methods, including Gardner-Wells tongs.

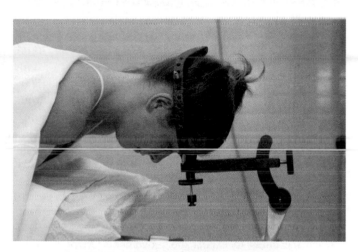

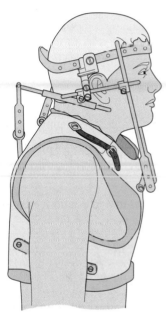

Figure 45–8 ■ The halo external fixation device.

secured with four pins inserted into the skull, two in the frontal bone and two in the occipital bone. The halo ring is then attached to a rigid plastic vest lined with sheepskin. Nursing interventions for the client using a halo fixation device are described in the box on the next page.

NURSING CARE

Both during the acute phase and the rehabilitative phase, the client with a SCI has complex needs that involve all members of the healthcare team. Because these injuries are more common in younger clients, consideration of lifelong effects on both the client and the family is essential. The nurse coordinates client care and develops and implements a care plan that is individualized to each client and family. The focus of the plan is to prevent the secondary complications of immobility and altered body functions, to promote self-care, and to educate the client and family. A Nursing Care Plan for a client with a SCI is found on page 1603.

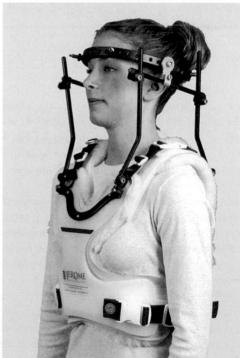

Figure 45–6 ■ Examples of traction or external fixation devices.

NURSING CARE OF THE CLIENT IN
Halo Fixation

- Maintain integrity of the halo external fixation device.
  a. Inspect pins and traction bars for tightness; report loosened pins to physician.
  b. Tape the appropriate wrench to the head of the bed for emergency intervention.
  c. Never use the halo ring to lift or reposition the client. *Loosening of the apparatus poses the risk of further damage to the cord. It is the responsibility of the nurse to maintain the integrity of the apparatus and the safety of the client.*
- Assess muscle function and skin sensation every 2 hours in the acute phase and every 4 hours thereafter.
  a. Assess motor function on a scale of 0 to 5, with 0 being no evidence of muscle contraction and 5 being normal muscle strength with full range of motion.
  b. Assess sensation by comparing touch and pain, moving from impaired to normal areas, and testing both the right and left sides of the body.
  Monitoring muscle function and skin sensation allows early identification of potential neurologic deficits.
- Monitor pin sites each shift and follow hospital policy for pin care. Here are some general guidelines.
  a. Assess pin sites for redness, edema, and drainage.
  b. Depending on policy, clean each pin site with a sterile applicator dipped in hydrogen peroxide, apply a topical antibiotic and cover with sterile 2-inch split gauze squares.
  Organisms can enter the body through the pin-insertion site; assessments and care are provided to detect signs of and prevent infection.
- Maintain skin integrity.
  a. Turn the immobile client every 2 hours.
  b. Inspect the skin around edges of the vest every 4 hours.
  c. Change the sheepskin liner when it is soiled and at least once each week.
  These interventions prevent skin injury and irritation.

Health Promotion

Health promotion for SCI primarily involves preventing injuries. Nurses can provide valuable information in the community and in the workplace to prevent SCI. Programs that focus on wearing seat belts and using approved infant seats and child booster chairs in automobiles can do much to help decrease the number of SCIs each year. Educational programs that promote workplace safety and farm safety should include information to prevent falls and how to use heavy equipment safely.

Assessment

The following data are collected through the health history and physical examination (see Chapter 43 ∞). Further focused assessments are described with nursing interventions in the next section.

- *Health history:* Time, location, and type of event-causing injury; location, duration, quality, and intensity of pain; dyspnea; sensation; paresthesia.
- *Physical examination:* Vital signs, motor strength, movement, spinal reflexes, bowel sounds, bladder distention.

Nursing Diagnoses and Interventions

Because an SCI has many possible effects, many nursing diagnoses may be appropriate. Nursing diagnoses discussed in this section focus on problems with physical mobility, respirations, dysreflexia, bowel and bladder elimination, sexual dysfunction, and self-esteem.

Impaired Physical Mobility

After the initial period of spinal shock and areflexia, the client regains spinal reflex activity and muscle tone that is not under the control of higher centers. Clients with injuries above the level of T12 experience involuntary spastic movements of skeletal muscles. These movements reach a peak about 2 years after the injury and then gradually subside (Porth, 2005). Spasms impair the ability to carry out the activities of daily life and work. In addition, the paraplegia or quadriplegia increases the potential for impaired skin integrity, thrombophlebitis, and contractures.

The goals of care for clients with impaired mobility related to a spinal cord injury are to reduce the effects of spasticity and to prevent complications involving the skin, the cardiovascular system, and joint function.

- Perform passive ROM exercises for all extremities at least twice a day. Identify stimuli that cause spastic movements and either avoid the stimuli (such as certain exercises) or teach the client to expect the movements. *ROM exercises help prevent contractures and stretch spastic muscles, promoting rehabilitation.*
- Maintain skin integrity by turning every 2 hours, assessing pressure points at least once each shift, and using a special bed if necessary. The client may be placed on a regular or special bed, such as a kinetic bed. *Immobility compresses soft tissues and promotes the development of decubitus ulcers. The lack of sensory warning mechanisms and of voluntary motor control of skin dermatomes further increases the risk for altered skin integrity. Special beds allow movement or turning while keeping the spinal column in alignment.*
- Assess the lower extremities each shift for manifestations of thrombophlebitis. Observe for redness and for increased heat every shift; measure thigh and calf circumference daily. If antiembolic stockings (TEDs) are ordered, remove for 30 to 60 minutes each shift. Assess for skin impairment and provide skin care while TEDs are removed. *Clients with neurologic deficits are at high risk for deep venous thrombosis as a result of immobility, vasomotor dysfunction, and decreased venous return with venous stasis. Antiembolic stockings help to prevent the pooling of blood in the lower extremities and increase venous return, lessening the risk for venous stasis and thrombus formation.*

NURSING CARE PLAN   A Client with an SCI

Jim Valdez, a 19-year-old college sophomore, is admitted to the hospital by ambulance following an automobile crash. His family (father, mother, and sister) live 100 miles away and cannot visit often, although they are very concerned. On admission to the hospital, a CT scan of the spine shows a fracture and partial laceration of the cord at the C7 level. Mr. Valdez is in halo traction. One night, he tells the nurse, "I wish I had just died when I got hurt. I don't think I can stand to live like this."

ASSESSMENT

When Mr. Valdez is admitted to the intensive care unit, he has flaccid paralysis involving all extremities. He has no sensation below the clavicle or in portions of his arms and legs. His bladder is distended and bowel sounds are absent. Other assessment findings include BP 90/56, P 50, T 97°F (36.1°C), arterial blood gases pH 7.4, Pao_2 96, $Paco_2$ 37, Sao_2 96%. Oxygen per nasal cannula is given at 2 L/min, and halo traction is applied. A Foley catheter is inserted into his bladder, and a nasogastric tube is inserted and attached to low-pressure continuous suction.

After 7 days, Mr. Valdez is moved from the intensive care unit to the neurosurgical unit for continuing care and planning for transfer to a rehabilitation hospital in his home town. His vital signs have stabilized and are normal for his age; respirations and oxygenation are normal. Other neurologic assessments remain the same.

DIAGNOSES

- *Impaired Physical Mobility* related to paralysis of lower and upper extremities
- *Bowel Incontinence* related to lack of voluntary sphincter control
- *Dysfunctional Grieving* related to denial of loss.

EXPECTED OUTCOMES

- Be actively involved in exercise programs.
- Have a soft, formed stool every second or third day.
- Verbally express his grief to parents and staff.

PLANNING AND IMPLEMENTATION

- Conduct passive exercises on all extremities four times a day.
- Provide progressive mobilization by initially raising the head of the bed 90 degrees (repeat two to three times during the first

day of movement); if blood pressure remains normal, dangle for 5 minutes before transferring him to a chair.
- His usual time for a bowel movement is after breakfast; schedule retraining program for that time.
- Encourage a diet high in fiber and fluids. Likes whole-wheat bread, orange juice, and cola; does not like water.
- Promote grief work by providing time to express feelings. Explain to the family that his denial and anger are part of the grieving process.
- Determine food likes and dislikes and order preferred foods from the menu. Encourage his friends to bring in his favorite foods periodically.
- Take and record weight every third day, using the bed scales.

EVALUATION

By the time Mr. Valdez is transferred to the rehabilitation hospital he is looking forward to learning how to use special equipment and getting his own motorized wheelchair. He is able to sit up in a chair without dizziness or hypotension. The use of ordered stool softeners combined with a high-fiber diet and fluid intake of 2000 to 3000 mL per day has maintained bowel elimination. Mr. Valdez and his parents have spent 3 hours talking about their feelings related to the accident and the future. Although the discussion is emotionally difficult, all three say they now feel much better. Mr. Valdez still has episodes of angry outbursts and tears, but he is more optimistic about what can be done and believes he can finish college. He selects foods from the menu each day and eats most of his meals, but he especially enjoys the times his friends bring in pizza or hamburgers.

CRITICAL THINKING IN THE NURSING PROCESS

1. Considering Mr. Valdez's age and developmental level, do you think his emotional responses to his injury were appropriate?
2. Issues of sexuality are obviously important for the client with a spinal cord injury. How would you approach Mr. Valdez about this topic?
3. What would be your response as a male or female nurse if Mr. Valdez would allow only male nurses to provide care?
4. Outline a teaching program to help Mr. Valdez meet long-term urinary elimination needs.

See Evaluating Your Response in Appendix C.

PRACTICE ALERT
Removing TED stockings each shift not only promotes healthy skin but also lets the nurse assess skin integrity.

Impaired Gas Exchange

Injuries at the level of T1 to T7 leave the phrenic nerve intact, but the innervation of intercostal muscles is affected, compromising respiratory function. In addition, because the abdominal muscles are paralyzed, the client cannot expel secretions by coughing. Clients with cord injuries at C3 or above have paralysis of the respiratory muscles and cannot breathe without a ventilator.

- Monitor vital capacity and respiratory effectiveness, assessing for tachycardia, restlessness, Pao_2 less than 60 mmHg, $Paco_2$ greater than 50 mmHg, and vital capacity less than 1 L. *Clients with cervical cord injuries frequently require ventilatory support because of reduced vital capacity and inability to expel secretions by coughing.*

PRACTICE ALERT
Changes in ABGs and vital capacity signal respiratory insufficiency.

- Monitor for signs of ascending edema of the spinal cord, including difficulty in swallowing or coughing, respiratory stridor, use of accessory muscles of respiration, bradycardia, and increased motor and sensory loss. *Hemorrhage and edema can further impair respiratory function.*

■ Help the client to cough, as follows: Place the hand between the umbilicus and xiphoid process and push in and up as the client exhales and coughs. *The client who is unable to cough effectively and has decreased ventilatory capacity may develop atelectasis, pneumonia, and respiratory failure.*

Ineffective Breathing Patterns

Respiratory function is impaired in the client with SCI in the cervical and thoracic levels if the diaphragm (innervated at C3 to C5), the intercostal muscles (innervated at T1 to T7), and the abdominal muscles are affected. In clients with injury at higher levels, assisted ventilation and a tracheostomy are necessary; when the injury is at lower levels, the client's ability to take a deep breath and cough is diminished. The goal of nursing interventions is to maintain normal respiratory rate (12 to 20 breaths per minute) and to prevent pulmonary complications such as atelectasis and pneumonia.

■ Assess respiratory rate, rhythm, and depth every 4 hours (or more frequently if needed). Auscultate breath sounds as a part of respiratory assessment. *Injury to the cord in the cervical or thoracic regions can decrease respiratory function and increase the risk for respiratory problems.*

PRACTICE ALERT
Auscultate the lungs for crackles and wheezes.

■ Monitor results of oxygen saturation with pulse oximetry and ABG studies. *ABG studies provide information about gas exchange; decreasing pH, oxygen, and oxygen saturation levels, and increasing carbon dioxide levels signal respiratory acidosis.*

■ Administer supplemental oxygen as prescribed. *Oxygen saturation must be maintained at 100% with supplemental oxygen to prevent hypoxemia and secondary SCI in all acute SCI clients.*

■ Help the client turn, cough, and deep breathe at least every 2 hours. Use assisted coughing as necessary. *Paralysis of intercostal or abdominal muscles decreases the ability to expel secretions by coughing; retained secretions increase the risk for pneumonia. The inability to breathe deeply may result in atelectasis.*

■ Increase fluids given by mouth to 3000 mL per day (if oral intake is approved), according to client preference for type of liquids and predicated on the client's ability to swallow. *Increased fluid intake thins secretions, which can more easily be expelled and expectorated.*

Dysreflexia

Autonomic dysreflexia is an emergency that requires immediate assessment and intervention to prevent complications of extremely high blood pressure (loss of consciousness, seizure, and even death).

■ Elevate the head of the client's bed and remove TEDs or sequential compression boots. *These measures increase pool-*

ing of blood in the lower extremities and decrease venous return, thus decreasing blood pressure.

■ Assess blood pressure every 2 to 3 minutes while at the same time assessing for stimuli that initiated the response (such as a full bladder, impacted stool, or skin pressure). *The most serious danger in dysreflexia is elevated blood pressure, which could precipitate a stroke, myocardial infarction, dysrhythmias, or seizures. If the client has a Foley catheter, ensure that there are no kinks in the tubing. If the client does not have a Foley catheter, drain the bladder with a straight catheter. If manifestations persist, assess for a fecal impaction. If an impaction is present, insert Nupercaine cream into the anus, wait 10 minutes, and manually remove the impaction.*

PRACTICE ALERT
Blood pressure readings may be as high as 300/160.

■ If blood pressure remains dangerously elevated, the physician may prescribe intravenous administration of diazoxide (Hyperstat). Other medications that may be used include nifedipine (Procardia) and hydralazine (Apresoline). *Diazoxide is an antihypertensive drug used in emergency situations to lower blood pressure in adults with dangerously high readings. Nifedipine and hydralazine are peripheral vasodilators that are administered to decrease the elevated blood pressure.*

PRACTICE ALERT
It is important to closely monitor for hypotension following administration of these medications, especially if the stimulus for the dysreflexia has been removed.

Impaired Urinary Elimination and Constipation

Depending on the level of the injury, the client with a SCI may have alterations in bowel and bladder function. Clients with injuries to the cord at or above the S2 to S4 levels will have a neurogenic bladder, with deficits in control of micturition. Voluntary and involuntary bowel control is affected in the client with a lower motor neuron injury. Both bowel and bladder retraining are possible; if not, some form of assisted elimination is necessary. Although an indwelling catheter may be used in the acute phase of care, the goal is to reestablish a catheter-free state.

■ Monitor for manifestations of a full bladder. *Overdistention stretches the bladder and can lead to backflow of urine into the ureters and kidney; stasis of urine in an incompletely emptied bladder increases the risk for infection.*

PRACTICE ALERT
A distended bladder can be palpated over the lower abdomen above the symphysis pubis.

■ Teach client to use trigger voiding techniques prior to straight catheterization. These techniques include stroking the inner thigh, pulling the pubic hair, tapping on the abdomen over the bladder, and (in females) pouring warm water over the vulva. *These trigger voiding techniques stimulate parasympathetic nerve fibers to cause reflex activity and may facilitate voiding.*

- Teach self-catheterization to clients who will be able to carry out the procedure alone or with minimal assistance (Procedure 45–1). *Straight catheterization at regular intervals is part of bladder training because periodic distention and relaxation of the muscles of the bladder promote reflex bladder activity. In addition, self-care fosters independence.*

- Monitor residual urine throughout the bladder retraining program. *A residual urine amount of less than 80 mL after a triggered voiding is considered satisfactory.*

- Institute a bowel retraining program as follows:
  - Assess usual patterns of bowel elimination to establish best times for individualized program.
  - Maintain a high-fluid, high-fiber diet
  - Use stool softeners as prescribed; rectal suppositories and enemas may be used 30 minutes after meals to stimulate stronger peristalsis and facilitate evacuation.
  - Maintain upright position if at all possible and ensure privacy.
  - If client is unable to evacuate, digital stimulation or manual removal on a regular basis may be the most effective long-term management.

A bowel retraining program to regulate the bowel through reflex activity may be instituted in clients with upper motor neuron injuries. The client with a lower motor neuron injury loses the defecation reflex, and bowel retraining is more difficult (if not impossible).

Sexual Dysfunction

Sexual intercourse is often still possible for the client with an SCI. In men, the general rule is that the higher the level of injury the greater the potential to have reflexogenic erections, although ejaculation or orgasm may not occur, and fertility is usually lower as a result of a lack of temperature control of the testes. However, ejaculation may be stimulated and the sperm used to inseminate the client's partner, so that fatherhood is a possibility. Men who have sacral-level injuries do not have reflexogenic erections but may have psychogenic erections. They are also more likely to remain fertile.

Women with SCI generally do not have sensation during sexual intercourse, but pregnancy is possible. However, pregnant women with an SCI are at increased risk for autonomic dysreflexia during labor and delivery. Birth control options should be discussed prior to discharge from the acute care setting.

A client with an SCI may be deeply concerned about alterations in sexual function. These concerns may lead to lowered self-esteem, altered self-image, or changes in feelings about being an attractive and desirable person. Assess concerns and provide a

---

PROCEDURE 45–1 CLIENT SELF-CATHETERIZATION

Self-catheterization on an intermittent basis (usually a part of self-care at home) is a clean rather than a sterile procedure. The hands should be washed before and after the procedure, and the urinary meatus should be cleaned by washing with soap and water.

FEMALE SELF-CATHETERIZATION

- Attempt to void. If urine is not of sufficient quantity (at least 100 mL) or if you cannot void at all, do self-catheterization. *A large amount of residual urine means that more frequent catheterizations (every 4 to 6 hours) are necessary.*
- While sitting on the wheelchair or the commode, locate the urethra. Visualize the urethra by looking in a mirror, or palpate the urethra with a fingertip. *Visualization or palpation of the meatus is necessary for proper catheter insertion.*
- Lubricate the meatus with a water-soluble lubricant. *Lubrication facilitates the insertion of the catheter and reduces trauma to tissues.*

- Take a deep breath and insert the catheter tip 2 to 3 inches or until urine flows. *The catheter enters the bladder more easily when the sphincter is relaxed. The deep breath relaxes the sphincter. The female urethra is 1½ to 2½ inches long.*
- Hold the catheter securely and allow urine to drain until the flow stops. *Withdrawing and reinserting the catheter increase the risk of infection.*
- Withdraw the catheter and wash it with soap and water. Store the catheter in a clean container. *The catheter can be reused until it is too soft or too hard to be directed into and through the urinary meatus. Clean rather than sterile technique is usually used for self-catheterization at home.*

MALE SELF-CATHETERIZATION

- Attempt to void. If urine is not of sufficient quantity (e.g., less than 100 mL) or if you cannot void at all, do self-catheterization. *A large amount of residual urine means that more frequent catheterizations (every 4 to 6 hours) are necessary.*
- Sit either on the commode or in the wheelchair. Hold the penis with slight upward tension and extend it to its full length. *Extending the penis straightens the urethra.*
- Lubricate the catheter from the tip to about 6 inches downward. *Lubrication is especially important for male catheterization because of the length of the urethra.*
- Take a deep breath and insert the catheter 6 to 7 inches or until urine flows. *The catheter enters the bladder more easily when the*

sphincter is relaxed. The deep breath relaxes the sphincter. The male urethra is about 6 inches long.
- Hold the catheter securely and allow urine to drain until flow has stopped. *Withdrawing and reinserting the catheter increase the risk of infection.*
- Withdraw the catheter and wash it with soap and water. Store the catheter in a clean container. *The catheter can be reused until it is too soft or too hard to be directed into and through the urethra. Clean rather than sterile technique is usually used for self-catheterization at home.*

- Nonpharmacologic methods of pain management include relaxation techniques, guided imagery, distraction, hypnosis, and music. Joining a support group may be an effective intervention in coping with and managing pain.
- Clients may be referred to a physical therapist for education about body mechanics and back-strengthening exercises. Nurses should have the client demonstrate the exercises to reinforce teaching.

THE CLIENT WITH A SPINAL CORD TUMOR

Spinal cord tumors may be benign or malignant, primary or metastatic. They may arise at any level of the spinal column. Of all spinal cord tumors, 50% are thoracic, 30% are cervical, and 20% are lumbosacral. They constitute about 0.5% to 1% of all tumors (Hickey, 2003). Tumors of the spinal cord are seen equally in men and in women, and they most often occur between the ages of 20 and 60. They are rarely seen in the older adult.

Classification

Spinal cord tumors are classified by anatomic location as either intramedullary or extramedullary tumors. Intramedullary tumors, which make up about 10% of spinal tumors, arise from within the neural tissues of the spinal cord; those that occur include astrocytomas, ependymomas, glioblastomas, and medulloblastomas (Tierney et al., 2005). Extramedullary tumors arise from tissues outside the spinal cord, with commonly occurring tumors including neurofibromas, meningiomas, sarcomas, chordomas, and vascular tumors.

Extramedullary tumors are further categorized as intradural (arising from the nerve roots or meninges within the subarachnoid space) or extradural (arising from epidural tissue or the vertebrae outside the dura).

Tumors of the spinal cord are also classified as either primary or secondary (metastatic). Primary tumors, arising from the epidural vessels, spinal meninges, or glial cells, have an unknown cause. Secondary tumors are metastatic in origin, most commonly the result of malignancies of the lung, breast, prostate, gastrointestinal tract, or uterus.

Pathophysiology

Depending on their anatomic location, spinal cord tumors result in pathologic changes as a result of compression, invasion, or ischemia secondary to arterial or venous obstruction. Extramedullary tumors (whether benign or malignant) alter normal function through compression of the spinal cord, with destruction of white matter and eventual filling of the space around the spinal cord. Cord compression interferes with normal blood flow and membrane potentials, altering afferent and efferent motor, sensory, and reflex impulses. Compression of the spinal cord also causes edema, which can ascend the cord and cause further neurologic deficits. Intramedullary tumors both compress and invade. As the tumor grows within the cord, the cord also enlarges and distorts the white matter.

Manifestations

The manifestations of a spinal cord tumor depend on the anatomic location, level of occurrence, type of tumor, and spinal nerves involved. General manifestations of a spinal cord tumor include pain, motor and sensory deficits, changes in bowel and/or bladder elimination, and changes in sexual function. Specific manifestations by anatomic level are outlined in the box below.

Pain is often the first manifestation of a spinal cord tumor. It is caused by compression of the spinal cord, tension on the spinal nerves, or tumor attachment to the proximal dura (the covering of the spinal cord). The pain may be either localized or radicular. Localized pain is felt when pressure is applied over the spinous process of the involved area; this type of pain often accompanies metastatic tumors involving the vertebrae. Radicular pain is felt along the course of a nerve as a result of compression, irritation, or tension of a nerve root. The pain is often made worse by any activity that causes intraspinal pressure, such as sneezing or coughing.

Motor manifestations resulting from a spinal cord tumor include paresis and paralysis below the level of the tumor, spasticity, and hyperactive reflexes. The Babinski reflex may be positive. These deficits are the result of involvement of the corticospinal tracts.

Many different sensory manifestations may occur, depending on the location and level of the tumor. Lateral tumor growth and compression affect the lateral spinothalamic tracts, causing pain, numbness, tingling, and coldness. If the tumor involves

---

MANIFESTATIONS of Spinal Cord Tumors

CERVICAL CORD TUMORS
- Ipsilateral arm motor involvement, followed by ipsilateral and contralateral leg involvement, followed by contralateral arm involvement
- Paresis of the arms and legs
- Stiffness of the neck
- Paraplegia
- Pain in the shoulders and arms
- Hyperactive reflexes

THORACIC CORD TUMORS
- Paresis and spasticity of one leg, followed by paresis and spasticity of the other leg
- Pain in the back and chest
- Positive Babinski reflex
- Bowel and bladder dysfunction
- Sexual dysfunction

LUMBOSACRAL CORD TUMORS
- Paresis and spasticity of one leg, followed by paresis and spasticity of the other leg
- Pain in the lower back, radiating to the legs and perineal area
- Loss of sensation in the legs
- Bowel and bladder dysfunction
- Sexual dysfunction
- Decreased or absent ankle and knee reflexes

the posterior columns, the senses of vibration and proprioception of body parts are affected.

Bladder and bowel elimination and sexual function are often affected. Bowel elimination deficits include constipation that may progress to paralytic ileus. Initial bladder elimination deficits include frequency, urgency, and difficulty voiding. The deficits may progress to urinary retention and a neurogenic bladder. In addition, the male client may be impotent.

Syringomyelia is a complication of some spinal cord tumors. In this condition, a fluid-filled cystic cavity forms in the central intramedullary gray matter. This syndrome causes pain, motor weakness, and spasticity.

INTERDISCIPLINARY CARE

The medical management of the client with a spinal cord tumor focuses first on diagnosis. Treatment depends on the type of tumor, its location, and the client's condition.

Diagnosis

The client with a spinal cord tumor undergoes many of the same diagnostic tests as does the client with a ruptured intervertebral disk. The tests used to identify the tumor include x-rays, CT scans, MRI, and myelogram (see Chapter 43 ∞). A lumbar puncture of the client with a spinal cord tumor will demonstrate CSF that is commonly xanthochromic (having a yellow color), has increased protein, has few to no cells, and clots immediately (this cluster of findings is called Froin's syndrome).

Medications

The client with a spinal cord tumor is given medications to relieve pain and control edema. If the pain is severe and the result of a metastatic tumor, an epidural catheter may be inserted for narcotic analgesic administration. Pain management for clients with a spinal cord tumor is provided by narcotic analgesics (see Chapter 9 ∞). Steroids, such as dexamethasone (Decadron), are administered to control edema of the cord.

Surgery

Intramedullary and intradural tumors are surgically excised when possible. Advances in microsurgical techniques and laser surgery have increased the possibility of tumor excision. Metastatic tumors may be partially excised to reduce cord compression; rapidly growing metastatic lesions may require surgical decompression to preserve motor, bowel, or bladder function.

The surgical excision is made through a laminectomy. The client with a tumor involving more than two vertebrae often has a spinal fusion and may also have rods inserted to stabilize the spinal column.

Radiation Therapy

Radiation therapy is used to treat metastatic spinal cord tumors for several different reasons. It may be used on an emergency basis to treat the client with rapidly progressing neurologic deficits. It may be used to reduce pain. Radiation may also be used following surgical excision of as much tumor mass as possible.

Radiation of the spinal cord may cause the development of radiation-induced myelopathy. This complication of radiation exposure occurs over time, with manifestations of a *Brown-Séquard syndrome* (weakness or paralysis on one side of the body and loss of sensation on the opposite side) developing 12 to 15 months after therapy. The manifestations may progress to paraplegia, sensory loss, and loss of bowel and bladder control (Hickey, 2003).

NURSING CARE

Nursing care for the client with a spinal cord tumor is individualized in accordance with the type of tumor and the type of treatment. The client with a benign tumor that is removed by surgery has different healthcare needs than the client with a metastatic tumor, even though they may have similar neurologic deficits. The client with a spinal cord tumor (regardless of type) requires nursing care to monitor for neurologic changes, to provide pain management, and to manage motor and sensory deficits in order to preserve quality of life.

The assessments and nursing interventions for the client with a spinal cord tumor are similar to those described for the client with SCI or who is undergoing surgery for a ruptured intervertebral disk. Following surgical treatment, the client may be transferred to a rehabilitation center or may go home for the recovery period. Referrals for home care, occupational therapy, and physical therapy often help the client regain functional abilities. Teach family members how to move the client in the bed and from the bed to a chair. Also teach them how to provide physical care, care for any appliances (such as an indwelling catheter), and prevent or treat constipation.

- If safety is a concern (such as turning on the stove and forgetting it), suggest using alternatives such as a microwave. Program emergency numbers into the telephone. Ask client to consider a Life-Line telephone program. *These measures can increase safety.*
- Suggest using cues, such as an alarm on a watch or a pocket computer, to trigger actions at designated times. *Cues are often helpful when memory loss is a problem.*

Chronic Confusion

Clients with AD often have memory deficits that make functioning in a nonstructured environment difficult. Many of the nursing interventions for this diagnosis need to be modified over time as the client continues to lose cognitive function.

- Label rooms, drawers, and other items as needed. *Visual cues promote the highest possible degree of independence for the client.*
- Remove potential hazards (such as sharp knives or potentially harmful liquids or chemicals) from the environment. *Ensuring safety is a critical factor in providing care.*
- Keep environmental stimuli to a minimum: Decrease noise levels; speak in a calm, low voice; and take an unhurried approach. *Minimizing sensory input and maintaining a calm manner may decrease anxiety.*
- Begin each interaction by identifying self and calling client by name. See Box 46–1 for other communication techniques. *These techniques provide information for the client with memory loss.*
- Limit questions to those that require a simple yes or no response. *Questions need to be appropriate to the client's ability as decision making and verbal skills decline.*
- Orient to the environment, person, and time as able; place large, easy-to-read calendars and clocks in the client's line of vision. Make references to the season or day of the week when conversing with the client. *Orient the client according to his or her level of ability; orienting to precise time may not be possible in the later stages of AD.*
- Provide boundaries by placing red or yellow tape on the floor. *Boundaries help the client stay within safe areas.*

PRACTICE ALERT
Red and yellow are more easily seen by older adults.

- Provide continuity in nursing staff. *This not only promotes consistency of care for the client but also allows the nurse to determine more accurately changes in the client's condition.*
- Repeat explanations simply and as needed to decrease anxiety. *Loss of short-term memory leads to loss of a point of reference; eventually, AD clients think they are experiencing everything for the first time.*

Anxiety

Managing the AD client's behaviors associated with anxiety, restlessness, and confusion is a major challenge confronting nurses and caregivers. Frequently, clients are relatively calm in the morning hours, only to experience increasing periods of agitation in the afternoon and evening hours. The AD client may even waken from the night's sleep with confusion, fearfulness, or panic attacks.

- Monitor for early behaviors of fatigue and agitation. *Early assessment of problems results in prompt intervention to promote rest or to remove the client from the situation causing anxiety.*
- Remove from situations that are causing increased anxiety, such as noisy activities involving large groups. *High-stimulus situations may increase anxious feelings and agitation.*
- Keep daily routine as consistent as possible. *Providing a structured day enhances feelings of familiarity and decreases stress.*
- Schedule rest periods or quiet times throughout the day. *Fatigue contributes to anxiety and lowers the ability to tolerate stress.*
- Provide quiet activities, such as listening to favorite music, in the afternoon or early evening. *Quiet activities may help decrease sundowning.*
- If confusion and agitation persist or escalate, assess for physical causes such as decreased oxygenation, infections, fatigue, constipation, and electrolyte imbalance. *Physical factors can increase agitation in clients with AD.*
- Use therapeutic touch or gentle hand massage. *These activities induce relaxation and have a calming effect.*

Hopelessness

As the client and family recognize the effect of AD on their lives, they may feel a sense of hopelessness. They may not have the coping skills to deal effectively with the diagnosis and anticipated problems. The increasingly degenerative, irreversible nature of the disorder tends to diminish hope; only the ability to adapt to the many problems can restore it.

- Assess the client's and family's response to the diagnosis and understanding of AD; encourage expression of feelings. *Understanding the client/family's perspective enables the nurse to dispel myths about AD.*

BOX 46–1 Communicating with the Client with AD

- Face the client and talk directly to him or her; call the client by name.
- When first approaching the client, identify yourself.
- Use simple sentences and words with few syllables.
- Speak in a calm, low voice.
- Ask one question at a time. Use questions that require only a yes or no response.
- Keep nonverbal communication relaxed and parallel to the verbal communication.
- Avoid giving the impression of being in a hurry; try to have a relaxed approach.
- Observe for anxiety—wringing hands, pacing, darting eye movements—and alter your approach to decrease anxiety.
- Avoid arguing with clients; do not insist on orienting client to reality; the client's point of reference may not be based in reality.
- Give plenty of time for the client with AD to process what you are trying to say; do not expect clients to perform skills beyond their abilities.
- Repeat explanations in simple terms.

- Provide realistic information about the disorder; provide information at the client/family's level of understanding. *Client and family may need to have separate sessions. Factual information provides a foundation for decision making.*
- Avoid criticizing or judging expressed feelings. *An environment accepting of the expression of real feelings promotes both further expression of feelings and willingness to discuss other issues.*
- Support positive family bonds and enhance communication among family members; promote mutual positive regard. *Strong family relationships can provide direction for living and convey a willingness to share the burden.*
- Encourage the client to make as many decisions as possible. *Self-determination enhances a feeling of control over a situation and may give a sense of hope.*
- Encourage the client and family to seek spiritual guidance that previously inspired hope. *The client's church is a legitimate support system. Belief in God can inspire hope beyond present circumstances.*

Caregiver Role Strain

Most caregivers of clients with AD are spouses or other family members. Because AD is a chronic and eventually debilitating disorder, caregivers may feel overwhelmed by their responsibilities. The caregiving spouse faces not only the responsibility for the client's multiple physical demands but also economic and psychosocial stressors. An area that must be discussed is the ability and safety of the client in driving an automobile. Although it may be necessary, the loss of independence represented by the loss of the ability to drive may further trigger anxiety and anger. Fear of the future, loss of income, loss of companionship and a mate—combined with fatigue—make the caregiver vulnerable. Caregivers may become physically and mentally exhausted and socially isolated because of the overwhelming responsibilities of providing total care to the incapacitated family member.

- Teach the caregivers self-care techniques, such as taking rest periods and avoiding fatigue. *Fatigue adds to stress and potentially leads to poor decision making.*
- Have the caregivers list and regularly take part in physical activities they enjoy, such as walking or swimming. *Regular physical exercise decreases stress.*
- Refer the caregivers to local AD support groups. Suggest books pertinent to the subject. *Explicit suggestions in locating support systems and providing specific information promotes coping.*
- Refer the caregivers to Meals-on-Wheels, home health, respite care, and other community services. *Community agencies can relieve some of the daily care burdens, thus providing time for other activities. Programs that support caregivers have been shown to delay nursing home placement.*
- Ensure the family knows that hospice care is available during the end stages of AD. *Hospice services can support the family during this difficult time.*

Using NANDA, NIC, and NOC

Chart 46–1 shows links between NANDA nursing diagnoses, NIC, and NOC when caring for the client with AD.

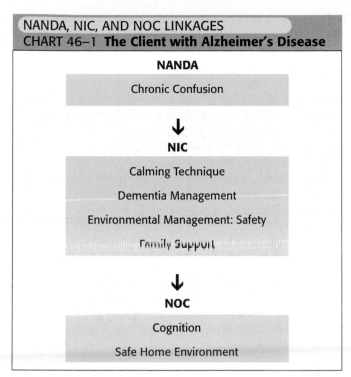

NANDA, NIC, AND NOC LINKAGES
CHART 46–1 **The Client with Alzheimer's Disease**

NANDA

Chronic Confusion

↓

NIC

Calming Technique

Dementia Management

Environmental Management: Safety

Family Support

↓

NOC

Cognition

Safe Home Environment

Data from *NANDA's Nursing Diagnoses: Definitions & Classification 2005–2006* by NANDA International (2003), Philadelphia; *Nursing Interventions Classification (NIC)* (4th ed.) by J. M. Dochterman & G. M. Bulechek (2004), St. Louis, MO: Mosby; and *Nursing Outcomes Classification (NOC)* (3rd ed.) by S. Moorhead, M. Johnson, and M. Maas (2004), St. Louis, MO: Mosby.

Community-Based Care

Teaching for clients and families centers initially on explaining the disorder and exploring available support systems. Anticipate the need to reexplain the disorder and its consequences, because clients and families may be in shock or denial during the initial period of the disease.

In addition to explaining the anticipated changes with AD, suggest practical solutions to identified problems. It is important to evaluate both the client and caregivers; interventions must be appropriate for the family's situation and resources. Maintaining the least restrictive environment that promotes safety for the client is a major goal of teaching. Using memory cues, such as labeling drawers to indicate the specific types of clothing and labeling rooms, can help orient the client and foster independence. Consistency in the environment and daily routine is an essential part of care. Emphasizing realistic expectations means adjusting care and communication techniques to the client's level of ability.

Address the following topics for home care of the client and for the caregiver:

- Support groups and peer counseling are helpful in handling caregiver stress.
- A person with AD who is confused or agitated is not comfortable and is usually frightened.
- Plan care that matches the person's level of coping, using a consistent routine.
- Provide regular rest periods to decrease the client's stress and fatigue (these do not increase nighttime wandering).

- Plan care for the caregiver. Periodic adult day care or respite care during the initial stages, with plans for increasing assistance to meet the client's daily needs as the disease progresses, may be sufficient. Referrals to the appropriate agency for long-term care, including skilled nursing facilities, may be indicated. Family members may need help adjusting to the idea of extended care but may be relieved to relinquish the physical care needs.
- Suggest the following resources:
  - Alzheimer's Association
  - Alzheimer's Disease and Related Disorders Association
  - Alzheimer's Disease Education and Referral Center
  - National Institute of Neurological Disorders and Stroke.

THE CLIENT WITH MULTIPLE SCLEROSIS

Multiple sclerosis (MS) is a chronic demyelinating neurologic disease of the CNS (brain, optic nerves, and spinal cord), associated with an abnormal immune response to an environmental factor. The manifestations of MS vary according to the area of the nervous system affected. The initial onset may be followed by a total remission, making diagnosis difficult. In about 60% of clients, MS is characterized by periods of exacerbation, when manifestations are highly pronounced, followed by periods of remission, when manifestations are not obvious. The end result, however, is progression of the disease with increasing loss of function.

Incidence and Prevalence

The onset of MS is usually between 20 and 50 years of age, with a peak at age 30. MS is the most prevalent CNS demyelinating disorder, and is a leading cause of neurologic disability in young adults. Although all races are affected, MS is primarily a disease of people of northern European ancestry; however, MS does occur in people of African, Asian, and Hispanic descent. A definite genetic factor has not been established but studies suggest that genetic factors may make some individuals more susceptible than others (National MS Society, 2005).

FAST FACTS

Multiple Sclerosis

- Approximately 400,000 people in the United States have MS; the incidence is 2.5 million worldwide.
- Females are affected two times more often than males, and the incidence is highest in young adults.
- The disease occurs more commonly in temperate climates, including the northern United States. This association is established by approximately age 15, and moving to or from a temperate climate after that age does not change it.

Source: National MS Society, 2005; Porth, 2005.

Pathophysiology

MS is believed to occur as a result of an autoimmune response to a prior viral infection in a genetically susceptible person. The infection, which is thought to occur early in life, activates T cells. T cells usually move in and out of the CNS across the blood–brain barrier, but for an unknown reason, they remain in the CNS in people with MS. The T cells facilitate infiltration by other leukocytes, and an inflammatory process follows. Inflammation destroys myelin and oligodendrocytes (myelin-producing cells), leading to axon dysfunction.

Myelin sheaths are fatty, segmented wrappings that normally protect and insulate nerve fibers and increase the speed of transmission of nerve impulses. In multiple sclerosis, these myelin sheaths of the white matter of the spinal cord, brain, and optic nerve are destroyed in patches, called *plaques,* along the axon (see *Pathophysiology Illustrated* on pages 1628–1629). The demyelination of nerve fibers slows and distorts the conduction of nerve impulses and sometimes results in the total absence of impulse transmission. The neurons usually affected by MS are located in the spinal cord, brainstem, cerebral and cerebellar areas, and the optic nerve.

Both plaques and diffuse lesions form as demyelinating lesions. Plaques typically are scattered through the white matter of the CNS, although they may extend into adjacent gray matter. Early manifestations are the result of inflammatory edema in and around the plaque and partial demyelination. These manifestations typically disappear within weeks after the initial episode. With progression of the disease, the demyelination and plaque formation result in scarring of glia (*gliosis*) and degeneration of axons. Continued loss of function leads to permanent disability, usually over about 20 years.

There are four classifications of MS: relapsing-remitting, primary progressive, secondary progressive, and progressive-relapsing (Box 46–2). Most individuals with MS present with the relapsing-remitting type.

Various stressors have been suggested as triggers for MS. These stressors include febrile states, pregnancy, extreme physical exertion, and fatigue. These precipitating factors can also cause a relapse of the manifestations during the course of the disease.

Manifestations

The manifestations of MS vary according to the areas destroyed by demyelination and the affected body system (see *Multisystems Effects of MS* on page 1630). Fatigue is one of the most disabling manifestations, and affects almost all clients

---

BOX 46–2 Classifications of Multiple Sclerosis

Relapsing-remitting: The most common clinical course of MS, characterized by exacerbations (acute attacks) with either full recovery or partial recovery with disability.

Primary progressive: Steady worsening of disease from the onset with occasional minor recovery.

Secondary progressive: Begins as with relapsing-remitting, but the disease steadily becomes worse between exacerbations.

Progressive-relapsing: This rare form continues to progress from the onset but also has exacerbations.

with MS. The manifestations, categorized by the established syndromes of MS, are listed in the box below.

Brief attacks of manifestations are described as short lived or paroxysmal. Short-lived attacks of neurologic deficits indicate the appearance or worsening of manifestations. Conditions that cause short-lived attacks include (1) minor increases in body temperature or serum calcium concentrations (both increase the leakage of current through demyelinated neurons) and (2) functional demands that exceed conduction capacity. Paroxysmal attacks are sensory or motor manifestations that occur abruptly and last for only seconds or minutes; the manifestations are paresthesias, dysarthria and ataxia, and tonic head turning. Paroxysmal attacks, which may occur many times a day, result from the direct transmission of nerve impulses between adjacent demyelinated axons.

INTERDISCIPLINARY CARE

Management of the client with MS varies according to the severity of the manifestations. The focus is on retaining the optimal level of functioning possible, given the degree of disability. Rehabilitation—physical, occupational/vocational, and psychosocial is a cornerstone of an interdisciplinary approach to treatment. During exacerbations, the focus of interventions shifts to controlling manifestations and quickly returning to remission.

Diagnosis

Diagnosis of MS is challenging because the disease does not present uniformly. A diagnosis requires that the client have one of the following: (1) two or more exacerbations separated by 1 month or more and lasting more than 24 hours, followed by recovery; (2) a history of repeated exacerbations and remissions with or without complete recovery, followed by progressively more severe manifestations lasting for 6 months or more; or (3) slowly increasing manifestations for at least 6 months.

Diagnostic tests vary with the presenting complaints. Magnetic resonance imaging (MRI) with findings of lesions is the most definitive test available; however, it is only one of several laboratory and diagnostic tests that may be performed when establishing the diagnosis. Other tests (described in Chapter 43 ∞) include:

- Cerebrospinal fluid (CSF) analysis reveals an increased number of T lymphocytes that are reactive with antigens, indicating the presence of an immune response in the client (but is not specific to MS). Of MS patients, 80% have elevated levels of immunoglobulin G (IgG) in the CSF.
- CT scan of the brain shows atrophy and white matter lesions. In about 25% of clients with MS, enlarged ventricles are visible on CT.
- Positron emission tomography (PET) scan measures brain activity. In MS clients, the scan reveals areas with changes in glucose metabolism.
- Evoked response testing of visual, auditory, or somatosensory impulses may show delayed conduction.

Medications

Medications slow the progression of MS and decrease the number of attacks. (See the Medication Administration box on page 1631.) Medications are used for a variety of reasons, including to treat manifestations, to modify the course of the disease, or to interrupt the progression of the disease.

The medications used during an exacerbation are aimed at decreasing inflammation to inhibit manifestations and induce remission. Frequently, a combination of adrenal corticosteroid hormone (ACTH) and glucocorticoids is used to decrease inflammation and suppress the immune system. Immunosuppressive agents, including azathioprine (Imuran) and cyclophosphamide (Cytoxan), are also used. Interferon and glatiramer acetate are used to reduce exacerbations in clients with relapsing-remitting MS. Interferon alpha, beta, and gamma (Roferon-A, Intron A, Wellferon, Infergen, Avonex or Rebif, Betaseron, Actimmune) enhance immune function, while glatiramer acetate (Copaxone) stimulates parts of the myelin basic protein to reduce the relapse rate of MS. Both drugs are given by injection and are usually well tolerated.

Other medications treat the manifestations of MS. Anticholinergics are administered for bladder spasticity; cholinergics

---

MANIFESTATIONS of Multiple Sclerosis

MIXED OR GENERALIZED TYPE (50% OF CASES)
- Visual deficits, with visual blurring, fogginess, or haziness; impaired color perception, decreased central visual acuity, area of diminished vision in the visual fields, acquired color vision deficit (especially to red and green), and an altered pupillary reaction to light.
- Brainstem lesions (cranial nerves III to XII) with nystagmus, dysarthria, deafness, vertigo, vomiting, tinnitus, facial weakness, decreased sensation, diplopia and eye pain; and cognitive dysfunctions involving concentration, short-term memory, word finding, and planning.
- Mood alterations are manifested as depression more often than euphoria.

SPINAL TYPE (25% OF CASES)
- Weakness and/or numbness in one or both extremities (most often the legs).
- Upper motor neuron involvement is manifested by stiffness, slowness, weakness (spastic paresis).
- Bladder dysfunctions include urgency, hesitancy, and incontinence.
- Bowel dysfunction is most often seen as constipation.
- Neurogenic impotence is noted.

CEREBELLAR TYPE (5% OF CASES)
- Manifestations of nystagmus, ataxia, and hyptonia.

AMAUROTIC FORM (5% OF CASES)
- Blindness

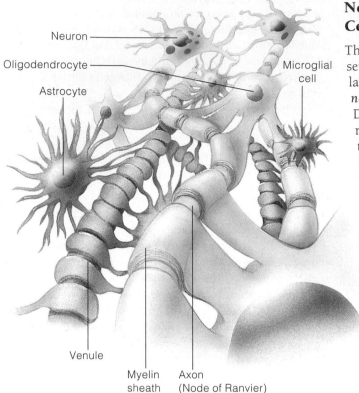

Neuron

Oligodendrocyte

Astrocyte

Microglial cell

Venule

Myelin sheath

Axon (Node of Ranvier)

Normal Anatomy of the Central Nervous System

The central nervous system (CNS) is composed of several cell types arranged in a dense, interconnected lattice. The basic functional cell of the CNS is the *neuron*, which transmits electrochemical impulses. Dendrites, thin projections extending from the neuron body, receive impulses that are passed down the neuronal axon for transmission to other cells. Myelin, a lipid-protein substance, surrounds the axons, insulating them and speeding nerve impulse transmission.

Neurons are surrounded by a network of cells:

- *Astrocytes* support neurons and connnect them to surrounding capillaries and venules.
- *Microglia* are motile phagocytic cells.
- *Oligodendrocytes* wrap concentric layers of myelin around nearby axons.

Acute Attack

Multiple sclerosis (MS) is a demyelinating disease in which axonal myelin in the central nervous system is eroded, destroyed, and replaced by scar tissue.

An autoimmune process apparently triggered by genetic and environmental factors is believed to cause inflammation of venules in the CNS. This disrupts the blood–brain barrier, allowing lymphocytes to enter CNS tissue. These lymphocytes proliferate and produce IgG, an antibody that attacks and damages myelin and causes the release of inflammatory chemicals and edema. As the inflammation subsides, the myelin regenerates and manifestations of the disease subside.

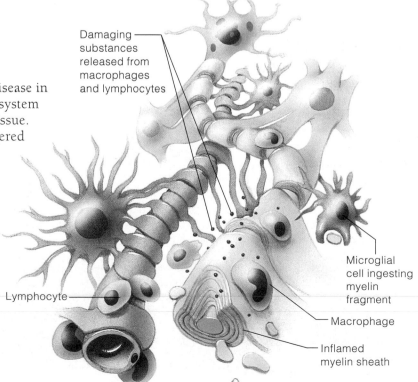

Damaging substances released from macrophages and lymphocytes

Microglial cell ingesting myelin fragment

Lymphocyte

Macrophage

Inflamed myelin sheath

Chronic Lesion

After repeated inflammatory attacks, myelin is irreparably damaged. Segments of axons become totally demyelinated and may degenerate. Astrocytes proliferate in damaged regions of the CNS (a process called *gliosis*), forming plaques. The plaques are scattered throughout the CNS, appearing as gray or pinkish lesions. The relapsing-remitting character of MS and the scattered areas of damage within the CNS account for the variable nature of MS manifestations.

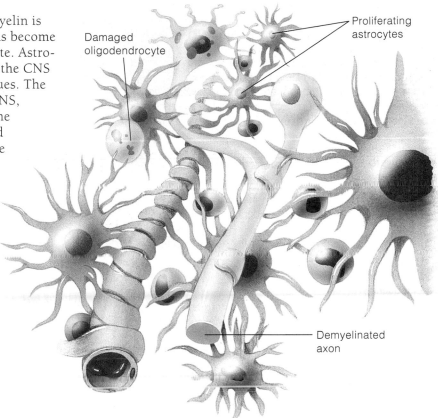

Damaged oligodendrocyte

Proliferating astrocytes

Demyelinated axon

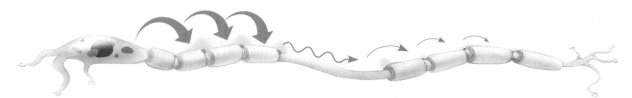

Abnormal Nerve Impulse Transmission

In an undamaged neuron, nerve impulses travel down the axon by "leaping" from one node of Ranvier to the next, thus greatly increasing the speed of impulse transmission. When nerve impulses travel down an axon damaged by MS, they are significantly slowed and weakened as they pass across the surface of demyelinated areas. Impulses may be blocked entirely when axons degenerate. The weakening or interruption of the transmission of nerve impulses and plaque formation within the CNS cause the manifestations of MS, including extremity weakness, paresthesias, visual disturbances, bladder dysfunction, and vertigo.

are given if the client has a problem with urinary retention related to flaccid bladder. Depression is treated with antidepressant drugs.

Surgery

Surgery may be indicated for clients who experience severe spasticity and deformity. However, physical therapy can prevent most severe problems. Foot drop from severe plantar flexion can be relieved with an Achilles tenotomy, a surgical procedure in which the Achilles tendon is transected.

Nutrition and Fluids

Several diets involving manipulation of fats are currently under investigation. Clients with MS may be overweight because of their inability to ambulate; depression may contribute to the problem because people who are depressed tend to eat more. Ideally, the client should maintain a weight as close as possible to that recommended for the client's height and body type.

As MS progresses, the client's ability to prepare food and eat is compromised. Changes in muscle tone, tremor, weakness, and ataxia all contribute to nutritional problems. Dysphagia also is a common problem. The diet must be adapted to accommodate changes in the client's ability to chew and swallow.

Rehabilitation

Physical and rehabilitative therapies are tailored to the client's level of functioning. The long-term goal is to enable the client to retain as much independence as possible. One major intervention is to maintain and increase existing muscle strength.

Spasticity is managed with stretching exercises, gait training, and braces, splints, or other assistive devices. To maintain balance, the client is encouraged to widen the base of support by standing with the feet slightly further apart. Walkers and canes may be weighted to provide support and balance for the ataxic client.

An interdisciplinary approach to rehabilitation will provide supportive services: speech therapy for problems with phonation, occupational therapy to maintain strength in the upper extremities and carry out ADLs, and occupational counseling. Referrals to a urologist are indicated for problems with urinary incontinence, urinary tract infections, retention, and impotence. Consultation with a respiratory therapist may be needed if the client develops chronic respiratory infections from inability to cough, move secretions, or breathe deeply, especially with increased debilitation.

NURSING CARE

Because the disease most often affects young adults in the prime of life, the psychosocial and economic effect can be devastating. People with MS have to make adjustments to the body image changes while simultaneously adapting to the altered relationships and decreased earnings usually encountered with the disease. A once-healthy spouse becomes wheelchair bound; a person once independent may eventually become dependent for even the most basic ADLs. The unpredictable course of MS is a challenge for long-term planning. A Nursing Care Plan for the client with MS is given on the next page.

Health Promotion

Following an overview of the disorder, the client needs to understand how to prevent fatigue and exacerbations. Teach the client to avoid stress, extremes of cold and heat, high humidity, physical overexertion, and infections. Because pregnancy can exacerbate manifestations, counseling about this risk is indicated. Also, address preventive measures to avoid risk of respiratory and urinary tract infections.

Assessment

Collect the following data through the health history and physical examination (see Chapter 43 ∞):

- *Health history:* History of childhood viral illnesses, geographical residence when a child, exposure to physical or emotional stressors (pregnancy/delivery, extremes of heat), medications, symptom onset, severity of manifestations.
- *Physical assessment:* Affect, mood, speech, eye movements, gait, tremors, vision and hearing, reflexes, muscle strength and movement, sensation.

Nursing Diagnoses and Interventions

Interventions for the client with MS vary with the acuity of exacerbations and the presenting problems. Many nursing diagnoses relate to the inability to perform ADLs, for example, *Self-Care Deficit* and *Impaired Home Maintenance*. Others reflect problems with musculoskeletal changes or altered nerve conduction, for example, *Impaired Physical Mobility, Ineffective Breathing Pattern, Constipation,* and *Functional Urinary Incontinence*. The nursing diagnoses discussed in this section are *Fatigue* and *Self-Care Deficit*.

Fatigue

Fatigue is defined by NANDA as an overwhelming sustained sense of exhaustion and decreased capacity for physical and mental work at the usual level. Fatigue affects every aspect of the MS client's life: the ability to remain independent and perform self-care, sexual function, mobility, airway clearance, and ultimately self-concept and coping. A great deal of teaching is needed to help the client and family understand fatigue and how to adapt. Clients and families need assistance managing fatigue in a society in which energy is highly valued.

- Assess degree of fatigue and identify contributing factors. *Fatigue is a subjective experience that needs to be evaluated thoroughly before planning can begin.*
- Arrange daily activities to include rest periods. *Rest is essential to manage feelings of fatigue; periods of relaxation may help replenish energy reserves.*

> **PRACTICE ALERT**
> *It is important to remember that the fatigue from chronic illnesses such as MS is very different from being "tired," and that rest and sleep may not result in improvement.*

- Ask the client to consider which activities are really necessary and to set priorities. *Prioritizing activities promotes independence and self-control.*

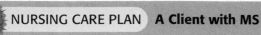

NURSING CARE PLAN   A Client with MS

George McMurphy, a 45-year-old from northern Minnesota, was diagnosed with MS approximately 5 years ago. He states that he probably had mild symptoms as long ago as 10 years. He works as a manager for a large grocery store chain near his home. He lives at home with his wife and two children, ages 12 and 15. Recently, Mr. McMurphy has had increasing problems with urinary incontinence, lack of energy, weakness, extreme fatigue, and altered mobility from spasticity in his leg muscles. He also has a fever, chest congestion, and a cough productive of green sputum. He is admitted to the hospital for evaluation and treatment of pneumonia and exacerbation of his MS.

ASSESSMENT

Denise Miller, RN, primary care nurse, is assigned to care for Mr. McMurphy. His major complaint is the inability to "bring up all this sputum; I feel rotten from being so congested. I hate not being able to get to work and for my wife having to tend to my personal needs." Vital signs are as follows: BP 134/84, P 94, R 30, T 102°F (38.8°C). Mr. McMurphy is admitted for an acute exacerbation of the disorder, probably triggered by pneumonia. He will be treated with ACTH and intravenous antibiotics during this admission.

DIAGNOSES

- *Ineffective Airway Clearance* related to lung infection and thick mucus
- *Activity Intolerance* related to fatigue and spasticity
- *Self Care Deficit: Toileting, Feeding, and Grooming* related to muscle weakness

EXPECTED OUTCOMES

- Be able to clear airway.
- Have breath sounds clear to auscultation and pulse oximetry readings above 95%.
- Be able to ambulate using assistive devices, if needed.
- Perform self-care activities without becoming overly fatigued and tired.
- Verbalize methods to adapt daily routine to his level of tolerance.

PLANNING AND IMPLEMENTATION

- Initiate pulmonary hygiene measures (e.g., incentive spirometry, turning, deep breathing and coughing, breathing exercises, and postural drainage) at least every 2 hours. Assess lung sounds, oxygen saturation, and ability to clear airway.

- Teach the importance of maintaining an oral fluid intake of at least 2000 mL per day to prevent tenacious sputum and urinary tract infections. Teach signs and symptoms of urinary and respiratory infections.
- Encourage participation in decision making about care.
- Assist with ADLs only as needed, based on level of fatigue and muscle weakness.
- Plan self-care activities so that they are performed during periods of peak level of energy; intersperse rest periods throughout the day.
- Refer to an MS support group.
- Refer to physical and occupational therapists for counseling regarding control of spasticity and possible splinting of spastic muscles.
- Consult a urologist for assessment of bladder incontinence; teach intermittent catheterization. Alternatively, the use of an external condom catheter may be indicated.

EVALUATION

Mr. McMurphy is discharged 3 days following admission. He states that he feels stronger; on discharge, he has no problem clearing his airway. Although he continues to pace his activities to avoid fatigue, his muscle strength and "tiredness" have improved. He is able to complete ADLs unassisted.

Pulmonary function has returned to normal prehospitalization levels: ABGs and pulse oximetry are within normal limits. Both Mr. McMurphy and his wife have listed several ways to modify their daily routine to allow more rest and decreased stress. Follow-up visits to his primary care physician have been arranged, and they have been provided with information about the local MS support group.

CRITICAL THINKING IN THE NURSING PROCESS

1. Describe approaches the nurse could take to ensure that Mr. McMurphy does not exceed his activity tolerance.
2. Develop a teaching plan for Mr. McMurphy to help prevent future respiratory infections.
3. Develop a care plan for Mr. McMurphy for the nursing diagnosis *Risk for Injury* related to fatigue, muscle weakness, and spasticity.

See Evaluating Your Response in Appendix C.

- Suggest performing tasks in the morning hours. *Biorhythm studies indicate that people usually have greater energy reserves in the morning hours and diminished reserves in the afternoon.*
- Advise to avoid temperature extremes, such as hot showers or exposure to cold. *Maintaining a relatively constant body temperature may avoid exacerbation of the disorder. Heat can delay impulse transmission across demyelinated nerves, which contributes to fatigue.*
- Refer to the appropriate professionals to manage fatigue: stress management groups, support groups, occupational or physical therapist, as indicated. *Support groups and therapy can facilitate self-management and improve coping.*

Self-Care Deficit

Clients with MS may need assistance with bathing, toileting, dressing, grooming, and feeding. The help needed can range from minimal guidance to total dependence. The client's ability to perform self-care activities is the gauge by which family members and caregivers need to adjust assistance. Self-care encompasses both the decisions about care and the provision of care; most clients are capable of making decisions even after physical limitations prevent physical self-care. The need to maintain self-determination cannot be overemphasized and must be incorporated into each intervention. As the client with MS ages, there may be even more need for teaching to provide self-care, as described in the Nursing Research box on the next page.

NURSING CARE PLAN A Client with PD

Walter Avneil, age 78, was diagnosed with PD at age 64. His wife died 5 years ago and he has no other family living. Mr. Avneil worked for more than 40 years as a mechanic in a large factory. He is a resident of a long-term care facility. During his last clinic visit for a review of his medications, the following assessment was made.

ASSESSMENT

White male with history of PD for the past 14 years. Skin oily and damp. Tremors in both hands and the lips. Gait is slow and shuffling, with a forward leaning posture. Speech slow and slurred. Face expressionless. Has lost 10 lb since last visit 3 months ago. Has been on levodopa with carbidopa since diagnosis. States major problems are "eating problems, bowel problems, walking problems."

DIAGNOSIS

- *Constipation* related to lack of exercise, decreased food intake, and effects of medications
- *Impaired Verbal Communication* related to lip tremors, slow/slurred speech, and facial muscle involvement of PD
- *Imbalanced Nutrition: Less than Body Requirements* related to difficulty swallowing and chewing
- *Impaired Physical Mobility* related to rigidity and bradykinesia

EXPECTED OUTCOMES

- Have a soft stool at least every other day.
- Practice exercises provided by speech therapist twice a day.
- Increase number of calories, fluids, and fiber in diet provided at long-term facility.
- Improve joint mobility and ability to ambulate.

PLANNING AND IMPLEMENTATION

- Discuss problems with bowel elimination with staff at long-term facility; suggest increasing fluids to 3000 mL per day and also increasing fiber in the diet with oatmeal for breakfast, and more fruits and vegetables at meals.
- Encourage exercises provided by speech therapist to improve speech and swallowing. If these are not effective, make a referral for another evaluation.

- Discuss diet plan with dietitian at the long-term care facility, including consistency of foods and number of calories. Suggest dietitian be a part of swallowing evaluation by the speech therapist.
- Refer for physical therapy and occupational therapy for a program to improve gait and joint mobility, and to decrease risk of falling.

EVALUATION

In a return visit 3 months later, Mr. Avneil reports that "my bowels are working better." He has gained 7 lb, and the staff report that this is related to multiple factors, including practicing his swallowing exercises, getting more exercise that stimulated his appetite, and changing his diet to six small meals a day of soft or pureed foods. The staff is offering him liquids at meals and snack times, and he usually drinks all they give him. His speech is not much improved. His posture and gait are somewhat better, and he is doing the exercises provided by the physical therapist and occupational therapist. Mr. Avneil's functional abilities have improved so much that the staff is considering training sessions specific to care of residents with PD.

CRITICAL THINKING IN THE NURSING PROCESS

1. Although Mr. Avneil did not mention it, the staff reports that he is frustrated by not being able to dress himself. What suggestions could you make to facilitate his independence?
2. Mr. Avneil spends most of his time alone, although he enjoys the company of the other residents. List assessments and interventions you might provide to increase his diversional activity.
3. The loss of his wife and the debilitating effects of his disease increase Mr. Avneil's risk for the nursing diagnosis of *Chronic Sorrow*. What might you suggest the long-term staff do to reduce this risk?

See Evaluating Your Response in Appendix C.

- *Health history:* Brain trauma, stroke, infection, exposure to heavy metals or carbon monoxide, medication and drug use, incontinence, constipation, weight loss, sweating, sleep problems, muscle pain, mood.
- *Physical assessment:* Affect; appearance; speech, scalp, eyelashes, and skin; drooling; tremor; coordination; posture; gait; muscle rigidity; mental status.

Nursing Diagnoses and Interventions

Clients with PD have complex and, ultimately, multisystem needs. Deficits in mobility and self-care are common. Psychosocial needs may include problems related to *Ineffective Coping*, *Powerlessness*, and *Disturbed Body Image*. Refer to the nursing care sections throughout this chapter for discussions of fatigue, self-care deficit, ineffective airway clearance, and other pertinent diagnoses. This section focuses on the nursing diagnoses related to impaired physical mobility, impaired verbal communication, imbalanced nutrition, and disturbed sleep pattern.

Impaired Physical Mobility

Clients with PD have impaired mobility for several reasons, including tremors, gait pattern disturbances, and alterations in body positioning, such as forward bending of the trunk. Poor self-esteem may contribute to the client's lack of motivation and willingness to be mobile.

- Suggest referral to a physical therapist to develop an individualized exercise program. *A program specific to the client supplies motivation as well as helping the client maintain muscle tone, flexibility, and mobility.*
- Request the physical therapist teach caregivers how to do ROM exercises at least twice a day, emphasizing the trunk, neck, arms, hips, and legs. *Maintaining joint mobility promotes better function and strength, improving gait pattern. Consistent ROM exercises can prevent contractures.*
- Ask caregivers to ambulate the client at least four times a day if possible. *Exercise fosters independence and self-esteem.*

- Recommend assistive devices, such as lift chairs, canes, splints, or braces, as indicated. *Adaptive equipment improves balance, protects joints, and promotes proper anatomic positioning.*
- To promote mobility and safety:
  - Slightly elevate the back legs of chairs and raise the toilet seat to help rise from a sitting position to a standing position.
  - Wear shoes with Velcro closures.
  - Remove potential hazards, such as unanchored throw rugs.
  - Install handrails and nonskid surfaces in bath tubs and showers.
  - Ensure adequate lighting throughout the home and in outside areas, especially in areas where transfers are common.
  Safety measures prevent potential complications that may result from falls or other accidents and promote self-esteem through self-care.

> ## PRACTICE ALERT
> *Parkinson's disease is a disorder common in older adults, who are at greater risk for falls resulting from orthostatic hypotension, osteoporosis, poor vision, and other problems causing disorientation and confusion, such as Alzheimer's disease.*

Impaired Verbal Communication

Diminished vocal amplitude and loss of muscular control can impair the client's ability to speak. Both caregivers and family members must remember to give clients enough time for self-expression; an unhurried approach is recommended. Seek input from family members when determining alternative methods of communicating with the client.

- Assess current communication abilities in speech, hearing, and writing. *Communication involves both sending and receiving messages.*
- Develop methods of communication appropriate to coordination abilities, such as a magic slate; flash cards with common phrases; pointing to objects. *Individualizing a method of communication decreases anxiety and isolation.*
- Suggest referral to a speech pathologist to develop oral exercises and interventions that will facilitate speaking. *The muscles of speech and swallowing are affected by the Parkinson's disease process.*
- Remind client to speak more loudly, if possible. *A low, monotonous voice is characteristic of the client with Parkinson's disease.*

Imbalanced Nutrition:
Less than Body Requirements

Tremors, altered gait, and impaired chewing and swallowing can cause nutritional problems in the client with PD. As the disorder progresses, interventions for ensuring optimal nutrition need to be adapted to the client's functional abilities. Assess the client's swallow reflex before starting any feeding program. During the initial stages of the disorder, some clients may have the nursing diagnosis *Imbalanced Nutrition: More than Body Requirements* if kilocalorie intake exceeds energy expenditure.

- Assess nutritional status and self-feeding abilities; suggest referral to an occupational or speech therapist, if needed. *An initial assessment of abilities ensures that interventions are personalized to the client's current functional abilities.*
- Teach caregivers how to prepare foods of proper consistency as determined by swallowing function. *The client may aspirate food that is too liquid.*
- Weigh weekly. *Early recognition of weight loss allows for intervention.*
- Teach eating methods to decrease tremors, such as holding a piece of bread in the hand that is not holding an eating utensil. *Nonintention tremor may be reduced through purposeful activity.*
- Encourage diet that is high in bulk and fluids. *Several anti-Parkinson's medications and inactivity can cause constipation.*

Disturbed Sleep Pattern

Rigidity and weakness can cause clients with Parkinson's disease to lose the ability to move and change positions during sleep. The resulting discomfort causes periods of wakefulness. Medications to treat Parkinson's disease contribute to sleep pattern disturbance; for example, levodopa can cause vivid dreams. Nurses can help accurately assess the sleep pattern disturbance and in planning interventions to improve or increase sleep time.

- Assess sleep pattern and existing conditions that may affect sleep, such as depression or pain. *Clients experiencing anxiety, depression, and dementia have a difficult time falling asleep and may wake up more at night.*

> ## PRACTICE ALERT
> Remember to assess pain status; lack of adequate pain control may interfere with sleep.

- Explain the disease process and the effects of decreased dopamine on the sleep–wake cycle. *Depending on the dosage, levodopa causes less REM sleep and deep sleep.*
- Review the client's medication. *Bromocriptine and levodopa, especially if used with an anticholinergic, can cause vivid dreams. Other medications (diuretics, theophylline, hypnotics) also may interfere with sleep.*
- Teach how to modify lifestyle activities that affect sleep:
  - Institute a routine of activities with limited rest periods during the day; avoid napping close to bedtime. Avoid strenuous exercise in the evening. *Daytime sleeping may contribute to decreased nighttime sleeping. Vigorous exercise just before bedtime may act as a stimulant.*
  - Incorporate diet modifications, such as limiting caffeine and alcohol intake. *Caffeine is a stimulant, and alcohol may cause early morning awakenings, increased daytime sleepiness, and nightmares.*
  - Drink a glass of milk before bedtime. *Milk contains L-tryptophan, which produces sedative effects by shortening the time taken to fall asleep (sleep latency).*
  - Adapt the environment to aid in sleep (e.g., darken the room and decrease noises). *Reducing environmental stimuli decreases external sleep disturbances.*

Using NANDA, NIC, and NOC

Chart 46–3 shows links between NANDA nursing diagnoses, NIC, and NOC when caring for the client with PD.

Community-Based Care

It is important for both the client and the family to maintain independence and self-care as long as possible. To maintain function and quality of life, the following topics should be addressed:

- Realistic expectations
- Equipment suppliers
- Home environment conducive to using equipment
- Referrals to speech therapist, occupational therapist, physical therapist, and dietitian
- Gait training and exercises for improving ambulation, speech, swallowing, and self-care
- Increased fluid intake of 3000 mL/day and increased fiber in every meal
- Stool softeners or laxatives as needed for bowel elimination
- Swallowing during eating and taking medications (Have suction equipment available and know the Heimlich maneuver if choking occurs.)
- Foods that can be easily swallowed (such as pureed or soft) and feed six small meals a day if possible

---

NANDA, NIC, AND NOC LINKAGES

CHART 46–3 **The Client with Parkinson's Disease**

NANDA

Impaired Physical Mobility

↓

NIC

Energy Management

Fall Prevention

Surveillance: Safety

Self-Care Assistance

↓

NOC

Coordinated Movement

Balance

Fall Prevention Behavior

Self-Care: Activities of Daily Living (ADL)

Data from *NANDA's Nursing Diagnoses: Definitions & Classification 2005–2006* by NANDA International (2003), Philadelphia; *Nursing Interventions Classification (NIC)* (4th ed.) by J. M. Dochterman & G. M. Bulechek (2004), St. Louis, MO: Mosby; and *Nursing Outcomes Classification (NOC)* (3rd ed.) by S. Moorhead, M. Johnson, and M. Maas (2004), St. Louis, MO: Mosby.

- Helpful resources:
  - American Parkinson's Disease Association
  - National Parkinson Foundation, Inc.
  - Parkinson's Disease Foundation
  - The National Institute of Neurological Disorders and Stroke.

THE CLIENT WITH HUNTINGTON'S DISEASE

Huntington's disease (HD) is a progressive, degenerative, inherited neurologic disease characterized by increasing dementia and chorea (jerky, rapid, involuntary movements). It is a single-gene autosomal-dominant inherited disease that causes localized death of neurons of the basal ganglia (Porth, 2005). The exact cause is unknown, but postmortem studies have demonstrated a decrease in gamma-aminobutyric acid (GABA), an inhibitory neurotransmitter in the basal ganglia. There is also a decrease in acetylcholine levels, suggesting that the manifestations are the result of an imbalance in dopamine and acetylcholine. HD is a familial disease; each child of an HD parent has a 50% chance of inheriting the HD gene and, if so, will eventually develop the disease (NINDS, 2005f). There is no cure for the disease. Huntington's disease causes progressive chorea, speech problems, and dementia.

Because the client is usually asymptomatic until age 30 to 40, he or she may already have passed the gene to the next generation. The psychologic effect is devastating to clients and their families. The family not only experiences guilt from passing the disease from one generation to the next, but also is faced with the overwhelming long-term care needs of those affected. It is common for several family members to have the disease.

Pathophysiology

Huntington's disease causes destruction of cells in the caudate nucleus and putamen areas of the basal ganglia. Other areas of the brain, such as the frontal lobes, may selectively atrophy. Several neurotransmitters and their receptors are decreased, including GABA and acetylcholine. The neurotransmitter dopamine is not affected in Huntington's disease, but the decrease in acetylcholine results in a relative excess of dopamine in the basal ganglia. Whereas in Parkinson's disease a deficit of dopamine causes slow movement or lack of movement, in Huntington's disease the opposite occurs: There is a relative excess of dopamine, causing excessive, uncontrolled movement.

Manifestations

Manifestations and complications primarily involve abnormal movement and progressive dementia (see the box on the next page). The progression and sequence of manifestations varies somewhat; however, initially the psychologic manifestations are more debilitating than the choreiform (rapid and jerky) movements.

Early signs of personality change include severe depression, memory loss with decreased ability to concentrate, emotional lability, and impulsiveness. The client experiences frequent mood swings ranging from uncontrollable periods of anger to

MANIFESTATIONS AND COMPLICATIONS
of Huntington's Disease

MOTOR EFFECTS

Early
- Restlessness
- "Fidgety" feeling
- Minor gait changes—unsteady on feet
- Posture and positioning disturbances, frequent falls
- Inability to keep the tongue from protruding
- Slurred speech with poor articulation
- Complications: increasing problem with self-care activities, such as bathing, grooming, eating

Late
- Chorea—severely altered gait with irregular, uncontrollable movement; shoulders shrug arrhythmically
- Facial grimacing—raising of eyebrows, uncontrollable protrusion of the tongue
- Dysphagia
- Unintelligible speech
- Impaired diaphragmatic movement
- Complications: immobility, aspiration, choking, and, eventually, total dependence, poor oxygenation, emaciation, and cachexia

PSYCHOSOCIAL EFFECTS

Early
- Irritability
- Outbursts of rage alternating with euphoria
- Depression
- Complication: suicide

Late
- Decreasing memory
- Loss of cognitive skills
- Eventual dementia
- Complication: total dependence

apathy. Eventually, signs of dementia, including disorientation, confusion, and lack of sense of time, become evident and interfere with self-care.

Motor manifestations usually parallel personality and mood changes. The motor manifestations worsen with environmental stimuli and emotional stress but are absent when the client is sleeping. Initially, movement problems are described as "fidgeting" or restlessness, followed by progressive worsening of abnormal movements. The choreiform movements, which begin in the face and arms and then involve the entire body, are manifested by facial grimaces, tongue protrusion, jerky movement of the distal arms or legs, and a rhythmic, lurching gait that almost resembles a dance. (The term *chorea* comes from *choreia,* the Greek word meaning "dance.") Gait changes cause uncoordinated movements and contribute to frequent falls.

The muscles of swallowing, chewing, and speaking are affected, leading to dysphagia and dysarthria and associated problems with communication and nutrition. The client's constant movement and difficulty in swallowing contribute to

weight loss and eventual cachexia. Breathing is impaired because the diaphragm is unable to move effectively.

The manifestations slowly progress over approximately 15 to 20 years after initial manifestations appear. Prognosis is poor, with inevitable debilitation and total dependence. Death usually results from aspiration pneumonia or another infectious process.

INTERDISCIPLINARY CARE

There is no cure for Huntington's disease, and treatment addresses the disease's manifestations. Nurses provide care to clients with Huntington's disease in a variety of community settings. Initially, clients and families can manage care needs at home, but as the disease progresses, the client requires constant supervision, such as that provided in day care facilities. Eventually, skilled long-term care is needed. Clients who develop acute problems may be hospitalized until the crisis is managed. Because of the inevitable total multisystem debilitation of clients with Huntington's disease, nurses and other caregivers face many challenges.

Diagnosis
Genetic testing is the only test available to diagnose clients suspected of having Huntington's disease. Both blood and amniotic fluid may be tested for the presence of a gene mutation on chromosome 4 using DNA analysis. The test can predict with 95% accuracy which offspring have the disease.

Medications
The following medications are given for the manifestations of Huntington's disease:
- Antipsychotics, specifically phenothiazines and butyrophenones, are effective in Huntington's disease because they block dopamine receptors in the brain. The therapeutic goal is to restore the balance among the neurotransmitters.
- Antidepressants are prescribed in the early stage of the disease; however, medications are no substitute for intense follow-up counseling for clients and families.

NURSING CARE

Nurses are faced with a multitude of challenges when caring for families who have Huntington's disease, including physiologic, psychosocial, and ethical problems. Physiologic problems are related to the progressive and eventually debilitating nature of the disease. Psychosocial concerns occur as a result of the client's personality and mental changes, the family's responsibility for providing care, and the guilt implicit in a genetically transmitted disease. Ethical difficulties relate to the genetic nature of the disease: DNA testing for the marker on chromosome 4 can determine whether the person is a carrier of the disease before he or she begins to exhibit manifestations. Children of people with Huntington's disease are thus faced with the choice of finding out whether they will eventually be affected. If they choose not to be tested, they may pass the disease on to yet another generation; and if a fetus is affected, they may face the decision of whether to undergo an abortion.

Nursing Diagnoses and Interventions

Initially, much of the nursing care focuses on teaching about the disease, psychologic support, and genetic counseling. As manifestations become more severe, nursing considerations center on problems related not only to immobility and altered nutrition, but also to the increasing self-care deficits. Families and clients experiencing Huntington's disease face many psychosocial issues. Nurses must be prepared to listen actively as well as to provide comfort and encouragement throughout the lengthy illness. There are many possible nursing diagnoses for the client with Huntington's disease; this section focuses on nursing diagnoses related to aspiration, nutrition, skin integrity, and communication.

Risk for Aspiration

Uncoordinated movements and swallowing and chewing problems put the client at high risk for aspiration.

- Maintain in an upright position while the client eats; support the head. *Proper positioning may prevent aspiration during mealtime.*
- Teach the Heimlich maneuver to caregivers and family members. *Aspiration is a real possibility; caregivers must be prepared to reestablish the client's airway.*
- Provide food that is thick enough to manage, such as thick soups, mashed potatoes, stews, or casseroles. *These foods are more readily tolerated and manipulated by the tongue than liquids.*
- Make sure food is swallowed before giving another spoonful of food. *The automatic phase of swallowing may be disrupted in the client with Huntington's disease; providing adequate time and smaller bites may improve the ability to manipulate foods.*
- Provide a calm, relaxing eating environment. *Stress worsens choreiform movements and inappropriate behaviors.*

Imbalanced Nutrition:
Less than Body Requirements

Clients with Huntington's disease have unpredictable choreiform movements of the extremities and decreased ability to control muscles involved with chewing and swallowing. Families and caregivers are challenged to provide sufficient calories to maintain the client in positive nitrogen balance.

- Evaluate current weight and nutritional status, including serum prealbumin and transferrin levels. *Establishing a baseline is crucial for meeting individual caloric, protein, vitamin, and mineral needs.*
- Assess ability to swallow and manipulate eating utensils. *Aspiration is an ever-present danger that must be avoided; utensils may need to be adapted to client's abilities, if client is able to assist at all.*
- Continue feeding even if the client physically turns away from the meal. *Involuntary choreiform movements should not be interpreted as a refusal to eat.*
- Provide high-kilocalorie, nutritious foods and sufficient snacks; request input from a dietitian. *The constant movement of Huntington's disease increases caloric requirements.*

- Avoid milk; provide frequent oral hygiene. *Milk tends to thicken secretions. Decreasing thick secretions may improve ability to swallow and enable the client to ingest more calories.*

Impaired Skin Integrity

Skin integrity is only one component of the client's general need for protection and avoidance of injury. Several factors increase the risk for impaired skin integrity, including poor nutritional status, eventual total immobility, and incontinence.

- Evaluate the skin for actual and potential areas of breakdown. *Establishing a baseline is necessary to modify care and provide prophylactic protection of high-risk pressure areas.*
- Determine nutritional status, especially serum prealbumin level and vitamin, mineral, and kilocalorie intake. *Optimal nutritional status and positive nitrogen balance help prevent skin breakdown and formation of pressure ulcers.*
- Turn and inspect the skin at least every 2 hours, giving special consideration to areas that are most prone to breakdown, such as heels and coccyx. *Pressure points are particularly susceptible to skin breakdown.*
- Provide ROM exercises on a regular schedule in the daytime. *Movement stimulates circulation, which provides oxygenation and allows nutrients to reach muscles and skin.*
- Keep the skin clean and dry; pay particular attention to the perineal area if incontinent. *Skin in close proximity to the perineal area, such as the sacral area, is highly susceptible to breakdown due to exposure to wet, acidic urine and fecal material.*
- Place on an alternating-pressure mattress with foot board. *Decreasing pressure on bony prominences and preventing shearing forces serve to prevent skin breakdown.*
- Pad side rails and headrests of special chairs; have the client wear a football-type helmet. *The client's violent movements can cause trauma to the head and extremities.*

Impaired Verbal Communication

The inability to control muscles related to speech, swallowing, and facial movement contributes to problems of verbal communication. Because Huntington's disease affects fine motor movement, especially the distal portion of the extremities, the hands are not effective in communication. As the disease progresses, mental abilities are also compromised, making both receptive and expressive communication impossible.

- Choose alternative methods of communication while the client is able to participate. *Anticipatory planning may facilitate communication and decrease anxiety.*
- Continue to incorporate therapeutic communication techniques, even though client is not responsive: Maintain eye contact, use touch, and talk directly to the client rather than to others in the room. *These techniques enhance the individual's dignity and worth.*
- Seek input from family about client's usual preferences and how they are communicated; be alert for subtle cues. *Nonverbal communication techniques may be individualized and more readily recognized by the family member or caregiver who usually provides care.*

- Continue talking to the client, even though there is no apparent response. *Hearing may not be impaired, even though the client cannot speak.*

Community-Based Care

Clients with Huntington's disease and their families may know how devastating the illness is because they may have cared for a parent or other close family member who had the illness. Many families are overwhelmed with just the thought of the physical and psychosocial debilitation that the disease brings. Fear, anxiety, and hopelessness leading to depression are common reactions. Teaching ways to cope effectively with the psychosocial and physical changes is an integral part of the nurse's responsibilities. Referrals to appropriate agencies, such as adult day care centers, the Huntington's Disease Foundation, and local support groups or a psychologist should be part of the nursing plan.

Another aspect of client teaching concerns the genetic transmission of Huntington's disease; refer clients and family members to a geneticist. Nurses are frequently involved with clarifying information, especially concerning the transmission, course of illness, and prognosis. A caring, sensitive approach is crucial. Information about transmission of an autosomal-dominant trait is discussed in Chapter 8 ∞ .

THE CLIENT WITH AMYOTROPHIC LATERAL SCLEROSIS

Amyotrophic lateral sclerosis (ALS), or *Lou Gehrig's disease,* is a rapidly progressive and fatal degenerative neurologic disease characterized by weakness and wasting of muscles under voluntary control, without any accompanying sensory or cognitive changes. The name is derived from the pathophysiologic processes of muscle atrophy (*amyotrophy*) resulting from lower motor neuron involvement and sclerosis of the corticospinal tract in the lateral column of the spinal cord resulting from upper motor neuron involvement. Death results in 2 to 5 years after onset of the manifestations (although some people live 10 years or more), usually due to respiratory failure.

ALS is the most common motor neuron disease in the United States. As many as 20,000 people in the United States have ALS, and approximately 5000 new cases are diagnosed each year. In up to 90% to 95% of cases, the disease occurs at random without clearly associated risk factors. About 5% to 10% of all cases are inherited in what is termed familial ALS (NINDS, 2005a).

Most people are between 40 and 60 years of age at diagnosis; the incidence is higher in men in the earlier ages but becomes equal with women after menopause. Most of the health problems a client with ALS encounters are related to swallowing and managing secretions, communication, and dysfunction of the muscles used in respiration.

Pathophysiology

ALS results from the degeneration and demyelination of both upper and lower motor neurons in the anterior horn of the spinal cord, brainstem, and cerebral cortex. Death of the motor neurons results in axonal degeneration, demyelination, glial proliferation, and scarring along the corticospinal tract. In the early stages of the disease, surviving motor neurons sprout new branches to reinnervate affected muscle fibers, preserving muscle strength. However, when more than half of the lower motor neurons are affected, reinnervation fails and weakness is evidenced.

Although the pathogenesis of ALS is not clear, abnormal glutamate metabolism and hydrogen peroxide production are being studied. Echovirus RNA has also been isolated in spinal cord tissue in some clients with nonfamilial ALS. Environmental factors, excess intracellular calcium, and antibodies to calcium channels are also being researched.

Manifestations

The initial manifestations may relate to dysfunction of upper motor neurons, lower motor neurons, or both. Dysfunction of upper motor neurons results in spastic, weak muscles with increased deep tendon reflexes. Dysfunction of lower motor neurons results in muscle flaccidity, paresis (weakness), paralysis, and atrophy.

Weakness and paresis are common early manifestations. The weakness may initially affect only one muscle group. Manifestations vary according to the particular muscle group involved; *fasciculations* (twitching) of involved muscles are common in the early stage of the disorder. With the loss of muscle innervation, the muscles atrophy, and paralysis results. Muscle mass decreases, and clients complain of progressive fatigue. Typically, the disease first affects the hands, then the shoulders, upper arms, and finally the legs.

Increasing brainstem involvement causes progressive atrophy of the tongue and facial muscles with eventual dysphagia and dysarthria. Emotional lability and loss of control occur, but dementia is not part of the pathologic progression of ALS. Vision, hearing, sensation, and cognitive ability usually remain intact. A summary of manifestations and complications is presented in the box on the next page.

INTERDISCIPLINARY CARE

Because many treatable disorders may cause manifestations similar to those that appear in the initial stage of ALS, a thorough evaluation is required. Once ALS is diagnosed, the primary goal is to support the client and family in meeting physical and psychosocial needs, particularly as the disease progresses.

Medical and nursing care for clients with ALS is primarily supportive. Referral for home health management is indicated. Occupational, physical, speech, and respiratory therapy are major supportive and rehabilitative treatments. As the disorder progresses and swallowing becomes ineffective, a gastrostomy tube may be necessary to provide adequate nutritional intake. Ventilatory assistance should be discussed with clients before the need occurs.

Diagnosis

There is no specific test to diagnose ALS. Rather, diagnosis is made based on manifestations and tests to rule out other diseases. A number of disorders may mimic early ALS, including

MANIFESTATIONS AND COMPLICATIONS of ALS

MUSCULOSKELETAL SYSTEM
- Weakness and fatigue
- "Heaviness" of legs
- Fasciculations
- Uncoordinated movements, loss of fine motor control in hands
- Spasticity
- Paresis
- Hyperreflexia
- Atrophy
- Problems with articulation
- Complications: paralysis, loss of ability to perform ADLs, total immobility, aspiration, loss of verbal communication

RESPIRATORY SYSTEM
- Dyspnea
- Difficulty clearing airway
- Complications: pneumonia, eventual respiratory failure

NUTRITIONAL EFFECTS
- Difficulty chewing
- Dysphagia
- Complication: malnutrition

EMOTIONAL EFFECTS
- Loss of control, lability
- Complication: depression

hyperthyroidism, hypoglycemia, compression of the spinal cord, toxic agents, infections, and neoplasms.

Medications

Riluzole (Rilutek), an antiglutamate, is the first medication developed to treat ALS. It inhibits the presynaptic release of glutamic acid in the CNS and protects neurons against the excitotoxicity of glutamic acid. This oral medication is administered without food at the same time each day. Clients are regularly monitored for liver function, blood count, blood chemistries, and alkaline phosphatase. They should be warned to report any febrile illness to their healthcare provider and to avoid alcohol.

NURSING CARE

Nursing care focuses on current health problems and on anticipating future difficulties. As with other disorders causing incapacitation and dependence, individualized nursing goals and interventions relate to decreasing complications, especially those associated with loss of muscular function and immobility; promoting independence to the extent possible; initiating referrals, particularly to a support group for both client and family; and providing physical and psychosocial support as indicated.

Of special consideration is planning for the client's eventual inability to communicate. Because the client's eye muscles and movements remain intact, signals can be prearranged before the loss of speech.

Nursing Diagnoses and Interventions

Two nursing diagnoses that frequently apply to clients with ALS are *Risk for Disuse Syndrome* and *Ineffective Breathing Pattern*.

Risk for Disuse Syndrome

Clients with ALS are at risk for developing problems associated with bed rest not only because they cannot move and reposition themselves, but also because they frequently have altered nutritional and hydration status. Nursing interventions focus on preventing skin breakdown and infections, such as urinary tract infections.

- Assess current condition for baseline parameters, particularly skin over bony prominences, lung sounds, and vital signs. *Understanding client's current condition allows accurate future assessment and realistic planning.*
- Assess skin; provide skin care, and obtain an alternating-pressure mattress. *Pressure points are at risk for breakdown; early detection is crucial to instituting appropriate care.*
- Institute active ROM exercises, as the client is able. Perform passive ROM exercises every 2 hours, when the client is turned. *Contractures can develop within a week because extensor muscles are weaker than flexor muscles.*
- Maintain positive nitrogen balance and hydration status: Monitor prealbumin levels, hemoglobin and hematocrit levels, and urine specific gravity. *Adequate protein is required to maintain osmotic pressure and prevent edema; positive nitrogen balance promotes optimal body functioning.*
- Monitor for manifestations of infection; for example, assess urine, especially if a urinary catheter is present. *Urinary catheters place clients at high risk for sepsis; bed rest places the client at greater risk for urinary stasis.*

PRACTICE ALERT
Urinary tract infection is indicated by cloudy, foul-smelling urine, pain on urination, fever, and general malaise.

Ineffective Breathing Pattern

As the muscle weakness of ALS continues, clients become less able to breathe. The respiratory muscles are affected, and clients eventually may require ventilatory assistance. The nurse must initiate measures to support the existing respiratory effort.

- Obtain a baseline assessment of breathing pattern, air movement, and oxygen saturation. *Assessments indicating the client's current condition provide data to plan individualized interventions.*
- Turn at least every 2 hours. *Movement enhances the ability to move pulmonary secretions and prevents stasis.*
- Elevate the head of the bed at least 30 degrees, suction as indicated, and provide oxygen. *This supports ventilation and enhances lung expansion as the client's condition changes.*
- Monitor temperature and lung sounds routinely; obtain sputum culture as indicated. *Early detection of a possible infectious process leads to prompt treatment.*

Community-Based Care

Initial teaching centers on explaining the disease process, expected course, and prognosis. Referral to a social worker to determine home care needs and financial assistance is helpful. Counseling and referrals to a home health agency, dietitian, and physical, speech, and occupational therapists can help the family meet the client's changing needs and abilities. The realistic anticipation of needs cannot be overemphasized.

As the client becomes more debilitated, family members or other care providers focus on preventing complications. For example, family members need to know how to suction the client and perform the Heimlich maneuver to prevent aspiration. Teaching the family how to prevent problems related to immobility is a primary consideration for the nurse.

Another focus of teaching is basic care needs, such as care required to meet elimination needs. Teach families methods to establish a bowel routine, considerations related to a urinary catheter, and the need to promptly report manifestations of an infection.

Throughout the early stage and continued care of the client and family with ALS, much consideration is given to psychosocial concerns. Depression, anger, and denial may be initial reactions; refer the client and family to an ALS support group, social worker, psychologist, or psychiatrist as indicated.

PERIPHERAL NERVOUS SYSTEM DISORDERS

Many etiologic agents are responsible for peripheral nervous system disorders. Autoimmune disorders, viruses, environmental toxins such as heavy metals, and nutritional deficiencies can affect the peripheral nervous system.

THE CLIENT WITH MYASTHENIA GRAVIS

Myasthenia gravis is a chronic autoimmune neuromuscular disorder characterized by fatigue and severe weakness of skeletal muscles. Clients experience periods of remission and exacerbation, and mild forms of the disorder exist. Weakness may remain limited to a few muscle groups, especially the ocular muscles, or may become generalized with all muscles eventually becoming weakened.

Women are affected three times more frequently than men. The age of onset for most clients is between ages 20 and 30 (Porth, 2005). Treatment with anticholinesterase medications has greatly improved the prognosis and symptom management.

Pathophysiology

The axons of motor neurons divide as they enter skeletal muscles, and each axonal ending forms a neuromuscular junction. Although the axonal ending and the muscle fiber are extremely close, they are separated by the synaptic cleft. The transmission of nerve impulses from the nerve to the muscles occurs at the neuromuscular junctions. The neurotransmitter acetylcholine is released from the axonal ending, crosses the synaptic cleft, attaches to acetylcholine receptors on the muscle fiber, and stimulates the muscle.

In myasthenia gravis, antibodies destroy or block neuromuscular junction receptor sites, resulting in a decreased number of acetylcholine receptors. Structural changes also result in diminished acetylcholine uptake. The net result is a decrease in the muscle's ability to contract despite a sufficient amount of acetylcholine. A comparison of a normal neuromuscular junction and one affected by myasthenia gravis is shown in Figure 46–4 ■.

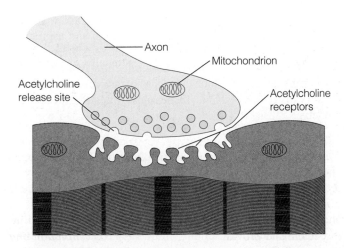

A Normal neuromuscular junction

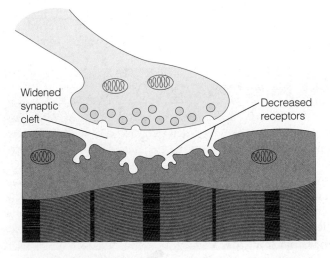

B Myasthenia gravis

Figure 46–4 ■ *A,* A normal neuromuscular junction and *B,* one showing the changes seen in myasthenia gravis. These changes interfere with the transmission of nerve impulses to the muscle.

In about 75% of clients with myasthenia gravis, the thymus gland, which is usually inactive after puberty, continues to produce antibodies because of hyperplasia of the gland or because of tumors. It is believed that the thymus is a source of autoantigen that triggers an autoimmune response in myasthenia gravis. The exact mechanism and reason for the thymus gland's antibody production are unknown.

Myasthenia gravis is sometimes associated with a tumor of the thymus, thyrotoxicosis (hyperthyroidism), rheumatoid arthritis, and lupus erythematosus. The disorder is often diagnosed when a client seeks treatment for a coincidental infection that exacerbates manifestations. Exacerbations may also occur before the menstrual period and during or soon after pregnancy.

Manifestations

The manifestations of myasthenia gravis correspond to the muscles involved. Initially, the eye muscles are affected and the client experiences either diplopia (unilateral or bilateral double vision) or ptosis (drooping of the eyelid) (Figure 46–5 ■). Next, the facial, speech, and mastication muscles become weak, and clients may have periods of dysarthria and dysphagia. Fatigue is evident even when the client tries to eat a meal; the muscles of chewing tire, and the client is forced to stop eating momentarily. A smile becomes a snarl or grimace, and the voice is weak with a muffled nasal quality. Problems performing fine motor movements of the hands, such as writing, appear early in the disease.

As the disease progresses, the muscles of the neck and extremities are affected. When the muscles of the neck become affected, the head juts forward. Deep tendon reflexes are usually normal, however, even in weak muscles. Fatigue and weakness are exacerbated with stress, fever, overexertion, and exposure to heat and are relieved by rest. Manifestations vary on a daily basis. Manifestations and complications of myasthenia gravis are listed in the box on this page.

Complications

Complications are directly related to the degree of muscle weakness and the specific muscles involved. For example, when the pharyngeal and palatal muscles are affected, the client cannot manage swallowing and may aspirate food or flu-

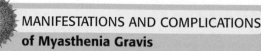

MANIFESTATIONS AND COMPLICATIONS
of Myasthenia Gravis

OCULAR AND FACIAL
- Ptosis
- Diplopia
- Facial weakness
- Dysphagia
- Dysarthria
- Complications: difficulty closing eyes, aspiration, impaired communication and nutrition

MUSCULOSKELETAL
- Weakness and fatigue
- Decreased function of hands, arms, legs, and neck muscles
- Complications: inability to perform ADLs and self-care activities, complications related to immobility, myasthenic and cholinergic crises

RESPIRATORY
- Weakening of intercostal muscles
- Decrease in diaphragm movement
- Breathlessness and dyspnea
- Poor gas exchange
- Complications: decreasing ability to walk, eat, and perform other ADLs, pneumonia

NUTRITIONAL
- Inability to chew and swallow
- Decreasing ability to move tongue
- Impairment of fine motor movements: inability to feed self
- Complications: weight loss, dehydration, malnutrition, aspiration

ids. The client is at increased risk for pneumonia because weakness of the diaphragm and muscles of respiration compromises gas exchange. Clients with myasthenia gravis can develop life-threatening emergencies, including myasthenic crisis and cholinergic crisis.

Myasthenic Crisis

Myasthenic crisis is a sudden exacerbation of motor weakness putting the client at risk of respiratory failure and aspiration. Myasthenic crisis most often is due to undermedication, missed doses of medication, or a developing infection. Manifestations of myasthenic crisis include tachycardia, tachypnea, severe respiratory distress, dysphagia, restlessness, impaired speech, and anxiety.

Cholinergic Crisis

Cholinergic crisis is the result of overdosage with the anticholinesterase (cholinergic) medications used to treat myasthenia gravis. Gastrointestinal manifestations, severe muscle weakness, vertigo, and respiratory distress are signs of cholinergic crisis. Both types of crises are emergency, life-threatening situations; clients frequently require ventilatory assistance. Differentiation is based on the client's response to edrophonium chloride (Tensilon). In myasthenic crisis the test is positive, and in cholinergic crisis the test is negative (see the discussions that follows under Diagnosis).

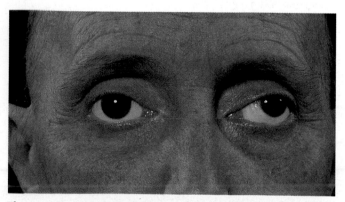

Figure 46–5 ■ In myasthenia gravis, the client experiences unilateral weakness of the facial muscles. Note the drooping of one eyelid.

Source: Custom Medical Stock Photo, Inc.

INTERDISCIPLINARY CARE

Care of the client with myasthenia gravis focuses on providing appropriate treatment, preventing complications, and supporting the client and family in meeting physical and psychosocial needs, especially as the disease progresses.

Diagnosis

Diagnostic tests are conducted following a thorough history and physical examination, with special attention to the facial, oculomotor, laryngeal, and respiratory muscles. Diagnostic tests include the anticholinesterase (Tensilon) test, nerve stimulation studies, and an analysis of antiacetylcholine receptor antibodies.

In the Tensilon test, the client is injected with edrophonium chloride (Tensilon), a short-acting anticholinesterase. Clients with myasthenia gravis show a significant improvement in muscle strength that lasts approximately 5 minutes. This test is also used to differentiate myasthenic crisis (caused by insufficient medication, so the client shows improvement with the drug) from cholinergic crisis (caused by overmedication, so the client does not show improvement).

Single-fiber electromyography can detect delayed or failed neuromuscular transmission in muscle fibers supplied by a single nerve fiber. Serum assay of circulating acetylcholine receptor antibodies, if increased, is diagnostic of myasthenia gravis with a sensitivity of 80% to 90%.

Medications

The primary group of medications used to treat myasthenia gravis is the anticholinesterases. These drugs act at the neuromuscular junction and allow acetylcholine to concentrate at the receptor sites, thus promoting muscle contraction. Pyridostigmine (Mestinon) is the most commonly used acetylcholinesterase inhibitor for myasthenia gravis. The client's decrease in manifestations guides dosage.

Immunosuppression with glucocorticoids, typically prednisone, is another pharmacologic therapy aimed at improving muscle strength. Clients must be aware of the need to stay on the drug at the prescribed dose to determine the least amount required for efficacy. If clients do not respond to prednisone alone, it may be combined with other immunosuppressive agents, such as cyclosporine or azathioprine (Imuran). Medications used to treat myasthenia gravis are discussed in the Medication Administration box below.

Surgery

Approximately 75% of clients with myasthenia gravis have dysplasia of the thymus gland. Therefore, thymectomy is often

---

MEDICATION ADMINISTRATION   The Client with Myasthenia Gravis

ANTICHOLINESTERASES/CHOLINESTERASE INHIBITORS
Neostigmine (Prostigmin)
Ambenonium (Mytelase Caplets)
Pyridostigmine (Mestinon, Regonol)
For diagnosis: edrophonium chloride (Tensilon)

Cholinesterase inhibitors are used in myasthenia gravis to enhance the effects of acetylcholine at the remaining skeletal muscle receptors. Cholinesterase inhibitors do not cure or change the underlying pathophysiologic processes, but they can provide effective, lifelong improvement of symptoms. Because the cholinesterase inhibitors are nonselective, the neuromuscular, muscarinic, and ganglionic junctions are each affected.

Adjusting the dose to obtain maximum benefit with minimal side effects is a major consideration when administering cholinesterase inhibitors. Initially, small doses are given followed by incremental increases until optimal muscle strength is obtained. The dose may need to be adjusted when activities result in symptoms of undermedication, such as increased ptosis. Severe undermedication results in myasthenic crisis. Although a sustained release form of pyridostigmine is available for bedtime use, it should not be used during the day because of its inconsistent absorption.

Cholinesterase inhibitors should not be administered to clients experiencing obstruction of the intestinal or urinary tract. Caution is advised when administering these drugs to clients with asthma, hyperthyroidism, bradycardia, or peptic ulcer disease. Cholinesterase inhibitors can cross the placenta; reproductive counseling is indicated.

Nursing Responsibilities
- Obtain a baseline assessment of muscle strength and abilities, concentrating on swallowing and ptosis.
- Administer the medication parenterally if the client has dysphagia. Check the dose of the medication carefully when changing from oral to parenteral routes.
- Evaluate the effectiveness of the medication and document the response, for example, time when fatigue occurs in relation to activities.
- Promptly recognize and respond to manifestations of excessive stimulation of muscarinic receptors: excess salivation, urinary urgency, bradycardia, gastrointestinal hypermotility, diaphoresis. Atropine can be administered to combat these manifestations. Respiratory depression and failure can occur and require mechanical ventilation.
- Have a muscarinic antagonist (e.g., physostigmine) readily available to treat poisoning.

Health Education for the Client and Family
- Balancing symptom control with dosage is crucial; record time of dose and response in a journal. Note the time of day when fatigued and any adverse effects, such as excess salivation, sweating, slow heartbeat, and diarrhea.
- Take the medication about 30 minutes prior to meals to enhance swallowing and chewing.
- Report manifestations of myasthenic crisis immediately: severe muscle weakness, fast heartbeat, restlessness, difficulty breathing, increasing difficulty swallowing or speaking.
- Report slow heartbeat, increased salivation or sweating, and/or decreased blood pressure immediately.
- Review possible causes of myasthenic crisis: physical or emotional stress, infection, or reduction in the medication dosage.
- Wear or carry Medic-Alert identification.

NURSING CARE OF THE CLIENT HAVING A Thymectomy

PREOPERATIVE CARE

■ Reinforce the physician's explanation of the procedure, and prepare the client for chest tubes and tracheostomy. *Realistic preparation of what to expect postoperatively encourages compliance and allays anxiety.*

■ Anticipate the need for alternative communication. *The client may have a tracheostomy; preoperative planning facilitates communication after surgery.*

■ Allow sufficient time for questions. *Thymectomy is a major surgery requiring either a thoracotomy and sternal split or transcervical approach. The client is usually anxious, and adequate time must be allocated to preoperative instruction.*

POSTOPERATIVE CARE

■ Provide meticulous pulmonary hygiene: turning, deep breathing, and coughing at least every 2 hours; use an incentive spirometer. *Regardless of surgical approach, measures are aimed at preventing pulmonary complications of atelectasis and pneumonia.*

■ Clients with a thoracotomy and sternal split procedure will require care of the anterior chest tube. Observe for complications; such as pneumothorax. *Air may enter the thoracic cavity—be alert for sudden chest pain and dyspnea, decreased breath sounds, and early signs of shock, such as restlessness.*

■ Manage pain with scheduled analgesic therapy. *Maintaining a therapeutic blood level of analgesic provides better pain control than waiting until the client requests medication, as on a prn basis.*

recommended for clients younger than 60. The two surgical approaches used are the transcervical approach, which is considered less invasive, and the transsternal approach. The latter approach allows a more extensive removal of the gland; however, it also poses more potential complications because it involves splitting the sternum.

Preoperatively, clients may be tapered from steroid therapy. Usually, pyridostigmine is administered to prevent muscular manifestations during the perioperative period. Postoperative nursing care focuses on preventing complications and controlling pain. Nursing implications for the client undergoing thymectomy are presented in the box on this page. Remission is obtained in about 40% of clients but may take several years to achieve. Refer to Chapter 38 ∞ for care of

the client having a thoracotomy and chest tubes. A tracheostomy may be required when the diaphragm or intercostal muscles are involved.

Plasmapheresis

Plasma exchange in myasthenia gravis may be used in conjunction with other therapies; for example, it may be performed prior to surgical intervention. The goal of therapy is to remove the antiacetylcholine receptor antibodies, thus improving severe muscle weakness, fatigue, and other manifestations. The procedure is frequently performed when respiratory muscle involvement is evident. See Figure 46–6 ■ and the box below for nursing care of the client having a plasmapheresis.

NURSING CARE OF THE CLIENT TREATED WITH Plasmapheresis

PREPROCEDURE CARE

■ Teach about the procedure and what to expect, including what the machine looks like, the need for arterial and venous insertion sites, and the length of time of the procedure (2 to 5 hours). *Giving information, answering questions, and addressing concerns decrease anxiety.*

■ Check with physician about holding medications until after the procedure. *Medications may be removed from the body as an incidental part of the plasmapheresis process.*

■ Assess vital signs and weight. *Baseline parameters are necessary to evaluate for fluid imbalances and response to therapy.*

■ Assess CBC, platelet count, and clotting studies. *Clients undergoing plasmapheresis are at high risk for anemia and coagulation problems secondary to hemolysis of cells.*

■ Check blood type and crossmatch for replacement blood products. *Hypersensitivity reactions can occur, and close monitoring is important.*

CARE DURING AND AFTER THE PROCEDURE

■ Observe for dizziness or hypotension. *Hypovolemia is a complication of plasma exchange, especially during the proce-*

dure when up to 15% of the client's blood volume is in the cell separator.

■ Apply pressure dressing to access site(s). *Direct pressure helps decrease or prevent bleeding.*

■ Monitor for infection and bruises at the intravenous port site. *The site of vascular access is at risk for complications and must be routinely and carefully assessed for signs of infection and for bleeding or hematoma formation.*

■ Monitor electrolytes and signs of electrolyte loss. Report imbalances, and replace electrolytes as ordered. Observe for circumoral tingling, Chvostek's and Trousseau's signs if calcium levels are low, and cardiac dysrhythmias and leg cramps if potassium levels are low. *Hypocalcemia and hypokalemia may occur. Hypocalcemia occurs because the anticoagulant citrate dextrose binds with calcium.*

■ Reevaluate preprocedure laboratory data, especially CBC, platelet count, and clotting times. *The cell-separating process can damage cells; anticoagulation is part of the procedure.*

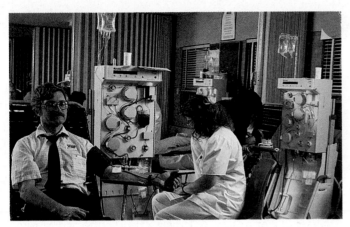

Figure 46–6 ■ Plasmapheresis is a procedure used to separate the blood's cellular components from plasma. About 50 mL per minute is withdrawn to the centrifuge in the plasmapheresis machine. The plasma is replaced with donor plasma or colloids and returned to the client.

Courtesy of Baxter Healthcare Corporation.

NURSING CARE

Because avoiding fatigue is a major part of teaching, it is important to incorporate interventions to enhance rest and conserve energy (Box 46–4). For example, suggest sitting while preparing meals and while performing hygiene and grooming. Anticipating problems, such as impaired communication, and developing alternative solutions can be helpful in promoting independence. A Nursing Care Plan for the client with myasthenia gravis is given on the next page.

Nursing Diagnoses and Interventions

Nursing care of clients with myasthenia gravis focuses not only on present problems but also on anticipated needs. Preventing myasthenic and cholinergic crises and providing psychologic support to clients and families are two important aspects of care. Individualized care depends on the specific therapy instituted. This section discusses the nursing diagnoses related to ineffective airway clearance and impaired swallowing; other nursing diagnoses that commonly apply, such as *Fatigue*, are addressed in other sections of this chapter.

Ineffective Airway Clearance

The underlying causes of ineffective airway clearance for the person with myasthenia gravis include poor cough mechanism, decreased rib cage expansion, diminished diaphragm movement, and decreased expiratory effort. The following interventions require particular attention if the client undergoes a thymectomy.

- Assist with turning, deep breathing, and coughing at least every 2 hours. Teach proper coughing techniques; use an incentive spirometer every 2 hours while the client is awake. *Position changes promote lung expansion; coughing helps clear secretions from the tracheobronchial tree.*
- Place in a semi-Fowler's position. *This position expands the lungs and alleviates pressure from the diaphragm, especially important considerations if the client is obese.*
- Maintain hydration status and monitor for dehydration; use a humidifier as needed. If needed, teach family how to perform percussion, postural drainage, and suction. *Interventions to liquefy secretions, such as ensuring a daily fluid intake of up to 2500 mL (perhaps via feeding tube or parenteral route), help the client mobilize and expectorate sputum.*
- Monitor lung sounds, the rate and character of respirations, and pulse oximetry readings at least every 4 hours or as indicated by client's condition. *Frequent assessments are critical to early identification of ineffective respirations and oxygenation of tissues.*

Impaired Swallowing

Clients with myasthenia gravis have weakness of the laryngeal and pharyngeal muscles involved with swallowing. Alterations in swallowing place the client at risk for poor nutrition as well as for possible aspiration. Family members need to be included in teaching, particularly the person who prepares and assists with meals.

- Assess the ability to safely manage various consistencies of foods; consult with a speech therapist for evaluation. *Dysphagic clients are at risk for aspiration; matching food consistency to the client's ability to swallow enhances safety.*
- Plan meals to promote medication effectiveness. *Pyridostigmine should be given 30 minutes before the meal to provide optimal muscle strength for swallowing and chewing.*
- Have the client eat slowly, using small bites of food. Schedule meals during periods when the client is adequately rested; develop a daily schedule incorporating rest periods. *Fatigue may add to dysphagia, putting the client at greater risk for aspiration.*
- If necessary, give cues while eating, such as "Chew your food thoroughly; swallow." *Keeping client focused may enhance swallowing.*
- Teach caregivers the Heimlich maneuver and how to suction. *Knowing specific measures to take in case of aspiration decreases both the client's and family's anxiety and promotes confidence in managing potential problems.*

Community-Based Care

Teaching for the client and family with myasthenia gravis focuses on prevention and recognition of crisis situations,

---

BOX 46–4 Client and Family Teaching: Myasthenia Gravis

- Schedule periods of rest and avoid stress; conserve energy when possible.
- Avoid cigarette smoke, alcohol, and beverages with quinine (e.g., tonic water).
- Take medications as prescribed. If manifestations change, consult the physician; the dose may need to be adjusted.
- Avoid extremes of temperature; an environment that is too hot or too cold may cause an exacerbation of myasthenia gravis.
- Avoid people with upper respiratory infections; infections can result in an exacerbation and extreme weakness.

NURSING CARE PLAN   A Client with Myasthenia Gravis

Kirsten Avis, a 44-year-old homemaker and mother of two teenage sons, was diagnosed with myasthenia gravis 2 years ago. She takes an anticholinesterase medication, pyridostigmine (Mestinon), four times a day. Over the past month she has been experimenting with decreasing the dose of her pyridostigmine because she has "felt so good." She was prescribed 60 mg of pyridostigmine three times a day before meals and one-half of a long-acting 180-mg pyridostigmine tablet at night.

Three days ago, she began having chills and fever and her myasthenic symptoms became markedly worse. Mrs. Avis is easily fatigued and has been experiencing increasing weakness, bilateral ptosis, and mild dysphagia in the late afternoon and evenings. She is admitted to the hospital.

ASSESSMENT

Lela Silva, RN, is caring for Mrs. Avis. Physical examination of Mrs. Avis reveals severe muscle weakness bilaterally in her hands, arms, and thorax. Her voice is nasal, and she speaks slowly; the longer she speaks, the more difficult it becomes to understand her. She is anxious and dyspneic. Her complaints of weakness, dysphagia, dysarthria, problems with mobility, and ptosis are more pronounced later in the day. Vital signs are as follows: BP 138/88, P 88, R 28, T 102.4°F (39°C).

Some improvement in muscle weakness is noted following a restful night's sleep; however, the respiratory distress is more evident, and Mrs. Avis is increasingly restless. She is moved to the intensive care unit for advanced monitoring and possible ventilatory assistance. The medical diagnosis is myasthenic crisis secondary to pulmonary infection.

DIAGNOSES

- *Impaired Gas Exchange* related to ineffective breathing pattern and muscle weakness
- *Risk for Aspiration* related to difficulty swallowing
- *Fatigue* related to increased energy needs from muscular involvement

EXPECTED OUTCOMES

- Pulse oximetry readings will be maintained at 92% or above.
- No aspiration will occur.
- Will verbalize decreasing fatigue when performing ADLs.
- Will state the correct method of medication dosing and demonstrate how she will maintain schedule.

PLANNING AND IMPLEMENTATION

Mrs. Avis's manifestations improve following administration of edrophonium chloride (Tensilon) to verify myasthenic crisis. She is placed on oxygen by mask and suctioned as needed; equipment for possible intubation and ventilation is made readily available. She is placed in a semi-Fowler's position, and vital signs are assessed every 5 minutes during the acute exacerbation. The nurses in the intensive care unit remain in constant attendance throughout the crisis period and provide explanations to Mrs. Avis in an effort to decrease her stress and to avoid further severity of manifestations.

Three days after the crisis period, Mrs. Avis is moved to a progressive nursing care unit. Nurses follow up on teaching her the manifestations of both myasthenic and cholinergic crises. They discuss the need to wear Medic-Alert identification and review medication administration techniques with Mrs. Avis. The nurses emphasize in particular that Mrs. Avis must not split time-released medications.

Within 5 days, Mrs. Avis's condition stabilizes, and her weakness decreases sufficiently to allow discharge home. Although her temperature has returned to normal and her respiratory status has improved, she still has a productive cough. Oral antibiotics are prescribed for 2 weeks, after which she will have a follow-up visit with her primary care provider. She is instructed to seek treatment promptly if respiratory symptoms or temperature indicate recurrence of infection.

EVALUATION

Mrs. Avis is discharged without developing aspiration pneumonia or any symptoms of aspiration. Her airway was maintained throughout the myasthenic crisis, and her pulse oximetry readings remained above 92% once oxygen therapy was initiated. On discharge, pulse oximetry is above 95% without oxygen therapy. Mrs. Avis states that her fatigue and weakness have significantly improved.

Both Mrs. Avis and her husband are able to explain the difference between myasthenic and cholinergic crises and to identify methods to avoid both problems. Mrs. Avis correctly relates her proper medication regimen and makes an appointment for a follow-up visit with her physician.

CRITICAL THINKING IN THE NURSING PROCESS

1. What is the rationale for administering Tensilon to evaluate a myasthenic crisis?
2. Develop a plan to teach Mrs. Avis how to avoid fatigue when preparing and eating meals.
3. Develop a nursing care plan for Mrs. Avis for the nursing diagnosis *Ineffective Role Performance*.

See Evaluating Your Response in Appendix C.

---

understanding the disorder, and methods for coping with both physical and psychosocial problems. Setting realistic goals with the client and family provides opportunities for self-assessment and promotes active participation in rehabilitation.

Address the following topics:
- The importance of maintaining consistency in medication dosage and management
- Realistic expectations

- Methods to avoid fatigue and undue stress; specific measures for avoiding upper respiratory infections and exposure to extreme heat or cold
- Birth control measures or referral for counseling (Pregnancy can exacerbate manifestations; also, medications used to control myasthenia gravis, such as neostigmine bromide [Prostigmin], cross the placenta.)
- Referral to support groups
- Helpful resources such as the Myasthenia Foundation.

THE CLIENT WITH GUILLAIN-BARRÉ SYNDROME

Guillain-Barré syndrome (GBS) is an acute inflammatory demyelinating disorder of the peripheral nervous system characterized by an acute onset of motor paralysis (usually ascending). The classification of Guillain-Barré subtypes includes acute inflammatory demyelinating polyradiculoneuropathy, acute axonal motor neuropathy, and acute motor and sensory axonal neuropathy.

Guillain-Barré syndrome is one of the most common peripheral nervous system disorders, affecting about 3500 people in the United States and Canada each year (Porth, 2005). The cause is unknown, but precipitating events include a respiratory or gastrointestinal viral or bacterial infection 1 to 3 weeks prior to the onset of manifestations, surgery, viral immunizations, and other viral illnesses. In 60% of cases, *Campylobacter jejuni* is identified as the cause of the preceding infection. Approximately 80% to 90% of clients with GBS have a spontaneous recovery with little or no residual disabilities.

The disease is characterized by progressive ascending flaccid paralysis, accompanied by paresthesias and numbness. About 20% of clients have respiratory involvement to the point that ventilatory assistance is required. GBS is often a medical emergency.

Pathophysiology

The primary pathophysiologic process in GBS is the destruction of myelin sheaths covering the axons of peripheral nerves. The demyelination is thought to be the result of both a humoral- and cell-mediated immunologic response. The loss of myelin results in poor conduction of nerve impulses, causing sudden muscle weakness and loss of reflex response. Other manifestations occur when nerve conduction to various muscles is interrupted. The stages of Guillain-Barré syndrome and their usual manifestations are presented in Box 46–5.

Manifestations

Muscles, sensory nerves, and cranial nerves are commonly affected in clients with GBS. Most people experience symmetric muscle weakness, initially in the lower extremities. The weakness and sensory loss then ascends to the upper extremities, torso, and cranial nerves. Sensory involvement includes severe pain, paresthesia, and numbness. Cognition and level of consciousness are not affected. Facial nerve involvement results in the inability to change facial expressions and close the eyes. Muscles involved with chewing, swallowing, and speaking may be affected.

Paralysis of intercostal and diaphragmatic muscles may alter respiratory function. These clients require ventilatory assistance and supportive care. Involvement of the autonomic nervous system is characterized by fluctuating blood pressure, cardiac dysrhythmias and tachycardia, paralytic ileus, syndrome of inappropriate antidiuretic hormone secretion, and urinary retention.

The weakness usually plateaus or improves by the fourth week. Strength then improves slowly over weeks or months. Women who have had Guillain-Barré syndrome are at increased risk for relapse in the first trimester of pregnancy.

BOX 46–5 Stages of Guillain-Barré Syndrome

I. Acute Stage
- Characterized by severe and rapid weakness, especially in the lower extremities; loss of muscle strength progressing to quadriplegia and respiratory failure; decreasing deep tendon reflexes; decreasing vital capacity; paresthesias, numbness; pain, especially nocturnal; facial muscle involvement (inability to wrinkle forehead or change expressions).
- Involvement of the autonomic nervous system manifested by bradycardia, sweating, fluctuating blood pressure (notably hypotension) which may last for 2 weeks.

II. Stabilizing/Plateau Stage
- Occurs 2 to 3 weeks after initial onset.
- Marks the end of changes in condition; characterized by a "leveling off" of symptoms.
- Generally, the labile autonomic functions stabilize.

III. Recovery Stage
- May take from several months to 2 years.
- Marked by improvement in symptoms.
- Generally, muscle strength and function return in descending order.

INTERDISCIPLINARY CARE

Interventions during the acute phase (1 to 3 weeks) focus primarily on ensuring oxygenation via ventilatory assistance and preventing complications from immobility. Rehabilitation time to regain muscle strength and function varies; most people return to full presyndrome muscle function within 6 months to 2 years.

Care of the client with GBS requires a team approach. From the initial acute phase through rehabilitation, many members of the healthcare team are involved. An accurate and rapid diagnosis is needed to ensure prompt supportive treatment, particularly if there is respiratory involvement combined with widespread paralysis.

Diagnosis

Diagnosis of GBS is made after a thorough history and clinical examination. It must be differentiated from several disorders, among them influenza, heavy metal poisoning, Lyme disease, and cranial hemorrhage. Diagnosis is made based on manifestations, history of a recent viral infection, elevated CSF protein levels, and EMG studies reflecting decreased nerve conduction. Although there is no specific test to diagnose this syndrome, several findings support and confirm the diagnosis.

Medications

No medications are available for the specific treatment of Guillain-Barré syndrome. Other medications may be prescribed to provide support or prophylaxis, or to combat concurrent problems; for example, antibiotics may be prescribed for urinary tract or respiratory infections. Morphine is commonly administered to control muscle pain. Anticoagulation therapy is usually instituted to prevent thromboembolic complications, such as deep venous thrombosis and pulmonary embolism, which are associated with prolonged bed rest. If hypotension is a problem, vasopressors are prescribed.

Surgery

Tracheostomy is performed if respiratory failure occurs. Clients who need ventilatory support are usually able to be weaned after 2 to 3 weeks, but the time frame varies greatly. When the client's vital capacity reaches 8 to 10 mL/kg, he or she may be weaned from the ventilator (Hickey, 2003). Insertion of a temporary pacemaker may be indicated for bradycardia.

Plasmapheresis

Plasma exchange has been beneficial, particularly when performed within the first 2 weeks of the syndrome's development. Antibodies are removed, and immunosuppressive agents are administered concurrently. Clients typically have five exchanges during an 8- to 10-day period.

Nutrition and Fluids

Nutritional support for the client who is immobilized for prolonged periods of time is crucial. Maintaining positive nitrogen balance, ensuring sufficient fluid intake and electrolyte balance, and ensuring recommended caloric intake are goals of therapy. When swallowing problems occur, total parenteral nutrition may be indicated if feeding via a nasogastric or gastrostomy tube is ineffective.

Physical and Occupational Therapy

Long-term physical and occupational therapy are crucial to recovery. Clients with Guillain-Barré syndrome usually require prolonged rehabilitation care, which begins during the acute phase and focuses on preventing complications and limiting the effects of immobility. The severe muscle atrophy and loss of muscle tone require that clients relearn many functions and skills, such as walking. Compromise in respiratory function may delay physical rehabilitation; clients need positive reinforcement when they make even small gains in their progress. Continued attention to pain control is essential because paresthesia and pain can interfere with physical therapy.

NURSING CARE

Many of the nursing interventions for clients with this syndrome involve monitoring neurologic function, preventing problems of immobility, ensuring adequate hydration and nutrition, and promoting respiratory function. Anticipating needs of both the client and family is an important aspect of care. For example, developing an alternative method of communication before it is necessary may decrease anxiety. It is important that nursing care focus on preventing complications that may be fatal by following a rigorous predetermined schedule for turning and respiratory care (e.g., coughing, deep breathing, suctioning), using strict aseptic technique, and providing continuous psychosocial support.

Nursing Diagnoses and Interventions

Anxiety and powerlessness are major nursing considerations. The client is almost always admitted to the ICU for care, and is mentally alert but suddenly mute, ventilator dependent, and immobile. Refer to previous nursing care sections in this chapter for interventions related to anxiety, imbalanced nutrition, impaired swallowing, impaired verbal communication, and ineffective airway clearance. This section focuses on the nursing diagnoses related to pain and risk for impaired skin integrity.

Acute Pain

Pain experienced with Guillain-Barré syndrome varies. Frequently, there is a "stocking–glove" pattern, with pain in the hands, feet, and legs. Pain and tenderness in muscles can be severe; interventions must be individualized to client needs. The intense pain combined with altered sensations leads to anxiety; nursing interventions can make a difference in breaking the cycle of increasing pain that leads to increased anxiety and in turn causes more pain.

- Listen to the description of pain; determine presence of triggers or a pattern. *Acknowledging the client's perception of pain is a basis for treatment; listening establishes trust.*
- Use a pain scale for determining extent of pain. *Consistent measurement is essential to evaluate degree of pain and effectiveness of intervention.*
- Use complementary therapies to help manage pain:
  - Application of heat/cold
  - Guided imagery
  - Relaxation techniques
  - Massage.
  Presenting options for managing pain gives the client control over the situation and helps reduce anxiety. Noninvasive interventions may augment the therapeutic benefit of medications.
- Provide analgesics as indicated; administer on a regular schedule rather than waiting until pain becomes severe. *Anticipating and managing pain before it becomes severe decreases anxiety and averts the cycle of increased anxiety leading to increased pain.*
- Monitor for side effects of analgesics, particularly respiratory depression; assess respirations and lung sounds. Perform routine pulmonary care measures and monitor for aspiration. *Clients with Guillain-Barré syndrome have weakened thoracic muscles; frequent respiratory monitoring is indicated.*

Risk for Impaired Skin Integrity

During the acute and plateau stages of Guillain-Barré syndrome, clients are at risk for problems related to immobility and malnutrition. Impaired skin integrity is one such problem. Preventing areas of skin breakdown is important. Prophylactic interventions will help ensure that ingested protein and calories are used to maintain ideal body weight and other body functions rather than to heal an avoidable problem. Implicit in interventions is maintenance of adequate nutrition.

- Inspect bony prominences and provide skin care at least every 2 hours. Reposition the client and clean, dry, and lubricate the skin as needed. *These activities stimulate circulation and ensure even distribution of body weight; baseline observations allow discovery of early signs of altered integrity.*

- Pad bony prominences, such as sacral area, heels, and elbows. *This decreases shearing tears on these pressure points.*
- Use an alternating-pressure mattress or water bed. *Relieving pressure stimulates circulation and promotes oxygenation of tissues.*
- Monitor for incontinence and provide thorough skin care following each episode of incontinence. *Urine is caustic to the skin, and the moisture promotes skin breakdown.*

Community-Based Care

Clients and family members are frequently stunned by the rapid deterioration of function and fear that the paralysis will be permanent. Regularly reinforce teaching because the client's high anxiety level may interfere with listening and understanding. When possible, include the client and family in decision making; for example, seek their input when planning a daily schedule of care that incorporates various therapies.

Teaching the rationales for preventive measures reinforces the client's and family's understanding and may promote compliance during the lengthy rehabilitation. For example, because of autonomic nerve involvement, clients need to be monitored for cardiac dysrhythmias and taught to avoid changing position suddenly to prevent orthostatic hypotension.

Referrals to appropriate therapists are a component of anticipating needs; speech, nutritional, occupational, and physical therapists are an integral part of rehabilitation. Another focus of care is teaching both the client and family; incorporate explanations for interventions aimed at promoting self-care. For further information, refer the client and family to the Guillain-Barré Syndrome Foundation, International.

CRANIAL NERVE DISORDERS

Disorders of the cranial nerves may be caused by intracranial trauma or by pathologic processes. The pairs of cranial nerves, described in Chapter 43 ∞, are numbered in the order in which they arise in the brain and are named according to their anatomic characteristic or primary function. The most common cranial nerve disorders are those affecting the trigeminal (cranial nerve V) and the facial (cranial nerve VII) nerves. These disorders, discussed in the following sections, result primarily in pain or loss of sensory or motor function.

THE CLIENT WITH TRIGEMINAL NEURALGIA

Trigeminal neuralgia, also called *tic douloureux,* is a chronic disease of the trigeminal cranial nerve (V) that causes severe facial pain. The trigeminal nerve has three divisions: the ophthalmic, the maxillary, and mandibular (Figure 46–7 ■). The ophthalmic division supplies the forehead, eyes, nose, temples, meninges, paranasal sinus, and part of the nasal mucosa. The maxillary division supplies the upper jaw, teeth, lip, cheeks, hard palate, maxillary sinus, and part of the nasal mucosa. The mandibular division supplies the lower jaw, teeth, lip, buccal mucosa, tongue, part of the external ear, and the meninges. Sensory fibers of the nerve conduct impulses for touch, pain, and temperature; motor fibers innervate the temporal and masseter muscles used for chewing and lateral movement of the jaw. The maxillary and mandibular divisions are the divisions of the trigeminal nerve affected in almost all cases of this disorder.

Trigeminal neuralgia occurs more commonly in middle-age and older adults and affects women more often than men.

Pathophysiology

The actual cause of trigeminal neuralgia is unknown; however, contributing factors include irritation from flulike illnesses, trauma or infection of the teeth or jaw, and pressure on the nerve by an aneurysm, a tumor, or arteriosclerotic changes of an artery close to the nerve (Hickey, 2003).

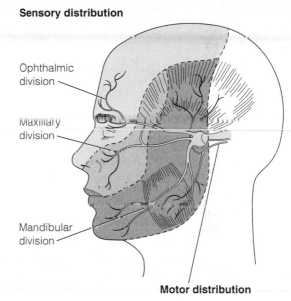

Sensory distribution

Ophthalmic division

Maxillary division

Mandibular division

Motor distribution

Figure 46–7 ■ Sensory and motor distribution of the trigeminal nerve. The three sensory divisions are ophthalmic, maxillary, and mandibular.

Stimulating specific areas of the face, called *trigger zones,* may initiate the onset of pain. These trigger zones usually parallel the distribution of the nerve and typically follow a track leading from just over the eyebrow to the ridge of the cheekbone, along the nasolabial fold, around the corner of the mouth, and down the side of the chin. The episodes of pain are initiated by many factors, including light touch, eating, swallowing, talking, sneezing, shaving, chewing gum, brushing the teeth, or washing the face. Other factors that may trigger a pain episode include changes in temperature and exposure to wind. In an attempt to control the pain, clients may refuse to wash, shave, eat, or talk.

The episodes of pain may recur for several weeks or months. The disease then spontaneously goes into remission, and the client is free of pain for periods lasting from days to years. As the client grows older, the remissions tend to become shorter, and a dull ache may be present between episodes of acute pain.

Manifestations

Trigeminal neuralgia is characterized by brief (lasting a few seconds to a few minutes), repetitive episodes of sudden severe (usually unilateral) facial pain. The pain may occur as often as hundreds of times a day to as infrequently as a few times a year. The pain is experienced over the surface of the skin. It most often begins near one side of the mouth and rises toward the ear, eye, or nostril on the same side of the face. Clients describe the pain as stabbing or lightning-like and often respond to the pain by wincing or grimacing.

INTERDISCIPLINARY CARE

There are no specific diagnostic tests for trigeminal neuralgia. The disorder is diagnosed by the characteristic location and type of pain. The disorder is treated by pharmacologic or surgical interventions.

Medications

The drug most useful in controlling the pain is the tricyclic anticonvulsant carbamazepine (Tegretol). If carbamazepine is ineffective, other medications such as the anticonvulsants phenytoin (Dilantin) or gabapentin (Neurontin) or the skeletal muscle relaxant baclofen (Lioresal) may be used. These drugs are administered to decrease paroxysmal afferent impulses and stop the pain. Drugs in this category may cause side effects of dizziness, nausea, and drowsiness. Liver function, bone marrow function, and blood levels of the medications should be monitored on a regular basis.

Surgery

If medications do not control the pain, surgical procedures may be performed, including various types of *rhizotomy,* the surgical severing of a nerve root. Closed surgical interventions by percutaneous rhizotomy involve inserting a needle through the cheek into the foramen ovale at the base of the brain and partially destroying the trigeminal nerve with glycerol (an alcohol), by radiofrequency-induced heat, or by balloon compression of the trigeminal ganglion. These procedures carry less risk and result in shorter hospital stays than do open procedures, but there is a possibility of recurrence of pain. Following surgery, the client may have some facial numbness, but there usually is no residual paralysis. The involved side of the face is insensitive to pain. The client will have some loss of facial sensation (e.g., to temperature and/or touch) and is at risk for loss of the corneal reflex. Closed procedures provide long-term pain relief and are well tolerated by the older adult. Nursing care of the client undergoing a percutaneous rhizotomy is presented in the box below.

It has been found that some structural abnormalities (such as an artery or vein compressing the nerve) may cause the neuralgia, and if so, decompression and separation of the blood vessel from the nerve root produce lasting relief of the pain (Tierney et al., 2005). The Jannetta procedure involves locating and lifting the involved vessel and placing a small piece of silicone sponge between the vessel and the nerve. Possible complications of the procedure include headache and facial pain.

NURSING CARE

Nursing care for the client with trigeminal neuralgia involves teaching self-management at home after medical or surgical intervention. Primary client concerns are managing pain, maintaining nutrition, and preventing injury.

Nursing Diagnoses and Interventions

Interventions for managing pain and improving nutritional intake are addressed here; teaching to prevent injury following surgery is discussed under client and family teaching.

Acute Pain

The client with trigeminal neuralgia has excruciating pain and often avoids ADLs and socializing with others in an attempt to

---

NURSING CARE OF THE CLIENT HAVING A   Percutaneous Rhizotomy

POSTOPERATIVE CARE

- Follow routine postoperative interventions for clients having surgery (see Chapter 4 ∞).
- Monitor cranial nerve function every 2 to 4 hours:
  a. Assess the corneal reflex by lightly touching the cornea with a wisp of cotton. If the reflex is intact, the client will blink. *Severing the ophthalmic division of the trigeminal nerve destroys the corneal reflex and leaves the cornea at risk for dryness and injury.*
  b. Assess the facial nerve by asking the client to blow out the cheeks, wrinkle the forehead, frown, wink, and close both eyes tightly. Test taste by placing bitter, salty, and sweet substances on the anterior portion of the tongue. *Facial weakness is evidenced by changes in movement in the involved side of the face. The facial nerve also innervates the anterior two-thirds of the tongue.*

  c. Assess the function of the oculomotor muscles by asking the client to follow your finger through the cardinal positions of vision (see Chapter 47 ∞). *The eyes should move together; alterations in movement indicate an abnormal response.*
  d. Assess the motor portion of the trigeminal nerve by asking the client to clench the teeth while you palpate the tightness of the contracted masseter and temporal muscles. *Loss of motor function is indicated by loss of bulk and tightness of these muscles.*
  e. Apply as prescribed; an ice pack to the jaw on the operative site. *Cold decreases bleeding and swelling.*
  f. Teach the client to avoid rubbing the eye on the involved side. *Loss of the corneal reflex removes protection because the client no longer has the sensation of pain in the involved eye. Rubbing the eye could cause corneal abrasions.*

prevent the onset of pain. Pain management is fully discussed in Chapter 9 ∞. Nursing interventions for pain in clients with this disorder focus on strategies for self-management.

- Identify factors that trigger an attack, and discuss strategies to avoid these precipitating factors. *Most clients can clearly identify trigger zones and triggering factors. Identification is the first step in pain control.*
- Determine usual response to pain. *Sensitivity and reaction to pain are influenced by previous experiences with pain and by age, gender, emotional factors, and cultural background.*
- Assess factors that affect the ability to influence pain tolerance, including the knowledge and cause of the pain, the meaning of the pain, the ability to control the pain, cultural background, and support systems. *Pain tolerance, which is the duration and intensity of pain a person is willing to endure, differs greatly among individuals and may also vary within particular clients in different situations.*
- Monitor the effects of the medication prescribed for the neuralgia. *If the prescribed medication does not provide relief, other medications or methods of treatment may be used to control the pain.*

Risk for Altered Nutrition: Less than Body Requirements

Clients often refuse to eat during periods of pain attacks, fearing that the movements of chewing may precipitate the pain. In addition, the chronic nature of the illness often causes depression, which may depress the appetite.

- Monitor dietary intake and weight at each visit, and ask the client to keep a weekly weight record. *Ongoing assessments are necessary for early detection of nutritional deficiencies.*
- Discuss the temperature and consistency of foods eaten, and suggest referral to a dietitian if necessary. *Hot or cold foods may trigger an attack; soft, warm, or cool foods are less likely to act as triggers.*
- Suggest chewing on the unaffected side of the mouth. *Chewing on the unaffected side is less likely to trigger an attack of pain and so facilitate food intake.*
- If unable to tolerate oral food, tube feedings may be necessary. *Adequate kilocalories and nutrients for metabolic processes are essential.*

Community-Based Care

The client with trigeminal neuralgia who is receiving medical treatment and providing self-care at home requires teaching about the disease process, the medication(s) being taken, and ways to reduce the incidence of attacks or pain. Diet teaching and assistance with self-management of pain are also important. For example, if the home setting is drafty and attacks of pain are triggered by wind blowing across the face, it may be necessary to encourage the client to put weather stripping around windows and doors. To prevent injury to affected areas, the topics in the Meeting Individualized Needs box below should be addressed.

THE CLIENT WITH BELL'S PALSY

Bell's palsy, also called *facial paralysis,* is a disorder of the seventh cranial (facial) nerve, characterized by unilateral paralysis of the facial muscles. The facial nerve is primarily a motor nerve that supplies all the muscles associated with expression on one side of the face. The sensory component innervates the anterior two-thirds of one side of the tongue.

This disorder can occur at any age but is seen most often in adults between 20 and 60. The incidence is equal in men and women. Eighty percent of clients recover completely within a few weeks to a few months (and three-fourths recover without any treatment). Of those remaining, 15% recover some function but have some permanent facial paralysis; these clients are usually older, have diabetes mellitus, or have more severe manifestations, such as vertigo, a sensitivity to noise, and deep head pain.

Pathophysiology

The exact cause of the disorder is unknown, although inflammation of the nerve and a relationship to the herpes simplex virus have been suggested (Tierney et al., 2005).

Manifestations

The onset of Bell's palsy is usually sudden and almost always involves one side of the face. Pain behind the ear or along the jaw may precede the paralysis. The client initially notices

---

MEETING INDIVIDUALIZED NEEDS   Teaching for Home Care of Trigeminal Neuralgia

EYE CARE
- Do not rub the eyes; use artificial tears four times a day if the eyes are dry or irritated.
- Wear an eye patch at night.
- Wear protective sunglasses or goggles when outside, when working in dusty areas, when mowing the lawn, and when using any type of spray material (e.g., hair spray, cleaning materials, paint, insecticides).
- Remember to blink frequently.
- Check your eyes for redness or swelling each day.
- Schedule regular eye examinations.

FACE AND MOUTH CARE
- Chew on the unaffected side of the mouth.
- Avoid eating hot foods or drinking hot liquids.
- After every meal, brush your teeth and inspect the inside of your mouth for food that may collect between the gums and cheek.
- Have regular dental examinations; you will not be able to feel pain associated with gum infection or tooth decay.
- Use an electric razor to shave the face.
- Protect your face from very cold or windy conditions.

numbness or stiffness of one side of the face that distorts the appearance. As the disease progresses, the distortion becomes more obvious, and the face appears asymmetric. The facial paralysis causes the entire side of the face to droop, and the client cannot wrinkle the forehead, close the eye, or pucker the lips on the affected side. When the client attempts to smile, the lower facial muscles are pulled to the opposite side of the face. Some clients have only mild manifestations, whereas others have complete facial paralysis (Figure 46–8 ■). Clients often believe they have had a stroke. Manifestations of Bell's palsy are listed in the box on this page.

INTERDISCIPLINARY CARE

There are no definitive laboratory or diagnostic tests for Bell's palsy, nor are there any specific treatments. Treatment includes medications and physical therapy. Recent studies have shown that antiviral drugs such as acyclovir combined with an anti-inflammatory drug such as prednisone may be effective by lim-

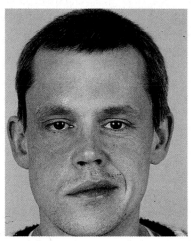

Figure 46–8 ■ The client with Bell's palsy shows the typical drooping of one side of the face.
Source: NIH/Phototake NYC.

MANIFESTATIONS   of Bell's Palsy

- Paralysis of the facial muscles on one side of the face
- Paralysis of the upper eyelid with loss of the corneal reflex on the affected side
- Loss or impairment of taste over the anterior portion of the tongue on the affected side
- Increased tearing from the lacrimal gland on the affected side

---

iting damage to the nerve. Physical therapy to stimulate the facial nerve and help maintain muscle tone may help prevent permanent contractures before recovery takes place. Moist heat applied to the affected side of the face may decrease pain.

NURSING CARE

Although clients provide self-care at home, the nurse plays a key role in teaching the client and family about the disease and how to prevent injury and maintain nutrition. The client is often anxious about his or her appearance and may require counseling if any deficits in facial expression become permanent. The following topics should be addressed:

- Use artificial tears four times a day to lubricate the eye; wear an eye patch or tape the eye shut at night. Wear sunglasses or goggles when outside, when working in dusty conditions, and when using any type of spray.
- Massage combined with warm, moist heat often is effective in relieving the pain.
- A soft diet that does not require chewing and six small meals a day are helpful. Chew slowly on the unaffected side and avoid hot foods. Clean the mouth and carefully inspect the area between the gums and cheek for food after each meal.
- As function returns, practice wrinkling the forehead, closing the eyes, blowing air out of the puckered mouth, and whistling for 5 minutes three or four times a day.

DISORDERS RESULTING FROM INFECTIONS AND NEUROTOXINS

A variety of disorders of the nervous system may have infectious or toxic causes. Although these disorders are not common, those included here require significant nursing care when they do occur.

THE CLIENT WITH CREUTZFELDT-JAKOB DISEASE

Creutzfeldt-Jakob disease (CJD) (also called *spongiform encephalopathy*) is a rapidly progressive, degenerative, neurologic disease that causes brain degeneration without inflammation. The disease is transmissible and progressively fatal. The causative agent is believed to be an abnormal form of a cellular glycoprotein known as the prion protein. Transmission of the agent is by direct contamination with infected neural tissue, such as during eye and brain surgery. The injection of contaminated human growth hormone from cadaveric pituitaries has also been implicated.

A different form of the disease, called *new variant CJD (vCJD)* is also a rare, degenerative, fatal brain disorder, but is not the same as the classic form of CJD. New variant CJD, referred to as "mad-cow disease," is believed to result from consumption of cattle products contaminated with bovine spongiform encephalopathy (BSE). This form primarily affects young adults. Because the illness is fatal and is associated with infected cattle, severe restrictions have been placed on the importation of cattle, sheep, and goats and on products from these animals from countries in which BSE is known to exist.

The disease occurs worldwide, but clusters occur in several areas, more often in England, Chile, and Italy. The incidence is approximately 1 or 2 cases per 1 million population (Centers for Disease Control and Prevention [CDC], 2005). Classic CJD affects adults over the age of 50; vCJD affects younger adults. The median age of death for people with classic CJD is 68 years. In contrast, the median age of death with vCJD is 28 years.

Pathophysiology

Creutzfeldt-Jakob disease is characterized by degeneration of the gray matter of the brain. The spongiform degeneration (involving the formation of tiny holes and resembling a sponge) produces severe dementia, myoclonus (muscle contractions), and characteristic changes in brain waves. On autopsy or biopsy of brain tissue, the brain shows loss of neurons and a proliferation of astrocytes (indicating destruction of nearby neurons).

Manifestations

The disease has characteristic stages and manifestations. The onset is characterized by memory changes, an exaggerated startle reflex, sleep disturbances, and nervousness. The person then experiences rapid deterioration in motor, sensory, and language function. Tremors, hyperreflexia, rigidity, and a positive Babinski reflex are often present, and confusion progresses to dementia in almost all cases. Clients in the terminal state are comatose and exhibit decorticate and decerebrate posturing. The median duration of illness for CJD is 4 to 5 months; the median duration of illness for vCJD is 13 to 14 months (CDC, 2005).

INTERDISCIPLINARY CARE

No specific treatment is available to stop or slow the progression of CJD. Collaborative interventions focus on the disease's manifestations. The disease is diagnosed by a thorough neurologic examination, specific EEG changes, and a CT scan. However, the final diagnosis of CJD can be made only by postmortem examination. It is often difficult to differentiate this disease from Alzheimer's disease, especially in the early stages.

NURSING CARE

The nurse may identify the manifestations of Creutzfeldt-Jakob disease when conducting a health history and total physical assessment. Include questions about familial history, cultural and geographic risk, and high-risk occupations or procedures in the history. Assessment of mental function, reflexes, and cranial nerve function may provide information to assist in diagnosis.

Nursing care focuses on maximizing comfort, preventing injury, preventing transmission, and providing support. The following guidelines are useful in designing the plan of care:

- Although comfort is difficult to assess in clients with impaired cognitive function, interventions that provide a quiet environment and analgesia are important.
- Communication is essential, even if the client is unable to respond.
- Institute seizure precautions, and pad side rails.
- Provide skin care, changes in position, and pressure-relief mattresses to decrease the risk of pressure ulcers, venous stasis, and pneumonia.
- Use standard precautions for blood and body fluids when providing care. Disinfect surfaces with a solution of 5% bleach. Sterilize contaminated equipment by autoclave, or soak in 5% bleach solution for 1 hour. Label all specimens as biohazardous. Teach staff members and family members

guidelines for care, including careful hand washing. It is not necessary to place the client in isolation, however.
- Provide time for family members to verbalize grief and loss, which may be manifested as anger and frustration with the healthcare system.
- Provide information to family members about all procedures and the plan of care.
- Refer family members to sources of support, such as social services and the appropriate clergy.

THE CLIENT WITH POSTPOLIOMYELITIS SYNDROME

Postpoliomyelitis syndrome is a complication of a previous infection by the poliomyelitis virus. This disease was epidemic in the 1940s and 1950s, but has largely been eradicated through immunization with oral live trivalent virus vaccine. However, it is thought that nearly 50% of the estimated 1.63 million people in the United States who had the disease are reexperiencing manifestations of the acute illness (NINDS, 2005g). These people have struggled for years to rehabilitate themselves and lead productive lives. Now, as they reach retirement age, they are again experiencing manifestations which may be physically and psychologically incapacitating.

The poliomyelitis virus destroys some of the motor cells of the anterior horn cells of the spinal cord, causing neuromuscular effects that range from mild to severe flaccid paralysis and atrophy. The primary cause of death is respiratory arrest (Tierney et al., 2005).

Manifestations of motor neuron degeneration and weakness may emerge 10 to 40 years after the initial infection. Most clients with postpoliomyelitis syndrome initially had a more severe case of polio and required hospitalization, contracted the disease after the age of 10, required ventilator assistance for respiration, and had paralysis in all four extremities. The incidence is slightly higher in women. As the population ages, it is projected that the number of older adults with postpoliomyelitis syndrome will increase.

Pathophysiology

The pathophysiologic process in postpoliomyelitis syndrome is not known.

Manifestations

The manifestations of postpoliomyelitis syndrome include fatigue, muscle and joint weakness, loss of muscle mass, respiratory difficulties, and pain. The manifestations are most often seen in muscles affected by the initial infection, but new muscle groups may also be affected. In addition to neuromuscular manifestations, the client may experience cold intolerance, dizziness, headaches, urinary incontinence, and sleep disorders.

INTERDISCIPLINARY CARE

Postpoliomyelitis syndrome is diagnosed by a previous history of polio and the current manifestations. Diagnostic studies of nerve conduction, muscle strength, and pulmonary function determine current physical status. Treatment addresses the manifestations, and often involves physical therapy and pulmonary rehabilitation programs.

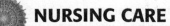 NURSING CARE

The client with postpoliomyelitis syndrome faces the challenge of unexpected physical changes. Clients are often anxious about how others will react or what the future holds. Respiratory dysfunction may result in the need for oxygen. Muscular weakness and decreased pulmonary function may make walking difficult, if not impossible. Activities of daily living, independent self-care, and careers are threatened.

Many clients have not fully recovered psychologically from having polio and may respond to a recurrence of manifestations with denial and disbelief. Older clients may not know they had polio as children. Nurses are responsible for assessing and identifying the manifestations of postpoliomyelitis syndrome. It is essential to question middle to older adults about a past history of polio when conducting the health history and to ask specific questions about manifestations that the client may be experiencing.

The nurse individualizes teaching to meet the physical and psychosocial needs of the client and family. Provide candid explanations, and teach the client how to prevent fatigue, promote optimal respiratory function, meet self-care needs, modify ADLs, and maintain safety. Follow-up care with nurses, physicians, physical therapists, respiratory therapists, and counselors is indicated. Referral to a support group can make a positive difference in the client's and family's ability to cope with the disorder.

THE CLIENT WITH RABIES

Rabies is a rhabdovirus infection of the central nervous system transmitted by infected saliva that enters the human body through a bite or an open wound. If untreated, rabies is a fatal viral encephalitis that causes 30,000 to 70,000 deaths worldwide each year. In the United States, 25,000 to 40,000 people are treated annually for exposure to rabid or potentially rabid animals (Hankins & Rosekrans, 2004). This is a critical illness that almost always causes death if untreated. The rabies virus is carried by both wild and domestic animals, including bats, skunks, foxes, raccoons, cats, and dogs. After an incubation period that may last from 10 days to many years (norm is 3 to 7 weeks), the virus travels to the brain of the infected animal via the nerves. It multiplies and migrates to the salivary glands.

Pathophysiology

The client with rabies usually has a history of an animal bite but may also become infected through an abrasion or open wound that is exposed to the infected saliva. The virus spreads from the wound to local muscle cells and then invades the peripheral nerves. It eventually travels to the central nervous system. The incubation period in humans varies according to the severity and location of the bite. For example, bites on the face may result in manifestations in 10 days to a few weeks, whereas bites on the lower extremities may incubate for as long as 1 year.

Manifestations

The manifestations occur in stages. During the initial, or prodromal, stage, the site of the wound is painful and then exhibits various paresthesias. The infected person is anxious, irritable, and depressed. General manifestations of infection (such as headache, loss of appetite, and sore throat) may appear. The person may also have increased sensitivity to light and sounds, and the skin is especially sensitive to changes in temperature.

The prodromal stage is followed by an excitement stage. The infected person has periods of excitement that alternate with periods of quiet. Attempts to drink cause such painful laryngospasms that the person refuses to drink (a phenomenon called *hydrophobia*). Large amounts of thick, tenacious mucus are present. The client experiences convulsions, muscle spasms, and periods of apnea. If untreated, death occurs approximately 7 days from the onset of manifestations and is usually due to respiratory failure.

INTERDISCIPLINARY CARE

Animals that bite are kept under observation, if possible, for 7 to 10 days to detect rabies manifestations. Sick animals should be euthanized and their brains examined for presence of the rabies virus, which is detected by fluorescent antibody testing. The blood of an infected person can also be tested with the same diagnostic study to demonstrate the presence of rabies antibodies.

NURSING CARE

Nursing care for clients with rabies is provided in an intensive care unit, with the client in a quiet, darkened room to decrease stimulation as much as possible. The client requires interventions to maintain the airway, maintain oxygenation, and control seizures. Standard precautions are essential, because the rabies virus is present in the saliva of the client. If an open wound of a healthcare provider is contaminated with infected saliva, the provider must receive postexposure immunizations.

Health Promotion

Client and family teaching focuses on the importance of immunizing pets, providing proper care of wounds, seeking immediate medical attention for animal bites, and obtaining treatment after any suspicious bite.

Because the untreated disease is almost always fatal, the best intervention is prevention. Preventive activities follow:

- Immunize household dogs and cats; immunize people who are exposed to animals.
- Local treatment of animal bites and scratches:
  - Carefully and thoroughly clean and flush wounds with soap and water to remove the saliva and dilute the viral exposure.
  - Immediately take the person with the bite for emergency treatment.
- Postexposure care:
  - Rabies immune globulin (RIG) is administered for passive immunization. Up to 50% of the globulin is infiltrated around the wound, and the rest is administered intramuscularly. At the same time, an inactivated human diploid cell vaccine (HDCV) is administered intramuscularly, with 1 mL given on the day of exposure and on days 3, 7, 14, and 28 after exposure (Tierney et al., 2005). RIG and HDCV should never be given in the same syringe or at the same site. Local and mild systemic reactions include itching, tenderness, headaches, muscle aches, and nausea.
  - If RIG is not available, equine rabies antiserum may be administered after testing the client for horse serum sensitivity.

THE CLIENT WITH TETANUS

Tetanus, more commonly called *lockjaw*, is a disorder of the nervous system caused by a neurotoxin elaborated by *Clostridium tetani*. This anaerobic bacillus lives in the soil. Spores of the bacillus enter the body through open wounds contaminated with dirt, street dust, or feces (animal or human). The wounds may result from punctures, scratches or abrasions, bee stings, abortions, surgery, trauma, burns, or intravenous drug use. Incidence is highest among people who have never been immunized, older adults whose immunity has been lost, and women. The majority of cases occur in people over age 50. Tetanus has a high mortality rate, with death occurring in over 40% of all cases. Contaminated lesions of the head and face are more dangerous than those in other parts of the body.

Pathophysiology

When the spores of *C. tetani* enter the open wound, they germinate and produce a toxin called tetanospasmin. The incubation period averages 8 to 12 days but can range from 5 days to 15 weeks (Tierney et al., 2005). The toxins are absorbed by the peripheral nerves and carried to the spinal cord, where they block the action of inhibitory enzymes at spinal synapses and interfere with transmission of neuromuscular impulses. As a result, even minor stimuli cause uncontrolled muscle spasms.

Manifestations

The manifestations begin with pain at the site of the infection. The infected person has stiffness of the jaw and neck and dysphagia. There is often profuse perspiration and drooling from increased salivation. As the infection progresses, the person experiences hyperreflexia, spasms of the jaw muscles (*trismus*) or facial muscles, and rigidity and spasms of the abdominal, neck, and back muscles. Generalized tonic seizures are caused by even minor stimuli, and the person assumes a typical opisthotonic position during the seizures: The head is retracted, the back is arched, and the feet are extended. The muscle spasms are painful. The person may be unable to breathe from spasms of the glottis and respiratory muscles. Despite these physical effects, the client has no change in mental status.

The complications of tetanus include urinary retention and airway obstruction from the spasms. Cardiac and respiratory failure are late, life-threatening complications.

INTERDISCIPLINARY CARE

There are no specific diagnostic tests for tetanus; diagnosis is based on manifestations. Tetanus is completely preventable by active immunization. Immunization for children includes tetanus toxoid, administered as part of the diphtheria-pertussis-tetanus (DPT) immunization series. In adults, immunization is obtained by administering tetanus toxoid as two doses 4 to 6 weeks apart, with a third dose in 6 to 12 months. All individuals should have a booster dose every 10 years throughout life or at the time of a major injury if the last booster dose was given more than 5 years prior to the injury.

If a wound is contaminated or if the person's immunization status is uncertain, passive immunization with tetanus immune globulin is administered. Active immunization with tetanus toxoid is begun at the same time. The wound is carefully and thoroughly debrided and antibiotics administered.

The client with tetanus requires intensive care in an area of minimal stimulation. Penicillin is administered to help destroy the toxin-producing organism. Muscle spasms and seizures are controlled by chlorpromazine (Thorazine) or diazepam (Valium), often combined with a sedative. Anticoagulants may be prescribed to prevent venous thrombosis. In severe cases, seizures and spasms are controlled with paralysis by a curare-like medication, and airway obstruction is managed by mechanical ventilation.

NURSING CARE

Nursing care for the client with tetanus is intensive and focuses on assessments and interventions to promote safety, prevent injury, maintain nutrition, and maintain pulmonary and cardiovascular function. The client usually requires in-hospital care for 2 to 5 weeks. The nursing care plan commonly includes the following:

- Place in a quiet, darkened room to decrease stimuli that cause muscle spasms and seizures.
- Provide only necessary physical care, and do so during periods of maximal sedation to decrease tactile stimulation that causes muscle spasms.
- Maintain oxygenation through mechanical ventilator and frequent suctioning of secretions.
- Maintain intravenous access for the administration of fluids and medications.
- Administer prescribed antibiotics, anticonvulsants, and sedatives. In the case of cardiovascular complications, administer prescribed beta-adrenergic blocking agents such as propranolol (Inderal).
- Provide adequate nutrition through prescribed nutritional support, such as total parenteral nutrition.
- Monitor respiratory and cardiovascular status and provide immediate interventions for respiratory or cardiovascular failure.
- Monitor fluid and electrolyte status. Ensure adequate fluid intake to maintain hydration and urinary output.
- Monitor urinary output, which should be maintained at 1.5 to 2 L per day.
- Monitor for the hazards of immobility, including constipation, pneumonia, deep venous thrombosis, and pressure ulcers.

Health Promotion

Tetanus is a preventable disorder, and nurses have a major role in promoting immunizations for all children and for educating adults about the need for booster doses. The older population is especially at risk for never having been immunized or for letting immunizations lapse. Information for this age group can be provided through activities such as community health fairs and programs at senior citizen groups.

It is also necessary to teach the proper care of wounds. All wounds, no matter how small, should be thoroughly washed with soap and water. All foreign material should be carefully flushed out or removed from a wound, and medical care should be sought for wounds that are more extensive or contaminated.

THE CLIENT WITH BOTULISM

Botulism is food poisoning caused by ingestion of food contaminated with a toxin produced by the bacillus *Clostridium*

8 What drug classification is the medication used to treat ALS?
1. dopamine agonist
2. anticholinergic
3. anti-inflammatory
4. antiglutamate

9 You are preparing a teaching plan for a client with Bell's palsy. What information would you include?
1. "You will experience severe facial pain during attacks."
2. "The disease affects your muscles so you can't walk."
3. "One side of your face will not move normally."
4. "Be sure to boil all home-canned foods before eating them."

10 How can the nurse prevent tetanus?
1. Teach safe food preparation techniques.
2. Promote immunizations for adults and children.
3. Demonstrate proper disposal of soiled dressings.
4. Promote immunization of household pets.

See Test Yourself answers in Appendix C.

BIBLIOGRAPHY

Acello, B. (2003). Handling an unwelcome comeback: Postpolio syndrome. *Nursing, 33*(11), Hospital Nursing: 32hn1–2, 32hn5.

Alzheimer's Disease Education & Referral Center. (2003). *Alzheimer's disease fact sheet.* Retrieved from http://www. alzheimers.org/pubs/adfact.html

Alzheimer's Foundation of America. (2005). *About dementia.* Retrieved from http://alzfdn.org/dementia/index.shtml

American Academy of Neurology. (2005). *Alzheimer's disease guidelines: A summary for patients, family and friends.* Retrieved from http://www.aan.com

Brown, C. (2003). Surgical treatment of trigeminal neuralgia. *AORN Journal, 78*(5), 743–744, 745, 748–750.

Centers for Disease Control and Prevention. (2005). *CJD (Creutzfeldt-Jakob disease, classic; vCJD).* Retrieved from http://cdc.gov/ncidod/dvrd/cjd/index.htm

Cheung, J., & Hocking, P. (2004). The experience of spousal carers of people with multiple sclerosis. *Qualitative Health Research, 14*(2), 153–166.

Dochterman, J., & Bulechek, G. (2004). *Nursing interventions classification (NIC)* (4th ed.). St. Louis, MO: Mosby.

Finlayson, M., Van Denend, T., & Hudson, E. (2004). Aging with multiple sclerosis. *Journal of Neuroscience Nursing, 36*(5), 245–251, 259.

Frock, T., & McCaffrey, R. (2005). Clinical case report. Postauricular pain with Bell's palsy. *Nurse Practitioner: American Journal of Primary Health Care, 30*(4), 58–61.

Gerdner, L., & Hall. G. (2001). Chronic confusion. In M. Maas, K. Buckwalter, M. Hardy, T. Tripp-Reimer, M. Titler, & J. Specht (Eds.), *Nursing care of older adults: Diagnoses, outcomes, & interventions* (pp. 421–441). St. Louis, MO: Mosby.

Hamilton, R., Bowers, B., & Williams, J. (2005). Disclosing genetic test results to family members. *Journal of Nursing Scholarship, 37*(1), 18–24.

Hankins, D., & Rosekrans, J. (2004). Overview, prevention, and treatment of rabies. *Mayo Clinic Proceedings, 79*(5), 671–676.

Hickey, J. (2003). *The clinical practice of neurological and neurosurgical nursing* (4th ed.). Philadelphia: Lippincott.

Holland, J., & Madonna, M. (2005). Nursing grand rounds: Multiple sclerosis. *Journal of Neuroscience Nursing, 37*(1), 15–19.

Huntington's Disease Society of America. (2004). *FAQ's.* Retrieved from http://www.hdsa.org/site/ PageServer?pagename=help_info_ed_faq

Improving the odds for avoiding dementia in advanced age. (2004). *Critical Care Nurse, 24*(5), 8–12.

Kee, J. (2006). *Handbook of laboratory and diagnostic tests with nursing implications* (6th ed.). Upper Saddle River, NJ: Prentice Hall.

Mini-mental state exam. (1975). *Journal of Psychiatric Research, 12,* 189–198.

Moorhead, S., Johnson, M., & Maas, M. (2003). *Nursing outcomes classification (NOC)* (3rd ed.). St. Louis, MO: Mosby.

Moyer, D. (2005). Hallmarks of Alzheimer's advances. *Nursingmatters, 16*(3), 8–9.

NANDA International. (2005). *Nursing diagnoses: Definitions & classification 2005–2006.* Philadelphia: Author.

National Institute of Neurological Disorders and Stroke. (2005a). *Amyotrophic lateral sclerosis fact sheet.* Retrieved from http://www.ninds.nih.gov/disorders/amyotrophiclateral sclerosis/detail_amyotrophiclateralsclerosis_pr.htm

_____. (2005b). *Bell's palsy fact sheet.* Retrieved from http://www.nih.gov/disorders/bells/detail_bells.htm

_____. (2005c). *Deep brain stimulation for Parkinson's disease information page.* Retrieved from http://www. ninds.nih.gov/disorders/deep_brain_stimulation/ deep_brain_stimulation_pr.htm

_____. (2005d). *Multiple sclerosis: Hope through research.* Retrieved from http://www.ninds.nih.gov/ disorders/multiple_sclerosis/detail_multiple_sclerosis.htm

_____. (2005e). *NINDS Guillain-Barré syndrome information page.* Retrieved from http://www.ninds.nih. gov/disorders/gbs?gbs_pr.htm

_____. (2005f). *NINDS Huntington's disease information page.* Retrieved from http://www.ninds.nih. gov/disorders/huntington/huntington.htm

_____. (2005g). *NINDS post-polio syndrome information page.* Retrieved from http://www.ninds. nih.gov/disorders/post_polio/post_polio.htm

_____. (2005h). *Parkinson's disease information page.* Retrieved from http://www.ninds.nikg.gov/disorders/ parkinsons_disease/parkinsons_disease.htm

_____. (2005i). *The dementias: Hope through research.* Retrieved from http://www.ninds.nih.gov/ disorders/alzheimersdisease/detail/alzheimersdisease_ pr.htm

National MS Society. (2005). *Just the facts: 2005–2006.* Retrieved from http://www.nationalmssociety.org/ Brochures-Just%20the.asp

National Parkinson Foundation. (2005a). *About Parkinson disease.* Retrieved from http://www.parkinson.org

_____. (2005b). *Parkinson primer.* Retrieved from http://www.parkinson.org/site/pp.asp?c=9dJFLPwB&b= 71354

O'Maley, K., O'Sullivan, J., Wollin, J., Barras, M., & Brammer, J. (2005). Teaching people with Parkinson's disease about their medication. *Nursing Older People, 17*(1), 14–16, 18, 20.

Parkinson's Disease Foundation, Inc. (2005). *Parkinson's disease: An overview.* Retrieved from http://www.pdf.org/ AboutPD/index.cfm

Porth, C. M. (2005). *Pathophysiology: Concepts of altered health states* (7th ed.). Philadelphia: Lippincott.

Richman, D., & Agius, M. (2003). Treatment of autoimmune myasthenia gravis. *Neurology, 61*(12), 1652–1661.

Rubin, R. (2005). Communication about sexual problems in male patients with multiple sclerosis. *Nursing Standard, 19*(24), 33–37.

Seman, D. (2003). "Listen with the ears of your heart." *Nursing Homes Long Term Care Management, 52*(9), 34, 36–40.

Sheff, B. (2005). Combating infection. Mad cow disease and vCJD: Understanding the risks. *Nursing, 35*(2), 74–75.

Sulton, L. (2001). Caring for the patient with Guillain-Barré syndrome. *Nursing, 31*(10), 32cc1–2, 32cc4, 32cc6.

Tierney, L., McPhee, S., & Papadakis, M. (Eds.). (2005). *Current medical diagnosis & treatment* (45th ed.). New York: McGraw-Hill.

Wilkinson, J. (2005). *Prentice Hall nursing diagnosis handbook with NIC interventions and NOC outcomes* (8th ed.). Upper Saddle River, NJ: Prentice Hall.

Wilson, B., Shannon, M., & Stang, C. (2006). *Prentice Hall nurse's drug guide 2006.* Upper Saddle River, NJ: Prentice Hall.

UNIT 13 BUILDING CLINICAL COMPETENCE
Responses to Altered Neurologic Function

Functional Health Pattern: Cognitive-Perceptual

■ Think about clients with cognitive-perceptual problems for whom you have cared in your clinical experiences.

- What were the clients' major medical diagnoses (e.g., traumatic brain injury, spinal cord injury, stroke, aneurysm)?
- What manifestations did each of these clients have? (Were these manifestations similar or different?
- How did each of these clients respond to interaction with you as you provided care for them? Was it difficult for them to remember the identity of visitors or family members, that they were in a hospital, the correct year? Was their speech affected (aphasia)? Did the family indicate that the client took longer than normal to "find the words" in conversation? Were their words "jumbled" or confused when they spoke?

■ The neurologic system regulates and integrates all body functions, mental abilities, and emotions. It is made up of the central nervous system and peripheral nervous system. These two components are made up of two types of cells: neurons (which receive and transmit information) and neuroglia (which protect and support the neurons). The Cognitive-Perceptual Pattern includes functional abilities such as language, memory, judgment, decision making, and sensation. The pathophysiologic factors affecting cognition and perception are:

- Decreased blood flow to and ischemia of neurons (e.g., stroke, ruptured intracranial aneurysm or arteriovenous malformation, spinal cord injury, increased intracranial pressure, cerebral edema)
- Direct injury to neurologic tissues from trauma or compression (e.g., traumatic brain injury, skull fractures, increased intracranial pressure, spinal cord injury, herniated intervertebral disk, brain tumors, spinal cord tumors)
- Alterations in the electrical activity of cerebral neurons (epilepsy)
- Infections of the neurologic system (e.g., meningitis, encephalitis, rabies, tetanus, botulism)
- Degeneration or alteration of neurons, supporting neurologic structures, or neurotransmitters (e.g., Alzheimer's disease, multiple sclerosis, Parkinson's disease, Huntington's disease, amyotrophic lateral sclerosis, myesthenia gravis, Guillain-Barré syndrome, cranial nerve disorders).

■ One example of the pathophysiologic effects of neurologic disorders, increased intracranial pressure (a response to many disorders of and injuries to the brain) causes cell damage and death and can lead to transient or permanent manifestations such as:

- *Altered level of consciousness* (with decreasing circulation to and oxygenation of neurons → decreased cellular metabolism → Na-K pump failure → edema damage to the RAS)
- *Aphasia or dysphagia* (resulting from changes in the complex neurologic pathways in the speech center through ischemia, decreased oxygen and blood circulation, cell death, and the toxins released by dying cells)
- *Seizures* (seizure threshold is exceeded → abnormal neuronal activity remains localized or spreads to involve the entire brain → causing local or generalized effects).

■ Priority nursing diagnoses within the Cognitive-Perceptual Pattern that may be appropriate for clients with neurologic disease or injury include:

- *Ineffective Tissue Perfusion: Cerebral* as evidenced by level of consciousness changes, cognitive defects, and inaccurate interpretation of stimuli including confusion, comprehension, problem solving, abstraction, and memory deficits
- *Impaired Verbal Communication* as evidenced by inability/difficulty in speaking or understanding spoken or written words
- *Powerlessness* as evidenced by expressions of frustration regarding inability to control their illness, recovery rate, or care
- *Acute Confusion* as evidenced by restlessness, hallucinations, disorientation, anxiety.

■ Two nursing diagnoses from other functional health patterns often are a high priority for the client with neurologic disease or injury:

- *Impaired Swallowing* (Nutritional-Metabolic)
- *Impaired Physical Mobility* (Activity-Exercise)

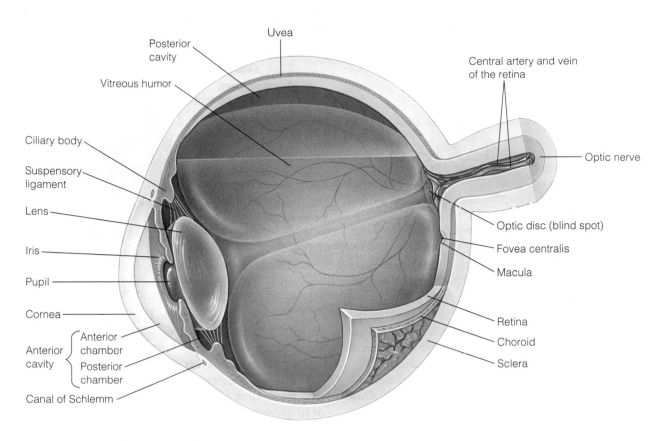

Figure 47–3 ■ Internal structures of the eye.

formed and drained to maintain a relatively constant pressure of from 15 to 20 mmHg in the eye. The canal of Schlemm, a network of channels that circles the eye in the angle at the junction of the sclera and the cornea, is the drainage system for fluid moving between the anterior and posterior chambers. Aqueous humor provides nutrients and oxygen to the cornea and the lens.

Internal Chamber

The intraocular structures that lie in the internal chamber of the eye are the lens, the posterior cavity and vitreous humor, the ciliary body, the uvea, and the retina.

The lens is a biconvex, avascular, transparent structure located directly behind the pupil. It can change shape to focus and refract light onto the retina. The posterior cavity lies behind the lens. It is filled with a clear gelatinous substance, the vitreous humor, which supports the posterior surface of the lens, maintains the position of the retina, and transmits light. The uvea, also called the vascular tunic, is the middle layer of the eyeball. This pigmented layer has three components: the iris, ciliary body, and choroid. The ciliary body encircles the lens, and along with the iris, regulates the amount of light reaching the retina by controlling the shape of the lens. Most of the uvea is made up of the choroid, which is pigmented and vascular. Blood vessels of the choroid nourish the layers of the eyeball. Its pigmented areas absorb light, preventing it from scattering within the eyeball.

The retina is the innermost lining of the eyeball. It has an outer pigmented layer and an inner neural layer. The outer layer, next to the choroid, serves as the link between visual stimuli and the brain. The transparent inner layer is made up of millions of light receptors in structures called rods and cones. Rods enable vision in dim light as well as peripheral vision. Cones enable vision in bright light and the perception of color. The optic disc, a cream-colored round or oval area within the retina, is the point at which the optic nerve enters the eye. The slight depression in the center of the optic disc is called the physiologic cup. Located laterally to the optic disc is the macula, a darker area with no visible blood vessels. The macula contains primarily cones. The fovea centralis is a slight depression in the center of the macula that contains only cones and is a main receptor of detailed color vision.

The Visual Pathway

The optic nerves are cranial nerves formed of the axons of ganglion cells. The two optic nerves meet at the optic chiasma, just anterior to the pituitary gland in the brain. At the optic chiasma, axons from the medial half of each retina cross to the opposite side to form pairs of axons from each eye. These pairs continue as the left and right optic tracts (Figure 47–4 ■). The crossing of the axons results in each optic tract carrying information from both eyes. The left optic tract carries visual information from the lateral half of the retina of the left eye and the medial half of the retina of the right eye, whereas the right optic tract carries visual information from the lateral half of the retina of the right eye and the medial half of the retina of the left eye.

The ganglion cell axons in the optic tracts travel to the thalamus and synapse with neurons, forming pathways called op-

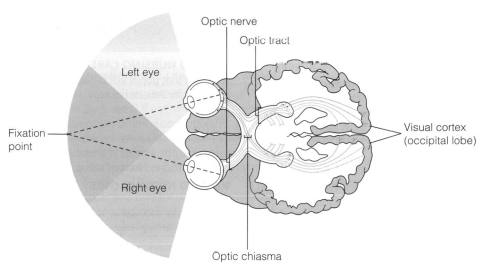

Figure 47–4 ■ The visual fields of the eye and the visual pathways to the brain.

tic radiations. The optic radiations terminate in the visual cortex of the occipital lobe. The nerve impulses that originated in the retina are interpreted here.

The visual fields of each eye overlap considerably, and each eye sees a slightly different view. Because of this overlap and the crossing of the axons, information from both eyes reaches each side of the visual cortex, which then fuses the information into one image. This fusion of images accounts for the ability to perceive depth; however, depth perception depends on visual input from two eyes that both focus well.

Refraction

Refraction is the bending of light rays as they pass from one medium to another medium of different optical density. As light rays pass through the eye, they are refracted at several points: as they enter the cornea, as they leave the cornea and enter the aqueous humor, as they enter the lens, and as they leave the lens and enter the vitreous humor. At the lens, the light is bent so that it converges at a single point on the retina. This focusing of the image is called **accommodation**. Because the lens is convex, the image projected onto the retina (the real image) is upside down and reversed from left to right. This real image is coded as electric signals that are sent to the brain. The brain decodes the image so that the person perceives it as it occurs in space.

The eyes are best adapted to see distant objects. Both eyes fix on the same distant image and do not require any change in accommodation. For people with emmetropic (normal) vision, the distance from the viewed object at which the eyes require no accommodation is 20 ft (6 m). This point is called the far point of vision. To focus for near vision, the eyes must instantly accommodate the lens, constrict the pupils, and converge the eyeballs. Accommodation is accomplished by contraction of the ciliary muscles. This contraction reduces the tension on the lens capsule so that it bulges outward to increase the curvature. This change in shape also achieves a shorter focal length, another requirement for focusing close images on the retina. The closest point on which a person can focus is called the near point of vision; in young adults with normal vision this is usu-

ally 8 to 10 inches (20 to 25 cm). Pupillary constriction helps eliminate most of the divergent light rays and sharpens focus. **Convergence** (the medial rotation of the eyeballs so that each is directed toward the viewed object) allows the focusing of the image on the retinal fovea of each eye.

ASSESSING THE EYES

Structures and functions of the eyes are assessed by findings from diagnostic tests, a health assessment interview to collect subjective data, and a physical assessment to collect objective data.

Diagnostic Tests

The results of diagnostic tests of the structure and functions of the eyes are used to support the diagnosis of a specific injury, disease, or vision problem; to provide information to identify or modify the appropriate medications or assistive devices used to treat the disease or problem; and to help nurses monitor the client's responses to treatment and nursing care interventions. Diagnostic tests of the eye, especially for vision testing, are most often conducted in a healthcare provider's office. Diagnostic tests to assess the structure and functions of the eyes are described in the Diagnostic Tests table on the next page and summarized in the following bulleted list. More information is included in the discussion of specific injuries or diseases in Chapter 48 ∞.

■ Refractive errors (with prescription for corrective lenses) are evaluated by retinoscopy and/or refractometry. Pupils must be dilated for accurate diagnosis.

■ Tonometry is used to identify and evaluate increased intraocular pressure, characteristic of glaucoma.

■ A CT scan may be used to identify foreign objects or tumors of the eye.

Regardless of the type of diagnostic test, the nurse is responsible for explaining the procedure and any special preparation needed, for assessing any medication use that might affect the outcome of the tests, for supporting the client during the examination as necessary, for documenting the procedures as appropriate, and for monitoring the results of the tests.

TABLE 47–1 Age-Related Changes in the Eye

AGE-RELATED CHANGE	SIGNIFICANCE
The lens: ■ ↓ elasticity, decreasing focus and accommodation for near vision (presbyopia). ■ ↑ density and size, making lens more stiff and opaque. ■ Yellowing of the lens and changes in the retina affect color perception.	Most older adults require corrective lenses to accommodate close and detailed work. Increased opacity leads to the development of cataracts. As cataracts develop, they increase sensitivity to glare and interfere with night vision.
The cornea: ■ Fat may be deposited around the periphery and throughout the cornea. ■ ↓ corneal sensitivity.	A partial or complete white circle may form around the cornea (*arcus senilis*). Lipid deposits in the cornea cause vision to be blurred. Decreased sensitivity increases the risk of injury to the eye.
The pupil: ■ ↓ size and responsiveness to light pupil; sphincter hardens.	Increased light perception threshold and difficulty seeing in dim light or at night means increased light is needed to see adequately.
The retina and visual pathways: ■ Visual fields narrow. ■ Photoreceptor cells are lost. ■ Rods work less effectively. ■ Macular degeneration is a risk. ■ Depth perception is distorted. ■ Adaptation to dark and light takes longer.	Peripheral vision is decreased and central vision may be lost from macular degeneration. Increased risk of falls as a result of changes in depth perception and adaptation to changes in light. Vision progressively declines with age.
The lacrimal apparatus: ■ ↓ reabsorption of intraocular fluid. ■ ↓ production of tears.	Increased risk of developing glaucoma, and eyes feel and look dry.
The posterior cavity: ■ Debris and condensation become visible. ■ Vitreous body may pull away from the retina.	Vision is blurred and distorted, and "floaters" are often seen by the older person.

grid, forming squares (boxes) that measure 5 mm. There is a black dot in the center of the grid. The Amsler grid is useful for identifying early changes in vision from macular degeneration and diabetes mellitus. To use the Amlser grid, ask the client to hold the grid at normal reading distance (about 12 to 14 inches), cover one eye, and stare at the center dot. Ask the client if any of the lines look crooked or bent, if any of the boxes are different in size or shape, and if any of the lines are wavy, missing, blurry, or discolored. Repeat with the other eye. The test should be conducted before the pupils are dilated, and the client should be wearing their best correction.

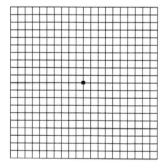

Figure 47–5 ■ The Amsler grid.

EYE AND VISION ASSESSMENTS

Vision Assessment

Visual acuity is assessed with an eye chart such as the Snellen chart or the E chart for testing distance vision and the Rosenbaum chart for testing near vision. The Snellen chart contains rows of letters in various sizes, with standardized numbers at the end of each row. The number at the end of the row indicates the visual acuity of a client who can read the row at a distance of 20 feet. (If the client is unable to read or does not read English, you can use the E chart to test visual acuity.) The top number at the end of the row is always 20, representing the distance between the client and the chart. The bottom number is the distance (in feet) at which a person with normal vision can read the line. A person with normal vision can read the row marked 20/20. To conduct the assessment, ask the person to stand 20 feet from the chart in a well-lit area. Ask the client to cover one eye with an opaque cover (Figure 47–6 ■). Then ask the client to read each row of letters, moving from largest letters to the smallest ones that the client can see. Measure visual acuity in the other eye in the same way, and then assess visual acuity while the client has both eyes uncovered. You may test the client who wears corrective lenses with and without the lenses.

The Rosenbaum chart is held at a distance of from 12 to 14 inches from the eyes, with visual acuity measured in the same manner as with the Snellen chart (Figure 47–7 ■). A gross estimate of near vision may also be assessed by asking the person to read from a magazine or newspaper.

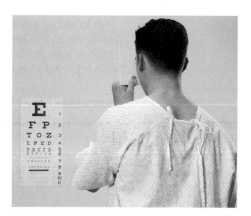

Figure 47–6 ■ Testing distant vision using the Snellen eye chart.

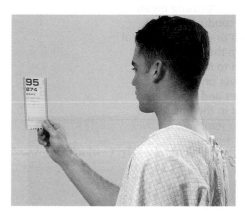

Figure 47–7 ■ Testing near vision using Rosenbaum eye chart.

Technique/Normal Findings	Abnormal Findings
Assess distant vision, using the Snellen or E chart. *When standing 20 feet from the chart, the client can read the smallest line of letters with or without corrective lenses (recorded as 20/20).*	■ Changes in distant vision are most commonly the result of **myopia** (nearsightedness). For example, a reading of 20/100 indicates impaired distance vision. A person has to stand 20 feet from the chart to read a line that a person with normal vision could read 100 feet from the chart.
Assess near vision, using a Rosenbaum chart or a card with newsprint held 12 to 14 inches from the client's eyes. *Normal near visual acuity is 14/14 with or without corrective lenses.*	■ Changes in near vision, especially in clients over age 45, can indicate **presbyopia**, impaired near vision resulting from a loss of elasticity of the lens related to aging. In younger clients, this condition is referred to as **hyperopia** (farsightedness).

Eye Movement Assessment

Assess the cardinal fields of vision to gain information about extraocular eye movements. Ask the client to follow a pen or your finger while keeping the head stationary. Move the pen or your finger through the six fields one at a time, returning to the central starting point before proceeding to the next field (Figure 47–8 ■). *The eyes should move through each field without involuntary movements.*

■ Failure of one or both eyes to follow the object in any given direction may indicate extraocular muscle weakness or cranial nerve dysfunction.
■ An involuntary rhythmic movement of the eyes, **nystagmus**, is associated with neurologic disorders and the use of some medications.

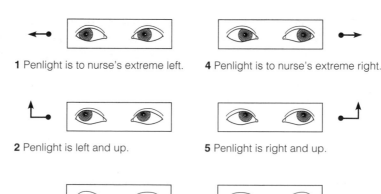

1 Penlight is to nurse's extreme left.   **4** Penlight is to nurse's extreme right.

2 Penlight is left and up.   **5** Penlight is right and up.

3 Penlight is left and down.   **6** Penlight is right and down.

Figure 47–8 ■ The six cardinal fields of vision.

Technique/Normal Findings	Abnormal Findings
Inspect the iris. *The iris is normally round, flat, and evenly colored.*	■ Lack of clarity of the iris may indicate a cloudiness of the cornea. ■ Constriction of the pupil accompanied by pain and circumcorneal redness indicates acute iritis.
Internal Eye Assessment Assess internal structures of the eye by using the ophthalmoscope, an instrument that allows visualization of the lens, the vitreous humor, and the retina. Box 47–1 provides guidelines for using the ophthalmoscope.	
Inspect for the red reflex. *The red reflex should be clearly visible.*	■ Absence of a red reflex often indicates improper position of the ophthalmoscope, but also may indicate total opacity of the pupil by a cataract or a hemorrhage into the vitreous humor.
Inspect the lens and vitreous body. *The lens should be clear.*	■ A cataract is an opacity of the lens, often seen as a dark shadow on ophthalmoscopic examination. It may be due to aging, trauma, diabetes, or a congenital defect.
Inspect the retina. *There should be no visible hemorrhages, exudate, or white patches.*	■ Areas of hemorrhage, exudate, and white patches may be a result of diabetes or long-standing hypertension.
Inspect the optic disc. *The optic disc should be round to oval in shape with clear, well-defined borders.*	■ Loss of definition of the optic disc, as well as an increase in the size of the physiologic cup, is seen in papilledema from increased intracranial pressure.
Inspect the blood vessels of the retina. *The retinal blood vessels should be distinct.*	■ Glaucoma often results in displacement of blood vessels from the center of the optic disc due to increased intraocular pressure. ■ Hypertension may cause a narrowing of the vein where an arteriole crosses over. ■ Engorged veins may occur with diabetes, atherosclerosis, and blood disorders.
Inspect the retinal background. *The retina should be a consistent red-orange color, becoming lighter around the optic disc.*	■ Variations in color or a pale color overall may indicate disease.
Inspect the macula. *The macula should be visible on the temporal side of the optic disc.*	■ Absence of the fovea centralis is common in older clients. It may indicate macular degeneration, a cause of loss of central vision.
Palpate over the lacrimal glands, puncta, and nasolacrimal duct. *There should be no tenderness, drainage, or excessive tearing.*	■ Tenderness over any of these areas or drainage from the puncta may indicate an infectious process. (Wear gloves if you see any drainage.) ■ Excessive tearing may indicate a blockage of the nasolacrimal duct.

ANATOMY, PHYSIOLOGY, AND FUNCTIONS OF THE EARS

As a sensory organ, the ears have two primary functions, hearing and maintaining equilibrium. Anatomically, each ear is divided into three areas: the external ear, the middle ear, and the inner ear (Figure 47–10 ■). Each area has a unique function. All three are involved in hearing, but only the inner ear is involved in equilibrium.

The External Ear

The external ear consists of the auricle (or pinna), the external auditory canal, and the tympanic membrane.

The auricles are elastic cartilage covered with thin skin. They contain sebaceous and sweat glands and sometimes hair. Each auricle has a rim (the helix) and a lobe. The auricle serves to direct sound waves into the ear.

The external auditory canal, which is about 1 inch (2.5 cm) long, extends from the auricle to the tympanic membrane. The canal is lined with skin that contains hair, sebaceous glands, and ceruminous glands. The external auditory canal serves as a resonator for the range of sound waves typical of human speech and increases the pressure that sound waves in this frequency

BOX 47-1 Guidelines for Using the Ophthalmoscope

The ophthalmoscope has a head and a handle. (See the figure below.) The head contains a focus wheel (also called a lens selector dial) located on the side, lenses of varying magnification, and an opening through which the eye structures are visualized. The focus wheel adjusts the lens refraction, which is measured in diopters. The diopter measurements range from 0 to +40 when the lens is rotated clockwise, and from 0 to −25 when the lens is rotated counterclockwise. By moving the focus wheel, the examiner can converge or diverge light rays to visualize the retina.

The handle usually contains batteries that can be recharged.

Before the examination, explain the procedure to the client. Assemble the ophthalmoscope. Wash your hands and wear disposable gloves if the client has any drainage from the eyes. Darken the room (to allow the pupils of the client to dilate), and ask the client to look straight ahead, focusing on a fixed point such as an object on the wall. Hold the ophthalmoscope in one hand, resting the index finger on the focus wheel (see the figure at right).

1. Turn on the ophthalmoscope light, and set focus wheel to 0 diopters. Hold the ophthalmoscope in your right hand with your index finger on the focus wheel. Standing in front of the client, position yourself at a 15-degree angle to the client's line of vision.
2. Hold the opening of the ophthalmoscope up to your right eye and direct the light toward the client's right eye from a distance of about 12 inches.
3. As the beam of light falls on the client's pupil, observe for the red reflex, which appears as a sharply outlined orange glow from within the pupil. This glow is the reflection of the light from the retina.
4. Move closer to the client, turning the focus wheel clockwise toward the positive numbers as needed to maintain clear focus.
5. Examine the lens and the vitreous body, both of which should be clear.
6. Gradually rotate the focus wheel counterclockwise toward the negative numbers as needed, focusing on a structure of the retina (such as the disc or a blood vessel). Turn the focus wheel until the image is clear. Examine the structures of the retina as follows:
   a. The optic disc (see the accompanying figure). Assess for size, shape, color, distinct margins, and the physiologic cup. The disc is round to slightly oval and about 1.5 mm in diameter. It has a yellow to pink color that is lighter than the retina itself. The margins should be sharp and clear. The physiologic cup is a small depression that occupies about one-third of the optic disc, lying temporal to the center of the disc.
   b. The vessels of the retina. Assess for color, arteriolar light reflex, ratio of arterioles to veins, and arteriovenous crossings. The arterioles are red, brighter than the veins,

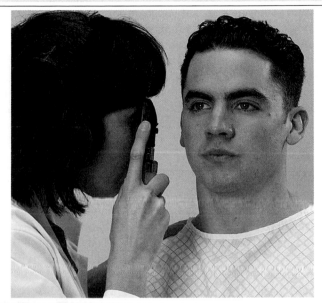

Technique for holding an ophthalmoscope.

and about one-fourth smaller. The arterioles normally have a narrow light reflex from the center of each vessel; veins do not have this light reflex. The ratio of arterioles to veins is usually 2:3 or 4:5. The vessels normally cross and become smaller toward the periphery.
   c. The retinal background. Assess color and changes in color. The retina is normally reddish orange and regular in color.
   d. The macula. Assess size and color. To assess the macula, ask the client to look directly into the ophthalmoscope light. The macula is temporal to the optic disc, appears slightly darker than the retina, and has no visible vessels. The fovea centralis may be seen as a bright spot of light. Because looking directly into the light causes some discomfort, conduct this portion of the examination last. The macula is often difficult to visualize.
7. Using the same technique, examine the left eye.

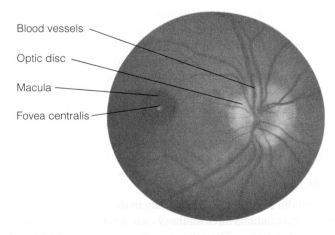

Blood vessels

Optic disc

Macula

Fovea centralis

The optic disc.

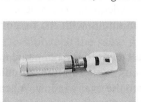

An ophthalmoscope.

Source: Don Wong/Science Source/Photo Researchers, Inc.

SAMPLE DOCUMENTATION
Assessment of the Ear

22-year-old male with complaints of "having some problems hearing these days." States he often listens to music in his car "as loud as it will go" and uses ear phones at home so he does not bother other family members. Ears are normally placed bilaterally; skin smooth without lesions. Small amount of dark brown cerumen present in ear canals. Tympanic membranes gray and shiny. No bulging or retraction noted. Whisper test: Unable to repeat back words spoken by examiner. Weber's test: Sound lateralized to left ear. Rinne test: BC ≥ AC. No tenderness noted when mastoids palpated. Referred to ear clinic for further evaluation.

provider's office. Diagnostic tests to assess the structure and functions of the ears are described in the Diagnostic Tests table below and summarized in the following bulleted list. More information is included in the discussion of specific injuries or diseases in Chapter 48 ∞ .

- Audiometry is used to evaluate and diagnose conductive and sensorineural hearing loss.
- Electrical activity of the auditory nerve may be evaluated by using an auditory evoked potential (AEP) or an auditory brainstem response (ABR).
- Vestibular system function is evaluated with a caloric test. If no nystagmus occurs during the test, further testing for brain lesions is conducted.

Regardless of the type of diagnostic test, the nurse is responsible for explaining the procedure and any special preparation needed, for assessing for any medication use that might affect the outcome of the tests, for supporting the client during the examination as necessary, for documenting the procedures as appropriate, and for monitoring the results of the tests.

Genetic Considerations

When conducting a health assessment interview and a physical assessment, it is important for the nurse to consider genetic influences on health of the adult. Several diseases of the ears have a genetic component. During the health assessment interview, ask about a family history of congenital deafness, deafness associated with a thyroid goiter, or tumors of the auditory nerve.

During the physical assessment, assess for any manifestations that might indicate a genetic disorder (see the Genetic Considerations box below). If data are found to indicate genetic risk factors or alterations, ask about genetic testing and refer for appropriate genetic counseling and evaluation. Chapter 8 ∞ provides further information about genetics in medical-surgical nursing.

Health Assessment Interview

The health history assessment to collect subjective data about the ears and hearing may be part of a health screening, may focus on a chief complaint (such as hearing problems or pain in

GENETIC CONSIDERATIONS
Ear Disorders

- Deafness (hearing loss) is a common disorder that is seen from newborns to those of old age. About 1 in 1000 infants have a profound hearing loss, with about half being genetic in origin (NIH, 2003b). Early diagnosis is important to facilitate language and social skill development in adults.
- Penred syndrome is an inherited disorder that accounts for as much as 10% of hereditary deafness. The deafness is usually accompanied by a thyroid goiter.
- Neurofibromatosis, a rare inherited disorder, is characterized by the development of acoustic neuromas (benign tumors of the auditory nerve) and malignant central nervous system tumors.

DIAGNOSTIC TESTS of Ear Disorders

NAME OF TEST Audiometry

PURPOSE AND DESCRIPTION Used to evaluate and diagnose conductive and sensorineural hearing loss. Client sits in soundproof room and responds by raising a hand when sounds are heard.

RELATED NURSING CARE No special preparation is needed.

NAME OF TEST Auditory evoked potential (AEP)

PURPOSE AND DESCRIPTION Used to identify electrical activity of the auditory nerve. Electrodes are placed on various areas of the ear and on the forehead and a graphic recording is made.

RELATED NURSING CARE No special preparation is needed.

NAME OF TEST Auditory brainstem response (ABR)

PURPOSE AND DESCRIPTION Measures electrical activity of the auditory pathway from inner ear to brain to diagnose brainstem pathology, stroke, and acoustic neuroma.

RELATED NURSING CARE No special preparation is needed.

NAME OF TEST Caloric test

PURPOSE AND DESCRIPTION Used to assess vestibular system function. Cold or warm water is used to irrigate the ear canals one at a time and the client is observed for nystagmus (repeated abnormal movements of the eyes). Normally, the nystagmus occurs opposite to the ear being irrigated. If no nystagmus occurs, the client needs further testing for brain lesions.

RELATED NURSING CARE Assess client for use of alcohol, central nervous system depressants, and barbiturates. These chemicals may alter the test results.

the ear), or may be part of a total health assessment. If the client has a problem involving one or both ears, analyze its onset, characteristics and course, severity, precipitating and relieving factors, and any associated symptoms, noting the timing and circumstances. For example, you may ask the following questions:

- Have you noticed any difficulty hearing high-pitched sounds, low-pitched sounds, or both?
- When did you first notice the ringing in your ears?
- Is your workplace very noisy? If so, do you wear protective ear equipment at work?

Throughout the examination, be alert to nonverbal behaviors (such as inappropriate answers or requests to repeat statements)

that suggest problems with ear function. Explore changes in hearing, ringing in the ears (*tinnitus*), ear pain, drainage from the ears, or the use of hearing aids. When taking the history, ask about trauma, surgery, or infections of the ear as well as the date of the last ear examination. In addition, ask the client about a medical history of infectious diseases, such as meningitis or mumps, as well as the use of medications that may affect hearing. Because ear problems tend to run in families, ask about a family history of hearing loss, ear problems, or diseases that could result in such problems. If the client has a hearing aid, ascertain the type and assess measures for its care.

Interview questions categorized by functional health patterns are found in the Functional Health Pattern table below.

FUNCTIONAL HEALTH PATTERN INTERVIEW The Ear

Functional Health Pattern	Interview Questions and Leading Statements
Health Perception-Health Management	■ Describe your hearing. Rate it on a scale of 1 to 10, with 10 being excellent hearing. Is it the same in both ears? If not, which ear is better? ■ Describe your current hearing problems. How have these been treated? ■ Do you use ear medications? What type and how often? ■ Have you ever had ear surgery? Describe. ■ Describe the type of hearing aid that you use. Are you satisfied with this appliance? How do you care for it? ■ Describe how you care for your ears each day. ■ When was your last ear examination? Have you ever had your hearing tested? ■ Do you listen to loud music? Do you use ear phones when you listen to loud music?
Nutritional-Metabolic	■ Do you have any swelling or tenderness in the ears or drainage from the ears?
Activity Exercise	■ Does your hearing problem interfere with your usual activities of daily living? Explain. ■ Do you wear protective earplugs when you take part in activities that increase the risk of injury to your ears (such as at work or when operating machinery at home)?
Sleep-Rest	■ Does your ear problem interfere with your ability to rest or sleep (for example, from pain)? If so, what do you do?
Cognitive-Perceptual	■ Do you have pain in or around your ears? Have you ever had ringing in your ears? If so, describe its location, intensity, what makes it worse, and how long it lasts. How do you treat it? ■ Do you have difficulty hearing conversations, either in person or on the telephone? Do you have trouble hearing the television? Do you have difficulty hearing when you are in crowds or there is background noise? ■ Have you noticed your hearing is different in each ear? ■ Do you have buzzing, ringing, or crackling noises in one or both ears? Explain. ■ Do you ever feel dizzy?
Self-Perception-Self-Concept	■ Has this problem with your ears affected how you feel about yourself?
Role-Relationships	■ How has having this condition affected your relationships with others? ■ Has having this condition interfered with your ability to work? Explain. ■ Has anyone in your family had problems with ear disease? Explain.
Sexuality-Reproductive	■ Has this condition interfered with your usual sexual activity?
Coping-Stress-Tolerance	■ Has having this condition created stress for you? If so, does your health problem seem to be more difficult when you are stressed? ■ Have you experienced any kind of stress that makes the condition worse? Explain. ■ Describe what you do when you feel stressed.
Value-Belief	■ Describe how specific relationships or activities help you cope with this problem. ■ Describe specific cultural beliefs or practices that affect how you care for and feel about this problem. ■ Are there any specific treatments that you would not use to treat this problem?

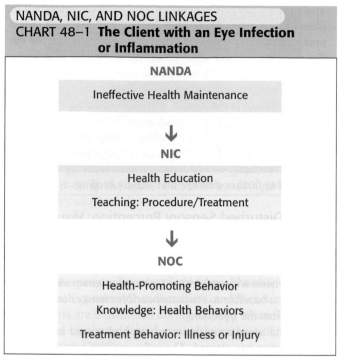

NANDA, NIC, AND NOC LINKAGES
CHART 48–1 **The Client with an Eye Infection or Inflammation**

NANDA

Ineffective Health Maintenance

↓

NIC

Health Education

Teaching: Procedure/Treatment

↓

NOC

Health-Promoting Behavior

Knowledge: Health Behaviors

Treatment Behavior: Illness or Injury

Data from *NANDA's Nursing Diagnoses: Definitions & Classification 2005–2006* by NANDA International (2005), Philadelphia; *Nursing Interventions Classification (NIC)* (4th ed.) by J. M. Dochterman & G. C. Bulechek (2004), St. Louis, MO: Mosby; and *Nursing Outcomes Classification (NOC)* (3rd ed.) by S. Moorhead, M. Johnson, and M. Maas (2004), St. Louis, MO: Mosby.

abrasions, injury to its deeper layers can delay healing or result in scarring.

Physiology Review

The cornea has three major layers: the outermost epithelium, which consists of five or six layers of cells that are constantly being renewed; the stroma, which makes up 90% of corneal tissue; and the single-cell thickness endothelium adjacent to the aqueous humor of the anterior chamber. The cornea is avascular tissue; the central cornea is dependent on atmospheric oxygen to meet its metabolic needs. Because there is no blood supply, immune defenses have difficulty fending off infections of the cornea.

Pathophysiology and Manifestations

Light enters the eye through the normally clear cornea. As light passes through the curved cornea, it is bent or *refracted* onto the lens, which then focuses the light on sensory cells of the retina. A change in the curvature of the cornea or in its clarity affects the ability of the eye to clearly focus; as a result, vision is distorted or blurred. Refractive errors such as nearsightedness, farsightedness, and astigmatism are common. Corneal scarring or ulceration are two major causes of blindness worldwide.

Refractive Errors

Refractive errors are the most common problem affecting visual acuity; they result from an abnormal curvature of the cornea or an altered shape of the eyeball. People with *emmetropia* (normal vision) see near and far objects clearly because light rays focus directly on the retina. In **myopia** (near-

sightedness) the curvature of the cornea is excessive or the eyeball is elongated, causing the image to focus in front of the retina instead of on it. Objects in close range are seen clearly and those at a distance are blurred. The eyeball is too short in **hyperopia** (farsightedness), causing the image to focus behind the retina. People with this condition see objects clearer at a distance than those close to them.

FAST FACTS
- The prevalence of myopia decreases with aging, from an estimated 36.4% of Americans ages 40 to 49 affected (15.5 million) to 17.5% of people ages 80 and older (1.6 million).
- In contrast, the prevalence of hyperopia increases with aging, affecting an estimated 3.1% of Americans ages 40 to 49 (1.5 million) and 23.6% of people ages 80 and older (2.2 million) (NEI, 2004).

Astigmatism develops due to an irregular or abnormal curvature of the cornea. Instead of the round, even curvature of the normal cornea, the cornea curves more in one direction than the other in astigmatism, resembling the back of a spoon. As a result, light rays focus on more than one area of the retina, distorting both near and distance vision.

Keratitis

Keratitis is inflammation of the cornea. When the inflammatory process involves both the conjunctiva and the cornea, the term *keratoconjunctivitis* may be used. Keratitis may be caused by infection, hypersensitivity reactions, ischemia, tearing defects, trauma, and impaired innervation of the cornea. Scarring that occurs as a result of keratitis is a leading cause of blindness worldwide (Porth, 2005).

Keratitis is described as either nonulcerative or ulcerative. In *nonulcerative keratitis,* all layers of corneal epithelium are affected, but remain intact. Viral infections, tuberculosis, and autoimmune disorders such as lupus erythematosus may cause nonulcerative keratitis. *Ulcerative keratitis,* in contrast, affects the epithelium and stroma of the cornea, leading to tissue destruction and ulceration. Bacterial conjunctivitis (e.g., *Staphylococcus, S. pneumoniae, Chlamydia*) may lead to ulcerative keratitis.

Keratitis commonly causes tearing, discomfort ranging from a gritty sensation in the eye to severe pain, decreased visual acuity, and *blepharospasm* (spasm of the eyelid and inability to open the eye). A discharge may be present, especially if the conjunctiva is also inflamed. Corneal ulceration may be visible on direct examination.

Corneal Ulcer

A **corneal ulcer**, local necrosis of the cornea, may be caused by infection, exposure trauma, or the misuse of contact lenses. A frequent cause is bacterial infection following trauma or contact lens overuse. Herpes viruses, including herpes simplex and herpes zoster, are a leading cause of ulcerative corneal disease. Corneal ulcers may also complicate bacterial conjunctivitis, trachoma, gonorrhea, and other acute infections. Clients who are immunosuppressed because of disease or drug therapy are at particular risk for developing corneal ulcers due to infection.

In corneal ulceration, a portion of the epithelium and/or stroma is destroyed. Ulcers may be superficial or deep, penetrating underlying layers and posing a risk of perforation. Fibrous tissue may form during healing, resulting in scarring and opacity of the cornea. Perforation can lead to infection of deeper eye structures or extrusion of eye contents. Partial or total vision loss may result.

Corneal Dystrophies

A corneal dystrophy is accumulation of cloudy material in part or parts of the normally clear cornea, potentially affecting visual acuity. Corneal dystrophies typically are inherited disorders that progress gradually and affect both eyes. *Keratoconus*, progressive thinning of the cornea, is the most common corneal dystrophy. It typically affects teenagers and young adults. In keratoconus, the center of the cornea thins and bulges outward, affecting the shape of the cornea and its ability to focus light on the lens of the eye. In most cases, the thinning stabilizes over time; up to 20% of clients, however, eventually require corneal transplant (NEI, 2005a).

INTERDISCIPLINARY CARE

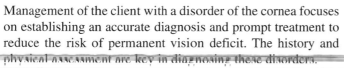

Management of the client with a disorder of the cornea focuses on establishing an accurate diagnosis and prompt treatment to reduce the risk of permanent vision deficit. The history and physical assessment are key in diagnosing these disorders.

Although many eye disorders can be treated in the community, the client with a severe corneal infection or ulcer may require hospitalization. Corneal ulcers are medical emergencies, requiring prompt referral to an ophthalmologist for treatment. Pressure dressings may be applied to both eyes for comfort and to reduce the risk of perforation and loss of eye contents.

Diagnosis

Visual acuity is tested on all clients presenting with refractory or corneal disorders. See Chapter 47 ∞ for more information about testing visual acuity. The following tests may be ordered to identify the cause and extent of eye infections or inflammations:

- *Fluorescein stain* with slit-lamp examination allows visualization of any corneal ulcerations or abrasions, which appear green with staining.
- *Conjunctival* or *ulcer scrapings* are examined microscopically or cultured to identify the organisms.

Additional laboratory testing such as blood counts or antibody titers may be used to identify any underlying infectious or autoimmune processes.

Medication

Infectious processes are treated with antibiotic or antiviral therapy as appropriate. Topical anti-infectives applied as either eyedrops or ointment may include erythromycin, gentamicin, penicillin, bacitracin, sulfacetamide sodium, amphotericin B, or idoxuridine. For severe infections, central ulcers, or cellulitis, anti-infectives may be administered by subconjunctival injection and/or systemic intravenous infusion. Corticosteroids may be prescribed for keratitis related to systemic inflamma-

tory disorders or trauma; however, it is important to avoid their use with local infections to avoid suppressing the immune and inflammatory responses.

Corrective Lenses

Corrective lenses, either in the form of eyeglasses or contact lenses, generally are prescribed to restore visual acuity for clients with refractive errors such as myopia, hyperopia, and astigmatism. Specially fitted contact lenses to reduce vision distortion are ordered for clients with keratoconus. Because contact lenses are a risk factor for corneal infection and ulcers, teaching appropriate care is vital (see Box 48–1).

Surgery

LASER EYE SURGERY Laser eye surgery is commonly performed to correct refractive errors such as myopia, hyperopia, and astigmatism. In these surgeries, a laser is used to permanently change the shape of the cornea. In most cases, the need to use corrective lenses is reduced or eliminated. Several surgical procedures are available:

- Laser *in situ* keratomileusis (LASIK)
- Photorefractive keratectomy (PRK)
- Laser epithelial keratomileusis (LASEK)
- Laser thermokeratoplasty (LTK).

These procedures reshape the cornea using laser technology to remove a thin layer of epithelial cells or to shrink and reshape the cornea. Candidates for laser vision correction surgery should be in good health and must have adequate corneal thickness such that perforation is not a risk.

Following surgery, clients may experience a temporary loss of contrast sharpness (images do not appear as crisp as with corrective lenses), over- or undercorrection of visual acuity, dry eyes, or temporarily decreased night vision with halos, glare, and starbursts. Diffuse lamellar keratitis (DLK) is a rare complication of surgery that, while treatable, can lead to vision impairment if not identified and treated early.

Phototherapeutic keratectomy (PTK) provides an alternative to corneal transplant in treating corneal dystrophies, scars, and some infections. In this procedure, diseased corneal tissue is vaporized and surface irregularities corrected with little trauma to surrounding tissue. Healing occurs rapidly.

CORNEAL TRANSPLANT Once the cornea has become scarred and opaque, no treatment can restore its clarity. The first successful corneal transplant (or *keratoplasty*), replacement of diseased cornea by healthy corneal tissue from a donor, was performed in 1906. Current corneal transplant procedures have a success rate of approximately 80% (NEI, 2005a).

Corneas are harvested from the cadavers of uninfected adults who were under the age of 65 and who died as a result of acute trauma or illness. After harvesting, the cornea can be stored in a tissue-culture medium for up to 4 weeks before being used as a graft. Corneal transplantation is usually an elective surgery, although emergency transplantation may be required for perforation of the cornea.

Corneal transplant may be either lamellar or penetrating. In a lamellar keratoplasty, the superficial layer of cornea is removed and replaced with a graft. The anterior chamber remains intact.

Health Promotion

Although glaucoma cannot be prevented, its severity and potentially deleterious permanent effects can be limited with early visual screening. The nurse assumes an important role in educating the public about the risk factors for glaucoma such as increased age, and the higher incidence in African Americans and Asians. All people over the age of 40 are encouraged to receive an eye examination every 2 to 4 years, including tonometry screening. Those with a predominant family history should be evaluated more frequently, every 1 to 2 years. After the age of 65, yearly ophthalmologic examinations are recommended.

Assessment

Collect the following data through a health history and physical examination (see Chapter 47 ∞).

- *Health history:* Family history; presence of altered vision, halos, and excessive tearing; sudden, severe eye pain; use of corrective lenses; most recent eye examination.
- *Physical examination:* Distant and near vision, peripheral fields, retina for optic nerve cupping.

Nursing Diagnoses and Interventions

Nursing care planning focuses on problems associated with the temporary or permanent visual impairment, the resultant increased risk for injury, and the psychosocial problems of anxiety and coping.

Disturbed Sensory Perception: Visual

Whether glaucoma and resulting impaired vision is the client's primary problem or a preexisting condition in a client with another disorder, it must be a primary consideration in nursing care planning.

- Address by name and identify yourself with each interaction. Orient to time, place, person, and situation as indicated. State the purpose of your visit. *The client with impaired vision must rely on input from the other senses. A lack of visual cues increases the importance of verbal ones. For example, the client with impaired vision cannot see the nurse checking an intravenous infusion and needs a verbal explanation of who is in the room and why. When the client's normal daily routine is disrupted by illness or hospitalization, additional sensory input such as a radio, television, and explanations of the routine and activities are useful to maintain the client's orientation.*
- Provide any visual aids that are routinely used. Keep them close, making sure that the client knows where they are and can reach them easily. *Easy access encourages the client to use these items and enhances the ability to provide self-care.*
- Orient to the environment. Explain the location of the call bell, personal items, and the furniture in the room. If able, tour client's room, including the bathroom and sink. *Clients with visual impairments are usually very capable of providing self-care in a known environment.*
- Provide other tools or items that can help compensate for diminished vision:
  a. Bright, nonglare lighting
  b. Books, magazines, and instructions in large print

  c. Books on tape
  d. Telephones with oversize pushbuttons
  e. A clock with numbers and hands that can be felt
- Assist with meals by:
  a. Reading menu selections and marking choices.
  b. Describing the position of foods on a meal tray according to the clock system, for example, "On the plate, the peas are at 9 o'clock, the mashed potatoes at 1 o'clock, and the chicken breast at 6 o'clock. The milk glass is at 2 o'clock on the tray above the plate, and coffee is at 11 o'clock."
  c. Placing the utensils in a readily accessible position.
  d. Removing lids from containers, buttering the bread, and cutting meat, as needed.
  e. If the visual impairment is new or temporary, the client may need feeding or continued assistance during the meal.
  Providing assistance during eating is important to maintain the client's nutritional status. The client may be ashamed of needing help or embarrassed to request it and may respond by not eating or by claiming not to be hungry.
- Assist with mobility and ambulation as needed:
  a. Have the client hold your arm or elbow, and walk slightly ahead as a guide. Do not hold the client's arm or elbow.
  b. Describe the surroundings and progress as you proceed. Warn in advance of potential hazards, turns, and steps.
  c. Teach to feel the chair, bed, or commode with the hands and the back of the legs before sitting.
  These measures help ensure the client's safety while providing for mobility and helping prevent complications associated with immobility.
- If the vision loss is unilateral and recent, provide instructions related to unilateral vision loss and change in depth perception:
  a. Caution about the loss of depth perception and teach safety precautions, such as reaching slowly for objects and using visual cues as to distance, especially when driving.
  b. Teach to scan, turning the head fully toward the affected side to identify potential hazards and looking up and down to compensate for the loss of depth perception.
  The client with a unilateral vision loss is often unaware of its effect on peripheral vision and depth perception.

Risk for Injury

Whether the client is experiencing a sudden loss of vision due to acute angle-closure glaucoma or significant visual impairment due to inadequately managed chronic glaucoma, both are at an increased risk for injury. Clients who have had surgical interventions for glaucoma are at even greater risk.

- Assess ability to perform ADLs. *Clients may be reluctant to request assistance, believing that they should be able to perform these familiar tasks. Careful assessment and provision of needed assistance help prevent injury and maintain the client's self-esteem.*
- Notify housekeeping and place a sign on the client's door to alert all personnel not to change the arrangement of the client's room. *The client with impaired vision is at high risk for falling when in an unfamiliar environment. It is important to maintain a safe, familiar room when the client is hospitalized.*

- Raise two or three side rails on the client's bed. *Raised rails remind clients to ask for assistance before ambulating in an unfamiliar environment.*
- Discuss possible adaptations in the home to help the client remain as independent as possible and prevent falls or other injuries. *Often minor changes in the home environment, such as removing scatter rugs and small items of furniture, allow the client to navigate safely in this already familiar environment.*

PRACTICE ALERT
Keep traffic area free of clutter to reduce the risk for injury in clients with impaired vision.

Anxiety

The actual or potential loss of sight threatens the client's self-concept, role functioning, patterns of interaction, and, potentially, environment. The client with impaired vision who functions well in a familiar environment will feel anxious in the unfamiliar setting of a hospital or care facility.

- Assess for verbal and nonverbal indications of level of anxiety and for normal coping mechanisms. Repeated expressions of concern or denial that the vision change will affect the client's life indicate anxiety. Nonverbal indicators include tension, difficulty concentrating or thinking, restlessness, poor eye contact, and changes in vocalization (rapid speech, voice quivering). Physical indicators include tachycardia, dilated pupils, cool and clammy skin, and tremors. *The client may not recognize this feeling as anxiety. Identifying and acknowledging the anxiety state can help the client recognize and deal with it.*
- Encourage to verbalize fears, anger, and feelings of anxiety. *Verbalizing helps externalize the anxiety and allows fears to be addressed.*
- Discuss perception of the eye condition and its effects on lifestyle and roles. *Discussion provides an opportunity to correct misperceptions and introduce alternative activities and assistive devices for clients with visual impairments.*
- Introduce yourself when entering the room, explain all procedures fully before and as they are being performed, and use touch to convey proximity and caring. *The client with impaired vision must rely on the other senses to make up for the loss of sight. Because the client cannot see what you are doing, complete explanations of even simple tasks such as refilling a water glass help to relieve anxiety.*
- Identify coping strategies that have been useful in the past and adapt these strategies to the present situation. *Previously successful coping strategies may be employed to increase the client's sense of control.*

Using NANDA, NIC, and NOC

Chart 48–2 shows links between NANDA nursing diagnoses, NIC, and NOC when caring for the client with glaucoma.

Community-Based Care

Clients with glaucoma require teaching about lifetime strategies for managing the disease at home. They need to under-

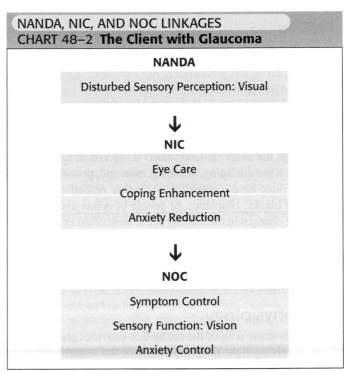

NANDA, NIC, AND NOC LINKAGES
CHART 48–2 The Client with Glaucoma

NANDA

Disturbed Sensory Perception: Visual

↓

NIC

Eye Care

Coping Enhancement

Anxiety Reduction

↓

NOC

Symptom Control

Sensory Function: Vision

Anxiety Control

Data from *NANDA's Nursing Diagnoses: Definitions & Classification 2005–2006* by NANDA International (2005), Philadelphia; *Nursing Interventions Classification (NIC)* (4th ed.) by J. M. Dochterman & G. M. Bulechek (2004), St. Louis, MO: Mosby; and *Nursing Outcomes Classification (NOC)* (3rd ed.) by S. Moorhead, M. Johnson, and M. Maas (2004). St. Louis, MO: Mosby.

stand the importance of lifetime therapy to control the disease and prevent blindness. If a permanent visual impairment has resulted, the client needs information on achieving the maximum possible independence while maintaining safety. The following topics should be discussed with the client and family:

- Prescribed medications including proper way to instill eyedrops
- Importance of not taking certain prescription and over-the-counter medications without consulting a physician
- Periodic eye examinations with intraocular pressure measurement
- Risks, warning signs, and management of acute angle-closure glaucoma
- Possible surgical options
- Community resources, such as Visually Impaired Society, local library, and transportation services
- Helpful resources:
  - National Glaucoma Foundation
  - Young and Under Pressure Glaucoma Foundation
  - Glaucoma Research Foundation
  - Prevention of Blindness Society.

THE CLIENT WITH AGE-RELATED MACULAR DEGENERATION

The leading cause of legal blindness and impaired vision in people over the age of 65 is age-related **macular degeneration** (AMD) (Prevent Blindness America, 2002).

a very thin bony plate separates mastoid air cells from the brain. Fortunately, this complication is rare since the advent of effective antibiotic therapy for treating otitis media.

Manifestations

Manifestations of acute mastoiditis usually develop approximately 2 to 3 weeks after an episode of acute otitis media and include recurrent earache and hearing loss on the affected side. The pain is persistent and throbbing; tenderness is present over the mastoid process (behind the ear). It may also be red and inflamed. Swelling of the process can cause the auricle of the ear to protrude more than normal. Fever may be accompanied by tinnitus and headache. Profuse drainage from the affected ear may be noted.

INTERDISCIPLINARY CARE

In addition to the manifestations of acute mastoiditis, loss of septa between mastoid air cells may be noted on radiologic examination. Acute mastoiditis is treated aggressively with antibiotic therapy. Intravenous ticarcillin-clavulanate (Timentin) and gentamicin may be used initially, with therapy tailored to the specific organism once culture results are obtained. Antibiotics are continued for at least 14 days. Infections that do not respond to medical therapy or that pose a high risk of spreading to the brain may necessitate *mastoidectomy*, surgical removal of the infected mastoid air cells, bone, and pus, and inspection of the underlying dura for possible abscess. The extent of tissue destruction determines the extent of surgery required. In a modified mastoidectomy, as much tissue is preserved as possible to avoid disruption of hearing. A radical mastoidectomy involves removal of middle ear structures including the incus and malleus as well as the diseased portions of the mastoid process. Unless reconstruction is performed at the time of surgery, this surgery results in conductive hearing loss. **Tympanoplasty,** surgical reconstruction of the middle ear, can restore or preserve hearing.

NURSING CARE

Prevention is the primary focus of collaborative and nursing care related to mastoiditis. Adequate, effective antibiotic treatment of acute otitis media prevents mastoiditis in nearly all instances.

Following surgical intervention, carefully assess the wound and drainage for evidence of infection or other complications. The client's hearing may be temporarily or permanently affected, depending on the extent of the surgery. If the client has impaired hearing in the unaffected ear as well, develop a means of communication with the client prior to surgery. If the hearing is preserved in the unaffected ear, position the client with that ear toward the door. Speak slowly and clearly; do not shout or speak unusually loudly. Be sure that family and staff know about the client's hearing loss and use appropriate communication techniques. Assist the client with ambulation initially, because dizziness and vertigo are not unusual following surgery.

Nursing care of the client having ear surgery is discussed in the box on the next page.

Community-Based Care

When teaching about acute mastoiditis, stress the importance of complying with the prescribed antibiotic therapy and recommendations for follow-up. Instruct the client and family to report any adverse reactions to the primary care provider so that therapy can be adjusted. Teach the client and family how to change the surgical dressing using aseptic technique. Provide referrals to appropriate community agencies for the client with a new hearing loss resulting from mastoiditis or its treatment.

THE CLIENT WITH CHRONIC OTITIS MEDIA

Chronic otitis media involves permanent perforation of the tympanic membrane, with or without recurrent pus formation. Changes in the mucosa and bony structures (ossicles) of the middle ear often accompany chronic otitis media. It usually is the result of recurrent acute otitis media and eustachian tube dysfunction, but may also result from trauma or other diseases.

Marginal perforations, which usually occur in the posterior-superior portion of the tympanic membrane, are associated with more complications than central perforations. With marginal perforations, squamous epithelium may migrate from the ear canal into the middle ear, where it begins to desquamate and accumulate, forming a *cholesteatoma* (a cyst or mass filled with epithelial cell debris). Its incidence is highest in children and young adults. The desquamating epithelium continues to accumulate and remains infected, producing collagenases (enzymes) that destroy adjacent bone. The inflammatory process impairs the blood supply to the stapes, causing its destruction and conductive hearing loss. Cholesteatomas are benign and slow-growing tumors, which can enlarge to fill the entire middle ear. Untreated, the cholesteatoma can progressively destroy the ossicles and erode into the inner ear, causing profound hearing loss.

Systemic antibiotics are prescribed for exacerbations of purulent otitis media. Tympanic membrane perforation is repaired with a tympanoplasty to restore sound conduction and the integrity of the middle ear. A cholesteatoma may require delicate surgery for its removal. If at all possible, radical mastoidectomy with removal of the tympanic membrane, ossicles, and tumor is avoided.

As with other complications of acute otitis media, a priority of nursing care is prevention of chronic otitis media and cholesteatoma. Clients with chronic otitis media need to understand various treatment options and their risks and benefits, as well as the long-term risk of not treating a perforated tympanic membrane. They are also taught how to instill eardrops, to clean the external auditory meatus, and to not irrigate the ear when the tympanic membrane is perforated or if they think it might be.

If surgical treatment of chronic otitis media will affect the client's hearing, include this information in preoperative teach-

NURSING CARE OF THE CLIENT HAVING Ear Surgery

PREOPERATIVE CARE

- Review Chapter 4 ∞ for routine preoperative care.
- Assess hearing or verify documentation of preoperative hearing assessment. *These data are important in evaluating the results of the surgical procedure.*
- Establish a means of communication to be used after surgery. *Hearing may be impaired after surgery.*
- Explain that blowing of the nose, coughing, and sneezing are restricted postoperatively to prevent pressure changes in the middle ear and potential disruption of the surgical site. Keeping the mouth open during a cough or sneeze minimizes pressure changes in the middle ear. *Providing teaching and the opportunity to practice before surgery promotes cooperation in the postoperative period.*

POSTOPERATIVE CARE

- Review Chapter 4 ∞ for routine postoperative care.
- Assess for bleeding or drainage from the affected ear. *Infection and hemorrhage are possible complications.*
- Administer antiemetics as ordered to prevent vomiting. *Vomiting may increase the pressure in the middle ear, disrupting the surgical site.*
- Elevate the head of bed and position the client on the unaffected side. *This position minimizes the pressure in the middle ear.*
- Assess for vertigo or dizziness, especially with ambulation or movement in bed. Avoid unnecessary movements such as turning. Take measures to ensure safety during ambulation. *Surgery on the ear may disrupt equilibrium, increasing the risk of falling.*

- Assess hearing postoperatively. Stand on the unaffected side to communicate and use other measures such as written messages as needed for effective communication with the client with impaired hearing. Reassure the client that decreased hearing acuity immediately after surgery is expected. *Hearing improvement, if an expected result of the ear surgery, typically does not occur until earplugs are removed and edema and drainage at the operative site have resolved. If no reconstruction of the middle ear is done or the cochlea is involved, permanent hearing loss in the affected ear may be an expected result.*
- Remind to avoid coughing, sneezing, or blowing the nose. *These increase pressure in the middle ear.*

Health Education for the Client and Family

- Provide instructions for home care:
  a. To prevent contamination of the ear canal, avoid showers, shampooing, and immersing the head until the physician says you can do so.
  b. Keep the outer earplug clean and dry, changing it as needed. Do not remove inner ear dressing until instructed to do so by the physician.
  c. Avoid blowing the nose; if you need to cough or sneeze, keep the mouth open.
  d. Do not swim or dive without physician approval. Check with your doctor regarding air travel.
  e. Meclizine hydrochloride (Antivert) or other antiemetic/antihistamine medication may be necessary for up to 1 month following surgery.
  f. Fever, bleeding, increased drainage, increased dizziness, or decreased hearing after discharge may indicate a complication. Notify the physician if any of these occur.

---

ing. Teach the client and family how to use alternative means of communication if this will be necessary postoperatively. When an assistive device is ordered, teach the client and a family member about its use.

THE CLIENT WITH OTOSCLEROSIS

Otosclerosis is a common cause of conductive hearing loss. Abnormal bone formation in the osseous labyrinth of the temporal bone causes the footplate of the stapes to become fixed or immobile in the oval window. The result is a conductive hearing loss.

Otosclerosis is a hereditary disorder with an autosomal dominant pattern of inheritance. It occurs most commonly in Caucasians and in females. The progressive hearing loss typically begins in adolescence or early adulthood and seems to be accelerated by pregnancy. Although both ears are affected, the rate of hearing loss is asymmetric. Because bone conduction of sound is retained, the client may be able to use the telephone but have difficulty conversing in person. Tinnitus may also be associated with otosclerosis.

On examination, a reddish or pinkish-orange tympanic membrane may be noted because of increased vascularity of the middle ear. The Rinne test (Chapter 47 ∞) shows bone sound conduction to be equal to or greater than air conduction, an abnormal finding.

Clients with otosclerosis may choose conservative treatment, relying on a hearing aid to improve their ability to hear and interact with others. Sodium fluoride may be prescribed to slow bone resorption and overgrowth. Surgical treatment involves a stapedectomy and middle ear reconstruction or a stapedotomy. A *stapedectomy* is a microsurgical technique for removing the diseased stapes. A metallic prosthesis is then inserted, with one end connected to the incus and the other inserted into the oval window. *Stapedotomy* involves creation of a small hole in the footplate of the stapes and insertion of a wire or platinum ribbon prosthesis. An argon, KTP, or CO_2 laser may be used for surgery. Surgery usually restores hearing for the client with otosclerosis.

Education and referral of the client to appropriate community agencies are important nursing care priorities for the client with otosclerosis. For the client who chooses surgical treatment, nursing care is similar to that for other clients undergoing ear surgery. The following nursing diagnoses may be appropriate:

- *Risk for Injury* related to hearing loss or postoperative vertigo
- *Disturbed Sensory Perception: Auditory* related to bony sclerosis of the stapes

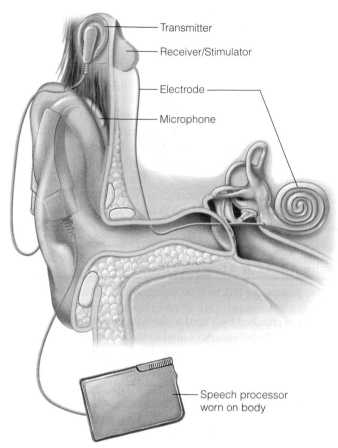

- Transmitter
- Receiver/Stimulator
- Electrode
- Microphone
- Speech processor worn on body

Figure 48–18 ■ A cochlear implant for sensorineural hearing loss.

send these impulses to the electrodes for transmission to the brain.

Cochlear implants provide sound perception but not normal hearing. The client is able to recognize warning sounds such as automobiles, sirens, telephones, and doors opening or closing. They also receive stimuli to alert them to incoming communication so they can focus on the person speaking. Many clients learn to interpret perceived sounds as words, especially when the hearing loss is acquired as an adult.

NURSING CARE

In planning and implementing nursing care for the client with a hearing deficit, the type and extent of hearing loss, the client's adaptation to the loss, and the availability of assistive hearing devices are considered, as well as the client's ability and willingness to use assistive devices.

Health Promotion

Healthcare personnel can be instrumental in preventing hearing loss through education. It is important to promote environmental noise control and the use of ear protection. The Occupational Safety and Health Administration requires ear protection for work environments that consis-

tently exceed 85 decibels. Teaching for primary prevention focuses on the following:

- Care of the ears and ear canals, including cleaning and treatment of infection
- Not placing hard objects into the ear canal
- Use of plugs to protect the ears during swimming or diving
- Avoiding intermittent or frequent exposure to loud noise
- Monitoring for side effects with ototoxic medications
- Hearing evaluation when hearing difficulty is present.

Assessment

- *Health history:* Perceived ability to hear; effect of hearing loss on function and lifestyle; risk factors such as use of ototoxic medications; upper respiratory tract or frequent ear infection; noise exposure; presence of vertigo, tinnitus, unsteadiness, or imbalance.
- *Physical examination:* Apparent perception of normal speech; inspection of external ear, tympanic membrane; whisper, Rinne, and Weber tests; tests of balance and cranial nerve function.

Nursing Diagnoses and Interventions

This section focuses on the problems of having a hearing deficit, impaired communication, and social isolation for the client who is hearing impaired.

Disturbed Sensory Perception: Auditory

Whether the client's hearing deficit is partial or total, impaired sound perception is the primary problem. The client needs to understand what causes the deficit and what to expect for the future. Nursing interventions focus on maximizing available hearing and preventing further deterioration to the extent possible.

- Encourage to talk about the hearing loss and its effect on activities of daily living. *Hearing loss affects each individual in a different way. The client may be denying the extent of the deficit or grieving the loss. Listening and providing support encourage the client to develop coping strategies.*
- Provide information about the type of hearing loss. Refer to an audiologist for evaluation of the hearing loss and possible exploration of amplification devices. *With improved understanding of the deficit, the client can plan ways to compensate.*
- Replace batteries in hearing aids regularly and as needed. *Hearing aid batteries last approximately 1 week. If a battery is old or has been improperly stored, the life may be reduced further.*
- If the hearing aid has a toggle switch for microphone/ telephone, be sure it is in the appropriate position. *This ensures proper amplification with the hearing aid.*

PRACTICE ALERT
Check hearing aids for patency, cleaning out cerumen as necessary.

Impaired Verbal Communication

A hearing deficit impairs the client's ability to receive and interpret verbal communication. A hearing loss affects the client's

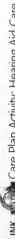

ability to follow conversations, use the telephone, and enjoy television or other forms of entertainment.

- Use the following techniques to improve communication:
  a. Wave the hand or tap the shoulder before beginning to speak.
  b. If the client wears corrective lenses, ensure that they are clean, and encourage the client to wear them.
  c. When speaking, face your client and keep your hands away from your face.
  d. Keep your face in full light.
  e. Reduce the noise in the environment before speaking.
  f. Use a low voice pitch with normal loudness.
  g. Use short sentences and pause at the end of each sentence.
  h. Speak at a normal rate, and do not overarticulate.
  i. Use facial expressions or gestures.
  j. Provide a magic slate for written communication.
  Individuals with hearing impairments often lip-read, making good visibility of the speaker's face necessary. Excessive environmental noise interferes with the ability to perceive the message. Higher tones are typically lost with presbycusis and other types of hearing loss. Using short sentences and pausing give the client time to interpret the message. Overarticulating makes it more difficult to follow the flow and to lip-read. Nonverbal cues and written messages enhance the client's understanding.
- Be sure hearing aid is properly placed, is turned on, and has fresh batteries. *The client may not be aware that the hearing aid is not functioning well.*
- Do not place intravenous catheters in the dominant hand. *The client may need to use that hand to write.*
- Rephrase sentences when there is difficulty understanding. *Hearing losses may affect different sound tones, making some words more difficult to comprehend. Using alternative words and phrases may increase the client's ability to perceive the message.*
- Repeat important information. *The nurse makes sure that the client understands the information.*
- Inform other staff about the client's hearing deficit and effective strategies for communication. *Consistent use of effective strategies for communication decreases the client's frustration.*

Social Isolation

The client with impaired hearing often becomes socially isolated. This isolation may be self-imposed because of difficulty communicating, especially in a group. Often, however, the isolation comes about gradually and without intention. The client finds social settings such as family dinners or community gatherings increasingly difficult. Friends and family become frustrated trying to communicate with someone who has a hearing impairment, and invitations to participate in social activities dwindle.

- Identify the extent and cause of the social isolation. Help to differentiate the reality of the isolation and its cause from the client's perception of isolation. *Clients with impaired hearing may be unaware that they are isolated. Identifying factors that contribute to isolation may provide the needed impetus*

to remedy the hearing loss. Clients may also experience paranoid thinking as a result of impaired communication and believe that friends and family have purposely begun to avoid interactions.

- Encourage to interact with friends and family on a one-to-one basis in quiet settings. *Clients with impaired hearing are more successful in understanding conversations that take place in small groups and quiet settings.*
- Treat with dignity and remind friends and family that a hearing deficit does not indicate loss of mental faculties. *Inappropriate responses due to a hearing deficit can cause others to perceive the client as "stupid" or demented.*
- Involve in activities that do not require acute hearing, such as checkers and chess. *The client has an opportunity to interact socially without the stress of straining to hear.*
- Obtain a pocket talker or encourage the client and family to do so.
- Refer the client to an audiologist for evaluation and possible hearing-aid fitting
- Refer to resources such as support groups and senior citizen centers. *These groups provide new social outlets.*

Using NANDA, NIC, and NOC

Chart 48–4 illustrates linkages between NANDA nursing diagnoses, NIC, and NOC for the client with a hearing deficit.

Community-Based Care

Teaching for home and community-based care for the client with hearing loss focuses on managing the deficit and developing coping strategies. Referral to an audiologist for evaluation of the deficit and the usefulness of a hearing aid may be

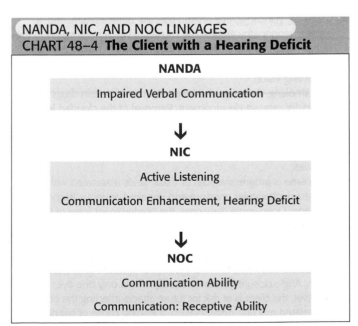

NANDA, NIC, AND NOC LINKAGES
CHART 48–4 The Client with a Hearing Deficit

NANDA

Impaired Verbal Communication

↓

NIC

Active Listening

Communication Enhancement, Hearing Deficit

↓

NOC

Communication Ability

Communication: Receptive Ability

Data from *NANDA's Nursing Diagnoses: Definitions & Classification 2005–2006* by NANDA International (2005), Philadelphia; *Nursing Interventions Classification (NIC)* (4th ed.) by J. M. Dochterman & G. M. Bulechek (2004), St. Louis, MO: Mosby; and *Nursing Outcomes Classification (NOC)* (3rd ed.) by S. Moorhead, M. Johnson, and M. Maas (2004), St. Louis, MO: Mosby.

Although the reproductive organs in men and women are very different, they do share common functions: enabling sexual pleasure and reproduction. The reproductive organs, in conjunction with the neuroendocrine system, produce hormones important in biologic development and sexual behavior. Parts of the reproductive organs also enclose and are integral to the function of the urinary system. The assessment of the reproductive and urinary systems is often difficult for both the nurse and the client and requires sensitivity on the part of the nurse when asking questions about topics that the client may be hesitant to talk about. Skill in conducting physical examinations of an area of the body usually considered private is also required.

ANATOMY, PHYSIOLOGY, AND FUNCTIONS OF THE MALE REPRODUCTIVE SYSTEM

The male reproductive system consists of the paired testes, the scrotum, ducts, glands, and penis (Figure 49–1 ■). The breasts are part of the male reproductive system, and are also assessed. The location and functions of the male reproductive organs are summarized in Table 49–1.

The Breasts

The male breast is comprised primarily of an areola (circular pigmented area) and a small nipple. These lie over a thin disk of undeveloped breast tissue that may not be overtly different from surrounding tissue. Approximately one in three men have a firm area of breast tissue 2 cm or larger; the limits of normal size of this area have not been established (Bickley & Szilagyi, 2007).

The Penis

The penis is the genital organ that encloses the urethra (see Figure 49–1). It is homologous to the clitoris of the female. The penis is composed of a shaft and a tip called the glans, which is covered in the uncircumcised man by the foreskin (or prepuce). The shaft contains three columns of erectile tissue: The two lateral columns are called the corpora cavernosa, and the central mass is called the corpus spongiosum.

Erection occurs when the penile masses become filled with blood in response to a reflex that triggers the parasympathetic nervous system to stimulate arteriolar vasodilation. The erection reflex may be initiated by touch, pressure, sights, sounds, smells, or thoughts of a sexual encounter. After ejaculation, the arterioles vasoconstrict, and the penis becomes flaccid.

The Scrotum

The scrotum is a sac or pouch made of two layers. The outer layer is continuous with the skin of the perineum and thighs. The inner layer is made of muscle and fascia. The scrotum hangs at the base of the penis, anterior to the anus, and regulates the temperature of the testes. The optimum temperature for sperm production is about 2 to 3 degrees below body temperature. When the testicular temperature is too low, the scrotum contracts to bring the testes up against the body. When the testicular temperature is too high, the scrotum relaxes to allow the testes to lie further away from the body.

The Testes

The testes develop in the abdominal cavity of the fetus and then descend through the inguinal canal into the scrotum. They are homologous to the female's ovaries. These paired organs are each about 1.5 inches (4 cm) long and 1 inch (2.5 cm) in diameter. They are suspended in the scrotum by the spermatic cord. Each is surrounded by two coverings: an outer tunica vaginalis and an inner tunica albuginea. Each testis is divided into 250 to 300 lobules, with each lobule containing one to four seminiferous tubules. The testes produce sperm and testosterone.

The seminiferous tubules are responsible for sperm production. Leydig's cells (or interstitial cells) lie in the connective tissue surrounding the seminiferous tubules and produce testosterone.

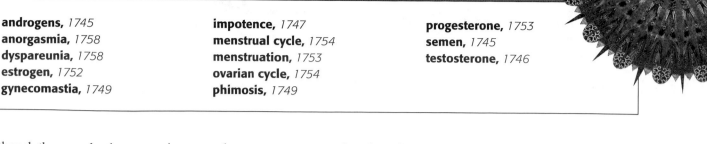

Figure 49–1 ■ The male reproductive system.

TABLE 49–1 Location and Function of the Male Reproductive Organs

MALE REPRODUCTIVE ORGAN	LOCATION	FUNCTION
Penis	Attached to front and sides of the pubic arch. Proximal, ventral surface is directly continuous with the scrotum.	Excretes semen and urine. Deposits sperm in female reproductive tract.
Scrotum	Hangs from body at root of penis.	Contains testes, epididymis, and portions of the vas (ductus) deferens.
Testes	In the scrotal sac.	Produce sperm and testosterone.
Epididymis	Posterolateral to upper aspect of each testis.	Stores sperm. Promotes sperm maturation. Transports sperm to vas deferens.
Vas deferens (ductus deferens)	Between the epididymis and the seminal vesicle forming the ejaculatory duct.	Stores sperm. Transports sperm
Urethra	Begins at bladder and passes through prostate and penis.	Serves as passageway for urine or semen.
Prostate gland	Encircles the urethra at the neck of the bladder.	Contributes to ejaculatory volume. Enhances sperm motility and fertility.
Seminal vesicles	Lie on posterior bladder wall.	Contribute to ejaculatory volume. Contain nutrients to sustain sperm and prostaglandins to facilitate sperm motility.
Bulbourethral (Cowper's) glands	Inferior to the prostate.	Secrete mucus into urethra. Neutralize traces of acidic urine in the urethra.

The Ducts and Semen

The seminiferous tubules lead into the efferent ducts and become the rete testis. From the rete testis, 10,000 to 20,000 efferent ducts join the epididymis, a long coiled tube that lies over the outer surface of each testis. The epididymis is the final area for the storage and maturation of sperm. When a man is sexually excited, the epididymis contracts to propel the sperm through the vas deferens to the ampulla, where the sperm are stored until ejaculation.

The seminal vesicles at the base of the bladder produce about 60% of the volume of seminal fluid. Seminal fluid is also made of secretions from the accessory sex organs, the epididymis, the prostate gland, and Cowper's glands. Seminal fluid nourishes the sperm, provides bulk, and increases its alkalinity. (An alkaline pH is essential to mobilize the sperm and ensure fertilization of the ova.) Sperm mixed with this fluid is called **semen**. Each seminal vesicle joins its corresponding vas deferens to form an ejaculatory duct, which enters the prostatic urethra. During ejaculation, seminal fluid mixes with sperm at the ejaculatory duct and enters the urethra for expulsion.

The total amount of semen ejaculated is 2 to 4 mL, although the amount varies. The total ejaculate of a healthy male contains from 100 to 400 million sperm.

The Prostate Gland

The prostate gland is about the size of a walnut. It encircles the urethra just below the urinary bladder (see Figure 49–1). It is made of 20 to 30 tubuloalveolar glands surrounded by smooth muscle. Secretions of the prostate gland make up about one-third of the volume of the semen. These secretions enter the urethra through several ducts during ejaculation.

Spermatogenesis

Spermatogenesis is the series of physiologic events that generate sperm in the seminiferous tubules. This process begins with puberty and continues throughout a man's life, with several hundred million sperm produced each day.

The inner layer of the seminiferous tubules consists of sustentacular cells (or Sertoli's cells), which contain the spermatocytes and sperm in different stages of development. Sertoli's cells secrete a nourishing fluid for the developing sperm, as well as enzymes that help convert spermatocytes to sperm. The events in spermatogenesis, which takes 64 to 72 days, are as follows:

1. The spermatogonia (sperm stem cells) undergo rapid mitotic division. As these cells multiply, the more mature spermatogonia divide into two daughter cells. These daughter cells grow and become the primary spermatocytes (and eventually become sperm).
2. Primary spermatocytes divide by meiosis to form two smaller secondary spermatocytes, which in turn divide to form two spermatids. This process occurs over several weeks.
3. The spermatids elongate into a mature sperm cell with a head and a tail. The head contains enzymes essential to the penetration and fertilization of the ova. The flagellar motion of the tail allows the sperm to move. The sperm cells then move to the epididymis to mature further and develop motility.

Male Sex Hormones

The male sex hormones are called **androgens**. Most androgens are produced in the testes, although the adrenal cortex also

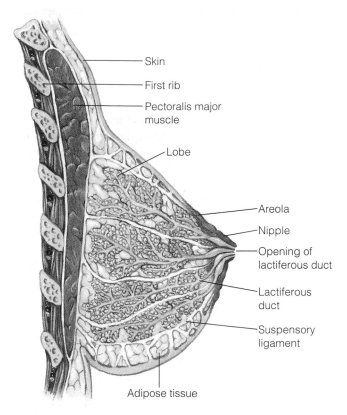

Figure 49–4 ■ Structure of the female breast.

anus. The labia minora, located between the clitoris and the base of the vagina, are enclosed by the labia majora. They are made of skin, adipose tissue, and some erectile tissues. They are usually light pink and hairless.

The area between the labia is called the vestibule, and contains the openings for the vagina and the urethra as well as the

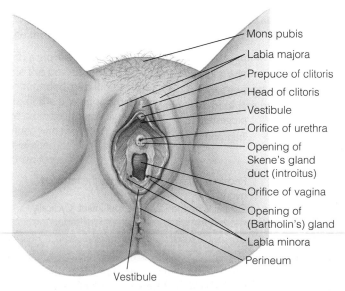

Figure 49–5 ■ The external organs of the female reproductive system.

Bartholin's glands. Skene's glands open onto the vestibule on each side of the urethra. Bartholin's and Skene's glands secrete lubricating fluid during the sexual response cycle prior to menopause.

The clitoris is an erectile organ analogous to the penis in the male. It is formed by the joining of the labia minora. Like the penis, it is highly sensitive and distends during sexual arousal.

The vaginal opening, called the introitus, is the opening between the internal and the external genitals. Prior to intercourse or trauma, the introitus is surrounded by a connective tissue membrane called the hymen.

The Internal Organs

The vagina and cervix, uterus, fallopian tubes, and ovaries are the internal organs of the female reproductive system (Figure 49–6 ■). The ovaries are the primary reproductive organs in women and also produce female sex hormones. The vagina, uterus, and fallopian tubes serve as accessory ducts for the ovaries and a developing fetus.

The Vagina and Cervix

The vagina is a fibromuscular tube about 3 to 4 inches (8 to 10 cm) in length located posterior to the bladder and urethra and anterior to the rectum. The upper end contains the uterine cervix in an area called the fornix. The walls of the vagina are membranes that form folds, called rugae. These membranes are composed of mucous-secreting stratified squamous epithelial cells. The vagina serves as a route for the excretion of secretions, including menstrual fluid, an organ of sexual response, and as a passageway for the birth of an infant.

The walls of the vagina are usually moist and maintain a pH ranging from 3.8 to 4.2. This pH is bacteriostatic and is maintained by the action of estrogen and normal vaginal flora. **Estrogen** stimulates the growth of vaginal mucosal cells so that they thicken and have increased glycogen content. The glycogen is fermented to lactic acid by Döderlein's bacilli (lactobacilli that normally inhabit the vagina), slightly acidifying the vaginal fluid.

The cervix projects into the vagina and forms a pathway between the uterus and the vagina. The uterine opening of the cervix is called the internal os; the vaginal opening is called the external os. The space between these openings, the endocervical canal, serves as a route for the discharge of menstrual fluid, the entrance for sperm, and expulsion of the infant during birth. The cervix is a firm structure, protected by mucus that changes consistency and quantity during the menstrual cycle and during pregnancy.

The Uterus

The uterus is a hollow pear-shaped muscular organ with thick walls located between the bladder and the rectum. It has three parts: the fundus, the body, and the cervix. It is supported in the abdominal cavity by the broad ligaments, the round ligaments, the uterosacral ligaments, and the transverse cervical ligaments. The uterus receives the fertilized ovum and provides a site for growth and development of the fetus.

The uterine wall has three layers. The perimetrium is the outer serous layer that merges with the peritoneum. The my-

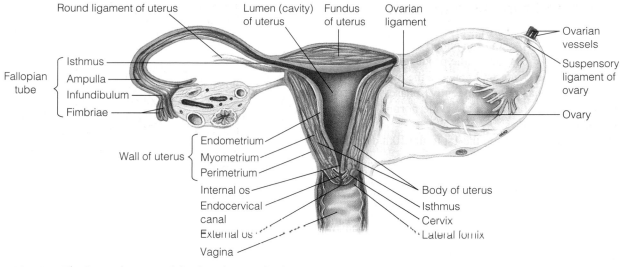

Figure 49–6 ■ The internal organs of the female reproductive system.

ometrium is the middle layer and makes up most of the uterine wall. This layer has muscle fibers that run in various directions, allowing contractions during **menstruation** (the periodic shedding of the uterine lining in a woman of childbearing age who is not pregnant) or childbirth, and expansion as the fetus grows. The endometrium lines the uterus; its outermost layer is shed during menstruation.

The Fallopian Tubes

The fallopian tubes are thin cylindrical structures about 4 inches (10 cm) long and 2.5 inches (1 cm) in diameter. They are attached to the uterus on one end and are supported by the broad ligaments. The lateral ends of the fallopian tubes are open and made of projections called fimbriae that drape over the ovary. The fimbriae pick up the ovum after it is discharged from the ovary.

The fallopian tubes are made of smooth muscle and are lined with ciliated, mucous-producing epithelial cells. The movement of the cilia and contractions of the smooth muscle move the ovum through the tubes toward the uterus. Fertilization of the ovum by the sperm usually occurs in the outer portion of a fallopian tube.

The Ovaries

The ovaries in the adult woman are flat, almond-shaped structures located on either side of the uterus below the ends of the fallopian tubes. They are homologous to the male's testes. They are attached to the uterus by a ligament and are also attached to the broad ligament. The ovaries store the female germ cells and produce the female hormones estrogen and progesterone. A woman's total number of ova is present at her birth.

Each ovary contains many small structures called ovarian follicles. Each follicle contains an immature ovum, called an oocyte. Each month, several follicles are stimulated by follicle-stimulating hormone (FSH) and luteinizing hormone (LH) to mature. The developing follicles are surrounded by layers of follicle cells, with the mature follicles called graafian follicles. The graafian follicles produce estrogen, which stimulates the devel-

opment of endometrium. Each month in the menstruating woman, one or two of the mature follicles eject an oocyte in a process called ovulation. The ruptured follicle then becomes a structure called the corpus luteum. The corpus luteum produces both estrogen and progesterone to support the endometrium until conception occurs or the cycle begins again. The corpus luteum slowly degenerates, leaving a scar on the surface of the ovary.

Female Sex Hormones

The ovaries produce estrogens, progesterone, and androgens in a cyclic pattern. Estrogens are steroid hormones that occur naturally in three forms: estrone (E_1), estradiol (E_2), and estriol (E_3). Estradiol is the most potent and is the form secreted in greatest amount by the ovaries. Although estrogens are secreted throughout the menstrual cycle, they are at a higher level during certain phases of the cycle, as discussed shortly.

Estrogens are essential for the development and maintenance of secondary sex characteristics; and in conjunction with other hormones, they stimulate the female reproductive organs to prepare for growth of a fetus. Estrogens are responsible for the normal structure of skin and blood vessels. They also decrease the rate of bone resorption, promote increased high-density lipoproteins, reduce cholesterol levels, and enhance the clotting of blood. Estrogens also promote the retention of sodium and water.

Menopause, a normal physiologic process, occurs as a result of the gradual decrease and final cessation of estrogen production by the ovaries. Menstruation ceases and the tissues that had been supported by estrogen change. Long-term effects of estrogen deprivation increase the risk of osteoporosis and cardiovascular disease. Menopause is discussed fully in Chapter 51 ∞.

Progesterone primarily affects the development of breast glandular tissue and the endometrium. During pregnancy, progesterone relaxes smooth muscle to decrease uterine contractions. It also increases body temperature. Androgens are responsible for normal hair growth patterns at puberty and may also have metabolic effects.

DIAGNOSTIC TESTS   of the Female Reproductive System

SCREENING TESTS, SMEARS, AND CULTURES

NAME OF TEST   Papanicolaou smear (Pap test)

PURPOSE AND DESCRIPTION   Conducted to diagnose malignant and premalignant lesions of the cervix; assess the effects of hormone replacement; identify viral, bacterial, fungal, and parasitic conditions; and to evaluate response to chemotherapy or radiation therapy to the cervix. Cells are obtained during a pelvic examination, with a wooden spatula, a cotton swab, or an endocervical brush. The sample collected may be smeared on a glass slide or put into a special liquid preservative and then the cells in suspension are processed onto a slide. The cells are then stained and examined.

RELATED NURSING CARE   Explain that the test should be done during a time when the woman is not menstruating, and that she should not have intercourse, douche, or use vaginal medications for 36 hours prior to the examination. Ask the woman to void prior to the examination.

NAME OF TEST   HPV test
(HPV DNA test, genital human papilloma test)

PURPOSE AND DESCRIPTION   Routinely used as a screening tool for human papillomavirus (HPV) in women after the age of 30. Conducted in conjunction with a pelvic examination and Pap smear. A finding of "low-grade changes" on the Pap smear with HPV indicates the likely presence of HPV and the need for further testing. A positive test for HPV indicates the presence of a high risk for cancer type of HPV, but does not specify which type is present.

RELATED NURSING CARE   Explain that the test should be done during a time when the woman is not menstruating, and that she should not have intercourse, douche, or use vaginal medications for 36 hours prior to the examination. Ask the woman to void prior to the examination.

NAME OF TEST   Chlamydia

PURPOSE AND DESCRIPTION   Performed to screen for or diagnose chlamydial infections. A swab of cells from the infected area is taken and either smeared on a slide and analyzed or cultured. Although usually taken from the urethra, vagina, or cervix, cultures may also be taken from the throat and rectum.

RELATED NURSING CARE   Assess if the woman is pregnant or has enlargement of inguinal lymph nodes. Withhold antibiotics (if prescribed) until after obtaining the specimen. Instruct not to douche before the examination. If the test is positive, request the names of all sexual partners and emphasize need for treatment to eradicate the infection.

NAME OF TEST   Gonorrhea culture

PURPOSE AND DESCRIPTION   A culture is performed to evaluate for gonorrhea. A swab is used to collect a sample of discharge from the infected area (cervix, urethra, anus, or throat), smeared on a slide, and a Gram stain is conducted to identify the organism (*N. gonorrhoeae*). A urine sample is used in some tests.

RELATED NURSING CARE   No special preparation is needed. Instruct not to douche before the examination. If the test is positive, request the names of all sexual partners and emphasize need for treatment to eradicate the infection.

NAME OF TEST   Trichomonas, Bacteria, Candidae (yeast)

PURPOSE AND DESCRIPTION   A culture is performed to identify vaginal organisms or blood cells. A specimen of vaginal discharge is obtained with a swab, placed in solution, and examined under the microscope immediately after it is collected (referred to as a wet-mount).

RELATED NURSING CARE   Request not to douche before the examination.

NAME OF TEST
■ Venereal Disease Research Laboratory (VDRL)
■ Rapid plasma reagin (RPR)
■ Fluorescent treponemal antibody absorption (FTA-ABS)

PURPOSE AND DESCRIPTION   These blood tests are conducted to screen for syphilis. Positive findings can be made within 1 to 2 weeks after primary lesion appears or 1 to 4 months after the initial infection. The FTA-ABS is considered the most accurate, and is often used if findings from the VDRL or RPR are questionable.

RELATED NURSING CARE   No special preparation is needed. If test is positive, request the names of all sexual partners and emphasize need for treatment to eradicate the infection.

NAME OF TEST   Syphilis (dark-field examination)

PURPOSE AND DESCRIPTION   A specimen is obtained from a lesion believed to be caused by syphilis (*Treponema pallidum*) and examined under the microscope.

RELATED NURSING CARE   No special preparation is needed. If test is positive, request the names of all sexual partners and emphasize need for treatment to eradicate the infection.

BREAST EXAMINATIONS

NAME OF TEST   Mammogram

PURPOSE AND DESCRIPTION   Used to detect tumors in the breast. Breasts are flattened in the mammography machine and low-dose x-rays are taken.

RELATED NURSING CARE   Ask the woman not to apply body powder or underarm deodorant prior to the test.

DIAGNOSTIC TESTS of the Female Reproductive System (continued)

NAME OF TEST Breast ultrasound

PURPOSE AND DESCRIPTION This examination uses high-frequency sound waves passing through tissues to detect masses in the breast. May be performed if lesions are identified in a mammogram.

RELATED NURSING CARE No special preparation is needed.

NAME OF TEST Breast biopsy
- Fine-needle aspiration
- Core needle biopsy
- Vacuum-assisted mammotome
- Large core surgical biopsy
- Open surgical biopsy

PURPOSE AND DESCRIPTION
- A fine-needle aspiration is conducted to withdraw fluid from cysts, and may be used to sample cells from masses in the breast. A 22- to 25-gauge needle is used to collect five to six samples of fluid or cells.
- A core needle biopsy is conducted to obtain a sample of tissue from a solid mass or calcium deposits in the breast. A 10-, 11-, or 12-gauge needle is used to collect five to six tissue samples.
- A vacuum-assisted mammotome is primarily used to evaluate calcifications. An 11- or 14-gauge needle is inserted through a small (1/4-inch) incision and 8 to 10 samples are removed.
- A large core surgical biopsy is performed to evaluate breast masses or calcification identified with a mammogram but nonpalpable. An incision is made and a 5- to 20-mm cylinder of breast tissue (about the size of a wine cork) is removed.
- An open surgical biopsy is performed to evaluate breast masses, hard-to-reach lesions, multiple lesions, and masses with calcifications. A 1.5- to 2-inch incision is made and a golf ball size (or larger) area of tissue is removed.

RELATED NURSING CARE For all types, wearing a bra, applying ice packs, and mild analgesics decrease discomfort postprocedure.
- Explain that, depending on the physician, some procedures may be performed with or without a local anesthetic.
- Explain that a local anesthetic is used, but no stitches are required for a core needle biopsy or mammotome.
- Explain that a local anesthetic will be administered and stitches will be used to close the incision for a large-core biopsy.
- Explain that a general anesthetic is usually used and that the incision will require stitches and leave a scar for an open surgical biopsy.

TESTS OF THE INTERNAL REPRODUCTIVE SYSTEM

NAME OF TEST Ultrasound (abdominal, vaginal)

PURPOSE AND DESCRIPTION Used to detect the presence of space-occupying lesions, such as fibroid tumors, cysts, abscesses, and neoplasms. The abdomen is coated with transducing gel, and a graphic visualization is made. For a vaginal ultrasound, a transducer is covered with a condom or vinyl glove coated with transducer gel and then introduced into the vagina.

RELATED NURSING CARE Explain need to increase intake of fluids and tell the woman not to void until the test is completed to ensure a full bladder (this lifts the pelvic organs higher in the abdomen and improves visualization).

NAME OF TEST Hysterosalpingogram

PURPOSE AND DESCRIPTION Used to diagnose causes of infertility and abnormalities of the uterus or fallopian tubes. A contrast medium is instilled through the cervix, through the uterus, and out the fallopian tubes while x-rays are taken.

RELATED NURSING CARE Assess for allergy to seafood (iodine) or previous contrast media. Explain that the procedure is briefly painful.

NAME OF TEST Colposcopy

PURPOSE AND DESCRIPTION Conducted to further study abnormal Pap tests, and as screening for women exposed to intrauterine DES. A binocular microscope is used to directly visualize the cervix.

RELATED NURSING CARE No special preparation is needed.

NAME OF TEST Conization, loop electrosurgical excision of transformation zone (LEETZ), loop electrosurgical excision procedure (LEEP)

PURPOSE AND DESCRIPTION A conization, LEETZ, or LEEP is performed to remove cervical tissue for evaluation (most often for cervical cancer). A cone-shaped area of tissue surrounding the cervical os is removed.

RELATED NURSING CARE Explain that the procedure requires general anesthesia. Postoperative self-care includes rest for 2 to 3 days. Explain that minor vaginal bleeding and discharge are expected for several days after the procedures; perineal pads (not tampons) should be used. Sexual intercourse should be avoided until discharge stops. Notify physician of increased bleeding or signs of infection (pain, foul-smelling discharge, fever) occur.

NAME OF TEST Endometrial biopsy

PURPOSE AND DESCRIPTION Performed to identify endometrial hyperplasia or endometrial cancer. The cervix is cleaned and tissue is obtained transcervically from the endometrium either by curettage or vacuum aspiration.

RELATED NURSING CARE Explain that the procedure is briefly painful, and causes vaginal bleeding. Advise to use perineal pads, and avoid tampons and sexual intercourse while bleeding.

(continued)

DIAGNOSTIC TESTS of the Female Reproductive System (continued)

NAME OF TEST Cervical biopsy

PURPOSE AND DESCRIPTION Performed for women when Pap test results indicate possible cervical cancer or cervical intraepithelial neoplasia (CIN) and for screening for women at high risk for vaginal and cervical cancers from intrauterine exposure to DES. Cervix is cleaned and a sample of tissue is taken for analysis.

RELATED NURSING CARE Explain that minor vaginal bleeding and discharge are expected for several days after the procedures; perineal pads (not tampons) should be used. Sexual intercourse should be avoided until discharge stops. Notify physician of increased bleeding or signs of infection (pain, foul-smelling discharge, fever) occur.

NAME OF TEST Laparoscopy

PURPOSE AND DESCRIPTION This examination is conducted to visualize the organs in the peritoneal cavity (uterus, fallopian tubes, ovaries); to withdraw fluid for analysis; and to perform a tubal ligation. A fiber-optic scope is inserted through small abdominal incisions and carbon dioxide is inserted into the peritoneal cavity for better visualization.

RELATED NURSING CARE Ask the woman to void prior to the examination and explain that a general anesthetic will be used. Explain that shoulder pain is common after the procedure (referred pain from the retained carbon dioxide gas); that some vaginal bleeding may occur and the woman should use a perineal pad; and to report excess bleeding, pain, or signs of infection to the physician.

Health Assessment Interview

A health assessment interview to determine problems with the female reproductive system may be conducted during a health screening, may focus on a chief complaint (such as severe menstrual cramping), or may be part of a total health assessment. Women may be embarrassed to discuss health problems or concerns involving their reproductive organs; it is important for the nurse to ask questions in a nonthreatening, matter-of-fact manner. Consider the psychologic, social, and cultural factors that affect sexuality and sexual activity. Use words that the woman can understand, and do not be embarrassed or offended by the words she uses. The woman may perceive the interview as less threatening if the discussion begins with more general questions and then progresses to specific questions, and if questions are asked in a way that gives the woman permission to describe behaviors and manifestations. For example, first ask a female client about menstrual and childbirth histories before asking questions about sexually transmitted infections.

The focused interview for the female reproductive system is usually extensive. However, the questions may in many instances be tailored to the specific health problem of the woman. As with the assessment of other body systems, analyze and document the onset of the problem, its duration, frequency, precipitating and relieving factors, any associated symptoms, treatment, self-care, and outcome. For example, ask the woman:

- Have you noticed vaginal bleeding after intercourse?
- Does over-the-counter medication relieve the vaginal itching and discharge?
- Have you had any fever or abdominal pain with this vaginal infection?

Ask about menstrual history, obstetric history, use of contraceptives, sexual history, use of medications, and reproductive system examinations. Also assess the use of condoms during intercourse; unprotected sexual intercourse increases the risk of sexually transmitted infections, including HIV infection. Also ask about smoking; a history of smoking increases the risk of circulatory problems in the woman taking oral contraceptives. Smoking also increases the risk for cancer of the cervix.

Chronic illnesses may affect the function of the female reproductive system. Diabetes mellitus increases the risk of vaginal infections and vaginal dryness, both of which interfere with sexual pleasure. Chronic heavy menstrual flow may result in anemia. Thyroid and adrenal disorders may affect secondary sex characteristics, the menstrual cycle, and the ability to become pregnant.

Obtaining any family history of cancer is important. The risk for endometrial cancer is higher in women with a family history of endometrial, breast, or colon cancer; the risk for ovarian cancer is higher in women with a family history of ovarian or breast cancer; and the risk for breast cancer is higher in women with a family history of breast cancer. Exposure to DES *in utero* increases the risk of cancer of the cervix and vagina. Exposure to asbestos poses a risk of cancer of the ovary. The risk for breast cancer is also greater if the woman has a history of fibrocystic disease.

Carefully explore any history of vaginal bleeding and vaginal discharge. Ask about the onset of vaginal bleeding, any related factors, the color (pink, red, dark red, brown), the character (thin, watery, presence of mucus, size and number of clots), the amount (spotting, how many pads or tampons in a specific amount of time), and relationship to menstrual cycle. Regarding vaginal discharge, ask about the onset, color (white, green, gray), character (thin, thick, curdlike), odor, itching, and rash.

Questions about sexuality may include sexual preference, number of sexual partners; history of **anorgasmia** (absence of orgasm), **dyspareunia** (painful intercourse), or other problems with intercourse; history of sexual trauma; use of condoms or other contraceptives; and current level of sexual satisfaction.

Interview questions categorized by functional health patterns are listed in the Functional Health Pattern Interview table on the next page.

FUNCTIONAL HEALTH PATTERN INTERVIEW The Female Reproductive System

Functional Health Pattern	Interview Questions and Leading Statements
Health Perception-Health Management	■ Have you ever had problems with your reproductive organs (ovaries, tubes, uterus, vagina) or with menstruation or menopause? Explain. If so, how was this problem treated? ■ Do you routinely take any prescribed or herbal medications for symptoms of menopause? If so, what and when do you take it? ■ Did you ever take hormone replacement therapy for menopausal symptoms? ■ Do you practice breast self-examination? When and how often do you do this? ■ Have you noticed any lumps in your breasts or discharge from your nipples? Describe, if so. ■ Have you ever had a breast examination or mammogram? When was your last one? How often do you have these? ■ When was your last gynecologic examination? Pap smear? How often do you have these done? ■ Do you use birth control? If so, what do you use? ■ What do you do to provide self-care if you have mood swings or menstrual cramps? ■ Have you ever had a sexually transmitted infection or an infection of the reproductive organs? What was it? How was it treated? ■ Do you use douches or vaginal sprays? If so, what type and how often? ■ Do you smoke? If so, how much and for how long?
Nutritional-Metabolic	■ Do you notice a change in your appetite right before your menstrual period? ■ Have you gained weight recently? If so, why do think this happened? ■ Describe your usual food intake for a 24-hour period.
Elimination	■ When was your last menstrual period? ■ At what age did you start/end having menstrual periods? ■ Describe the length, amount of flow, and clotting with your menstrual periods. Do you ever have bleeding between your menstrual periods? If so, describe the type and amount. ■ Describe any unusual vaginal discharge you have had (color, consistency, odor, itching, or rash). ■ Have you noticed any changes in urination (frequency, urgency, burning)? ■ Have you noticed changes in bowel elimination during your menstrual periods?
Activity-Exercise	■ Describe your usual activities of daily living. ■ Have you noticed any change in activity or energy during your menstrual period? ■ Have you noticed any change in activity or energy since menopause (if applicable)? If so, how?
Sleep-Rest	■ How long do you sleep at night? ■ Do night sweats wake you? ■ Do menstrual cramps ever wake you at night?
Cognitive-Perceptual	■ Do you have pain or other symptoms (such as headache, mood swings, irritability, bloating, constipation, diarrhea, and/or breast tenderness) before your menstrual period? Describe. What do you do about this? ■ Do you have cramping before or during your menstrual period? Describe the type of cramping, how long it lasts, and what you do to be more comfortable. ■ Do you ever have vaginal itching, pain, burning, or dryness? If so, is it affected by sexual intercourse? Does dryness interfere with intercourse?
Self-Perception-Self-Concept	■ Has this problem affected how you feel about yourself as a woman? ■ Do you believe your needs for intimacy and affection are being met?
Role-Relationships	■ How has having this condition affected your relationships with others? ■ Has having this condition interfered with your ability to work? Explain. ■ Has anyone in your family had problems with breast or ovarian cancer? Explain.
Sexuality-Reproductive	■ Are you currently in a sexual relationship? If so, has this condition interfered with your usual sexual activity? How long have you been with your current partner? Have you had any other partners during this time? ■ What is your sexual preference? ■ Has having this problem affected your relationship with your spouse or sexual partner? ■ Have you ever been pregnant? How many times? Have you ever had a miscarriage? ■ Do you practice birth control? If so, what do you use? ■ Do you ensure that your partner of the opposite gender uses a condom every time you have intercourse? ■ Do you use a vaginal condom?

(continued)

FUNCTIONAL HEALTH PATTERN INTERVIEW	The Female Reproductive System (continued)
Functional Health Pattern	**Interview Questions and Leading Statements**
Coping-Stress-Tolerance	■ Has having this condition created stress for you? If so, does your health problem seem to be more difficult when you are stressed? ■ Have you experienced any kind of stress that makes the condition worse? Explain. ■ Describe what you do when you feel stressed.
Value-Belief	■ Describe how specific relationships or activities help you cope with this problem. ■ Describe specific cultural beliefs or practices that affect how you care for and feel about this problem. ■ Are there any specific treatments that you would not use to treat this problem?

Physical Assessment

Physical assessment of the female reproductive system usually is conducted as part of a scheduled screening (e.g., for an annual Pap smear) or for a specific reproductive health problem. If conducted as part of a total physical assessment, this is usually the final system to be assessed. The nurse must feel comfortable with the examination of clients of the opposite gender; if either the nurse or the client is not comfortable, a nurse of the same gender should be asked to conduct this part of the assessment.

The female reproductive system is assessed by inspection and palpation. Ask the woman to void before having the examination. Prior to the examination, collect all necessary equipment and explain the techniques to the woman to decrease anxiety. Put on disposable gloves before beginning the examination and wear them throughout the examination. Ask the woman to remove her clothing and put on a gown. Ensure that the examining room is private and warm.

The female reproductive system is assessed by inspection and palpation. Explain the procedures for the examination thoroughly and in a matter-of-fact way to decrease anxiety and embarrass-ment. If the woman is unfamiliar with her reproductive organs, charts may be used to demonstrate the parts that will be examined. Carefully explain the procedure for the examination, and show the speculum to the woman. The assessment may be done with the woman in the sitting or supine position to examine the breasts and in the lithotomy position to assess the external genitalia and internal organs. Expose only those body parts being examined to preserve modesty. Normal age-related findings for the older woman are summarized in Table 49–4.

The examination usually begins with examination of the breasts with the woman in the sitting and supine positions. The nurse then helps the woman move to the lithotomy position on the examining table, with the feet in the stirrups and the buttocks even with the foot of the table. Older or frail women may not be able to tolerate this position. In this case, the woman is examined in the supine position. Although the entire examination is described here, the internal examination is conducted only by a nurse with advanced practice in the procedure. However, nurses are often asked to assist with the examination and should be able to explain the examination to a woman.

TABLE 49–4 Age-Related Changes in the Female Reproductive System

AGE-RELATED CHANGE	SIGNIFICANCE
Breasts ■ Atrophy, with sagging of breast tissue ■ Linear strands may appear from shrinkage and fibrotic changes	Although aging does not cause breast cancer, the incidence rises in older women; age-related changes may make finding tumors more difficult.
External Genitalia ■ Labia flatten, and vulvar adipose tissue and hair decrease. ■ ↓ collagen and adipose tissues in the vaginal canal, resulting in loss of rugae, shortening and narrowing of vaginal canal. ■ ↓ vaginal lubrication, epithelium becomes thinner and avascular. ■ More alkaline pH of vagina. ■ Cervix becomes smaller.	Vagina is more easily irritated, increasing the risk of vaginal infections. Lubricants are necessary for comfortable intercourse.
Internal Organs ■ Uterus shrinks. ■ Fallopian tubes shrink and shorten. ■ Ovaries are smaller and thicker. ■ With menopause, hormone production of estrogen decreases. ■ Loss of estrogen may cause pelvic floor muscles to weaken. ■ Loss of estrogen causes changes throughout the body, including loss of skin tone (wrinkling) and growth of facial hair.	With the completion of menopause, the menstrual cycles end and the woman is infertile. Weakening of the pelvic floor muscles may contribute to involuntary incontinence with increased intra-abdominal pressure (as with coughing and sneezing). Skin is dry and thin.

FEMALE REPRODUCTIVE SYSTEM ASSESSMENTS

Technique/Normal Findings	Abnormal Findings

Breast Assessment

Inspect both breasts simultaneously with the woman seated in the following positions: arms at sides, arms overhead, hands pressed on hips, leaning forward. Inspect breast size, symmetry, contour, skin color, texture, venous patterns, and lesions. Lift the breasts, and inspect the lower and lateral aspects. *Breasts normally vary in size and shape, and one breast may normally be larger than the other. Color should be consistent with the skin tone and texture smooth. There should be no redness, swelling, prominent veins, or lesions.*

- Retractions, dimpling, and abnormal contours suggest benign lesions, but may also suggest malignancy.
- Thickened, dimpled skin with enlarged pores (called peau d'orange, orange peel, or pig skin) and unilateral venous patterns are also associated with malignancy.
- Redness may be seen with infection or carcinoma.

Inspect the areolae and nipples. *The color of the areolae should be consistent with the woman's skin color (ranging from dark pink to dark brown), and Montgomery tubercles may be present. The nipples should be equal bilaterally in size, centrally located in each breast, and free of lesions or discharge. Nipples are usually everted, but may normally be inverted or flat.*

- Peau d'orange may be noted first in the areola.
- Recent unilateral inversion of the nipple or asymmetry in the directions in which the nipples point suggests cancer.

Palpate both breasts, axillae, and supraclavicular areas. Figure 49–8 ■ illustrates a possible pattern for breast palpation. Various palpation patterns may be used as long as every part of each breast is palpated, including the axillary tail (also called tail of Spence), which is the breast tissue that extends from the upper outer quadrant toward and into the axillae. Ask the woman to assume a supine position with a small pillow under the shoulder and the arm over the head, and repeat the systematic palpation sequence. Describe identified masses by location, size, shape, consistency, tenderness, mobility, and delineation of borders. *Breasts should feel smooth, firm, and elastic, without palpable masses. Prior to the menstrual cycle, there may be increased nodularity and tenderness.*

- Tenderness may be related to premenstrual fullness, fibrocystic disease, or inflammation. Tenderness may also indicate cancer.
- Nodules in the tail of the breast may be enlarged lymph nodes.
- Hard, irregular, fixed unilateral masses that are poorly delineated suggest carcinoma.
- Bilateral, single or multiple, round, mobile, well-delineated masses are consistent with fibrocystic breast disease or fibroadenoma.
- Swelling, tenderness, erythema, and heat may be seen with mastitis.

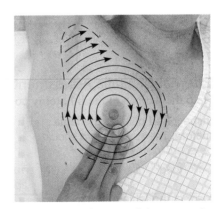

Figure 49–8 ■ Possible pattern for palpation of the breast.

and reproductive issues. Although chances of a cure are excellent, the long-term effect on quality of life may be extensive, requiring a change in life goals.

Deficient Knowledge

The nurse often initiates and reinforces teaching about what to expect after radical orchiectomy. The man's knowledge about surgery is assessed, and postoperative routines such as early ambulation are explained (see Chapter 4 ∞).

- Explain pain control methods. In addition to the usual analgesics used to control postoperative incisional pain, ice bags may be applied to the scrotum. A scrotal support provides relief, especially when the client ambulates. *Surgery results in incisional pain, and the scrotum is tender and slightly swollen.*
- Teach the manifestations of complications. The incision is closed with Steri-Strips or staples, and, although rare, wound dehiscence is possible. If the incision gapes open, or if there is bleeding beyond slight oozing after 24 hours, the man should call the surgeon. Another rare complication is a hematoma in the scrotum caused by bleeding from the spermatic cord stump. Rapid onset of scrotal edema is a sign of this problem. *Because the man is usually discharged early, complications may not become apparent until he is at home.*

Ineffective Sexuality Patterns

The effect of testicular cancer and its treatment on sexual and reproductive function is varied. If the man has a retroperitoneal lymph node dissection, severing of the sympathetic plexus may result in retrograde ejaculation or failure to ejaculate. Infertility may be caused by ejaculation disorders, surgery, chemotherapy, or radiation therapy.

- Assess the man's prediagnosis sexual function. To assess this area, the nurse must establish an atmosphere of openness and permission to discuss sexual concerns. After the initial shock of the diagnosis, men report intense concern about sexual and reproductive issues, which can be relieved only by information. *Knowledge of the man's usual sexual function can guide teaching.*
- Discuss the possibility of preserving sperm in a bank prior to treatment. *This option may help relieve the man's fears about his ability to father children in the future, but must be completed prior to initiating treatment with surgery, chemotherapy, or radiation therapy.*
- Help coping with feelings about altered sexual function and appearance. Explain that testicular implants can be inserted to preserve appearance. *Many clients, regardless of whether they are in a significant relationship, deeply grieve the loss of the ability to father children. It is important to maintain body image despite disfiguring surgery.*

Community-Based Care

Families need to be included in teaching for a variety of reasons. If the man is of reproductive age, his partner will have significant anxiety and will require information. For the teenager, parents need information about the effect on sexual function and are often very involved in postoperative care. The man needs the support of the people he loves, and knowledgeable loved ones can give effective support.

Provide teaching and reinforcement of the need for follow-up, especially if the retroperitoneal lymph nodes were not surgically explored. For men with a risk for recurrence, surveillance with periodic physical examinations, chest x-ray films, tumor markers, and CT scans of the retroperitoneal nodes could continue for a minimum of 5 years and possibly 10 years after orchiectomy.

DISORDERS OF THE PROSTATE GLAND

THE MAN WITH PROSTATITIS

Prostatitis is a term used to refer to different types of inflammatory disorders of the prostate gland. *Prostatodynia* is a condition in which the client experiences the symptoms of prostatitis but shows no evidence of inflammation or infection. Manifestations of prostatitis and prostatodynia are summarized in the box on the next page.

Pathophysiology and Manifestations

The National Institutes of Health have defined four types of prostatitis: acute bacterial prostatitis, chronic bacterial prostatitis, chronic prostatitis/pelvic pain syndrome, and asymptomatic inflammatory prostatitis. Men with asymptomatic inflammatory prostatitis have no subjective symptoms, but are diagnosed when a biopsy or prostatic fluid examination is conducted.

Acute Bacterial Prostatitis

Acute bacterial prostatitis is most often caused by an ascending infection from the urethra or reflux of infected urine into the ducts of the prostate gland. The organism most often responsible for the infection is *E. coli;* other causative organisms include *Pseudomonas, Klebsiella,* and *Chlamydia.*

Manifestations of acute bacterial prostatitis include increased temperature, malaise, muscle and joint pain, urinary frequency and urgency, dysuria, and urethral discharge. The man often experiences dull, aching pain in the perineum, rectum, or lower back. On rectal examination, the prostate is enlarged and painful.

Chronic Bacterial Prostatitis

Men with chronic bacterial prostatitis often present with a history of recurrent urinary tract infections. The causative organisms are most often *E. coli, Proteus,* or *Klebsiella.* Calculi may form in the prostate and contribute to the chronicity of the problem.

The manifestations of chronic bacterial prostatitis include urinary frequency and urgency, dysuria, low back pain, and perineal discomfort. Epididymitis may be associated with the prostatitis.

Chronic Prostatitis/Chronic Pelvic Pain Syndrome

This type of prostatitis is both the most common and the least understood of the syndromes (NKUDIC, 2003b). The two

MANIFESTATIONS of Prostatitis and Prostatodynia

Acute Bacterial Prostatitis
- Onset (may be abrupt): obstruction, irritation, or pain upon voiding; frequency; and urgency
- Positive cultures of infectious organism
- Nonurinary symptoms: chills, fever, low back and pelvic floor pain

Chronic Bacterial Prostatitis
- Urinary symptoms sometimes similar to those of the acute form, except less sudden, less dramatic, or even absent
- Positive cultures of causative organism not always obtainable

Chronic Prostatitis
- Perineal, suprapubic, low back, or genital pain
- Irritation upon voiding
- Postejaculatory pain
- Negative cultures of organisms

Prostatodynia
- Pelvic, low back, or perineal pain
- Irritation or obstruction upon voiding
- No evidence of inflammation in the prostate
- No urinary tract infection
- Normal prostatic secretions

types (inflammatory and noninflammatory) are based on the presence of white blood cells in the prostatic fluid.

- *Inflammatory prostatitis* is believed to be an autoimmune disorder, but the actual cause is unknown. Men with this type of prostatitis have low back pain; urinary manifestations; pain in the penis, testicles, scrotum, lower back, and rectum; decreased libido; and painful ejaculations. They do not have bacteria in their urine, but do have abnormal inflammatory cells in prostatic secretions.
- *Noninflammatory prostatitis* (prostatodynia) has manifestations similar to those of inflammatory prostatitis, but no evidence of urinary or prostatic infection or inflammation can be found. The cause is not known, but is believed to be the result of a problem outside the prostate gland, such as obstruction of the bladder neck.

INTERDISCIPLINARY CARE

Diagnosis
It is often difficult to diagnose prostatitis. Urine and prostatic secretion examination and cultures are obtained to determine the presence and type of blood cells and bacteria. X-ray studies and ultrasound to visualize pelvic structures also may be useful.

Medications
Bacterial prostatitis is treated with appropriate antibiotics. Men with the chronic form must take antibiotics for a much longer period, often up to 4 months, and may still relapse as soon as the antibiotic is discontinued. Nonbacterial prostatitis does not usually respond satisfactorily to drug therapy, although relief

from symptoms is possible. Nonsteroidal anti-inflammatory drugs are useful for pain, and anticholinergics may reduce voiding symptoms. Prostatodynia is treated symptomatically to relieve muscle tension, usually with alpha-adrenergic blocking agents or muscle relaxants.

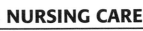

NURSING CARE

Teaching for the man with prostatitis focuses on symptom management. Men with acute and chronic bacterial prostatitis should be taught to increase fluid intake to around 3 L daily and to void often. These measures help decrease irritation when voiding. Regular bowel movements help ease the pain associated with defecation. Local heat, such as sitz baths, may be helpful to relieve pain and irritation. It is important to teach the man to finish the course of antibiotic therapy. Men with chronic prostatitis/chronic pelvic pain syndrome need to know that the condition is not contagious and does not cause cancer (Porth, 2005). Referral sources for information include the National Kidney and Urologic Diseases Information Clearinghouse, the American Foundation for Urologic Disease, and the Prostatitis Foundation.

THE MAN WITH BENIGN PROSTATIC HYPERPLASIA

Benign prostatic hyperplasia (BPH), an age-related, nonmalignant enlargement of the prostate gland, is a common disorder of the aging male. The prostate, very small at birth, grows at puberty, and reaches adult size around age 20. Benign hyperplasia (increased number of cells) begins at 40 to 45 years of age, and continues slowly through the rest of life. It is estimated that more than one-half of all men over age 60 have BPH (Porth, 2005). The problem that brings men to a healthcare provider is the associated urinary dysfunction.

Risk Factors
Although the exact cause of BPH is unknown, risk factors include:
- Age
- Family history
- Race (highest in African Americans and lowest in native Japanese)
- Diet high in meat and fats.

Pathophysiology
The two necessary preconditions for BPH are age of 50 or greater and the presence of testes. Men who are castrated before puberty do not develop BPH. The androgen that mediates prostatic growth at all ages is dihydrotestosterone (DHT), which is formed in the prostate from testosterone. Although androgen levels decrease in aging men, the aging prostate appears to become more sensitive to available DHT. Estrogen, produced in small amounts in men, appears to sensitize the prostate gland to the effects of DHT. Increasing estrogen levels associated with aging or a relative increase in estrogen related to testosterone levels may contribute to prostatic hyperplasia.

which is produced during the luteal phase of the menstrual cycle, also is markedly reduced.

Manifestations

As estrogen decreases, various tissues are affected. The breast tissue, body hair, skin elasticity, and subcutaneous fat decrease. The ovaries and uterus become smaller, and the cervix and vagina also decrease in size and become pale in color. These changes may result in problems with vaginal dryness, dyspareunia, urinary stress incontinence, urinary tract infections (UTIs), and vaginitis. Vasomotor instability often results in hot flashes, palpitations, dizziness, and headaches. Other problems resulting from vasomotor instability include insomnia, frequent awakening, and perspiration (night sweats). The woman may experience irritability, anxiety, and depression as a result of these events.

Long-term estrogen deprivation results in an imbalance in bone remodeling and osteoporosis, leading to fractures and kyphosis. The risk for cardiovascular diseases increases in response to an increase in atherosclerosis (from an increase in the LDL-to-HDL cholesterol ratio). Manifestations of the perimenopausal period are listed in the box below. These manifestations vary widely. Some women experience severe symptoms, others experience moderate symptoms, and some women experience few or no symptoms.

INTERDISCIPLINARY CARE

Care of the woman experiencing menopausal symptoms focuses on relieving symptoms and minimizing postmenopausal health risks.

Diagnosis

As estrogen secretion diminishes, levels of follicle-stimulating hormone (FSH) and luteinizing hormone (LH) rise and remain elevated. A woman who had not menstruated for 1 full year or who has an increased FSH blood level is considered menopausal (Porth, 2005).

MANIFESTATIONS of the Perimenopausal Period

- Menstrual cycles become erratic. Menstrual flow varies widely in amount and duration and eventually ceases.
- Vaginal, vulval, and urethral tissues begin to atrophy.
- Vaginal pH rises, predisposing the woman to bacterial infections.
- Vaginal lubrication decreases, and vaginal rugae decrease in number. This may result in dyspareunia, injury, and fungal infections.
- Vasomotor instability due to a decrease in estrogen may result in hot flashes and night sweats. A hot flash starts in the chest and moves upward toward the face and may last from seconds to several minutes.
- Psychologic symptoms may include moodiness, nervousness, insomnia, headaches, irritability, anxiety, inability to concentrate, and depression.

Medications

Although controversial, hormone replacement therapy (HRT) may be prescribed to alleviate severe manifestations of menopause, but only for a limited amount of time and only after a woman has been provided with known risks. HRT may include estrogen alone for women who have had a hysterectomy, or a combination of estrogen and progestin. The addition of progestin stimulates monthly shedding of the interuterine lining, decreasing the risk of uterine cancer. HRT relieves hot flashes and night sweats and decreases problems of vaginal dryness and urogenital tissue atrophy, which can lead to painful intercourse and urinary incontinence. Long-term HRT may increase the risk for breast cancer, ovarian cancer, stroke, heart attacks, and venous thrombosis (Tierney et al., 2004). However, women who have had a hysterectomy and take estrogen alone do not have an increased risk of breast cancer (Health & Science, 2006).

Selective estrogen receptor modulators (SERMs) such as raloxifene (Evista) and triphenylethylene (Tamoxifen) bind to estrogen receptors and exert site-specific effects in different target tissues. Tamoxifen and toremifene (a derivative of tamoxifen) have a beneficial effect on bone mineral density and serum lipids and decrease the risk of invasive breast cancer in women at high risk. They also provide an alternative to HRT for preventing osteoporosis.

Alternative and Complementary Therapies

As a result of the controversy surrounding the use of HRT, nontraditional or alternative therapies have become more popular. The following complementary therapies are examples of those used by menopausal women to reduce associated discomforts (ARHP, 2005b; Mayo Clinic, 2004):

- Acupuncture
- Biofeedback
- Massage
- Herbs: *Cimcifuga racemosa* (black cohosh), Vitex agnus castii (chaste tree), *Rehmannia*, ginseng, Chinese tonic of He Shou Wu, dong quai, golden seal, flaxseed, and evening primrose
- Supplements: vitamin E, soy protein (soy is high in plant estrogens)
- Meditation and yoga.

 ## NURSING CARE

Nursing care during and after the menopausal period focuses on minimizing the symptoms associated with hormonal changes, reducing the risk of cardiovascular disease, cancer, and osteoporosis, and educating the woman about lifestyle changes important to health and well-being.

Health Promotion

The American Cancer Society recommends a cancer-related checkup every year after the age of 40. This checkup includes examination for cancers of the thyroid, ovaries, lymph nodes, oral cavity, and skin. Other important checkups include screening for cervical, breast, and colorectal cancer. Health counseling should also include information about alcohol and tobacco use, sun exposure, diet and nutrition, exercise, risk factors, sexual practices, and environmental and occupational exposures. It is important to discuss the benefits of rest and exercise, as well as a diet that includes fruits, vegetables, and fiber. In addition, suggest the following resources for further information:

- National Institute on Aging
- Centers for Disease Control and Prevention
- North American Menopause Society
- Association of Reproductive Health Professionals
- Women's Health Initiative
- National Women's Health Information Center.

Assessment

Collect the following data through the health history and physical examination. When assessing the older woman, be aware of normal changes with aging, as outlined in Chapter 49 ∞.

- *Health history:* Problems with urinary frequency, urgency, or incontinence; menstrual history; sexual history; dyspareunia; use of alcohol, nicotine, and drugs; medications, sleep patterns, hot flashes, night sweats, changes in emotional responses.
- *Physical assessment:* Height and weight, posture, vital signs, breast examination, pelvic examination, abdominal assessment.

Nursing Diagnoses and Interventions

Although each nursing care plan must be individualized, interventions often focus on problems with lack of information, sexuality, self-esteem, and a disturbed body image.

Deficient Knowledge

Because menopausal manifestations vary widely, it is difficult to predict their effect on an individual woman. However, the well-informed woman is better prepared to deal with whatever symptoms she experiences.

- Discuss physiologic manifestations, such as hot flashes and night sweats. *The underlying cause of hot flashes is not known (Porth, 2005). Many physiologic effects of menopause are amenable to nonpharmacologic methods of relief, such as lifestyle changes.*

PRACTICE ALERT

When hot flashes occur at night and are accompanied by perspiration, they are called night sweats. Night sweats often interfere with normal sleep patterns, leading to increased fatigue and irritability.

- Provide information about dietary recommendations. The recommended daily intake of calcium for women over 50 is 1200 mg. *Some women need to use calcium supplements or calcium-containing antacid tablets to meet this requirement.*
- Emphasize the importance of weight-bearing exercise. *Weight-bearing exercise reduces the rate of bone loss, helps maintain optimum weight, and reduces cardiovascular risk.*

- Provide information about the benefits and risks of HRT. Not every woman will need or want it. *Every woman needs to understand both the risks and the benefits before deciding whether to use HRT.*
- Encourage the woman to obtain yearly mammograms, clinical breast examinations, and Pap tests, and to perform monthly breast self-examination (BSE) at the same day each month. *The increased risk for cancer of the breast and pelvic reproductive organs makes self-examination and healthcare provider screening during and after menopause even more important.*

Ineffective Sexuality Pattern

Vaginal dryness and atrophy, together with the emotional effect of menopause, can interfere with sexual expression and satisfaction. Suggesting measures to help the woman and her partner cope with these changes can enable them to continue or resume a mutually satisfying sexual relationship.

- Encourage expression of feelings and concerns about how menopause is changing her sex life. *Midlife and older women may not be comfortable in discussing their intimate sexual behavior.*
- Suggest ways to increase vaginal lubrication, such as spending more time in foreplay and/or using water-soluble gels (e.g., Replens) for vaginal lubrication. *A more leisurely approach to sexual activity can be mutually gratifying for both the woman and her partner. Use of water-soluble gels can prevent vaginal pain and irritation and improve the quality of the sexual experience.*

PRACTICE ALERT

Plant estrogens, found in food such as brown rice, corn, green beans, lemon and orange peels, and tofu, are mildly estrogenic and may improve vaginal dryness.

- Explain that as women age, it may take longer for vaginal lubrication and orgasm to occur. *This information is important to prevent the woman from believing something is wrong with her, or her partner believing he or she is no longer interesting or sexually exciting.*

Situational Low Self-Esteem

Each woman responds to the aging process in her own way, and most women have coping skills that adequately equip them to deal with the gradual changes associated with aging. Among the factors that may provoke a self-esteem disturbance are the loss of youth, a sense of emptiness as children leave home, and the need to redefine one's self-concept and roles as parenting becomes less important. Women who place a high value on their physical attractiveness may experience a painful psychologic response to the physical changes of menopause.

- Encourage expression of fears and concerns related to changes in interpersonal and family functions. *Many women associate aging with "uselessness" and unattractiveness.*
- Suggest volunteer activities or employment for the woman who has extra time. *This enables the woman to feel that she is still a contributing member of society. Volunteering for activities involving young people can help reduce anxiety about*

Alternative and Complementary Therapies

Alternative and complementary therapies the woman with PMS may find helpful focus on diet, exercise, relaxation, and stress management:

- A diet high in complex carbohydrates with limited simple sugars and alcohol is recommended to minimize reactive hypoglycemia, which can contribute to the manifestations of PMS.
- Reduced sodium intake helps minimize fluid retention. Increased intake of calcium (1200 mg per day), magnesium (200 mg per day), vitamin B$_6$ (50 to 100 mg per day), and vitamin E (400 international units per day) may be helpful (Mayo Clinic, 2004).
- Caffeine is restricted to reduce irritability.
- Herbal remedies include black cohosh, ginger, chaste tree berry, and evening primrose oil. Natural progesterone creams, derived from wild yams and soybeans, relieve manifestations in some women (Mayo Clinic, 2004). Discussion about these alternative therapies with the healthcare provider is recommended.
- Exercise is beneficial, but adequate rest also is necessary.
- Techniques for relaxation and stress management include deep abdominal breathing, meditation, muscle relaxation, and guided imagery.

 NURSING CARE

Nursing Diagnoses and Interventions

Nursing care for the woman with PMS focuses on relieving manifestations. Most women experiencing PMS require interventions to manage pain and enhance coping.

Acute Pain

The woman with PMS may have pain from headache (including migraine), menstrual cramps, excessive fluid retention, breast swelling, joint and muscle pain, and backache.

- Teach effective pharmacologic and nonpharmacologic self-care measures to relieve pain: application of heat, relaxation techniques (such as breathing exercises, imagery techniques, or meditation), and exercise. *Heat relieves muscle spasms and dilates blood vessels, increasing blood supply to the pelvis and uterine muscles. Relaxation and exercise aid the release of naturally produced pain relievers called endorphins.*
- Review daily activities and suggest ways to balance rest periods and activity. *During rest periods, energy and oxygen requirements decrease, increasing the amount of energy and oxygen available to muscles.*
- Review manifestations and, if possible, correlate these with dietary patterns and activity levels. Encourage the woman to keep a diary of PMS manifestations. *Maintaining a diary of PMS manifestations, activity, and foods eaten can provide data to identify modifiable causes of discomfort.*
- If appropriate, suggest sexual activity as a way to lessen menstrual cramps. *Orgasm may help relieve dysmenorrhea.*

Ineffective Coping

Many women experience wide mood swings during episodes of PMS, sometimes exhibiting self-destructive or aggressive behaviors toward others. These mood swings can interfere with a woman's ability to manage her responsibilities at home or at work.

- Encourage the woman to keep a journal of her menstrual cycle and to document her mood changes in the 7 to 10 days prior to menstruation. *Recognizing the signs and timing of PMS is the first step in developing methods to cope with the problem.*
- Explore possible ways to rearrange or reschedule activities when experiencing PMS. *Planning ahead enables the woman to assume more control and promotes coping methods.*
- Explore what, if any, self-care measures have helped cope with mood alterations in the past. *Encourage healthful coping mechanisms, such as relaxation techniques and exercise. Some women may rely on alcohol or other drugs during PMS, which only exacerbate the manifestations.*

Community-Based Care

Teach the woman and family that PMS is not caused by a pathologic process but is a physiologic response to hormonal changes of the menstrual cycle. With an understanding of the condition, the woman is better able to manage anxiety and to become actively involved in techniques to reduce the manifestations. Teaching should also include dietary measures, relaxation techniques and exercise, stress reduction techniques, and support systems.

THE WOMAN WITH DYSMENORRHEA

Dysmenorrhea (pain or discomfort associated with menstruation) is experienced by a significant number of menstruating women. *Primary dysmenorrhea* occurs without specific pelvic pathology, and is most often seen in girls who have just begun menstruating, becoming less severe after the mid-20s or giving birth. *Secondary dysmenorrhea* is related to identified pelvic disease.

Pathophysiology

In primary dysmenorrhea, excessive production of prostaglandins stimulates uterine muscle fibers to contract. As the muscles contract, uterine circulation is compromised, resulting in uterine ischemia and pain. These contractions can range from mild cramping to severe muscle spasms. Psychologic factors, such as anxiety and tension, may contribute to dysmenorrhea. Secondary dysmenorrhea is related to underlying organic conditions that involve scarring or injury to the reproductive tract. Endometriosis, fibroid tumors, pelvic inflammatory disease, or ovarian cancer may result in painful menses.

Manifestations

Manifestations of primary dysmenorrhea (see the box on the next page) may be severe enough to disrupt activities of daily living, sexual function, and even fertility.

INTERDISCIPLINARY CARE

Care of the woman with menstrual pain focuses on identifying the underlying cause, reestablishing functional capacity, and managing pain.

- Abdominal pain beginning with onset of menses and lasting 12 to 48 hours
- Pain radiating to lower back and thighs
- Headache
- Nausea
- Vomiting
- Diarrhea
- Fatigue
- Breast tenderness

A careful history and physical assessment are performed to rule out any underlying organic cause of dysmenorrhea. If no organic cause can be found, the diagnosis is primary dysmenorrhea. In addition, attitudes and expectations about menstruation and lifestyle disruption are identified and explored.

Diagnosis

Various diagnostic tests are performed to identify structural abnormalities, hormonal imbalances, and pathologic conditions that could cause menstrual pain. Diagnostic tests are described in Chapter 49 ∞.

Diagnosis is made based on findings from a pelvic examination and diagnostic procedures, including a Papanicolaou (Pap) smear and cervical and vaginal cultures, ultrasound of the pelvis and vagina, and CT scan or MRI to detect structural abnormalities, malignancy, or infections. Laboratory tests used to assess possible causes of dysmenorrhea are as follows:

- FSH and LH levels to assess the function of the pituitary gland. The results are correlated with the time of the menstrual cycle.
- Progesterone and estradiol levels to assess ovarian function.
- Thyroid function tests (T_3 and T_4) to assess thyroid function.

Laparoscopy is used to diagnose structural defects and blockages caused by scarring, endometriosis, tumors, and cysts (Figure 51–1 ■). See the box below for nursing care of the woman having a laparoscopy. A dilation and curettage (D&C) of the uterus may be performed to obtain tissue for evaluation

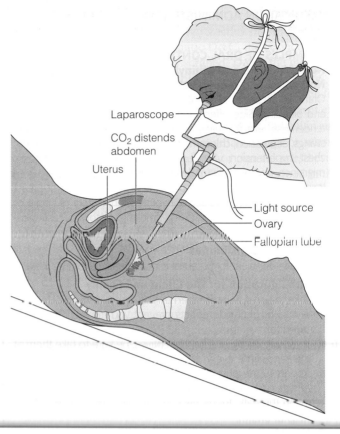

Figure 51–1 ■ Laparoscopy. In this surgical procedure, a flexible, lighted instrument (laparoscope) is inserted through a periumbilical incision. Laparoscopy allows visualization of the pelvic cavity.

or to relieve dysmenorrhea and heavy menstrual bleeding. (This procedure is discussed later in this chapter.)

Medications

Dysmenorrhea may be treated with analgesics, prostaglandin inhibitors such as NSAIDs, or oral contraceptives (see the Medication Administration box on the next page).

Alternative and Complementary Therapies

The complementary therapies listed for the woman with PMS may also be useful for the woman with dysmenorrhea. Other

---

NURSING CARE OF THE WOMAN HAVING A Laparoscopy

PREOPERATIVE CARE
- Instruct the woman to empty the bladder prior to the surgical procedure.
- Explain to the woman that referred shoulder pain or expulsion of gas through the vagina may occur postoperatively. *During the procedure, the woman's abdomen is insufflated with carbon dioxide gas to distend the abdomen and facilitate visualization of the pelvic organs. The surgical table is then tilted so that the intestines will fall away from the pelvic organs. Some carbon dioxide gas may remain in the abdomen after the procedure.*

- Explain that pain should be minimal. Instruct the woman to report excessive pain to the nurse or physician at once. *Excessive pain signals infection or other postoperative complication.*

POSTOPERATIVE CARE
- Apply a perineal pad. Teach the woman proper perineal hygiene, emphasizing the need to change pads at least every 4 hours. Keep a pad count. *Proper perineal hygiene reduces the risk of postoperative infection. Pad count is an indication of blood loss.*
- Assess for excessive vaginal bleeding. *Minor bleeding is normal; excessive bleeding may indicate hemorrhage.*

Hysterectomy may involve either an abdominal or a vaginal approach. The choice depends on the underlying disorder, the need to explore the abdominal cavity, and the preference of the surgeon and woman. Nursing care of the woman undergoing a hysterectomy is described in the box below.

Abdominal hysterectomy is performed when a preexisting abdominal scar is present, when adhesions are thought to be present, or when a large operating field is necessary. For example, the woman with endometriosis is more likely to have an abdominal hysterectomy because endometrial tissue implants that may be present on other abdominal organs need to be removed. The surgical incision may be either longitudinal, made in the midline from umbilicus to pubis, or a *Pfannenstiel incision,* also known as the bikini cut.

Vaginal hysterectomy, removal of the uterus through the vagina, is desirable when the uterus has descended into the vagina or if the urinary bladder or rectum have prolapsed into the vagina. Vaginal hysterectomy leaves no visible abdominal scar. Laparoscopy-assisted vaginal hysterectomy (LAVH) is most often performed.

NURSING CARE

DUB usually causes the woman anxiety. Her self-image, sexuality, or reproductive capacity may be threatened, and she may fear the possibility of cancer. She may be embarrassed to discuss her menstrual history and hygiene practices.

Nursing Diagnoses and Interventions

Interventions for the woman with DUB commonly address problems with anxiety and sexual function.

Anxiety

The anxiety associated with abnormal uterine bleeding can be intense. Until the cause of the bleeding is identified and has been addressed, the woman may fear cancer or other life-threatening conditions.

- Discuss the results of tests and examinations with the woman. *This allows for open exchange of information.*
- Provide information about the causes, treatments, risks, long-term effects of treatments, and prognosis. *This allows the woman to assume responsibility for her own health and become involved in her own treatment plan.*

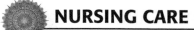

NURSING CARE OF THE WOMAN HAVING A Hysterectomy

PREOPERATIVE CARE

- Assess the woman's understanding of the procedure. Provide explanation, clarification, and emotional support as needed. Reassure that the anesthesia will eliminate any pain during surgery and that medication will be administered postoperatively to minimize discomfort. *The woman who understands about the procedure to be performed and what to expect after surgery will be less anxious.*
- Cleanse the abdominal and perineal area, and, if ordered, shave the perineal area.
- If ordered, administer a small cleansing enema and ask the woman to empty her bladder. *This precaution helps prevent contamination from the bowel or bladder during surgery.*
- Administer preoperative medications as ordered.
- Check the chart to ensure that the consent form has been signed.

POSTOPERATIVE CARE

- Assess for signs of hemorrhage. *Hemorrhage is more common after vaginal hysterectomy than after abdominal hysterectomy.*
- Monitor vital signs every 4 hours, auscultate lungs every shift and measure intake and output. *These data are important indicators of hemodynamic status and complications.*
- Once the catheter has been removed, measure the amount of urine voided.
- Assess for complications, including infection, ileus, shock or hemorrhage, thrombophlebitis, and pulmonary embolus.
- Assess vaginal discharge; instruct the woman in perineal care.
- Assess incision and bowel sounds every shift.
- Encourage turning, coughing, deep breathing, and early ambulation.
- Encourage fluid intake.

- Teach to splint the abdomen and cough deeply. Teach the use of the incentive spirometer.
- Instruct to restrict physical activity for 4 to 6 weeks. Heavy lifting, stair climbing, douching, tampons, and sexual intercourse should be avoided. The woman should shower, avoiding tub baths, until bleeding has ceased. *Infection and hemorrhage are the greatest postoperative risks; restricting activities and preventing the introduction of any foreign material into the vagina helps reduce these risks.*
- Explain to the woman that she may feel tired for several days after surgery and needs to rest periodically.
- Explain that appetite may be depressed and bowel elimination may be sluggish. *These are aftereffects of general anesthesia, handling of the bowel during surgery, and loss of muscle tone in the bowel while empty.*
- Teach the woman to recognize signs of complications that should be reported to the physician or nurse:
  a. Temperature greater than 100°F (37.7°C)
  b. Vaginal bleeding that is greater than a typical menstrual period or is bright red
  c. Urinary incontinence, urgency, burning, or frequency
  d. Severe pain.
- Encourage the woman to express feelings that may signal a negative self-concept. Correct any misconceptions. *Some women believe that hysterectomy means weight gain, the end of sexual activity, and the growth of facial hair.*
- Provide information on risks and benefits of hormone replacement therapy, if indicated. *If the ovaries have also been removed, the woman is immediately thrust into menopause and may want or need hormone replacement therapy.*
- Reinforce the need to obtain gynecologic examinations regularly even after hysterectomy.

- Evaluate coping strategies and psychosocial support systems. Teach coping strategies if indicated. *The possibility of surgery or cancer represents a crisis for the woman and her support system. Support groups can provide assistance for the woman through crisis intervention.*

Sexual Dysfunction

The woman with DUB may be unwilling to express herself sexually, particularly if bleeding is frequent or heavy. Additionally, fatigue may prevent her from participating in sexual activity.

- Offer information about engaging in sexual activity during menstruation. Explain that conception is possible during this time and that orgasm may help relieve symptoms. *Some women mistakenly believe that birth control measures are unnecessary during menstruation. Orgasm causes a release of tension and vascular congestion and frequently provides at least temporary relief of symptoms.*
- Provide an opportunity for the expression of concerns related to alterations in lifestyle and sexual functioning. *Some women have had a prolonged period of sexual abstinence related to DUB. Allowing women to verbalize concerns can assist them in working collaboratively with the healthcare provider to minimize the impact of illness and optimize function.*
- Encourage frequent rest periods. *This conserves energy and may allow sexual activities to resume.*

- Provide information about alternative methods of sexual expression. *Methods of sexual expression other than vaginal intercourse may satisfy the needs of both partners.*

PRACTICE ALERT

If the nurse is not comfortable with frank discussions about sexual activities, referral is indicated.

Community-Based Care

Provide support, appropriate reassurance, and information to help the woman and her family better understand her disorder and the therapeutic interventions indicated. Teaching also includes self-care measures that help minimize the effects of DUB on the daily functioning of the woman. The following topics should be included:

- Administration and side effects of prescribed medications, including iron
- The need to maintain a balanced diet, increasing iron-rich foods such as eggs, beans, liver, beef, and shrimp (Inform the woman that while orange juice may improve the absorption of iron, foods high in calcium and oxalic acid, such as spinach, may reduce its absorption.)
- Importance of maintaining a fluid intake of 2000 to 3000 mL a day
- The need to immediately report recurring episodes of DUB, particularly in postmenopausal women, to the healthcare provider.

STRUCTURAL DISORDERS

Structural disorders of the female reproductive system include displacement disorders and fistulas.

THE WOMAN WITH A UTERINE DISPLACEMENT

The uterus may be displaced within the pelvic cavity or may descend into the vaginal canal. Displacement of the uterus within the pelvic cavity is classified according to the direction of the displacement (Figure 51–2 ■):

- *Retroversion* of the uterus is a backward tilting of the uterus toward the rectum.
- *Retroflexion* involves a flexing or bending of the uterine corpus in a backward manner toward the rectum.
- *Anteversion* is an exaggerated forward tilting of the uterus.
- *Anteflexion* is a flexing or folding of the uterine corpus upon itself.

Prolapse of the uterus into the vaginal canal can vary from mild to complete prolapse outside of the body. First-degree, or mild, prolapse involves a descent of less than half the uterine corpus into the vagina. Second-degree, or marked, prolapse involves the descent of the entire uterus into the vaginal canal, so that the cervix is at the introitus to the vagina. Third-degree prolapse, or *procidentia*, is complete prolapse of the uterus outside the body, with inversion

of the vaginal canal (Figure 51–3 ■). Prolapse of the uterus is often accompanied by *cystocele* (herniation of the bladder into the vagina) or *rectocele* (herniation of the rectum into the vagina).

Pathophysiology

Displacement or prolapse of the uterus, bladder, or rectum can be a congenital or an acquired condition. Congenital tilting or flexion of the uterus is rare. More commonly, tilting or flexion disorders in which the uterus remains within the pelvic cavity are related to the scarring and inflammation of pelvic inflammatory disease, endometriosis, pregnancy, and tumors.

Downward displacement of the pelvic organs into the vagina results from weakened pelvic musculature, usually attributable to stretching of the supporting ligaments and muscles during pregnancy and childbirth. Unrepaired lacerations from childbirth, rapid deliveries, multiple pregnancies, congenital weakness, or loss of elasticity and muscle tone with aging may contribute to these disorders.

Manifestations

The manifestations of displacement disorders are listed on page 1807.

leading to incontinent leakage of urine through the vagina. A *rectovaginal fistula* (less common) is an abnormal opening between the rectum and vagina, causing incontinent leakage of stool or flatus through the vagina.

Fistulas between the bladder and the vagina (vesicovaginal) or between the rectum and the vagina (rectovaginal) may develop as a complication of childbirth, gynecologic or urologic surgery, or radiation therapy for gynecologic cancer. Cancer of the bladder is sometimes involved. The woman with a vaginal fistula often presents with a complaint of involuntary leakage of urine or flatus and symptoms of infection.

Interdisciplinary Care

Fistulas are diagnosed by pelvic examination. Diagnosis of a vesicovaginal fistula can be made by instilling dye into the urinary bladder through a catheter and observing the vagina for leakage. If no leakage is detected, a tampon or vaginal pack is inserted into the vagina, and the woman is asked to ambulate. If an abnormal opening is present, the tampon will absorb the dye. Dye may also be injected intravenously because it is excreted by the kidneys. Urine and vaginal cultures may be performed to rule out infections. Antibiotics are administered if infection is present.

A small vaginal fistula may resolve spontaneously. Otherwise, surgery is performed after inflammation has subsided, often a period of several months. Rarely, in the presence of a large, highly inflamed rectovaginal fistula, a temporary colostomy is performed, allowing inflammation and irritation to subside (see Chapter 26 ∞).

Nursing Care

Nursing care for the woman with repair of a vaginal fistula is similar to that for the woman with a displacement disorder. Teaching is an important component of nursing care. Stress the importance of careful perineal cleansing to reduce irritation and prevent further tissue breakdown. Suggest perineal irrigation or sitz baths for cleansing. Perineal pads or special underwear may be used to absorb urine or fecal drainage. For the woman with a rectovaginal fistula, provide information about avoiding gas-forming foods to minimize embarrassment from odor.

DISORDERS OF FEMALE REPRODUCTIVE TISSUE

Both benign and malignant tissue disorders affect the female reproductive system. Benign tumors and cysts include Bartholin's gland cysts, cervical polyps, endometrial cysts and polyps, ovarian cysts, and uterine leiomyomas (fibroids). Endometriosis is a condition in which endometrial tissue implants outside the uterus in various locations in the pelvic cavity. Malignant tumors of reproductive tissue include cervical cancer, endometrial cancer, ovarian cancer, and vulvar cancer.

THE WOMAN WITH CYSTS OR POLYPS

A *cyst* is a fluid-filled sac. A *polyp* is a highly vascular solid tumor attached by a pedicle or stem. Cysts or polyps of the female reproductive system can occur in the vulva, cervix, endometrium, or ovaries.

Pathophysiology

Following are different types of female reproductive tissue cysts and polyps:

- *Bartholin's gland cysts* are the most common cystic disorder of the vulva. These cysts are caused by the infection or obstruction of Bartholin's gland.
- *Cervical polyps* are the most common benign cervical lesion in women of reproductive age. These polyps tend to occur in women over age 40 who have borne several children and have a history of using oral contraceptives. It is possible that cervical polyps develop from endocervical hyperplasia. The polyp develops at the vaginal end of the cervix, has a stem, and is highly vascular.
- *Endometrial cysts and polyps* are caused by endometrial overgrowth and are often filled with old blood (the dark color leads to the label "chocolate cysts"). Endometrial cysts are the result of endometrial implants on the ovary and are associated with endometriosis. Endometrial polyps, in contrast, are intrauterine overgrowths, similar to cervical polyps, and usually have a stalk.
- *Ovarian cysts* are classified as follicular cysts and corpus luteum cysts. Follicular cysts develop as a result of failure of the mature follicle to rupture or failure of an immature follicle to reabsorb fluid after ovulation. Corpus luteum cysts develop as a result of increased hormone secretion by the corpus luteum after ovulation. Most functional cysts regress spontaneously within two or three menstrual cycles.
- *Polycystic ovarian syndrome* (POS, also known as *Stein-Leventhal syndrome*) is an endocrine disorder characterized by an excess of androgens and a long-term lack of ovulation. The exact cause is unknown. As a part of the disease, as many as 8 to 10 cysts form in the ovaries from a failure to release ovum. Manifestations include amenorrhea or irregular menses, hirsutism, obesity, acne, hypertension, sleep apnea, and infertility. Women with POS often have insulin resistance and are at increased risk for early-onset type 2 diabetes, as well as heart disease, breast cancer, and endometrial cancer.

Manifestations and Complications

The causes and manifestations of benign cysts and polyps of the female reproductive system are presented in Table 51–1. Complications associated with these disorders include infection, rupture, infertility, hemorrhage, and recurrence.

INTERDISCIPLINARY CARE

Care focuses on identifying and correcting the disorder and preventing its recurrence. A careful history and physical examination are performed, including inspection and visualization.

TABLE 51–1 Benign Cysts and Polyps of the Female Reproductive System

SITE	TYPE	ETIOLOGIC ORIGIN	MANIFESTATIONS
Ovary	Functional cysts	Ovulation—include follicular cysts and corpus luteum cysts	May resolve spontaneously; can cause pain, menstrual irregularity, or amenorrhea
	Polycystic ovarian syndrome	Unknown; possible hypothalamic-pituitary dysfunction	Hirsutism, obesity; amenorrhea or irregular menses; hyperinsulinemia; infertility
Vulva	Bartholin cysts	Obstruction or infection of Bartholin's gland	Pain, redness, perineal mass, dyspareunia
Endometrium	Chocolate cysts	Endometrial overgrowth; filled with old blood	
	Endometrial polyps	Unknown	Bleeding between periods
Cervix	Cervical polyps	Unknown	Bleeding after intercourse or between periods

Examination of the reproductive tract reveals the presence of most cysts and polyps. The menstrual history may reveal menstrual irregularities.

Diagnosis

Diagnostic tests that may be used to diagnose cysts and polyps of the female reproductive system include a laparoscopy to visualize ovarian cysts, an ultrasound or x-ray to differentiate cysts from solid tumors, and a pregnancy test when luteal cysts are suspected. Laboratory analysis will demonstrate elevated LH and testosterone levels, as well as a reverse in FSH/LH in the woman with polycystic ovary syndrome (POS).

Medications

Antibiotics are used to treat infection or abscess, and oral contraceptives are used to promote regression of functional ovarian cysts. Clomiphene (Clomid, Serophene) may be prescribed to stimulate ovulation in the woman with POS who wishes to become pregnant. Dexamethasone (Decadron) suppresses ACTH and adrenal androgens, and may be added to increase the likelihood of ovulation.

Surgery

Cervical polyps are visible through a vaginal speculum and usually are removed with a clamp, using a twisting motion. To remove endometrial cysts or polyps, a transcervical approach is used. The specimen is sent to the laboratory for evaluation, and chemical or electrical cauterization is applied after cyst removal. For Bartholin's gland cysts and any abscesses, the lesion is incised and drained, and a drainage device is left in place. Follicular cysts may be punctured through laser surgery, or a wedge resection of the ovary may be performed to restore ovulation. Rarely, *oophorectomy* (removal of the ovary) is performed if the cysts are very large.

NURSING CARE

Nursing care focuses on relieving pain and preventing recurrence and complications. Address the following topics for self-care at home:
- The condition, its treatment, and measures to relieve pain
- The importance of keeping follow-up appointments
- Manifestations of infection (for postsurgical care) and the need to notify the physician should they occur

- If cervical polypectomy is performed, advise use of external pads for 1 week. The woman must be able to state the signs of excessive bleeding and recognize that saturating more than one pad in an hour indicates the need for immediate follow-up.
- The importance of long-term follow-up care for the woman with POS.

THE WOMAN WITH LEIOMYOMA

Leiomyomas *(fibroid tumors)* are benign tumors that originate from smooth muscle of the uterus. They are the most common form of pelvic tumor, believed to occur in 1 of every 4 or 5 women older than 35 years of age (Porth, 2005). Fibroids are seen more often and grow more rapidly in African American women.

Pathophysiology

The actual cause of fibroid tumors is not clearly understood, but there is a strong association with estrogen stimulation. Fibroid tumors usually develop in the uterine corpus, and may be intramural, subserous, or submucous (Figure 51–4 ■):
- *Intramural fibroid tumors* (the most common type) are embedded in the myometrium. They usually present as an enlargement of the uterus.
- *Subserous fibroid tumors* lie beneath the serous lining of the uterus and project into the peritoneal cavity. They may become pedunculated (on a stem) and displace or compress other tissues, such as the ureter or bladder.
- *Submucous fibroid tumors* lie beneath the endometrial lining of the uterus. They displace endometrial tissue and are more likely to cause bleeding, infection, and necrosis than the other types.

Manifestations

Small tumors may be asymptomatic. The rate of growth varies, but they may increase in size during pregnancy or with use of oral contraceptives or HRT. Large fibroid tumors can crowd other organs, leading to pelvic pressure, pain, dysmenorrhea, menorrhagia, and fatigue. Depending on the location of the tumor, constipation and urinary urgency and frequency may occur. Most fibroid tumors shrink with menopause.

Nursing Diagnoses and Interventions

Interventions for pain, discussed previously, are also appropriate for the woman with endometriosis. A priority diagnosis for the young woman with this disorder is anxiety related to the risk for loss of reproductive function.

Anxiety

Anxiety about the unsure prognosis related to infertility is a particular problem for young women who plan to have a family in the future.

■ Encourage expression of fears and anxiety about infertility, and answer questions honestly. *Knowledge helps relieve anxiety and fear.*
■ Provide information on fertility awareness methods, including measurement of basal body temperature and other techniques for recognizing ovulation. *Understanding these techniques helps the woman and her partner optimize the conditions for conception.*

Using NANDA, NIC, and NOC

Chart 51–1 shows links between NANDA nursing diagnoses, NIC, and NOC when caring for the client with endometriosis.

Community-Based Care

Explain the cause of the disorder and the various treatment options, including their side effects. Discuss fertility awareness methods and the risks and benefits of long-term use of oral contraceptives. Stress the importance of exercise, smoking cessation, and weight control. If surgical treatment is chosen, provide preoperative and postoperative teaching.

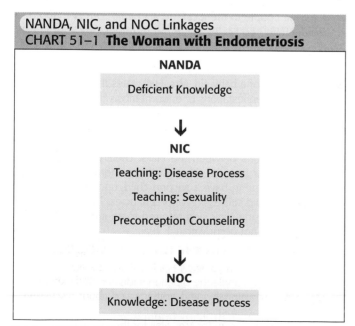

NANDA, NIC, and NOC Linkages
CHART 51–1 **The Woman with Endometriosis**

NANDA

Deficient Knowledge

↓

NIC

Teaching: Disease Process

Teaching: Sexuality

Preconception Counseling

↓

NOC

Knowledge: Disease Process

Data from *NANDA's Nursing Diagnoses: Definitions & Classification 2005–2006* by NANDA International (2003), Philadelphia; *Nursing Interventions Classification (NIC)* (4th ed.) by J. M. Dochterman & G. M. Bulecheck (2004), St. Louis, MO: Mosby; and *Nursing Outcomes Classification (NOC)* (3rd ed.) by S. Moorhead, M. Johnson, and M. Maas (2004), St. Louis, MO: Mosby.

THE WOMAN WITH CERVICAL CANCER

Cancer of the cervix is the second most common cancer in women worldwide, and the 14th most common in women in the United States (the lower number is primarily the result of screening with Pap tests). The incidence is greater in black women than in white women.

> **FAST FACTS**
> **Cervical Cancer**
> ■ The American Cancer Society (ACS, 2006d) estimates that there will be more than 10,000 new cases of cervical cancer each year, resulting in nearly 4000 deaths annually.
> ■ Nearly 100% of women with cervical cancer have evidence of cervical infection with human papillomavirus (HPV) (see Chapter 52 ∞).
> ■ The FDA recently approved HPV testing as an adjunct to cervical cancer screening.

Effective screening with the Pap smear test and treatment have reduced the death rate by 55% during the last 30 years, although the death rates for blacks continues to be more than two times that of whites (ACS, 2006c). The age of diagnosis is usually between 50 and 55 years; however, cervical cancer begins to appear in women in their 20s.

Risk Factors

Risk factors for cervical cancer include infection of the external genitalia and anus with HPV, first intercourse before 16 years of age, multiple sex partners or male partners with multiple sex partners, a history of sexually transmitted infections, and infection with HIV. The most important risk factor is infection with HPV. Other risk factors include smoking and poor nutritional status, family history of cervical cancer, and exposure to diethylstilbestrol (DES) *in utero*.

Pathophysiology

Most cervical cancers (90%) are squamous cell carcinomas that begin as neoplasia in the cervical epithelium. *Precancerous dysplasia (cervical intraepithelial neoplasia [CIN], cervical carcinoma in situ)* is estimated to occur in one of eight women before the age of 20 and is often associated with HPV infection. Studies have also found a strong association with reproductive infections with *Chlamydia trachomatis*. (These infections are discussed in Chapter 52 ∞ .) The precursor lesions may spontaneously regress (60%), persist (30%), or progress and undergo malignant change (10%). Only about 1% become invasive (Porth, 2005). Systems of grading of dysplastic changes in the cervix use the term *cervical intraepithelial neoplasia (CIN)* or the Bethesda system (Table 51–2). Carcinoma *in situ* is localized; invasive cancer spreads to deeper layers.

Cancer *in situ* most often develops in the transformation zone where the columnar epithelium of the cervical lining meets the squamous epithelium of the outer cervix and vagina. Squamous cell cancers spread by direct invasion of accessory structures, including the vaginal wall, pelvic wall, bladder, and rectum. Although metastasis is most frequently confined to the

TABLE 51–2 Classification Systems for Pap Smears

DYSPLASIA/NEOPLASIA	CIN (CERVICAL INTRAEPITHELIAL NEOPLASIA)	BETHESDA SYSTEM	NUMERICAL
Benign	Benign	■ Normal	1
Benign with inflammation	Benign with inflammation	■ Normal	2
		■ Atypical squamous cells of undetermined significance (ASC-US)	
Moderate dysplasia	CIN I	■ Low-grade squamous intraepithelial lesion (SIL)	3
Severe dysplasia	CIN II	■ High-grade SIL	3
Carcinoma *in situ*	CIN III	■ High-grade SIL	4
Invasive cancer	Invasive cancer	■ Invasive cancer	5

pelvic area, distant metastasis may occur through the lymphatic system.

Manifestations

Preinvasive cancer is limited to the cervix and rarely causes manifestations. Invasive cancer causes vaginal bleeding after intercourse or between menstrual periods, and a vaginal discharge that increases as the cancer progresses. These changes are subtle, and may be more readily noticed by the postmenopausal woman. Manifestations of advanced disease include referred pain in the back or thighs, hematuria, bloody stools, anemia, and weight loss.

INTERDISCIPLINARY CARE

The goals of treatment are to eradicate the cancer and minimize complications and metastasis. The type of treatment depends on the degree of malignant change, the size and location of the lesion, and the extent of metastasis.

Diagnosis

Diagnostic tests used to diagnose cervical cancer include a Pap smear, colposcopy, and cervical biopsy (see Chapter 49 ∞ for further information about these procedures). A loop diathermy technique (loop electrosurgical excision procedure [LEEP]) allows simultaneous diagnosis and treatment of dysplastic lesions found on colposcopy. This procedure is performed in the health provider's office, using a wire for both cutting and coagulation during excision of the dysplastic region of the cervix. An MRI or CT of the pelvis, abdomen, or bones may be performed to evaluate the spread of the tumor.

Medications

Chemotherapy is used for tumors not responsive to other therapy, tumors that cannot be removed, or as adjunct therapy if metastasis has occurred (see Chapter 14 ∞).

Surgery

When combined with colposcopy, laser surgery is a viable treatment method provided that the cancer is limited to the cervical epithelium. Cryosurgery, which involves the use of a probe to freeze tissue, causing necrosis and sloughing, is also used for noninvasive lesions. Conization (Figure 51–5 ■) is performed to treat microinvasive carcinoma when colposcopy cannot define the limits of the invasion. For invasive lesions, hysterectomy or radical hysterectomy (removal of the uterus, fallopian tubes, lymph nodes, and ovaries) is performed.

A *pelvic exenteration*, the removal of all pelvic contents, including the bowel, vagina, and bladder, is performed if the cancer recurs without involvement of the lymphatic system. An anterior exenteration is the removal of the uterus, ovaries, fallopian tubes, vagina, bladder, urethra, and lymphatic vessels and nodes. An ileal conduit is created for excretion of urine (see Chapter 29 ∞). A posterior exenteration is the removal of the uterus, ovaries, fallopian tubes, bowel, and rectum. A colostomy is created for excretion of feces (see Chapter 26 ∞).

Radiation Therapy

Radiation therapy is used to treat invasive cervical cancer. External radiation beam therapy and intracavity cesium irradiation can be used. Radiation is discussed in Chapter 14 ∞ .

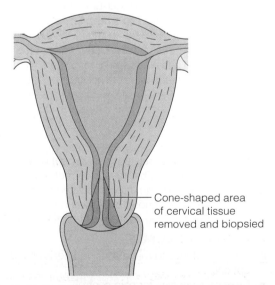

Cone-shaped area of cervical tissue removed and biopsied

Figure 51–5 ■ Conization, the surgical removal of a cone-shaped section of the cervix, is used to treat microinvasive carcinoma of the cervix.

chemotherapy, or surgery, as indicated. Preoperative teaching focuses on postoperative expectations, including management of urinary or fecal diversion, if indicated (see Chapter 26 ∞ and 29 ∞). Help the woman and family recognize signs of infection and understand the importance of follow-up care. In addition, suggest the following resources:

- American Cancer Society
- National Cancer Institute
- Women's Cancer Network.

THE WOMAN WITH ENDOMETRIAL CANCER

Endometrial cancer is the most frequently diagnosed pelvic cancer in the United States. The ACS (2006a) estimates that each year approximately 41,000 women are diagnosed with endometrial cancer, and more than 7000 die annually from this disease. The incidence is higher in white women than in black women, but the mortality rate is nearly twice as high in black women. Most endometrial cancer is diagnosed in postmenopausal women, with the peak incidence in the late 50s and early 60s, with only a 2% to 5% incidence in women younger than 40 (Porth, 2005). When diagnosed and treated early in the disease, the 5-year survival rate is about 90%.

Risk Factors

A significant risk factor for endometrial cancer is prolonged estrogen stimulation. Other factors that increase risk are obesity, anovulatory menstrual cycles, decreasing ovarian function (as from menopause), estrogen-secreting tumors, and unopposed estrogen (e.g., estrogen therapy without progesterone). Medical conditions that may alter estrogen metabolism and increase the risk of endometrial cancer are diabetes mellitus, hypertension, and POS (Porth, 2005). Tamoxifen, a drug that blocks estrogen receptor sites and is used to treat breast cancer, has a weak estrogenic effect on the endometrium, and is also a risk factor.

Endometrial cancer is the most commonly inherited gynecologic cancer. A family history of hereditary nonpolyposis colon cancer (HNPCC) may mean that a woman has an inherited mutation that is a mismatch of repair genes, and has a 60% risk of endometrial cancer (Porth, 2005).

Pathophysiology

Most endometrial malignancies are adenocarcinomas that are slow to grow and metastasize. These cancers develop in the glandular cells or endometrial lining of the uterus (the same tissue that is shed each month during a normal menstrual period). Endometrial hyperplasia (excessive growth) is a precursor of endometrial cancer. These tumors tend to grow slowly in the early stages.

Tumor growth usually begins in the fundus, invades the vascular myometrium, and spreads throughout the female reproductive tract. Metastasis occurs by means of the lymphatic system, through the fallopian tubes to the peritoneal cavity, and to the rest of the body via the bloodstream. Target areas for metastasis include the lungs, liver, and bone. The International Federation of Gynecology and Obstetrics (FIGO) classification of endometrial cancer is presented in Table 51–3.

Manifestations

The major manifestation of endometrial hyperplasia or overt endometrial cancer is abnormal, painless vaginal bleeding. In menstruating women, this bleeding is manifested as menorrhagia or metrorrhagia. In postmenopausal women, any bleeding is abnormal. Later manifestations include pelvic cramping, bleeding after intercourse, and lower abdominal pressure. In advanced disease, lymph node enlargement, pleural effusion, abdominal masses, and ascites may be present.

INTERDISCIPLINARY CARE

The goals of care for the woman with endometrial cancer are to eradicate the cancer and minimize complications and metastasis.

Diagnosis

Tests used to diagnose cancer of the endometrium include a vaginal or transvaginal ultrasound, used to determine endometrial thickening, which may indicate hypertrophy or malignant changes, or an endometrial biopsy or a dilation and curettage (D&C) to provide a definitive diagnosis (see Chapter 49 ∞ for further information and nursing care). Other tests to determine the extent of the disease include chest x-ray, intravenous urography, cystoscopy, barium enema, sigmoidoscopy, MRI, and bone scans.

Medications

Although the treatment of choice for primary endometrial carcinoma is surgery, progesterone therapy may be used for recurrent disease. About one-third of women respond favorably, primarily those with well-differentiated tumors. Chemotherapy is less effective than other forms of therapy, although cisplatin or combination chemotherapy may be used for women with disseminated disease.

Surgery

After the diagnosis is confirmed, a total abdominal hysterectomy and bilateral salpingo-oophorectomy is performed for stage I cancer. A radical hysterectomy with node dissection is performed if the disease is stage II or beyond.

TABLE 51–3 FIGO Staging Classification for Endometrial Cancer

STAGE	DESCRIPTION
I	Tumor limited to endometrium or myometrium
II	Endocervical glandular involvement or invasion of cervical stroma
III	Metastasis or invasion of serosa, adnexae, vagina, and pelvic or para-aortic lymph nodes
IV	Tumor invasion of bladder or bowel mucosa; distant metastases

Radiation Therapy

Treatment with external and internal radiation may be performed as a preoperative measure or as adjuvant treatment in advanced cases.

NURSING CARE

Health Promotion

All perimenopausal and postmenopausal women need annual pelvic examinations. The ACS recommends that at the time of menopause all women be informed of the risks and manifestations of endometrial cancer, and strongly encouraged to report any unexpected bleeding or spotting to their healthcare provider. Those in high risk groups are advised to have endometrial biopsies every 2 years, beginning at age 35. In addition, control of diseases such as diabetes mellitus and hypertension decrease the risk of endometrial hyperplasia.

Assessment

Collect the following data through a health history and physical examination (see Chapter 49 ∞):

- *Health history:* Abnormal vaginal bleeding, menstrual history, use of estrogen (without progesterone) to treat menopausal symptoms, breast cancer treated with tamoxifen, childbearing status, presence of chronic illnesses, family history of hereditary nonpolyposis colon cancer.
- *Physical assessment:* Height and weight, pelvic examination, abdomen, lymph glands.

Nursing Diagnoses and Interventions

Nursing care involves helping the woman deal with the physical and psychologic effects of a potentially life-threatening illness, make informed decisions, and minimize the adverse effects of therapy. Pain relief is a key component of care, as is grief work on the part of the woman and family. Encourage the woman to perform self-care and resume normal activities of daily living.

Acute Pain

Total abdominal hysterectomy can involve severe and prolonged pain, not only from the surgical incision but also from the manipulation of internal organs during surgery. Abdominal viscera are highly vascular and easily bruised by handling.

- Administer analgesics as ordered. *Analgesics provide pain relief and promote early ambulation.*
- Encourage ambulation. *Ambulation facilitates the expulsion of flatus, which can cause distention as well as discomfort.*
- Apply heat to the abdomen, and recommend that the woman use a heating pad at home. *Heat dilates blood vessels, increasing blood supply to the pelvis, decreasing pain.*

Disturbed Body Image

For many women, the side effects of cancer treatment can be almost as difficult and painful as the disease itself. Although side effects of the different therapies vary among individuals, the woman's body image and quality of life are always affected. Such side effects as alopecia (hair loss), nausea, vomiting, fatigue, diarrhea, stomatitis, and surgical scarring disturb body image.

- Review the side effects of the treatment regimen proposed, and assist the woman to develop a plan to deal with these effects. *This promotes a sense of control.*
- Remind the woman and family that side effects are usually manageable and may be temporary. *Over-the-counter agents can be used to alleviate stomatitis. Frequent rest periods can relieve fatigue. Medications can be prescribed for nausea, vomiting, and diarrhea.*

Ineffective Sexuality Pattern

Altered sexuality may result from a feeling of unattractiveness, fatigue, or pain and discomfort. The woman's partner may fear that sexual activity will be harmful.

- Encourage expression of feelings about the effect of cancer on their lives and sexual relationship. *Verbalizing feelings helps relieve stress and maximizes relaxation.*
- Suggest that the couple explore alternative sexual positions and coordinate sexual activity with rest periods and times that are relatively free from pain. *This creates a more favorable environment for satisfying sexual activity.*

Community-Based Care

Provide information about the specific treatment and prognosis for the cancer. Explain the expected side effects of radiation implant therapy (see Chapter 14 ∞). Pain control measures are also an essential part of the teaching plan (see Chapter 9 ∞). The resources listed for the woman with cervical cancer are also appropriate for the woman with endometrial cancer.

THE WOMAN WITH OVARIAN CANCER

Ovarian cancer is the fourth most common gynecologic cancer in women in the United States. Approximately 20,000 women are diagnosed with ovarian cancer and an estimated 15,000 deaths result each year (ACS, 2006a). The incidence increases with age, peaking in women between the ages of 40 and 80 years; half of all cases are in women over 65 years of age (Porth, 2005). Ovarian cancer is more common in white women than in black women, and mortality rate is highest in whites.

Risk Factors

Family history is a significant risk factor, with a 50% risk of developing the disease if two or more first- or second-degree relatives have site-specific ovarian cancer. Other types of inherited risk are breast-ovarian cancer syndrome (first- and second-degree relatives have both breast and ovarian cancer) and family cancer syndrome (Lynch syndrome II), in which male or female relatives have a history of colorectal, endometrial, ovarian, pancreatic, or other types of cancer (Porth, 2005). The breast cancer susceptibility genes *BRAC1* and *BRAC2* are implicated in 5% to 10% of hereditary ovarian cancers.

Risk factors also include having no children or giving birth after age 35, exposure to talc or asbestos, endometriosis, pelvic inflammatory disease, and living in a Western civilized country. Protective factors include long-term contraceptive use, having a child before the age of 25, tubal ligation, breast-feeding, and hysterectomy (Martin, 2005).

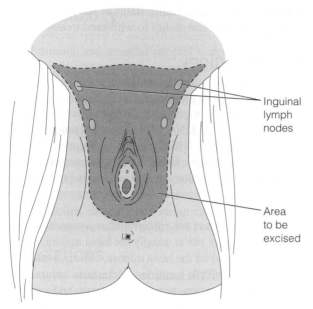

Figure 51–6 ■ Vulvectomy for vulvar carcinoma. A radical vulvectomy involves removal of the vulva, labia majora, labia minora, clitoris, prepuce, subcutaneous tissue, and regional lymph nodes.

Inguinal lymph nodes

Area to be excised

performed if invasion is suspected. This procedure involves removal of all the tissue in a simple vulvectomy, as well as the subcutaneous tissue and regional lymph nodes.

NURSING CARE

Nursing care is similar to that for the woman with endometrial cancer. The woman fears death as the ultimate outcome as well as the possible pain and suffering that surgery and other treatments may cause. Radical surgery represents a great loss to women of all ages.

Nursing Diagnoses and Interventions

Disruption of perineal tissues is a priority problem for these women.

Impaired Tissue Integrity

The woman who has undergone a vulvectomy is at high risk for infection and impaired healing because of proximity of the surgical site to urinary and anal orifices. In addition, the women are often older and may have age-related changes in healing and immune function.

■ Teach the woman and/or her partner or other family member the procedure for irrigation of the vulvectomy. If neither is able to perform this procedure, arrange for home health nursing. *Irrigation helps prevent skin breakdown and infection.*

■ After irrigation, apply dry heat using a heat lamp positioned about 18 inches from the area; emphasize safety precautions, including use of a low-wattage bulb (40 to 60 watts). *Dry heat helps promote healing and comfort.*

■ Provide information on maintaining a diet high in protein, iron, and vitamin C. *These nutrients promote collagen formation and wound healing.*

Community-Based Care

Explain the association between STIs such as HPV (genital warts) and cancer of the vulva. Provide information about safer sex practices such as abstinence, limiting the number of sexual partners, and using condoms (male or female). Explain that early diagnosis and treatment of STIs and other irritative conditions of the external genitalia may reduce the risk of developing vulvar cancer. Teaching for the woman undergoing a vulvectomy should emphasize the potential for skin breakdown, particularly with radiation therapy. Explain that removal of lymph nodes leads to lymphedema and that recurrent cellulitis and sexual dysfunction are common complications of vulvar cancer.

DISORDERS OF THE BREAST

Breast disorders are common conditions that primarily affect women (disorders of the male breast are discussed in Chapter 50 ∞). When a woman discovers a breast lump, her first response is often fear: of breast cancer, of losing her breast, and perhaps of losing her life. Because American society views the breast as a significant component of feminine beauty, any problem that threatens the breast often strikes at the core of a woman's self-image.

Nurses play a critical role in the care of women experiencing breast disorders by providing education, support, and advocacy. Part of the nurse's role is educating women about normal breast tissue, common benign breast disorders, available screening techniques and risk factors for breast cancer, and breast self-examination.

THE WOMAN WITH A BENIGN BREAST DISORDER

Benign breast disorders occur frequently in women and may be a source of anxiety. Changes in a woman's breast tissue often correspond to hormonal changes of the menstrual cycle. Most women notice increased tenderness and lumpiness prior to menses. (For this reason, it is best to perform breast self-examination (BSE) 7 to 10 days after the beginning of the menstrual period.) Breast tissue changes in response to hormonal, nutritional, physical, and environmental stimuli. Benign breast disorders include fibrocystic breast changes, fibroadenomas, intraductal papillomas, duct ectasia, fat necrosis, and mastitis (Table 51–6).

Pathophysiology and Manifestations

Fibrocystic Changes

Fibrocystic changes (FCC) (*fibrocystic breast disease*) is the physiologic nodularity and breast tenderness that increases and decreases with the menstrual cycle. An estimated 50% to 80% of all women experience some of these changes, which include fibrosis, epithelial proliferation, and cyst formation. FCC is most common in women 30 to 50 years of age, and is rare in postmenopausal women who are not taking hormone replacement (Porth, 2005).

TABLE 51-6 Summary of Common Breast Disorders

CONDITION	AGE	PAIN	NIPPLE DISCHARGE	LOCATION	CONSISTENCY AND MOBILITY	DIAGNOSIS AND TREATMENT
Duct ectasia	35 to 55 years; median age 40	Burning around nipple	Sticky, multicolored; usually bilateral	No specific location	Retroareolar mass with advanced disease	Open biopsy; local excision of diseased portion of breast
Fibroadenoma	15 to 39 years; median age 20	No	No	No specific location	Mobile, firm, smooth, well-delineated mass	Mammography, surgical or needle biopsy; excision of the tumor
Fibrocystic changes (FCC)	20 to 49 years; median age 30 (may subside with menopause)	Yes	May occur	Upper outer quadrant	Bilateral multiple lumps influenced by the menstrual cycle	Needle aspiration; observation; biopsy if there is an unresolved mass or mammographic changes
Intraductal papilloma	35 to 55 years; median age 40	Yes	Serous or sanguineous; usually unilateral from one duct	No specific location	Usually soft, poorly delineated mass	Pap smear of nipple discharge; biopsy; wedge resection
Mastitis, acute	Childbearing years	Tenderness, pain	No	No specific location	Generalized redness of overlying skin	Antibiotic therapy; incision and drainage if mastitis progresses to an abscess
Mastitis, chronic	Any age	Tenderness, pain; headache; high fever	No	No specific location	Generalized redness and swelling	Antibiotics, usually penicillin
Fat necrosis	Any age	Tenderness	No	No specific location	Firm, irregular, palpable	Surgical biopsy to rule out cancer

FCC includes many different lesions and breast changes. The more common nonproliferative form does not increase the risk for breast cancer. The proliferative form, accompanied by giant cysts and proliferative epithelial lesions, does increase the risk for breast cancer.

Nonproliferative changes may be cystic or fibrous. Cystic change refers to the dilation of ducts in the subareolar, lobular, or lobe areas. Cysts often go unnoticed unless pain and tenderness is associated with menses. Fibrous changes are infrequent but can occur during the menstrual years. A firm, palpable mass, 2 to 3 cm in size, is typically located in the upper outer breast quadrant following an inflammatory response to ductal irritation.

Women with fibrocystic changes experience bilateral or unilateral pain or tenderness in the upper, outer quadrants of their breasts, and report that their breasts feel particularly thick and lumpy the week prior to menses. Nipple discharge may be pres-ent. Pain is due to edema of the connective tissue of the breast, dilation of the ducts, and some inflammatory response; some women report an increase in breast size. Multiple, mobile cysts may form, usually in both breasts (Figure 51–7 ■). Fluid aspirated from these cysts ranges in color from milky white to yellow, brown, or green. If the fluid is tinged with blood, there is reason to suspect malignancy.

Intraductal Disorders

An *intraductal papilloma* is a tiny, wartlike growth on the inside of the peripheral mammary duct that causes discharge from the nipple. The discharge may be clear and sticky or bloody. When more than one of these growths is present, the condition is called *intraductal papillomatosis*. This condition is most common in women in their 30s and 40s. The lesion must be investigated to rule out malignancy.

TABLE 51–7 **Staging of Breast Cancer**

STAGE	TUMOR	NODE	METASTASIS
0	Tis-Carcinoma *in situ* or Paget's disease of the nipple	N0-No regional lymph node metastasis	M0-No evidence of distant metastasis
I	T1-Tumor no larger than 2 cm	N0	M0
IIA	T0-No evidence of primary tumor T1	N1-Metastasis to movable ipsilateral axillary nodes	M0
	T2-Tumor no larger than 5 cm	N0	M0
IIB	T2	N1	M0
	T3-Tumor larger than 5 cm	N0	M0
IIIA	T0 T1 T2	N2-Metastasis to ipsilateral fixed axillary nodes	M0
	T3	N1	M0
		N2	M0
IIIB	T4-Tumor of any size with direct extension to chest wall or skin	Any N	M0
	Any T	N3-Metastasis to ipsilateral internal mammary lymph nodes	M0
IV	Any T	N0 and N1	M1-Distant metastasis

some women report a burning or stinging sensation. Many women with breast cancer have no manifestations, and their tumors are detected by mammography. However, most breast cancers are found by the women themselves (during BSE or a shower) or by their partners during sexual activity.

INTERDISCIPLINARY CARE

Diagnosis of breast cancer begins with detection, either detection of asymptomatic lesions discovered through screening or symptomatic lesions discovered by the woman. Any palpable mass requires evaluation. Once the diagnosis is made, a number of treatment options are available. The choice of treatment depends on several factors, such as the stage of the cancer, the age of the woman, and the woman's preferences.

Diagnosis

Early detection of breast cancer is possible with clinical breast examination (CBE) and mammogram (see Chapter 49 ∞ for further information). Mammography can detect breast tumors 2 years before they reach palpable size; most of these tumors have been present for 8 to 10 years. Although controversy exists about the ability of screening mammography to improve mortality rates for women under 50, the ACS recommends annual mammograms beginning at age 40 and CBE at least every 3 years for women in their 20s and 30s.

Other diagnostic tests include a percutaneous needle biopsy to define a cystic mass or fibrocystic changes and provide specimens for cytologic examination, and a breast biopsy. In aspiration biopsy or fine-needle aspiration biopsy, a needle is used to remove cells or fluid from the breast lesion (Figures 51–8A and B ■). The types of breast biopsy and related nursing care are described in Chapter 49 ∞. In many

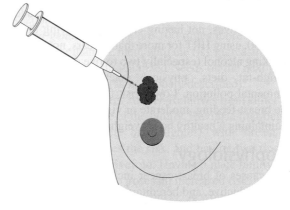

A Aspiration biopsy

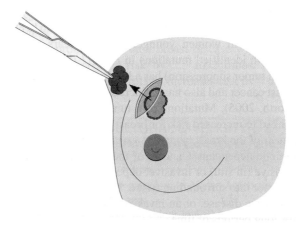

B Excisional biopsy

Figure 51–8 ■ Types of breast biopsy. *A,* In an aspiration biopsy, a needle is used to aspirate fluid or tissue from the breast. *B,* In an excisional biopsy, tissue from the breast lesion is removed surgically.

facilities, fine-needle aspiration biopsies are performed using a stereotactic biopsy device; mammography and a computer are used to guide the needle.

Medications

Tamoxifen citrate (Nolvadex) is an oral medication that interferes with estrogen activity. It is used to treat advanced breast cancer, as an adjuvant for early-stage breast cancer, and as a preventive treatment for women at high risk of developing breast cancer. Nursing implications for tamoxifen are presented in the Medication Administration box below.

Immunotherapy, using trastuzumab (Herceptin), is used to stop the growth of breast tumors that express the HER2/neu receptor (which binds an epidermal growth factor that contributes to cancer cell growth) on their cell surface. This drug is a recombinant DNA-derived monoclonal antibody that binds to the receptor, inhibiting tumor cell proliferation.

Chemotherapy has become the standard of care for the majority of breast cancer cases with axillary node involvement. In late metastatic disease, chemotherapy becomes the primary treatment to prolong the woman's life. Chemotherapy is discussed in Chapter 14 ∞. Adjuvant (additional) systemic therapy following primary treatment for early-stage breast cancer refers to the administration of chemotherapy and other pharmacologic agents. This type of therapy has been widely studied; its use reduces the rates of recurrence and death from breast cancer. For example, the drug Avastin, when combined with chemotherapy to treat metastatic breast cancer, has extended cancer-free survival; and Femara (an aromatase inhibitor) has reduced the risk of recurrence after surgery (in some cases more effectively than tamoxifen).

Surgery

Until recently, the treatment of choice for breast cancer was a radical mastectomy. The trend now is toward more conservative surgery combined with chemotherapy, hormone therapy, or radiation, depending on the stage of the tumor and the age of the woman.

MASTECTOMY There are various types of mastectomy for breast cancer. *Radical mastectomy* is the removal of the entire affected breast, the underlying chest muscles, and the lymph nodes under the arms. *Simple mastectomy* is the removal of the complete breast only. *Segmental mastectomy* or *lumpectomy* (Figure 51–9A ■) is the removal of the tumor and the surrounding margin of breast tissues. *Modified radical mastectomy* is the removal of the breast tissue and lymph nodes under the arm (axillary node dissection), leaving the chest wall muscles intact (Figure 51–9B). See the next page for the nursing care of a woman having a mastectomy.

Axillary node dissection is generally performed during surgery for all invasive breast carcinoma to stage the tumor. Because this surgery can cause **lymphedema** (accumulation of fluid in the soft tissues of the arm caused by removal of lymph channels), nerve damage, and adhesions, and because of the role of the lymph nodes in immune system function, nonsurgical methods of detecting lymph node involvement are being used. Sentinel node biopsy prior to a node dissection is conducted by injecting a radioactive substance or dye into the region of the tumor. The dye is carried to the first (sentinel) lymph node to receive lymph from the tumor and would therefore be the node most likely to contain cancer cells if the cancer had metastasized. If the sentinel node is positive, more nodes are removed. If it is negative, further node evaluation is usually not indicated.

LUMPECTOMY Breast conservation surgery (*lumpectomy*) may be defined as excision of the primary tumor and adjacent breast tissue followed by radiation therapy. Many women are candidates for this procedure; however, women who have multicentric breast neoplasms and those who have large tumors in relation to their breast size are examples of unsuitable candidates. Selection of women for this procedure is guided by the need for local control of the lesion, cosmetic results, and personal preference.

BREAST RECONSTRUCTION After a mastectomy, some women may choose to have their breast reconstructed. They report that surgical reconstruction of the breast simplifies their lives and restores a sense of body integrity. Other women choose to use a removable breast prosthesis, and some women are comfortable without reconstruction or a prosthesis.

MEDICATION ADMINISTRATION Tamoxifen

TAMOXIFEN (NOLVADEX)
Tamoxifen is the most widely prescribed breast cancer drug, commonly given to prevent recurrence of estrogen-positive breast cancer in postmenopausal women. It inhibits tumor growth by blocking the estrogen receptor sites of cancer cells. Tamoxifen increases a woman's risk of developing endometrial cancer, deep venous thrombosis (DVT), and pulmonary embolism.

Nursing Responsibilities
- Assess for potential contraindications to therapy.
- Assess liver function tests; tamoxifen may interfere with liver function.

Health Education for the Client and Family
- If in childbearing years, use a nonhormonal, barrier form of contraception; tamoxifen has adverse effects on the developing fetus.
- Take the drug as prescribed until the physician indicates otherwise.
- Side effects such as hot flashes, vaginal dryness, irregular periods, and weight gain are commonly experienced by women taking tamoxifen.
- Do not smoke while taking tamoxifen; smoking further increases the risk of DVT.
- Promptly report any abnormal vaginal bleeding (nonmenstrual bleeding, bleeding after menopause) to your primary care provider.

CHAPTER 52 Nursing Care of Clients with Sexually Transmitted Infections

LEARNING OUTCOMES

- Explain the incidence, prevalence, characteristics, and prevention/control of sexually transmitted infections (STIs).

- Compare and contrast the pathophysiology, manifestations, interdisciplinary care, and nursing care of genital herpes, genital warts, vaginitis, chlamydia, gonorrhea, syphilis, and pelvic inflammatory disease.

- Explain the risk factors for and complications of STIs.

- Discuss the effects and nursing implications of medications and treatments used to treat STIs.

CLINICAL COMPETENCIES

- Assess functional health status of clients with STIs and monitor, document, and report abnormal manifestations.

- Determine priority nursing diagnoses and select and implement individualized nursing interventions for clients with STIs.

- Administer topical, oral, and injectable medications knowledgeably and safely.

- Integrate interdisciplinary care into care of clients with STIs.

- Provide teaching appropriate for prevention, control, and self-care of STIs.

- Revise plan of care as needed to provide effective interventions to promote, maintain, or restore functional health status to clients with STIs.

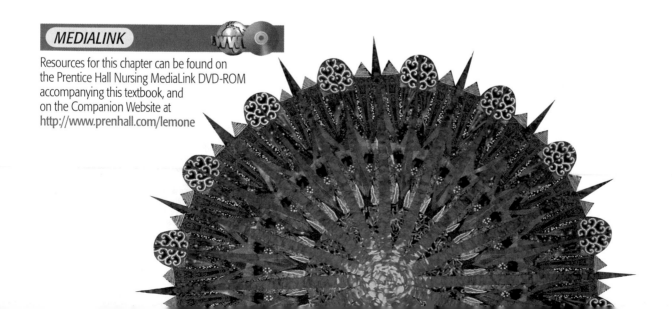

MEDIALINK

Resources for this chapter can be found on
the Prentice Hall Nursing MediaLink DVD-ROM
accompanying this textbook, and
on the Companion Website at
http://www.prenhall.com/lemone

bacterial vaginosis, *1842*
candidiasis, *1842*
chancre, *1847*
chlamydia, *1844*
dyspareunia, *1844*

genital herpes, *1838*
genital warts, *1840*
gonorrhea, *1845*
pelvic inflammatory disease (PID), *1850*

sexually transmitted infections (STIs), *1837*
syphilis, *1846*
trichomoniasis, *1843*

Infections transmitted by vaginal, oral, and anal intimate contact and intercourse are referred to as **sexually transmitted infections (STIs)**. Infections transmitted by sexual intercourse are also labeled as *sexually transmitted diseases (STDs)* or *venereal diseases*. STIs also include systemic diseases (such as tuberculosis, hepatitis, and HIV/AIDS) that can be transmitted from an infected person to a partner. This chapter discusses STIs that involve the urogenital system. Vaginal infections are included in this chapter because they are also included in the CDC (2006) treatment guidelines.

OVERVIEW OF SEXUALLY TRANSMITTED INFECTIONS

Sexually transmitted infections include those caused by bacteria, *Chlamydiae*, viruses, fungi, protozoa, and parasites. Portals of entry for these agents of transmission include the mouth, genitalia, urinary meatus, anus, rectum, and skin. STIs have many consequences, and nurses have the responsibility of teaching sexually active clients how to prevent STIs, regardless of their gender, age, or sexual orientation. Nurses have a critical role in the prevention of STIs by teaching clients about these diseases, their prevention, treatment, and potential complications.

Incidence and Prevalence

STIs have reached epidemic proportions in the United States and are on the increase worldwide. They are the most frequent infections encountered by professionals in the field of reproductive health, and occur in more than half of all people at some point in their life (American Social Health Association [ASHA], 2005).

FAST FACTS

STIs
- More than 65 million people in the United States are estimated to have a viral STI, with 15 million new cases occurring each year.
- One in two sexually active persons will contract an STI by age 25.
- More than $8 billion is spent each year to diagnose and treat STIs and their complications. This figure does not include HIV.

Source: American Social Health Association (2005).

Women and infants are disproportionately affected by STIs. Many STIs are more easily transmitted from a man to a woman than from a woman to a man. Women often experience few early manifestations of the infection, delaying diagnosis and treatment. Furthermore, women are at greater risk for complications of STIs such as pelvic inflammatory disease (PID) and genital cancers.

Several factors help explain the escalating incidence of STIs. The so-called sexual revolution of the 1960s and 1970s, fueled by "the pill" and the freedom from unplanned pregnancy, led to a more permissive attitude about sexuality and increases in sexual activity and the number of sexual partners. In addition, since oral contraceptives were introduced to American women in 1961, they have replaced the condom as a birth control method for many couples. However, oral contraceptives do not protect against STIs, a fact of increasing importance.

STIs affect men and women of all ages, backgrounds, and socioeconomic levels. The incidence of STIs is highest in young adults ages 15 to 24 and in minorities. Drug abuse, unprotected sexual activity, and sexual activity with multiple partners also are associated with increased incidence of STIs (Dixon, 2004). A further factor in the increasing incidence is that young people are becoming sexually active at an earlier age, marrying later, and divorce is more common. As a result, sexually active people today are more likely to have multiple sex partners in their lifetime and are potentially at risk for STIs (National Institute of Allergy and Infectious Diseases, 2003).

The emergence of HIV/AIDS has created a kind of "epidemiologic synergy" among all STIs. Other STIs, such as syphilis, herpes simplex virus (HSV), and chancroid, facilitate the transmission of HIV/AIDS, and the immune suppression caused by HIV potentiates the infectious process of other STIs. In fact, individuals who are infected with STIs are at greater risk of acquiring HIV if they are exposed to the virus. This is the result of several factors: Genital ulcers create a portal of entry for HIV, nonulcerative STIs increase the concentration of cells in genital secretions that can be targets for HIV, and infection with both an STI and HIV results in an increased likelihood of having HIV in genital secretions and semen.

Characteristics

Although STIs are caused by various organisms, they have several characteristics in common:
- Most can be prevented by the use of latex condoms.
- They can be transmitted during both heterosexual and homosexual activities, including non-penetrating intimate exposure.
- For treatment to be effective, sexual partners of the infected person must also be treated.
- Two or more STIs frequently coexist in the same client.

The complications of STIs in women include PID, ectopic pregnancy, infertility, chronic pelvic pain, neonatal illness and

✳ NURSING CARE

In planning and implementing nursing care for the client with genital herpes, the nurse needs to consider both short-term and long-term implications. Although the immediate priority is symptom relief and prevention of further transmission, the client needs assistance to deal with the life-changing diagnosis of a chronic disease.

Nursing Diagnoses and Interventions

Nursing diagnoses discussed in this section focus on pain and sexual dysfunction.

Acute Pain

Herpetic lesions are very painful and can become infected. Because the virus resides in the nerve ganglia, pain may also occur in the legs, thighs, groin, or buttocks. Although acyclovir diminishes the pain of herpes and accelerates the healing process, additional measures can relieve the discomfort further.

- Teach how to keep herpes blisters clean and dry. A solution of warm water, soap, and hydrogen peroxide (if lesions are not open) can be used to cleanse the lesions two or three times daily. Burrow's solution (a liquid containing aluminum sulfate, acetic acid, precipitated calcium carbonate, and water) can also be used. Lesions should be dried using a hair dryer turned to a cool setting. It is important to wear loose cotton clothing that will not trap moisture; and to avoid wearing panty hose and tight jeans. *Keeping the lesions clean and dry reduces the possibility of secondary infection and speeds the healing process.*
- For dysuria, suggest pouring water over the genitals while urinating. Drinking additional fluids also helps dilute the acidity of the urine; however, fluids that increase acidity, such as cranberry juice, should be avoided. *These measures dilute the acid content of urine and thereby reduce the burning sensation.*
- Suggest the use of sitz baths (with tepid water) for 15 to 30 minutes several times a day. *The warm water is soothing and decreases pain from ulcers and an irritated urethral meatus. It also facilitates wound healing.*

Sexual Dysfunction

Clients who learn that they are infected with an incurable STI may believe they can no longer have a normal sex life. Fortunately, many people have learned to live with and manage genital herpes without infecting their partners or their children.

- Provide a supportive, nonjudgmental environment for the client to discuss feelings and ask questions about what this diagnosis means to future sexual relationships. *Feelings of guilt, shame, and anger are natural responses to such a diagnosis and can lead to a total avoidance of sexual intimacy.*
- Offer information about support groups and other resources for people with herpes such as the National Herpes Information Hotline. *Information about how others cope with this disease can offset feelings of shame and hopelessness.*

Community-Based Care

Health teaching for clients with genital herpes involves helping them manage this chronic disease with the least possible disruption in lifestyle and relationships. Understanding the disease process and factors that affect it helps the client regain a sense of control and see the potential for future sexual intimacy without transmission of infection. The following topics should be addressed:

- How to recognize prodromal symptoms of recurrence and factors that seem to trigger recurrences (such as emotional stress, acidic food, sun exposure)
- The need for abstinence from sexual contact from the time prodromal symptoms appear until 10 days after all lesions have healed
- If lesions become infected, use of topical acyclovir (Painful lesions can be protected with sterile petroleum jelly or aloe vera gel.)
- Use of latex condoms due to viral shedding at any time and careful hygiene practices (such as not sharing towels or other personal items) even during latency periods.

THE CLIENT WITH GENITAL WARTS

Genital warts (*condylomata acuminata*), caused by the human papillomavirus (HPV) are the most common infectious genital infections in the United States, and are considered epidemic. Genital warts are chronic and, in many people, largely asymptomatic. Currently, they are incurable.

Women are at greater risk for HPV genital infections because they have a larger mucosal surface area exposed in the genital area. Most HPV infections are asymptomatic or unrecognized. An estimated 20 million Americans are infected with the virus, and up to 6.2 million new cases are diagnosed annually (CDC, 2006).

FAST FACTS
Genital HPV Infection
- At least 50% of sexually active men and women acquire genital HPV infection at some point in their lives.
- By age 50, at least 80% of women will have acquired genital HPV infection.
- Most people with a genital HPV infection do not know they are infected; most women are diagnosed by abnormal Pap tests.

Source: CDC (2004).

Although the majority of infected people are asymptomatic, others experience frequent recurrences. Other than recurrences, men are not likely to experience serious physical complications of genital warts. Women, however, face concerns about the increased risk of cervical cancer, with HPV DNA having been identified in almost all cervical cancers worldwide and in approximately 50% to 80% of vaginal, vulvar, and anogenital cancers (Porth, 2005).

Pathophysiology

Genital warts are caused by HPV and are transmitted by vaginal, anal, or oral–genital contact. The incubation period is 6 weeks to 8 months (Porth, 2005).

Manifestations

Although some people with HPV may not have manifestations, others exhibit characteristic lesions: single or multiple painless, soft, moist, pink or flesh-colored swellings in the vulvovaginal area, perineum, penis, urethra, anus, groin, or thigh (Figure 52–2 ■). In women, the growths may be in the vagina or on the cervix and be apparent only during a pelvic examination.

The four types of genital warts are as follows:

- *Condyloma acuminata:* cauliflower-shaped lesions that appear on moist skin surfaces such as the vagina or anus
- *Keratotic warts:* thick, hard lesions that develop on keratinized skin such as the labia major, penis, or scrotum
- *Papular warts:* smooth lesions that also develop on keratinized skin
- *Flat warts:* slightly raised lesions, often invisible to the naked eye, that also develop on keratinized skin.

INTERDISCIPLINARY CARE

Treatment is directed at removal of the warts, relief of symptoms, and health teaching to reduce the risk of recurrence and future transmission. Infection with HPV is considered chronic; however, research has shown that for about 90% of women, cervical HPV becomes undetectable within 2 years (CDC, 2004).

Genital and anal warts are diagnosed primarily by clinical appearance. A HPV DNA test is specific for diagnosis in women. There are no HPV tests for men.

Medications

Topical agents used to treat genital warts include podofilox and imiquimod (both can be applied by the client) or podophyllin and trichloroacetic acid (provider-administered treatments). Podophyllin (Condylox, Podofin) is contraindicated during pregnancy and can have side effects in any client, ranging from nausea, diarrhea, and lethargy to paralysis and coma (see the Medication Administration box on the next page). Gardasil is a vaccine developed to prevent genital warts, precancerous geni-

tal lesions, and cervical cancer due to HPV. It is administered by 3 intramuscular injections given over a 6-month period. As HPV is so closely associated with cervical cancer, a federal advisory panel has recommended that the vaccine be targeted for females, aged 9 to 26. The vaccine does not protect against an existing HPV infection.

Other Treatments

Genital warts may also be removed by cryotherapy, electrocautery, laser vaporization, or surgical excision. Carbon dioxide laser surgery is becoming increasingly common for removal of extensive warts.

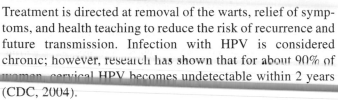

NURSING CARE

Health promotion activities for adults of all ages should include information about the causes, treatments, and prevention of HPV infections.

Nursing Diagnoses and Interventions

Nursing interventions are primarily directed toward problems with deficient knowledge, fear, and anxiety.

Deficient Knowledge

HPV is spread by contact with infectious lesions or secretions, with up to 70% of genital warts spread by people who do not know they have the infection. Although there is no known cure, it is essential to prevent secondary infections.

- Discuss the need for prompt treatment and the necessity for sexual abstinence until lesions have healed, or using a condom while lesions are present. *This reduces the risk of reinfection and further transmission of the disease. Some studies have found that using condoms promotes the regression of HPV lesions in both men and women (ASHA, 2005).*
- Discuss the increased risk of cervical cancer and the importance of an annual Pap smear. *Understanding the risk, the client will be more motivated to seek annual screening.*
- Stress the importance of thorough handwashing. *Handwashing is essential to prevent the spread of HPV.*

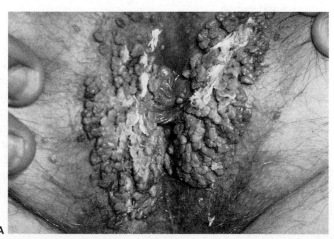
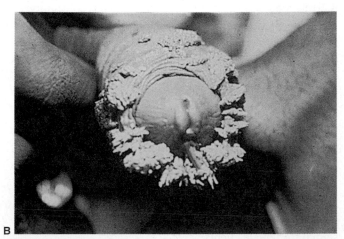

Figure 52–2 ■ Genital warts (condyloma acuminatum) on the A, vulva and B, penis.
Source: Kenneth Greer/Visuals Unlimited; National AV Center

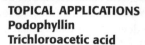

MEDICATION ADMINISTRATION **The Client with Genital Warts**

TOPICAL APPLICATIONS
Podophyllin
Trichloroacetic acid
Although cryotherapy using liquid nitrogen or a cryoprobe is more commonly used to treat genital warts, podophyllum preparations are sometimes used. Podophyllin is applied topically to the warts by the physician once weekly for 3 to 5 weeks.

Podophyllin is contraindicated during pregnancy; the alternative is cryotherapy. Podophyllin is also contraindicated in cervical, urethral, oral, or anorectal warts. It is important to avoid contact of podophyllin resin with the eyes.

Adverse effects of podophyllin include local irritation, severe ulceration of surrounding tissue, nausea, diarrhea, lethargy, paralysis, and coma.

Nursing Responsibilities
- Establish baseline data, including mental status, vital signs, and weight.

- Document and report any existing lesions (genital, anal, or oral).
- Cover the tissue surrounding the warts with petrolatum or a paste of baking soda and water to protect the tissue from the caustic treatment solution.

Health Education for the Client and Family
- Wash off the treated area thoroughly within 1 to 4 hours after the first application; gradually increase this period to 6 to 8 hours after the second and subsequent applications.
- Return for regular treatment until warts are gone.
- Refer partners for examination and any necessary treatment.
- Report any adverse effects (nausea, diarrhea, local irritation, lethargy, numbness)
- Avoid sexual activity until you and your partners have been free of disease for 1 month.
- Use condoms to prevent future infections.
- Return for an annual Pap smear.

Fear

Surgery engenders some degree of fear in most clients: fear of the procedure itself and of pain and possible complications. Surgery or cryotherapy in the genital area involves all of these fears plus fear of possible impaired sexual function.

- Allow the client to express specific fears and feelings about the procedure. Explain the procedure, approximate recovery time, possible complications and ways to avoid them, and ways to cope with complications that do occur. *Knowing what to expect reduces the client's fear and helps the client feel a greater sense of control.*
- Explain that the procedure is performed with a local anesthesia. *Being awake during surgery gives the client a greater sense of participation in the treatment process.*

Anxiety

The woman with an HPV infection faces an increased risk of infection of her neonate during delivery. The neonatal infection can range from asymptomatic to widely disseminated fatal disease. Transmission occurs during passage through the birth canal. The risk is highest during the first episode of infection.

- Discuss with women of childbearing age that cesarean delivery can prevent transmission of infection to the neonate. In women without manifestations of recurrence, vaginal delivery is possible. *Understanding that infection of the neonate can be prevented helps relieve anxiety.*

Community-Based Care

Health teaching emphasizes the need for the client and infected partners to return for regular treatment until lesions have resolved, and to use condoms to prevent reinfection. Because of the increased risk of cervical cancer, annual Pap smears are essential for female clients.

THE CLIENT WITH A VAGINAL INFECTION

The vagina may be infected by yeasts, protozoa, or bacteria. These infections can be sexually transmitted, but the male partner does not usually have manifestations of the infection. Risk factors include the use of hormonal contraceptives or broad-spectrum antibiotics, obesity, diabetes, pregnancy, unprotected sexual activity, and multiple sexual partners. Manifestations of vaginal infections are outlined in Table 52–1.

Preventive measures include educating women about personal hygiene practices and safer sex. Women need to avoid frequent douching and wearing nylon underwear and/or tight pants. Unprotected sexual activity, particularly with multiple partners, increases the risk of vaginal infections.

Pathophysiology and Manifestations

Alterations in pH, changes in the normal flora, and low estrogen levels are conducive to the development of vaginal infections. When conditions are favorable, microorganisms invade the vulva and vagina.

Bacterial Vaginosis

Bacterial vaginosis (nonspecific vaginitis) is the most common cause of vaginal infection in women of reproductive age. *Gardnerella vaginalis* is one of the causative organisms, but others are also implicated. The relationship of sexual activity to this infection is not clear. The primary manifestation is a vaginal discharge that is thin and grayish-white, and has a foul, fishy odor. Complications include PID, preterm labor, premature rupture of the membranes, and postpartum endometritis (Porth, 2005). The infection is treated with oral or intravaginal antibacterial agents.

Candidiasis

Candidiasis (moniliasis or yeast infection) is caused by the organism *Candida albicans*, which has several strains of dif-

TABLE 52–1 Vaginal Infections

INFECTION	TYPE OF DISCHARGE	TYPICAL MANIFESTATIONS	NURSING CARE
Candidiasis (*Monilia,* yeast)	Thick white patches adhering to cervix and vaginal wall, resembling cottage cheese; little odor	Itching of vulva and vaginal area, redness, painful intercourse	Teach perineal hygiene and proper use of vaginal applicators. Instruct the client to complete the entire treatment.
Simple vaginalis (bacterial vaginosis, *Gardnerella* vaginosis)	Thin, white, "milklike," or gray with fishy odor, especially when mixed with potassium hydroxide	None to mild itching or burning in vulvar area; clue cells on microscopic examination	Teach proper perineal hygiene. Instruct client to complete treatment. Teach client relationship of infection to PID.
Trichomoniasis	Frothy, yellow or white, foul odor	Burning and itching of vulva	Teach perineal hygiene.
Atrophic vaginitis (senile vaginitis)	Thin, opaque discharge, occasionally blood tinged, odorless; pale, smooth, thin, dry vaginal walls	Painful intercourse, itching, vaginal dryness	Counsel client on symptoms of menopause and sexual techniques to minimize trauma.

ferent virulence. Candida organisms are part of the normal vaginal environment in up to 50% of women (Porth, 2005), causing problems only when they multiply rapidly. When increased estrogen levels, antibiotics, diabetes mellitus, fecal contamination, or other factors alter the normal vaginal flora, the organism proliferates, resulting in a yeast infection. The manifestations include an odorless, thick, cheesy vaginal discharge. This is often accompanied by itching and irritation of the vulva and vagina, dysuria, and dyspareunia (Figure 52–3 ■). Uncircumcised men may develop a yeast infection over the glans penis, manifested by itching and dysuria. The infection is treated with oral or intravaginal antifungal agents.

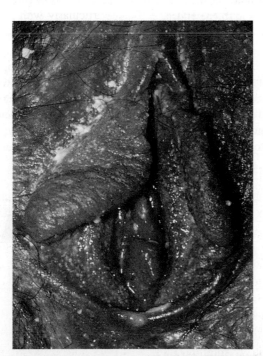

Figure 52–3 ■ Yeast infection on female genitalia.

Trichomoniasis

Trichomoniasis is caused by *Trichomonas vaginalis,* a protozoan parasite. It is the most common curable STI in young, sexually active women. An estimated 7.4 million new cases occur each year in both men and women (CDC, 2004). Symptoms usually appear in 5 to 28 days of exposure. It most commonly infects the vagina in women and the urethra in men. Most men are asymptomatic, but when symptomatic may complain of dysuria and urethral discomfort. Women have a frothy, green-yellow vaginal discharge with a strong fishy odor, often accompanied by itching and irritation of the genitalia. A woman with HIV who becomes infected has an increased risk of transmitting HIV to her sex partner. Trichomoniasis is treated with a single oral dose of metronidazole or tinidazole.

INTERDISCIPLINARY CARE

Interdisciplinary care focuses on identifying and eliminating the infection and preventing recurrence.

Diagnosis

Diagnostic tests vary with the suspected organism. Cervical cultures are examined to diagnose the causative organism. Trichomonas is identified by microscopically examining a specimen of vaginal discharge in saline. Ten percent potassium hydroxide is used to identify spores and filaments of candida. Diagnostic tests are described in Chapter 49 ∞.

Medications

The pharmacologic treatment varies with the organism as previously described. The sexual partner of a woman with a trichomonas infection must also be treated to prevent reinfection. Some antifungal agents are available without prescription, which can lead to self-medication with the incorrect agent or allow repeated infections to go unreported.

NURSING CARE

Nursing care focuses on teaching the client and, if necessary, her sexual partner to comply with the treatment regimen, use safer sex practices, and prevent future transmission of the infection. Careful history taking may also reveal high-risk sexual practices that require intervention, particularly if the client has had repeated infections. The initial presenting symptom for many HIV-positive women is vaginal candidiasis, which may not respond to over-the-counter treatments. Treatment with some antibiotics destroys normal vaginal flora, resulting in superinfection with yeast.

Nursing Diagnoses and Interventions

Although each nursing care plan must be individualized, nursing diagnoses that often apply to clients with vaginal infections are deficient knowledge and acute pain.

Deficient Knowledge

Many women are unaware of the causes of vaginal infections and the self-care measures to prevent and treat these infections. If possible, both the woman and her sexual partner should be taught the information.

- Explain the transmission of the infection. Many infections are transmitted most easily during menstruation; some can also be transmitted by towels or other inanimate objects, or by certain types of sexual activity. *A frank discussion of disease transmission and prevention with the woman and her partner can reduce the risk of reinfection.*
- The need to complete the course of treatment. *Many infections are asymptomatic in one partner. Incomplete treatment allows for recurrence of the infection and reinfection of the partner.*

Acute Pain

The symptoms of vaginitis can include dysuria, painful excoriation or ulceration of tissue, and painful intercourse (**dyspareunia**). Often these symptoms can be relieved by relatively simple self-care measures. See Box 52–2 for additional comfort measures.

- Suggest the use of cool compresses. *Cool compresses relieve itching.*
- Recommend sitz baths to alleviate discomfort. *Sitz baths cleanse the perineal area and the warmth is soothing to inflamed, irritated skin and membranes.*
- Wear cotton underwear. *Cotton absorbs moisture and allows better air circulation than other types of material.*
- If infected with trichomonas avoid sexual contact until treatment is completed. *Treatment of the infected woman and her partner as well as sexual abstinence are necessary to facilitate healing and to prevent reinfection.*

Community-Based Care

Teaching focuses on eradicating the infection, preventing further disease transmission, and relieving discomfort associated with the condition. Educating the client and her partner(s) about safer sex and improved genital hygiene practices can reduce the incidence of recurrence.

BOX 52–2 Self-Care Comfort Measures

- Do not wear panty hose; wear loose fitting pants or skirts.
- Double-rinse underwear; do not use fabric softener on underwear.
- Do not use bubble bath, perfumed soaps, or feminine hygiene products.
- Use 100% cotton menstrual pads and tampons.
- Use white, unscented toilet paper.
- Use a water-soluble lubricant for intercourse.
- Apply ice or a frozen blue gel pack wrapped in a towel to the vulva after intercourse to relieve burning.
- Rinse vulva with cool water after voiding and intercourse.

THE CLIENT WITH CHLAMYDIA

Chlamydia are a group of STIs, caused by *Chlamydia trachomatis,* a bacterium that behaves like a virus, reproducing only within the host cell. The bacterium is spread by any sexual contact and to the neonate by passage through the birth canal of an infected mother. The infections caused by chlamydia include acute urethral syndrome, nongonococcal urethritis, mucopurulent cervicitis, and PID.

Chlamydia is the most commonly reported bacterial STI in the United States, affecting an estimated 2 to 3 million people each year (CDC, 2004). Of that number, three of every four reported cases occurred in people under age 25. Risk factors for chlamydia are listed in Box 52–3.

Because chlamydia is asymptomatic in most women until the uterus and fallopian tubes have been invaded, treatment may be delayed, resulting in devastating long-term complications. Nearly a third of men with urethral chlamydia are also asymptomatic. Chlamydia is a leading cause of preventable blindness in the newborn.

Pathophysiology

Chlamydia trachomatis is an intracellular bacterial pathogen that resembles both a virus and a bacteria. The organism enters the body as an elementary body, a form in which it is capable of entering uninfected cells. The infection begins when the organism enters a cell and changes into a reticulate body. The reticulate body divides within the cell, bursting the cell and infecting adjoining cells.

Manifestations

The incubation period is from 1 to 3 weeks; however, chlamydia may be present for months or years without producing no-

---

BOX 52–3 Risk Factors for Chlamydial Infection

- Personal or partner history of STI
- Pregnancy
- Adolescent sexual activity
- Oral contraceptive use
- Unprotected sexual activity
- Multiple sexual partners

ticeable symptoms in women. Chlamydia typically invades the same target organs as gonorrhea (cervix and male urethra) and results in similar manifestations (dysuria, urinary frequency, and discharge). Clients may be asymptomatic; however, they are still potentially infectious.

Complications

If a chlamydial infection in women is not treated, it ascends into the upper reproductive tract, causing such complications as PID, which includes endometritis and salpingitis. Chronic pelvic pain may result. These infections are a major cause of infertility and ectopic pregnancy, a potentially life-threatening disorder in women. Complications of chlamydial infections in men include epididymitis, prostatitis, sterility, and Reiter's syndrome. Routine screening for sexually active adolescents and young adults has been suggested by the CDC to minimize these serious complications in asymptomatic people (Porth, 2005).

INTERDISCIPLINARY CARE

C. trachomatis is treated with medications to eradicate the infection. Its prevalence, particularly in younger populations, makes widespread screening necessary if the disease is to be controlled. Because chlamydia is often asymptomatic, treatment is often begun on a presumptive basis.

Diagnosis

The diagnostic tests that may be ordered include Gram stain of discharge from the female endocervix and urethra or from the male urethra to look for poly-morphonuclear leukocytes (considered evidence of infection).

Tests for antibodies to chlamydia such as the direct fluorescent antibody (DFA) test and an enzyme-linked immunosorbent assay (ELISA), as well as polymerase chain reaction (PCR) or ligase chain reaction (LCR) tests, are highly sensitive and specific tests performed on cervical and urethral swab specimens. However, nucleic acid amplification tests (NAATs), also performed on cervical and urethral swab specimens, have become the diagnostic method of choice (Porth, 2005).

Medications

The antibiotic recommended by the CDC for chlamydial infections in men and nonpregnant women is azithromycin (Zithromax), orally in a single dose, or doxycycline (Adoxa, Apo-Doxy), orally for 7 days. Both sexual partners must be treated at the same time or prior to resuming sexual intercourse.

NURSING CARE

Nursing care of the client with chlamydia focuses on eradication of the infection, prevention of future infections, and management of any chronic complications. Nursing diagnoses for the client with chlamydia are the same as for clients with any STI. Interventions are similar to those discussed later in the chapter for gonorrhea and previously for genital herpes.

Community-Based Care

Health teaching for the client with chlamydia centers on the need to comply with the treatment regimen, refer partners for examination and necessary treatment, and the use of condoms to avoid reinfection. If the infection has progressed to PID (discussed later), the client needs additional information on self-care and health promotion. The CDC recommends annual screening for chlamydia for clients who are young, sexually active, and do not use condoms correctly with every act of sexual intercourse.

THE CLIENT WITH GONORRHEA

Gonorrhea, also known as "GC" or "the clap," is caused by *Neisseria gonorrhoeae*, a gram-negative diplococcus. Gonorrhea is the most common *reportable* communicable disease in the United States. The CDC (2004) estimates that approximately 700,000 new cases occur annually, with the rate of reported gonorrhea increasing.

Gonorrhea rates for African Americans are 30% higher than for non-Hispanic whites. Other risk factors include residence in large urban areas, being transients, early onset of sexual activity, multiple serial or consecutive sex partners, drug use, prostitution, and previous gonorrheal or concurrent STI infection.

Pathophysiology

The causative organism of gonorrhea is a pyogenic (pus-forming) bacteria that causes inflammation characterized by purulent exudate. Humans are the only host for the organism. Gonorrhea is transmitted by direct hetero- and homosexual intercourse and during delivery as the neonate passes through the birth canal. The portal of entry can be the genitourinary tract, eyes, oropharynx, anorectum, or skin. The incubation period is 2 to 7 days after exposure. The organism initially targets the female cervix and the male urethra. Without treatment, the disease ultimately disseminates (spreads widely) to other organs. In men, gonorrhea can cause acute, painful inflammation of the prostate, epididymis, and periurethral glands and can lead to sterility. In women, it can cause PID, endometritis, salpingitis, and pelvic peritonitis.

Manifestations

Manifestations of gonorrhea in men include dysuria and serous, milky, or purulent discharge from the penis. Some men also experience regional lymphadenopathy. About 20% of men and 80% of women remain asymptomatic until the disease is advanced. Women with symptoms experience dysuria, urinary frequency, abnormal menses (increased flow or dysmenorrhea), increased vaginal discharge, and dyspareunia.

Anorectal gonorrhea is seen most often in homosexual men. The manifestations include pruritus, mucopurulent rectal discharge, rectal bleeding and pain, and constipation. Gonococcal pharyngitis occurs primarily in homosexual or bisexual men or heterosexual women after oral sexual contact (fellatio) with an infected partner. The manifestations include fever, sore throat, and enlarged lymph glands.

Complications

The complications of untreated gonorrhea in both men and women may be permanent and serious. They include:

- PID in women, leading to internal abscesses, chronic pain, ectopic pregnancy, and infertility
- Blindness, infection of joints, and potentially lethal infections of the blood in the newborn, contracted during delivery
- Epididymitis and prostatitis in men, resulting in infertility and dysuria
- Spread of the infection to the blood and joints
- Increased susceptibility to and transmission of HIV.

INTERDISCIPLINARY CARE

The goals of treatment for the client with gonorrhea include eradication of the organism and any coexisting disease, and prevention of reinfection or transmission. It is important to emphasize the importance of taking all medications as prescribed and abstaining from sexual contact until the infection is cured in both client and partners. Condom use to prevent future infections is essential, particularly for pregnant women whose partners may be infected.

Diagnosis

Diagnosis of gonorrhea is based on cultures from the infected mucous membranes (cervix, urethra, rectum, or throat), examination of urine from an infected person, and a Gram stain to visualize the bacteria under the microscope. Testing for other STIs (especially chlamydia and syphilis) at the same time is recommended. Pregnant women are routinely screened during their first prenatal visit. Diagnostic tests are described in Chapter 49 ∞.

Medications

Because of the many penicillin-resistant strains of *N. gonorrhoeae,* an alternative antibiotic, such as ciprofloxacin (Cipro) or ofloxacin (Floxin), is used to treat gonorrhea. Fluoroquinolone therapy (such as with ciprofloxacin or levofloxacin) is often prescribed because it is inexpensive, oral, and single dose. However, because of increased prevalence of fluoroquinolone-resistant *N. gonorrhoeae* in Asia, the Pacific Islands, and California, this therapy is no longer recommended for use in treating gonorrhea in those areas. A single dose of oral azithromycin (Zithromax) or a 7-day course of oral doxycycline (Vibramycin, Vivox) usually is added to treat any coexisting chlamydial infection. All sexual partners within 60 days before diagnosis of the infection also need to be treated.

NURSING CARE

In planning and implementing care for the client with gonorrhea, the nurse considers the possible coexistence of other STIs such as syphilis and HIV, the impact of the disease and its treatment on the client's lifestyle, and the likelihood of noncompliance. A Nursing Care Plan for the client with gonorrhea is on page 1847.

Nursing Diagnoses and Interventions

Nursing diagnoses discussed in this section focus on noncompliance and impaired social interaction.

Noncompliance

Although one-time treatment with the recommended antibiotic is highly effective in curing gonorrhea, noncompliance with the doxycycline regimen may leave any coexisting chlamydial infection unresolved. Noncompliance with recommendations for abstinence, follow-up, or condom use fosters a high rate of reinfection. Failure to refer partners for examination and treatment also leads to reinfection.

- Reinforce the need to take all medications as directed and keep follow-up appointments to be sure no reinfection has occurred. Discuss the prevalence of gonorrhea and the potential complications if it is not cured. *The client who understands the complications of incomplete or failed treatment is more likely to comply with the medication regimen.*
- Discuss the importance of sexual abstinence until the infection is cured, referral of partners, and condom use to prevent reinfection. *Understanding that cure is possible and reinfection is avoidable helps the client cope with the disease and its treatment and is likely to increase compliance*
- Explain to women that condoms must be used during treatment, even if other methods of birth control are used. *Oral contraceptives increase the alkalinity of the vaginal pH, facilitating the growth of the gonococcal bacteria, and intrauterine devices alter the endometrial barrier, favoring persistent gonococcal infections (Blair, 2004).*

Impaired Social Interaction

Diagnosis of any STI can make clients feel "dirty," ashamed, and guilty about their sexual behaviors, and unworthy to be with others.

- Provide privacy, confidentiality, and a safe, nonjudgmental environment for expression of concerns. Help the client understand that gonorrhea is a consequence of sexual behavior, not a punishment, and that it can be avoided in the future. *Being treated with respect and privacy helps the client realize that the disease does not change an individual's worth as a person. This knowledge enhances the client's ability to relate to others.*

Community-Based Care

Health teaching focuses on helping clients understand the importance of (1) taking any and all prescribed medication, (2) referring sexual partners for evaluation and treatment, (3) abstaining from all sexual contact until the client and partners are cured, and (4) using a condom to avoid transmitting or contracting infections in the future. Clients also need to understand the need for a follow-up visit 4 to 7 days after treatment is completed.

THE CLIENT WITH SYPHILIS

Syphilis is a complex systemic STI caused by the spirochete *Treponema pallidum,* and it can infect almost any body tissue or organ. It is transmitted from open lesions during any sexual

NURSING CARE PLAN   A Client with Gonorrhea

Janet Cirit, a 33-year-old legal secretary, lives in a suburban Midwestern community. She is unmarried but dating a man named Jim Adkins, who lives in an adjacent suburb. Ms. Cirit visits her gynecologist because her periods have become irregular and she is experiencing pelvic pain and an abnormal amount of vaginal discharge. Recently she has developed a sore throat. The pelvic pain has begun to disrupt her sleeping pattern, and she is concerned that she might have cancer because her mother recently died of ovarian cancer.

ASSESSMENT

When Ms. Cirit arrives for her appointment at the gynecologist's office, Marsha Davidson, the nurse practitioner, interviews her. Ms. Davidson completes a thorough medical and sexual history, including questions about her menstrual periods, pain associated with urination or sexual intercourse, urinary frequency, most recent Pap smear, birth control method, history of STI and drug use, and types of sexual activity. Ms. Cirit reports her symptoms and her concern about ovarian cancer. She also indicates that she is taking oral contraceptives and therefore sees no need for her boyfriend to use a condom because she believes their relationship is monogamous.

Physical examination reveals both pharyngeal and cervical inflammation, and lower abdominal tenderness. Her temperature is 98.5°F (37.0°C). There are no signs or symptoms of pregnancy.

The gynecologist orders a Pap smear and cultures of the cervix, urethra, and pharynx to evaluate for gonorrhea and chlamydial infection. Blood is drawn for WBC. Test results are positive for gonorrhea and negative for chlamydia. The WBC is slightly elevated, indicating possible salpingitis. Because Mr. Adkins has been Ms. Cirit's only sexual partner, it is clear that he is the source of infection and needs to be treated as well.

DIAGNOSES

- *Acute Pain* related to the infectious process
- *Anxiety* related to fear about possible cancer
- *Situational Low Self-Esteem* related to shame and guilt because of having an STI

- *Ineffective Sexuality Patterns* related to the impaired relationship and fear of reinfection

EXPECTED OUTCOMES

- Experience relief of pain, indicating that the infection has been eradicated.
- Verbalize that she has nothing to be ashamed of and that she has been wise to seek treatment as soon as symptoms occurred.
- Verbalize that she will insist her partner use condoms during future sexual activity.

PLANNING AND IMPLEMENTATION

- Administer ceftriaxone IM as ordered.
- Emphasize the need for regular Pap smears and pelvic examinations because of the family history of ovarian cancer.
- Discuss feelings and concerns about the diagnosis of gonorrhea. Stress that such a diagnosis does not reflect on one's self-worth as a person.
- Teach how to talk with a future sexual partner about condom use.

EVALUATION

A week later during her follow-up visit, Ms. Cirit states that she is feeling much better and sleeping well at night since the pain has ended. She has terminated her relationship with Mr. Adkins and is considering joining a health club in the hope of increasing her level of fitness and perhaps meeting someone new.

CRITICAL THINKING IN THE NURSING PROCESS

1. How are Ms. Cirit's manifestations related to the infectious process of gonorrhea?
2. Should the nurse have suggested that Ms. Cirit also be tested for HIV? Why or why not?
3. Develop a care plan for Ms. Cirit for the nursing diagnosis *Impaired Social Interaction*.
   See Evaluating Your Response in Appendix C.

---

contact (genital, oral–genital, or anal–genital). The organism is highly susceptible to heat and drying, but can survive for days in fluids; thus, it may also be transmitted by infected blood or other body fluid such as saliva. The incubation period ranges from 10 to 90 days, averaging 21 days. If not treated appropriately, syphilis can lead to blindness, paralysis, mental illness, cardiovascular damage, and death. Syphilis often occurs with one or more other STIs, such as HIV/AIDS or chlamydial infection.

Although in 1996 the rate of syphilis infection reached its lowest level in many years, it remains a significant problem in certain geographic regions, and among specific populations such as African Americans. Rates also remain high in many urban centers, with higher infection rates found in drug users, transients, and the homeless. The incidence of primary and secondary syphilis is highest in people 20 to 39 years of age, with the incidence in women decreasing. However, the rate of syphilis among men having sex with men (MSM) is increasing (CDC, 2004).

Pathophysiology

Any break in the skin or mucous membrane is vulnerable to invasion by the spirochete. Once it has entered the system, the spirochete is spread through the blood and lymphatic system. Congenital syphilis is transferred to the fetus through the placental circulation.

Manifestations

Syphilis is generally characterized by three clinical stages: primary, secondary, and tertiary. Each stage has characteristic manifestations (see the box on page 1848). The client with syphilis also may experience a latency period when no signs of the disease are evident.

Primary Syphilis

The primary stage of syphilis is characterized by the appearance of a **chancre** (Figure 52–4 ■) and by regional enlargement of lymph nodes; little or no pain accompanies these warning signs. The chancre appears at the site of inoculation (such as the genitals,

MANIFESTATIONS of Syphilis

REPRODUCTIVE

Primary
- Genital chancre (may be internal in female)

Secondary
- Condyloma lata

INTEGUMENTARY SYSTEM

Secondary
- Rash on palms of hands and soles of feet

Tertiary
- Granulomatous lesions involving mucous membranes and skin

GASTROINTESTINAL SYSTEM

Secondary
- Anorexia
- Oral mucous patches

NEUROLOGIC SYSTEM

Secondary
- Asymptomatic
- Headache
- Meningitis
- Cranial neuropathies

Tertiary
- Asymptomatic
- Neurosyphilis
- Personality changes, hyperactive reflexes, Argyll Robertson pupil, decreased memory, slurred speech, optic atrophy
- Tabes dorsalis
- Seizures, hemiparesis, hemiplegia

MUSCULOSKELETAL SYSTEM

Secondary
- Arthralgia
- Bone and joint arthritis
- Myalgia
- Periostitis

Tertiary
- Gummas

CARDIOVASCULAR SYSTEM

Tertiary
- Aortic insufficiency
- Aortic aneurysm
- Stenosis of openings to coronary arteries

RENAL SYSTEM

Secondary
- Glomerulonephritis
- Nephrotic syndrome

OTHER

Primary
- Regional lymphadenopathy

Secondary
- Generalized lymphadenopathy
- Fever
- Malaise
- Hepatitis
- Alopecia

anus, mouth, breast, fingers) 3 to 4 weeks after the infectious contact. In women, a genital chancre may go unnoticed, disappearing within 4 to 6 weeks. In both primary and secondary stages, syphilis remains highly infectious, even if no symptoms are evident.

Secondary Syphilis

Manifestations of secondary syphilis may appear any time from 2 weeks to 6 months after the initial chancre disappears. These symptoms can include a skin rash, especially on the palms of the hands or soles of the feet, mucous patches in the oral cavity; sore throat; generalized lymphadenopathy; condyloma lata (flat, broad-based papules, unlike the pedunculated structure of geni-

tal warts) on the labia, anus or corner of the mouth; flulike symptoms; and alopecia. These manifestations generally disappear within 2 to 6 weeks, and an asymptomatic latency period begins.

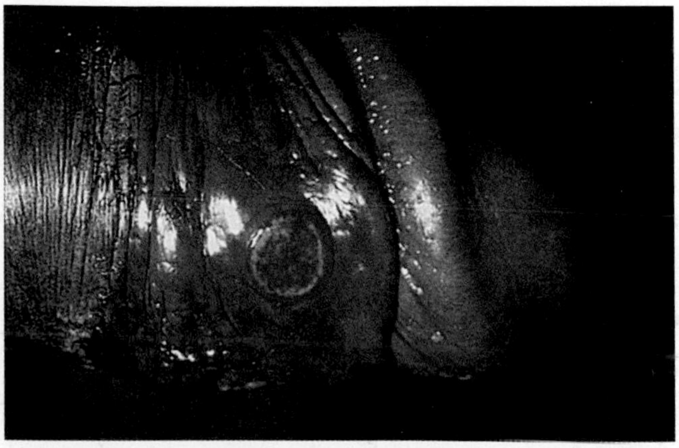

Latent and Tertiary Syphilis

The latent stage of syphilis begins 2 or more years after the initial infection and can last up to 50 years. During this stage, no symptoms of syphilis are apparent, and the disease is not transmissible by sexual contact. It can be transmitted by infected blood, however; thus, all prospective blood donors must be screened for syphilis. In two-thirds of all cases, the latent stage persists without further complications. Unless treated, the remaining one-third of infected people progress to late-stage or tertiary syphilis. In the presence of HIV infection, disease progression seems to be more rapid.

Two types of late-stage syphilis occur. Benign late syphilis, of rapid onset, is characterized by localized development of infiltrating tumors (*gummas*) in skin, bones, and liver, generally responding promptly to treatment. Of more insidious onset is a diffuse inflammatory response that involves the central nervous system and the cardiovascular system. Though the disease can still be treated at this stage, much of the cardiovascular and central nervous system damage is irreversible.

INTERDISCIPLINARY CARE

The goals of treatment are to inactivate the spirochete and educate the client about how to prevent reinfection or further transmission. Treatment includes antibiotic therapy and identi-

Figure 52–4 ■ Chancre of primary syphilis on the penis.

Source: Biophoto Associates/Photo Researchers, Inc.

fication and referral of partners for testing and treatment if necessary, follow-up testing, and education about condom use to prevent reinfection of self and transmission of disease to partners. In addition, clients should be screened for chlamydial infection and advised to have an HIV test.

Diagnosis

Diagnosis of syphilis is complex because it mimics many other diseases. A careful history and physical examination are obtained, as well as laboratory evaluations of lesions and blood. Diagnostic tests are described in Chapter 49 ∞.

The VDRL (Venereal Disease Research Laboratory) and RPR (rapid plasma reagin) blood tests measure antibody production. People with syphilis become positive about 4 to 6 weeks after infection. However, these tests are not specific for syphilis, and other diseases may also cause positive results. Additional tests are required for definitive diagnosis.

The FTA-ABS (fluorescent treponemal antibody absorption) test is specific for *T. pallidum* and can be used to confirm VDRL and RPR findings. It may be used for clients whose clinical picture indicates syphilis but who have negative VDRL results. In immunofluorescent staining a specimen is obtained from early lesions or aspiration of lymph nodes and is specially treated and examined microscopically for the presence of *T. pallidum*. Darkfield microscopy involves examining a specimen from the chancre for the presence of *T. pallidum* using a darkfield microscope.

Medications

The treatment of choice for all stages of syphilis in adults is penicillin G, given intramuscularly (IM) in a single dose. Clients allergic to penicillin are given oral doxycycline or tetracycline for 28 days.

Treatment of syphilis may result in a severe reaction called the *Jarisch-Herxheimer reaction*, involving fever, musculoskeletal pain, tachycardia, and sometimes hypotension. This is not a reaction to the penicillin itself, but to the sudden and massive destruction of spirochetes by the penicillin and the resulting release of toxins into the bloodstream. The Jarisch-Herxheimer reaction generally begins within 24 hours of treatment and subsides in another 24 hours. Treatment should not be discontinued unless symptoms become life threatening.

NURSING CARE

In planning and implementing nursing care for the client with syphilis, the nurse needs to consider the client's age, lifestyle, access to health care, and educational level. Although each client has individualized needs, nursing diagnoses for the client with syphilis would be the same as for any client with an STI. A Nursing Care Plan for a client with syphilis is on the next page.

Nursing Diagnoses and Interventions

Nursing diagnoses discussed in this section focus on risk for injury, anxiety, and self-esteem.

Risk for Injury

If syphilis is not diagnosed and treated promptly and effectively, it can have devastating effects on all body systems, particularly the neurologic and cardiovascular systems, eventually leading to a painful death.

- Teach the importance of taking any prescribed medication. *Taking the prescribed antibiotic is important to ensure eradication of the infecting organism.*
- Encourage referral of any sexual partners for evaluation and any necessary treatment. *Without treatment of both partners, reinfection can occur or the disease may be transmitted to other people through sexual activity.*
- Teach abstinence from sexual contact until client and partners are cured and to use condoms to prevent future infections. *Abstinence until the organism is eradicated prevents reinfection. Condoms provide barrier protection, reducing the risk of infection during sexual activity.*
- Emphasize the importance of returning for follow-up testing at 3- and 6-month intervals for early syphilis, and 6- and 12-month intervals for late latent syphilis. *Follow-up testing is performed to ensure eradication of the disease.*
- Provide information about manifestations of reinfection. *Successful treatment of the disease does not prevent possible subsequent infections.*

Anxiety

The diagnosis of syphilis understandably causes the client anxiety, not only about personal well-being but about the well-being of partners and, in the expectant woman, her fetus.

- Emphasize that syphilis can be effectively treated, preventing the serious complications of late-stage disease. *This information provides a sense of control and helps decrease anxiety.*
- Teach the pregnant client that taking medications as directed and returning each month for follow-up testing will help ensure the well-being of her baby. *Knowing that treatment can reduce the risk to her baby relieves anxiety and possibly increases compliance.*

Low Self-Esteem

Living with any chronic disease can be damaging to a person's self-esteem. However, the client with syphilis needs additional support to cope with the stigma of this kind of infection. Unfortunately, the populations most affected by STIs often lack family and other social support networks.

- Create an environment where the client feels respected and safe to discuss questions and concerns about the disease and its effect on the client's life. *Being treated with respect helps enhance self-esteem.*
- Provide privacy and confidentiality. *Clients are often embarrassed to discuss the intimate details of their sex lives.*
- Let clients know that the nurse and other healthcare providers care about them and the successful treatment of their disease. *Feeling valued enhances self-esteem.*

Community-Based Care

Education is an essential part of nursing care for the client with any STI, and syphilis is no exception. The nurse emphasizes that

NURSING CARE PLAN   A Client with Syphilis

Eddie Kratz, age 22, works as bellman at a large hotel. For the past year, he has shared a small apartment with Maria Jones, who is 5 months pregnant with his child. Although he intends to marry Ms. Jones before the baby is born, he has continued a previous relationship with a woman named Justine Simpson. His sexual activities with Ms. Simpson have increased in frequency as Ms. Jones's pregnancy has advanced. Recently Mr. Kratz has noticed a swelling in his groin and a sore on his penis.

ASSESSMENT

When Mr. Kratz comes to the community clinic, he is interviewed by the NP, Sally Morovitz. She takes a thorough medical and sexual history, including questions about drug use, allergies, difficulty with urination, urinary frequency, itching or discharge from the penis, recent sexual activities, precautions taken against infection, history of STIs, and sexual function. She determines that Mr. Kratz has been having unprotected sex with both Ms. Jones and Ms. Simpson. He believes that Ms. Jones is not having sex with anyone except him, but he is not sure.

Physical assessment reveals a classic syphilitic chancre on the shaft of the penis and regional lymphadenopathy. A specimen of exudates from the chancre is sent for darkfield examination. Ms. Morovitz discusses with Mr. Kratz the likelihood that he has syphilis and the need to tell both Ms. Jones and Ms. Simpson so that they can be tested and, if necessary, treated. Ms. Morovitz also suggests that Mr. Kratz be tested for HIV since he has been having unprotected sex with two women, at least one of whom may be sexually active with other partners. He agrees, and blood is drawn for an ELISA test. Darkfield analysis of the chancre exudate confirms the diagnosis of syphilis; the ELISA results are negative for HIV.

DIAGNOSES

- *Risk for Injury* to the client, his partners, and the infant, related to the disease process
- *Ineffective Health Maintenance* related to a lack of knowledge about the disease process, its transmission, and the need for treatment
- *Interrupted Family Processes* related to the effects of the diagnosis of syphilis on the couple's relationship
- *Anxiety* related to the effects of the infection on the unborn child

EXPECTED OUTCOMES

- Prompt treatment will cure the syphilis.

- Verbalize understanding for the need to abstain from sexual contact during treatment, complete all medications, return for follow-up visits, and use condoms to prevent reinfection.
- Verbalize ability to cope with the effect of diagnosis and treatment on the relationship.
- Verbalize decreased anxiety following education and treatment.

PLANNING AND IMPLEMENTATION

- Administer IM injection of penicillin G as ordered.
- Discuss the importance of abstaining from sexual activity until he and his partners are cured, and of using condoms to prevent reinfection.
- Explain the need to return for follow-up testing in 3 months and again at 6 months. Provide a copy of the STI prevention checklist, and document that reminders need to be sent at 3- and 6-month intervals.
- Notify sexual partners that they need to come to the clinic for testing.
- Refer to a social worker for counseling about the effect of the disease on their relationship.
- Teach the couple about the importance of treatment to the health of their infant.

EVALUATION

At the 3-month follow-up visit, the chancre on Mr. Kratz's penis has healed, and he reports that he is using a condom any time he has sex. Ms. Jones has also tested positive for syphilis and negative for HIV, so she, too, is given penicillin G, and verbal and written follow-up instructions, including follow-up until the infant is born. The couple is meeting every other week with the social worker and say that their relationship is improving. Ms. Simpson has received similar test results and is given a prescription for doxycycline because she is allergic to penicillin.

CRITICAL THINKING IN THE NURSING PROCESS

1. What manifestations might a client with early syphilis experience?
2. List some appropriate questions for taking a sexual history when you suspect the presence of one or more STIs.
3. How might you counsel Mr. Kratz to help him break the news of the diagnosis to Ms. Jones?

See Evaluating Your Response in Appendix C.

---

syphilis is a chronic disease that can be spread to others even though no symptoms are evident. Address the following topics:

- Taking all prescribed medication
- Referring sexual partners for evaluation and treatment
- Abstaining from all sexual contact as recommended by CDC guidelines
- Using a condom to avoid transmitting or contracting infections in the future
- The need for follow-up testing (at 3 and 6 months for clients with primary or secondary syphilis, and at 6 and 12 months for those with late-stage disease). If clients are HIV positive,

follow-up visits are recommended 1, 2, 3, 6, 9, and 12 months after treatment.

THE CLIENT WITH PELVIC INFLAMMATORY DISEASE

Pelvic inflammatory disease (PID) is a term used to describe infection of the pelvic organs, including the fallopian tubes (*salpingitis*), ovaries (*oophoritis*), cervix (*cervicitis*), endometrium (*endometritis*), pelvic peritoneum, and the pelvic vascular system. PID can be caused by one or more infectious agents, including *Neisseria gonorrhoeae, Chlamydia trachomatis, Escherichia coli,* and *Mycoplasma hominis. N. gonorrhoeae* and *C. trachomatis* are responsible for as much as 80% of PID; dual infection with both agents is common.

PID is not a reportable disease in the United States; however, it is estimated that about 1 million women experience PID each year. As a result of the infection, more than 100,000 women become infertile and a large proportion of the ectopic pregnancies occurring each year are the result of PID (CDC, 2004). The disease may also cause pelvic abscesses and chronic abdominal pain.

Sexually active women ages 16 to 24 years are most at risk. Risk factors include a history of sexually transmitted infection (especially gonorrhea and chlamydia), bacterial vaginosis, multiple sexual partners, douching, and previous PID. Barrier contraceptive devices such as condoms reduce the risk of PID.

The prognosis depends on the number of episodes, promptness of treatment, and modification of risk-taking behaviors. Prevention includes educating women, especially young women, regarding the causes and transmission of infection and methods of self-protection, such as avoiding unprotected sexual activity.

Pathophysiology

Pelvic inflammatory disease is usually polymicrobial (caused by more than one microbe) in origin, with gonorrhea and chlamydia being common causative organisms. Pathogenic microorganisms enter the vagina and travel to the uterus during intercourse or other sexual activity. They can also gain direct access to the uterus during childbirth, abortion, or surgery of the reproductive tract. The organisms ascend from the endocervical canal to the fallopian tubes and ovaries.

Manifestations

Manifestations of PID include fever, purulent vaginal discharge, severe lower abdominal pain, and painful cervical movement. However, the manifestations may be so mild that the infection is not recognized.

Complications

Complications include pelvic abscess, infertility, ectopic pregnancy, chronic pelvic pain, pelvic adhesions, dyspareunia, and chronic pelvic pain. Abscess formation is common.

INTERDISCIPLINARY CARE

The goals of treatment are to eliminate the infection and prevent complications and recurrence. The physical examination may reveal abdominal, adnexal, and cervical pain.

Diagnosis

Tests used in the diagnosis of PID may include a CBC with differential, which will show a markedly elevated WBC, and an increased sedimentation rate. If a laparoscopy or laparotomy is done, it may reveal inflammation, edema, or hyperemia of the fallopian tubes, or tubal discharge and, possibly, generalized pelvic involvement, abscesses, and scarring.

Medications

Combination antibiotic therapy with at least two broad-spectrum antibiotics administered IV or orally is the typical treatment for PID. If PID is not acute, outpatient antibiotic therapy is prescribed. In acute cases, however, the client may be hospitalized. Analgesics are given, and antibiotics and fluids are administered intravenously. Commonly prescribed antibiotics include parental cefoxitin (Mefoxin), or clindamycin (Cleocin), plus gentamicin (Garamycin) or doxycycline (Vibramcin). Nursing implications for antibiotics are discussed in Chapter 12 ∞.

Surgery

The surgeon may insert a drain into an abscess, if present, and remove any adhesions. If the client does not respond to conservative therapy, surgical removal of the uterus, fallopian tubes, and ovaries may be necessary.

NURSING CARE

The goals of nursing care are to treat the infection and to prevent complications, such as scarring and infertility. The client who is hospitalized maintains bed rest in the semi-Fowler's position to promote drainage and to localize the infectious process in the pelvic cavity.

Nursing Diagnoses and Interventions

Nursing diagnoses that apply to the client with PID include a risk for injury and deficient knowledge.

Risk for Injury

PID can have severe, even life-threatening, complications. Scarring of fallopian tubes can lead to ectopic pregnancy or pelvic abscess. Infertility is a common complication, as are recurrent or chronic PID, chronic abdominal pain, pelvic adhesions, premature hysterectomy, and depression. The woman who has severe infection and manifestations may be hospitalized for treatment.

- Administer antibiotic therapy as ordered, and monitor closely for adverse effects. *Antibiotics used in acute PID are potent agents; some can have serious side effects.*
- Practice thorough hand washing and strict adherence to universal precautions when handling perineal pads and linens. Appropriate disinfection of bedpans, toilet seats, linens, and utensils is also important. *These practices help avoid disseminating the infection to others.*

Deficient Knowledge

PID is most common in young women, who often do not understand their own anatomy and physiology or sexually transmitted infections. Diagnosis and treatment of PID offer an opportunity to increase that understanding, thereby preventing complications and recurrent infection.

- Explain how infection is spread and what measures to take to prevent future infection. *Understanding can improve compliance with treatment regimens and perhaps change high-risk behavior.*

- Explain the need to complete the treatment regimen and the importance of follow-up visits. If the client or partner fails to take all of the medication as prescribed, the infection may not be completely cured. *Noncompliance and recurrence are common, particularly if follow-up appointments are not kept.*
- Teach proper perineal care, especially wiping from front to back. *This reduces transmission of fecal organisms to reproductive tissues and reduces the incidence of urinary tract infections.*
- Caution the client about using tampons. Instruct the client to change tampons or pads at least every 4 hours. *Menstrual flow and other discharges provide a favorable environment for microorganisms to multiply.*
- Provide information about safer sex practices and family planning. Instruct the client to remove diaphragms within 6 hours after use. IUDs are contraindicated. Latex condoms offer the most effective protection against infection. *These measures help prevent recurrence of infection.*
- Teach the client to report any unusual vaginal discharge or odor to the healthcare provider. *Treatment is most effective early in the disease process.*

Community-Based Care

Provide general information related to sexually transmitted infections. Teach measures to eradicate the infection and prevent recurrence, and help the client deal with the physical and psychosocial implications of treatment, including possible infertility. Inform the client that the patency of the fallopian tubes can be evaluated after several menstrual cycles; this delay allows for complete resolution of the inflammatory process.

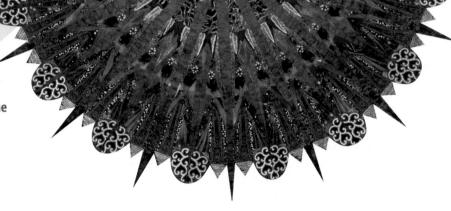

EXPLORE MediaLink

Prentice Hall Nursing MediaLink DVD-ROM
Audio Glossary
NCLEX-RN® Review

Animation
Gonorrhea

COMPANION WEBSITE www.prenhall.com/lemone
Audio Glossary
NCLEX-RN® Review
Care Plan Activity: Gonorrhea
Case Studies
Pelvic Inflammatory Disease
Syphilis
Teaching Plans
Risk of Cancer with HPV
Singles and Safer Sex
MediaLink Applications
HPV
HPV Prevention
Links to Resources

CHAPTER HIGHLIGHTS

- Sexually transmitted infections (STIs) are infections transmitted by sexual contact, including vaginal, oral, and anal intercourse. STIs affect women and infants more than men, and are more common in people who have multiple sex partners, abuse drugs, and are of lower socioeconomic status.
- STIs can coexist in the same person and can be transmitted by either heterosexual or homosexual sexual contact. Effective treatment mandates that both sex partners be treated. Most STIs can be prevented by using latex condoms.
- Genital herpes, caused by an infection with an HSV virus, is a commonly occurring STI in teens and young adults. There is no cure and treatment is primarily symptomatic. Nursing care is directed toward relieving the pain of the lesions, mitigating sexual dysfunction, and relieving anxiety.
- Genital warts, caused by the human papilloma virus (HPV), are a chronic, incurable STI. They are manifested by warts of various forms, or may be present without manifestations. Infection with

HPV poses a major risk for cervical cancer. A vaccine against the virus is recommended.
- Urogenital infections include vaginal infections (bacterial vaginosis, candidiasis, and trichomoniasis), chlamydia, gonorrhea, syphilis, and pelvic inflammatory disease (PID).
- Chlamydia, occurring most in young adults under age 25, is a bacterial infection that can spread to the uterus and fallopian tubes in women, causing PID, infertility, and ectopic pregnancy. Untreated chlamydia in men may result in epididymitis, prostatitis, sterility, and Reiter's syndrome.
- Gonorrhea (caused by a bacteria) and syphilis (caused by a spirochete) affect both men and women, and may infect the newborn as it moves through the birth canal in an untreated woman. Syphilis, if untreated, exists in the body in three stages, with the third stage lasting up to 50 years. Both of these STIs are treated with antibiotics. Nursing care focuses on education, preventing injury from complications, relieving anxiety, and supporting self-esteem.

■ PID is an infection of the female pelvic organs, and may be caused by one or more infectious agents. Sexually active young women between the ages of 16 and 24 are most at risk. The prognosis depends on the number of episodes, promptness of treatment, and modification of risk-taking behaviors. The goals of nursing care are to treat the infection and prevent complications.

TEST YOURSELF NCLEX-RN® REVIEW

1 Which population is most often affected by STIs?
1. men
2. women and infants
3. adolescent males
4. older adults

2 Which of the following statements would indicate a client understands teaching to treat an STI?
1. "My sex partner and I must both take medications."
2. "I know I can never have sex again."
3. "I will douche after every sexual encounter with my partner."
4. "My sex partner does not have an infection, so won't need medications."

3 You are teaching a male client information about using condoms to prevent STI. What topics would you include? (Select all that apply.)
1. Use a new condom with each sex act.
2. Ensure a small amount of air in the tip.
3. Use oil-based lubricants, such as petroleum jelly.
4. Handle carefully to ensure no damage.
5. Withdraw when the penis is erect.

4 You are assessing a young male. He has both blisters and ulcerations on the shaft of his penis. What is his most likely medical diagnosis?
1. chlamydia
2. gonorrhea
3. genital warts
4. genital herpes

5 Of the following statements about genital warts, which one is **not** true?
1. The infection is caused by a yeast organism.
2. The infection can be spread by any type of intercourse.
3. The infection may be transmitted to the fetus.
4. The infection cannot be cured.

6 You are counseling a young woman with an HPV genital infection. What screening test would you recommend she have every year?
1. breast exam and mammogram
2. stool for occult blood
3. CBC to detect anemia and infection
4. pelvic exam and Pap smear

7 Which of the following manifestations would most commonly be elicited during a health history for a woman with a vaginal infection?
1. pain
2. itching
3. nausea
4. diarrhea

8 You are teaching a woman with an STI who has severe genital discomfort. What is one simple recommendation that may relieve the discomfort?
1. Wear nylon panty hose.
2. Cut fingernails short.
3. Wear cotton underwear.
4. Have sex more frequently.

9 The infective organism responsible for gonorrhea *initially targets* what body parts?
1. male urethra and female cervix
2. female vulva and vagina
3. male prostate
4. male and female external genitalia

10 Which of the following would you teach a client about syphilis?
1. Syphilis is caused by a virus.
2. Syphilis is a local genital infection.
3. Syphilis is a systemic infection.
4. Syphilis has no effect on the developing fetus.

See Test Yourself answers in Appendix C.

BIBLIOGRAPHY

Ali, M., Cleland, J., & Shah, I. (2004). Condom use within marriage. A neglected HIV intervention. *Bulletin of the World Health Organization, 82*(3), 180–186.

American Social Health Association. (2005). *Facts & answers about STDs: Statistics.* Retrieved from http://www.ashastd.org/stdfaqs/statistics.html

Anderson, M., Klink, K., & Cohrssen, A. (2004). The rational clinical examination: Evaluation of vaginal complaints. *Journal of the American Medical Association, 291*(11), 1368–1379.

Ashcroft, T. (2004). Clinical preventative services for men: Information for women's health care providers. *AWHONN LIFELINES, 8*(6), 528–533.

Blair, M. (2004). Sexually transmitted diseases: An update. *Urology Nursing, 24*(6), 467–473.

Centers for Disease Control and Prevention. (2004). *STD general information (PID, syphilis, trichomoniasis, human papillomavirus, genital herpes, HPV, chlamydia).* Retrieved from http://www.cdc.gov/std.htm

_____.(2006). Treatment guidelines for sexually transmitted diseases. Retrieved from http://www.cdc.gov/std/treatment.htm

Drop-in service cuts wait for STI clinic. (2005). *Nursing Times, 101*(10), 9.

Farley, T., Cohen, D., Kahn, R., Lolis, S., Johnson, G., & Martin, D. (2003). The acceptability and behavioral effects of antibiotic prophylaxis for syphilis prevention. *Sexually Transmitted Diseases, 30*(11), 844–849.

Jungmann, E. (2004). Clinical evidence concise. Genital herpes. *American Family Physician, 70*(5), 912–914, 813–815.

Klebanoff, M., Schwebke, J., Zhang, J., Nansel, T., Yu, K., & Andrews, W. (2004). Vulvovaginal symptoms in women with bacterial vaginosis. *Obstetrics and Gynecology, 104*(2), 267–272.

NANDA International. (2005). *Nursing diagnoses: Definitions and classification 2005–2006.* Philadelphia.

National Institute of Allergy and Infectious Diseases, National Institutes of Health. (2003). *An introduction to sexually transmitted infections.* Retrieved from http://niaid.nih.gov/factsheets/stdinfo.htm

Ness, R., Hillier, S., Kip, K., Soper, D., Stamm, C., McGregor, J., et al. (2004). Bacterial vaginosis and risk of pelvic inflammatory disease. *Obstetrics and Gynecology, 104*(4), 761–769.

Phrma. (2005). *New medicines in development.* Retrieved from http://www.phrma.org/newmedicines/

newmedsdb/drugs.cfm?indicationcode=Prevention+of+Human+Pap...

Porth, C. M. (2005). *Pathophysiology: Concepts of altered health states* (7th ed.). Philadelphia: Lippincott.

Snapshot. New trends in STDs in the U.S. (2005). *Contraceptive Technology Update, March.* STD Quarterly, 4.

STD rates soaring: HPA promotes "safe, responsible sex." (2005, January). *RCM Midwives Journal, P.* 2.

Sterk, C., Klein, H., & Elifson, K. (2004). Predictors of condom-related attitudes among at-risk women. *Journal of Women's Health, 13*(6), 676–688.

Tierney, L. M., McPhee, S. J., & Papadakis, M. A. (Eds.). (2004). *Current medical diagnosis & treatment* (43rd ed.). Stamford, CT: Appleton & Lange.

What is the role of herpes virus serology in sexually transmitted disease screening? (2005). *Evidence-Based Practice, 8*(2), 4.

Young men not included in chlamydia testing. (2005). *Practice Nurse, 29*(3), 10l.

Wilson, B., Shannon, M., & Stang, C. (2005). *Nurse's drug guide 2005.* Upper Saddle River, NJ: Prentice Hall.

Case Study

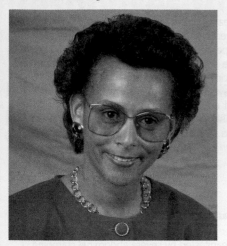

Eva Gibson, a 43-year-old married housewife with two children, had a routine annual mammogram that revealed a mass in the left breast. She has a family history of breast cancer with her mother and a maternal aunt having breast cancer. She was admitted to outpatient surgery for an incisional biopsy, with results of invasive lobular carcinoma. An MRI was performed, which indicated that four axillary glands have been infiltrated with cancer. She was admitted to the hospital and a modified radical mastectomy on the left side is performed. Postoperatively, she is admitted to the chemotherapy unit. Vital signs are T 98.5°F, P 65, R 14, BP 110/68. She has a dressing on the left chest that is dry and intact and the JP drain is intact for suction. Her left arm is elevated on two pillows. The decision has been made to start radiation and chemotherapy treatments as soon as possible.

The pathophysiology of breast cancer is a mutation of breast tissue cells related to hormones and mutations of tumor suppressor genes. Abnormal cell growth occurs. Cancer cells create a factor that stimulates blood vessels to grow into the tumor. Cancer cells invade the blood vessels and travel through the bloodstream or through the lymphatic system to other sites. Manifestations of breast cancer include nontender lump in the breast, abnormal nipple discharge, rash around the nipple area, nipple retraction, edema, dimpling of the skin, or change in position of the nipple. Some women report a burning or stinging sensation in the breast or nipple pain. Complications of breast cancer are metastasis to bone, brain, lung, liver, skin, and lymph nodes, and death.

Based on the client's surgery of modified radical mastectomy and treatment with radiation and chemotherapy, the nursing diagnosis of *Risk for Infection* is appropriate for planning care for Mrs. Gibson.

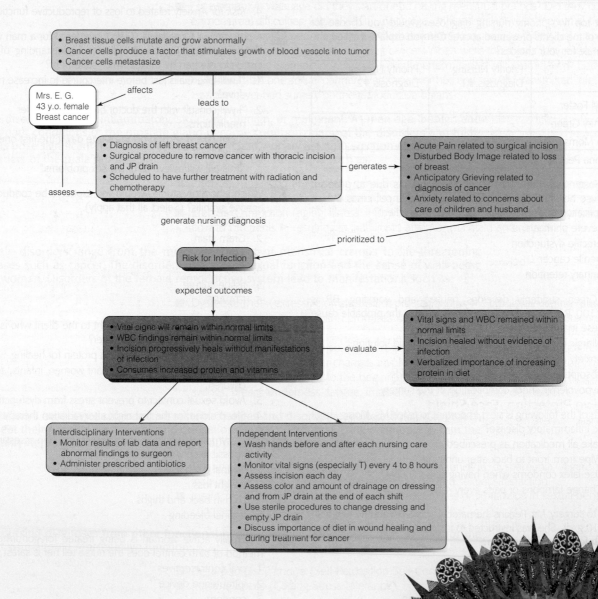

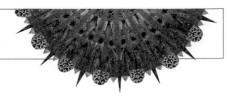
Standard precautions are designed to reduce the risk of transmission of microorganisms from both recognized and unrecognized sources of infection. They are the primary strategies for preventing nosocomial infections within institutions, and are important to protect healthcare workers as well. Standard precautions apply to (1) blood; (2) all body fluids, secretions, and excretions except sweat, regardless of whether or not they contain visible blood; (3) nonintact skin; and (4) mucous membranes. Standard precautions are applied to all clients receiving care in hospitals, regardless of their diagnosis or presumed infection status. These precautions are specifically designed for hospitals; however, they also may be implemented in extended and long-term care facilities, and to a more limited extent in providing home care or in other community-based care settings.

Hand Washing

- Wash your hands (a) after touching blood, body fluids, secretions, excretions, and contaminated items, whether or not gloves are worn; (b) immediately after removing gloves, even if gloves appear to be intact; (c) between contacts with clients; and (d) when otherwise indicated to prevent transfer of organisms to other clients. You may need to wash your hands between tasks and procedures on the same client to prevent cross-contaminating different body sites.
- Use soap and warm water for hand washing when hands are visibly dirty or contaminated with blood or other body fluids.
- If hands are not visibly soiled, use an alcohol-based hand rub for routinely decontaminating hands in all other situations.

Gloves

- Wear clean, nonsterile gloves when touching blood, body fluids, secretions, excretions, and contaminated items.
- Put on clean gloves just before touching mucous membranes and nonintact skin.
- Change your gloves between tasks and procedures on the same client after contacting material that may contain a high concentration of microorganisms.
- Wear gloves for all invasive procedures such as performing venipuncture or other vascular or surgical procedures.
- Wear gloves if you have cuts, scratches, or other breaks in the skin.
- Remove gloves promptly after use, before touching noncontaminated items and surfaces, and before going to another client; wash hands immediately after removing gloves.

Mask, Eye Protection, Face Shield

Wear a mask and eye protection or a face shield to protect mucous membranes of your eyes, nose, and mouth during procedures and client care activities that are likely to generate splashes or sprays of blood, body fluids, secretions, or excretions.

Gown

Wear a gown (clean, disposable) to protect your skin and prevent soiling of clothing during procedures and client care activities that are likely to generate splashes or sprays of blood, body fluids, secretions, or excretions. Remove soiled gowns promptly, washing your hands immediately after gown removal.

Equipment

Handle used client care equipment that is soiled with blood, body fluids, secretions, and excretions in a way that prevents exposing your skin and mucous membranes, contaminating your clothing, and transferring microorganisms to other clients or environments. Ensure that reusable equipment is cleaned and appropriately reprocessed before using for the care of another client.

Environmental Control

Follow hospital procedures for routine care, cleaning, and disinfecting environmental surfaces, beds, bed rails, bedside equipment, and other frequently touched surfaces.

Linen

Handle and transport linens soiled with blood, body fluids, secretions, and excretions in a manner that prevents exposing your skin and mucous membranes, contaminating your clothing, and transferring microorganisms to other clients and environments. Place soiled linen in leakage-resistant bags at the location where it is used.

Occupational Health and Bloodborne Pathogens

- Take care to prevent injuries when using needles, scalpels, and other sharps; when handling sharp instruments after procedures; when cleaning used instruments; and when disposing of used needles.
- Never recap used needles, manipulate them using both hands, or handle them in a manner that directs the point of a needle toward any part of your body. If it is necessary to protect the needle prior to disposal, use a one-handed "scoop" technique or mechanical device to hold the needle sheath.
- Do not remove used needles from disposable syringes by hand; do not bend, break, or otherwise manipulate used needles by hand.
- Place used disposable syringes and needles, scalpel blades, and other sharp items in appropriate puncture-resistant containers located as close as practical to the area in which the items were used.
- Place reusable syringes and needles in a puncture-resistant container for transport to the reprocessing area.
- Use mouthpieces, resuscitation bags, or other ventilation devices as an alternative to mouth-to-mouth resuscitation methods whenever possible.

Client Placement

Place clients who contaminate the environment or who do not (or are not expected to) assist in maintaining appropriate hygiene or environmental control (e.g., an ambulatory, confused client with fecal incontinence) in a private room.

Sources. *Centers for Disease Control and Prevention. (2002). Guidelines for hand hygiene in health-care settings: Recommendations of the Healthcare Infection Control Practices Advisory Committee and the HICPAC/SHEA/APIC/IDSA Hand Hygiene Taskforce. MMWR, 51(RR-16), 1–56; Hospital Infection Control Practices Advisory Committee. (1997). Part II. Recommendations for isolation precautions in hospitals. Atlanta: Public Health Service, U.S. Department of Health and Human Services, Centers for Disease Control and Prevention.*

greatest risk for falls and injury in the home due to sensory problems including vision loss, unsteady gait, loss of sensation to hot and cold, and loss of sense of smell and taste to identify spoiled food. Substance abuse is more important to address with the young adult and adolescent population, as well as family roles and tasks. Treating acute illness is something all populations may benefit from, but not nearly as vital to seniors as accident prevention in the home.

10. **Answer: 3, 4 Rationale:** Recognizing that dying is a part of living is part of adjusting to aging and recognizing the bodily changes that occur as a result of aging. Coping with loss is part of the grieving process that the widowed spouse must endure as the result of death of a loved one. Although coping with the lack of privacy may occur if they move in with other family members, that is not what is being addressed here. Planning for retirement may be part of what is happening, but is not what is occurring in this setting. Relating to kin may also be occurring, but is not pertinent to this situation.

Chapter 3: Community-Based and Home Care of the Adult Client

1. **Answer: 3 Rationale:** Although all of the choices listed in this question are part of community-based nursing care, the primary focus is individual and family health. Interventions that deal with the function and health of the community are based on individual and family needs.

2. **Answer: 1 Rationale:** Access to healthcare services may be more challenging for rural residents due to transportation issues. Urban residents often have easier access to public transportation to obtain healthcare services. Age and gender of residents, family tasks and values, and ability to follow directions are similar between urban and rural residents.

3. **Answer: 2 Rationale:** Parish nursing is often organized through church services, also known as a faith community. Although some of the services may include respite care, day care, or block nursing, these are not the only services parish nursing may offer clients.

4. **Answer: 4 Rationale:** Respite care provides assistance to full-time caregivers and helps relieve some of the stress associated with this huge responsibility. Although this may be one of the services parishes or block nursing may provide, the official term is respite care. Day care is reserved for children or adults in need of supervision outside of the home, whereas respite care often takes place in the home.

5. **Answer: 1, 3, 4 Rationale:** Mrs. Jones, who cannot live independently at home due to a broken hip, would benefit from home care. A home health aide can assist her with activities of daily living, and a physical therapist may help her with improving her mobility. Miss Ace should not require home care services as her illness is self-limiting and she should be more independent very soon. Mr. Strip would benefit from home care, as he is terminal and wishes to die at home. Hospice care would be an excellent choice. Miss Taylor would benefit from home care as she lives alone and may not be completely independent due to her major abdominal surgery. Mr. Wines is not in need of home care as weakness due to arthritis is not an appropriate reason, further we do not know if he lives alone or not.

6. **Answer: 4 Rationale:** Home care nurses must advocate for their clients by having all necessary paperwork to provide care, which includes advance directives, living wills, and durable power of attorney. Although home care nurses may also func-

tion as providers of direct care, coordinator of services, and educators, these are not part of the role discussed above.

7. **Answer: 4 Rationale:** The registered nurse is the person responsible for care coordination. This is done with the initial visit to assess the individual's need of services and will continue to be evaluated on an ongoing basis. The physician orders services, but leaves the scope of services up to the agency to determine the need. The social worker makes the initial contact with the agency to determine access. The home health aide assists with normal activities.

8. **Answer: 1 Rationale:** Medicare is the largest single reimbursement source for home care. Medicaid, private insurance, and self-pay also provide reimbursement, but not in as great a scope as Medicare.

9. **Answer: 2 Rationale:** Hand washing is the most important factor to help prevent infection in the home. Although it is also important for home care nurses to perform needs assessments regarding fire and smoke detector function, fall prevention, and proper medication administration, the only education factor to prevent the spread of infection is hand washing.

10. **Answer: 4 Rationale:** A treatment form is needed in order to receive reimbursement from insurance. Family member approval is not needed for reimbursement. Completion of agency forms is important for communication between agency personnel, but not for reimbursement. A physician order is needed to start the process of home care, but not for reimbursement of services.

Chapter 4: Nursing Care of Clients Having Surgery

1. **Answer: 2 Rationale:** The nurse's primary responsibility to informed consent is serving as a witness to the client signature on the consent form. It is the physician's responsibility to define the risks and benefits of surgery, as well as explain the right to refuse treatment or withdraw consent, and advise the client and family about what is needed for diagnosis. The nurse may reinforce all of these issues, but they primarily fall under the role of the physician.

2. **Answer: 4 Rationale:** Obtaining a preoperative blood pressure is necessary to provide a baseline for post-operative care. This helps assess for any post-operative blood loss or hemorrhaging. This has no legal requirement issue and is not necessary for induction with anesthesia or preventing atelectasis.

3. **Answer: 3 Rationale:** Nonsteroidal anti-inflammatory drugs potentiate analgesia and reduce inflammation caused from surgery. They do not stimulate appetite, increase amnesia, or improve renal function.

4. **Answer: 2 Rationale:** A high protein diet is important to help with healing post-operatively. Low-fat, high fiber may also be important; however, the most important factor is high protein.

5. **Answer: 4 Rationale:** Neurovascular assessments are important to assess for any complications of surgery such as a blood clot after knee surgery. Urinary pH is not important. Rebound tenderness and Chvostek's sign are not part of post-operative assessments for knee surgery.

6. **Answer: 3 Rationale:** Medications must be reordered post-operatively, as the needs may have changed as a result of surgery. It is not a nursing responsibility to determine if decreasing the dose is needed or to withhold until anesthesia wears off.

7. **Answer: 4 Rationale:** Anesthetic agents cause paralysis and block sympathetic nervous system control. This blocks signs and symptoms of hypoglycemia and could prevent recognition of the condition.

8. **Answer: 3 Rationale:** It is expected that pain is a result of any surgical procedure. Clients may not exhibit signs and symptoms of pain initially due to effects of anesthesia. Medications should be provided regularly to help maintain adequate pain control and help promote rapid recovery.

9. **Answer: 4 Rationale:** The metal OR tables have no cushioning and the OR environment is often kept cooler. The client has to be positioned appropriately for the procedures. This can cause pressure areas to boney prominences. Since the skin of elderly clients is less elastic and more fragile, skin tears may result. The lower temperature in the OR environment can decrease skin circulation. This, compounded with the positioning and the predisposing risks of skin impairment, can cause pressure sores and joint pain.

10. **Answer: 4 Rationale:** Hypothermia can result from the OR environment and prolonged exposure during this period. Anesthesia blocks sympathetic nervous system stimulation, preventing the client from shivering to help increase body temperature. Thus, it is necessary for the nurse to intervene in order to help increase the body temperature.

Chapter 5: Nursing Care of Clients Experiencing Loss, Grief, and Death

1. **Answer: 3 Rationale:** Only the person experiencing loss can evaluate their experiences. This is very individualized and cannot be judged by others. Although cultural values and support of friends and family may impact loss, many other factors affect the ability to cope with loss.

2. **Answer: 4 Rationale:** Denial is often the first stage of grief. Although the different stages of grief do not really go in order, denial is an exception. This is often the first reaction, and the client may go back to denial when going through the grieving process.

3. **Answer: 2 Rationale:** A strong support system of friends and family is extremely important in helping one through the grieving process and to cope with loss. The client does not expect those in their support system to fix their situation but to simply provide moral support and listen for when he/she is ready to talk. Each individual will go through the grieving process in his or her own way and on his or her own time.

4. **Answer: 1 Rationale:** Culture is what dictates the rituals of mourning. This does not replace the grieving process, but is simply part of acceptance in the process. The individual will continue to grieve for the loss in his or her own way. Culture simply provides a pathway to express the loss.

5. **Answer: 2 Rationale:** A living will expresses the exact wishes of a client regarding expectations for medical care. It addresses what the client is willing to or not willing to endure to sustain life. This takes the decision from other family members and provides the client with peace of mind in knowing his/her wishes will be followed.

6. **Answer: 3 Rationale:** Hospice care is for clients suffering from terminal illnesses. Hospice is designed to meet the needs of the client's end-of-life care by providing quality to the time that remains. Although Hospice Homes exist, hospice represents a model of nursing care more than a location.

7. **Answer: 4 Rationale:** We as nurses develop partnerships with our clients regarding their care. End-of-life care is no exception. It is necessary to respect the client's wishes and withhold pain medications. Other methods of pain control can be suggested such as relaxation therapy, therapeutic touch, or positioning for comfort.

8. **Answer: 1 Rationale:** Comatose clients cannot see. As circulation becomes more impaired, sense of touch is diminished. In many near death experiences, clients have recalled hearing the voices of those taking care of them. It is thought that the sense of hearing is the last sense to go before death occurs.

9. **Answer: 3 Rationale:** It is important to continue to manage pain at all times of life, especially in end-of-life care. Terminal illnesses cause great pain and the goal of hospice nursing is to help provide quality to the client's remaining time including helping the client to maintain comfort and be as free of pain as possible.

10. **Answer: 2 Rationale:** The open-ended statement of acknowledging to the woman "This must be a difficult time for you"" is the best choice. This provides the woman to opportunity to express her feelings, recognizing the nurse's willingness to listen.

Chapter 6: Nursing Care of Clients with Problems of Substance Abuse

1. **Answer: 2 Rationale:** The minimum level of alcohol in the blood to consider the individual to be intoxicated is 0.08%. The allowable blood alcohol level for driving in some states is 0.1%, but this has now been lowered to 0.08% in many states.

2. **Answer: 1 Rationale:** Asking a client how many days a week he/she drinks alcoholic beverages is very general. It does not force the client into a defensive "no" answer. It provides an avenue for discussion, which could lead to more specific information.

3. **Answer: 4 Rationale:** Clients suffering from chronic alcoholism have significant malnutrition issues. Thiamine depletion can cause neurological problems and cognitive impairment, known as Wernicke-Korsakoff syndrome. Wernicke's encephalopathy is the acute stage of the disease and Korsakoff's psychosis is the chronic stage of the disease. Thiamine replacement can help prevent this from occurring.

4. **Answer: 3 Rationale:** Alcohol and CNS depressants present the greatest risk during withdrawal due to concerns of seizures and delirium tremens. The brain becomes overly excited since the receptors are no longer being blocked. Delirium tremens from alcohol withdrawal has a mortality rate of 1-5%.

5. **Answer: 2 Rationale:** Clients who suffer from alcoholism feel a sense of enjoyment when they start drinking. Antabuse takes away this pleasant sensation and replaces it, causing physical illness and intense vomiting. Antabuse prevents the breakdown of alcohol if taken while the person is drinking. The goal in taking away the enjoyment of drinking and replacing it with this negative reinforcement is to decrease the desire to drink and help facilitate recovery.

6. **Answer: 3 Rationale:** Clients reporting effective pain control are receiving their needed medications. If clients were consistently reporting poor pain control, this would be more of a cause for concern.

7. **Answer: 2 Rationale:** The smoking rates for women have not steadily declined since the 1950s. In fact, this population has had a rise in the smoking rate.

8. **Answer: 4 Rationale:** It is a good idea for clients to wear a medic alert bracelet while on naltrexone. This medication blocks opiate receptors in the brain that trigger the feelings of pleasure experienced when taking alcohol or narcotics. In case of emergency medical treatment, it is important for caregivers to know the client is taking naltrexone to prevent administration of any narcotics.

9. **Answer: 1 Rationale:** Identifying alternative ways of dealing with stressful situations is key. It is unrealistic to think the craving will

go away. The craving will always be there. It is more important to understand how to cope. Focusing on the past will not help solve the problems of the future, it just causes unnecessary pain and encourages feelings of failure and inadequacy. Avoiding using alcohol or drugs is needed. It is not possible to limit to only one.

10. **Answer: 3 Rationale:** *Ineffective Denial* is the best choice. 1. is not an option since nutrition is often imbalanced due to malnutrition, not excess food intake. 2. is not an option since clients often are not taking vitamins or supplements and even if they do, it would not cause fluid overload. 4. is not an option since there is no infectious process present.

Chapter 7: Nursing Care of Clients Experiencing Disasters

1. **Answer: 3 Rationale:** Emergencies are not controlled. Disasters do not only result from man-made errors, but can be caused by nature. Disasters often involve multiple services and agencies working together.

2. **Answer: 3 Rationale:** Nurses are an integral part in assisting with disasters. However, they do not serve in a leadership role in the command center. Their role is in assisting with triage and in meeting the emergency healthcare needs of those injured or involved in the disaster.

3. **Answer: 4 Rationale:** Reverse triage is necessary when there are limited resources to care for multiple people injured in a disaster. This is so the majority of people can be helped with the resources currently available.

4. **Answer: 3 Rationale:** It is important to recognize that a client whose primary language is not English may not read in his or her primary language. This can create a significant problem when providing health education. It is important to have someone translate all information to the client and have the client explain what has been taught in order to ensure proper understanding of the information.

5. **Answer: 3 Rationale:** PPE should lessen the likelihood of occupational injury and/or illness, but proper precautions also must be taken to ensure safety. This can be as simple as proper hand washing after removing gloves, or following isolation guidelines.

6. **Answer: 2 Rationale:** Decontamination cannot begin in the hot zone as this is the area of greatest contamination. It is important to decontaminate the area outside of the hot zone to prevent its spread.

7. **Answer: 1 Rationale:** A dirty bomb is a bomb that carries a radiological signature and can cause contamination and radiation poisoning.

8. **Answer: 2 Rationale:** Radiation sickness is the direct result of exposure to ionizing radiation, which causes cellular mutation. This condition must be treated rapidly or death may result as the cells continue to mutate and die.

9. **Answer: 3 Rationale:** Older adults have individual needs. Some may be more independent than others regarding the degree of support needed in emergencies, whereas others may require multiple resources and support in an evacuation.

10. **Answer: 4 Rationale:** Nurses often are so involved in caring for others they tend to neglect themselves. In disaster situations, nurses may also suffer from loss while caring for others. As a result the nurse may feel overwhelmed and be as traumatized as those for whom he/she is caring.

Chapter 8: Genetic Implications of Adult Health Nursing

1. **Answer: 2 Rationale:** In an autosomal dominant condition, you only need one of the genotypes to have the condition. An autosomal dominant condition is not a sex-linked disease and is not found on the x or y chromosomes.

2. **Answer: 1, 3 Rationale:** Fabry disease is an x-linked genetic disorder. Since the male provides the y chromosome to a male offspring, the male cannot pass on this disease to male offspring. The female can pass this disorder on. Also, which grandmother (maternal or fraternal) is not stated, and if the grandmother was not affected, she could be a carrier since her brother had the disease.

3. **Answer: 4 Rationale:** It is a nurse's responsibility to explain what is involved in genetic testing. It is not the nurse's responsibility to discuss potential outcomes, as this is the responsibility of the genetic counselor.

4. **Answer: 1, 4 Rationale:** Breast cancer at this early an age is most likely to have a genetic component that makes the client more likely to have this condition. A brother's unexpected infertility can be cause for alarm in many genetic conditions.

5. **Answer: 5 Rationale:** Mitochondrial mutations are only passed from the mother. This is because mitochondria are primarily found in ova and not sperm. This is considered a matrilineal pattern of inheritance. An affected female will pass the condition on to her children; however, an affected male will not.

6. **Answer: 1, 2 Rationale:** Performing a family history assessment helps the nurse know what is important to focus on regarding health promotion and maintenance when planning. This is necessary in order to individualize the treatment plan to best meet the needs of the client and family. This also provides the opportunity to encourage preventative and prophylactic treatments to promote wellness. This is not done to determine specific genotypes, but family and environmental influences on health behavior.

7. **Answer: 3 Rationale:** It is not important to include all details for all those included in the pedigree. It is more important to know cause of death, chronic illness, and age. The paternal side of the family is usually placed on the left and the maternal on the right. A minimum of three generations should be included and labeled appropriately. The proband should be marked with an arrow and a "P" so it is easy to identify.

8. **Answer: 1, 2, 4 Rationale:** Minor physical anomalies are simply visual. However, an ASD is a functional defect, which can impair activity and cause severe complications, as the client gets older.

9. **Answer: 2, 3 Rationale:** Certification status is appropriate as it explains that the results of the testing can be considered reliable. CLIA88 = Clinical Laboratory Improvement Amendment 88 (this is the year the law was amended) is an accreditation for certification, and contains a full list of the certifications for the laboratory. This is done on a yearly basis. It is important to explain that a mutation panel can address the most common gene alterations, but not all.

10. **Answer: 2, 4 Rationale:** Often tests will be ordered at the initial visit to look at chromosome studies. Once the results are received, the client will be informed of the findings. The role of the genetic healthcare provider is to present the client with accurate information to make informed decisions and provide information about the natural history of the condition.

Chapter 9: Nursing Care of Clients Experiencing Pain

1. **Answer: 2 Rationale:** Chronic pain, pain that has been ongoing for more than six months, is the most appropriate answer. Acute pain is sudden in onset and has not been ongoing for

more than six months. Referred pain is pain that originates in another location. Somatic pain is considered to be psychological in origin.

2. **Answer: 1 Rationale:** It is very important to provide medication to prevent pain and to help keep pain from getting worse rather than waiting until it does get bad. Pain causes release of chemical mediators that attach to pain receptors, causing pain to be more intense, difficult to treat, and get in control.

3. **Answer: 2 Rationale:** NSAIDs are known to cause problems with gastric ulcerations. Taking an NSAID for years can cause significant problems with erosion.

4. **Answer: 4 Rationale:** Transdermal pain medications are most effective when placed on the upper torso. This is because the medication is absorbed through the surface of the skin and returned to the heart, where circulation is better than in distal extremities.

5. **Answer: 3 Rationale:** This statement is most appropriate as the nurse is asking for a description of the pain, which addresses the quality.

6. **Answer: 2 Rationale:** An overdose can occur as clients can become over-sedated and develop respiratory depression.

7. **Answer: 2 Rationale:** Constipation, nausea, and sedation are all very common side effects of opioid analgesia. The narcotic slows down peristalsis, causing constipation and nausea. Sedation is caused from the opioids crossing the blood-brain barrier.

8. **Answer: 2 Rationale:** Oral opioid analgesia is the recommended route for chronic pain.

9. **Answer: 4 Rationale:** The equivalent dose of an oral drug compared to the intravenous preparation of the same drug is often significantly less effective. It may take about five times the dose to equal the IV dose.

10. **Answer: 4 Rationale:** Clients treated for chronic pain may need additional pain management strategies to help manage breakthrough pain, acute pain, and end-of-dose pain. In addition to chronic pain, clients often have flares of acute pain. As the pain medication wears off, there may be breakthrough pain or end-of-dose pain.

Chapter 10: Nursing Care of Clients with Altered Fluid, Electrolyte, and Acid-Base Balance

1. **Answer: 1 Rationale:** Ringer's solution is an Isotonic, balanced electrolyte solution that can expand plasma volume and help restore electrolyte balance. Hypertonic solutions such as 10% dextrose and 3% sodium chloride pull interstitial and intracellular fluid into the vascular system, leading to cellular dehydration. A hypotonic solution such as 0.45% sodium chloride may be used to treat cellular dehydration.

2. **Answer: 4 Rationale:** In fluid volume deficit, there is less volume in the vascular system, which decreases venous return and cardiac output, leading to manifestations of dizziness, orthostatic hypotension and flat neck veins. The heart rate increases and the blood pressure falls. Dyspnea and crackles usually are associated with excess fluid volume; headache and muscle cramps are often due to electrolyte imbalance, not fluid loss.

3. **Answer: 1, 3, 4 Rationale:** Frequent neurological checks are necessary as hypernatremia draws water out of brain cells, causing them to shrink. As the brain shrinks, tension is placed on cerebral vessels, which may cause them to tear and bleed. Hypernatremia affects mental status and brain function (including orientation to time, place and person), as can rapid correction of hypernatremia. Fluid replacement is the primary treatment for hypernatremia. Maintaining intravenous access is necessary for administration of fluids and possible emergency medications. There is no reason to limit visit length.

4. **Answer: 2 Rationale:** Hypokalemia affects nerve impulse transmission, including the transmission of cardiac impulses. The client may develop ECG changes and atrial or ventricular dysrhythmias. Although hypokalemia can lead to muscle weakness and activity intolerance, bedrest generally is unnecessary.

5. **Answer: 4 Rationale:** Calcium should be taken with a full glass of water to allow maximum absorption. It is more effectively absorbed when taken on an empty stomach and the prescribed doses spaced throughout the day.

6. **Answer: 1 Rationale:** A positive Chvostek's sign indicates increased neuromuscular excitability, commonly associated with both hypomagnesia and hypocalcemia. Additional manifestations of hypomagnesemia include confusion, hallucinations, and possible psychoses. Administration of magnesium sulfate helps restore magnesium balance and neuromuscular function.

7. **Answer: 1 Rationale:** The pH is indicative of acidosis (less than 7.35), and the bicarbonate level is low (less than 22 mEq/L), indicating bicarbonate deficit as cause of the acidosis. In addition, the $PaCO_2$ is low (less than 35 mmHg), indicating respiratory compensation for the excess acid.

8. **Answer: 1, 3, 5 Rationale:** The slow respiratory rate leads to inadequate alveolar ventilation. As a result, carbon dioxide is not effectively eliminated from the blood, causing it to accumulate. This increases carbonic acid levels, leading to respiratory acidosis, as indicated by the low pH and high $PaCO_2$. Excess carbon dioxide causes vasodilation, leading to warm, flushed skin, particularly in acute respiratory acidosis.

9. **Answer: 1 Rationale:** Gastric suctioning removes highly acidic gastric secretions, increasing the alkalinity of body fluids. Chloride, the primary anion in extracellular fluid, also is lost through gastric suction, causing the kidneys to retain bicarbonate to restore the balance between positively and negatively charged ions in the body.

10. **Answer: 3 Rationale:** The client is demonstrating classic manifestations of respiratory alkalosis, a potential complication of mechanical ventilation when the rate or volume of ventilations are too high. Arterial blood gases provide the data necessary to confirm and treat this problem.

Chapter 11: Nursing Care of the Client Experiencing Trauma and Shock

1. **Answer: 4 Rationale:** Although all of the choices can be sources of injury or death in adults of all ages, motor vehicle accidents remain the leading cause of injury. As people become more aware of the need for seatbelts and other safety considerations, the fatality rate of motor vehicle accidents decreases.

2. **Answer: 1 Rationale:** Airway obstruction is the first and foremost risk to assess for, as this represents the ABCs of life support. A = airway, B = breathing, C = circulation. Although all of the other choices can also be present, a patent airway must be the number one priority for survival.

3. **Answer: 2 Rationale:** Assessing airway patency is the first step in the ABCs of life support. Although the rest of the choices listed are important to assess also, the first and foremost intervention is the airway patency.

4. **Answer: 3 Rationale:** The most severe reaction is decreasing blood pressure and dyspnea.

5. **Answer: 2 Rationale:** The endotoxins released from bacteria in septic shock stimulate the release of vasoactive proteins causing peripheral vasodilation and decreased peripheral resistance.

6. **Answer: 1 Rationale:** Direct pressure to the wound is the best method to manage uncontrolled bleeding. If 1. is ineffective, then it is necessary to consider the other options. However, in the field, 1. is definitely the first choice.

7. **Answer: 1 Rationale:** Trauma is defined as injury to human tissues from the transfer of energy. It is not specific to intentional or accidental. It simply addresses tissue injury. Knowing the type of energy can help understand the severity of tissue injury.

8. **Answer: 4 Rationale:** Weight gain is not a risk from a blood transfusion.

9. **Answer: 2 Rationale:** Widespread vasodilation can cause distributive shock as the blood pressure drops dangerously due to the very low peripheral vascular resistance. A hypersensitivity reaction will cause anaphylactic shock, not distributive shock.

10. **Answer: 4 Rationale:** Ultimately there is a systemic imbalance between oxygen supply and demand. Sufficient cardiac output is not shock, insufficient cardiac output is. Hemorrhage is a cause of one of the types of shock, but does not define shock. Abnormal blood pressure may be either high or low.

Chapter 12: Nursing Care of Clients with Infections

1. **Answer: 3 Rationale:** Natural passive immunity is the result of a gamma globulin infusion following exposure to hepatitis A. This type of immunity is short-lived and usually lasts only about four weeks. This is considered "borrowed immunity."

2. **Answer: 2 Rationale:** Enlarged lymph nodes are a common physical finding of a systemic infection, as the immune system is actively trying to fight this infection. Lymph node enlargement is stimulated by full activation of the immune system. Pain and erythema can be a symptom of a local infection, but these are not specific to systemic symptoms. A decreased heart rate is a late symptom of shock, not simply a systemic infection.

3. **Answer: 4 Rationale:** Although the exact mechanism of action is unknown, aspirin inhibits prostaglandin synthesis. This can serve many purposes including producing analgesia, anti-inflammatory and anti-pyretic effects, and inhibit platelet aggregation.

4. **Answer: 1 Rationale:** A "left shift" is commonly referred to when there is an increase in band neutrophils. This is to be expected when the body is mounting a response to a bacterial infection. This occurs when the bone marrow is stimulated to rapidly produce more white blood cells. The bone marrow starts churning out increased quantities of immature white blood cells, otherwise known as bands.

5. **Answer: 2 Rationale:** Contact precautions are the form of isolation recommended for an MRSA wound. This requires a gown to be worn for any direct client contact and gloves to be worn upon entering the room. Good hand washing is essential after removing gloves, as the gloves do not ensure cleanliness of the hands.

6. **Answer: 1 Rationale:** The T cells of the immune system adapt to kill intracellular organisms. These can be viral-infected cells, cancer cells, or foreign tissue. This is part of humoral immunity and is a cell-mediated response. All of the other choices are occurring outside of the cells.

7. **Answer: 1 Rationale:** Thrombocytosis is best explained as increased platelets. This causes platelet aggregation and increases clot formation.

8. **Answer: 4 Rationale:** When there is a nursing diagnosis "Risk for Infection," this can pertain to the client, caregivers, or other clients. It addresses the possibility that the client cannot fight infection, the staff is potentially at risk for developing an infection from the infected client, or the other clients are at risk for becoming infected from the infected client.

9. **Answer: 4 Rationale:** When administering antibiotics, the nurse must be aware of potential hypersensitivity reactions. It is important to monitor for any hypersensitivities in addition to providing education about the infection, antibiotic, and any potential side effects of treatment.

10. **Answer: 3 Rationale:** Wearing gloves, gowns, and goggles when coming in contact with contaminated body fluids is considered to be a standard procedure.

Chapter 13: Nursing Care of Clients with Altered Immunity

1. **Answer: 4 Rationale:** Anaphylaxis occurs as the direct result from a Type 1 hypersensitivity reaction. The body has IgE circulating, which is specific to a certain allergen. Allergen re-exposure causes this cascade leading to anaphylaxis.

2. **Answer: 1 Rationale:** An acute tissue rejection episode is the most common and treatable type of rejection. It occurs between four days and three months after the transplant. Symptoms can include fever and tenderness over the liver, and elevated liver enzymes and bilirubin levels.

3. **Answer: 3 Rationale:** These symptoms are indicative of a respiratory infection. Of the choices listed, pneumocystis carinii is the choice that causes the respiratory infection known as PCP.

4. **Answer: 4 Rationale:** When a client tests positive for HIV, this means that antibodies to the AIDS virus are present in the blood. HIV does not equal AIDS. It is important for the nurse to be able to explain the difference between HIV and AIDS to the client. AIDS is diagnosed when the CD4 count drops below 200. The client needs to understand that AIDS could develop in the future, especially without treatment.

5. **Answer: 2 Rationale:** Leukopenia can be an adverse reaction of Retrovir. As Retrovir can cause bone marrow suppression and pancytopenia, CBCs should be done on a routine basis, in addition to other lab work to assess the t-cell levels plus any other warranted lab work.

6. **Answer: 2 Rationale:** Of all of the choices available, the allergen prick testing has the lowest risk of anaphylaxis associated with it. This is because there is the smallest amount of allergen entering the bloodstream. This is also the most accurate way to assess for allergies as the wheal and flare will only occur with the allergens that are positive.

7. **Answer: 2 Rationale:** When hypersensitivity is suspected it is important to avoid any further exposure to the potential cause. The best way to do this is by replacing all tubing and attaching a new line primed with NS.

8. **Answer: 2 Rationale:** Protease inhibitors and nucleoside analogs are associated with serious metabolic problems such as elevated cholesterol and triglycerides, insulin resistance and diabetes mellitus, and changes in body fat composition. These can be very distressing to clients.

9. **Answer: 4 Rationale:** The priority when initiating or changing HIV drug therapy regimens is the client's willingness to adhere

to the drug regimen. This is due to the high resistance to therapy associated when clients choose to discontinue treatment with their anti-viral medications. Since the side effects can be difficult and challenging to overcome, many clients are not willing to continue with their therapy.

10. **Answer: 4 Rationale:** Antithymocyte globulin (ATG) is used to induce immunosuppression immediately following a transplant. Its purpose is to bind with the peripheral lymphocytes and mononuclear cells to remove them from circulation and prevent them from being able to reject the new organ.

Chapter 14: Nursing Care of Clients with Cancer

1. **Answer: 3 Rationale:** Metastasis occurs when cells from a primary tumor site travel through the lymphatic system or bloodstream to find a secondary target.

2. **Answer: 1 Rationale:** One of the many qualities those of us in nursing possess is the ability to listen. Often, when clients are dealing with a difficult diagnosis with a questionable future, this quality helps the client to cope. Encouraging the client to express his feelings about the cancer diagnosis is the most valuable and powerful intervention that could be offered. It is important to document on the chart the client's report of difficulty sleeping and tenseness in order to communicate with other staff, but this is not the primary intervention. It also may be a good idea to obtain an order for medication for sleep from the physician, but again, this is not the best primary intervention. Offering an antianxiety drug may be helpful, but this is not the primary need.

3. **Answer: 3 Rationale:** It is important not to rub or scratch the treated skin areas, as this can cause irritation to the surface of the skin as well as breaks in the skin. Rubbing may also wipe off the ink markings, which are important landmarks to ensure that the radiation treatments are directed to the correct location.

4. **Answer: 2 Rationale:** Providing an antiemetic prior to chemotherapy is an excellent preventative treatment to prevent nausea and vomiting following chemotherapy. This helps to improve the quality of life the client has while in treatment. We know that feeling very ill can increase symptoms of depression; thus, providing the antiemetic prior to the chemotherapy can improve Ms. Smith's general outlook.

5. **Answer: 3 Rationale:** Although all of these choices can be a result of chemotherapy, the one that is directly affected with bone marrow suppression is a low platelet count of 50,000. A fever can also be caused from the degree of neutropenia, as Ms. Smith is not able to fight infection. However, the most correct answer remains c.

6. **Answer: 3 Rationale:** Chemotherapy is not cell type specific. It simply targets cells that are rapidly dividing, which can be both cancer cells and healthy cells. It is important to understand that as normal cells are destroyed, this can cause other symptoms such as mucositis, hair loss, and bone marrow suppression.

7. **Answer: 1 Rationale:** External radiation therapy is when the radiation is initiated outside of the body, directed towards the client, and is set to deliver to a certain depth for a specified period of time. This exposure is meant to destroy the cancer cells the radiation comes into direct contact with.

8. **Answer: 2 Rationale:** Tumor lysis syndrome can cause high levels of uric acid. Clients are often treated with allopurinal to help excrete the uric acid in the urine. Also, electrolyte imbalances may occur and need to be monitored and replaced as needed. Often the client may suffer from low potassium, phosphorus, and calcium levels. This can cause a multitude of problems including severe life-threatening arrhythmias.

9. **Answer: 3 Rationale:** The S phase is when DNA replication occurs. This is when the cell is beginning mitosis and the chromosomes multiply from 23 to 46. They then migrate towards each axis in preparation for division of the cell.

10. **Answer: 1 Rationale:** Oncogenes are genes that stimulate cell growth. These genes require something to activate them in order to cause this reaction to occur.

Chapter 15: Assessing Clients with Integumentary Disorders

1. **Answer: 2 Rationale:** There are many layers to the skin. The layer that has the most glands and hair follicles located in it is the dermis. The epidermis is on top of this layer and the stratum spinosum and stratum basale are beneath the dermis.

2. **Answer: 3 Rationale:** Melanin is the pigment found in skin that protects the skin from the sun. This is the pigment responsible for tanning. It is also the source of malignancy in malignant melanoma.

3. **Answer: 1, 2 Rationale:** Inspection is the first assessment technique to check the skin surface. This is done by simply looking at the skin for any abnormalities or imperfections. The next assessment step is to palpate any areas of the skin that appear abnormal in order to get a better understanding of depth and size of any lesions. This is also a way to assess if the abnormality causes any pain or discomfort.

4. **Answer: 1 Rationale:** Erythema often occurs as a result of increased body temperature. This occurs when the capillaries in the skin dilate to release some of the heat caused from the increased body temperature.

5. **Answer: 3 Rationale:** Often new soap can cause skin irritation and itching. It is important to determine if there is anything that has changed to cause this irritation. This is the easiest variable to assess.

6. **Answer: 1 Rationale:** A decreased skin turgor is a sign of dehydration. This is often referred to as "tenting." By pinching the skin gently, when you release the skin, a small tent remains before flattening out.

7. **Answer: 4 Rationale:** Edema begins in the distal extremities. The best place to assess for this is the ankle area. By pressing the fingertip into the skin and releasing it, you can determine the severity of edema by seeing how deep the pitting goes after removing your fingertips. This is often categorized on a scale of one to four.

8. **Answer: 4 Rationale:** Lichenification is a condition in which the skin cells multiply causing what appears to be thickened and calloused skin. The skin often has a rough and leathery appearance to it. This condition is common in clients suffering from chronic dermatitis.

9. **Answer: 2 Rationale:** Although aging skin is known to bruise easier, a greater concern would be the possibility of elder abuse. It is extremely important for the nurse making the home visit to assess for this in order to provide support and assistance to the older woman and caregiver.

10. **Answer: 3 Rationale:** Head lice cause small white eggs to be found attached to the hair shaft, very close to the scalp. These are called nits and are the eggs of the lice. After using an anti-lice shampoo, it is necessary to carefully comb these out of the hair.

Chapter 16: Nursing Care of Clients with Integumentary Disorders

1. **Answer: 3 Rationale:** Xerosis is a skin condition in which the skin appears very dry and roughened. It is important to help remoisturize the skin. The best way to do this is to apply a moisturizing agent to the skin after bathing. Blotting dry with a towel and then applying a moisturizer will help lock in the moisture from the bath and help nourish the skin.

2. **Answer: 1 Rationale:** Nevi are the skin lesions that need to be monitored for changes. These lesions can become malignant and need to be monitored for any change. The ABCDE of nevi include A-abnormal border, B-black, C-color change, D-diameter, E-elevation.

3. **Answer: 4 Rationale:** Psoriasis causes abnormal growth and division of epidermal cells, causing keratosis. The use of ultraviolet light therapy helps to slow down this cellular division, which decreases the lesions and keratosis associated with psoriasis.

4. **Answer: 2 Rationale:** Pregnancy causes many changes in the body. Included in this is that the vaginal tissue is more prone to yeast infections. During pregnancy there is often an increase in vaginal secretions. Yeast is an opportunistic organism that grows best in warm, dark moist environments such as the vagina.

5. **Answer: 4 Rationale:** This condition is most likely shingles, which is a type of varicella infection. It is important to assess if the client has any degree of natural immunity to varicella. The easiest way to determine this is to know if the client has ever had chickenpox. This can help to determine if the shingles will only be isolated to this dermatome or if the client is at risk for a more severe infection and may need to be started on antiviral therapy.

6. **Answer: 2 Rationale:** It is a myth that only dirty people get lice. Major infestations often occur in areas where many are in close proximity of each other, especially in the public school setting. Lice are a parasite and are found in the hair and scalp of humans.

7. **Answer: 1 Rationale:** People with fair skin, blond hair, and freckles are at increased risk for non-melanoma skin cancers. People meeting this description should have yearly skin checks to assess for any changes in nevi or other lesions.

8. **Answer: 1 Rationale:** A change in the color or size of a nevus is cause for concern when evaluating for the possibility of melanoma. This falls under the ABCDE of skin checks.

9. **Answer: 2 Rationale:** Clients who are bedridden are at increased risk for pressure sores and skin tears. Skin tears may occur as a result of the shearing force of pulling a client up in bed. Skin assessments should be done each shift and appropriate interventions for preventing skin breakdown implemented as needed.

10. **Answer: 3 Rationale:** Dermabrasion is a skin treatment that helps to reduce the appearance of acne scarring and other skin imperfections. Often these treatments are done on a regular basis for clients in a plastic surgery clinic.

Chapter 17: Nursing Care of Clients with Burns

1. **Answer: 3 Rationale:** In the emergent phase of burn management, it is important to monitor electrolyte levels frequently. Initially the client is at risk for fluid and electrolyte imbalances, especially for decreased serum potassium levels. This can cause an increased risk for arrhythmias.

2. **Answer: 4 Rationale:** A full thickness burn is not painful, as the nerves have also been affected from the burn. In this situation, pain is not a good sign. It tells the nurse that the depth of the burn goes beyond the nerves. Superficial, superficial partial thickness, and deep partial thickness burns will still be very painful to the client, as the nerves remain intact or exposed.

3. **Answer: 4 Rationale:** The larger the surface area of the burn and the deeper the burn, the more at risk the client is for burn shock. A high-voltage electrical accident will cause a deeper burn and since this scenario explains that >50% of the body is affected, this places the client at the highest risk.

4. **Answer: 2 Rationale:** Silvadene cream can cause neutropenia. It is important for the nurse to monitor the client's WBC count daily to assess for any changes, which could indicate neutropenia. Although this is the most important intervention, it is also important to keep the client as comfortable as possible. Premedicating is definitely not a bad idea, as burn dressing changes can be very painful and the Silvadene will help debride the burn.

5. **Answer: 2 Rationale:** The Parkland Formula uses lactated Ringer's solution, administered at 4 mL × kg × % TBSA burn, with 50% of the total volume infused in the first eight hours, and the remaining 50% over the next 16 hours. This would be $4 \times 70 \times 50\% = 14,000 \times 50\% = 7,000$.

6. **Answer: 1 Rationale:** Urine output is the most sensitive indicator of fluid resuscitation success. A decrease in urine output is seen in dehydration and a recovery from dehydration is seen with an increase in urine output.

7. **Answer: 4 Rationale:** A decreased left radial pulse is cause for alarm in this type and location of burn. This can be the first symptom seen in compartment syndrome and is a surgical emergency.

8. **Answer: 2 Rationale:** The Rule of Nines is a method of quickly estimating the percentage of TBSA affected by a burn injury. It is most useful in emergency situations but is not accurate for estimating TBSA in adults who are short, obese, or very thin. Anterior trunk = 18%, perineum = 1%, left arm = 9%. These are added together to = 28%.

9. **Answer: 1, 3, 5, 6 Rationale:** Teaching injury prevention is a very important job in nursing. Burns are a common injury in the home. It is important to help older adults understand ways to help prevent burns. Wearing close-fitting clothing when cooking can help prevent shirtsleeves or scarves from catching on fire. The water temperature of the water heater should not be set above 120 degrees. This can help prevent burns from water scalding. Installing anti-scald devices can also help prevent water burns. As older adults often have decreased olfactory senses, having a neighbor routinely check for the odor of gas can help prevent fires.

10. **Answer: 3 Rationale:** A 15% carbon monoxide level would cause only mild symptoms of dizziness at this stage. Later stages with higher levels will cause the remaining symptoms of the skin color change, drowsiness, and hypotension.

Chapter 18: Assessing Clients with Endocrine Disorders

1. **Answer: 2 Rationale:** ADH, antidiuretic hormone, helps to concentrate urine, which would decrease the urine output. The ADH causes the distal tubules in the kidney to reabsorb water, which will concentrate the urine.

2. **Answer: 3 Rationale:** Testing for Trousseau's sign is done by inflating a blood pressure cuff above the antecubital area, higher than the systolic blood pressure, for two to five minutes. A positive test causes carpal spasm and the fingers and hand will contract on the arm where the blood pressure cuff is inflated.

3. **Answer: 1 Rationale:** Excessive amounts of glucocorticoids cause symptoms of immunosuppression. The glucocorticoids

are natural steroids, which cause immunosuppression. These are hormones, which affect carbohydrate metabolism. Glucocorticoids include cortisol and cortisone and are released in times of stress. Any significant excess of these can depress the inflammatory response and inhibit the effectiveness of the immune system.

4. **Answer: 3 Rationale:** When assessing the endocrine system, it is important to look for signs and symptoms of diabetes. One of the first symptoms is polydypsia, which is increased thirst. Asking clients if they have noticed any change in their thirst can help to address this symptom.

5. **Answer: 2 Rationale:** Palpating the thyroid gland can assess the size and consistency of the gland. This is important to check when assessing for goiters, enlargement, or nodules.

6. **Answer: 2 Rationale:** Assessment for Chvostek's sign is done by tapping a finger in front of the ear, at the angle of the jaw. A positive sign causes facial grimacing with repeated contractions of the facial muscle. A normal sign shows no grimacing.

7. **Answer: 4 Rationale:** TSH is thyroid-stimulating hormone. This is a hormone, which is supposed to stimulate the thyroid gland to function. When the TSH level is high, the thyroid is not functioning enough, known as hypothyroidism. When the TSH level is very low, this is a condition known as hyperthyroidism.

8. **Answer: 3 Rationale:** The thyroid gland is the only endocrine organ that can be palpated during an exam. It is located behind the thyroid cartilage of the trachea and the edges of the gland can often be palpated on either side of the trachea. The pancreas is found deep in the abdominal cavity. The liver is behind the rib cage, but the edge of the liver can often be palpated at the base of the rib cage. The pituitary gland is located in the brain.

9. **Answer: 2 Rationale:** Rough, dry skin is often found in clients with hypothyroidism. The skin temperature is also often cool.

10. **Answer: 4 Rationale:** Thyroid function can be assessed by testing deep tendon reflexes. Increased deep tendon reflexes are seen in hyperthyroidism. Decreased deep tendon reflexes are seen in hypothyroidism.

Chapter 19: Nursing Care of Clients with Endocrine Disorders

1. **Answer: 1 Rationale:** An antibody attaches to TSH receptors in the thyroid and causes increased production. There is no infectious agent, allergen, or genetic link.

2. **Answer: 3 Rationale:** Oral administration of radioactive iodine concentrates in the thyroid gland and damages or destroys thyroid cells decreasing TH levels. There is no effect on vascularity of the thyroid but hypothyroidism can be created with this therapy.

3. **Answer: 3 Rationale:** The body tries to produce more hormones by simply producing more cells that produce that hormone. TH is not increased, it is decreased. Dietary iodine has no effect on thyroid enlargement.

4. **Answer: 4 Rationale:** Persons who take corticosteroids for treatment of rheumatoid arthritis for long periods are at increased risk for developing Cushing's syndrome since it is the result of increased stimulation of the adrenal cortex.

5. **Answer: 2 Rationale:** A client with the diagnosis of Addison's disease will be stressed by infection and an additional dose of steroids may be needed to prevent crisis. Therefore clients are urged to carry injectable cortisone and a syringe at all times.

6. **Answer: 2 Rationale:** Irritability occurs as the brain and nerve cells become edematous as the blood volume expands.

7. **Answer: 2 Rationale:** Clients with this disorder are at risk for pathological fractures of the bones because of the decreased density of the bone.

8. **Answer: 3 Rationale:** Clients with hypercalcemia will demonstrate decreased bowel sounds related to the decreased neuromuscular excitability with increased calcium. Clients also will have increased urinary output, a negative Chvostek's sign, and decreased deep tendon reflexes.

9. **Answer: 4 Rationale:** In 98% of clients with increased ACTH levels and Addison's disease the exposed and unexposed skin is deeply suntanned or bronzed.

10. **Answer: 1 Rationale:** With a sudden stoppage of steroids, the adrenal cortex cannot recuperate rapidly enough to increase production because it has been suppressed with exogenous steroids. Therefore steroids are gradually decreased and clients weaned to allow endogenous steroid production to resume.

Chapter 20: Nursing Care of Clients with Diabetes Mellitus

1. **Answer: 1 Rationale:** 95% of clients diagnosed with type 1 diabetes mellitus have the genetic markers with DR3 & DR 4 antigens on chromosome 6 of the leukocyte antigen system. This indicates increased susceptibility to develop diabetes type 1. Obesity in adolescence is more indicative of type 2 diabetes. Diabetic women usually produce a baby weighing more than ten pounds, not underweight babies. Elevation of glucagons would occur in hypoglycemia, not hyperglycemia.

2. **Answer: 3 Rationale:** Increased glucagon levels and deficit of insulin increases the liver's production of ketone bodies and increased release of free fatty acids. With this process, bicarbonate production is decreased and it cannot buffer so metabolic acidosis occurs.

3. **Answer: 4 Rationale:** There is an increased risk of developing type 2 diabetes in the older population (over 65) with a decrease in the calorie need and especially with the decrease of exercise.

4. **Answer: 3 Rationale:** With diabetes often the client will state changes in sensation of the feet caused by impaired nerve function. The client may complain of numbness or tingling.

5. **Answer: 3 Rationale:** Checking the feet daily is important. Someone needs to look at all surfaces and between toes for any breaks in skin integrity or changes in cellular makeup. The other three answers are all on the *do not do* list of diabetic foot care.

6. **Answer: 3 Rationale:** Since it is clear, Lantus (glargine) could be confused with regular insulin. Regular insulin is short acting in 4-6 hours and Lantus is long acting in 24-28 hours. Confusing these two insulins could be extremely harmful to client. Lantus should not be mixed with other insulins or given IV.

7. **Answer: 3 Rationale:** Only regular insulin can safely be administered intravenously for diabetic ketoacidosis. Subcutaneous injection is recommended for all other insulins.

8. **Answer: 3 Rationale:** HgbA1C levels 7-9% show that the glucose level has been elevated or erratic over this period of time.

9. **Answer: 3 Rationale:** No intermediate- or long-acting insulin is given the day of surgery since dietary intake post-operatively is uncertain. IV glucose (5%) and regular insulin in equally divided doses will compensate for the increase in serum glucose until the client is eating and drinking normally.

10. **Answer: 4 Rationale:** The abdomen absorbs insulin the fastest. After the abdomen the order is deltoid, thigh, and lastly, hip.

Chapter 21: Assessing Clients with Nutritional and GI Disorders

1. **Answer: 1 Rationale:** Bile is necessary for emulsifying and absorption of fats.

2. **Answer: 3 Rationale:** Catabolism is the breakdown of complex structures into simpler forms. Anabolism is the combining of simple molecules to form complex structures. Metabolism is the biochemical reactions within the cells—anabolism and catabolism.

3. **Answer: 2 Rationale:** Animal products are considered complete proteins in that they meet the body's requirements for tissue building and maintenance. Fruits and vegetables are missing at least one essential amino acid. Butter and oils are sources of fat.

4. **Answer: 2 Rationale:** Vitamin K is an essential element for blood clotting and, without sufficient levels, bleeding can occur. Vitamin K does not affect the other answers.

5. **Answer: 4 Rationale:** A 24-hour dietary intake recall will demonstrate quantities and patterns of food intake that would be important in the nutritional assessment of a client.

6. **Answer: 4 Rationale:** An elevated amylase indicates that the pancreatic enzymes are digesting their own tissues. Cheliosis is the breakdown of tissues of the corner of the mouth due to vitamin B deficiency. Gastric reflux is related to the esophagus and will not produce elevation in enzymes. Gallstones are associated with potential elevation of the bilirubin test.

7. **Answer: 1 Rationale:** The condition of the client's teeth, possible difficulty for her to chew comfortably, and her dry mouth because of decreased production of saliva in the older adult may cause a nutritional deficit because she will tend to eat food that is easier to chew and swallow. She may not eat enough protein.

8. **Answer: 1 Rationale:** The liver is located in the right upper quadrant with the border palpated below the rib cage when the client takes a deep breath.

9. **Answer: 4 Rationale:** In client with ascites of the liver of more than 500 mL, a method of determining fluid presence is palpating dullness in the abdomen in the supine position and then on the right side. The presence of dullness moving in these two positions indicates ascites with shifting dullness pattern.

10. **Answer: 3 Rationale:** Palpation of the abdomen is done last in order to avoid influencing bowel peristalsis or cause pain that could end the exam. The order of assessment is observe, auscultate, percuss, and palpate.

Chapter 22: Nursing Care of Clients with Nutritional Disorders

1. **Answer: 3 Rationale:** The lack of regular exercise in daily life means less expenditure of energy, therefore nutrients are stored as fat. Research has shown that adopted children's weight is related to their biological parents. "Fast foods" are a contributing factor. Allergies are not related to obesity.

2. **Answer: 2 Rationale:** This response informs the client of the calorie-pound relationship and involves the client in the planning strategies to improve and maintain weight loss.

3. **Answer: 1 Rationale:** Recent weight loss is the most prevalent finding in protein-calorie malnutrition. Skinfold thickness is decreased and the client demonstrates lethargy and drowsiness.

4. **Answer: 3 Rationale:** Small-bore feeding tubes displace easily. Accurate placement is evaluated by aspirating contents and checking the pH. In the stomach the pH is <4. None of the other methods are as accurate or supported by research.

5. **Answer: 4 Rationale:** An identified contributing factor to anorexia is family pressure. Family therapy commonly is an important part of the interdisciplinary treatment plan. The caloric intake and weight gain is unrealistic for these clients.

6. **Answer: 2 Rationale:** A BMI greater than 25 and central obesity as indicated by a waist-hip ratio of 1 or greater are associated with a higher risk for hypertension, elevated lipid levels, heart disease and stroke. These conditions have the greatest impact on health over time.

7. **Answer: 4, 5 Rationale:** Because this drug causes dry mouth and potential for constipation, fluids are important to maintain function. The drug is intended to be taken along with a restricted calorie diet for weight loss. The drug is taken only once a day not with each meal, so a skipped meal doesn't matter. There are no guidelines about alcohol consumption in drug reference manuals. Drowsiness is not a problem because this drug will increase stimulation and may in fact interfere with sleep.

8. **Answer: 1, 2, 4, 5 Rationale:** There are many contributing factors that influence nutrition in the home-bound older adult such as inability to shop for nutritional foods, ability to afford and to prepare nutritional food. There are also psychosocial issues of depression and loneliness since eating is a social affair, this could well influence the amount and proportion of caloric intake. Arranging for food to be brought to the client and for the client to be transported to a senior center for a meal may solve the weight loss issue and no further interventions may be necessary.

9. **Answer: 4 Rationale:** Beginning oral intake of nutrients as soon as possible after surgery is the best way to prevent malnutrition. Aggressive pain management may have the opposite effect—it may decrease appetite or sedate the client , interfering with food intake. While IV fluids may be necessary to maintain fluid volume, most do not contain adequate calories to maintain nutritional status. Daily weights often are more reflective of fluid volume status than of nutritional status.

10. **Answer: 1 Rationale:** One of the postoperative complications with gastric bypass surgery is an anastomotic leak causing peritonitis. These symptoms could be related to this condition and the surgeon needs to be notified.

Chapter 23: Nursing Care of Clients Experiencing Upper GI Disorders

1. **Answer: 4 Rationale:** The use of tobacco and drinking alcohol are the two primary risk factors for oral cancers. The others are not risk factors for oral cancer.

2. **Answer: 2, 5 Rationale:** Placing the head of the bed on blocks and avoiding lying down for at least 3 hours after eating will help prevent backflow of gastric content into the esophagus by decreasing the pressure on the lower esophageal sphincter. GERD is a chronic disease that can affect not only lifestyle, but also cause changes in the esophageal mucosa and integrity. Drug therapy may be prolonged. Chocolate and peppermint may aggravate the problem.

3. **Answer: 1 Rationale:** The most common contributing factor to acute stress gastritis is the interruption of the integrity of the gastric lining by gastric irritants such as aspirin and/or NSAIDs. A period of gastric rest, followed by a slow progression to regular dietary intake is advised. There is no indication for bland foods or regular endoscopy. The discussion of consuming fully cooked food is indicated in cases of gastric upset from toxins.

4. **Answer: 4 Rationale:** A peptic ulcer is an interruption of the integrity of the gastric lining; perforation is the most lethal complication of this process. It produces inflammation, infection and possibly shock. While the other nursing diagnoses will be present and need to be addressed at some point, disrup-

tion of the integrity of the gastrointestinal tissue is the highest priority.

5. **Answer: 3 Rationale:** Frequent small meals with solid foods or liquids, not both, are effective in controlling the hyperosmolar problem of dumping syndrome. Proteins and fats slow down the gastric emptying, whereas simple carbohydrates may rapidly enter the duodenum, increasing the risk for dumping syndrome.

6. **Answer: 2 Rationale:** Bright bleeding from the mouth could indicate perforation of the esophageal wall or vessel rupture by invasion of tumor. The other symptoms are manifestations of esophageal cancer but are not an emergency requiring immediate action.

7. **Answer: 1 Rationale:** These symptoms indicate a possible hypersensitivity response to the antibiotics. Anaphylaxis could occur, this is an emergency situation. The other answers are indeed included in the client teaching for taking antibiotics.

8. **Answer: 3 Rationale:** The discomfort of stomatitis is aggravated by eating; viscous lidocaine to reduce mouth pain is important to promote nutrition. Mouthwashes contain alcohol and may produce more pain and damage. Selection of foods that are appealing and smoking cessation are not the priority in this instance.

9. **Answer: 3 Rationale:** Maintaining patency of the nasogastric tube following gastric surgery is vital to prevent pressure gastric distension and pressure on the suture line. Irrigating gently with NS, if ordered, is the appropriate action. If unable to open tube, notify surgeon. Charting the finding without action is harmful to the client. Repositioning nasogastric tubes following gastric surgery is done by the surgeon.

10. **Answer: 3, 4, 5 Rationale:** Severe pain may be a manifestation of perforation of the ulcer. Oral food and fluids are withheld to prevent vomiting and prepare for possible surgery. The client is placed in Fowler's position to localize drainage to the pelvic area, and the physician notified to ensure prompt diagnosis and treatment. Administering additional IV dose of proton pump inhibitor has no benefit. Narcotics may mask the symptoms and should not be administered.

Chapter 24: Nursing Care of the Client Experiencing Gallbladder, Liver, and Pancreatic Disorders

1. **Answer: 1 Rationale:** Right upper quadrant pain following ingestion of a fatty meal is the typical symptom experienced by clients with choleliathiasis. Jaundice and ascites are symptoms of liver failure. Heartburn and acid reflux are symptoms of gastroesophageal reflux disease (GERD).

2. **Answer: 1, 4 Rationale:** Acute cholecystitis usually develops from a stone obstructing the cystic duct preventing release of bile from the gallbladder. High fatty foods like gravies and peanut butter stimulate contraction of the obstructed gallbladder, causing pain. Temperature and severe upper abdominal pain may be symptoms of acute peritonitis resulting from rupture of the necrotic gallbladder.

3. **Answer: 3 Rationale:** Hepatitis A is transmitted by oral-fecal route from an infected person handling food, water, fish or through direct-contact without washing hands before handling food or after using the bathroom. Hepatitis A immunization is not a cost-effective prevention measure. Testing for hepatitis A antigen on employment will not prevent spread of the disease by a newly infected current employee. Hepatitis A rarely is transmitted by blood and body fluids.

4. **Answer: 4 Rationale:** Hepatitis C is transmitted through contact with blood or body fluids. Clients with this disease must

understand the importance of refraining from donating blood and using barrier protection (condoms) during sex is important. The client should avoid hepatic toxins such as acetaminophen and alcohol. Biopsies are usually done for cirrhosis. There are antiviral medications used for the treatment of hepatitis but a long life is not guaranteed.

5. **Answer: 2 Rationale:** The hepatitis A virus can be transmitted before manifestations of the disease (including jaundice) develop, therefore it is important to identify people who have had direct contact with the newly diagnosed client. Hepatitis A is not transmitted through sexual contact. Immunization for hepatitis A is only recommended in certain areas, not for the general public.

6. **Answer: 2 Rationale:** Maintaining a patent airway is of highest priority. Placing the client in Fowler's position may prevent aspiration of blood and should be the primary action. The other activities may be needed but are a lesser priority

7. **Answer: 3 Rationale:** It is important to empty the bladder prior to the paracentesis to make sure the bladder is not punctured during the procedure. It is not necessary for the client to abstain from eating or drinking, rather the client needs to maintain fluid volume prior to the procedure. The physician will do the scrub before inserting the needle. Flatus is not related to paracentesis.

8. **Answer: 1 Rationale:** The nurse should assess bowel sounds and palpate for tenderness since spontaneous bacterial infection can develop with ascites producing fever and worsening encephalopathy. Headache and nuccal rigidity are associated with meningitis. Neck vein distention is associated with right-sided heart failure. Abdominal girth and shifting dullness are important in monitoring progress of ascites, not infection.

9. **Answer: 3 Rationale:** In women, the most common contributing factor to development of acute pancreatitis is a gallstone obstructing the duct, so this is an appropriate response. Pancreatitis usually develops from an immediate toxin or obstruction, not a delayed one. There is no association between pancreatitis and smoking. Clients who use IV drugs are susceptible to hepatitis, not pancreatitis.

10. **Answer: 4 Rationale:** Maintaining a patent nasogastric tube is vital to prevent accumulation of gastric secretions and pressure on the anastomoses created in Whipple's procedure. Smoking cessation is not a priority at this time. Turning and coughing will prevent respiratory complications but this is less important than suture line integrity. Ambulation will prevent thrombosis, but suture line integrity is of utmost importance.

Chapter 25: Assessing Clients with Bowel Elimination Disorders

1. **Answer: 2 Rationale:** The small intestine is where the nutrients and vitamins are absorbed.

2. **Answer: 4 Rationale:** The large intestine's function is to absorb water, salts, and vitamins, and then eliminate undigested substances. Hormones and bile used in digestion come from other parts of the digestive system. Breakdown of lipids, proteins, and carbohydrates occur in the small intestine.

3. **Answer: 1 Rationale:** The appendix is an extension of the surface of the cecum. The others are all parts of the large intestine but not attached to the appendix.

4. **Answer: 3 Rationale:** Internal hemorrhoids occur with impaired venous return during evacuation of stool or increased abdominal pressure in pregnancy causing distension of veins of the anus.

5. **Answer: 4 Rationale:** A client with an ostomy should have questions answered about the consistency of the stool. This

information may indicate location of the opening within the intestinal tract and demonstrate how the bowel is functioning. The other three answers do not give valuable information for a client with an ostomy.

6. **Answer: 4 Rationale:** A stool specimen will supply the opportunity to directly exam the feces and detect presence of intestinal parasites. The other tests are used for other purposes and are invasive and expensive.

7. **Answer: 2 Rationale:** Polyps have been documented as increased risk factors for developing cancer, therefore removal is indicated to prevent neoplastic cell development.

8. **Answer: 4 Rationale:** By listening with a stethoscope, you will hear the soft sounds produced by movement through the intestines every 5-15 seconds. Inspection will identify shapes and contour, palpation will assist with size of masses, and percussion will identify locations of masses.

9. **Answer: 3 Rationale:** Melena is the term used to describe black, tarry stools. Occult blood is the presence of blood in stool that is not obvious. Hematemesis is the vomiting of blood. Steatorrhea is foul smelling, high fat content stool.

10. **Answer: 3 Rationale:** The absence of bowel sounds on the first post operative day after bowel surgery is a normal expectation because the assault during surgery causes peristalsis to stop temporarily. No further action is indicated at this time.

Chapter 26: Nursing Care of Clients with Bowel Disorders

1. **Answer: 2 Rationale:** The nurse must first assess the number, frequency, and water content of stools to confirm the diagnosis of diarrhea, and estimate fluid and electrolyte loss. The client needs to ingest fluids as long as nausea and vomiting are not present, and slowly increase to solid foods. Enterotoxins' possibility should be identified. Anti-diarrhea medications are reserved for use for rectal tissue comfort.

2. **Answer: 3 Rationale:** Once the diagnosis of appendicitis is confirmed, the client should be prepared for surgery quickly before perforation or necrosis develops to decrease chance of complications. The client is kept NPO and no foreign substances are introduced into the intestinal tract. Intravenous fluids will be necessary, since the client is NPO, to maintain vascular volume and electrolyte balance as well as to administer antibiotic solutions.

3. **Answer: 1 Rationale:** Sulfasalazine makes the client susceptible to sunburn so a sunscreen should be used while outside. The drug is best tolerated when taken with meals. Fluid intake is recommended to be around 2000 mL per day. There is no mention of vitamin C supplementation while on this drug.

4. **Answer: 4 Rationale:** The symptoms reported by the client are the definition of steatorrhea. Hematochezia is bright blood in the stool. Frequent, mucus-filled stools are symptomatic of inflammatory bowel disease. These symptoms are not early signs of colorectal cancer; for example, change in bowel habits, narrow stools, diarrhea, or constipation.

5. **Answer: 2 Rationale:** The recommendation for client health with this familial history of cancer is to monitor to identify polyps and tumors early. Research has proven a direct genetic link of polyps and cancer development (20%). CEA is used to monitor treatment and detect reoccurrence and is not a screening tool in early tumor development. Dietary fiber is not the only contributing factor to cancer prevention and should be integrated into the regular diet.

6. **Answer: 4, 5, 7 Rationale:** The documentation and frequent measuring of nasogastric output will help maintain vascular volume with replacement of fluids, and the color will indicate if drainage is normal. Measuring abdominal girth will assist in determining if increased intestinal distension is occurring.

7. **Answer: 4 Rationale:** It is most important to maintain the patency of the nasogastric tube to remove gastric secretions and air that may apply pressure to the anastomosis site and cause failure of the suture line. Keeping the stomach decompressed is important to prevent vomiting that could also cause damage to the anastomosis site.

8. **Answer: 2 Rationale:** Popcorn can cause obstruction to the diverticular opening and set up the environment to initiate diverticulitis. The other foods are recommended for control of stool bulk, decreasing intraluminal pressure, and reduction of spasms associated with diverticular disease.

9. **Answer: 1, 3, 5, 6 Rationale:** Fresh fruits and vegetables, whole wheat bread, and bran cereal supply roughage and fiber in diet that can assist in the evacuation of fecal material and lessen the possibility of developing diverticulum, the incidence of which is high in this age group. Adequate liquid is important to prevent hard, formed stools that are difficult to pass. Taking daily laxatives can decrease the normal bowel reflexes. Colace can be administered safely either in the morning or at nighttime.

10. **Answer: 2 Rationale:** Abdominal adhesions following surgery usually obstruct only one section of the small bowel. The other three do not cause bowel obstruction, they may prevent obstruction.

Chapter 27: Assessing Client with Urinary Disorders

1. **Answer: 4 Rationale:** The nephrons are the working units of the kidney that produce urine. Located within the medulla, the pyramids collect the blood. The ureters transport the urine to the bladder.

2. **Answer: 4 Rationale:** ADH is increased to limit the excretion of water in the urine to maintain fluid balance. The other hormones do not affect fluid balance.

3. **Answer: 3 Rationale:** Creatinine clearance is a test that determines the filtering ability of the glomeruli and the blood circulation to them. Therefore, if the clearance is decreased, the glomeruli are damaged or the circulation is slowed. The other tests do not measure GFR.

4. **Answer: 3 Rationale:** The prostate surrounds the male urethra. The other organs are within the abdominal cavity.

5. **Answer: 2 Rationale:** Nocturia is defined as two or more voidings during the night. Polyuria is excessive urine production. Dysuria is painful urination. Hematuria is blood in the urine.

6. **Answer: 1 Rationale:** The contrast media used in IVPs cause some adverse reactions in clients that are allergic to iodine or products containing iodine. Shellfish contain iodine.

7. **Answer: 3 Rationale:** Collecting a urine specimen allows the examiner to assess the urine for color, odor, and clarity before the exam. By collecting a specimen the client has emptied the bladder. Deep breathing may help the client relax during the exam. The client with a full bladder would possibly make the exam uncomfortable.

8. **Answer: 1 Rationale:** Anesthetic agents used during surgery may cause problems with initiating voiding. Palpation will determine if the bladder is distended. Gastric assessments are not needed here.

9. **Answer: 4 Rationale:** Urinary incontinence is not considered a normal process in aging.

10. **Answer: 2 Rationale:** Skin turgor is the best assessment technique to determine hydration of clients. The other assessment techniques are not measurements of hydration status.

Chapter 28: Nursing Care of Clients with Urinary Disorders

1. **Answer: 2 Rationale:** The form of birth control, especially for those using a diaphragm and spermicidal gel, can alter the vaginal flora and increase the risk of UTIs. The reoccurrence time factor of the UTI is too long to be a failure to complete antibiotic treatment the first time. The other answers are not related to UTIs.

2. **Answer: 1, 3, 4 Rationale:** The nurse needs to inform the client that a urine culture in ten days is done to ensure antibiotic therapy was effective; in a peri-menopausal woman vaginal cream may maintain tissue integrity to prevent bacterial colonization of perineal tissues; instructions on cleansing may prevent further infections. The other two answers are invasive tests and may not be necessary for this client since three UTIs per year in a sexually active woman is considered normal.

3. **Answer: 4 Rationale:** Increasing fluid intake to 3,000 mL per day will produce enough urine to prevent stone-forming salts from concentrating sufficiently to precipitate. Calcium supplement will not prevent stones, it may contribute. Monitoring pH of urine or an indwelling catheter will not prevent stone formation.

4. **Answer: 3 Rationale:** These are manifestations of renal colic and possible ureteral obstruction. Prompt diagnosis and treatment is vital to prevent hydroureter and hydronephrosis should the ureter be completely obstructed. Although pain management and collection of the stone are important, prevention of hydronephrosis is of highest priority. Residual urine is not expected in this scenario.

5. **Answer: 1 Rationale:** Bladder cancer is two times more prevalent in smokers than non-smokers. While occupational exposure to dyes and chemicals are identified as risk factors for bladder cancers, home exposure is not. Caffeine intake and urinary retention are not identified risk factors for bladder cancer.

6. **Answer: 2 Rationale:** Painless hematuria is the usual presenting manifestation of bladder cancers and should be evaluated quickly for best outcome.

7. **Answer: 3 Rationale:** The client with a newly created continent ileal diversion will have to demonstrate self-catheterization since this is the only way to empty the continent ileal diversion. There is no collection device in this surgical procedure. Urine may normally appear cloudy since the ileum continues to produce mucus. Identification of risk factors is not necessary since the bladder has been removed.

8. **Answer: 3 Rationale:** Stress incontinence should not be viewed as a normal result of aging, rather as a treatable problem. Pelvic floor muscle exercises strengthen perineal muscles, increasing urinary sphincter control and will reduce the incidence of incontinence. Artificial sweeteners have been identified as bladder irritants contributing to urge incontinence, but have less impact on stress incontinence.

9. **Answer: 1 Rationale:** Inability to retain urine long enough to reach the toilet following perception of the need to urinate is characteristic of urge incontinence. Caffeine and artificial sweeteners are bladder irritants, causing instability of the detrusor muscle and aggravating manifestations. Restricting intake of fluids containing these substances in the evening reduces nocturia. While the other measures may be indicated for other types of incontinence, they are of lower priority or not indicated for urge incontinence.

10. **Answer: 4 Rationale:** Catheterizing the client every three to four hours with a straight catheter prevents over distension of the bladder and the increased risk for infection associated with an indwelling catheter. During spinal shock, the bladder does not empty in response to stretch or other reflexes. Measuring residual urine is not indicated at this time.

Chapter 29: Nursing Care of the Client with Kidney Disorders

1. **Answer: 2 Rationale:** The GFR tends to decrease with aging, decreasing drug excretion and increasing the risk for toxicity. Administering smaller doses less frequently reduces the risk, but the client needs continued monitoring for manifestations of digoxin toxicity.

2. **Answer: 3 Rationale:** The adult form of polycystic kidney disease (PKD) is transmitted in an autosomal dominant pattern. Each child has a 50% chance of inheriting the disease. Only 10% of PKD clients are due to new genetic mutation.

3. **Answer: 2 Rationale:** The most common cause of acute glomerulonephritis is an abnormal immune response to beta-hemolytic streptococcus A infection, usually strep throat. Urinary tract infection, contrast media or illicit drug use are not generally implicated in development of glomerulonephritis.

4. **Answer: 1 Rationale:** Soy or animal proteins are complete proteins necessary for growth and tissue maintenance. Complete proteins are preferred when total protein intake is restricted, as in acute glomerulonephritis. Although bed rest may be recommended during the acute phase of the disorder, activities may be resumed during recovery. Dialysis would not be indicated for this client at this time so a device is not needed. Sodium may be restricted if edema is severe or the client is hypertensive, but fluid intake is individually determined, based on fluid volume status.

5. **Answer: 4 Rationale:** Postoperatively, it is important to monitor separately all drainage device volumes to determine function of each catheter or drain, and prevent hydronephrosis. Because of the location of the incision, cough suppression increases the risk of retained respiratory secretions and pneumonia. Catheters may be irrigated only when necessary and by physician's order to reduce the risk of tissue damage and infection.

6. **Answer: 1 Rationale:** Ischemia is the most common cause of acute renal failure (ARF), therefore maintaining fluid volume, cardiac output, and renal output are the highest priority nursing interventions to prevent renal failure.

7. **Answer: 3 Rationale:** Nephrotoxic drugs, including over-the-counter products, can produce further damage to the kidney cells and should be avoided. Depending on urinary output, fluid intake generally is not restricted during the recovery phase of ARF. Vegetable proteins are not complete proteins, therefore are not recommended if protein intake is restricted.

8. **Answer: 1, 3 Rationale:** Weight and orthostatic vital signs are indicators of fluid volume status and electrolyte balance. Laboratory tests are monitored to evaluate the effects of treatment. Restriction of fluid and food during dialysis is not necessary and may contribute to decreased fluid volume.

9. **Answer: 2 Rationale:** The client's ability to state renal replacement therapies indicates understanding of treatment options and the ability to make informed decisions on treatment. Clients may be able to live independently, or with the assistance of a part-time caregiver. Home hemodialysis would require a helper for safety reasons to monitor the client's response. Hospice Care is not necessarily needed for ESRD.

10. **Answer: 4 Rationale:** Cloudy urine could be a symptom of an infection. Prompt treatment is vital to preserve integrity of the transplanted organ in an immunosuppressed client. Recording the finding is insufficient, action must be taken. The nurse does

not increase the intravenous flow rate without a physician's order. Irrigation of the urinary catheter would introduce the possibility of contaminates into an immunosuppressed client.

Chapter 30: Assessing the Client with Heart Disorder

1. **Answer: 3 Rationale:** Coronary circulation supplies the heart with blood. Systemic circulation supplies the body. The pulmonary circulation supplies blood to the lungs and alveoli. The hepatic circulation supplies the liver.
2. **Answer: 4 Rationale:** Definition of cardiac output is the amount of blood pumped by the ventricles in 1 minute. Heart rate is how many times per minute the cardiac cycle occurs. Ventricular contraction is the number of times the ventricles contract. Stroke volume is the measurement of blood volume ejected with each ventricular contraction.
3. **Answer: 2 Rationale:** The coronary arteries are filled during systole when the ventricles contract so it would be prior to ventricular relaxation.
4. **Answer: 3 Rationale:** Hemorrhage would decrease the total volume of blood and venous return, which would decrease stroke volume and likewise cardiac output.
5. **Answer: 1 Rationale:** Action potential is the movement of ions across cell membranes causing electrical impulses that stimulate cardiac muscle contraction.
6. **Answer: 3 Rationale:** Since pain is subjective, a numerical rating scale assesses what the client's perception of pain intensity is. The other answers do not assess intensity.
7. **Answer: 1 Rationale:** This is the only exercise test listed. The others are not conducted during exercise.
8. **Answer: 1 Rationale:** This is the location of the apex of the heart and can be assessed at left midclavicular, 5th intercostals space on most clients.
9. **Answer: 2 Rationale:** Bradycardia is defined as pulse rate < 60 beats per minute. Tachycardia is >100 beats per minute. Hypertension and hypotension relate to blood pressure not pulse rate.
10. **Answer: 2 Rationale:** S1 is the closing of the A-V valves, the mitral, and the tricuspid valves. They are located at the apex of the heart.

Chapter 31: Nursing Care of Clients with Coronary Disorders

1. **Answer: 3 Rationale:** Stopping smoking decreases the risk of coronary heart disease by 50%. The others are contributing factors but the effects are not as significant as smoking cessation.
2. **Answer: 1 Rationale:** These symptoms could indicate myopathy, a serious potential complication of statin drugs that needs to be reported promptly.
3. **Answer: 2 Rationale:** Stable angina is predictable and it is associated with increased activity and relieved by rest and nitrates.
4. **Answer: 4 Rationale:** Re-establishing coronary blood flow and cardiac tissue perfusion within 20–45 minutes is imperative to minimize damage to the myocardium.
5. **Answer: 2 Rationale:** The cardiac catheter used to insert the stent is usually inserted via the femoral artery, a large, high-pressure vessel. The leg is maintained in extension for a prescribed period after the procedure to reduce the risk of bleeding, hematoma formation, or clot formation at the insertion site. No chest tubes are needed as the pleural cavity remains intact. IV lines are maintained for medication administration as indicated. Because the stent re-establishes myocardial blood flow, narcotic analgesics rarely are required.

6. **Answer: 4 Rationale:** Relieving pain in AMI decreases sympathetic nervous system stimulation and cardiac work. Pain relief is of highest priority, although the other goals also are appropriate for the client with AMI.
7. **Answer: 1 Rationale:** Fibrinolytic therapy, administered to restore myocardial perfusion, disrupts the clotting cascade and can lead to potentially serious bleeding. Establishing bleeding precautions is vital to preserve physiologic integrity.
8. **Answer: 3 Rationale:** A CK of 320 U/L, four times the normal level, is indicative of muscle tissue damage; in the client with acute chest pain, it often indicates acute myocardial infarction.
9. **Answer: 2 Rationale:** Mobitz type II AV block often is associated with a large anterior MI and a high mortality rate. Pacemaker therapy may be necessary to maintain effective ventricular contractions and cardiac output.
10. **Answer: 1 Rationale:** Sinus bradycardia may be well tolerated in some clients. Assessment is important before treating. However, if decreased mental status and hypotension is present, intervention is necessary.

Chapter 32: Nursing Care of Clients with Cardiac Disorders

1. **Answer: 1 Rationale:** Normal ejection fraction is 60%; an ejection fraction of 25% indicates severe impairment of ventricular function.
2. **Answer: 3 Rationale:** Interdisciplinary treatment goals for the client with heart failure are to reduce the cardiac workload and improve pump effectiveness. Loss of excess fluid, as indicated by weight loss, reduces cardiac work. The drop in heart rate and reduced pulmonary vascular congestion are indicative of improved cardiac pump.
3. **Answer: 2, 4, 5 Rationale:** In left ventricular failure, the cardiac output falls and pressure in the pulmonary vascular system increases. This leads to fatigue, increasing dyspnea, and crackles in the lung bases. Jugular vein distention is associated with right ventricular heart failure. Chest pain is not a common manifestation of heart failure.
4. **Answer: 4 Rationale:** Calibrating and leveling the system during each shift ensures accuracy and consistency of measurements. The intravenous line should be secured to the client, not the bed linens, to offer movement without tension on the lines. The arterial flush solution will not work with only gravity, it must be under pressure to prevent back-up from high pressure of the artery. Dampening of wave form would be expected during wedge pressure measurements.
5. **Answer: 2 Rationale:** Morphine is given intravenously to relieve anxiety; it also is a venous vasodilator, reducing venous return and cardiac work.
6. **Answer: 1 Rationale:** A pericardial friction rub, a grating sound, is a characteristic sign of pericarditis so it is expected, but should be documented in the client's record. No further action is indicated.
7. **Answer: 4 Rationale:** Effective treatment for acute infective endocarditis requires long-term intravenous antibiotic therapy to eliminate the infecting organisms. One week of treatment is too short for cure, it is a serious condition and potentially life-threatening. Transplantation would not be an option during the infective process since the infection would affect the transplanted organ as well unless eliminated.
8. **Answer: 3 Rationale:** Murmurs are created by turbulant blood flow through valves. The murmur of mitral valve stenosis would be heard during diastole (when blood is flowing through the stenotic valve from the atrium to the ventricle) at the apex of

the heart. Muffled heart sounds are are not characteristic of valvular disorders; S3 and S4 heart sounds are associated with fluid volume overload and heart failure.

9. **Answer: 2 Rationale:** Anticoagulant therapy to prevent clot formation is necessary following insertion of a mechanical valve. Biologic valve replacement does not require anti-rejection medication; these valves, however, are less durable, lasting only 10–15 years. Prosthetic valve endocarditis is a risk following both mechanical and biologic valve replacements.

10. **Answer: 1 Rationale:** In hypertrophic cardiomyopathy, symptoms may not develop until the demand for oxygen increases, such as with athletes during activity, causing sudden death due to a ventricular dysrhythmia. This type of cardiomyopathy is not a filling problem but rather an obstruction to ejection of blood to the body to meet oxygen demand.

Chapter 33: Assessing Clients with Hematologic, Peripheral Vascular, and Lymphatic Disorders

1. **Answer: 4 Rationale:** Arterioles have major control of blood pressure.

2. **Answer: 3 Rationale:** Fatigue would indicate that the body's tissues are not receiving adequate oxygenation. O2 is carried by the hemoglobin molecule on the RBC; if RBC numbers are very low there are insufficient numbers to carry adequate oxygen to meet demands.

3. **Answer: 2 Rationale:** Platelet plug formation is the first step in clotting. If the count is low , fewer platelets are available for clotting, therefore with tissue injury, platelets are not available and bruising occurs.

4. **Answer: 4 Rationale:** The middle layer of the arteries are thicker than in veins, made of smooth muscle that allows the arteries to expand and contract with the heart as it relaxes and contracts with each beat.

5. **Answer: 1 Rationale:** The thickness of the blood will affect the ability of the blood to flow through the vessels thus increasing the peripheral vascular resistance.

6. **Answer: 2 Rationale:** The lymphatic vessels form a network with the cardiovascular system at the capillary beds to collect and drain excess tissue fluid.

7. **Answer: 2 Rationale:** Auscultating with the bell will identify soft sounds such as the carotid arteries and identify any bruits. Inspecting for movement or absence is not precise since carotid movement may not be visible in some clients. Palpation should be done with light pressure so blood flow is not obscured. Percussion of the carotid artery is not recommended.

8. **Answer: 3 Rationale:** A murmuring or blowing sound is the definition of a bruit. The other terms are related to cardiac rhythm assessment.

9. **Answer: 1 Rationale:** The definition of lymphedema is swelling of a body part as the result of obstruction. Lymphadenopathy indicates abnormal enlargement of the lymph nodes, not necessarily a body part. Atrophic change means a change in size. Central cyanosis is oxygen deprivation.

10. **Answer: 4 Rationale:** Notify the physician immediately, these manifestations indicate a severe decrease in perfusion to the leg, and cells are dying from lack of blood flow.

Chapter 34: Nursing Care of Clients with Hematologic Disorders

1. **Answer: 3 Rationale:** Red blood cells and the hemoglobin they contain carry oxygen to the tissues; in anemia, the oxygen-carrying capacity of blood is reduced, leading to exertional dyspnea. Hematocrit of 45% is elevated slightly, not decreased. A pulse rate of 140 would not be expected in moderate anemia. WBC level is unrelated to anemia.

2. **Answer: 1 Rationale:** a. During gastric resection, intrinsic factor production may decrease, leading to vitamin B_{12} deficiency anemia with associated neurologic deficits such as numbness and tingling of extremities. The other answers are not related to nutritional deficiency anemias.

3. **Answer: 2 Rationale:** Prior to bone marrow transplant, chemotherapy or total body irradiation is used to destroy leukemic cells in the bone marrow. Normal blood cells also are destroyed, causing significant risk for infection and bleeding. The other diagnoses, while appropriate, are of lower priority.

4. **Answer: 1, 3, 5 Rationale:** AML causes both neutropenia and thrombocytopenia, with resulting increased risk for infection and bleeding. A private room and oral hygiene help reduce infection risk, and a soft, bland diet reduces trauma to oral mucosal membranes. Leukemia is not communicable; airborne infection control measures are unneccessary. Rectal temperatures are avoided to protect rectal mucosal integrity.

5. **Answer: 1 Rationale:** This question demonstrates a non-verbalized concern. The correct response is open-ended and allows the client to state more specifically what he is concerned about. The other answers assume what the client wishes to discuss.

6. **Answer: 3 Rationale:** Multiple-drug chemotherapy regimes are effective at different phases of the cell cycle, allowing lower doses of individual drugs to decrease adverse effects and more effective tumor destruction. While adverse effects and destruction of normal cells may be reduced, this regime does not eliminate them.

7. **Answer: 4 Rationale:** A new onset of severe pain may signal a pathological fracture and needs to be reported.

8. **Answer: 2 Rationale:** A platelet count of 60,000/mm^3 is significantly low (normal 150,000-450,000/mm^3), increasing the risk of bleeding and bruising with minor trauma.

9. **Answer: 1 Rationale:** The most common form of classic hemophilia is transmitted as an x-linked recessive disorder passed from mother to son, therefore the daughter may be a carrier. The other answers are incorrect.

10. **Answer: 4 Rationale:** A platelet infusion replaces those platelets used in the abnormal clotting process of DIC. Platelets do not replace clotting factors or increase the oxygen-carrying capacity of the blood. Promotion of intravascular clotting is not a desired effect.

Chapter 35: Nursing Care of Clients with Peripheral Vascular Disorders

1. **Answer: 3 Rationale:** Hypertension generally is asymptomatic. Follow-up evaluation and treatment is necessary to reduce long-term effects of the disorder.

2. **Answer: 1 Rationale:** While lasagna made with whole-grain pasta, low-fat cheese, and vegetables or lean meats would be allowed, this answer demonstrates the need for additional teaching.

3. **Answer: 2, 4 Rationale:** First-dose hypotension and orthostatic hypotension are potential adverse effects of this drug, as is persistent cough. The drug should be taken in the morning to reduce potential nocturia. Potassium supplements are not recommended unless prescribed by the physican. Hypertension treatment may be life-long.

4. **Answer: 1 Rationale:** These symptoms indicate a possible arterial occlusion. This is an emergency; immediate intervention is necessary to preserve the extremity.

5. **Answer: 4 Rationale:** Endovascular approach on an 86-year-old client would mean less surgical risk and faster recovery.
6. **Answer: 4 Rationale:** Clients with peripheral atherosclerosis may have paresthesias and decreased hair on the affected extremity. Pallor is associated with elevation of the affected extremity, and the blood pressure may be lower in the affected extremity.
7. **Answer: 2, 3, 1, 4, 5 Rationale:** First, nicotine causes vasoconstriction, further decreasing blood flow; next, daily skin inspections looking for breaks in integrity to prevent infections; then, maintaining feet by regular cleansing, cotton socks, and protecting feet by wearing shoes; fourth, regular daily exercise to develop collateral circulation; and fifth, weight loss if necessary to keep client mobile.
8. **Answer: 2 Rationale:** Anticoagulant therapy will be continued after discharge; understanding the importance of follow-up care and monitoring for adverse effects is vital. Sitting in a straight chair is not recommended as it impairs venous return; progressive exercise is recommended to promote venous return. While a low-fat, low-cholesterol diet is a good idea, it will not prevent future venous thrombosis.
9. **Answer: 1 Rationale:** Elevating the legs and wearing elastic stockings may relieve the discomfort associated wtih varicose veins. Significant symptoms, recurrent superficial venous thrombosis, or stasis ulcers are the primary indications for surgical treatment of varicose veins.
10. **Answer: 3 Rationale:** Careful skin and foot care is a high priority to prevent skin breakdown and potential infection.

Chapter 36: Assessing Clients with Respiratory Disorders

1. **Answer: 4 Rationale:** The apex or top of the lungs is located just below the clavicle.
2. **Answer: 3 Rationale:** Simple diffusion at the respiratory membrane is where gases dissolved in substances move from higher concentration to one of lower concentration.
3. **Answer: 4 Rationale:** Pulmonary capillaries cover the external surface of the alveoli. The other answers are above the alveoli in the lungs.
4. **Answer: 1 Rationale:** As the body temperature rises the bond between oxygen and hemoglobin decreases so less oxygen binds and unloading is enhanced.
5. **Answer: 2 Rationale:** Thoracentesis is the removal of fluid around the lung by placing a needle in the pleural space and extracting the excess fluid.
6. **Answer: 3 Rationale:** To identify a genetic risk of respiratory disease, during an interview the nurse would ask about lung cancer in the family.
7. **Answer: 2 Rationale:** Wheezes are continuous musical sounds heard in the chest. Crackles and rales are discontinuous sounds, and with murmurs, are heard in the cardiac assessment.
8. **Answer: 4 Rationale:** If the client had a lung removed, breath sounds would be absent from that side because without air movement no sound would be generated.
9. **Answer: 3 Rationale:** While auscultating the lungs, the client should take slow deep breaths to allow adequate time for air to go into and out of the lung. Breathing through the mouth amplifies the sound, making it easier to hear.
10. **Answer: 2 Rationale:** Decreased diaphragmatic movement on the left side should be documented; it is an expected outcome with pneumothorax on the left since air movement and diaphragm movement would be decreased.

Chapter 37: Nursing Care of Clients with Upper Respiratory Disorders

1. **Answer: 4 Rationale:** Over-the-counter nasal spray is the best choice to relieve URI symptoms in the client with hypertension, since its effects are local, not systemic. The duration of use is limited to prevent rebound. Many systemic decongestants such as pseudoephedrine elevate the blood pressure. Antibiotics are not effective against viral infections. Vitamin C and zinc lozenges have not been demonstrated to be more effective than placebo in studies.
2. **Answer: 2 Rationale:** Yearly influenza vaccinations are the most effective way of preventing flu and pneumonia in this group. Handwashing will prevent spread to others once the person has developed the flu. The clients should maintain optimum health through exercise all-year-round.
3. **Answer: 1 Rationale:** Completion of the antibiotic medication is the most important in order to cure the bacterial infection and prevent reoccurrence. The other answers will assist but are not the most important.
4. **Answer: 3 Rationale:** Posterior nasal packing obstructs the nares and may compromise oxygenation. While the other interventions are important for comfort, facilitating oxygenation has higher priority.
5. **Answer: 4 Rationale:** Fracture of other facial bones may accompany nasal fracture, damaging the dura and causing spinal fluid leak. A positive glucose indicates the presence of spinal fluid, indicates a need to initiate appropriate treatment to prevent infection. The other responses are inappropriate to preserve physiologic integrity.
6. **Answer: 3, 5, 6 Rationale:** The manifestations of sleep apnea include daytime sleepiness, elevated BP, and complaints of morning headache. Oxygen saturation levels may fall while asleep, not while awake. Confusion, dementia, and an enlarged tongue are not related to obstructive sleep apnea.
7. **Answer: 1 Rationale:** Persistent voice hoarseness may be the first sign of a laryngeal tumor, necessitating follow-up diagnostic testing. While smoking is a risk factor for laryngeal cancer, the question does not help differentiate hoarseness due to an acute infection from laryngeal cancer.
8. **Answer: 3 Rationale:** With stage I laryngeal cancer, radiation can cure the cancer, and preserve the voice. This cancer does metastasize to other areas.
9. **Answer: 4, 5, 2, 1, 3 Rationale:** Maintaining airway patency is of highest priority. The head may need additional support because of the removal of neck muscles. Frequent, small meals help meet metabolic needs; swallowing may be difficult and the effort may produce fatigue. Regaining speech will require practice and assistance from a speech therapist. Loss of the voice will result in grieving; encouraging expression of feelings can facilitate gradual acceptance of the loss.
10. **Answer: 2 Rationale:** When providing tracheostomy care, the nurse secures clean ties before removing soiled ones to prevent accidental dislodgement of the tube. Sterile scissors are not necessary. Sterile technique is used to clean the phlange of the outer cannula; iodine antiseptic interferes with healing, and is avoided.

Chapter 38: Nursing Care of Clients with Ventilation Disorders

1. **Answer: 1 Rationale:** Unless oxygenation is compromised by the inflammatory process, the sputum specimen is obtained first. Oxygen therapy is then initiated, the IV established, and antibiotic therapy started. Providing food is of lower priority.

2. **Answer: 1, 4, 5, 2, 3 Rationale:** Overall gray skin color and bluish tinge to lips indicate hypoxemia; supplemental oxygen is highest priority. Second, raise the head of the bed to promote chest expansion and alveolar ventilation. Assessment of oxygen saturation and breath sounds provide important information to be provided to the physician.

3. **Answer: 3 Rationale:** A 9 mm induration is a positive result in a client with HIV disease. Induration of 10–15 mm would be considered positive in the other instances.

4. **Answer: 2 Rationale:** When teaching a client who is taking INH, the nurse needs to include information on adverse effects such as numbness and tingling of extremities to the doctor. The other answers reflect adverse responses to other drugs used in treatment of TB.

5. **Answer: 3 Rationale:** Smoking cessation is important with the diagnosis of lung cancer to prevent further damage from the chemicals in the cigarettes. The other answers contain statements that either erase all hope or contain unreasonable expectations since lung cancer metastasis early, and survival rates are low at five year interval.

6. **Answer: 3, 4 Rationale:** Chest tube drainage that is red, free-flowing, and exceeds 70mL/hour indicates hemorrhage and must be reported. Vital signs and level of consciousness are measured to evaluate cardiac output and hemodynamic stability. Chest tube drainage devices are never emptied to maintain system integrity; placing pressure on the insertion site will not reduce internal bleeding.

7. **Answer: 1 Rationale:** The client having a thoracentesis needs to sit upright, leaning forward during the procedure to spread the rib cage for easier placement of the needle. The client should hold his breath while needle is inserted to prevent damage to lung tissues. After the procedure, activity may be resumed as tolerated. Coughing during fluid aspiration is not recommended to avoid displacing the needle.

8. **Answer: 4 Rationale:** A client with a fractured rib would be urged to use a small pillow to splint the area when coughing to reduce the movement of rib cage, and pain.

9. **Answer: 2 Rationale:** A respiratory rate of 36 indicates respiratory distress, and is of greatest concern.

10. **Answer: 1 Rationale:** Tension pneumothorax displaces structures in the mediastinum, including the great vessels. Cardiac output may be severely compromised, resulting in inadequate oxygen delivery and nutrients to cells and tissues.

Chapter 39: Nursing Care of Clients with Gas Exchange Disorders

1. **Answer: 2 Rationale:** Ineffective airway clearance is the highest priority because it impairs alveolar ventilation and the exchange of oxygen and carbon dioxide at the capillaries, decreasing the blood and tissue oxygen levels.

2. **Answer: 1 Rationale:** The physician needs to be informed because this indicates increasing fatigue and impending respiratory failure. The other answers do not address the immediate need of the client.

3. **Answer: 3 Rationale:** Rinsing the mouth after using an MDI reduces systemic absorption and adverse effects of the drug. The bronchodilator drug is used before the anti-inflammatory to facilitate its delivery to distal lung tissues.

4. **Answer: 1 Rationale:** Development of a barrel chest due to air trapping is an expected finding in COPD. Confusion, lethargy, and low oxygen saturation levels indicate respiratory failure. Pitting edema may indicate heart failure or an untreated problem.

5. **Answer: 3 Rationale:** During an acute exacerbation of COPD, keeping the SaO_2 above 90% is an appropriate goal. COPD is a progressive disease, lost lung function cannot be regained, nor is it likely ABGs will return to normal values. Smoking cessation, not reduction, is vital.

6. **Answer: 4 Rationale:** In some clients with COPD, decreased arterial oxygen concentrations drive respirations. Administered O_2 may decrease the drive to breathe, however, many clients with COPD require supplemental oxygen.

7. **Answer: 1, 2, 4, 5 Rationale:** Thick, tenacious, milky white sputum and fever indicate possible infection. Difficulty coughing up mucus and increased shortness of breath and fatigue indicate potential early symptoms of respiratory failure. Bulky, fatty stools are an expected finding in clients with cystic fibrosis.

8. **Answer: 2 Rationale:** These symptoms may indicate pulmonary embolism. Oxygen is administered to support gas exchange and tissue oxygenation. While elevating the head of the bed supports ventilation, it may be contraindicated by the type of skeletal traction. Homan's sign may provide information about venous thrombosis, but is not a priority action at this time. The analgesic is of lower priority than oxygen, and may depress the respiratory drive.

9. **Answer: 1 Rationale:** Restlessness and tachypnea are early signs of respiratory failure caused by hypoxemia and stimulation of the respiratory center. The other answers are late symptoms of failure.

10. **Answer: 4 Rationale:** Patent airways are necessary to maintain effective alveolar ventilation and gas exchange. The other options do not promote airway clearance and alveolar ventilation.

Chapter 40: Assessing Clients with Musculoskeletal Disorders

1. **Answer: 3 Rationale:** Long bones have two broad ends that are called epiphyses. The other types of bones do not have the epiphyses.

2. **Answer: 1 Rationale:** Abduction is the term for moving an extremity away from the midline of the body. Adduction is moving the extremity towards the midline of the body. Extension is straightening an extremity. Flexion is bending a joint in an extremity.

3. **Answer: 1 Rationale:** Clients with gout have increased serum uric acid and if medication for treating gout is effective the serum level of uric acid should be decreased. Rheumatoid factor is used to diagnose rheumatoid arthritis. The other answers are not related to gout.

4. **Answer: 4 Rationale:** Women in their 60s are usually postmenopausal, this is when they are at risk for decreased bone density as well as for fractures due to osteoporosis.

5. **Answer: 3 Rationale:** With decreased bone mass and decreased calcium absorption, the bones become brittle and at risk for fractures. The other answers are not related to bone mass or calcium absorption.

6. **Answer: 2 Rationale:** When assessing facial muscle strength the nurse would ask the client to stick out his tongue. This would test cranial nerve IX.

7. **Answer: 4 Rationale:** Crepitation is the grating sound as the joint moves. Arthritis and synovitis are medical conditions. Crackles are lung sounds.

8. **Answer: 3 Rationale:** The ballottement test indicates fluid in the knee joint. The other answers are not in the knee.

9. **Answer: 2 Rationale:** Scoliosis is the term used to describe a lateral curve in the spine. Lordosis is an exaggerated forward curvature of the lumbar spine. Kyphosis is an abnormal protuberance of the thoracic spine.

10. **Answer: 1 Rationale:** Pain and limited mobility are the most common symptoms of musculoskeletal disorders.

Chapter 41: Nursing Care of Clients with Musculoskeletal Trauma

1. **Answer: 2 Rationale:** Ice used on a sprained ankle immediately after injury will cause vasoconstriction of the blood vessels to decrease edema and pain. Ice will not affect WBCs or BP and pulse.
2. **Answer: 3 Rationale:** A client with a compound fracture means bone has broken the skin, which is the first line of defense against bacterial invasion. The client is now at risk for infection either from trauma or during surgery.
3. **Answer: 3 Rationale:** Pale, cold fingers of an older woman with a cast could indicate decreased circulation to the hand. The other answers indicate favorable indications in this situation.
4. **Answer: 4 Rationale:** Calcium deposits in the fracture site allows callus to begin to form and healing occurs.
5. **Answer: 2 Rationale:** The client who is cyanotic and lacks sensation in the toes indicates decreased circulation and pressure on nerve, if not relieved soon permanent damage could occur. While the other answers are usual nursing activities they do not address the emergent need in this situation.
6. **Answer: 2 Rationale:** Clients with deep vein thrombosis of the lower extremity need the respiratory system to be monitored carefully for complications of emboli.
7. **Answer: 2 Rationale:** Clients who have suffered musculoskeletal injuries have soft tissue damage, muscle spasm and swelling causing acute pain. The other nursing diagnoses are not as common.
8. **Answer: 1 Rationale:** During the first 24 hours after amputation the remaining extremity is elevated above the level of the heart to promote venous return and decrease swelling.
9. **Answer: 4 Rationale:** Phantom limb pain is experienced by a majority of amputees especially in the early postoperative period.
10. **Answer: 4 Rationale:** The amputated finger should be wrapped in a clean cloth, put in a plastic bag and place on ice to preserve tissue—not directly on ice, which could cause tissue frostbite. This will preserve the amputated finger so that it can be surgically reattached.

Chapter 42: Nursing Care of Clients with Musculoskeletal Disorders

1. **Answer: 2 Rationale:** Risk for falls is the most significant nursing diagnosis in terms of long-term disability because falls that would result in no injury to the healthy adult may cause fractures in the osteoporotic client.
2. **Answer: 4 Rationale:** Most clients with osteoarthritis use NSAIDs for control of discomfort from disease. The other three categories are not utilized in osteoarthritis.
3. **Answer:2 Rationale:** Clients with gout have increased serum levels of uric acid. The other lab tests are not affected by gout.
4. **Answer: 3 Rationale:** In clients with osteoporosis and osteomalacia, fractures are a potential complication because of lack of calcium intake and vitamin D intake.
5. **Answer: 1 Rationale:** In clients complaining of knee pain, being overweight by thirty pounds is indicative of an increased risk for osteoarthritis. None of the other answers are an increased risk for developing OA.
6. **Answer: 3 Rationale:** By monitoring vital signs, hemoglobin and hematocrit, the nurse can determine early if the fluid volume is deficient, caused by excessive bleeding, or if blood supply to extremity is compromised.

7. **Answer: 1 Rationale:** Fever and weight loss are found in clients with rheumatoid arthritis; not found in osteoarthritis.
8. **Answer: 3 Rationale:** In the nursing diagnosis *ineffective protection*, the most important intervention for the client with SLE would be to practice careful handwashing, since SLE clients are at risk for opportunistic and severe infection.
9. **Answer: 4 Rationale:** Most cases of Lyme disease occur when an infected tick remains embedded for at least 24 hours. Malaria/West Nile Fever are transmitted by mosquitoes. Droplet infection is primarily tuberculosis.
10. **Answer: 2 Rationale:** Septic arthritis is a medical emergency since if not diagnosed quickly and treatment begun, destruction of the affected joint may occur.

Chapter 43: Assessing Clients with Neurologic Disorders

1. **Answer: 4 Rationale:** The blood-brain barrier controls the environment within by allowing oxygen, carbon dioxide, lipids, glucose, and water into the capillaries but preventing urea, creatinine, toxins, proteins, and antibiotic entry.
2. **Answer: 3 Rationale:** The lower motor neurons maintain muscle tone and reflexes, any damage could result in loss of reflexes.
3. **Answer: 3 Rationale:** Cerebrospinal fluid (CSF) cushions the brain tissue and spinal cord, protects them from trauma, provides nourishment to the brain, and removes waste products.
4. **Answer: 1 Rationale:** The posterior spinal roots contain cells that discriminate fine touch sensations such as dull and sharp, therefore damage to these roots would mean the client would be unable to detect dull or sharp sensation.
5. **Answer: 1 Rationale:** The sympathetic division of the ANS has the purpose of preparing the body to handle stressful events, such as a near auto accident, by increasing heart rate, force of contraction, vasodilation of coronary arteries, and increased mental alertness.
6. **Answer: 2 Rationale:** Auscultation is not used in assessing the neurologic examination. Inspection is used to observe physical characteristics and mental condition. Percussion with a hammer checks reflexes. Muscles are palpated.
7. **Answer: 1 Rationale:** A cotton ball and a safety pin would be used to assess sensations of light dull and sharp on the face. The cotton ball would also be used to test corneal reflex.
8. **Answer: 4 Rationale:** In clients that are unconscious the corneal reflex is absent, so when the cornea is touched with a wisp of cotton, the client would not blink the way a conscious client would.
9. **Answer: 3 Rationale:** A tongue depressor is utilized on the posterior section of the tongue to illicit a gag reflex, testing cranial nerve IX.
10. **Answer: 2 Rationale:** In decorticate posturing the upper arms are close to the body, the elbows, wrists, and fingers are flexed, and the legs are extended with internal rotation.

Chapter 44: Nursing Care of Clients with Intracranial Disorders

1. **Answer: 4 Rationale:** Normally the RAS and cerebral hemispheres control respirations with a regular pattern however, when they are damaged, the lower brainstem responds to changes is $Paco_2$ resulting in irregular respiratory patterns.
2. **Answer: 2 Rationale:** The unconscious client with impaired gag or swallowing reflexes would be at risk for aspiration since saliva and any fluids taken by mouth could not be swallowed normally.
3. **Answer: 2 Rationale:** Osmotic diuretics increase the osmolarity of blood by excreting water and leaving solutes, as a result,

the water in the brain would be drawn into the vascular space. Osmotic diuretics would not be related to other answers.

4. **Answer: 3 Rationale:** Motor responses to a direct stimuli such as "squeeze my hand" are the best way to identify changes in mental status. These other answers would require an alert client, not one in a coma.

5. **Answer: 1, 2, 3 Rationale:** A client with an altered LOC would probably have blood glucose to check for hypoglycemia, electrolytes to check for metabolic disturbances, especially sodium, and toxicology to test for drug or alcohol toxicity. Since testing spinal fluid is invasive, it would not be done unless there were symptoms of meningeal irritation.

6. **Answer: 3 Rationale:** Serum osmolality would assess water and solute balance in the blood indicating the hydration status of the client. The other tests would not tell the hydration status.

7. **Answer: 1 Rationale:** Clients with perceived generalized seizures must have loss of consciousness or they are not considered generalized seizures. Tonic and clonic are movements that may not be present. Repetitive, non-purposeful movements are not associated with seizures.

8. **Answer: 3 Rationale:** In a client with a head injury that has fluid draining from the ear, the nurse must suspect a potential CSF leak and would test the drainage for glucose. That is present in CSF but not fluid from the ear.

9. **Answer: 4 Rationale:** Antiepileptic (AED) drugs are not a cure but rather they provide control of seizures or reduce seizure activity. The other answers are not related to use of AEDs.

10. **Answer: 1 Rationale:** All brain tumors are potentially lethal because they grow within a closed, confined space and can produce problems on the CNS.

Chapter 45: Nursing Care of Clients with Cerebrovascular and Spinal Cord Disorders

1. **Answer: 2 Rationale:** Numbness and tingling in the corner of the client's mouth that disappears within minutes or hours is a manifestation of temporary occlusion of the middle cerebral artery. The other manifestations are present with strokes, not TIAs.

2. **Answer: 1 Rationale:** Hypertension is the greatest risk factor for a stroke because it's sustained systolic and diastolic pressure causes damage to cerebral blood vessels with a 4–6X greater risk for stroke than clients without hypertension.

3. **Answer: 3 Rationale:** The motor pathways of the nervous system cross at the medulla and spinal cord meaning damage to the left cerebral vessel will demonstrate neurologic deficits on the right side, an effect called contralateral.

4. **Answer: 4 Rationale:** Tissue plasminogen activator is given within the first 3 hours of the ischemic stroke to cause fibrinolysis of the clot.

5. **Answer: 3 Rationale:** Preventing hypoxia and hypercapnia through administration of oxygen will prevent further ischemia of cerebral tissues and increase of intracranial pressure. The other answers are not related to this question.

6. **Answer: 1 Rationale:** In a client with spinal cord injury no impulses are transmitted between the brain and spinal cord and the cord does not function at all, producing spinal shock that may last from minutes to weeks or months.

7. **Answer: 2 Rationale:** Autonomic dysreflexia can be caused by kinked catheter tubing allowing the bladder to become full, triggering massive vasoconstriction below the injury site, producing the symptoms of this process. The other answers will not cause autonomic dysreflexia.

8. **Answer: 3 Rationale:** SCI at the C1-C4 level produces respiratory paralysis and the client will be unable to breathe on his own, so a ventilator will be necessary to maintain respiratory function.

9. **Answer: 1, 2, 4 Rationale:** Cortiocsteroids will be used to decrease cord edema. Vasopressors will be used to treat bradycardia or hypotension from spinal shock. Analgesics will be used to control pain. There is no reason to use antihistamines or antibiotics.

10. **Answer: 1, 3, 5 Rationale:** In teaching prevention of back injuries the nurse would incorporate principles of proper body mechanics, which are spread feet apart, use large leg muscles, and work as close to the object as possible. Bending from the waist to lift rather than sometimes rolling or pushing, will contribute to back injuries.

Chapter 46: Nursing Care of Clients with Neurologic Disorders

1. **Answer: 1, 2 Rationale:** Dementia is a general term used to describe the outcome of the death of neurons, and the cognitive and behavioral symptoms of AD. The other answers are incorrect.

2. **Answer: 3 Rationale:** Memory deficits are usually the first indication of AD, are subtle and may not be noticed by friends and family until the client exhibits unsafe behaviors. The other answers listed are symptoms in later stages of AD.

3. **Answer: 1 Rationale:** Fatigue affects all clients with MS regardless of type or severity. The other answers are not as pervasive.

4. **Answer: 3 Rationale:** Interferons are used to reduce exacerbations in clients with multiple sclerosis and enhance immune function. The other drugs or category of drugs are not used in treatment of MS.

5. **Answer: 4 Rationale:** When teaching a young adult with MS it is important to stress avoidance of extremes of heat and cold since maintaining a constant body temperature will decrease exacerbations of symptoms, and heat slows down transmission of nerve impulses.

6. **Answer: 2 Rationale:** Parkinson's disease symptoms appear when the brain cells not longer produce enough dopamine to inhibit acetylcholine, this produces uncoordinated motor movement.

7. **Answer: 3 Rationale:** With the gait changes, balance problems and possible orthostatic hypotension, clients with PD are at increased risk for falls. This safety issue needs to be addressed with the caregivers. The other answers are not accurate or not a major concern.

8. **Answer: 4 Rationale:** Antiglutamate is the drug classification used to treat ALS because it prevents the release of glutamic acid and protects against toxicity of neurons. The other drugs are not used to treat ALS.

9. **Answer: 3 Rationale:** When teaching clients about Bell's palsy, the nurse needs to tell the client that one side of the face will not move normally since the affected nerve supplies the muscles that produce expression on one side of the face. Pain in Bell's palsy may be present before the paralysis appears, not during. Bell's palsy affects only the facial area, not walking, and boiling foods is to prevent botulism.

10. **Answer: 2 Rationale:** The nurse can prevent tetanus by promoting tetanus immunization to adults and children, since this is the most effective way to prevent the disease from contaminated wounds. Older adults may not have had the immunization as a child, or may need a booster to keep up immunity. The other answers do not reflect prevention of tetanus.

Chapter 47: Assessing Clients with Eye and Ear Disorders

1. **Answer: 2 Rationale:** When the cornea is touched the client will blink as a mechanism to protect it from foreign objects entering.

2. **Answer: 4 Rationale:** Presbyopia develops in older adults as the lens of the eye looses its ability to adjust, requiring the client to hold papers further away in order to focus and read.

3. **Answer: 2 Rationale:** Tuning forks are used to assess the hearing acuity, if a deficit is present it will tell if the loss is conductive or sensorineural.

4. **Answer: 1 Rationale:** As the light enters the lens, the rays bend and is focused on a single point on the retina; this focusing is called accommodation.

5. **Answer: 4 Rationale:** Clients having a test of refraction will have the pupil dilated for better access to examine the internal structures.

6. **Answer: 3 Rationale:** Receptors within the inner ear maintain equilibrium by responding to changes in head position in order to coordinate body movements and balance.

7. **Answer: 1 Rationale:** The Snellen eye chart measures the client's ability to read letters at a standard distance of twenty feet. The client reads the smallest line, the numbers on the side would indicate visual acuity, e.g., 20/20, 20/30.

8. **Answer: 1 Rationale:** The examiner can whisper a word one or two feet behind the client, asking the client to repeat the word, this may provide a rough estimate of hearing acuity. The other tests are more specific and would be done after the client failed the whisper test.

9. **Answer: 2 Rationale:** The vestibular structures maintain balance. As the person ages this function may decrease and the client may be at risk for loosing balance and falling.

10. **Answer: 4 Rationale:** The examiner must have a normal visual field when assessing the visual field of a client because the examiner's field becomes the standard or norm. If the examiner does not have normal visual field then the results of this part of the exam would be inaccurate.

Chapter 48: Nursing Care of Clients with Eye or Ear Disorders

1. **Answer: 4 Rationale:** The highest priority for residents with moderate to severe hearing or vision impairment is safety.

2. **Answer: 2 Rationale:** In teaching a client with newly diagnosed glaucoma, the nurse emphasizes the importance of taking eye drops as prescribed on a continuing basis to control intraocular pressure and prevent vision loss.

3. **Answer: 3 Rationale:** Timolol is a beta adrenergic blocker that can decrease myocardial contractility and impair cardiac function in the client with heart failure.

4. **Answer: 4 Rationale:** The highest priority for a client with repeated attacks of vertigo and tinnitus is maintenance of safety. Sitting when an attack occurs reduces the risk of injury from falling.

5. **Answer: 1 Rationale:** Following eye surgery, clients are placed in semi-Fowler's or Fowler's position to reduce intraocular pressure and edema.

6. **Answer: 3 Rationale:** Immediate referral to an ophthalmologist is necessary because the symptoms suggest a detached retina. Immediate treatment is necessary to optimize sight restoration. The other answers do not address the seriousness of the situation.

7. **Answer: 1, 2, 3, 4, 5 Rationale:** All the assessments should be included because each provides information about infection and possible location in the ear.

8. **Answer: 4 Rationale:** The client's symptoms could be due to impacted cerumen. The nurse should inspect the ear canal for patency. Aging is a risk factor for cerumen impaction because there is less and it is harder and drier.

9. **Answer: 1 Rationale:** One-on-one social interactions in a quiet environment facilitate effective communication for the client with a severe hearing deficit.

10. **Answer: 2 Rationale:** Cataract removal is elective surgery, generally performed only when visual impairment interferes with activities of daily living.

Chapter 49: Assessing Clients with Reproductive System and Breast Disorders

1. **Answer: 3 Rationale:** In the male the testes produce the sperm and testosterone. The epididymis stores the sperm, the seminal vesicles and Cowper's glands produce the seminal fluid.

2. **Answer: 4 Rationale:** In the female, the clitoris is an erectile organ similar to the penis in the male. The others are not erectile tissue.

3. **Answer: 2 Rationale:** The explanation should begin with the prostate gland surrounding the urethra, as it grows larger it decreases the size of the opening. The client may not empty the bladder and need to urinate more frequently.

4. **Answer: 1 Rationale:** PSA is the diagnostic test used to diagnose and monitor prostate cancer. CBC & WBC monitor blood cells. VDRL is a diagnostic test for sexually transmitted diseases.

5. **Answer: 1 Rationale:** Transillumination is used if any swelling is noted during inspection. None of the other methods will be as helpful in detecting problems in the scrotum.

6. **Answer: 3 Rationale:** Estrogens reduce cholesterol levels but following menopause the estrogen level drops and cholesterol increases, putting the woman at risk for cardiovascular disease.

7. **Answer: 1 Rationale:** When women of reproductive age become pregnant, the embryo implants in the uterus and menstruation stops until after delivery.

8. **Answer: 4 Rationale:** Pap smears are used to detect cervical cancers and precancerous lesions of the cervix. Colposcopy is used after a pap test is abnormal. Mammograms are done to detect breast tumors. Culture is done if an infection is suspected.

9. **Answer: 3 Rationale:** Monthly breast exams done by the client utilize palpation to find any lumps or changes in breast tissues.

10. **Answer: 2 Rationale:** The Bartholin's gland would be palpated at the posterior section of the labia majora.

Chapter 50: Nursing Care of Men with Reproductive System and Breast Disorders

1. **Answer: 4 Rationale:** This is stated in an appropriate way to allow the client to feel free to ask any question about his sexual concerns. The other answers presume problems or contain judgmental attitudes.

2. **Answer: 2 Rationale:** In a health teaching session with young men, the nurse should tell them about retracting the foreskin while showering, and cleaning regularly to decrease the presence of collection of secretions under the foreskin, which has been show to increase the risk of penile cancer.

3. **Answer: 1 Rationale:** Sexually active men who have gonorrhea are especially susceptible to inflammation or infection of the epididymis. A sexually transmitted disease is not associated with the other conditions.

4. **Answer: 2 Rationale:** Testicular cancer commonly occurs between the ages of fifteen and forty. The incidence decreases with age, has a genetic predisposition in brothers and has no associate pain symptoms.

5. **Answer: 3 Rationale:** Men with chronic prostatitis should increase their fluid intake to 3L/day and void often to decrease the irritation when voiding. Cold showers and restricting fluids would be contraindicated, it would not help to relieve symptoms. A scrotal support, increased fiber intake, and avoiding sexual activity would not help discomfort.

6. **Answer: 2, 4 Rationale:** In digital rectal examination for BPH, the prostate is asymmetrical and enlarged while in prostate cancer the exam shows nodules and a fixed position. PSA is specific to the prostate and is released by both benign and malignant cells however, in BPH the amounts of the free form of PSA and complex PSA would be different. The other tests are not helpful in distinguishing cancer from BPH.

7. **Answer: 2 Rationale:** As the prostate enlarges around the urethra it begins to obstruct the outflow of urine from the bladder during urination causing problems with urinary retention, frequency and urgency. The other systems are not affected.

8. **Answer: 3 Rationale:** The nurse needs to notify the surgeon because dark red fluid with obvious clots and painful bladder spasms could indicate that the client may be hemorrhaging postoperatively and the doctor will need to know to direct next actions to keep the client safe. The other answers do not address the need for appropriate action.

9. **Answer: 1 Rationale:** Prostate cancer is the most common type of malignancy in American men and the second leading cause of death in North America.

10. **Answer: 4 Rationale:** Some studies have shown an increase in prostate cancer in societies with diets high in red meats and fats. Informing the community of this relationship could help members change their dietary habits to decrease the risk of prostate cancer.

Chapter 51: Nursing Care of Women with Reproductive System and Breast Disorders

1. **Answer: 1 Rationale:** The nurse acknowledging the problem stated by the client gives credence for the client, but because the nurse is uncomfortable addressing the issue herself, she refers the client to the physician to address her problem. The other answers would not be therapeutic responses.

2. **Answer: 2, 3, 4 Rationale:** Osteoporosis, cardiovascular disease, and fractures are all related to estrogen deprivation. Cervical and colon cancer have not been linked to decreased estrogen levels.

3. **Answer: 1200 Rationale:** This level can be achieved through diet and supplements if necessary.

4. **Answer: 1 Rationale:** Kegel exercises utilized in uterine displacement strengthens perineal muscle tone, minimizes urinary leakage, and the descent of the bladder into the vagina. These exercises do not have an affect on the other conditions.

5. **Answer: 2 Rationale:** A health-promotion seminar for reducing the risk of cervical cancer should contain information about safe sex methods that reduce the incidence of genital infections from HPV, which is the most important risk factor. The other answers are not risk factors of cervical cancer.

6. **Answer: 4 Rationale:** For a woman with PMS, the nurse would recommend a decrease in sodium intake to help minimize the fluid retention due to the increased production of aldosterone, which results in sodium retention and edema.

7. **Answer: 2 Rationale:** Endometrial implantations tend to atrophy and disappear after menopause since ovarian hormones no longer stimulate them.

8. **Answer: 1, 3, 4 Rationale:** A teaching plan for home care of a woman following an abdominal hysterectomy, should include no lifting to decrease chances of hemorrhage, report temperature > 100° F since this may be a sign of infection, and take regular rest periods since she may be tired for several days postoperatively. She should be told to take showers until bleeding stops and should be encouraged to splint abdomen so she may breathe and cough deeply to prevent respiratory complications of atelectasis.

9. **Answer: 4 Rationale:** Risk factors for breast cancer are doubled for the 64-year-old with a positive family history.

10. **Answer: 3 Rationale:** Anticipatory grieving is appropriate ND since she is losing a portion of her body. She is beginning to grieve for that loss by crying.

Chapter 52: Nursing Care of Clients with Sexually Transmitted Infections

1. **Answer: 2 Rationale:** Women and infants are disproportionally affected by STIs because women may not experience symptoms of the disease and pass the infection on to the infant through vaginal birth.

2. **Answer: 1 Rationale:** STIs must be treated by treating both partners to prevent reinfection from one to the other, since symptoms are not always demonstrated when the infection is present.

3. **Answer: 1, 4, 5 Rationale:** Topics of information when teaching a male to prevent an STI should include using a new condom with each sex act, careful handling to prevent damage to condom, and withdrawal from the vagina when the penis is erect, holding the condom against the base of the penis to prevent contamination of the penis. No air should be in the tip and oil-based lubricants should never be used.

4. **Answer: 4 Rationale:** Blisters and ulcers appear on the penis of clients infected with genital herpes. The other STIs do not have these characteristics.

5. **Answer: 1 Rationale:** The statement is untrue about genital warts being caused by a yeast infection, viruses cause them.

6. **Answer: 4 Rationale:** Women with HPV genital infection should be advised to have a pelvic exam and pap smears every year since this infection causes an increased risk in developing cervical cancer, and the annual exams would identify the cancer early.

7. **Answer: 2 Rationale:** Itching is the most common manifestation experienced by a woman with a vaginal infection.

8. **Answer: 3 Rationale:** When teaching a woman with an STI experiencing severe genital discomfort, a simple recommendation is to wear cotton underwear because it absorbs moisture and allows airflow better than other materials. Sex should be avoided until treatment is completed.

9. **Answer: 1 Rationale:** Initially the male urethra and female cervix is affected by the gonorrheal organism.

10. **Answer: 3 Rationale:** Syphilis is a systemic infection that is caused by a spirochete that can affect a developing fetus in multiple places, brain, bone, and eyes.

Evaluate Your Response: Cues for Critical Thinking Questions

Chapter 4: Nursing Care of Clients Having Surgery
A Client Having Surgery

1. Safety concerns include ambulating and not tripping over scatter rugs or clutter. See information in Chapter 3 on safety in the home.

2. Medications used to prevent an occurrence such as infection are called prophylactic medications. Her risks for infection are from the surgical wound and microvascular circulation in bone.

Teach her to take the complete course of antibiotics prescribed and the possible side effects of the antibiotic. Encourage her to notify the physician if side effects or adverse events occur.

3. When blood stops flowing, it clots. Her immobility is a concern and puts her at risk for thrombosis and emboli. She has a risk for bleeding secondary to the anticoagulant and should inform any health care providers such as dentists that she is taking the anticoagulant.

4. Consider the risk for osteoporosis in addition to the degenerative changes Mrs. Overbeck experienced. She will need calcium sources and vitamin D.

Chapter 5: Nursing Care of Clients Experiencing Loss, Grief, and Death
A Client Experiencing Loss and Grief

1. Review the physical manifestations of grief described in the chapter and compare and contrast those with the ones verbalized by Mrs. Rogers.

2. Consider the benefits of including Mrs. Rogers's daughter in a meeting of the staff. What type of questions would be most useful in making the daughter feel a part of the plan of care? Why would a statement such as, "Why don't you do more for your mother," be inappropriate?

3. Consider the losses Mrs. Rogers has experienced. Review the material in the chapter on responses to loss. Think about the reasons you would not say, "Oh, you have a lot to live for." Think of two or three questions or statements that would help you assess the reason why Mrs. Rogers said this to you.

Chapter 6: Nursing Care of Clients with Problems of Substance Abuse

1. Consider the interactions of prescribed or over-the-counter medications with alcohol. What if the client has not taken prescribed medications because of chronic alcoholism?

2. Review the effects of Anatbuse. Make a list of possible interactions and side effects.

3. *Imbalanced nutrition:* Less than body requirements is an appropriate nursing diagnosis when a client does not have sufficient nutritional intake to meet metabolic needs. What in Mr. Russell's history and physical assessment supports this diagnosis? What nutritional information should you provide?

Chapter 7: A Client Experiencing a Disaster

1. What action did Mr. Jones take that probably exacerbated his skin lesions? Review Table 7–1 for injuries related to natural disasters. Consider how Mr. Jones put himself at risk for infection. (See Chapter 12.) How could Mr. Jones have avoided exacerbating his skin lesions?

2. What other testing might you anticipate related to Mr. Jones's delayed healing? Since Mr. Jones has a history of elevated blood pressure that has not been consistently treated or monitored, cardiac status should be evaluated. Which tests are indicated? Also, could his decreased sensation and poor healing be related to cardiac impairment? Mr. Jones also has indentifying data in his history and physical to suggest diabetes. Identify this data, and tests that would be indicated.

3. What were the contributing factors to Mr. Jones's fever? Review risk factors for and causes and manifestations of infection in Chapter 12. Identify the factors that contributed to Mr. Jones's fever.

4. What life situations contributed to Mr. Jones's attitude about life? Consider Mr. Jones's environmental and personal situations. What information do you have about Mr. Jones that indicate a lack of interest in health maintenance? Are there signs of a change in outlook?

Chapter 9: Nursing Care of Clients in Pain
A Client with Chronic Pain

1. Review the factors that affect an individual's response to pain. What have you observed in your own family and friends, as well as clients for whom you have cared?

2. Reflect on the benefits and disadvantages of each alternative. Make your decision based on knowledge about pain and about medications for pain.

3. What factors in Ms. Akers's illness and treatment increase her risk for constipation? What would you include in the plan specific to fluid intake and diet?

Chapter 10: Nursing Care of Clients with Altered Fluid, Electrolyte, or Acid-Base Balance
A Client with Fluid Volume Excess

1. Review the homeostatic mechanisms that control fluid balance and cardiac output. Which mechanisms are employed in this situation?

2. Review the anatomy and physiology of the respiratory system, including cardiopulmonary blood flow. Think about the effects of the upper abdominal organs on respiratory function as well.

3. Use therapeutic communication techniques: What is behind the client's statement? How can you facilitate Mrs. Rainwater's involvement in care decisions?

4. Review the actions and precautions for diuretic therapy. Think about what the client needs to know in terms of timing, possible adverse effects, and other information about diuretic therapy.

A Client with Hypokalemia

1. Review the physiologic effects of potassium, especially its intracellular and neuromuscular effects.

2. Review the potential sites and causes of excess potassium loss.

3. Think about the effects of diuretics on potassium balance and the effects of hypokalemia on digitalis therapy. What is the primary indication for digitalis therapy and how does this contribute to the interaction of these three factors?

4. Review the section in Chapter 26 on constipation and its management.

A Client with Hyperkalemia

1. Review the causes and manifestations of hyperkalemia.

2. What are the potential effects of hyperkalemia on cardiac conduction? At what level of hyperkalemia are these likely to be seen?

3. Review collaborative treatment measures to rapidly reduce potassium levels. Why would these be used with a K1 of 8.5?

4. Think about the effects of anxiety on learning as you develop a plan to provide teaching to avoid future episodes of hyperkalemia. As you develop your plan, remember the potential long-term effects of chronic renal failure.

A Client with Acute Respiratory Acidosis

1. Review normal gas exchange across the alveolar-capillary membrane and the processes that drive this exchange. Then review the role that carbon dioxide plays as a potential acid.

2. Describe the effect of acidosis on mental function.

3. Consider risk factors for choking: alcohol consumption, taking large bites of food, inadequate chewing, and so forth.

Chapter 11: Nursing Care of Clients Experiencing Trauma and Shock
A Client with Multiple Injuries

1. The definition of *Deficient fluid volume* is decreased intravascular, interstitial, and/or intracellular fluid. Which of Mrs. Souza's vital signs would support this definition? What other assessments could you make that would further support this diagnosis?

2. Consider the physiology of cellular metabolism. How long do brain cells live without oxygen? What happens if circulation is improved but the airway is blocked?

3. What can cause restlessness? Consider comfort, elimination, oxygenation, emotional status, and immobility.

4. List the multiple possibilities for entry of pathogens into the human body. Would age and physical condition increase the risk? What about transmission from health care personnel?

A Client with Septic Shock

1. Review the pharmacologic effects of vasopressors. Consider the pathologic basis for septic shock and how these medications may be effective.

2. Review the content on respiratory acidosis in Chapter 10. What do these findings tell you? What is present in Ms. Huang's physical status that would cause these manifestations?

3. Review the content about colloidal intravenous solutions in the chapter. What would you expect them to do when they are administered? How does this correlate to cardiac output? How do you assess increased circulatory volume?

Chapter 12: Nursing Care of Clients with Infection
A Client with Acquired Immunity

1. Review the adult immunizations listed in this chapter. Consider the geographical area in which the client lives. For example, clients living in areas at risk for Lyme disease should check with their physician about the new Lyme disease vaccine.

2. Review the concept of acquired immunity and the discussion of immunization in this chapter. What affect could nonimmunized persons have on their family and community?

3. Identify possible systemic and local reactions associated with immunizations. List manifestations that the client should report to the primary caregiver.

Chapter 13: Nursing Care of Clients with Altered Immunity
A Client with HIV Infection

1. Considering Ms. Lu's age, how effective is her immune system? How could lifestyle factors affect immune status?

2. At this stage of Ms. Lu's diagnosis, would you expect the physician to order a viral load test? Why or why not?

3. You have been asked to discuss AIDS and safe sex practices to a group of high school freshmen. What information would you present to them?

4. What resources could you provide to Ms. Lu and her fiancé regarding their desire to have a child?

Chapter 14: Nursing Care of Clients with Cancer

1. Review content on altered nutrition in Chapter 22 and the content in this chapter on the nursing diagnosis Altered Nutrition: Less than Body Requirements. Make a list of diagnostic tests for malnutrition with normal values.

2. Consider the type of cancers Mr. Casey has been diagnosed as having. Where in the body do these malignancies commonly metastasize? What would cause the pain?

3. Review a pharmacology book for medications that increase appetite and make a list of those appropriate to Mr. Casey.

4. Sepsis is discussed in Chapter 6. Review the content in that chapter on septic shock and outline manifestations. Develop a plan of care for Mr. Casey that is structured by priority of nursing diagnoses.

Chapter 16: Nursing Care of Clients with Integumentary Disorders
A Client with Herpes Zoster

1. Consider environmental, economic, and language barriers. What agencies in your own city or state exist to provide help?

What can you do other than make referrals? If you do make a referral, to whom would it be?

2. Review skin assessment guidelines in Chapter 14. How would you determine that the lesions had not improved? What manifestations would indicate secondary infection of the lesions? What would you do next if the lesions are still very painful and have not improved?

3. *Ineffective role performance* is defined as patterns of behavior and self-expression that do not match the environmental context, norms, and expectations. Related factors include inadequate or inappropriate linkage with the health care system and poverty. Based on this information, what interventions would you use? How would you evaluate the effectiveness of your interventions?

A Client with Malignant Melanoma

1. List reasons why people do not seek health care. Do you believe nurses can effect change? If so, what community activities would be most effective?

2. Consider attitudes toward the possibility of future illnesses. How would this affect your plan? What do you believe would be most effective in teaching this age group?

3. Think about what you know about taking prescribed antibiotics as well as the side effects of antibiotic therapy. What would you suggest that Mr. Sanders do?

4. *Powerlessness* is the perception that one's own actions will not significantly affect an outcome. Is this a common response to the diagnosis of cancer? Consider types of communications and interventions that would allow greater decision making for Mr. Sanders.

Chapter 17: Nursing Care of Clients with Burns
A Client with a Major Burn

1. Review the effects of the major burn wound on the renal and gastrointestinal systems. What assessments would indicate effective fluid resuscitation?

2. What type of burns did Mr. Howard have on his arms? Consider the effect of compression on the peripheral vascular system. What assessments would you make to identify this complication?

3. Consider the type of pain the client has. What do you think might happen if the narcotics were given by other routes, such as oral or intramuscularly?

4. Review the effects of a major burn. Consider the damage to cell wall integrity and capillary beds. What effect does the shift of proteins and sodium have on intravascular volume?

Chapter 19: Nursing Care of Clients with Endocrine Disorders
A Client with Graves' Disease

1. What effect does increased TH have on metabolism and cardiac rate and stroke volume? How does this effect compare to that of sympathetic stimulation?

2. Consider the effect of elevating any body part, such as elevating your leg above heart level for a sprained ankle. How does this affect venous return?

3. You will need to consider Mrs. Manuel from both a medical and a surgical perspective. How would you teach her to care for her incision? With removal of most of the thyroid gland, what symptoms would you be sure she knew about? What should she do if these occur?

A Client with Hypothyroidism

1. Make a list of changes in body systems with aging and with decreased TH levels. How would you determine what assessment findings were abnormal?

2. Consider the effects of the following factors: weakness, fatigue, problems with memory. What would you recommend she do in her home to increase her safety?

3. Prepare a list of manifestations of hyperthyroidism. Be sure they are in terms a client would understand.

A Client with Cushing's Syndrome

1. Review Ms. Domico's lab results and compare them to normal results. What altered the findings in her case?
2. How many ways can you think of to assess fluid balance? Consider weight, I&O, and skin. What other assessments provide information?
3. How does fatigue differ from "just being tired"? Would increasing hours of sleep be an intervention you would include? Why or why not?

A Client with Addison's Disease

1. Review the functions of the hormones of the adrenal cortex in Chapter 18. Consider the effects of stress, and formulate your response with rationale.
2. Review content on fluid imbalance in Chapter 5. Make a list of assessments you might make that would indicate severe dehydration. What is the pathophysiology of fluid loss in the client with Addison's disease?
3. Review content on sodium and potassium in Chapter 5 and make a list of foods you would suggest Mr. Sardoff eat.

Chapter 2: Nursing Care of Clients with Diabetes Mellitus

A Client with Type 1 Diabetes

1. How do the increased urinary output and increased osmolarity of the blood plasma affect the fluid status of the body? What is the response of the body to decreased intravascular volume?
2. Consider the effects of nicotine on blood vessels. How would these effects, when combined with the pathologic effects of long-standing hyperglycemia, affect blood vessel walls?
3. Review the information about chronic illness in Chapter 2. Powerlessness is a perceived lack of control over a situation and/or one's ability to significantly affect an outcome. What types of statements by a client would help you make this nursing diagnosis?
4. Compare and contrast the developmental needs and tasks of the young adult and the older adult (see Chapter 2). Consider the teaching materials that might have to be adapted to physical changes in the older adult.

Chapter 22: Nursing Care of Clients with Nutritional Disorders

A Client with Obesity

1. Review the physiology of cholesterol formation in the body and the factors that affect this process.
2. Consider developmental stages and teaching strategies for adult learners.
3. Think about individual factors, family and support group influences, and cultural factors that may affect recommended weight loss and exercise strategies.

A Client with Malnutrition

1. Review the physiology of albumin and cholesterol formation in the body.
2. Review Mrs. Chow's diet and compare it to the food pyramid or recommendations for food intake to formulate your response.
3. Consider cultural influences and the client's preferred foods as you plan a diet that is high in calories and protein.

Chapter 23: Nursing Care of Clients with Upper Gastrointestinal Disorders

A Client with Oral Cancer

1. Review the major risk factors for oral cancer and identify the populations most likely to have these risk factors.

2. Work with your classmates to plan (and implement) an education program, considering the developmental/teaching needs of this group of young people.
3. Think about the possible causes for Mr. Chavez's refusal to talk (remember that assessment is the first step of the nursing process). How will you identify factors contributing to his behavior?

A Client with Peptic Ulcer Disease

1. Review the physiology of the gastric mucosal barrier and the pathogenesis of peptic ulcer disease, and the effect of *H. pylori* infection on these processes.
2. Review physiologic responses to stress in your physiology or nursing fundamentals text; compare and apply this information with the physiology of the gastric mucosal barrier and the pathophysiology of ulcer development.
3. Consider Mr. O'Donnell's occupation and schedule, as well as the prescribed medications and when each should be taken.
4. Using journal and text resources as well as your classmates, identify as many stress reduction techniques as possible. Then sort your list into those which could be used while working, and identify ways to effectively teach each technique.

A Client with Gastric Cancer

1. Review the healing process and the normal physiology of the stomach as you formulate your answer to this question.
2. Consider the surgery, immediate postoperative care, and what the client and family should expect in developing your teaching plan.
3. Review Chapter 14 and nursing care related to chemotherapy.
4. Again, review Chapter 14 for nursing care measures for clients with cancer; also review Chapter 22 for strategies to prevent and manage malnutrition.

Chapter 24: Nursing Care of Clients with Gallbladder, Liver, and Pancreatic Disorders

A Client with Cholelithiasis

1. Review the composition of gallstones, as well as the physiology of gallbladder function and bile. Research and discuss dietary practices of the Chickasaw tribe (or of Native Americans).
2. Review Chapter 4 for care related to a laparotomy (incision into the abdomen).
3. As you develop your plan, consider Mrs. Red Wing's culture, job, and family obligations.

A Client with Hepatitis A

1. In your plan, consider the transmission and pathophysiology of hepatitis A. Review developmental considerations when teaching clients to adapt your teaching to Mr. Johns's level.
2. Review the hepatitis table in this chapter, as well as the pathophysiology of hepatitis.
3. Review the hepatitis tables as well as standard precautions in Appendix A.
4. In your plan, consider the living situation (group home), the developmental level of the residents, and the resident care managers (largely unskilled). Work with your study or clinical group to develop this plan.

A Client with Alcoholic Cirrhosis

1. Review the anatomy and physiology of the liver and its circulation, as well as the pathophysiology of cirrhosis and its complications.
2. Consult your nutrition textbook as needed for foods that are high in calories but low in protein and sodium. When planning for limited protein intake, be sure to include high-quality proteins and limit intake of lower-quality proteins such as legumes.

3. Review the pathophysiology of hepatic encephalopathy to develop your responses to this question.
4. Review therapeutic communication skills; consult your nursing diagnosis and care planning text book as you develop this care plan.

A Client with Acute Pancreatitis
1. Review Chapter 6 for assessment data indicative of alcohol withdrawal.
2. Review both the pathophysiology of acute pancreatitis and the acute inflammatory process.
3. Consult your nutrition textbook or the American Dietetic Association web site.
4. Consult your nursing care planning textbook to develop this care plan.

Chapter 26: Nursing Care of Clients with Bowel Disorders
A Client with Acute Appendicitis
1. Review the acute inflammatory response to an infectious process and the role WBCs play in the immune response.
2. Review Chapter 4. Consider factors such as incision size, abdominal muscle disruption, and manipulation of the bowel in developing your response.
3. Consider points such as pain management, resumption of activities, incision care, and potential complications in developing your teaching plan. Consider the client's education and developmental stage as well.
4. Review the effects of anxiety on recovery and learning. Identify nursing measures to reduce situational anxiety.

A Client with Ulcerative Colitis
1. Review normal functions of the small and large intestine. Review the usual location of an ileostomy. Review fluid volume deficit in Chapter 10 for manifestations and assessment data.
2. Think about the effect of chronic blood loss and review the effect of malnutrition on the hemoglobin and hematocrit.
3. Review the home care section of inflammatory bowel disease for teaching points to include.
4. Review nursing care for the client with diarrhea, as well as the procedure for ileostomy care.

A Client with Colorectal Cancer
1. Review peripheral innervation and impulse transmission in your anatomy and physiology textbook; think about how nerves in the rectal region are disrupted in an abdominoperineal resection. Also review the phantom pain phenomenon in Chapter 9.
2. Compare elimination through a colostomy with "normal" bowel elimination through the anus. How do they differ in terms of the passage of flatus?
3. Review Procedure 26–1. Also review the procedure for administering an enema in your fundamentals or skills textbook.
4. Review this nursing diagnosis in your nursing diagnosis or nursing care planning handbook; be sure to individualize your plan to Mr. Cunningham's situation and needs.

Chapter 28: Nursing Care of Clients with Urinary Tract Disorders
A Client with Cystitis
1. Consider risk factors for UTI as well as factors affecting Mrs. Waisanen's immune function.
2. Consider the indications for short-course antibiotic therapy and the indications for conventional therapy. Think about factors such as cost, compliance, and the risk for adverse effects, as well as how antibiotics work to eradicate bacteria.
3. Identify why *Ineffective health maintenance* may be an appropriate nursing diagnosis for Mrs. Waisanen and the individual factors contributing to this diagnosis as you plan care.

A Client with Urinary Calculi
1. Review the risk factors for urinary lithiasis.
2/3. Using the medications section of interdisciplinary care for the client with urinary calculi in this chapter and your pharmacology textbook or drug handbook, review analgesia for the client with renal colic and the intended and adverse effects of the drugs given to Mr. Leton.

A Client with a Bladder Tumor
1. Review the physiology of the bladder and the risk factors for urinary tract tumors.
2. Review Mr. Hussain's health history for possible contributing factors.
3. See Chapter 6 for nursing care of clients with problems of substance abuse.
4. Use your nursing care planning and nursing diagnoses textbooks to identify possible outcomes and interventions for *Sexual dysfunction*.

A Client with Urinary Incontinence
1. Review the desired and adverse effects of the prescribed medications.
2. Review the effects of menopause and estrogen deficiency on perineal tissues.
3. Review Mrs. Giovanni's physical examination findings and risk factors for UTI.
4. Identify factors that may contribute to *Situational low self-esteem* in Mrs. Giovanni and nursing measures to address this diagnosis.

Chapter 29: Nursing Care of Clients with Kidney Disorders
A Client with Acute Glomerulonephritis
1. Review Chapter 12 and the use of antibiotics to treat infection.
2. Review Mr. Chang's history and the risk factors for acute glomerulonephritis.
3. Review the diagnostic tests used to differentiate different forms of glomerulonephritis.

A Client with Acute Renal Failure
1. Review common causes and the pathophysiology of acute renal failure.
2. Review the sections on peptic ulcer disease and stress gastritis in Chapter 23.
3. Consider the position requirements to maintain body and bone alignment in skeletal traction (Chapter 41).

A Client with End-Stage Renal Disease
1. Review the usual onset, pathophysiology, and long-term effects of type 1 and type 2 diabetes (Chapter 20).
2. Consider the effects of urea and ammonia (both neurologic toxins) on brain function.
3. Review the manifestations of uremia.
4. Consider the composition of the dialysate and its possible effect on blood glucose control.

Chapter 31: Nursing Care of Clients with Coronary Heart Disease
A Client with Coronary Artery Bypass Surgery
1. Identify Mr. Clements's modifiable risk factors as you develop your plan. What barriers might need to be overcome to implement strategies to reduce his risk factors?
2. What strategies can you use to overcome denial without creating hostility or impairing the client-nurse relationship?
3. Consider traditional family roles as well as those roles that are unique to these individuals. Identify measures you can use to enlist the spouse's support.

4. Think about therapeutic communications as you formulate your response. Will your age or gender potentially affect your ability to respond effectively to these concerns? Would referral to another health care provider be appropriate?

A Client with Acute Myocardial Infarction

1. Review immediate treatment measures for MI. Are other means available for reestablishing coronary artery perfusion? If you are in a rural area without immediate access to a cardiac catheterization lab, how will this affect your response?
2. Review the section of this chapter on dysrhythmias and their treatment. Research protocols for treating frequent PVCs in the post-MI client at your clinical facility.
3. Review the goals of cardiac rehabilitation and Mrs. Williams's individual risk factors as you develop your teaching plan.
4. Consider the value of using a therapeutic response to Mrs. Williams's statement concerning smoking. Also consider the risks associated with cigarette smoke. How can you respond without supporting Mrs. Williams's desire to smoke and without precipitating anger or resistance? Review Chapter 6.

A Client with Supraventricular Tachycardia

1. Review the effects of sympathetic and parasympathetic nervous system stimulation on cardiac function.
2. Review the section on supraventricular tachycardias, as well as the antidysrhythmic medications for other treatment options.
3. Use your pharmacology textbook as you develop your teaching plan.

Chapter 32: Nursing Care of Clients with Cardiac Disorders

A Client with Heart Failure

1. Review the prescribed medications and their interactions. Do not forget to consider Mr. Jackson's age in assessing his risk for toxicity and interactions.
2. Review therapeutic communications skills and the use of open-ended statements to evaluate the underlying message of Mr. Jackson's statement.
3. Review exercise recommendations for the client with heart failure as well as cardiac rehabilitation principles (Chapter 31).
4. Review the rationale for aspirin therapy in the client with CHD and its effects on platelets and clotting as you formulate your response.
5. Review Chapter 45 for causes of CVA and the section of Chapter 31 on atrial fibrillation.

A Client with Mitral Valve Prolapse

1. Review the pathophysiology and manifestations of MVP, as well as the general treatment measures for valve disorders.
2. Think about the effects of progressive conditioning on cardiac function.
3. Consider the anxiety associated with heart conditions and with a potentially progressive disorder that could affect childbearing and other life activities, as well as ultimately necessitate surgery.
4. Review the manifestations of MVP and of mitral regurgitation.

Chapter 34: Nursing Care of Clients with Hematologic Disorders

A Client with Anemia

1. Consider the effects of Mrs. Matthews's rapid weight loss on fluid balance, as well as the effects of tissue hypoxia on cardiac output.
2. Refer to this chapter and your nutrition text. Be sure to consider Mrs. Matthews's age in designing your menu.
3. Consider factors such as Mrs. Matthews's recent dietary history, the folic acid content of foods, and other pertinent factors in the history and physical assessment

4. In addition to general factors to consider for the older adult (don't forget transportation among other factors), also consider the possible effect of Mrs. Matthews's recent loss and the grieving process.

A Client with Leukemia

1. Review the physiology of white blood cells, and the immune and inflammatory responses.
2. Think about the risks created by hospitalization in terms of exposure to infection and invasive procedures.
3. Think about the effect of inability to perform self care on self-esteem, self-confidence, and perception of power and control.
4. Use information provided in the nursing care and home care sections of this chapter as well as in Chapter 12.
5. Use your nursing care planning and fundamentals texts to develop your care plan.

A Client with Hodgkin's disease

1. Review Chapter 14 and the effects of chemotherapy and radiation on cancerous cells. Think about the advantages of combining these two therapies in terms of short and long-term desired and adverse effects.
2. Consider the primary and potential risks for infection in community settings as you design your teaching plan. What teaching strategies will you use for a young adult with Mr. Quito's education and experience?
3. Review theories of development and the developmental tasks for the young adult.
4. Use your nursing fundamentals and nursing care planning texts for reference in developing your care plan.

A Client with Hemophilia

1. Review the pathophysiology of hemophilia and its effect on the clotting process.
2. Consider both the ABCs and Maslow's hierarchy of needs as you respond to this question.
3. Think about the genetic transmission of hemophilia. How might Mr. Cruise's hemophilia affect any children that he has? Grandchildren?
4. Review your nursing fundamentals book, nursing skills book, and intravenous therapy text to develop your teaching plan. Also consider previous learning and developmental levels.
5. Consult your nursing care planning text. Consider why this might be an appropriate nursing diagnosis for Mr. Cruise.

Chapter 35: Nursing Care of Clients with Peripheral Vascular and Lymphatic Disorders

A Client with Hypertension

1. Review Mrs. Spezia's assessment data and the risk factors for primary hypertension.
2. Review the pathophysiology of primary hypertension and of obesity (Chapter 22), as well as the relationship between hypertension and coronary heart disease.
3. Think about resources that are available in your community for homeless people. Talk to community health and social service agencies to identify additional resources.
4. Again, review Mrs. Spezia's assessment data, the pathophysiology of hypertension, and the long-term effects of stress.
5. Use your nursing care planning and nursing diagnosis textbooks to help develop your care plan.

A Client with Peripheral Atherosclerosis

1. Review treatments for peripheral atherosclerosis, as well as lifestyle measures for preventing and treating atherosclerosis and coronary heart disease (Chapter 31).

2. Compare the pathophysiology of peripheral atherosclerosis, intermittent claudication, and coronary heart disease (Chapter 31) to identify similarities and differences.
3. Review the actions of beta blockers and their role in angina prophylaxis.
4. Use your nursing care planning and nutrition textbooks to help develop your care plan.

A Client with Deep Vein Thrombosis
1. Review the pathophysiologic processes of venous thrombosis and inflammation as you develop your answer.
2. Think about questions you could ask for further information as well as potential resources for Mrs. Hipps.
3. Consider assessment data to evaluate Mrs. Hipps's limitations and resources, as well as community resources to help meet her needs.
4. Use your nursing diagnosis and care planning textbooks to develop your plan of care.

Chapter 37: Nursing Care of Clients with Upper Respiratory Disorders
A Client with Peritonsillar Abscess
1/2. Review the manifestations of upper respiratory infections and management of these disorders.
3. Think about the primary uses of the nose, mouth, and pharynx as you consider nursing diagnoses related to upper respiratory disorders.

A Client with Nasal Fracture
1. Consider other measures to restore the client's sense of control over the situation. Consider the potentially harmful effects of suction on the mucous membranes as well as possible infection control risks.
2. Review the implications and potential dangers of CSF leakage to help you develop your care plan.
3. Think about the benefits and drawbacks of immediate and delayed rhinoplasty.

A Client with Total Laryngectomy
1. Review the options for speech rehabilitation. If available, practice using a speech generator. Practice esophageal speech.
2. Use your nursing care planning and nursing diagnoses handbook to develop your care plan. Consider Mr. Tom's age, occupation, and marital status in your plan of care.
3. Review Chapter 4 for surgical nursing care interventions, as well as your nursing fundamentals textbook for wound care strategies.
4. Consider measures to promote airway clearance and ventilation of all lung fields.

Chapter 38: Nursing Care of Clients with Ventilation Disorders
A Client with Pneumonia
1. Review Mrs. O'Neal's assessment data and compare her history with identified risk factors for pneumonia.
2. Review normal immune and inflammatory responses and the role of white blood cells in these processes.
3. Review Chapter 11 and altered immune responses for the physiology and effects of anaphylactic shock.
4. Use your nursing care planning and nursing diagnosis textbooks to help develop your care plan.

A Client with Tuberculosis
1. Consider available resources for mentally ill clients, as well as community and public health resources. Consider measures to ensure compliance with the prescribed treatment.

2. Contact your local public health department, the discharge planner for your unit, or the social services department in your clinical facility to help identify available resources.
3. Use your nursing fundamentals text, the nursing care section under Pneumonia, and your nursing diagnosis or care planning handbook as you develop your care plan.

A Client with Lung Cancer
1. Review Chapter 14 and use your pharmacology text to research the effects of these drugs and the rationale for combination chemotherapy.
2. Use Chapter 14 and your pharmacology text to identify probable side effects of this treatment regimen. Then use your nursing care planning book to identify appropriate nursing diagnoses and interventions.
3. Review the pathophysiology and collaborative care sections for lung cancer to develop your response to this question.

Chapter 39: Nursing Care of Clients with Gas Exchange Disorders
A Client with COPD
1. Review the processes by which cigarette smoke inflicts damage on lung tissue. Use your pediatric and pathophysiology texts for additional information.
2. Review the physiology of the respiratory drive, as well as the effects of chronic elevated carbon dioxide levels in the blood.
3. Review the manifestations of COPD and its complications as well as the section of this chapter on respiratory failure.
4. Use your nursing diagnosis handbook to help identify appropriate goals and interventions for this nursing diagnosis.

A Client with ARDS
1. As you respond to this question, consider additional treatment measures for ARDS and respiratory failure. Also consider the potential long-term consequences and complications of intubation and mechanical ventilation. Discuss strategies for communicating with Ms. Adamson's family and supporting coping and decision-making by Ms. Adamson and her family in an instance such as this.
2. Think about the precipitating factors for ARDS and the factors that may precipitate respiratory failure in a client with COPD. Consider the probable overall respiratory and general health status of the individual affected by each of these conditions.
3. Review the precipitating factors for ARDS and discuss strategies to prevent them.
4. Use your nursing care planning book to identify appropriate goals and nursing interventions for this nursing diagnosis.

Chapter 41: Nursing Care of Clients with Musculoskeletal Trauma
A Client with a Hip Fracture
1. Consider Mrs. Carbolito's age and the fact that she is postmenopausal. What effect does estrogen have on bone health? What might have increased her risk for falls?
2. Review the principles of traction application. What purpose does it serve prior to surgery? What words could you use that she would understand? Think about the effects of trauma, pain, and suddenly finding oneself in a strange environment on listening and understanding verbal communications.
3. List how each of these manifestations would affect skin integrity, food intake, and bone healing.

A Client with a Below-the-Knee Amputation
1. Design a sequential plan for Mr. Rocke's self-care of the stump. Consider his readiness to learn and the complexity of the care.

3. Review the information on chemotherapy in Chapter 14. List the types of chemotherapy and its common side effects. Consider the classifications of medications that are used to treat these side effects.
4. What factors in the treatment of Mrs. Clemments treatment might disrupt the amount and quality of her sleep? What interventions might be used to improve her sleep pattern?

Chapter 52: Nursing Care of Clients with Sexually Transmitted Infections

A Client with Gonorrhea

1. What manifestations does Ms. Cirit have that are typical of the disease? Would you make other assessments? If so, what are they?
2. Review the discussion of HIV in Chapter 13. Do you believe it is true that infection with gonorrhea may increase the risk of HIV? If so, how would you explain this to Ms. Cirit?

3. *Impaired social interaction* is a state of aloneness or rejection experienced by an individual that is perceived as negative. What assessments of Ms. Cirit might support this diagnosis? What interventions and expected outcomes would you develop?

A Client with Syphilis

1. Describe the assessments you would expect to find in a man with early syphilis.
2. Consider topics such as number of sex partners, patterns of sexual activity, and use of safe sex practices. What other topics should be explored? How can you ask these questions without being embarrassed or embarrassing the client?
3. List possible statements you might make. Do you believe this is a nursing responsibility? If you do not feel comfortable with this topic, what could you do?

GLOSSARY

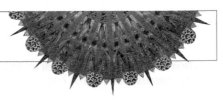

Abrasion Partial-thickness denudation of an area of integument, generally resulting from falls or scrapes.

Absence seizure (petit mal seizure) A type of generalized seizure characterized by a sudden brief cessation of all motor activity accompanied by a blank stare and unresponsiveness.

Accommodation The ability of the eye to adjust to variations in distance.

Achalasia Absence of peristalsis of the esophagus and high gastroesophageal sphincter pressure resulting in dilation and loss of tone in the esophagus.

Acidosis The condition in which the hydrogen ion concentration increases above normal (reflected in a pH below 7.35).

Acids A substance that releases hydrogen ions in solution.

Acne Disorder of the pilosebaceous (hair and sebaceous gland) structure, resulting in eruption of papules or pustules.

Acoustic neuroma or schwannoma Benign tumor of cranial nerve VIII.

Acquired immune deficiency syndrome (AIDS) A specific group of diseases or conditions that are indicative of severe immunosuppression related to infection with the human immunodeficiency virus.

Acquired immunity Immunity developed after exposure to a pathogen. See *Active immunity.*

Acromegaly Meaning literally "enlarged extremities," this is a condition resulting from excessive growth hormone secretion during adulthood.

Actinic keratosis Also called senile or solar keratosis, this is an epidermal skin lesion directly related to chronic sun exposure and photodamage.

Active immunity Production of antibodies or development of immune lymphocytes against specific antigens.

Active transport Movement of molecules across cell membranes and epithelial membranes against a concentration gradient; requires energy.

Acute coronary syndromes A general term used to describe the effects of coronary heart disease, including angina and myocardial infarction.

Acute gastritis A benign, self-limiting disorder associated with ingestion of gastric irritants such as aspirin, alcohol, caffeine, or foods contaminated with certain bacteria.

Acute illness An illness that occurs rapidly, lasts for a relatively short time, and is self-limiting.

Acute lymphoblastic leukemia (ALL) Abnormal proliferation of lymphoblasts in the bone marrow, lymph nodes, and spleen; the most common type of leukemia in children and young adults.

Acute myeloblastic leukemia (AML) Uncontrolled proliferation of myeloblasts (granulocyte precursors) and hyperplasia of bone marrow and the spleen; the most common acute leukemia in adults.

Acute myocardial infarction (AMI) Necrosis (death) of myocardial cells.

Acute pain Usually temporary, localized, and of sudden onset; it lasts for less than 6 months and has an identifiable cause, such as trauma, surgery, or inflammation.

Acute renal failure Abrupt onset of renal failure, often reversible.

Acute respiratory distress syndrome (ARDS) Noncardiac pulmonary edema and progressive refractory hypoxemia.

Acute tubular necrosis (ATN) A syndrome of abrupt and progressive decline in tubular and glomerular function.

Advance directive Also called a *living will*, this is a document in which a client formally states preferences for health care in the event that he or she later becomes mentally incapacitated and names a person who has durable power of attorney to serve as a substitute decision maker to implement the client's stated preferences.

Aesthetic surgery See *Cosmetic surgery.*

Afterload The force the ventricles must overcome to eject their blood volume; the pressure in the arterial system ahead of the ventricles.

Agnosia The inability to recognize one or more subjects that were previously familiar; agnosia may be visual, tactile, or auditory.

Agranulocytosis Severe neutropenia, with less than 200 cells/μm.

Alcoholic cirrhosis (Laënnec's cirrhosis) The end result of alcoholic liver disease.

Alkalosis The condition where the hydrogen ion concentration decreases below normal (reflected in a pH above 7.45).

Alleles Different forms of a gene or DNA occupying the same place on a pair of chromosomes; an allele for each gene is inherited from each parent.

Allergy A hypersensitivity response to environmental or exogenous antigens.

Allografts Grafts between members of the same species but who have different genotypes and HLA antigens. See also *Homograft.*

Alopecia Loss of hair; baldness.

Alzheimer's disease (AD) A form of dementia characterized by progressive, irreversible deterioration of the general intellectual functioning.

Amenorrhea Absence of menstruation.

Amputation Partial or total removal of a body part.

Amyotrophic lateral sclerosis (ALS) Progressive, degenerative neurologic disease characterized by weakness and wasting of the involved muscles, without any accompanying sensory or cognitive changes; also called *Lou Gehrig's disease.*

Analgesic A medication that reduces or eliminates the perception of pain.

Anaphylactic shock Shock resulting from a widespread hypersensitivity reaction (called *anaphylaxis*). The pathophysiology in this type of shock includes vasodilation, pooling of blood in the periphery, and hypovolemia with altered cellular metabolism.

involved; marked by uncontrolled growth and the spread of abnormal cells.

Candidiasis Infection of mucous membranes caused by *Candida albicans,* a yeast-like fungus.

Carbuncle A group of infected hair follicles.

Carcinogen Cancer-causing agent.

Carcinogenesis The production or origin of cancer.

Carcinoma A tumor arising from epithelial tissue.

Cardiac arrest Sudden failure of the heart to pump.

Cardiac cycle The contraction and relaxation of the heart during one heartbeat.

Cardiac index Cardiac output adjusted for body size.

Cardiac output (CO) The amount of blood pumped by the ventricles into the pulmonary and systemic circulations in 1 minute.

Cardiac rehabilitation A long-term program of medical evaluation, exercise, risk factor modification, education, and counseling designed to limit the physical and psychologic effects of cardiac illness and improve the client's quality of life.

Cardiac reserve The ability of the heart to respond to the body's changing need for cardiac output.

Cardiac tamponade Compression of the heart due to pericardial effusion, trauma, cardiac rupture, or hemorrhage.

Cardiogenic shock Shock that occurs when the heart's pumping ability is compromised to the point that it cannot maintain cardiac output and adequate tissue perfusion.

Cardiomegaly Enlargement of the heart.

Cardiomyopathy Primary abnormality of the heart muscle that affects its structural or functional characteristics.

Cardiovascular disease (CVD) Generic term for disorders of the heart and blood vessels.

Carpal tunnel syndrome Compression of the median nerve as a result of inflammation and swelling of the synovial lining of the tendon sheaths.

Carrier Any individual who carries a single copy of an altered gene or mutation for a recessive condition on one chromosome of a chromosome pair and an unaltered form of that gene on the other chromosome; a carrier generally is not affected by the gene alteration; on the average, each person in the general population is a carrier of five or six gene mutations for recessive disorders.

Catabolism Biochemical process involving the breakdown of complex structures into simpler forms.

Cataract Opacification (clouding) of the lens of the eye.

Celiac disease (celiac sprue, nontropical sprue) Chronic hereditary disorder characterized by sensitivity to the gliadin fraction of gluten, a cereal protein.

Cell cycle The four phases that occur during growth and development of a cell.

Cell-mediated (cellular) immune response Direct or indirect inactivation of antigen by lymphocytes.

Cellulitis A localized infection of the dermis and subcutaneous tissue.

Central pain Related to a lesion in the brain that may spontaneously produce high-frequency bursts of impulses that are perceived as pain.

Cerebral concussion Transient, temporary, neurogenic dysfunction caused by mechanical force to the brain.

Cerebral contusion Bruise on the surface of the brain.

Cerebral edema An increase in the volume of brain tissue due to abnormal accumulation of fluid.

Cerumen Earwax.

Chalazion Granulomatous cyst or nodule of the lid.

Chancre Hard, syphilitic primary ulcer.

Cheilosis Chemical peeling; the application of a chemical to produce a controlled and predictable injury that alters the anatomy of the epidermis and superficial dermis.

Chemotherapy Cancer treatment involving the use of cytotoxic medications to decrease tumor size, adjunctive to surgery or radiation therapy; or to prevent or treat suspected metastases.

Chlamydia A group of syndromes caused by *Chlamydia trachomatis,* a bacterium that behaves like a virus spreading within a host cell; spread by sexual contact and to the neonate by passage through the birth canal of an infected mother.

Cholecystectomy Removal of the gallbladder.

Cholecystitis Inflammation of the gallbladder, usually associated with stones in the cystic or common bile duct.

Cholelithiasis Formation of stones (calculi) within the gallbladder or biliary duct system.

Cholera Acute diarrheal illness caused by certain strains of *Vibrio cholerae.*

Chorea Jerky, rapid, involuntary movements.

Chromosome Genetic material carried by each cell; found in the cell nucleus.

Chronic bronchitis Excessive secretion of bronchial mucus characterized by a productive cough lasting 3 or more months in 2 consecutive years.

Chronic gastritis Disorders characterized by progressive and irreversible changes in the gastric mucosa.

Chronic lymphocytic leukemia (CLL) Proliferation and accumulation of small, abnormal, mature lymphocytes in the bone marrow, peripheral blood, and body tissues; least common type of the major leukemias.

Chronic myelogenous leukemia (CML) Abnormal proliferation of all bone marrow elements, usually associated with a chromosome abnormality (the Philadelphia chromosome).

Chronic obstructive pulmonary disease (COPD) Chronic air flow obstruction due to chronic bronchitis and/or emphysema.

Chronic renal failure Progressive renal tissue destruction with loss of entire nephron unit and function; renal mass decreases, and glomerular filtration, tubular secretion, and reabsorption deteriorate.

Chronic otitis media Condition involving permanent perforation of the tympanic membrane, with or without recurrent pus formation and often accompanied by changes in the mucosa and bony structures (ossicles) of the middle ear.

Chronic pain Prolonged pain, usually lasting longer than 6 months. It is not always associated with an identifiable cause and is often unresponsive to conventional medical treatment.

Chronic sorrow A cyclical, recurring, and potentially progressive pattern of pervasive sadness experienced in response to continual loss, throughout the trajectory of an illness or disability.

Chronic stump pain The result of neuroma formation, causing severe burning pain.

Chronic venous insufficiency A chronic disorder of inadequate venous return.

Chvostek's sign Contraction of the lateral facial muscles in response to tapping the face in front of the ear; caused by decreased blood calcium levels.

Chyme Thick, fluid mixture of food and gastric juices formed in the stomach during the digestive process.

Cirrhosis A progressive, irreversible disorder, eventually leading to liver failure; the end stage of chronic liver disease.

Client A term used instead of "patient" that is based on a philosophy that individuals are active participants in health and illness as well as consumers of healthcare services.

Closed fracture (simple fracture) Break in continuity of bone with skin still intact.

Clubbing Enlargement and blunting of the terminal portion of the fingers; associated with chronic hypoxemia.

Cluster headache A form of vascular headache predominantly experienced by men ages 20 to 40. The headache typically begins 2 to 3 hours after the person falls asleep.

Coagulation The process of creating a fibrin meshwork that cements blood components together to form an insoluble clot.

Code of ethics An established and agreed-on group of principles of conduct that provide a professional framework.

Cold sore See Herpes simplex.

Cold zone Considered the "safe zone" during a disaster, it is adjacent to the warm zone and is the area where a more in-depth triage of victims would occur; survivors may find shelter in this area, and command and control vehicles would be found here as well as the emergency transport vehicles.

Colectomy Surgical removal of the colon.

Collateral channels Connections between small arteries.

Collateral vessels Accessory pathways connected to the smaller arteries in the coronary system.

Colorectal cancer Malignant tumor arising from the epithelial tissues of the colon or rectum.

Colostomy Ostomy made in the colon.

Comedones Noninflammatory acne lesions.

Community-based care Centers on individual and family healthcare needs. The nurse practicing community-based care provides direct services to individuals to manage acute or chronic health problems and to promote self-care. The care is provided in the local community, is culturally competent, and is family centered.

Compartment A space enclosed by a fibrous membrane or fascia.

Compartment syndrome Condition in which excess pressure constricts the structures within a compartment, and reduces circulation to muscles and nerves.

Concussion Injury resulting from a violent jar, shake, or impact with an object.

Conjunctivitis Inflammation of the conjunctiva.

Consanguinity Related by having a common ancestor; close blood relationship.

Conscious sedation Anesthesia that provides analgesia and amnesia, but in which the client remains conscious. Clients are able to breathe independently and are cardiovascularly stable.

Consciousness A condition in which a person is aware of self and environment and is able to respond appropriately to stimuli; full consciousness requires both normal arousal and full cognition.

Constipation The infrequent (two or fewer bowel movements weekly) or difficult passage of stools.

Contact dermatitis Type of dermatitis caused by a hypersensitivity response or chemical irritation.

Continuous renal replacement therapy (CRRT) A form of hemodialysis in which blood is continuously circulated through a highly porous hemofilter from artery to vein or vein to vein.

Contractility The inherent capability of the cardiac muscle fibers to shorten.

Contracting The negotiation of a cooperative working agreement between the nurse and client that is continuously renegotiated.

Contracture Permanent shortening of connective tissue.

Contralateral deficit Manifestations of a stroke on the side of the body opposite the side of the brain that is damaged.

Contusion Superficial tissue injury resulting from blunt trauma, such as a kick or blow from an object, that causes the breakage of small blood vessels and bleeding into the surrounding tissue.

Conventional weapons Weapons such as bombs and guns that are used more frequently than nonconventional terrorist weapons.

Convergence Moving inward of the eyes to see an object close to the face.

Co-occurring disorders Concurrent diagnosis of a substance use disorder and a psychiatric disorder. One disorder can precede and cause the other, such as the relationship between alcoholism and depression.

Cor pulmonale Condition of right ventricular hypertrophy and failure that results from long-standing pulmonary hypertension.

Core competencies Standards that a profession agrees are essential for a person to be deemed competent in his or her field.

Corneal reflex Closure of eyelids (blinking) due to corneal irritation.

Coronary heart disease (CHD) Heart disease caused by impaired blood flow to the myocardium.

Coryza (rhinorrhea) Profuse nasal discharge.

Cosmetic surgery (aesthetic surgery) One of two fields within plastic surgery. Cosmetic surgery enhances the attractiveness of normal features.

Crackles Discontinuous lung sound heard by auscultation; can be fine or coarse. Produced by air passing over airway secretions or the opening of collapsed airways.

Crepitation A grating sound heard on movement of a joint.

Creutzfeldt-Jakob disease (CJD, spongiform encephalopathy) Rare, progressive neurologic disease that causes brain degeneration without inflammation.

Emphysema Destruction of the walls of the alveoli, with resulting enlargement of abnormal air spaces.

Empyema Accumulation of purulent exudate in the pleural cavity.

Encephalitis An acute inflammation of the parenchyma of the brain or spinal cord.

End of life The final days or weeks of life when death is imminent.

Endocarditis Inflammation of the endocardium.

Endometriosis A condition in which multiple, small implants of endometrial tissue develop throughout the pelvic cavity.

Endoscopy Inspection of organs or cavities of the body using an endoscope.

Endotoxins Found in the cell wall of gram-negative bacteria, endotoxins are released only when the cell is disrupted. They act as activators of many human regulatory systems, producing fever, inflammation, and potentially clotting, bleeding, or hypotension when released in large quantities.

End-stage renal disease The final stage of chronic renal failure in which the kidneys are unable to excrete metabolic wastes and regulate fluid and electrolyte balance adequately; characterized by a glomerular filtration rate of less than 5% of normal.

Enophthalmos Sunken appearance of the eyes.

Enteral nutrition Administration of liquid nutritional formulas to meet calorie and protein needs in clients unable to consume adequate food; also called *tube feeding.*

Enucleation Surgical removal of an eye.

Epicondylitis (tennis elbow, golfer's elbow) Inflammation of the tendon at its point of origin into the bone.

Epididymitis Infection or inflammation of the epididymis.

Epidural hematoma (extradural hematoma) A collection of blood between the dura and the skull.

Epilepsy Chronic seizure activity.

Epistaxis Nosebleed.

Erectile dysfunction Inability of the male to attain and maintain an erection sufficient to permit satisfactory sexual intercourse.

Erosive gastritis See *Stress-induced (erosive) gastritis.*

Erysipelas Infection of the skin most often caused by group A streptococci.

Erythema A reddening of the skin.

Erythropoiesis Red blood cell production.

Eschar Hard, leathery crust that covers a burn wound and harbors necrotic tissue.

Escharotomy Surgical removal of eschar from the torso or extremity to prevent circumferential constriction.

Esophageal varices Enlarged, thin-walled veins that form in the submucosa of the esophagus.

Esophagojejunostomy Removal of the entire stomach with anastomosis of the distal esophagus to the jejunum.

Estrogen Hormone produced by the ovary.

Ethics Principles of conduct. Ethical behavior is concerned with moral duty, values, obligations, and the distinction between right and wrong.

Euthanasia From the Greek for painless, easy, gentle, or good death, now commonly used to signify a killing prompted by a humanitarian motive.

Evisceration Protrusion of body contents through a surgical wound.

Exacerbation A period during chronic illness in which symptoms reappear.

Exfoliative dermatitis Inflammatory skin disorder characterized by excessive peeling or shedding of skin.

Exophthalmos Protrusion of the eyeballs.

Exotoxins Soluble proteins secreted into surrounding tissue by the microorganism. Exotoxins are highly poisonous, causing cell death or dysfunction.

External otitis Inflammation of the ear canal.

Extracapsular fractures Fractures of the trochanteric region.

Extracorporeal shock-wave lithotripsy (ESWL, transcutaneous shock-wave lithotripsy) Noninvasive technique for fragmenting kidney stones using shock waves generated outside the body.

Family Two or more persons joined by emotional closeness and shared bonds and who identify themselves as being part of a family.

Fasciculations Involuntary twitching.

Fasciectomy (fascial excision) Process of excising the wound to the level of fascia.

Fat embolism syndrome (FES) Characterized by neurologic dysfunction, pulmonary insufficiency, and a petechial rash on the chest, axilla, and upper arms due to fat globules lodged in the pulmonary vascular bed or peripheral circulation.

Fecal impaction A rock-hard or putty-like mass of feces in the rectum.

Fecal incontinence Loss of voluntary control of defecation.

Fecalith A hard mass of feces.

Fibrocystic changes (FCC) Physiologic nodularity and breast tenderness that increases and decreases with the menstrual cycle.

Fibroid tumors (uterine leiomyomata) Solid, pedunculated benign tumors.

Fibromyalgia (fibrositis) A common rheumatic syndrome characterized by musculoskeletal pain, stiffness, and tenderness.

Filtration The process by which water and dissolved substances (solutes) move from an area of higher hydrostatic pressure to an area of lower hydrostatic pressure.

Fistula Abnormal opening or passage between two organs or spaces that are normally separated or an abnormal passage to the outside of the body.

Flaccidity Decreased muscle tone in disease or trauma of the lower motor neurons.

Flail chest Free-floating segment of the chest wall, resulting from two or more consecutive ribs fractured in multiple places.

Flap A piece of tissue whose free end is moved from a donor site to a recipient site while maintaining a continuous blood supply through its connection at the base or pedicle.

Flatus Gas in the digestive tract.

Fluid resuscitation Replacement of the extensive fluid and electrolyte losses associated with major burn injuries.

Fluid volume deficit (FVD) A decrease in intravascular, interstitial, and/or intracellular fluid in the body.

Fluid volume excess (FVE) Excess extracellular fluid resulting from retention of both water and sodium in the body.

Folic acid deficiency anemia An anemia resulting from folic acid deficiency, a necessary nutrient for DNA synthesis and RBC maturation.

Folliculitis Bacterial infection of the hair follicle, most commonly caused by *Staphylococcus aureus.*

Fracture A break in a bone usually due to trauma.

Freestanding outpatient surgical facilities Surgical units independent of a hospital with or without financial connections to a hospital or healthcare organization.

Friction rub The sound heard when two dry surfaces are rubbed together.

Frostbite An injury of the skin from freezing.

Full-thickness burn A burn that involves all layers of the skin, including the epidermis, dermis, and epidermal appendages.

Fulminant hepatitis Hepatitis with a rapid and severe onset and course.

Furuncle Often called a boil, but also an inflammation of the hair follicle.

Fusiform excision The removal of a full thickness of the epidermis and dermis, usually with a thin layer of subcutaneous tissue.

Galactorrhea Lactation not associated with pregnancy or nursing.

Gastric lavage Irrigation of the stomach with large quantities of normal saline.

Gastric mucosal barrier A protective barrier consisting of lipids, bicarbonate ions, and mucous gel that protects the stomach lining from the damaging effects of gastric juices.

Gastric outlet obstruction Obstruction of the pyloric region of the stomach and duodenum that impairs gastric outflow; a potential complication of peptic ulcer disease.

Gastric ulcers Ulcers of the stomach lining, usually in the lesser curvature and antrum; more common in older adults.

Gastritis Inflammation of the stomach lining.

Gastroduodenostomy (Billroth I) Excision of the pylorus of the stomach with the anastomosis of the upper stomach to the duodenum; commonly used partial gastrectomy procedure.

Gastroenteritis Inflammation of the gastrointestinal tract; not a specific disease, but a group of syndromes or a collection of related manifestations.

Gastroesophageal reflux Backward flow of gastric contents into the esophagus.

Gastrointestinal reflux disease (GERD) The reflux of acidic gastric contents into the lower esophagus.

Gastrojejunostomy (Billroth II) Subtotal excision of the stomach with closure of the duodenum and side-to-side anastomosis of the jejunum to the stomach; commonly used partial gastrectomy procedure.

Gastroparesis Slowed gastrointestinal motility, which causes early satiety.

Gene A sequence of DNA on a chromosome that represents a fundamental unit of heredity; occupies a specific spot on a chromosome (gene locus).

Gene expression When the protein product of a gene is visible (for example, through the presence of a body structure or identifiable through biochemical tests such as insulin or phenylalanine levels).

General anesthesia Deep sedation, which includes analgesia and muscle paralysis. This type of anesthesia requires respiratory maintenance without the aid of the client's respiratory musculature.

Genital herpes (herpes simplex genitalis) An infection of the external genitalia caused by herpes simplex genitalis; transmitted by vaginal, anal, or oral–genital contact.

Genital warts (condyloma acuminatum, venereal warts) A sexually transmitted condition caused by the human papilloma virus.

Genotype The genes and the variations therein that a person inherits from his or her parents.

Germ cells Cells that give rise to a sperm or egg.

Gingivitis Inflamation of the gums, characterized by inflammation, redness, and bleeding.

Gland Tissue that synthesizes hormones.

Glaucoma Condition characterized by increased intraocular pressure of the eye and a gradual loss of vision.

Glomerular filtration rate (GFR) The rate at which plasma is filtered through the glomeruli of the kidney.

Glomerulonephritis Inflammation of the capillary loops of the glomeruli.

Glossitis Inflammation of the tongue.

Glucocorticoid A group of hormones secreted by the adrenal cortex; they regulate carbohydrate levels in the body.

Gluconeogenesis Formation of glucose from fats and proteins.

Glucose-6-phosphate dehydrogenase (G6PD) anemia Anemia due to a hereditary defect in RBC metabolism.

Glucosuria Excessive glucose in urine.

Glycogenolysis Breakdown of liver glycogen to glucose.

Goiter An enlarged thyroid gland. Enlargement results from both inadequate and excessive synthesis of thyroid hormones.

Gonorrhea (GC, clap) An infection caused by *Neisseria gonorrhoeae* that is transmitted by direct sexual contact or by delivery of a neonate by an infected mother.

Gout A syndrome that occurs from an inflammatory response to the production or excretion of uric acid resulting in high levels of uric acid in the blood (hyperuricemia) and in other body fluids, including synovial fluid.

Grief The emotional response to loss and its accompanying changes.

Grieving The internal process the person uses to work through the response to loss.

Guillain-Barré syndrome (GBS) Acute demyelinating disorder of the peripheral nervous system characterized by progressive, usually rapid muscle weakness and paralysis.

Gynecomastia Breast enlargement in men.

Hallucinogens Drugs that produce hallucinations.

Hallux valgus (bunion) The enlargement and lateral displacement of the first metatarsal.

Intraductal papilloma A tiny wartlike growth on the inside of the peripheral mammary duct that causes discharge from the nipple.

Intraoperative phase The time during surgery, from beginning to end.

Iron deficiency anemia The most common type of anemia; results from inadequate iron for optimal RBC formation.

Irritable bowel syndrome (IBS) A motility disorder of the gastrointestinal tract characterized by alternating periods of constipation and diarrhea.

Ischemia Deficient blood flow to tissue.

Ischemic Deprived of oxygen.

Islets of Langerhans Hormone-producing cells (alpha cells, beta cells, and delta cells) scattered through the pancreas.

Isograft Tissue transplant where the donor and recipient are identical twins.

Jaundice Yellow-to-orange color visible in the skin and mucous membranes; most often the result of a hepatic disorder.

Joint arthroplasty Reconstruction or replacement of a joint.

Kaposi's sarcoma (KS) A vascular malignancy (a tumor of the endothelial cells lining small blood vessels) that presents as vascular macules, papules, or violet lesions affecting the skin and viscera. It is often the presenting symptom of AIDS.

Keloid Elevated, irregularly shaped, progressively enlarging scar arising from excessive amounts of collagen in the stratum corneum during scar formation in connective tissue repair.

Keratitis Inflammation of the cornea.

Keratosis Any skin condition in which there is a benign overgrowth and thickening of the cornified epithelium.

Ketoacidosis A condition of very high blood glucose and insufficient insulin that results in accumulation of ketones and fatty acids in the blood and urine and diuresis.

Ketonuria The presence of ketones in the urine.

Ketosis An accumulation of ketone bodies produced during the oxidation of fatty acids.

Kindling Long-term changes in brain neurotransmission that occur after repeated detoxifications.

Kinesthesia The ability to perceive movement and sense of position.

Korotkoff's sounds Sounds heard during auscultation of blood pressure.

Korsakoff's psychosis Secondary dementia caused by thiamine (B₁) deficiency that may be associated with chronic alcoholism; characterized by progressive cognitive deterioration, confabulation, peripheral neuropathy, and myopathy.

Kussmaul's respirations Deep, rapid respirations associated with compensatory mechanisms.

Kwashiorkor protein energy undernutrition (protein energy malnutrition, PEM) Chronic protein deficiency with adequate calories to meet body needs.

Kyphosis Exaggerated thoracic curvature of the spine common in older adults.

Labyrinthectomy Surgical removal of the labyrinth.

Labyrinthitis Inflammation of the inner ear.

Laceration Open wound that results from sharp cutting or tearing. Injuries to the integument are at risk for contamination from dirt, debris, or foreign objects.

Lacunar strokes Thrombotic stroke of smaller cerebral blood vessels that causes tissue to slough off, leaving a small cavity in the brain tissue.

Laminectomy Removal of the lamina of the vertebrae.

Laparoscopic cholecystectomy Removal of the gallbladder using an endoscope.

Laryngectomy Removal of the larynx.

Laryngitis Inflammation of the larynx.

Leukemia ("white blood") A group of chronic malignant disorders of white blood cells and WBC precursors; characterized by replacement of bone marrow by malignant immature WBCs, abnormal immature circulating WBCs, and infiltration of malignant cells into other tissues.

Leukocytes Also called white blood cells, these are the primary cells involved in both nonspecific and specific immune system responses. These cells isolate the infecting organism or injury, destroy pathogens, and promote healing.

Leukocytosis An increase in the number of leukocytes in the blood (above 10,000/mm³), usually caused by infection.

Leukopenia Abnormal decrease of circulating leukocytes, usually below 5000/mm³; occurs when bone marrow activity is suppressed or when leukocyte destruction increases.

Leukoplakia Formation of white patches or spots on the mucous membranes or tongue; these lesions may become malignant.

Lichen planus Benign inflammatory disorder of the mucous membranes and skin.

Lift A more sustained thrust than normal.

Lipoatrophy Atrophy of subcutaneous tissue.

Liposuction A method of changing the contours of the body by aspirating fat from the subcutaneous layer of tissue.

Lithiasis Stone formation.

Lithotripsy Crushing of renal calculi.

Lobectomy Surgical removal of tumors in a single lobe of lung.

Locked-in syndrome Client is alert and fully aware of the environment, but is unable to communicate through speech or movement as a result of blocked efferent pathways to the brain.

Lordosis Increased lumbar curve.

Lower body obesity (peripheral obesity) A waist-to-hip ratio of less than 0.8.

Lung abscess Localized area of lung destruction or necrosis and pus formation.

Lung compliance Distensibility of the lungs.

Lyme disease An inflammatory disorder caused by a spirochete, *Borrelia burgdorferi,* which is transmitted primarily by ticks.

Lymphadenopathy The enlargement of lymph nodes (over 1 cm) with or without tenderness. It may be caused by inflammation, infection, or malignancy of the nodes or the regions drained by the nodes.

Lymphangitis Inflammation of a lymphatic vessel.

Lymphedema Extremity edema due to accumulated lymph; may be primary or secondary, resulting from inflammation, obstruction, or removal of lymphatic vessels.

Lymphocytes Lymphocytes account for 20% to 40% of circulating leukocytes. Lymphocytes are the principal effector and regulator cells of specific immune responses.

Lymphoid tissues Connective tissues containing lymphocytes; include tissues of the bone marrow, thymus, lymph nodes, and spleen.

Lymphomas Malignancy of lymphoid tissue.

Macrophages Monocytes mature into macrophages after settling into tissue. Macrophages are large phagocytes. They are important in the body's defense against chronic infections.

Macular degeneration Destructive changes in the macula due to injury or gradual failure of the outer pigmented layer of the retina (the retinal layer adjacent to the choroid), which removes cellular waste products and keeps the retina attached to the choroid.

Malabsorption A condition in which nutrients are ineffectively absorbed by the intestinal mucosa, resulting in their excretion in the stool.

Malignant hypertension A hypertensive emergency, marked by a diastolic pressure greater than 120 mmHg.

Malignant melanoma (cutaneous melanoma) Skin cancer that arises from melanocytes.

Malignant pain Pain associated with a life-threatening illness such as cancer but not limited to cancer pain.

Malnutrition Inadequate nutrient intake to meet body needs; may include deficiency of major nutrients (calories, carbohydrates, proteins, and fats) or micronutrients such as vitamins and minerals.

Manifestations Signs and symptoms of a disease or condition caused by alterations in structure or function.

Man-made disasters Either accidental or intentional, they are complex emergencies, technological disasters, material shortages, and other disasters not caused by natural hazards.

Marasmus (protein energy undernutrition) Insufficient protein and calorie intake to meet metabolic needs.

Mass casualty incidents Situations in which 100 or more casualties are involved, significantly overwhelming available emergency medical services, facilities, and resources.

Mastoidectomy Surgical removal of infected mastoid air cells.

Mastoiditis Bacterial infection of the mastoid process.

Maturity-onset diabetes of the young (MODY) Diabetes in young obese adults.

Mean arterial pressure (MAP) The average pressure in the arterial circulation throughout the cardiac cycle; the product of cardiac output and systemic vascular resistance (SVR).

Medical-surgical nursing The health promotion, health care, and illness care of adults, based on knowledge derived from the arts and sciences and shaped by knowledge (the science) of nursing.

Melanin Skin pigment that forms a protective shield to protect keratinocytes and nerve endings in the dermis from the damaging effects of ultraviolet light.

Melena Black, tarry stool that contains blood.

Ménière's disease Chronic disorder of unknown cause characterized by recurrent attacks of vertigo with tinnitus and a progressive unilateral hearing loss.

Meningitis Inflammation of the meninges of the brain and spinal cord.

Menopause Permanent cessation of menses.

Menorrhagia Excessive or prolonged menstruation.

Menstrual cycle Cyclic buildup of the uterine lining, ovulation, and sloughing of the lining occurring approximately every 28 days in nonpregnant females.

Menstruation Periodic shedding of the uterine lining in a woman of childbearing age who is not pregnant.

Metabolism Consisting of the breakdown of complex structures into simpler forms to produce energy (catabolism) and the combination of simpler molecules to produce and maintain more complex structures necessary to living organisms (anabolism).

Metaplasia A change in the normal pattern of differentiation such that dividing cells differentiate into cell types not normally found in that location in the body.

Metastasis Secondary tumor; the process by which spreading of malignant neoplasms occurs; the transfer of disease from one organ or part to another not directly connected with it.

Metrorrhagia Bleeding between menstrual periods; may be caused by hormonal imbalances, pelvic inflammatory disease, cervical or uterine polyps, uterine fibroids, or cervical or uterine cancer.

Microalbuminuria Protein in the urine.

Micturition Releasing urine from the urinary bladder (voiding).

Mild concussion Brain trauma resulting in a brief loss of consciousness that lasts from seconds to hours.

Minor trauma Injury to a single part or system of the body, usually treated in the hospital or emergency department.

Mitigation The action taken to prevent or reduce the harmful effects of a disaster on human health or property, it involves future-oriented activities to prevent subsequent disasters or to minimize their effects.

Mitral valve (bicuspid valve) Valve between the left atrium and ventricle in the heart; prevents blood from flowing backwards into the atrium.

Monosomic (monosomy) When one member of the chromosome pair is missing, for example, Turner syndrome (45, XO).

Morbid obesity Weight greater than 100% over ideal body weight.

Morton's neuroma A tumor-like mass formed within the neurovascular bundle of the intermetatarsal spaces.

Mosaicism A chromosome variation or abnormality that occurs after fertilization during mitosis at an early cell stage so not all cells are affected with the variation; for example, a child who is mosaic for Down syndrome will have some cells with two copies of chromosome 21 and some that have an extra chromosome 21.

Mourning The actions or expressions of the bereaved, including the symbols, clothing, and ceremonies that make up the outward manifestations of grief.

Pericarditis Inflammation of the pericardium.

Perioperative nursing A specialized area of nursing practice that incorporates the three phases of the surgical experience: preoperative, intraoperative, and postoperative.

Peripheral vascular disease (PVD) Impaired blood supply to peripheral tissues, particularly the lower extremities.

Peripheral vascular resistance (PVR) The opposing forces or impedance to blood flow as the arterial channels become more and more distant from the heart.

Peristalsis Alternating waves of contraction and relaxation of involuntary muscle.

Peritoneal dialysis Procedure in which electrolytes, waste products, and excess water are removed from the body by diffusion using the peritoneum surrounding the abdominal cavity as the dialyzing membrane.

Peritonitis Inflammation of the peritoneum.

Pernicious anemia Anemia resulting from failure to absorb dietary vitamin B_{12} due to lack of intrinsic factor.

Persistent vegetative state (PVS) Condition of complete unawareness of self and the environment.

Personal protective equipment (PPE) Equipment used for the protection of personnel including gloves, masks, goggles, gowns, and biologic disposal bags (red bags); may also include hoods, helmets, head gear, and impermeable suits.

Pertussis (whooping cough) A highly contagious acute upper respiratory infection cause by the bacterium *Bordetella pertussis*.

Phagocytosis A process by which a foreign agent or target cell is engulfed, destroyed, and digested. Neutrophils and macrophages, known as phagocytes, are the primary cells involved in phagocytosis.

Phantom limb syndrome (phantom pain) A confusing pain syndrome that occurs following surgical or traumatic amputation of a limb. The client experiences pain in the missing body part even though there is complete mental awareness that the limb is gone.

Pharyngitis Acute inflammation of the pharynx.

Phenotype The expression of a person's entire physical, biochemical, and physiologic makeup, as determined by the individual's genotype and environmental factors.

Phimosis Constriction of the foreskin so that it cannot be retracted over the glans penis.

Plasmapheresis (plasma exchange) Removal of the plasma component from whole blood.

Plastic surgery The alteration, replacement, or restoration of visible portions of the body, performed to correct a structural or cosmetic defect.

Platelets (thrombocytes) Cell fragments that have no nucleus and cannot replicate.

Pleural effusion Collection of excess fluid in the pleural space.

Pleuritis Inflammation of the pleura.

Pneumonectomy Removal of an entire lung.

Pneumonia Inflammation of the lung parenchyma (the respiratory bronchioles and alveoli).

Pneumothorax Results when air enters the pleural space due to blunt and penetrating injuries to the chest.

Polycystic kidney disease A hereditary disease characterized by cyst formation and massive kidney enlargement.

Polycythemia (erythrocytosis) Excess RBCs characterized by a hematocrit higher than 55%.

Polydipsia Excessive thirst.

Polymyositis A systemic connective-tissue disorder characterized by inflammation of connective tissue and muscle fibers leading to muscle weakness and atrophy.

Polyp Mass of tissue that arises from the bowel wall and protrudes into the lumen.

Polyphagia Excessive eating.

Polysubstance abuse The simultaneous use of many substances.

Polyuria A condition where increased blood volume increases renal blood flow, and the hyperglycemia acts as an osmotic diuretic, thereby increasing urine output.

Portal hypertension Elevated pressure in the portal venous system that causes rerouting of blood to adjoining lower pressure vessels.

Postconcussion syndrome Persistent headache, dizziness, irritability, insomnia, impaired memory and concentration, and learning problems following a concussion; may last for several weeks or up to 1 year.

Postoperative phase Period when a procedure or surgery has been completed and the client is recovering from the stress associated with the surgery.

Postpoliomyelitis syndrome A complication of a previous infection by the poliomyelitis virus.

Preload The amount of cardiac muscle fiber tension or stretch that exists at diastole, just before ventricular contraction.

Premenstrual syndrome (PMS) Complex of symptoms characterized by irritability, depression, edema, and breast tenderness preceding the monthly menses.

Preoperative phase Time when preparation of the client for surgery is conducted and completed.

Presbycusis Age-related loss of the ability to hear high-frequency sounds, may occur because of cochlear hair cell degeneration or loss of auditory neurons in the organ of Corti.

Presbyopia Impaired near vision resulting from a loss of elasticity of the lens related to aging.

Pressure ulcer Ischemic lesion of the skin and underlying tissue caused by external pressure that impairs the flow of blood and lymph.

Priapism Sustained, painful erection that lasts at least 4 hours and is not associated with sexual arousal.

Primary hypertension (idiopathic, essential) A persistently elevated systemic blood pressure.

Primary polycythemia (polycythemia vera) A neoplastic stem cell disorder characterized by overproduction of red blood cells and, to a lesser extent, white blood cells and platelets.

Progesterone Hormone produced by the ovary; works with estrogen to control the menstrual cycle.

Prostatitis Inflammation of the prostate gland.

Protein-calorie malnutrition (PCM) Deficient protein and calories to meet metabolic needs.

Proteinuria Abnormal proteins in the urine.

Pruritus Subjective itching sensation producing an urge to scratch.

Psoriasis Chronic, noninfectious skin disorder that is characterized by raised, reddened, round circumscribed plaques covered by silvery white scales.

Psychogenic pain Pain that is experienced in the absence of any diagnosed physiologic cause or event.

Ptosis Drooping of the eyelid.

Pulmonary edema An abnormal accumulation of fluid in the interstitial tissue and alveoli of the lung.

Pulmonary embolism Sudden occlusion of a pulmonary artery resulting in disruption of blood supply to the lung parenchyma.

Pulmonary hypertension Condition in which the pulmonary arterial pressure is elevated to an abnormal level.

Pulmonic valves One of the semilunar valves, separating the ventricles from the great vessels.

Pulse Rhythmic pressure wave that can be felt over an artery.

Pulse deficit Condition in which the radial pulse is less than the apical pulse, indicating weak, inefficient left ventricular contractions.

Pulse pressure The difference between the systolic and diastolic blood pressure.

Puncture wound Wound that occurs when a sharp or blunt object penetrates the integument.

Pupillary light reflex Reflex in which the pupil contracts in response to a bright light.

Pyelonephritis Upper urinary tract inflammation affecting the kidney and renal pelvis.

Pyoderma Purulent bacterial infection of skin.

Pyuria (bacteriuria) Pus in the urine.

Quadriplegia See *Tetraplegia*.

Quality assurance The process of ensuring quality control activities that evaluate, monitor, or regulate the standard of services provided to the consumer.

Rabies Viral (rhabdovirus) infection of the central nervous system transmitted by infected saliva that enters the human body through a bite or an open wound.

Radiation sickness One of the results of DNA mutation inside cells exposed to ionizing radiation.

Radiation therapy Therapy that uses radiation to kill a tumor, to reduce its size, to decrease pain, or to relieve obstruction.

Radiological dispersion bomb Also called a "dirty bomb," consists of a conventional explosive such as trinitrotoluene (TNT) packed with radioactive waste by-products from nuclear reactors that discharges deadly radioactive particles into the environment.

Raynaud's disease (Raynaud's phenomenon) Disorders characterized by episodes of intense vasospasm in the small arteries and arterioles of the fingers and possibly the toes.

Reactive arthritis (Reiter's syndrome) An acute, nonpurulent inflammatory arthritis that complicates a bacterial infection of the genitourinary or gastrointestinal tracts.

Rebound tenderness Pain that occurs with withdrawal or release of pressure applied during abdominal palpation.

Recessive A characteristic that is apparent only when two copies of the gene encoding it are present, one from the mother and one from the father.

Reconstruction The recovery aspect of disaster response; during this period restoration, reconstitution, and mitigation take place.

Red blood cell (RBCs, erythrocytes) Blood cells shaped like a biconcave disk that contain hemoglobin required for oxygen transport to body tissues; the most common type of blood cell.

Referral source A person recommending home care services and supplying the agency with details about the client's needs. The source may be a physician, nurse, social worker, therapist, or discharge planner.

Referred pain Pain that is perceived in an area distant from the site of the stimuli.

Reflex sympathetic dystrophy A group of poorly understood post-traumatic conditions involving persistent pain, hyperesthesias, swelling, changes in skin color and texture, changes in temperature, and decreased motion.

Reflux, urinary Backflow of urine toward the kidneys.

Refraction The bending of light rays as they pass from one medium to another medium of different optical density.

Refractory period A period in which myocardial cells are resistant to stimulation.

Regional anesthesia Anesthesia that desensitizes the area to be operated but does not involve the full central nervous system or cause sedation.

Regurgitation (valvular) Backflow of blood through an incompletely closed valve into the area it just left.

Rehabilitation The process of learning to live to one's maximum potential with a chronic impairment and its resultant functional disability.

Reiter's syndrome See *Reactive arthritis*.

Remission A period in which symptoms are not experienced even though the disease is still clinically present.

Renal artery stenosis Narrowing of the renal artery.

Renal colic Acute, severe, intermittent pain in the flank and upper outer abdominal quadrant generally associated with acute obstruction of a ureter and resulting ureteral spasm.

Renal failure A condition in which the kidneys are unable to remove accumulated metabolites from the blood, resulting in altered fluid, electrolyte, and acid–base balance.

Renal impairment (decreased renal reserve) A glomerular filtration rate of approximately 50% of normal with normal BUN and serum creatinine levels.

Renal insufficiency A glomerular filtration rate of 20% to 50% of normal with azotemia and some manifestations of renal failure.

Renal transplant The surgical insertion of a functioning kidney.

Renin–angiotensin mechanism Method of controlling the glomerular filtration rate by releasing chemicals that cause intense vasodilation of the afferent arterioles. Conversely, an increase in the flow of filtrate results in the promotion of vasoconstriction, decreasing the glomerular filtration rate.

Repolarization Restoration of the resting cell membrane potential following generation of an action potential.

Synovitis Inflammation of the synovial membrane lining the articular capsule of a joint.

Syphilis A sexually transmitted infection caused by a spirochete that may invade almost any body tissue or organ. It enters the body through a break in the skin or mucous membranes, and can be transferred to the fetus through the placental circulation.

Systemic lupus erythematosus (SLE) A chronic, inflammatory immune complex connective tissue disease.

Systemic sclerosis (scleroderma) Hardening of the skin; a chronic disease characterized by the formation of excess fibrous connective tissue and diffuse fibrosis of the skin and internal organs.

Systole A phase during which the ventricles contract and eject blood into the pulmonary and systemic circuits.

Systolic blood pressure This arterial pressure wave produced by ventricular contraction (systole) averages 120 mmHg in healthy adults.

T lymphocytes (T cells) Type of lymphocyte that matures in the thymus gland.

Tachycardia A heart rate exceeding 100 beats per minute.

Tachypnea Abnormally rapid respiratory rate.

Tendonitis Inflammation of a tendon.

Tension headache Poorly localized headache characterized by ill-defined bilateral head aching, tightness, pressure, or a viselike feeling.

Tension pneumothorax A condition in which an injury to the chest allows air to enter but not escape the pleural cavity.

Testicular torsion Twisting of the testes and spermatic cord.

Testosterone Male hormone produced in the testes.

Tetanus Disorder of the nervous system caused by a neurotoxin elaborated by *Clostridium tetani*.

Tetany Tonic muscular spasms.

Tetraplegia (formerly called quadriplegia) Injury to cervical segments of the cord thus impairing function of the arms, trunk, legs, and pelvic organs.

Thalassemia An inherited disorder of hemoglobin synthesis in which either the alpha or beta chains of the hemoglobin molecule are missing or defective.

Third spacing The accumulation and sequestration of trapped extracellular fluid in an actual or potential body space as a result of disease or injury.

Thoracentesis Invasive procedure in which fluid (or occasionally air) is removed from the pleural space with a needle.

Thoracotomy Incision of the chest wall to gain access to the lung for surgery.

Thrill Palpable vibration over the precordium or an artery.

Thromboangiitis obliterans (Buerger's disease) An occlusive vascular disease involving inflammation, spasm, and clot formation in small- and medium-sized peripheral arteries.

Thrombocytopenia A platelet count of less than 100,000 per milliliter of blood.

Thromboembolus A thrombus that breaks loose from the arterial wall.

Thrombophlebitis See *Venous thrombosis*.

Thrombotic cerebrovascular accident Cerebrovascular accident caused by occlusion of a vessel by a thrombus (a blood clot) on the interior wall of an artery.

Thrombus A blood clot that adheres to a vessel wall.

Tidal volume (TV) The amount of air (approximately 500 mL) moved in and out of the lungs with each normal, quiet breath.

Tinea capitis A fungal infection of the scalp.

Tinea corporis A fungal infection of the body.

Tinea pedis A fungal infection of the toenails and feet.

Tinnitus Perception of sound such as ringing, buzzing, or roaring in the ears.

Titration Administration of analgesics in small increasing or decreasing increments.

Tolerance A cumulative state in which a particular dose of a chemical elicits a smaller response than before. With increased tolerance, the individual needs higher and higher doses to obtain the desired effect.

Tonic-clonic seizures Alternating contraction (tonic phase) and relaxation (clonic phase) of muscles during seizure activity.

Tonsillitis Acute inflammation of the palatine tonsils.

Tophi Small white nodules in subcutaneous tissue composed of urate deposits resulting from gout.

Total colectomy Surgical removal of the entire colon.

Total gastrectomy Removal of the entire stomach.

Total hip arthroplasty (THA) Replacement of both the femoral head and the acetabulum.

Total parenteral nutrition (TPN) Intravenous administration of carbohydrates (high concentrations of dextrose), protein (amino acids), electrolytes, vitamins, minerals, and fat emulsions.

Toxic epidermal necrolysis (TENS) Rare, life-threatening disease in which the epidermis peels off the dermis in sheets, leaving large areas of denuded skin.

Toxic megacolon A condition characterized by acute motor paralysis and dilation of the colon.

Traction The application of a straightening or pulling force to return or maintain the fractured bones in normal anatomic position.

Transcutaneous electrical nerve stimulation (TENS) A unit that consists of a low-voltage transmitter connected by wires to electrodes that are placed by the client as directed by the physical therapist. The client experiences a gentle tapping or vibrating sensation over the electrodes. The client can adjust the voltage to achieve maximum pain relief.

Transdermal Medication absorbed through the skin without injection.

Transfusion An infusion of blood or blood components.

Transient ischemic attack (TIA) Brief period of localized cerebral ischemia that causes neurologic deficits lasting for less than 24 hours.

Transjugular intrahepatic portosystemic shunt (TIPS) Used to relieve portal hypertension and its complications of esophageal varices and ascites. A channel is created through the liver tissue using a needle inserted transcutaneously; an expandable metal stent is inserted into this channel, to allow blood to flow directly from the portal vein into the hepatic vein, bypassing the cirrhotic liver. The shunt relieves pressure in esophageal varices and allows better control of fluid retention with diuretic therapy. Generally is used as a short-term measure until liver transplant is performed.

Translocation The joining of a part of or a whole chromosome to another separate chromosome.

Traumatic brain injury (TBI) A traumatic insult to the brain capable of causing physical, intellectual, emotional, social, and vocational changes.

Tremors Rhythmic movement.

Triage Means "sorting." Triage is a continuous process in which client priorities are reassigned as needed treatments, time, and the condition of the clients change.

Tricuspid valve A valve between the right atrium and ventricle of the heart; prevents blood from flowing backwards into the atrium.

Trigeminal neuralgia (tic douloureux) A chronic disease of the trigeminal cranial nerve (cranial nerve V) that causes severe facial pain.

Triglycerides Molecules of glycerol with fatty acids used to transport and store fats in body tissues.

Trisomy Possessing three chromosomes instead of the usual two as in trisomy 21 or Down syndrome.

Trousseau's sign Contraction of the hand and fingers in response to occlusion of the blood supply by a blood pressure cuff; caused by decreased blood calcium levels.

Tuberculosis (TB) Chronic, recurrent infectious disease caused by *Mycobacterium tuberculosis;* usually affects the lungs, although any organ can be affected.

Tumor marker A protein molecule detectable in serum or other body fluids. This marker is used as a biochemical indicator of the presence of a malignancy.

Tympanoplasty Surgical reconstruction of the middle ear.

Type 1 diabetes One of two types of diabetes characterized by the destruction of beta cells, usually leading to absolute insulin deficiency.

Type 2 diabetes One of two types of diabetes the characteristics of which may range from predominantly insulin resistance with relative insulin deficiency to a predominantly secretory defect with insulin resistance. There is no immune destruction of beta cells.

Ulcer A lesion of the skin or mucous membranes.

Ulcerative colitis Chronic inflammatory bowel disorder of the mucosa and submucosa of the colon and rectum.

Ultrafiltration Removal of excess body water using a hydrostatic pressure gradient.

Uniform Anatomical Gift Act Legislation that requires people to be informed about their options related to organ donation.

Unilateral neglect State in which a client is unaware of and inattentive to one side of body.

Upper body obesity (central obesity) Excess intra-abdominal fat characterized by a waist-to-hip ratio greater than 1 in men and 0.8 in women.

Urea An end product of protein metabolism, and along with water the main constituent of urine.

Uremia Literally "urine in the blood"; the syndrome or group of symptoms associated with end-stage renal failure.

Ureteral stent Thin catheter inserted into the ureter to provide for urine flow and ureteral support.

Ureteroplasty Surgical repair of a ureter.

Urgency A sudden, compelling need to urinate.

Urinary calculi Calculi or "stones" in the urinary tract.

Urinary diversion Procedure to provide for urine collection and drainage following cystectomy. The most common urinary diversion is the ileal conduit.

Urinary drainage system The ureters, urinary bladder, and urethra.

Urinary incontinence Involuntary urination.

Urinary retention Incomplete emptying of the bladder.

Urolithiasis Development of stones within the urinary tract.

Urticaria Hives.

Vaccine Suspensions of whole or fractionated bacteria or viruses that have been treated to make them nonpathogenic.

Valsalva's maneuver Closing the glottis and contracting the diaphragm and abdominal muscles to increase intra-abdominal pressure to facilitate expulsion of feces.

Valvular heart disease Interference of blood flow to, within, and from the heart.

Vancomycin intermediate-resistant *Staphylococcus aureus* (VISA) A form of *S. aureus* with intermediate resistance to vancomycin.

Varicocele Dilation of the pampiniform venous complex of the spermatic cord.

Varicose veins Irregular, tortuous veins with incompetent valves.

Vasectomy Sterilization procedure in which a portion of the spermatic cord is removed.

Vasoconstriction Smooth muscle contraction that narrows the vessel lumen.

Vasodilation Smooth muscle relaxation that expands the vessel lumen.

Vasogenic shock See *Neurogenic shock.*

Venous thrombosis (thrombophlebitis) Blood clot (thrombus) formation on the wall of a vein, accompanied by inflammation of the vein wall and obstructed venous blood flow.

Vertigo Sensation of whirling or rotation.

Very low calorie diet (VLCD) A protein-sparing modified fast (400 to 800 kcal/day or less) under close medical supervision that may be used to treat significant obesity.

Vesicoureteral reflux Condition in which urine moves from the bladder back toward the kidney.

Visceral pain Pain arising from body organs. It is dull and poorly localized because of the low number of nociceptors.

Vital capacity The sum of TV (tidal volume) + IRV (inspiratory reserve volume) + ERV (expiratory reserve volume); approximately 4500 mL in healthy clients.

Vitamin B$_{12}$ deficiency anemia Anemia due to inadequate vitamin B$_{12}$ consumption or impaired absorption.

Vitiligo Abnormal loss of melanin in patches.

Acute arterial occlusion—*continued*
  nursing care
    assessment, 1185
    community-based care, 1185
    nursing diagnoses and interventions
      altered protection, 1185–86
      anxiety, 1185
      ineffective tissue perfusion: peripheral, 1185
  pathophysiology
    arterial embolism, 1184
    arterial thrombosis, 1184
Acute brain injury. *See* Traumatic brain injury
Acute bronchitis:
  interdisciplinary care, 1266
  manifestations, 1266
  nursing care, 1267
  pathophysiology, 1266
Acute chest syndrome, 1109
Acute cholecystitis, 698. *See also* Gallstones
Acute coronary syndrome (ACS):
  definition, 974
  interdisciplinary care
    diagnosis, 975–76
    medications, 976, 976*t*
    revascularization procedures
      coronary artery bypass grafting. *See*
        Coronary artery bypass grafting
      minimally invasive coronary artery
        surgery, 979
      percutaneous coronary revascularization,
        977, 977*f,* 978*t*
      transmyocardial laser revascularization, 979
  manifestations, 975
  Medication Administration, 976*t*
  Nursing Care Plan
    assessment, 983*t*
    critical thinking in the nursing process, 983*t*
    diagnoses, 983*t*
    evaluation, 983*t*
    expected outcomes, 983*t*
    planning and implementation, 983*t*
  pathophysiology, 974–75
  vs. stable angina and myocardial infarction, 975*t*
Acute disease, 22*t*
Acute gastritis, 677. *See also* Gastritis
Acute heart failure, 1027. *See also* Heart failure
Acute illness, 23. *See also* Illness
Acute infective endocarditis, 1045, 1046*t*. *See also*
  Endocarditis
Acute lymphocytic leukemia (ALL). *See also*
  Leukemia
  characteristics, 1119*t*
  interdisciplinary care
    diagnosis, 1123*t*
    treatment, 1119*t*, 1123*t*
  manifestations, 1119*t,* 1122
  pathophysiology, 1122
Acute myeloid leukemia (AML). *See also*
  Leukemia
  characteristics, 1119*t*
  FAB classification, 1121*t*
  interdisciplinary care
    diagnosis, 1123*t*
    treatment, 1119*t*, 1123*t*
    management, 1121
  manifestations, 1119*t*
  Nursing Care Plan
    assessment, 1125*t*
    critical thinking in the nursing process, 1125*t*
    diagnoses, 1125*t*
    evaluation, 1125*t*
    expected outcomes, 1125*t*
    planning and implementation, 1125*t*

pathophysiology, 1121, 1121*f*
  prognosis, 1121, 1121*t*
Acute myocardial infarction (AMI):
  vs. acute coronary syndrome and stable
    angina, 975*t*
  cocaine-induced, 984
  complications
    cardiogenic shock, 985. *See also* Cardiogenic
      shock
    dysrhythmias, 985. *See also* Cardiac
      dysrhythmias
    infarct extension, 985
    pericarditis, 985–86
    pump failure, 985. *See also* Heart failure
    structural defects, 985
  definition, 979
  incidence, 982
  interdisciplinary care
    diagnosis, 986–87, 987*t,* 988*f*
    immediate goals, 986
    medications
      ACE inhibitors, 988
      analgesia, 987
      anticoagulants, 988. *See also* Anticoagulants
      antidysrhythmics, 988, 1006*t*
      antiplatelets, 976*t,* 988
      beta-blockers, 988. *See also* Beta-blockers
      dopamine, 989
      fibrinolytic therapy, 987–88, 989*t*
    treatments
      cardiac rehabilitation, 990
      general considerations, 989
      intra-aortic balloon pump, 990, 990*f*
      revascularization procedures, 990. *See also*
        Coronary artery bypass grafting;
        Percutaneous coronary revascularization
      ventricular assist devices, 990
  manifestations, 984, 984*t,* 985*t*
  mortality rate, 982
  nursing care
    assessment, 992
    of client receiving fibrinolytic therapy, 989*t*
    community-based care, 994
    health promotion, 991
    nursing diagnoses and interventions
      acute pain, 992
      fear, 993–94
      ineffective coping, 993
      ineffective tissue perfusion, 992–93
    using NANDA, NIC, and NOC, 994, 994*t*
  Nursing Care Plan
    assessment, 991*t*
    diagnoses, 991*t*
    evaluation, 992*t*
    expected outcomes, 991*t*
    planning and implementation, 991*t*
  Nursing Research: lifestyle changes in
    women, 995*t*
  pathophysiology, 961*t,* 982–84
  risk factors, 982
Acute otitis media. *See* Otitis media
Acute pain, 173–74. *See also* Pain
Acute pancreatitis, 726–27, 727*t. See also*
  Pancreatitis
Acute proliferative glomerulonephritis. *See also*
  Glomerular disorders
  complications, 886–87
  manifestations, 886–87, 888*t*
  pathophysiology, 886, 886*f,* 887*t*
  prognosis, 887
Acute pyelonephritis, 848, 848*t. See also* Urinary
  tract infection
Acute rejection, 921

Acute renal artery thrombosis, 894
Acute renal failure:
  acute tubular necrosis, 901–2, 903*f*
  course and manifestations
    initiation phase, 902
    maintenance phase, 902
    recovery phase, 902
  definition, 899
  incidence, 899
  interdisciplinary care
    diagnosis, 904
    fluid management, 905
    goals, 902
    medications, 904–5, 905*t*
    nutrition, 906
    renal replacement therapy. *See* Dialysis
  intrarenal, 900*t,* 901–2
  nursing care
    assessment, 911
    community-based care, 913
    health promotion, 910–11
    Medication Administration, 905–6*t*
    nursing diagnoses and interventions
      deficient knowledge, 913
      excess fluid volume, 911
      imbalanced nutrition: less than body
        requirements, 911–12
    using NANDA, NIC, and NOC, 913, 913*t*
  Nursing Care Plan
    assessment, 912*t*
    critical thinking in the nursing process, 912*t*
    diagnoses, 912*t*
    evaluation, 912*t*
    expected outcomes, 912*t*
    planning and implementation, 912*t*
  pathophysiology, 899, 900, 900*t*
  physical assessment, 901*t*
  postrenal, 900, 900*t*
  prerenal, 900, 900*t*
  risk factors, 900
Acute respiratory distress syndrome (ARDS):
  causes, 1366, 1366*t*
  definition, 1365
  incidence, 1365
  interdisciplinary care
    diagnosis, 1366–67
    mechanical ventilation, 1367. *See also*
      Mechanical ventilation
    medications, 1367
    treatments, 1367
  manifestations, 1366
  mortality rate, 1365
  nursing care
    community-based care, 1372
    nursing diagnoses and interventions, 1367
      decreased cardiac output, 1367,
        1370–71
      dysfunctional ventilatory weaning
        response, 1371
    using NANDA, NIC, and NOC, 1371, 1371*t*
  Nursing Care Plan
    assessment, 1370*t*
    critical thinking in the nursing process, 1370*t*
    diagnoses, 1370*t*
    evaluation, 1370*t*
    expected outcomes, 1370*t*
    planning and implementation, 1370*t*
  pathophysiology, 1366, 1366*f,* 1368–69*t*
  in shock, 272
Acute respiratory failure:
  causes, 1353–54, 1354*f,* 1354*t*
  definition, 1353
  interdisciplinary care

airway management, 1355–56, 1357*t*
  diagnosis, 1355
  mechanical ventilation. *See* Mechanical ventilation
  medications, 1355
  nutrition and fluids, 1361
  oxygen therapy, 1355
  management, 1354–55
  manifestations, 1354*f*
  nursing care
    assessment, 1361
    community-based care, 1365
    endotracheal suctioning, 1363*t*
    health promotion, 1361
    nursing diagnoses and interventions
      anxiety, 1364–65
      impaired spontaneous ventilation, 1362
      ineffective airway clearance, 1362
      risk for injury, 1363–64
    using NANDA, NIC, and NOC, 1365, 1365*t*
  pathophysiology, 1354
  prognosis, 1355
Acute response, in asthma, 1322
Acute tissue rejection, 342, 343*t*
Acute tubular necrosis, 901–2, 903*f*. *See also* Acute renal failure
Acute viral rhinitis. *See* Upper respiratory disorders, viral infections
Acutrim. *See* Phenylpropanolamine
Acyclovir:
  Medication Administration, 322*t*, 658*t*
  in specific conditions
    Bell's palsy, 1658
    bone marrow transplant recipients, 344
    herpes infection, 359*t*, 452, 453, 658*t*, 1839
    viral encephalitis, 1566
Adalat. *See* Nifedipine
Adalimumab, 341, 1465
Addiction. *See also* Substance abuse
  definition, 103*t*, 179*t*
  fear of, 175
Addisonian crisis, 553–54
Addison's disease:
  addisonian crisis, 553–54
  definition, 553
  interdisciplinary care
    diagnostic tests, 524–25*t*, 554, 554*t*
    medications, 554, 555*t*
  manifestations, 553, 554*t*
  nursing care
    assessment, 529–30*t*, 554–55
    community-based care, 557
    health promotion, 554
    Medication Administration, 555*t*
    nursing diagnoses and interventions
      deficient fluid volume, 555–56
      risk for ineffective therapeutic regimen management, 556–57
  Nursing Care Plan
    assessment, 556*t*
    critical thinking in the nursing process, 556*t*
    diagnoses, 556*t*
    evaluation, 556*t*
    expected outcomes, 556*t*
    planning and implementation, 556*t*
  pathophysiology, 553
Adduction, 1386*t*
A-delta fibers, 171, 171*f*, 172
Adenocarcinoma:
  breast. *See* Breast cancer
  endometrial. *See* Endometrial cancer
  esophageal, 669. *See also* Esophageal cancer
  lung, 1309*t*. *See also* Lung cancer
  stomach, 688. *See also* Gastric cancer

Adenocard. *See* Adenosine
Adenoma, 800, 800*f*
Adenosine, 1006, 1006*t*
Adenosine triphosphate, 962
ADH. *See* Antidiuretic hormone
Adipex-P. *See* Phentermine
Adjustable gastric banding (AGB), 637, 637*f*
Adolescence, surgical risk and nursing implications, 58*t*
Adoxa. *See* Doxycycline
Adrenal glands:
  age-related changes, 529*t*
  anatomy, physiology, and functions, 520–21, 520*f*
  diagnostic tests, 524–25*t*
  disorders
    Addison's disease (adrenocortical insufficiency). *See* Addison's disease
    Cushing's syndrome (hypercortisolism). *See* Cushing's syndrome
    pheochromocytoma, 557
  hormones produced by, 519*t*, 520–21. *See also specific hormones*
Adrenalectomy:
  nursing care, 550*t*
  procedure, 550
Adrenaline. *See* Epinephrine
Adrenergic agonists (mydriatics), 1710*t*
Adrenergic neurotransmitters, 1505
Adrenergic stimulants (β₂-agonists), 1325, 1327*t*, 1355
Adrenergics (sympathomimetics), 278*t*, 1034*t*
Adrenocortical insufficiency. *See* Addison's disease
Adrenocorticotropic hormone (ACTH):
  abnormal, possible causes, 386*t*
  diagnostic tests, 380*t*, 525*t*, 549, 550, 550*t*
  excess. *See* Cushing's syndrome
  functions, 518
  laboratory tests, 380*t*
  Medication Administration, 1631*t*
  normal values, 386*t*, 525*t*
  in specific conditions
    cancer, 380
    multiple sclerosis, 1627, 1631*t*
Adrenomedullin, 1155
Adriamycin. *See* Doxorubicin
Adult polycystic kidney disease, 839*t*
Adult rickets. *See* Osteomalacia
Adults, 24, 25*t*. *See also* Middle adults; Older adults; Young adults
Advair. *See* Salmeterol/fluticasone
Advance directives:
  definition, 12
  ethical dilemmas, 12
  legal issues, 90
  Medicare/Medicaid requirements, 90–91
  types, 90
Advanced life support (ALS), 1016–17
Advil. *See* Ibuprofen
Advocate, nurse as, 14
Adynamic ileus. *See* Paralytic ileus
AED. *See* Automatic external defibrillator
Aerobes, 311*t*
AeroBid. *See* Flunisolide
Aesthetic surgery. *See* Cosmetic surgery
Aethoxysclerol, 478
Afferent, 894
AFP. *See* Alpha-fetoprotein
African Americans. *See* Blacks/African Americans
Afterload, 940, 1023, 1024*t*
AGB (adjustable gastric banding), 637, 637*f*
Agenerase. *See* Amprenavir
Agenesis, kidney, 883

Age-related macular degeneration (AMD):
  incidence, 1713–14
  interdisciplinary care, 1714
  manifestations, 1714, 1714*f*
  nursing care, 1714
  Nursing Research: effect on older adults, 1715*t*
  pathophysiology, 1714
Agglutination, 262
Aggrastat. *See* Tirofiban
Aging:
  as cancer risk factor, 370
  as coronary heart disease risk factor, 962–63
  functional changes with
    fluid and electrolyte balances, 202
    pain response, 175, 175*t*
  health and, 20
  physical status and
    middle adults, 27*t*. *See also* Middle adults
    older adults, 29*t*. *See also* Older adults
    young adults, 26*t*. *See also* Young adults
  surgical risk and nursing implications, 57*t*
Agnosia, 1582
Agranulocytosis, 1138
Agraphia, 1620
AHAs (alpha-hydroxy acids), 479
AIDS. *See* Acquired immunodeficiency syndrome
Airborne precautions, 323*t*
Airway management, in acute respiratory failure, 1355–56, 1356*f*, 1357*t*
Airway obstruction:
  in burns, 257, 499
  in trauma, 257–58, 257*f*
Airway resistance, 1216
Alanine aminotransferase (ALT), 386*t*
Alaska Natives, diabetes mellitus risk and incidence, 564*t*
Albendazole, 780*t*
Albenza. *See* Albendazole
Albinism, 426*t*, 427*t*
Albumin:
  serum. *See* Serum albumin
  for shock, 277, 279*t*
  as volume resuscitation therapy, 263*t*
Albumin 5%, 279*t*
Albumin 25%, 279*t*
Albuminar-5. *See* Albumin 5%
Albuminar-25. *See* Albumin 25%
Albuterol, 1327*t*
Albuterol/ipratropium, 1327*t*
Alcohol:
  abuse
    biologic factors, 104, 105
    complications, 108
    depression and, 103
    folic acid deficiency in, 1105
    genetic factors, 104, 104*t*
    hypertension and, 1157
    hypomagnesemia in, 233
    other drugs used with, 107*t*
    prevalence, 107
    screening tools, 116, 116*f*
    surgical risk and nursing implications, 57*t*
    treatment, 112
    underage, 107, 108*t*
    in young adults, 107, 108*t*
  characteristics, 107
  consumption
    cancer risk and, 372
    coronary heart disease risk and, 966
    in diabetes mellitus, 579
    effects, 108
    in hypertension, 1160
    osteoporosis risk and, 1434

Alcohol—*continued*
  overdose signs and treatment, 113*t*
  street names, 111*t*
  withdrawal, 108, 112, 113*t*
Alcoholic cirrhosis. *See also* Cirrhosis
  incidence, 710
  Nursing Care Plan, 721*t*
  pathophysiology, 710
Aldactone. *See* Spironolactone
Aldehyde dehydrogenase, in alcohol abuse, 105
Aldomet. *See* Methyldopa
Aldosterone:
  diagnostic test, 525*t*
  functions, 521
  normal values, 525*t*
  in potassium balance, 217
Alendronate:
  Medication Administration, 1442*t*
  in specific conditions
    hypercalcemia, 547
    osteoporosis, 1436
    Paget's disease, 1442, 1442*t*
Aleve. *See* Naproxen
Alfuzosin, 1779
ALG (antilymphocyte globulin), 344, 346*t*
Alkaline phosphatase (ALP):
  abnormal, possible causes, 386*t*
  in musculoskeletal system assessment, 1388*t*
  normal values, 386*t*, 728*t*
  in specific conditions
    osteomalacia, 1436*t*
    osteoporosis, 1436*t*
    Paget's disease, 1436*t*, 1442
    pancreatitis, 728*t*
Alkalis, 238
Alkalosis:
  definition, 238
  metabolic. *See* Metabolic alkalosis
  respiratory. *See* Respiratory alkalosis
Alkeran. *See* Melphalan
Alkylating agents, 390, 392*t*. *See also*
    Chemotherapy
ALL. *See* Acute lymphocytic leukemia
Allegra. *See* Fexofenadine
Alleles, 151
Allen test, 1096*t*
Allerest. *See* Phenylpropanolamine
Allergen, 276, 331
Allergic rhinitis, 1229
Allergy, 331. *See also* Hypersensitivity
Alloderm, 503
Allogeneic bone marrow transplant, 1124. *See also*
    Bone marrow transplant
Allograft, 342, 503
Allopurinol, 1445, 1446*t*
All-*trans* retinoic acid (ATRA), 1123*t*
Alopecia:
  causes, 435*t*
  from chemotherapy, 406
  definition, 435*t*
  interdisciplinary care, 482
  manifestations, 481, 482*f*
  medications causing, 482*t*
  nursing care, 482–83
  pathophysiology, 481
Alopecia areata, 482
Alopecia totalis, 482
Alopecia universalis, 482
ALP. *See* Alkaline phosphatase
Alpha cells, pancreas, 521, 564
Alpha interferon. *See also* Interferon(s)
  functions, 299*t*
  for hepatitis C, 708

for immune system enhancement, 396
for leukemia, 1125
production, 299*t*
Alpha Keri, 441*t*
Alpha-adrenergic antagonists. *See* Alpha-blockers
Alpha₁(α₁)-antitrypsin:
  deficiency, 1220*t*, 1331*t*, 1333–34
  normal values, 1334
  replacement therapy, 1334
Alpha-blockers:
  Medication Administration, 1161*t*
  in specific conditions
    benign prostatic hyperplasia, 1779
    hypertension, 1161*t*, 1163
    scleroderma, 1485
Alpha-fetoprotein (AFP):
  abnormal, possible causes, 384*t*, 386*t*
  normal values, 386*t*
  in testicular cancer, 1775
Alphagan. *See* Brimonidine
Alpha-glucoside inhibitors, 578*t*
Alpha-hydroxy acids (AHAs), 479
Alpha-thalassemia major, 1109. *See also*
    Thalassemias
Alprostadil, 1769
ALS. *See* Amyotrophic lateral sclerosis
ALS (advanced life support), 1016–17
ALT (alanine aminotransferase), 386*t*
Altace. *See* Ramipril
Altered level of consciousness:
  arousal, 1529–30
  coma states
    brain death, 265*t*, 1532
    definition, 1529*t*
    locked-in syndrome, 1532
    persistent vegetative state, 1532
    resources for families, 1531*t*
  interdisciplinary care
    diagnosis, 1532–33
    medications, 1533
    nutrition, 1533
    other treatments, 1533
    surgery, 1533
  motor responses, 1531
  nursing care
    nursing diagnoses and interventions
      impaired physical mobility, 1535
      ineffective airway clearance, 1534
      risk for aspiration, 1534
      risk for imbalanced nutrition: less than body
        requirements, 1535
      risk for impaired skin integrity, 1534–35
      support of the family, 1533–34
  pathophysiology, 1529
  prognosis, 1532
  pupillary and oculomotor responses,
    1531, 1531*f*
  respiration patterns, 1530, 1530*t*
  terminology, 1529*t*
AlternaGEL. *See* Aluminum hydroxide
Alternating current (AC), 488
Alternative therapies. *See* Complementary and
    alternative therapies
Aludrox, 666*t*
Aluminum hydroxide, 905, 919
Alupent. *See* Metaproterenol
Alveolar macrophages, 289
Alveoli, 1212*f*, 1213, 1216
Alzheimer's disease:
  characteristics, 1617–18
  familial, 1618
  genetic considerations, 1513*t*
  incidence, 1618

interdisciplinary care
  complementary and alternative therapies, 1621
  diagnosis, 1620–21
  medications, 1621, 1621*t*
manifestations
  stage 1, 1619, 1620*t*
  stage 2, 1619–20, 1620*t*
  stage 3, 1620, 1620*t*
nursing care
  assessment, 1623
  communication techniques, 1624*t*
  community-based care, 1625–26
  health promotion, 1621, 1623
  Medication Administration, 1621*t*
  nursing diagnoses and interventions
    anxiety, 1624
    caregiver role strain, 1625
    chronic confusion, 1624
    hopelessness, 1624–25
    impaired memory, 1623–24
    safety interventions, 1623*t*
    using NANDA, NIC, and NOC, 1625, 1625*t*
Nursing Care Plan
  assessment, 1622*t*
  critical thinking in the nursing process, 1623*t*
  diagnoses, 1622*t*
  evaluation, 1622–23*t*
  expected outcomes, 1622*t*
  planning and implementation, 1622*t*
pathophysiology, 1618–19, 1618*t*, 1619*f*
progression, 1618
risk factors, 1618
sporadic, 1618
warning signs, 1618
Amantadine:
  Medication Administration, 322*t*, 1637*t*
  in specific conditions
    influenza, 322*t*, 1234
    Parkinson's disease, 1637*t*, 1639
Amaryl. *See* Glimepiride
Amaurosis fugax, 1581
Ambenonium, 1649*t*
AMD. *See* Age-related macular degeneration
Amebaquine. *See* Iodoquinol
Amebiasis, 778, 778*t*
Amebic meningoencephalitis, 1565*t*
Amenorrhea, 1802. *See also* Dysfunctional uterine
    bleeding
American Burn Association:
  burn injury classification, 491*t*
  guidelines for transfer to burn center, 497–98
American Cancer Society (ACS):
  cancer prevention guidelines, 412*t*
  cancer screening guidelines, 401*t*
  cancer warning signs, 400*t*
American Indians. *See* Native Americans
American Nurses Association (ANA):
  Code of Ethics for Nurses, 11, 11*t*
  definition of nursing, 8
  do-not-resuscitate decisions, nursing care and, 91
  genetics nursing practice, scope and standards,
    148–49, 149*t*
  Standards of Practice and Professional
    Performance, 11*t*
AMI. *See* Acute myocardial infarction
Amidopyrine, 832*t*
Amikacin, 320*t*, 770
Amikin. *See* Amikacin
Amiloride HCl, 210*t*, 1033*t*
Amino acids, in gout treatment, 1445
Aminogluthemide, 550
Aminoglycosides, 320*t*, 1730
Aminophylline, 1326, 1327*t*

Amiodarone, 541, 1006*t*
Amitriptyline:
  Medication Administration, 1545*t*
  in specific conditions
    fibromyalgia, 1487
    headache, 1545*t*
  urine color changes caused by, 832*t*
AML. *See* Acute myeloid leukemia
Amlexanox oral paste, 657*t*
Amlodipine, 1162*t*
Amoxicillin:
  Medication Administration, 319*t*
  in specific conditions
    endocarditis prophylaxis, 1047*t*
    Lyme disease, 1477
    otitis media, 1722
    pneumonia, 1271*t*
Amoxicillin-clavulanate, 319*t*, 1280
Amoxil. *See* Amoxicillin
Amphetamines:
  abuse, 109. *See also* Methamphetamine
  for counteracting sedation, 189
  effects, 109
  for obesity, 633
  overdose signs and treatment, 113*t*
  street names, 111*t*
  withdrawal signs and treatment, 110, 113*t*
Amphiarthrosis, 1383*t*
Amphojel. *See* Aluminum hydroxide
Amphotec. *See* Amphotericin B
Amphotericin B:
  indications, 318
  Medication Administration, 450*t*
  in specific conditions
    conjunctivitis, 1694
    corneal infections, 1697
    fungal lung infections, 1295
    fungal meningitis, 1566
    fungal skin infections, 450*t*
Ampicillin:
  Medication Administration, 319*t*
  in specific conditions
    endocarditis prophylaxis, 1047*t*
    endocarditis treatment, 1046
    gastroenteritis, 776
    peritonitis, 770
    urinary tract infection, 849
Ampicillin/sulbactam, 1241
Amprenavir, 358
Ampulla of Vater, 726
Amputation:
  causes, 1421
  complications
    chronic stump pain, 1423
    contractures, 1423
    delayed healing, 1423
    infection, 1422–23
    phantom pain, 1423
  definition, 1421
  in diabetes mellitus, 590, 1421
  incidence, 1421
  interdisciplinary care
    diagnosis, 1423
    medications, 1423–24
    prosthesis, 1424
  levels of, 1421, 1422*f*
  nursing care
    assessment, 1424
    community-based care, 1426–27, 1427*t*
    health promotion, 1424
    nursing diagnoses and interventions
      acute pain, 1424
      disturbed body image, 1426

      impaired physical mobility, 1426
      risk for dysfunctional grieving, 1426
      risk for impaired skin integrity, 1425–26
      risk for infection, 1424–25
    using NANDA, NIC, and NOC, 1426, 1426*t*
  Nursing Care Plan
    assessment, 1425*t*
    critical thinking in the nursing process, 1425*t*
    diagnoses, 1425*t*
    evaluation, 1425*t*
    expected outcomes, 1425*t*
    planning and implementation, 1425*t*
  in peripheral vascular disease, 1421
  site healing, 1422, 1423*f*
  terminology, 1422*t*
  types, 1421–22
Amrinone, 1034*t*
Amsler grid, 1676, 1676*f*
Amyl nitrite, 111, 973*t*
Amylase, 612, 742. *See also* Serum amylase
Amyloid plaques, 1618
Amyotrophic lateral sclerosis (ALS):
  characteristics, 1645
  complications, 1646*t*
  genetic considerations, 1389*t*, 1513*t*
  incidence, 1645
  interdisciplinary care
    diagnosis, 1645–46
    medications, 1646
  manifestations, 1645, 1646*t*
  nursing care
    community-based care, 1647
    nursing diagnoses and interventions
      ineffective breathing pattern, 1646
      risk for disuse syndrome, 1646
  pathophysiology, 1645
Amyotrophy, 1645
ANA. *See* American Nurses Association
ANA (antinuclear antibody), 341, 1141
Anabolism, 307, 613
Anacobin. *See* Vitamin B$_{12}$, replacement therapy
Anaerobes, 311*t*
Anakinra, 341
Anal fissures, 820
Analgesics. *See also specific drugs*
  definition, 174
  narcotic. *See* Narcotic analgesics
  nonnarcotic, 178
  nonsteroidal anti-inflammatory drugs. *See*
    Nonsteroidal anti-inflammatory drugs
  urinary, 850*t*
  WHO ladder, 177, 177*f*
Anaphylactic shock:
  assessment, 279–80
  definition, 276, 332
  manifestations, 276, 276*t*
  pathophysiology, 276
Anaphylaxis:
  common triggers, 333*t*
  definition, 276
  epinephrine for, 337–38
  manifestations, 332
  pathophysiology, 332
Anaplasia, 374
Anaprox. *See* Naproxen sodium
Anasarca, 209
Anaspaz. *See* Hyoscyamine
Anastomosed, 978
Anbesol, 658*t*
Ancef. *See* Cefazolin
Ancobon. *See* Flucytosine
Androgen deprivation therapy, 1786, 1787*t*
Androgens, 1745

Anemia:
  aplastic. *See* Aplastic anemia
  assessment in light and dark skin, 426*t*
  from blood loss, 1103
  definition, 1076, 1102
  hemolytic
    acquired, 1109
    causes, 1106, 1106*t*
    definition, 1106
    glucose-6-phosphate dehydrogenase anemia,
      1106, 1109*t*
    racial/ethnic considerations, 1106*t*
    sickle cell anemia. *See* Sickle cell anemia
    thalassemias. *See* Thalassemias
  interdisciplinary care
    blood transfusion, 1111
    complementary therapies, 1111–12
    diagnosis, 1110–11
    focus for major anemias, 1110*t*
    medications, 1111, 1111*t*
    nutrition, 1111, 1111*t*
  manifestations, 1102–3, 1103*f*
  Multisystem Effects, 1104*t*
  nursing care
    assessment, 1112–13
    community-based care, 1114–15
    health promotion, 1112
    Medication Administration, 1112*t*
    nursing diagnoses and interventions
      activity intolerance, 1113–14
      impaired oral mucous membrane, 1114
      risk for decreased cardiac output, 1114
      self-care deficit, 1114
    using NANDA, NIC, and NOC,
      1114, 1115*t*
  nutritional
    folic acid deficiency. *See* Folic acid,
      deficiency
    iron deficiency. *See* Iron deficiency anemia
    vitamin B$_{12}$ deficiency. *See* Vitamin B$_{12}$,
      deficiency
  pathophysiology, 1102, 1103*t*, 1106
  in specific conditions
    after gastric resection, 691
    chronic renal failure, 916
Anergy, 300
Anesthesia:
  conscious sedation, 63–64
  definition, 61
  general, 61–63
  intraoperative awareness, 67
  regional, 63
Anesthesiologist, 65
Anesthetics, local. *See* Local anesthetics
Aneuploidy, 150*t*
Aneurysm:
  aortic. *See* Aortic aneurysm
  definition, 1170
  femoral, 1172
  intracranial. *See* Intracranial aneurysm
  manifestations, 1170
  pathophysiology, 1170, 1170*f*
  popliteal, 1172, 1172*f*
  types, 1170, 1592
Angina pectoris:
  vs. acute coronary syndrome and myocardial
    infarction, 975*t*
  course and manifestations, 970, 970*t*
  definition, 969
  interdisciplinary care
    diagnosis, 970–71, 971*f*
    medications, 973–74*t*
    nitrates, 971

Angina pectoris—*continued*
  nursing care
    assessment, 92
    community-based care, 974
    health promotion, 972
    Medication Administration, 973–74*t*
    nursing diagnoses and interventions
      ineffective tissue perfusion: cardiac, 972
      risk for ineffective therapeutic regimen
        management, 972, 974
  pathophysiology, 961*t*, 969–70
  severity classification, 970
  types, 969–70
Angioedema, 221
Angiography:
  in aortic aneurysm, 1173
  in cancer, 385
  cardiac. *See* Cardiac catheterization
  cerebral. *See* Cerebral angiogram
  in peripheral vascular disease, 1177
  principles, 385
  pulmonary. *See* Pulmonary angiography
  renal, 837*t*
Angiomas, 430*t*, 443
Angiotensin II receptor blockers (ARBs):
  Medication Administration, 1033*t*, 1161*t*
  in specific conditions
    heart failure, 1032, 1033*t*
    hypertension, 1161*t*, 1163
Angiotensin-converting enzyme (ACE) inhibitors:
  Medication Administration, 1033*t*, 1161*t*
  in specific conditions
    acute myocardial infarction, 988
    glomerular disorders, 891
    heart failure, 1032, 1033*t*
    hypertension, 1161*t*, 1163
    scleroderma, 1485
Angiotensinogen, 521
Angle-closure glaucoma. *See* Glaucoma
Anhydrosis, 589
Anion gap, 243, 243*f*
Anions, 196
Anisoylated plasminogen streptokinase activator
    complex (APSAC), 988
Ankle:
  fracture, 1416
  physical assessment, 1394*t*
Ankle-brachial blood pressure index (ABI), 965
Ankylosing spondylitis:
  definition, 1469
  genetic considerations, 1469
  incidence, 1469
  interdisciplinary care, 1470
  manifestations, 1470
  nursing care, 1470
  pathophysiology, 1470
Annuloplasty, 1060
Annulus, 1054
Anorectal abscess, 820
Anorectal disorders:
  anal fissure, 820
  anorectal abscess, 820
  anorectal fistula, 820–21
  hemorrhoids. *See* Hemorrhoids
  nursing care, 821
  pilonidal disease, 821
Anorectal fistula, 820–21
Anorexia, 380, 677
Anorexia nervosa:
  complications, 651*t*
  interdisciplinary care
    diagnosis, 651–52
    treatment, 652

manifestations, 650, 651*t*
  nursing care, 652
Anorexia-cachexia syndrome, 380, 380*f*
Anorgasmia:
  definition, 1758
  in health assessment interview, 1758
  nursing care, 1795
  pathophysiology, 1795
Anosmia, 1519*t*
Anovulation, 1802
ANP. *See* Atrial natriuretic peptide
Ansaid. *See* Flurbiprofen
Antabuse. *See* Disulfiram
Antacids:
  adverse/side effects, 685
  magnesium-containing, 236*t*
  Medication Administration, 666*t*
  preoperative use and nursing implications, 51*t*
  in specific conditions
    cirrhosis, 716
    gastritis, 666*t*
    gastroesophageal reflux disease, 665, 666*t*
    peptic ulcer disease, 666*t*, 685
Anteflexion, uterus, 1805, 1806*f*
Antegrade amnesia, 1559
Antegrade pyelography, 904
Anterior descending artery, 939*f*, 958
Anterior myocardial infarction, 984. *See also*
    Acute myocardial infarction
Anterior syndrome, 1597*t*. *See also* Spinal cord
    injury
Anteversion, uterus, 1805, 1806*f*
Anthralin, 444
Anthranilates, 465*t*
Anthranilic acids, 178*t*
Anthrax, 128*t*, 1293, 1294
Anthropometric assessment:
  body weight, 620–21*t*
  midarm circumference, 621*t*, 622*f*, 622*t*
  midarm muscle circumference, 622*t*
  triceps skinfold thickness, 621*t*
  waist-to-hip ratio, 622*t*
Antiandrogens, 1787*t*
Antibiotics. *See also specific drugs*
  antitumor, 391
  characteristics, 318
  for endocarditis prophylaxis, 1047*t*
  Medication Administration, 319–21*t*
  monitoring blood levels, 316
  Nursing Research: antibiotics regimens, 310*t*
  preoperative use and nursing implications, 62*t*
  resistant microorganisms, 313–14
  in specific conditions
    acne, 458
    acute bronchitis, 1266
    appendicitis, 767
    bacterial meningitis, 1566
    chlamydia, 1845
    diverticulitis, 816
    endocarditis, 1046
    epiglottitis, 1241
    gastroenteritis, 776
    glomerular disorders, 890
    gonorrhea, 1846
    H. pylori infection, 684
    lung abscess, 1280
    osteomyelitis, 1479
    otitis media, 1722
    pelvic inflammatory disease, 1851
    peritonitis, 770
    pharyngitis, 1239
    pneumonia, 1271–72, 1271*t*
    prostatitis, 1777

rheumatic fever, 1043
    skin disorders, 441*t*, 447
    urinary tract infection, 849
  as surgical risk factor, 58*t*
  topical. *See* Topical medications, antimicrobial
Antibodies:
  classes, 291
  definition, 291
  in immune response, 295–97, 296*f*, 297*f*
  monoclonal. *See* Monoclonal antibodies
  structure, 296, 297*f*
Antibody-mediated (humoral) immune response,
    291, 295–97, 296*f*, 297*f*
Anticholinergics:
  Medication Administration, 871*t*, 1327–28*t*
  preoperative use and nursing implications, 62*t*
  side effects, 871, 875
  in specific conditions
    acute respiratory failure, 1355
    asthma, 1326, 1327–28*t*
    diarrhea, 756*t*
    irritable bowel syndrome, 762
    neurogenic bladder, 871, 871*t*
    urinary incontinence, 875
    urinary retention, 869
Anticholinesterases. *See* Cholinesterase inhibitors
Anticipation, in genetics, 155
Anticipatory grieving, 86, 96
Anticoagulants:
  bleeding risk with, 1349
  Medication Administration, 1189–90*t*
  non-heparin, 1141
  in specific conditions
    acute arterial occlusion, 1184
    acute myocardial infarction, 988
    aortic aneurysm, 1173
    cardiomyopathy, 1067
    ischemic stroke, 1585
    pulmonary embolism, 1349
    pulmonary hypertension, 1353
    valvular heart disease, 1060
    venous thrombosis, 1188, 1189–90*t*
  as surgical risk factor, 58*t*, 59
Anticonvulsants. *See* Antiepileptic drugs
Antidepressants. *See also* Monoamine oxidase
      inhibitors; Selective serotonin reuptake
      inhibitors; Tricyclic antidepressants
  for eating disorders, 652
  for irritable bowel syndrome, 763
  for substance abuse/withdrawal treatment, 114*t*
  as surgical risk factor, 58*t*
Antidiarrheal medications, 756*t*, 762
Antidiuretic hormone (ADH):
  in blood pressure regulation, 1155
  in body fluid regulation, 201–2, 202*f*
  in cancer, 380
  for esophageal varices, 718
  functions, 520
  in heart failure, 1025
  laboratory tests, 380*t*
  in sodium balance regulation, 214
  in urine dilution/concentration, 834
Antidysrhythmics:
  for acute myocardial infarction, 988
  for cardiac dysrhythmias, 1005–6, 1006*t*
  Medication Administration, 1006*t*
Antiemetics, 62*t*, 672, 673*t*
Antiepileptic drugs:
  drug interactions with, 1551*t*
  Medication Administration, 1550*t*
  in specific conditions
    intracranial aneurysm, 1593
    pain management, 179

seizure disorders, 1550t
  substance abuse/withdrawal, 114t
  trigeminal neuralgia, 1656
Antifungal agents, 318, 450t, 658t
Antigen:
  characteristics, 290
  definition, 276, 290
  detection methods, 316, 317t
  immune response to, 290–91
  as tumor marker, 384, 384t
Antigen-binding fragment, 296, 297f
Antigen-presenting cells (APCs), 289. See also
    Dendritic cells
Antiglutamate, 1646
Antihemophilic factor, 1082t
Antihistamines:
  Medication Administration, 673t, 1230t
  in specific conditions
    hypersensitivity reactions, 337
    nausea and vomiting, 672, 673t
    upper respiratory infections, 1230, 1230t
Antihypertensives:
  in chronic renal failure, 919
  classes, 1160, 1163
  Medication Administration, 1161–62t
  regimens, 1163
  sites of action, 1160t
  as surgical risk factor, 58t
Antilymphocyte globulin (ALG), 344, 346t
Antimetabolites, 390, 1483t. See also Chemotherapy
Antimicrobials:
  antibiotics. See Antibiotics
  antifungal agents. See Antifungal agents
  antiparasitics. See Antiparasitic agents
  antivirals. See Antivirals
  classification, 318
  mechanisms of action, 318
  selecting, 318
  topical, in burns, 500, 500t
Antiminth. See Pyrantel pamoate
Antinuclear antibody (ANA), 341, 1141
Antiparasitic agents, 321, 321t
Antiplatelet drugs, 976t, 1177, 1585
Antiprotozoal agents, 780t
Antipsychotics, 1643
Antiretroviral nucleoside analogs, 356, 357t, 358
Antispas. See Dicyclomine
Antispasmodics, 1600t
Antistreptolysin A (ASO) titer:
  in glomerular disorders, 889
  in rheumatic fever, 1043
  in rheumatic heart disease, 1043t
Antithymocyte globulin (ATG), 344, 346t
Antituberculosis drugs:
  adverse effects, 1288, 1288t
  dosage, 1288t
  Medication Administration, 1288–89t
  prophylactic, 1287
  regimens, 1287–88
Antitumor antibiotics, 391
Antivert. See Meclizine
Antivirals. See also specific drugs
  characteristics, 318
  Medication Administration, 322t, 658t
  in specific conditions
    Bell's palsy, 1658
    influenza, 1234
    stomatitis, 658t
Antral irrigation, 1237
Anturane. See Sulfinpyrazone
Anus:
  anatomy and functions, 743, 743f
  physical assessment, 750f, 750t

Anxiety:
  levels of, 135t
  pain perception and, 176
  preoperative management, 61, 62t
Anzemet. See Dolasetron
Aorta:
  aneurysm. See Aortic aneurysm
  coarctation of, 1167
  dissection. See Aortic dissection
  physical assessment, 1098f, 1098t
Aortic aneurysm:
  abdominal, 1172
  dissection. See Aortic dissection
  interdisciplinary care
    diagnosis, 1173
    medications, 1173
    surgery, 1173, 1174f
  manifestations, 1170
  nursing care
    assessment, 1173–74
    community-based care, 1175–76
    nursing diagnoses and interventions
      anxiety, 1175
      risk for ineffective tissue perfusion, 1174–75
      risk for injury, 1175
    postoperative, 1174t
    preoperative, 1174t
  pathophysiology, 1170, 1170f
  thoracic, 1171–72, 1171t, 1172t
Aortic dissection:
  complications, 1171t, 1173
  manifestations, 1171t, 1172–73
  pathophysiology, 1171f
  risk factors, 1172
Aortic regurgitation. See also Valvular heart
    disease
  causes, 1058
  manifestations, 1059
  murmur characteristics, 1055t
  pathophysiology, 1058–59, 1058f
Aortic stenosis. See also Valvular heart disease
  manifestations, 1057–58
  murmur characteristics, 1055t
  pathophysiology, 1057, 1058f
Aortic valve, 937f, 938, 1054
APCs (antigen-presenting cells), 289. See also
    Dendritic cells
Aphasia:
  in Alzheimer's disease, 1620
  causes, 1518t
  definition, 1518t, 1583
  types, 1583
Aphonia, 1241
Aphthasol. See Amlexanox oral paste
Aphthoid lesion, 785
Aphthous ulcer, 657t. See also Stomatitis
Apical impulse, 952–53t, 953f
Aplastic anemia:
  interdisciplinary care, 1110t
  manifestations, 1110, 1138
  pathophysiology, 1109–10
  in sickle cell disease, 1109
  types, 1109
Apligraf, 504
Apnea:
  causes, 1223t
  definition, 1223t
  sleep, 1250. See also Obstructive sleep apnea
Apneustic breathing, 1530, 1530t
Apocrine sweat glands, 424
Apo-Doxy. See Doxycycline
Apo-K. See Potassium chloride
Appendectomy, 766f, 767

Appendicitis:
  complications, 767
  definition, 766
  interdisciplinary care
    diagnosis, 767
    medications, 767
    surgery, 767
  manifestations, 766
  nursing care
    assessment, 767
    community-based care, 768–69
    nursing diagnoses and interventions
      acute pain, 768
      risk for infection, 767–68
      using NANDA, NIC, and NOC, 768, 769t
    Nursing Care Plan
      assessment, 768t
      critical thinking in the nursing process, 768t
      diagnoses, 768t
      evaluation, 768t
      expected outcomes, 768t
      planning and implementation, 768t
  pathophysiology, 766, 766f
Appetite suppressants, 633, 634t
Apraclonidine, 1710t
Apraxia, 1582, 1620
Aprazone. See Sulfinpyrazone
Apresoline. See Hydralazine
APSAC (anisoylated plasminogen streptokinase
    activator complex), 988
Aquacare, 441t
Aquaphor, 441t
Aqueous humor, 1671–72
Aralen. See Chloroquine
Aramine. See Metaraminol
Arava. See Leflunomide
Arbovirus encephalitis, 1565, 1565t
ARBs. See Angiotensin II receptor blockers
Ardeparin, 1189t
ARDS. See Acute respiratory distress syndrome
Aredia. See Pamidronate
Areflexia, 1598
Argatroban, 1141
Aricept. See Donepezil
Aromatherapy, 1231
Around-the-clock (ATC) dosing, 181
Arousal, 1529–30. See also Altered level of
    consciousness
Arrhythmogenic, 985
Arsenic, as cancer risk factor, 372t
Artane. See Trihexyphenidyl
Arterial blood gases (ABGs):
  interpretation, 240t
  normal values, 240t, 1217t
  physiology, 1216, 1216f
  purpose and description, 1217t
  related nursing care, 1217t
  in specific conditions
    acid–base balance assessment, 239, 240t
    acute myocardial infarction, 986
    acute renal failure, 904
    acute respiratory distress syndrome, 1367
    acute respiratory failure, 1355
    altered level of consciousness, 1533
    asthma, 1324
    burns, 500
    chronic obstructive pulmonary disease, 1334
    fluid volume excess, 213
    gastroenteritis and diarrhea, 776t
    heart failure, 1027
    hypokalemia, 221
    increased intracranial pressure, 1538
    inhalation injury, 1306

Arterial blood gases (ABGs)—*continued*
  metabolic acidosis, 242t, 244
  metabolic alkalosis, 242t, 246
  pneumonia, 1271
  pulmonary edema, 1040
  pulmonary embolism, 1349
  respiratory acidosis, 242t, 247
  respiratory alkalosis, 242t, 250
  shock, 276–77
Arterial insufficiency, 426t
Arterial line (art line, A line), 1029–30
Arteries:
  anatomy, 1082, 1083f, 1085f
  assessment, 1094–95t
  cerebral, 1507, 1508f
  physiology, 1082, 1085
Arteriography, 837t, 1184
Arterioles, 1082
Arteriovenous fistula, 908, 909f
Arteriovenous graft, 908
Arteriovenous malformation:
  characteristics, 1595
  interdisciplinary care, 1595
  nursing care, 1595
  pathophysiology, 1595
ArthriCare. *See* Counterirritants
Arthritis. *See also* Osteoarthritis
  definition, 1433
  gouty. *See* Gout
  reactive. *See* Reactive arthritis
  rheumatoid. *See* Rheumatoid arthritis
  septic. *See* Septic arthritis
Arthrocentesis, 1387t
Arthropan. *See* Choline salicylate
Arthroscopy, 1387t, 1452
Asacol. *See* Mesalamine
Asbestos, as cancer risk factor, 372t
Asbestosis, 1345
Ascariasis, 781t
Ascending colon, 742f, 743
Ascending contrast venography, 1188
Aschoff bodies, 1042
Ascites:
  in cirrhosis, 711, 715t
  definition, 209, 704
  in fluid volume excess, 209
  in hepatocellular failure, 704
  in ovarian cancer, 1818t
  in pancreatitis, 727
  physical assessment, 626f, 626t
  treatment
    diuretics, 716, 717t
    paracentesis, 717, 718f, 719t
Ascorbic acid. *See* Vitamin C
Asian Americans:
  end-of-life practices, 89
  lactate deficiency incidence, 798t
  osteoporosis incidence, 1434, 1434t
  substance use, 105, 105t
  tuberculosis incidence, 1281t
ASO titer. *See* Antistreptolysin A (ASO) titer
Asparaginase, 1123t
Aspart, 571t
Aspartame, 579
Aspercreme. *See* Salicylates
Aspergillosis, 1294
Aspergillus, 1294
Asphyxiation, 1305
Aspiration pneumonia, 1270. *See also* Pneumonia
Aspirin:
  adverse/side effects, 1463
  effects, 306
  factors in selecting, 178t
  low-dose therapy

for angina, 972
contraindications, 968
for coronary heart disease risk reduction, 968
in diabetes mellitus, 576
for peripheral vascular disease, 1177
for stroke prevention, 1585t
Medication Administration, 179t, 976t
in specific conditions
  headache, 1546t
  rheumatoid arthritis, 1463–64, 1464t
  systemic lupus erythematosus, 1473
Assessment. *See also specific body systems*
  critical thinking skills in, 7t
  data collection in, 8
  overview, 8
  skills needed for, 8
Assist-control mode ventilation (ACMV), 1358, 1359t
Assistive listening device, 1731
Astereognosis, 1620
Asterixis, 715, 715f, 715t
Asthma:
  classification, 1323t
  cough-variant, 1324
  definition, 1321
  genetic considerations, 1220t
  incidence, 1321–22
  interdisciplinary care
    complementary therapies, 1326
    diagnosis, 1324
    disease monitoring, 1324
    medications
      administration, 1324, 1325t, 1327–28t
      anti-inflammatory agents, 1326, 1328t
      bronchodilators, 1325–26, 1327–28t
      leukotriene modifiers, 1326, 1328t
      stepwise approach, 1324, 1325t
    preventive measures, 1324
  manifestations, 1323, 1323t
  mortality rate, 1322
  nursing care
    assessment, 1326
    client teaching, 1325t
    community-based care, 1330
    health promotion, 1326
    Medication Administration, 1327–28t
    nursing diagnoses and interventions
      anxiety, 1329–30
      ineffective airway clearance, 1329
      ineffective breathing pattern, 1329
      ineffective therapeutic regimen management, 1330
  pathophysiology
    attack triggers, 1322
    overview, 1322, 1323f
    responses, 1322–23
  physiology review, 1322
  risk factors, 1321–22
Astigmatism, 1696
Astroblastoma, 1570t. *See also* Brain tumors
Astrocytes, 1628t
Astrocytoma, 1570t. *See also* Brain tumors
Asynchronous pacing, 1010t. *See also* Pacemakers
Asystole, 1015
Atacand. *See* Candesartan
Atarax. *See* Hydroxyzine
Ataxia, 1522t
Ataxic respirations, 1530, 1530t
ATC (around-the-clock) dosing, 181
Atelectasis:
  in acute respiratory distress syndrome, 1367
  causes, 1343
  definition, 1223t, 1343
  manifestations, 1343–44

nursing care, 1344
postoperative
  assessment findings, 76
  nursing care, 76
respiratory rate in, 1223t
treatment, 1344
Atenolol:
  Medication Administration, 973t, 1161t, 1545t
  in specific conditions
    acute myocardial infarction, 988
    angina, 973t
    headache, 1545t
    hypertension, 1161t
ATG (antithymocyte globulin), 344, 346t
Atherectomy, 977
Atherogenic, 959
Atheromas, 958, 959
Atherosclerosis:
  coronary artery. *See* Coronary heart disease
  definition, 1176
  genetic considerations, 1089t
  pathophysiology, 959, 960t
  peripheral. *See* Peripheral vascular disease
Athlete's foot, 448, 448f, 449
Ativan. *See* Lorazepam
Atopic dermatitis, 456–57, 457f. *See also* Dermatitis
Atorvastatin, 967t
ATRA (all-*trans* retinoic acid), 1123t
Atracurium besylate, 1356t
Atria, 938
Atrial fibrillation:
  causes, 1001
  ECG characteristics, 998t, 1001
  management, 998t
  manifestations, 1001
  stroke risk and, 1579
  in valvular heart disease, 1060
Atrial flutter:
  causes, 1001
  ECG characteristics, 998t, 1001
  management, 998t
  pathophysiology, 1001
  types, 1001
Atrial kick, 996
Atrial natriuretic peptide (ANP):
  in blood pressure regulation, 1155
  in body fluid regulation, 202
  in heart failure, 1025, 1027
  in sodium balance regulation, 214
Atrioventricular (AV) conduction blocks. *See also* Cardiac dysrhythmias
  causes, 1003
  ECG characteristics, 999t
  management, 999t
  manifestations, 1003
  pathophysiology, 996
Atrioventricular (AV) dissociation, 1003
Atrioventricular (AV) node, 941, 941f
Atrioventricular (AV) sequential pacing, 1009. *See also* Pacemakers
Atrioventricular (AV) valves, 938
Atromid-S. *See* Clofibrate
Atropa belladonna, 1326
Atrophic rhinitis, 1229
Atrophic vaginitis, 1843t
Atrophy, skin, 433t
Atropine sulfate:
  adverse/side effects, 869
  Medication Administration, 1327–28t
  preoperative use and nursing implications, 62t
  in specific conditions
    asthma, 1327–28t
    diarrhea, 756t
Atrovent. *See* Ipratropium bromide

Atypical pneumonia, 1269, 1270t. *See also* Pneumonia
Audiometry, 1684t, 1730
Auditory brainstem response, 1684t
Auditory evoked potential, 1684t
Augmentin. *See* Amoxicillin-clavulanate
Auranofin, 1465t
Auricles:
  anatomy, 1680, 1682f
  physical assessment, 1688
Aurothioglucose, 1465t
Auscultatory gap, 1092t
Autograft:
  in burns, 503, 503f
  definition, 342
  types, 342
Autoimmune disorders. *See also specific disorders*
  examples, 330t
  interdisciplinary care
    diagnosis, 340–41
    medications, 341
  nursing care
    community-based care, 341
    diagnoses, 341
  pathophysiology, 340
Autoimmune gastritis, 678
Autoinoculation, 1839
Autologous bone marrow transplant, 1124. *See also* Bone marrow transplant
Autologous peripheral blood stem cell transplant (PBSCT), 398, 1132, 1333t. *See also* Stem cell transplant
Automatic external defibrillator (AED):
  for cardiac arrest, 1016, 1016f
  for cardiac dysrhythmias, 1008, 1008t
Automaticity, 995
Automatisms, 1549
Autonomic dysreflexia, 1599
Autonomic nervous system:
  parasympathetic division. *See* Parasympathetic nervous system
  physiology, 1511
  sympathetic division. *See* Sympathetic nervous system
Autonomic neuropathies, 589
Autoregulation, 1580
Autosomal dominant inheritance, 153, 153f, 153t
Autosomal recessive inheritance, 153–54, 153f, 154t
Autosomes, 149
AV. *See* Atrioventricular
Avage. *See* Tazarotene gel
Avandia. *See* Rosiglitazone
Avapro. *See* Irbesartan
Avastin, 1825
Aveeno. *See* Oatmeal
Avian influenza, 1232t. *See also* Influenza
Avodart. *See* Dutasteride
Avonex. *See* Beta interferon
Avulsed fracture, 1401, 1402f
Axial loading, 1596f, 1597
Axid. *See* Nizatidine
Axilla:
  lymph node dissection, 1825
  physical assessment, 1749t, 1762f, 1762t
Axon, 1504, 1504f
Azacitidine, 1116
Azathioprine:
  adverse effects, 344
  Medication Administration, 345, 1474t, 1631t
  site of action, 344f
  in specific conditions
    inflammatory bowel disease, 786
    multiple sclerosis, 1627, 1631t

in organ transplantation, 344, 921
systemic lupus erythematosus, 1474t
Azelaic acid, 458
Azithromycin:
  Medication Administration, 320t
  in specific conditions
    chlamydia, 1845, 1846
    otitis media, 1722
    pneumonia, 1271t
Azmacort. *See* Triamcinolone acetonide
Azopt. *See* Brinzolamide
Azotemia, 886
AZT. *See* Zidovudine
Azulfidine. *See* Sulfasalazine

B

B cells. *See* B lymphocytes
B lymphocytes (B cells):
  in antibody-mediated immune response, 295, 295f
  development, 290, 290f
  functions, 288t
  location, 288t
Babinski reflex, 1524f, 1524t
Bacillary dysentery, 774t, 775
Bacillus anthracis, 128t, 1293
Bacillus Calmette-Guérin (BCG), 396, 863, 1287
Bacitracin, 441t, 1694, 1697
Back pain. *See* Low back pain
Backward effects, heart failure, 1026
Baclofen, 1600t, 1631t, 1656
Bacteria. *See also specific bacteria*
  characteristics, 311t
  in gastroenteritis, 774–75, 774t. *See also* Gastroenteritis
  in pneumonia, 1267t. *See also* Pneumonia
  in skin infections. *See* Skin infections/infestations, bacterial
  in urinary tract infections, 846. *See also* Urinary tract infection
Bacterial meningitis. *See also* Central nervous system infections
  complications, 1564
  manifestations, 1564, 1564t
  Nursing Care Plan
    assessment, 1567t
    critical thinking in the nursing process, 1567t
    diagnoses, 1567t
    evaluation, 1567t
    expected outcomes, 1567t
    planning and implementation, 1567t
  pathophysiology, 1564
Bacterial translocation, 496
Bacterial vaginosis, 1842, 1843t
Bactericidal agent, 318. *See also* Antibiotics
Bacteriostatic agent, 318. *See also* Antibiotics
Bactrim. *See* Trimethoprim-sulfamethoxazole
Bagging, 111
BAL (blood alcohol level), 108, 112
Balanced suspension traction, 1408, 1409f
Balanitis, 449t, 1749
Balanoposthitis, 1749
Balloon dilation, lower esophageal sphincter, 668, 668f,
Balloon tamponade, for esophageal varices, 718–19, 719f
Ballottement, 1395f, 1395t
Balnetar. *See* Coal tar derivatives
Balsalazide, 786
Banding, for esophageal varices, 718t
Bands, 288
Barbiturates:
  abuse, 108
  overdose signs and treatment, 113t

street names, 111t
withdrawal signs and treatment, 113t
Bariatric surgery:
  benefits, 637
  complications, 638
  diet following, 638t
  indications, 636
  procedures, 637–38, 637f
Barium enema, 744t, 758
Barium sulfate, 615t
Barium swallow. *See* Upper gastrointestinal (GI) series
Barotrauma, 1360
Bartholin's glands:
  cysts, 1808, 1809t
  location and function, 1751t, 1752, 1752f
  physical assessment, 1763f, 1763t
Basal cell cancer, skin, 462–63, 462t, 463f. *See also* Skin cancer
Basal metabolic rate (BMR), 631
Base excess (BE), 239, 240t
Base rate, 1010t
Bases, 238
Basic life support (BLS), 1016, 1016f, 1017t
Basilar fracture, skull, 1555, 1555t. *See also* Skull fracture
Basiliximab, 344, 345–46t
Basopenia, 307t
Basophilia, 307t
Basophils:
  abnormal, possible causes, 307t, 387t
  characteristics, 288
  development, 289f, 1077f
  functions, 288, 288t
  location, 288t
  normal values, 307t, 387t, 1118t
Baths, therapeutic, 441t
Battle's sign, 1555
B-cell lymphomas, 1130t. *See also* Non-Hodgkin's lymphoma
BCG (bacillus Calmette-Guérin), 396, 863, 1287
BCGLive. *See* Bacillus Calmette-Guérin
B-complex vitamins. *See* Vitamin B complex
B-DAST (Brief Drug Abuse Screening Test), 117
BE (base excess), 239, 240t
Beau's line, 436t
Becker's muscular dystrophy, 1459t
Beclomethasone dipropionate, 1328t
Beclovent. *See* Beclomethasone dipropionate
Bedoz. *See* Vitamin B₁₂, replacement therapy
Behavior modification:
  for eating disorders, 652
  for obesity, 636, 637t
Belladonna alkaloids, 756t
Bell's palsy:
  characteristics, 1657
  incidence, 1657
  interdisciplinary care, 1658
  manifestations, 1657–58, 1658f, 1658t
  nursing care, 1658
  pathophysiology, 1657
Benadryl. *See* Diphenhydramine
Benazepril, 1161t
Bence Jones proteins, 1136
Bendroflumethiazide, 210t
Benemid. *See* Probenecid
Bengay. *See* Counterirritants
Benicar. *See* Olmesartan
Benign prostatic hyperplasia (BPH):
  complications, 1778
  definition, 1777
  interdisciplinary care
    complementary and alternative therapies, 1781
    diagnosis, 1778

Benign prostatic hyperplasia (BPH)—continued
  medications, 1778–79
  minimally invasive procedures, 1781
  surgery
    laser, 1781
    minimally invasive, 1779
    open, 1779, 1779f
    transurethral, 1779, 1779f
  manifestations, 1778, 1778f, 1778t
  nursing care
    of client having prostatectomy
      perineal, 1781t
      postoperative, 1780t
      preoperative, 1780t
      retropubic, 1781t
      suprapubic, 1781t
      transurethral resection, 1780t
    community-based care, 1782
    discharge instructions after prostate
      surgery, 1783t
    nursing diagnoses and interventions
      deficient knowledge, 1781–82
      risk for imbalanced fluid volume,
        1782, 1782t
      risk for infection, 1782
      urinary retention, 1782
  pathophysiology, 1777–78
  risk factors, 1777
  urinary retention in, 869
Bentyl. See Dicyclomine
Benzocaine spray, 657
Benzodiazepines:
  abuse, 108
  overdose signs and treatment, 113t
  preoperative use and nursing implications, 62t
  street names, 111t
  for substance abuse/withdrawal treatment, 114t
  withdrawal signs and treatment, 113t
Benzophenones, 465t
Benzopyrene, as cancer risk factor, 372t
Benzoyl peroxide, 458
Benztropine, 1638t
Bepridil, 973–74t
Berberine, 701
Bereavement, 92
Bernstein (acid perfusion) test, 615t
Berry aneurysm, 1170, 1171f, 1592
Best disease, 1674t
Beta cells, pancreas:
  functions, 521, 564
  genetic defects, 566
  in type 1 diabetes mellitus, 565
Beta interferon, 299t, 1631t. See also Interferon(s)
β_2-agonists. See Adrenergic stimulants
Beta-amyloid, 1618
Beta-blockers:
  Medication Administration, 973t, 1006t,
    1161–62t
  in specific conditions
    acute myocardial infarction, 988
    angina, 971–72, 973t
    aortic aneurysm, 1173
    cardiac dysrhythmias, 1006, 1006t
    cardiomyopathy, 1067
    headache, 1545t
    heart failure, 1032
    hypertension, 1161–62t, 1163
  topical
    in glaucoma, 1709, 1710t
    Medication Administration, 1710t
Betagan. See Levobunolol
Beta-lactamase inhibitors, 320t
Betapace. See Sotalol

Betaseron. See Beta interferon
Beta-thalassemia major, 1109. See also
  Thalassemias
Beta-thalassemia minor, 1109. See also
  Thalassemias
Betaxolol, 1161t, 1710t
Bethanechol chloride, 869, 870, 871t
Bethesda system, 1813t
Betoptic. See Betaxolol
Bicarbonate (HCO_3^-):
  in body fluid compartments, 197f
  serum levels
    in gastroenteritis and diarrhea, 776t
    in metabolic acidosis, 242, 242t
    in metabolic alkalosis, 242t, 245
    normal values, 198t, 239, 240t
Bicarbonate-carbonic acid buffer system,
  238–39, 238f
Biceps reflex, 1523f
Bicitra. See Sodium citrate
Bicuspid valve, 937f, 938. See also Mitral valve
BiDil. See Hydralazine/isosorbide
Bifurcate, 959
Bigeminal pulse, 1094t
Biguanides, 578t
Bile, 612
Bile acid sequestrants, 967t, 968
Bilevel ventilation (BiPAP), 1358
Biliary colic, 698. See also Gallstones
Biliopancreatic diversion, 637
Bilirubin:
  direct (conjugated), 699t
  indirect (unconjugated), 699t
  serum (total). See Serum bilirubin
Billroth I (gastroduodenostomy), 689, 689f
Billroth II (gastrojejunostomy), 689, 689f
Bimatoprost, 1710t
Binge-eating disorder:
  complications, 651t
  interdisciplinary care
    diagnosis, 651–52
    treatment, 652
  manifestations, 651, 651t
  nursing care, 652
Biobrane, 503
Bioelectrical impedance, 632, 642, 644
Biofeedback:
  for nausea and vomiting, 672
  for pain management, 185
Biologic dressing, 503
Biological response modifiers (biologicals), 341
Biopsy:
  breast, 1755, 1757t, 1824, 1824f
  cervical, 1758t
  endometrial, 1757t
  endomyocardial, 1049
  kidney. See Renal biopsy
  liver, 617t, 716
  lung. See Lung biopsy
  lymph nodes. See Lymph nodes, biopsy
  myocardial, 1067
  prostate, 1746t
  skin, 428t
  types, 388t
  urease test, 684
Biosynthetic dressing, 503–4
Bioterrorism:
  agents, 128t, 314
  definition, 127
  surveillance, 127
Biotherapy, 396. See also Immunotherapy
Biotin, 609t
BiPAP (bilevel ventilation), 1358
Biperidin, 1638t

Bisacodyl, 759–60t
Bisco-Lax. See Bisacodyl
Bismuth subsalicylate, 685, 756t
Bisoprolol, 1161t
Bisphosphonates:
  Medication Administration, 1442t
  in specific conditions
    bony metastases, 181
    hypercalcemia, 232
    multiple myeloma, 1137
    osteoporosis, 1436
    Paget's disease, 1442, 1442t
Bitolterol, 1327t
Black cohosh, 1796, 1800
Black lung disease, 1345
Blacks/African Americans:
  asthma mortality rate, 1322
  breast cancer
    incidence and mortality, 1822t
    Nursing Research: improving diagnosis and
      treatment, 1829t
  cancer incidence and mortality rates, 369, 370t
  diabetes mellitus risk and incidence, 564t
  end-of-life practices, 89
  heart failure
    incidence, 1023t
    treatment, 1032
  hypertension prevalence, 963, 1157t
  inflammatory bowel disease incidence, 782t
  integumentary system, 427t
  lactate deficiency incidence, 798t
  obesity prevalence, 631t
  osteoarthritis, 1449t
  osteoporosis incidence, 1434, 1434t
  sickle cell anemia, 1106–7, 1106t, 1107t
  stroke risk factors, 1580t
  substance use, 105, 105t
  tuberculosis incidence, 1281t
Bladder:
  anatomy, physiology, and functions, 834–35,
    834f, 869
  cancer. See Bladder cancer
  physical assessment, 843t
Bladder cancer:
  incidence, 862
  interdisciplinary care
    diagnosis, 863
    medications, 863
    radiation therapy, 863
    surgery, 863, 863f, 863t, 864t
  manifestations, 863
  nursing care
    assessment, 865
    community-based care, 868
    health promotion, 865
    nursing diagnoses and interventions
      disturbed body image, 868
      impaired urinary elimination, 865–66
      risk for impaired skin integrity, 866–67
      risk for infection, 868
      stoma care, 868t
  Nursing Care Plan
    assessment, 867t
    critical thinking in the nursing process, 867t
    diagnoses, 867t
    evaluation, 867t
    expected outcomes, 867t
    planning and implementation, 867t
  pathophysiology, 861–62, 861f
  risk factors, 862
  staging, 863t
Bladder neck suspension:
  nursing care, 876t
  procedure, 875

Bladder retraining, 871
Blast injuries, 129t, 131
Blastomyces dermatitidis, 1294
Blastomycosis, 1294
Bleeding precautions, 722t
Bleeding time, 386t
Blenoxane. *See* Bleomycin
Bleomycin:
  adverse/side effects, 393t
  nursing implications, 393t
  in specific conditions
    bone tumors, 1483t
    laryngeal cancer, 1254
    testicular cancer, 1775
  target malignancies, 393t
Blepharitis, 1700
Blepharoplasty, 479
Blindness. *See* Vision, impairments
Blocadren. *See* Timolol
Blood. *See* Hematologic system
Blood alcohol level (BAL), 108, 112
Blood cultures, 316, 1046
Blood flow, 1082
Blood gases. *See* Arterial blood gases
Blood glucose:
  in altered level of consciousness, 1533
  diagnostic tests
    fasting blood sugar, 386t, 526t, 569
    fasting plasma glucose, 569
    glycosylated hemoglobin, 526t
    oral glucose tolerance test, 526t, 569
    perioperative, 60t
  homeostasis, 564, 565f
  self-monitoring, 570–71, 570f
Blood pool imaging, 1123
Blood pressure:
  age-related changes, 1091t
  assessment
    abnormal findings, 1092–93t. *See also*
      Hypertension; Hypotension
    guidelines, 1092t
    technique/normal findings, 1092–93t
  classification, 1156t
  definition, 1085, 1154
  factors affecting, 1092t, 1154–55, 1155f
  regulation, 1085, 1154
  segmental measurements, 1177
Blood transfusion:
  hypocalcemia and, 228
  Medication Administration, 264t
  nursing diagnoses and interventions, 339
  in specific conditions
    anemia from blood loss, 1111
    shock, 279
    trauma, 262
Blood types, 262, 263t, 336
Blood urea nitrogen (BUN):
  abnormal, possible causes, 386t
  normal values, 386t, 890t
  purpose and description, 835t
  related nursing care, 835t
  in specific conditions
    acute renal failure, 904
    chronic renal failure, 918
    glomerular disorders, 889–90, 890t
    neurogenic bladder, 870
    shock, 277
Blood–brain barrier, 1507
Blowout fracture, orbital, 1702
BLS (basic life support), 1016, 1016f, 1017t
Blueberry juice, for urinary tract infection, 851
Blunt trauma. *See also* Trauma
  definition, 256
  in disasters, 129t

effects, 256
  eyes, 1702
BMD (bone mineral density), 1387t
BMI (body mass index), 61t, 360, 632, 632t, 633t
BMR (basal metabolic rate), 631
BMT. *See* Bone marrow transplant
BNP. *See* Brain natriuretic peptide
Body fluids. *See also* Fluids and electrolytes
  composition, 195–96, 197f
  distribution, 196–97, 196f, 197f
  imbalances
    deficit. *See* Fluid volume deficit
    excess. *See* Fluid volume excess
  movement
    active transport, 200, 201f
    diffusion, 199–200, 200f
    filtration, 200, 200f
    osmosis
      definition, 198, 198f
      osmolarity and osmolality, 198
      osmotic pressure and tonicity, 198–99, 199f
  regulation
    antidiuretic hormone, 201–2, 202f
    atrial natriuretic peptide, 202
    kidneys, 201
    renin–angiotensin–aldosterone system,
      201, 202f
    thirst, 200–201, 201f
Body lice, 451
Body mass index (BMI), 61t, 630, 632, 632t, 633t
Body posture, 1391t
Body temperature, variations in surgery, 58t, 59
Body weight. *See also* Malnutrition; Obesity
  assessment, 620–21t
  gain, in fluid volume excess, 209, 211–12
  loss
    in fluid volume deficit, 205
    in malnutrition, 641
    in obesity
      calorie reduction requirements, 634
      maintaining, 638
      nutrient intake for, 635, 635t, 636t
    for monitoring fluid balance, 208t
Boggy, 1229
Boil. *See* Furuncle
Bolus, 610
Bone(s). *See also* Musculoskeletal system
  classification, 1380, 1382f
  healing
    factors affecting, 1403t
    phases, 1402, 1404–5t
  metabolic disorders
    gout. *See* Gout
    osteomalacia. *See* Osteomalacia
    osteoporosis. *See* Osteoporosis
    Paget's disease. *See* Paget's disease
  remodeling in adults, 1380–81
  of skeleton, 1381f
  structure, 1380, 1382f
  traumatic injury. *See* Fractures
  tumors. *See* Bone tumors
Bone density scans, 232, 1387t
Bone marrow:
  functions, 291
  procedure, 1124f
  tests
    in leukemia, 1123t
    in multiple myeloma, 1137
    in myelodysplastic syndrome, 1115
    nursing care, 1087t
    purpose and description, 1087t
    in thrombocytopenia, 1141
  transplant. *See* Bone marrow transplant
Bone marrow rescue, 1124

Bone marrow transplant (BMT):
  allogeneic, 1124
  autologous, 1124
  complications, 1124
  indications, 342t, 398
  for leukemia, 1124
  success rate, 342t
Bone mineral density (BMD), 1387t
Bone scan, 1387t
Bone tumors:
  classification, 1481–82
  incidence, 1482t
  interdisciplinary care
    diagnosis, 1482–83
    treatments
      chemotherapy, 1483, 1483t
      radiation therapy, 1483
      surgery, 1483
  manifestations, 1482, 1483t
  nursing care
    community-based care, 1484
    nursing diagnoses and interventions
      acute pain, chronic pain, 1484
      decisional conflict, 1484
      impaired physical mobility, 1484
      risk for injury, 1483–84
  pathophysiology, 1482
  sites, 1482t
  types, 1482t
Boniva. *See* Ibandronate sodium
Bony metastases, 181
Borborygmus (borborygmi), 624t, 748t, 751
Bordetella pertussis. See Pertussis
Borrelia burgdorferi, 1476–77
Bosentan, 1353
Botulinum toxin, 668, 1639
Botulism:
  characteristics, 1661–62
  interdisciplinary care, 1662
  manifestations, 1662
  nursing care, 1662
  pathophysiology, 1662
Bouchard's nodes, 1393, 1450
Boutonnière deformity, 1393, 1461, 1461f
Bowel disorders:
  acute infectious/inflammatory disorders
    appendicitis. *See* Appendicitis
    gastroenteritis. *See* Gastroenteritis
    helminthic disorders. *See* Helminthic disorders
    peritonitis. *See* Peritonitis
    protozoal infections. *See* Protozoal bowel
      infections
  anorectal
    anal fissure, 820
    anorectal abscess, 820
    anorectal fistula, 820–21
    hemorrhoids. *See* Hemorrhoids
    nursing care, 821
    pilonidal disease, 821
  assessment
    diagnostic tests, 743, 744–45t
    functional health pattern interview, 747t
    genetic considerations, 745, 746t
    health assessment interview, 745–46
    physical assessment
      abdomen, 747–48t
      anus and rectum, 750f, 750t
      inguinal area, 748
      overview, 746–47
      perianal area, 750t
      stool, 750–51t
    postoperative, 78–79
    sample documentation, 743
  Chapter Highlights, 821–22t

Bowel disorders—*continued*
Clinical Scenarios, 825*t*
inflammatory bowel disease. *See* Inflammatory bowel disease
intestinal motility disorders
constipation. *See* Constipation
diarrhea. *See* Diarrhea
fecal incontinence. *See* Fecal incontinence
neoplastic
colorectal cancer. *See* Colorectal cancer
polyps. *See* Polyps
postoperative assessment and nursing care, 78–79
structural and obstructive
diverticular disease. *See* Diverticular disease
hernia. *See* Hernia
intestinal obstruction. *See* Intestinal obstruction
Bowel sounds, 624*t*, 748*t*
Bowlby, theory of loss and grief, 85–86, 86*t*
BPH. *See* Benign prostatic hyperplasia
Brachial pulse, 1096*t*
Brachioradialis reflex, 1523*f*
Brachytherapy, 395, 396*t*, 1786. *See also* Radiation therapy
Bradycardia, 953*t*
Bradykinesia, 1635
Bradykinin, 170, 304*t*
Bradyphrenia, 1636
Bradypnea, 1223*t*
Brain. *See also* Neurologic system
anatomy, physiology, and functions
brainstem, 1506, 1506*t*
cerebellum, 1505*f*, 1506*t*
cerebrum, 1505–6, 1505*f*, 1506*f*, 1506*t*
diencephalon, 1506, 1506*t*
ventricles, 1506
cerebral function disorders
altered level of consciousness. *See* Altered level of consciousness
epilepsy. *See* Epilepsy
headache. *See* Headache
increased intracranial pressure. *See* Increased intracranial pressure
manifestations, 1528*t*
traumatic brain injury. *See* Traumatic brain injury
tumors. *See* Brain tumors
Brain abscess, 1565–66. *See also* Central nervous system infections
Brain attack. *See* Stroke
Brain death, 265*t*, 1532
Brain herniation, 1537–38, 1538*f*. *See also* Increased intracranial pressure
Brain natriuretic peptide (BNP):
in blood pressure regulation, 1155
in heart failure, 1025, 1027
Brain tumors:
classification, 1569, 1570*t*
incidence and prevalence, 1569
interdisciplinary care
diagnosis, 1571
medications, 1571, 1571*f*
radiation therapy, 1572
specialty procedures, 1572
surgery, 1571, 1571*f*
manifestations, 1569–70, 1569*t*
metastatic, 1569
nursing care
community-based care, 1575
nursing diagnoses and interventions
acute pain, 1574
anxiety, 1572
ineffective protection, 1574

risk for infection, 1572–74
situational low self-esteem, 1574–75
using NANDA, NIC, and NOC, 1575, 1575*t*
Nursing Care Plan
assessment, 1573*t*
critical thinking in the nursing process, 1573*t*
diagnoses, 1573*t*
evaluation, 1573*t*
expected outcomes, 1573*t*
planning and implementation, 1573*t*
pathophysiology, 1569
Brainstem, 1506, 1506*t*
Bran, 759*t*, 760
Brawny edema, 1200
BRCA1/BRCA2 genes, 1755*t*, 1817, 1823
Brc/abl gene:
in acute lymphocytic leukemia, 1122
in chronic myeloid leukemia, 1121
Breakthrough pain, 174. *See also* Pain
Breast:
biopsy, 1755, 1757*t*, 1824, 1824*f*
female
age-related changes, 1760*t*
anatomy, physiology, and functions, 1751, 1752*f*
benign disorders
fibrocystic changes, 1820–21, 1821*t*
interdisciplinary care, 1821*t*, 1822
intraductal, 1821–22, 1821*t*
manifestations, 1820–22, 1821*t*
nursing care, 1822
pathophysiology, 1820–22
cancer. *See* Breast cancer
diagnostic tests, 1755, 1756–57*t*
physical assessment, 1761–62*t*, 1761*f*
self-examination, 1829*t*
male
anatomy, 1744
disorders
cancer, 1790. *See also* Breast cancer
gynecomastia. *See* Gynecomastia
physical assessment, 1749*t*
Breast cancer:
Case Study, 1856*t*
genetic considerations, 1755*t*, 1758, 1823
incidence, 1822
interdisciplinary care
diagnosis, 1824–25, 1824*f*
medications, 1825, 1825*t*
radiation therapy, 1826–27
surgery
breast reconstruction, 1825–26, 1827*f*
lumpectomy, 1825
mastectomy, 1825, 1826*f*
manifestations, 1823–24, 1823*t*
nursing care
assessment, 1829
of client having a mastectomy, 1826*t*
of client having breast reconstruction, 1827*t*
community-based care, 1831, 1831*f*
health promotion, 1828, 1829*t*
nursing diagnoses and interventions
anticipatory grieving, 1830
anxiety, 1829–30
decisional conflict, 1830
disturbed body image, 1831
risk for infection, 1830
risk for injury, 1830–31
using NANDA, NIC, and NOC, 1831*t*
Nursing Care Plan
assessment, 1828*t*
critical thinking in the nursing process, 1828*t*
diagnoses, 1828*t*
evaluation, 1828*t*

expected outcomes, 1828*t*
planning and implementation, 1828*t*
pathophysiology, 1823
racial/ethnic considerations, 1822*t*
risk factors, 1822–23
screening guidelines, 401*t*
staging, 1824*t*
Breast reconstruction:
nursing care, 1827*t*
procedure, 1825–26, 1827*f*
Breast self-examination (BSE), 1829*t*
Breath odors, 623*t*
Breath sounds:
abnormal, 1226*t*
assessment, 1225–26*t*, 1225*f*
normal, 1225*t*
types, 1225*t*
Breathing. *See* Respiration
Brethaire. *See* Terbutaline
Brethine. *See* Terbutaline
Bretylium, 1006*t*
Bretylol. *See* Bretylium
Brevibloc. *See* Esmolol
Brevicon. *See* Norethindrone/ethinyl estradiol
Brief Drug Abuse Screening Test (B-DAST), 117
Brimonidine, 1709, 1710*t*
Brinzolamide, 1710*t*
Broca's aphasia, 1583
Broca's area, 1506*t*
Bromocriptine, 1638*t*, 1639
Brompheniramine, 1230*t*
Bronchi, 1212*f*, 1213
Bronchial provocation testing, 1324
Bronchiectasis, 1344
Bronchitis:
acute. *See* Acute bronchitis
chronic, 1331–32, 1332*t*. *See also* Chronic obstructive pulmonary disease
definition, 1266
Bronchodilators:
Medication Administration, 1327–28*t*
in specific conditions
asthma, 1325–26, 1327–28*t*
chronic obstructive pulmonary disease, 1334
cystic fibrosis, 1342
pneumonia, 1271–72
Bronchogenic carcinoma, 1308. *See also* Lung cancer
Bronchophony, 1226*t*
Bronchoplastic reconstruction, 1312*t*
Bronchopneumonia, 1268, 1268*t*, 1270*t*
Bronchoscopy:
laser, 1312*t*
nursing care, 1218–19*t*
purpose and description, 1218*t*, 1219
in specific conditions
lung cancer, 1312
pneumonia, 1271
Bronkometer. *See* Isoetharine
Bronkosol. *See* Isoetharine
Bronkotabs. *See* Theophylline
Brown-Séquard syndrome, 1597*t*, 1613. *See also* Spinal cord injury; Spinal cord tumors
Brudzinski's sign, 1524*t*, 1525*f*
Bruises. *See* Ecchymosis
Bruits:
abdominal, 624*t*, 749*t*, 1098*t*
carotid, 1094*t*
definition, 624*t*, 749*t*, 1094*t*
BSE (breast self-examination), 1829*t*
Buerger's disease. *See* Thromboangiitis obliterans
Bufferin. *See* Aspirin
Buffers, 238

Build Clinical Competence:
  activity-exercise pattern
    responses to altered cardiac function, 1071*t*
    responses to altered musculoskeletal function, 1497*t*
    responses to altered respiratory patterns, 1375*t*
    responses to altered tissue perfusion, 1205*t*
  cognitive-perceptual pattern
    responses to altered neurologic function, 1665*t*
    responses to altered visual and auditory function, 1737*t*
  elimination pattern
    responses to altered bowel elimination, 824*t*
    responses to altered urinary elimination, 929*t*
  health perception-health management pattern
    alterations in patterns of health, 143*t*
    dimensions of medical-surgical nursing, 49*t*
    pathophysiology and patterns of health, 416*t*
  nutritional-metabolic pattern
    responses to altered endocrine function, 600*t*
    responses to altered integumentary structure and function, 513*t*
    responses to altered nutrition, 735*t*
  sexuality-reproductive pattern
    responses to altered reproductive function, 1854*t*
Bulbourethral glands, 1745*t*
Bulge sign, 1395*f*, 1395*t*
Bulimia nervosa:
  complications, 651*t*
  interdisciplinary care
    diagnosis, 651–52
    treatment, 652
  manifestations, 650–51, 651*t*
  nursing care, 652
Bulk-forming agents, 759*t*
Bullous lesions, 431*t*
Bumetanide, 210*t*, 905*t*, 1033*t*
Bumex. *See* Bumetanide
Buminate 5%. *See* Albumin 5%
Buminate 25%. *See* Albumin 25%
BUN. *See* Blood urea nitrogen
Bunion, 1492, 1492*f*
Buprenex. *See* Buprenorphine HCl
Buprenorphine HCl, 182*t*
Burkitt lymphoma, 354, 1130*t*. *See also* Lymphomas
Burn shock, 495
Burns:
  Case Study, 515*t*
  causative agents, 488*t*
  Chapter Highlights, 511*t*
  classification
    depth
      characteristics, 489*t*
      full-thickness, 490, 490*f*
      partial-thickness, 490, 490*f*
      superficial, 489–90
    extent, 490–91, 491*f*, 491*t*, 492*f*
  definition, 487
  eyes, 1702
  incidence, 487
  interdisciplinary care
    diagnosis, 500
    emergency and acute
      fluid resuscitation, 499
      respiratory management, 257, 499
    medications
      antimicrobial, 500, 501*t*
      gastric hyperacidity prevention, 502
      pain control, 500
      tetanus prophylaxis, 502
    prehospital management
      stop burning process, 498
      support vital function, 498

stages
  acute, 498
  emergent/resuscitative, 497–98
  overview, 497*f*
  rehabilitative, 498
treatments
  biological and biosynthetic dressings, 503–4
  nutritional support, 505
  positioning, splints, and exercise, 504–5
  support garments, 505, 505*f*
  surgery, 502–3, 502*f*, 502*t*
  wound dressing, 504, 505*f*
  wound management, 504
minor, 493
in nuclear detonation, 130*t*, 131
nursing care
  assessment, 505–6
  community-based care, 510–11
  health promotion, 505
  interventions by stage, 506*t*
  Medication Administration, 501*t*
  nursing diagnoses and interventions
    acute pain, 508–9
    deficient fluid volume, 508
    imbalanced nutrition: less than body requirements, 509–10
    impaired physical mobility, 509
    impaired skin integrity, 506–8
    powerlessness, 510
    risk for infection, 509
  of older adults, 508*t*
  using NANDA, NIC, and NOC, 510, 511*t*
Nursing Care Plan
  assessment, 507*t*
  critical thinking in the nursing process, 507*t*
  diagnosis, 507*t*
  evaluation, 507*t*
  expected outcomes, 507*t*
  planning and implementation, 507*t*
Nursing Research: prevention of pressure ulcers in client with major burn, 510*t*
pathophysiology, 494
priority treatment, 488*t*
risk factors, 487
systemic effects
  cardiovascular
    cardiac rhythm alterations, 495
    hypovolemic shock, 495
    peripheral vascular compromise, 495
  gastrointestinal, 496
  immune, 496
  integumentary system, 494, 495*f*
  metabolic, 496–97
  overview, 494*f*
  respiratory, 495–96
  urinary, 496
types of injury
  chemical, 488–99, 499*t*
  electrical, 488
  radiation, 488
  thermal, 487, 488*t*
wound healing in, 493
Burr hole, 1560*f*, 1571, 1571*f*
Burrow's solution, 1194
Bursitis, 1394*t*, 1428. *See also* Repetitive use injury
Busulfan, 392*t*, 1704
Butazolidin. *See* Phenylbutazone
Butenafine, 450*t*
Butorphanol, 180*t*
Butyl nitrite, 111
Butyrophenones, 672
Byetta. *See* Exenatide

C
C fibers, 171, 171*f*
CA 15-3, 384*t*
CA 19-9, 384*t*
CA 125, 384*t*, 1818
Ca²⁺. *See* Calcium
CABG. *See* Coronary artery bypass grafting
Cachectic, 689
Cachexia, 380, 380*f*
Café coronary, 1249
Cafergot. *See* Ergotamine tartrate
Caffeine, 106
CAGE questionnaire, 116
Calan. *See* Verapamil
Calcimar. *See* Calcitonin
Calcipotriene, 444
Calcitonin:
  abnormal, possible causes, 384*t*, 386*t*
  functions, 520
  for hypercalcemia, 232, 547
  laboratory tests, 380*t*
  normal values, 386*t*
  for osteoporosis, 1436
  for Paget's disease, 1442
Calcium (Ca²⁺):
  abnormal, possible causes, 386*t*
  balance, 227, 227*f*
  in body fluid compartments, 197*t*
  in coagulation, 1082*t*
  foods high in, 230*t*, 858*t*
  functions, 227
  imbalances. *See* Hypercalcemia; Hypocalcemia
  limiting intake, in urinary calculi, 858, 858*t*
  in osteoporosis, 1434
  recommended daily intake, 610*t*
  serum levels. *See* Serum calcium
  supplements, 230*t*, 1437*t*
Calcium carbonate, 230*t*
Calcium channel blockers:
  Medication Administration, 973–74*t*, 1006*t*, 1162*t*, 1545–46*t*
  in specific conditions
    angina, 972, 973–74*t*
    aortic aneurysm, 1173
    cardiac dysrhythmias, 1006*t*
    headache, 1545–46*t*
    hypertension, 1162*t*, 1163
    intracranial aneurysm, 1593
    pulmonary hypertension, 1353
    scleroderma, 1485
    thromboangiitis obliterans, 1182
Calcium chloride:
  Medication Administration, 225*t*, 230*t*, 905–6*t*
  in specific conditions
    acute renal failure, 904, 905–6*t*
    hypocalcemia, 229
Calcium citrate, 230*t*
Calcium glubionate, 230*t*
Calcium gluceptate, 230*t*
Calcium gluconate:
  Medication Administration, 225*t*, 230*t*, 905–6*t*
  in specific conditions
    acute renal failure, 905–6*t*
    hyperkalemia, 224, 225*t*
    hypocalcemia, 229
Calcium lactate, 230*t*
Calcium polycarbophil, 759*t*
Calcium salts, 230*t*
Calcium stones, 856, 856*t*. *See also* Urinary calculi
Calculi:
  definition, 697, 838
  gallbladder. *See* Gallstones
  urinary. *See* Urinary calculi

Caldwell-Luc procedure, 1237
Caloric test, 1684t, 1727
Camey procedure, 865t
Camphorated tincture of opium, 756t
Campylobacter jejuni, 1653
Canal of Schlemm, 1672, 1672f
Canasa. *See* Mesalamine
Cancer:
  Chapter Highlights, 413t
  definition, 369
  etiology
    altered immune response, 379, 379t
    carcinogens
      chemicals, 372t, 375
      drugs and hormones, 375
      radiation, 375–76
      viruses, 374–75, 375t
    cellular characteristics, 376–77, 377t
    theories of carcinogenesis
      cellular mutations, 374
      oncogenes, 374
      tumor suppressor genes, 374
    tumor invasion and metastasis
      invasion, 377–78, 377f
      metastasis, 378–79, 378f, 378t
    types of neoplasms, 376, 376t
  incidence and mortality, 369
  interdisciplinary care
    diagnosis
      classification, 382, 383t
      cytologic examination, 382–83
      direct visualization, 385
      grading and staging, 382, 383t
      imaging, 384–85
      laboratory tests, 385, 386–87t
      psychologic support during, 387–88
      surgical procedures, 388t
      tumor markers, 383–84, 384t
    treatment
      biotherapy, 396, 398t
      bone marrow transplant. *See* Bone marrow
        transplant
      chemotherapy. *See* Chemotherapy
      complementary therapies, 398–99
      peripheral blood stem cell transplant. *See*
        Peripheral blood stem cell transplant
      photodynamic therapy, 398
      radiation therapy. *See* Radiation therapy
      surgery, 388–89, 388t
  manifestations, 405
  in middle adults, 27
  nursing care
    assessment
      focused interview, 400–402
      functional status scales, 401t
      physical assessment, 402–3, 402t, 403t
    community-based care
      hospice. *See* Hospice
      teaching, 412
    health education for the client and family
      prevention, 411–12, 412t
      rehabilitation and survival, 412
    health promotion, 400, 400t, 401t
    nursing diagnoses and interventions
      anticipatory grieving, 406
      anxiety, 403, 405
      disturbed body image, 405–6
      imbalanced nutrition: less than body
        requirements, 407–8
      impaired tissue integrity, 408–9, 409t
      risk for infection, 406–7
      risk for injury, 407, 407t
    nursing interventions for oncologic
      emergencies

        hypercalcemia, 410
        hyperuricemia. *See* Hypercalcemia
        obstructive uropathy, 410
        pericardial effusions and neoplastic cardiac
         tamponade, 409
        sepsis and septic shock, 410
        spinal cord compression, 410
        superior vena cava syndrome, 409, 410f
        syndrome of inappropriate diuretic
         hormone, 410
        tumor lysis syndrome, 410–11
    of older adults, 371t
    using NANDA, NIC, and NOC, 411, 411t
  Nursing Care Plan
    assessment, 403–4t
    critical thinking in the nursing process, 404t
    diagnoses, 404t
    evaluation, 404t
    expected outcomes, 404t
    planning and implementation, 404t
  pathophysiology, 372–74. *See also* Cell(s)
  physiologic and psychologic effects
    anorexia-cachexia syndrome, 380
    disruption of function, 379
    hematologic alterations, 379
    hemorrhage, 380
    infection, 379–80
    pain, 381, 399
    paraneoplastic syndromes, 380, 380t
    physical stress, 381, 382t
    psychologic stress, 381, 382t
  risk factors
    age, 370
    alcohol use, 372
    chemical exposure, 372t
    diet, 371
    gender, 370
    heredity, 370
    infection, 371
    interactions, 373f
    obesity, 372
    occupation, 371
    poverty, 370
    recreational drug use, 372
    stress, 370–71
    sun exposure, 372
    tobacco use, 371–72
  types
    bladder. *See* Bladder cancer
    bone. *See* Bone tumors
    breast. *See* Breast cancer
    cervical. *See* Cervical cancer
    endometrial. *See* Endometrial cancer
    esophageal. *See* Esophageal cancer
    gallbladder, 703
    gastric. *See* Gastric cancer
    larynx. *See* Laryngeal cancer
    liver, 723–24, 724t
    oral. *See* Oral cancer
    ovarian. *See* Ovarian cancer
    pancreas. *See* Pancreatic cancer
    penis, 1772
    prostate. *See* Prostate cancer
    skin. *See* Skin cancer
    testicular. *See* Testicular cancer
    thyroid, 546
  warning signs, 400t
Candesartan, 1033t, 1161t
Candida albicans. See Candidiasis
Candidiasis:
  in AIDS, 353, 359t
  definition, 449
  in diabetes mellitus, 592
  interdisciplinary care, 449–50, 450t

    manifestations, 449, 449f, 449t
    nursing care, 450
    oral. *See* Thrush
    risk factors, 449
    vaginal, 449t, 1842–43, 1843f, 1843t
Canker sore, 657t. *See also* Stomatitis
Cannabinoids, 672, 673t
Cannabis sativa, 107. *See also* Marijuana
CAPD (continuous ambulatory peritoneal
    dialysis), 920
Capillaries, 1082, 1085f
Capillary refill, 1095t
Caplan, theory of loss and grief, 86, 86t
Capnogram. *See* Exhaled carbon dioxide
Capoten. *See* Captopril
Capsaicin, 1326, 1451
Captopril, 1033t, 1161t
Captopril test, 895
Capture, pacemaker, 1010t
Caput medusae, 704, 715t
Capzasin. *See* Capsaicin
Carbamazepine:
  interaction with oral contraceptives, 1551t
  Medication Administration, 1550t
  in specific conditions
    seizures, 1550t
    trigeminal neuralgia, 1656
Carbapenems, 319t
Carbenicillin, 319t
Carbex. *See* Selegiline
Carbidopa-levodopa, 1637t, 1639
Carbohydrates:
  intake in diabetes mellitus, 576–77
  recommended daily intake, 606
  recommended dietary guidelines, 606t
  sources, 606
  use by body, 606, 607f
Carbon dioxide (CO_2). *See also* Exhaled carbon
    dioxide
  perioperative levels, significance and nursing
    implications, 60t
  transport from lungs, 1216–17
Carbon monoxide poisoning:
  assessment in light and dark skin, 426t, 1305
  in burns, 496
  interdisciplinary care, 499
  manifestations, 496t, 1305
  pathophysiology, 1305
Carbonic anhydrase inhibitors, 1703, 1710t
Carboplatin, 1254, 1819
Carboxyhemoglobin, 1306
Carbuncle, 447
Carcinoembryonic antigen (CEA), 384t, 386t
Carcinogenesis, 374. *See also* Cancer, etiology
Carcinogens, 372t, 374. *See also* Cancer, etiology
Cardene. *See* Nicardipine
Cardiac arrest, 1002, 1015. *See also* Sudden
    cardiac death; Ventricular fibrillation
Cardiac auscultation, 954–55t, 954f
Cardiac catheterization:
  in angina, 971
  in cardiomyopathy, 1067
  purpose and description, 943, 945t
  related nursing care, 945–46t
  in valvular heart disease, 1060
Cardiac conduction system, 941, 941f, 995
Cardiac cycle, 939–40, 939f
Cardiac dysrhythmias:
  in acute myocardial infarction, 985
  assessment, 953t
  atrioventricular (AV) conduction blocks
    causes, 1003
    ECG characteristics, 999t
    management, 999t

manifestations, 1003
pathophysiology, 996
classification, 996
definition, 219, 953, 985
in dilated cardiomyopathy, 1065
in heart failure, 1034
in hypokalemia, 219, 219f
interdisciplinary care
cardiac mapping and catheter ablation, 1012–13
carotid sinus massage, 1013
countershock
defibrillation, 1008
synchronized cardioversion, 1007, 1007t
diagnosis, 1004–5, 1004t
implantable cardioverter-defibrillator, 1009–10
medications, 1005–6, 1006t
pacemaker therapy. See Pacemakers
Valsalva maneuver, 1013
nursing care
assessment, 1014
community-based care, 1015
health promotion, 1014
Medication Administration, 1006t
nursing diagnoses and interventions, 1014–15
of older adults, 996t
Nursing Care Plan
assessment, 1013t
critical thinking in the nursing process, 1013t
diagnoses, 1013t
evaluation, 1013t
expected outcomes, 1013t
planning and implementation, 1013t
pathophysiology, 996
supraventricular
ECG characteristics, 997–98t
management, 997–98t
manifestations, 1000–1001
pathophysiology, 1000–1001
ventricular
causes, 1002–3
ECG characteristics, 998–99t, 1002–3
management, 998–99t
manifestations, 1002–3
pathophysiology, 996
Cardiac enzymes. See Cardiac markers
Cardiac index (CI), 941, 1031
Cardiac mapping, 1012
Cardiac markers:
in acute coronary syndrome, 975–76
in acute myocardial infarction, 986, 987t
in myocarditis, 1049
in pericarditis, 1051
in rheumatic heart disease, 1043t
in shock, 277
Cardiac monitoring:
in cardiac dysrhythmias, 1004
indications, 1004t
procedure, 1005t
Cardiac output (CO):
clinical indicators, 940
definition, 269, 940
in hypovolemic shock, 273f
normal values, 940
Cardiac rehabilitation, 990
Cardiac reserve, 940, 1023
Cardiac tamponade:
definition, 1050
in end-stage renal disease, 916
manifestations, 409, 1050, 1051t
nursing interventions, 409
pathophysiology, 1050, 1051f
Cardiac transplantation. See Heart transplant

Cardiac-specific troponin I (cTnI), 975–76, 986, 987t
Cardiac-specific troponin T (cTnT), 975–76, 986, 987t
Cardinal fields of vision, 1677, 1677f
Cardiogenic embolic stroke, 1581. See also Stroke
Cardiogenic shock:
in acute myocardial infarction, 985
assessment, 279
causes, 274
definition, 274
manifestations, 274, 274t
pathophysiology, 274
Cardiolite scan, 945t
Cardiomyopathy:
causes, 1063
dilated
management, 1065t
manifestations, 1065, 1065t
pathophysiology, 1063–65, 1065t
prognosis, 1065
hypertrophic
genetic considerations, 950t
management, 1065t
manifestations, 1065t, 1066
pathophysiology, 1065–66, 1065t
prognosis, 1066
interdisciplinary care
diagnosis, 1067
medications, 1067
surgery, 1067
mortality rate, 1063
nursing care, 1067–68
restrictive
manifestations, 1066
pathophysiology, 1066
prognosis, 1066
Cardiopulmonary bypass (CPB), 978, 979f
Cardiopulmonary resuscitation (CPR):
family presence during, 1066t
procedure, 1016, 1017t
Cardioquin. See Quinidine
Cardiovascular disease:
acute coronary syndrome. See Acute coronary syndrome
acute myocardial infarction. See Acute myocardial infarction
angina pectoris. See Angina pectoris
cardiogenic pulmonary edema. See Pulmonary edema, cardiogenic
cardiomyopathy. See Cardiomyopathy
Chapter Highlights, 1019t, 1068t
Clinical Scenarios, 1072t
coronary heart disease. See Coronary heart disease
definition, 958
dysrhythmias. See Cardiac dysrhythmias
endocarditis. See Endocarditis
heart failure. See Heart failure
incidence, 958
pericarditis. See Pericarditis
rheumatic heart disease. See Rheumatic fever/heart disease
risk factors in middle adults, 26–27
sudden cardiac death. See Sudden cardiac death
surgical risk and nursing implications, 57t
Cardiovascular system. See also Heart
age-related changes
in middle adults, 27t
in older adults, 29t
in young adults, 26t
postoperative complications
deep venous thrombosis, 75. See also Deep venous thrombosis
hemorrhage, 74–75

pulmonary embolism, 75. See also Pulmonary embolism
shock, 74. See also Shock
Cardioversion. See Defibrillation; Synchronized cardioversion
Carditis, 1042
Cardizem. See Diltiazem
Cardura. See Doxazosin
Caregiver:
family, burdens of, 45
nurse as, 12–13, 12f, 13t
Carisoprodol, 1491
Carotene, 425
Carotid arteries:
duplex study, 1515t
endarterectomy
nursing care, 1586t
procedure, 1586, 1586f
physical assessment, 1094t
Carotid sinus massage, 1013
Carpal spasm, 531t
Carpal tunnel syndrome, 1427–28. See also Repetitive use injury
Carrier testing, 156
Carriers, 153, 200
Carteolol, 1710t
Carter's Liver Pills. See Bisacodyl
Cartrol. See Carteolol
Carvedilol, 1161t
Cascara sagrada, 759–60t, 832t
Case Studies:
breast cancer, 1856t
burns, 515t
chronic obstructive pulmonary disease, 1377t
chronic renal failure, 931t
client with multiple trauma, 145t
diabetes mellitus, 602t
fracture, 1499t
glaucoma, 1739t
heart failure, 1073t
hypertension, 1207t
lung cancer, 418t
pelvic inflammatory disease, 51t
stroke, 1667t
ulcerative colitis, 826t
Caseation necrosis, 1281
Castor oil, 759–60t
Casts:
bivalving, 1419f
nursing care of client, 1410t
types, 1409–10, 1410f
Casts, urinary, 832t
Casualty management. See Disasters
Catabolism, 307, 613, 641
Catapres. See Clonidine
Cataracts:
incidence, 1704
interdisciplinary care
diagnosis, 1704
surgery, 1705, 1705f
manifestations, 1704, 1704f
nursing care
assessment, 1706
community-based care, 1706
health promotion, 1705
nursing diagnoses and interventions
decisional conflict: cataract removal, 1706
risk for ineffective therapeutic regimen management, 1706
Nursing Care Plan
assessment, 1711t
critical thinking in the nursing process, 1711t
diagnoses, 1711t
evaluation, 1711t

Cataracts—*continued*
expected outcomes, 1711*t*
planning and implementation, 1711*t*
pathophysiology, 1704
risk factors, 1704
Catecholamines. *See* Epinephrine; Norepinephrine
Catechol-*O*-methyltransferase (COMT) inhibitors, 1638*t*, 1639
Cathartic colon, 758
Catheter, urinary:
client self-catheterization procedure, 1605*t*
infections associated with, 848
for neurogenic bladder, 872, 1605*t*
nursing interventions, 852–53, 869–70
Nursing Research: insertion methods in male
client, 854*t*
Cations, 196
Caucasians/European Americans:
breast cancer incidence, 1822*t*
osteoarthritis, 1449*t*
osteoporosis incidence, 1434, 1434*t*
substance use, 105, 105*t*
testicular cancer incidence, 1774*t*
Caverject. *See* Alprostadil
Cavitation, 1280
CBC. *See* Complete blood count
CCPD (continuous cyclic peritoneal dialysis), 920
CCR5 gene, 152
CD antigen, 329
CD4 cells, 329, 352*t*, 355
CEA (carcinoembryonic antigen), 384*t*, 386*t*
Ceclor. *See* Cefaclor
Cecum, 743
Cefaclor, 319*t*, 1722
Cefazolin:
Medication Administration, 319*t*
preoperative use and nursing implications, 62*t*
in specific conditions
endocarditis, 1046
eye trauma, 1703
Cefepime, 319*t*
Cefobid. *See* Cefoperazone
Cefoperazone, 319*t*
Cefotaxime, 1566
Cefoxitin, 816, 1851
Ceftazidime, 319*t*
Ceftin. *See* Cefuroxime
Ceftriaxone:
Medication Administration, 319*t*
in specific conditions
endocarditis, 1046
epiglottitis, 1241
urinary tract infection, 849
Cefuroxime, 319*t*, 1241, 1477
Celebrex. *See* Celecoxib
Celecoxib, 1451
Celiac sprue (celiac disease), 746*t*, 796, 1106. *See also* Sprue
Cell(s):
differentiation, 373–74
division, 149–50
DNA, 149, 372–73, 373*t*. *See also* Genetics
mutations, 374
normal growth, 372–73
nucleus, 149
Cell cycle:
characteristics, 373
chemotherapeutic drugs and, 389, 389*f*
CellCept. *See* Mycophenolate mofetil
Cell-kill hypothesis, 390
Cell-mediated (cellular) immune response, 291
Cellular immune response. *See* Cell-mediated
(cellular) immune response

Cellular immunity. *See* Cell-mediated (cellular)
immune response
Cellulitis, 447, 447*f*
Central herniation, 1538, 1538*f*. *See also* Increased
intracranial pressure
Central nervous system (CNS). *See also*
Neurologic system
anatomy, physiology, and functions
blood–brain barrier, 1507
brain
brainstem, 1506, 1506*t*
cerebellum, 1505*f*, 1506*t*
cerebrum, 1505–6, 1505*f*, 1506*f*, 1506*t*
diencephalon, 1506, 1506*t*
ventricles, 1506
cerebral circulation, 1507, 1508*f*
cerebrospinal fluid
formation, 1506–7
functions, 1507
normal values, 1507*t*
limbic system, 1507
meninges, 1507, 1507*f*
neurons, 1628*t*
reticular formation, 1507
spinal cord, 1508–9, 1508*f*, 1509*f*
Central nervous system depressants:
abuse, 108
overdose signs and treatment, 113*t*
withdrawal signs and treatment, 113*t*
Central nervous system infections:
complications, 1564
Creutzfeldt-Jakob disease. *See* Creutzfeldt-Jakob
disease
encephalitis, 1565, 1565*t*
interdisciplinary care
diagnosis, 1566
medications, 1566
surgery, 1566
manifestations, 1564–65, 1564*t*
meningitis. *See* Meningitis
nursing care
assessment, 1567
community-based care, 1569
health promotion, 1567
nursing diagnoses and interventions
ineffective protection, 1568
risk for deficient fluid volume, 1568
using NANDA, NIC, and NOC, 1568, 1568*t*
Nursing Care Plan
assessment, 1567*t*
critical thinking in the nursing process, 1567*t*
diagnoses, 1567*t*
evaluation, 1567*t*
expected outcomes, 1567*t*
planning and implementation, 1567*t*
pathophysiology, 1563–66
postpoliomyelitis syndrome. *See*
Postpoliomyelitis syndrome
rabies. *See* Rabies
tetanus. *See* Tetanus
Central neurogenic hyperventilation, 1530, 1530*t*
Central obesity, 632
Central pain, 174. *See also* Pain
Central pain syndrome (CPS), 1582
Central sleep apnea, 1250
Central stroke pain, 1583
Central syndrome, 1597*t*. *See also* Spinal cord
injury
Central venous catheter, 277, 648
Central venous pressure (CVP):
in fluid volume deficit, 205
measuring with a manometer, 206*t*, 1030
normal values, 206*t*, 1030

Cephalexin, 319*t*
Cephalosporins:
Medication Administration, 319*t*
in specific conditions
bacterial meningitis, 1566
peritonitis, 770
pneumonia, 1271*t*
Cephulac. *See* Lactulose
Cerebellum, 1505*f*, 1506*t*
Cerebral angiogram:
in altered level of consciousness, 1532
in intracranial aneurysm, 1593
purpose and description, 1514*t*
related nursing care, 1514*t*
Cerebral edema, 1537. *See also* Increased
intracranial pressure
Cerebral oxygenation, 1560*t*
Cerebral perfusion pressure (CPP), 1560*t*
Cerebral vascular accident. *See* Stroke
Cerebrospinal fluid:
formation, 1506–7
functions, 1507
in multiple sclerosis, 1627
normal values, 1507*t*
Cerebrovascular accident. *See* Stroke
Cerebrovascular disorders:
arteriovenous malformation. *See* Arteriovenous
malformation
intracranial aneurysm. *See* Intracranial aneurysm
stroke. *See* Stroke
Cerebrum. *See also* Neurologic system
anatomy, physiology, and functions, 1505,
1505*f*, 1506*t*
manifestations of deteriorating function, 1528*t*
Certified registered nurse anesthetist (CRNA), 65
Cerubidine. *See* Daunorubicin
Cerumen:
characteristics, 424, 1682
impacted
interdisciplinary care, 1721
nursing care, 1721
pathophysiology, 1721
Cervical cancer:
classification systems, 1813*t*
incidence, 1812
interdisciplinary care
diagnosis, 1813
medications, 1813
radiation therapy, 1813
surgery, 1813, 1813*f*
manifestations, 1813
nursing care
assessment, 1815
community-based care, 1815–16
health promotion, 1814–15
nursing diagnoses and interventions
fear, 1815
impaired tissue integrity, 1815
using NANDA, NIC, and NOC, 1815, 1815*t*
Nursing Care Plan
assessment, 1814*t*
critical thinking in the nursing process, 1814*t*
diagnoses, 1814*t*
evaluation, 1814*t*
expected outcomes, 1814*t*
planning and implementation, 1814*t*
pathophysiology, 1812
prevention, HPV vaccine for, 1815
risk factors, 1812
screening guidelines, 401*t*, 1814
Cervical disk herniation, 1608. *See also* Herniated
intervertebral disk
Cervical intraepithelial neoplasia (CIN), 1812, 1813*t*

Cervical spine:
  immobilization, 260, 260f
  physical assessment, 1392t
Cervical traction, 1601, 1601f
Cervicitis, 1850
Cervix:
  anatomy and function, 1751t, 1752, 1753f
  biopsy, 1758t
  cancer. See Cervical cancer
  physical assessment, 1764–65t
  polyps, 1808, 1809t
Cesamet. See Nabilone
Cetirizine, 1230t
CFTR gene, 152
Chalazion, 1679, 1700, 1701f
Challenge testing, 1324
Chamomile tea, 679, 792
Champion Revised Trauma Scoring System, 260t
Chancre, 1847, 1848f
Chapter Highlights:
  bowel disorders, 821–22t
  burn injuries, 511t
  cancer, 413t
  cardiac disorders, 1019t, 1068t
  community-based and home care, 47–48t
  coronary heart disease, 1019t
  diabetes mellitus, 598t
  disasters, 141t
  endocrine disorders, 560t
  eye and ear disorders, 1734t
  female reproductive system disorders, 1833t
  fluid, electrolyte, and acid–base imbalances, 252
  gallbladder, liver, and pancreatic disorders, 733t
  genetics, 166t
  health and illness, 33t
  hematologic disorders, 1150t
  immune system, 366t
  infections, 325–26
  kidney disorders, 927t
  loss, grief, and death, 99t
  lower respiratory disorders, 1317–18t, 1372–73t
  male reproductive system disorders, 1790–91t
  medical-surgical nursing, 16t
  musculoskeletal disorders, 1494t
  musculoskeletal trauma, 1429–30t
  neurologic system disorders, 1614t, 1663t
  pain, 192t
  peripheral vascular disorders, 1202t
  sexually transmitted infections, 1852t
  skin disorders, 483–84t
  substance abuse, 122–23t
  surgery, 82t
  trauma and shock, 283–84t
  upper gastrointestinal disorders, 694t
  urinary system disorders, 880t
Charcot-Marie-Tooth syndrome, 1513t
Chaste tree, 1796, 1800
CHD. See Coronary heart disease
Cheilosis:
  in anemia, 1105, 1106
  definition, 622t
  nursing interventions, 1114
  in nutritional deficiencies, 622t
Chemical burns. See also Burns
  causative agents, 487–88, 488t
  in disasters, 130t
  eye, 1702
  prehospital management, 498
  priority treatment, 488t
Chemical menopause, 1795
Chemical peeling, 479
Chemical terrorism, 127
Chemotaxis, 289

Chemotherapy:
  classes
    alkylating agents, 390, 392t
    antimetabolites, 390, 392t, 1483t
    antitumor antibiotics, 391, 392–93t
    hormones and hormone antagonists, 391, 393–94t
    mitotic inhibitors, 391
    plant alkaloids, 391, 393t
  definition, 389
  effects, 391
  management of clients receiving, 394–95
  mechanisms of action, 389–90, 390f
  preparation and administration, 391, 394, 395f
  principles, 389–90
  in specific conditions
    bladder cancer, 863
    bone tumors, 1483, 1483t
    breast cancer, 1825
    colorectal cancer, 805
    endometrial cancer, 1816
    laryngeal cancer, 1254
    leukemia, 1123, 1123t
    lung cancer, 1312
    lymphoma, 1132
    multiple myeloma, 1137
    ovarian cancer, 1819
    testicular cancer, 1775
Chenix. See Chenodiol
Chenodiol, 699
Cherry angiomas, 443
Chest, physical assessment, 1223–24t
Chest injuries. See Thoracic trauma
Chest pain:
  in acute coronary syndrome, 975, 975t
  in acute myocardial infarction, 975t, 984
  in angina pectoris, 970, 975t
  assessment, 950t
Chest physiotherapy:
  in cystic fibrosis, 1342
  in pneumonia, 1272–73, 1273f, 1274f
Chest tubes:
  equipment, 1299f, 1300f
  in lung abscess, 1280
  nursing care, 1300t
  in pneumothorax, 1299
  procedure, 1299
Chest x-ray:
  in cardiac function assessment, 944t
  in preoperative assessment, 60
  in respiratory function assessment, 1218t
  in specific conditions
    acute respiratory distress syndrome, 1367
    aortic aneurysm, 1173
    cardiomyopathy, 1067
    chronic obstructive pulmonary disease, 1334
    heart failure, 1027
    inhalation injury, 1307
    lung cancer, 1311
    lymphoma, 1131
    pericarditis, 1051
    pneumonia, 1270
    pulmonary embolism, 1349
    rheumatic heart disease, 1043t
    severe acute respiratory syndrome, 1278
    tuberculosis, 1287
    valvular heart disease, 1060
Cheyne-Stokes respirations, 93, 1530, 1530t
Chinese culture, death rituals, 88
Chlamydia:
  cervical cancer risk and, 1812
  characteristics, 311t
  complications, 1845
  diagnostic test, 1756t

in epididymitis, 1773
incidence, 1844
interdisciplinary care
  diagnosis, 1845
  medications, 1845
manifestations, 1844–45
nursing care, 1845
pathophysiology, 1844
in reactive arthritis, 1470
risk factors, 1844t
Chlamydia pneumoniae, 1271t
Chlamydia trachomatis, 1693
Chloral hydrate, 108
Chlorambucil, 891, 1123t, 1137
Chlordiazepoxide, 114t
Chloride (Cl⁻):
  abnormal, possible causes, 386t
  in body fluid compartments, 197f
  normal values, 198t, 386t
  perioperative levels, significance and nursing implications, 60t
  recommended daily intake, 610t
  in sweat, for cystic fibrosis diagnosis, 1342
Chlorocon. See Chloroquine
Chloromycetin. See Chlorambucil
Chloroquine, 321, 778t
Chlorothiazide, 210t, 1033t
Chlorpheniramine, 1230t
Chlorphenoxamine, 1638t
Chlorpromazine:
  cataract formation and, 1704
  for tetanus, 1661
  urine color changes caused by, 832t
Chlorthalidone, 210t
Chlor-Trimeton. See Chlorpheniramine
Chlorzoxazone, 1600t
Chocolate cysts, 1808, 1809t
Cholangiography, 616t
Cholangitis, 698, 784–85
Cholecystectomy:
  nursing care, 700t
  Nursing Research: postoperative pain management, 700t
  procedure, 699
Cholecystitis, 698, 698t. See also Gallstones
Cholecystography, 616t
Cholecystotomy, 700
Choledochostomy, 700
Cholelithiasis, 697, 698. See also Gallstones
Cholera, 774t, 775
Cholesteatoma, 1724
Cholesterol:
  gallstone formation and, 697
  serum levels. See Serum cholesterol
  uses in body, 608
Cholesterol-lowering drugs, 967t, 968
Cholestyramine, 699, 967t
Choline magnesium trisalicylate, 178t, 1464
Choline salicylate, 178t
Cholinergic crisis, 1648
Cholinergic neurotransmitters, 1505
Cholinergics, 871t, 1621t
Cholinesterase inhibitors, 1621t, 1649, 1649t
Chondroma, 1482t
Chondrosarcoma, 1482t. See also Bone tumors
Chorea, 1643, 1643t
Choreiform movements, 1643
Choroid, 1672, 1672f
Chromium, 610t
Chromosomes:
  alterations
    diagnosing, 157
    in number, 150, 150t
    in structure, 150–51

Chromosomes—*continued*
homologous, 149
structure, 149, 150*f*
Chronic bronchitis, 1331–32, 1332*t*. *See also*
Chronic obstructive pulmonary disease
Chronic cholecystitis, 698. *See also* Gallstones
Chronic disease, 22*t*
Chronic gastritis, 677, 678. *See also* Gastritis
Chronic glomerulonephritis, 888–89. *See also*
Glomerular disorders
Chronic heart failure, 1027. *See also* Heart
failure
Chronic hepatitis, 706. *See also* Hepatitis
Chronic illness. *See also* Illness
definition, 23
family of client with, 33
responses to, 23–24
Chronic intermittent colitis, 784. *See also*
Inflammatory bowel disease
Chronic ischemic heart disease, 962
Chronic lymphocytic leukemia (CLL). *See also*
Leukemia
characteristics, 1119*t*, 1122
interdisciplinary care
diagnosis, 1123*t*
treatment, 1119*t*, 1123*t*
manifestations, 1119*t*, 1122
pathophysiology, 1122
Chronic myeloid leukemia (CML). *See also*
Leukemia
characteristics, 1119*t*, 1121
genetic considerations, 151, 1089*t*, 1121, 1122*f*
interdisciplinary care
diagnosis, 1123*t*
treatment, 1119*t*, 1123*t*
manifestations, 1119*t*, 1121
pathophysiology, 1121
Chronic obstructive pulmonary disease (COPD):
Case Study, 1377*t*
classification, 1332*t*
client teaching, 1341*t*
definition, 1330
genetic considerations, 1331*t*
incidence, 1330–31
interdisciplinary care
complementary therapies, 1335–36
diagnosis, 1333–34, 1333*f*
medications, 1334
oxygen therapy, 1335
smoking cessation, 1334
surgery, 1335
treatments, 1334–35
manifestations, 1332–33, 1332*t*, 1333*f*
mortality rate, 1331
nursing care
assessment, 1336
client teaching, 1341*t*
community-based care, 1340, 1341*t*
health promotion, 1336
nursing diagnoses and interventions
compromised family coping, 1339–40
decisional conflict: smoking, 1340
imbalance nutrition: less than body
requirements, 1339
ineffective airway clearance, 1336–39
using NANDA, NIC, and NOC, 1340, 1340*t*
Nursing Care Plan
assessment, 1338*t*
critical thinking in the nursing process, 1338*t*
diagnoses, 1338*t*
evaluation, 1338*t*
expected outcomes, 1338*t*
planning and implementation, 1338*t*
Nursing Research: physical activity benefits, 1335*t*

pathophysiology
chronic bronchitis, 1331–32
emphysema, 1332
overview, 1331, 1331*f*
risk factors, 1331
Chronic otitis media, 1724–25
Chronic pain, 174. *See also* Pain
Chronic pancreatitis, 727, 727*t*. *See also*
Pancreatitis
Chronic pyelonephritis, 848–49. *See also* Urinary
tract infection
Chronic rejection, 921–22
Chronic renal failure:
Case Study, 931*t*
causes, 913–14, 914*f*
definition, 899
genetic considerations, 839*t*
incidence, 913
interdisciplinary care
diagnosis, 918
medications, 918–19
nutrition and fluid management, 919
renal replacement therapies
dialysis, 919–20. *See also* Dialysis
kidney transplant. *See* Kidney transplant
manifestations and complications
cardiovascular, 916
dermatologic, 918
endocrine and metabolic, 918
fluid and electrolytes, 915–16
gastrointestinal, 916
hematologic, 916
immune system, 916
musculoskeletal, 918
neurologic, 916
Multisystem Effects, 917*t*
nursing care
assessment, 923
community-based care, 926
health promotion, 923
nursing diagnoses and interventions
disturbed body image, 925
imbalanced nutrition: less than body
requirements, 923, 925
ineffective tissue perfusion: renal, 923
risk for infection, 925
in older adults, 914*t*
Nursing Care Plan
assessment, 924*t*
critical thinking in the nursing process, 924*t*
diagnoses, 924*t*
evaluation, 924*t*
expected outcomes, 924*t*
planning and implementation, 924*t*
pathophysiology, 914–15, 915*f*, 915*t*
stages, 916*t*
Chronic sorrow, 97
Chronic tissue rejection, 342–43, 343*t*
Chronic venous insufficiency:
definition, 1194
interdisciplinary care, 1194–95
manifestations, 1194, 1194*f*, 1194*t*, 1195*t*
nursing care, 1195, 1196*t*
Nursing Research: rest periods for improved
healing, 1196*t*
in older adults, 1196*t*
pathophysiology, 1194
Chronulac. *See* Lactulose
Chvostek's sign, 229, 229*f*, 531*t*
Chylothorax, 1295
CI (cardiac index), 941, 1031
Cialis. *See* Tadalafil
Cibacalcin. *See* Calcitonin
Cigarette smoking. *See* Smoking

Ciliary body, 1672, 1672*f*
Cilostazol, 1177
Cimetidine:
Medication Administration, 665*t*
preoperative use and nursing implications, 62*t*
in specific conditions
gastritis, 678
gastroesophageal reflux disease, 665
pancreatitis, 728
CIN (cervical intraepithelial neoplasia), 1812, 1813*t*
Cingulate herniation, 1537, 1538*f*. *See also*
Increased intracranial pressure
Cipro. *See* Ciprofloxacin
Ciprofloxacin:
Medication Administration, 320*t*
in specific conditions
anthrax prophylaxis and treatment, 128*t*, 1294
diverticulitis, 816
epiglottitis, 1241
gastroenteritis, 776
gonorrhea, 1846
urinary tract infection, 849
Circle of Willis, 1508*f*
Circulating nurse, 65–66
Circumduction, 1386*c*
Circumferential aneurysm, 1170, 1170*f*
Circumflex artery, 939*f*, 958
Cirrhosis:
complications
ascites, 711
esophageal varices, 711
hepatorenal syndrome, 716
portal hypertension, 711
portal systemic encephalopathy, 715, 715*t*
splenomegaly, 711
spontaneous bacterial peritonitis, 716
definition, 710
incidence and mortality, 710
interdisciplinary care
diagnosis, 617*t*, 716
medications, 716, 717*t*
treatments
liver transplant. *See* Liver transplant
management of complications, 717–19
nutrition, 717
manifestations, 711, 715*t*
Multisystem Effects, 714*t*
nursing care
assessment, 720–21
health promotion, 720
Medication Administration, 717*t*
nursing diagnoses and interventions
community-based care, 723
disturbed thought processes, 722
excess fluid volume, 722
imbalanced nutrition: less than body
requirements, 723
impaired skin integrity, 723
inefficient protection, 722
using NANDA, NIC, and NOC, 723, 723*t*
Nursing Care Plan
assessment, 721*t*
critical thinking in the nursing process, 721*t*
diagnoses, 721*t*
evaluation, 721*t*
expected outcomes, 721*t*
planning and implementation, 721*t*
pathophysiology, 710–11, 712–13*t*
racial/ethnic considerations, 711*t*
types
alcoholic, 710, 711
biliary, 711
posthepatic, 711
Cisatracurium, 1356*t*

Cisplatin:
adverse/side effects, 394t, 1730
mechanisms of action, 390
nursing implications, 394t
in specific conditions
bone tumors, 1483t
laryngeal cancer, 1254
ovarian cancer, 1819
testicular cancer, 1775
target malignancies, 394t
Citrucel. See Methylcellulose
CIWA-Ar (Clinical Institute Withdrawal
Assessment of Alcohol–Revised), 112,
117, 118f
CK. See Creatine kinase
CK-MB. See Creatine kinase-MB
Cl⁻. See Chloride (Cl⁻)
Claforan. See Cefotaxime
Clarifying, 6
Clarithromycin, 320t
Claritin. See Loratadine
Clark staging, melanoma, 467, 468f
Classic migraine, 1543. See also Headache
Clavicle, fracture, 1412–13
Clavulanic acid sulbactam, 320t
Claw toe, 1492
Clemastine, 1230t
Cleocin. See Clindamycin
Client, 5
Climacteric, 1795. See also Menopause
Clindamycin:
for acne, 458
for endocarditis prophylaxis, 1047t
for epiglottitis, 1241
for lung abscess, 1280
for pelvic inflammatory disease, 1851
for peritonitis, 770
Clinical Institute Withdrawal Assessment of
Alcohol–Revised (CIWA-Ar), 112, 117, 118f
Clinical Opiate Withdrawal Scale (COWS), 117
Clinical Scenarios:
bowel elimination alterations, 825t
cardiac function alterations, 1072t
endocrine function alterations, 601t
home care, 50t
integumentary structure and function
alterations, 514t
musculoskeletal function alterations, 1498t
neurologic function alterations, 1666t
nutritional alterations, 736t
pathophysiology and patterns of health, 417t
patterns of health alterations, 144t
peripheral tissue perfusion alterations, 1206t
reproductive function alterations, 1855t
respiratory function alterations, 1376t
urinary elimination alterations, 930t
visual and auditory function alterations, 1738t
Clinoril. See Sulindac
Clitoris:
anatomy, 1751t, 1752, 1752f
physical assessment, 1763t
CLL. See Chronic lymphocytic leukemia
Clofibrate, 967t
Clomid. See Clomiphene
Clomiphene, 1809
Clonazepam, 1550t
Clones, 297
Clonidine, 1162t
Clopidogrel:
Medication Administration, 976t
in specific conditions
acute coronary syndrome, 976, 976t
peripheral vascular disease, 1177
stroke prevention, 1585

Clorotione, 441t
Closed (flap) amputation, 1421, 1422t. See also
Amputation
Closed (simple) fracture, 1401, 1402f. See also
Fractures
Closed pneumothorax, 1299. See also
Pneumothorax
Closed-loop obstruction, 811, 812, 812f. See also
Intestinal obstruction
Clostridium, 1407
Clostridium botulinum, 1661–62
Clostridium difficile:
colitis, 774t, 775
nosocomial infection, 313, 314
treatment, 314
Clostridium perfringens, 267
Clostridium tetani, 1661
Clotrimazole:
Medication Administration, 450t, 658t
troches, for thrush, 359t, 657t, 658, 658t
Clotting. See Coagulation
Cloxacillin, 447
Clubbing:
fingers, 1342, 1342f
nails, 436f, 436t
Cluster breathing, 1530t
Cluster headache, 1542t, 1543. See also Headache
CMG. See Cystometrogram
CML. See Chronic myeloid leukemia
CMV. See Cytomegalovirus
CNS. See Central nervous system
CO. See Cardiac output
CO₂. See Carbon dioxide
Coagulation:
definition, 1079
disorders
disseminated intravascular coagulation. See
Disseminated intravascular coagulation
hemophilia. See Hemophilia
thrombocytopenia. See Thrombocytopenia
factors, 1082t
stages
clot dissolution, 1081
clot retraction, 1080
fibrin clot formation, 1080, 1081f
platelet plug formation, 1080, 1080f
vessel spasm, 1080
Coagulation studies:
in disseminated intravascular coagulation, 1148
in hemophilia, 1144
in pulmonary embolism, 1349
Coal tar derivatives, 441t, 444
Coal worker's pneumoconiosis, 1345
Coarctation of the aorta, 1167
Cocaine:
characteristics, 108
effects, 108
myocardial infarction induced by, 984
overdose signs and treatment, 108, 113t
street names, 111t
topical, for epistaxis, 1243
use in pregnancy, 109
withdrawal signs and treatment, 113t
Coccidioides immitis, 1294
Coccidiomycosis, 1294
Coccidiosis. See Cryptosporidiosis
Cochlea, 1683, 1683f
Cochlear implant, 1731–32, 1732f
Code of ethics, 10. See also Nursing ethics, codes
Codeine, 62t, 180t, 182t
Codependence, 103t
Codylax. See Bisacodyl
Coenzyme Q10, 1036, 1621
Cogentin. See Benztropine

Cognex. See Tacrine hydrochloride
Cognition, 1529
Cognitive behavioral therapy, 110, 652
Cognitive function:
assessment, 1519t
health and, 19
impairments, special considerations in
disasters, 140
Cognitive-perceptual patterns:
altered neurologic function. See also Neurologic
system
Build Clinical Competence, 1665t
Clinical Scenarios, 1666t
altered visual and auditory function. See also
Ears; Eyes
Build Clinical Competence, 1737t
Clinical Scenarios, 1738t
NANDA nursing diagnoses, 1501t
Cogwheel rigidity, 1635
Colace. See Docusate
Colchicine, 1445, 1446t
Cold phase, septic shock, 275, 275t
Cold sore. See Herpes simplex
Cold zone, in disaster, 134t
Colectomy, 788, 789f
Colesevelam, 967t
Colestid. See Colestipol
Colestipol, 967t
Colitis:
functional. See Irritable bowel syndrome
ulcerative. See Ulcerative colitis
Collagen disorders. See Connective tissue disorders
Collagenase, 504
Collateral channels/vessels, 958, 984
Colles's fracture, 1413
Colloid solutions, 277–78, 279t
Colon, 742f, 743
Colonoscopy:
in bowel disorders, 745t
for colorectal cancer screening/diagnosis, 401t,
802, 803
in diverticular disease, 816
Colony-stimulating factors, 1123, 1139
Color Doppler echocardiography, 945t
Colorectal cancer:
complications, 802
incidence, 801
interdisciplinary care
chemotherapy, 805
diagnosis, 802–3
laser photocoagulation, 803
prevention, 802
radiation therapy, 805
screening, 401t, 802
staging, 803, 803t
surgery
colostomy. See Colostomy
local excision, 803
resection, 803
manifestations, 802
nursing care
assessment, 805
colostomy, 806t
community-based care, 808–9
health promotion, 805
nursing diagnoses and interventions
acute pain, 806–7
anticipatory grieving, 808
imbalance nutrition: less than body
requirements, 808
risk for sexual dysfunction, 808
postoperative, 804t
preoperative, 804t
using NANDA, NIC, and NOC, 808, 809t

Colorectal cancer—*continued*
  Nursing Care Plan
    assessment, 807*t*
    critical thinking in the nursing process, 807*t*
    diagnoses, 807*t*
    evaluation, 807*t*
    expected outcomes, 807*t*
    planning and implementation, 807*t*
  pathophysiology, 802, 802*f*
  risk factors, 801–2, 801*t*
Color-flow Doppler ultrasound, 1177
Colostomy:
  definition, 803
  dietary considerations, 806*t*
  double-barrel, 804, 805*f*
  Hartmann procedure, 805
  health assessment interview, 746
  levels and sites, 803–4, 804*f*
  nursing care, 806*t*
  sigmoid, 804
  transverse loop, 804
Colporrhaphy, 1806
Colposcopy, 1757*t*
Coma, 1529*t*. *See also* Altered level of
    consciousness
Comatose client, nursing care, 93
Combivent. *See* Albuterol/ipratropium
Combivir. *See* Lamivudine; Zidovudine
Comedones, 457
Comminuted fracture. *See also* Fractures
  characteristics, 1402*f*
  definition, 1401
  skull, 1555, 1555*t*. *See also* Skull fracture
Common cold. *See* Upper respiratory disorders,
    viral infections
Common migraine, 1543. *See also* Headache
Common wart, 452, 452*f*
Communicable disease, 22*t*
Communication accommodation theory, 65*t*
Community health care, 36
Community-based care, 36. *See also* Community-
    based nursing care
Community-based healthcare services:
  community centers and clinics, 37
  day care programs, 37
  Meals-on-Wheels, 38
  parish nursing, 37–38
Community-based nursing care:
  Chapter Highlights, 47–48*t*
  definition, 36
  end-of-life care, 97
  factors affecting health
    community healthcare structure, 37
    economic resources, 37
    environment, 37
    social support systems, 37
  pain management, 190, 190*t*
  postoperative, 80
  settings, 36*t*
  substance abuse, 120–21
Compartment syndrome:
  in burn injuries, 495
  manifestations, 1403, 1403*t*
  pathophysiology, 495, 1403
  treatment, 1406
Compazine. *See* Prochlorperazine
Compensation, in acid–base disorders, 241–42, 243*t*
Complement assay, 336, 341
Complement system, 294*t*
Complementary and alternative therapies:
  for asthma, 1326
  for benign prostatic hyperplasia, 1781
  for cancer, 398–99, 399*t*
  for chronic obstructive pulmonary disease, 1335

  for conjunctivitis, 1694–95
  for constipation, 760–61
  for coronary heart disease, 968, 968*t*
  for diarrhea, 755
  for gallstones, 701
  for gastritis, 679
  for gout, 1445
  for headache, 1544
  for heart failure, 1036
  for hepatitis, 709
  herbal supplements as surgical risk factor,
    58*t*, 59
  for hypertension, 1163
  for inflammatory bowel disease, 792
  for irritable bowel syndrome, 763
  for leukemia, 1125
  for lung cancer, 1313
  for menopausal symptoms, 1796
  for nausea and vomiting, 672
  for pain management
    acupuncture, 185
    biofeedback, 185
    cutaneous stimulation, 186
    distraction, 186
    hypnotism, 185
    relaxation, 185–86
  for pancreatitis, 728
  for peripheral vascular disease, 1178
  for urinary incontinence, 875–76
  for urinary tract infection, 851
Complete blood count (CBC):
  components, 1078*t*
  normal values, 1078*t*
  purpose and description, 1087*t*
  in specific conditions
    acute myocardial infarction, 986
    acute renal failure, 904
    anemias, 1110
    burns, 500
    chronic obstructive pulmonary disease, 1334
    chronic renal failure, 918
    disseminated intravascular coagulation, 1148
    leukemia, 1122, 1123*t*
    lymphoma, 1131
    multiple myeloma, 1137
    myelodysplastic syndrome, 1115
    pericarditis, 1051
    pharyngitis, 1239
    pneumonia, 1271
    rheumatic fever, 1043
    systemic lupus erythematosus, 1473
Complete fracture, 1402. *See also* Fractures
Complete heart block, 999*t*, 1003
Completed stroke, 1581
Complex partial seizures, 1549
Complex regional pain syndrome, 174
Compliance, 1023, 1024*t*, 1536
Compound (open) fracture, 1401, 1402*f*. *See also*
    Fractures
Compressed fracture, 1401, 1402*f*
Compression, 256
Compression sclerotherapy, 1197
Computed tomography (CT):
  abdomen
    adrenals, 526*t*
    in aortic aneurysm, 1173
    pancreas, 526*t*
  brain
    in altered level of consciousness, 1532
    in brain tumor, 1571
    client preparation, 1514*t*
    health education for the client and family, 1514*t*
    in multiple sclerosis, 1627
    purpose and description, 1514*t*

    related nursing care, 1514*t*
    in stroke, 1584
  in cancer, 384
  ear, 1727
  electron beam. *See* Electron beam computed
    tomography
  eye, 1674*t*
  gastrointestinal system, 616*t*
  heart, 945*t*
  kidneys, 837*t*, 857
  lungs
    in lung cancer, 1312
    in pulmonary embolism, 1349
  lymphatic system, 1088*t*
  musculoskeletal system, 1387*t*
  principles, 384
  sinuses, 1236
  thorax, 1218*t*
COMT (catechol-*O*-methyltransferase) inhibitors,
    1638*t*, 1639
Comtan. *See* Entacapone
Comtrex. *See* Phenylpropanolamine
Concentric plaque formation, 959
Concussion, 1558*t*, 1559. *See also* Traumatic brain
    injury
Condoms:
  female, 1838*t*
  male, 1838*t*
  in safer sex practices, 359, 361*t*, 1838*t*
Conduction system, heart, 941, 941*f*, 995
Conductive hearing loss, 1729–30. *See also*
    Hearing loss
Conductivity, 995*t*
Condyloma lata, 1848
Condylomata acuminata, 1841, 1841*f*. *See also*
    Genital warts
Condylox. *See* Podophyllin
Cones, 1672
Confusion, 1529*t*
Congenital disease, 22*t*
Congenital lymphedema, 1199*t*
Congenital nevi, 466
Congestive heart failure, 1022. *See also* Heart
    failure
Conization:
  purpose and description, 1757*t*, 1813, 1813*f*
  related nursing care, 1757*t*
Conjugated bilirubin, 699*t*
Conjunctiva, 1670
Conjunctivitis:
  acute, 1692–93
  causes, 1694*t*
  definition, 1692
  eye disorders
    nursing care
      assessment, 1695
      community-based care, 1695
      health promotion, 1695, 1695*t*
      nursing diagnoses and interventions, 1695
      using NANDA, NIC, and NOC, 1695, 1696*t*
  interdisciplinary care
    complementary and alternative therapies,
      1694–95
    diagnosis, 1694
    medications, 1694
  manifestations, 1693, 1694*f*
  nursing care
    assessment, 1695
    community-based care, 1695
    health promotion, 1695, 1695*t*
    nursing diagnoses and interventions
      risk for disturbed sensory perception:
        visual, 1695
      risk for infection, 1695

using NANDA, NIC, and NOC, 1695, 1696t
pathophysiology, 1692–94
Connective tissue disorders:
fibromyalgia. See Fibromyalgia
polymyositis. See Polymyositis
scleroderma. See Scleroderma
Sjögren's syndrome, 1486
systemic lupus erythematosus. See Systemic lupus erythematosus
Conscious sedation, 63–64
Consciousness, 1529. See also Altered level of consciousness
Consolidation, 1268
Constipation:
causes, 758t
definition, 743, 758
interdisciplinary care
complementary and alternative therapies, 760–61
diagnosis, 758
enemas, 760
medications, 758–59t
nutrition, 760
manifestations, 758
nursing care
assessment, 761
community-based care, 761–62
health promotion, 761
Medication Administration, 758–59t
nursing diagnoses and interventions, 761
in older adults, 761t
pathophysiology, 758
Constructive procedure, 54t
Contac. See Phenylpropanolamine
Contact dermatitis, 335, 456, 456f, 456t, 457
Contact inhibition, 376
Contact lenses, 1695t, 1697
Contact precautions, 323t
Continent ileal diversion, 864, 864f, 865t
Continent ileostomy, 789, 789f
Continuous ambulatory peritoneal dialysis (CAPD), 920
Continuous arteriovenous hemodialysis, 907t, 909f
Continuous arteriovenous hemofiltration, 907t
Continuous cyclic peritoneal dialysis (CCPD), 920
Continuous positive airway pressure (CPAP):
in acute respiratory failure, 1355
characteristics, 1358, 1359t
nasal, for obstructive sleep apnea, 1250, 1251f
Continuous renal replacement therapy (CRRT), 906, 907–8, 907t
Continuous venovenous hemodialysis, 907t
Contractibility, 1383
Contractility, 940, 995, 1024
Contracting, 42
Contractures:
after amputation, 1423
in burn injuries, 490, 490f, 504
definition, 1423
Volkmann's, 1406, 1413
Contralateral deficit, 1580
Contrast venography, 1188
Control zone, in disaster, 134t
Contusions:
cerebral, 1557. See also Traumatic brain injury
musculoskeletal, 259, 259f, 1399
pulmonary, 1303. See also Thoracic trauma
Conventional weapons, 127
Convergence, 1673, 1678t
Co-occurring disorders, 103, 103t
Cooley's anemia, 1109. See also Thalassemias
Coordination, assessment, 1523f, 1523t
Copaxone. See Glatiramer acetate
COPD. See Chronic obstructive pulmonary disease

Copolymer-1. See Glatiramer acetate
Copper, 610t
Cor pulmonale, 1352–53
Cordarone. See Amiodarone
Cordotomy, 184, 185f
Core competencies:
for healthcare professionals, 5, 5t
for nurses responding to mass casualty incidents, 126, 126t
Core needle biopsy, breast, 1757t
Coreg. See Carvedilol
Corgard. See Nadolol
Corlopam. See Fenoldopam
Cornea:
age-related changes, 1676t
anatomy, physiology, and functions, 1671, 1672f, 1696
assessment, 1679
disorders. See Corneal disorders
transplant. See Corneal transplant
Corneal arcus, 1679
Corneal disorders:
dystrophies, 1697
interdisciplinary care
corrective lenses, 1697
disease, 1697
medications, 1697
surgery, 1697–98. See also Corneal transplant
keratitis, 1696
manifestations, 1697–98
nursing care
assessment, 1698
of client having eye surgery
health education for the client and family, 1699t
postoperative care, 1699t
preoperative care, 1699t
community-based care, 1700
health promotion, 1698
nursing diagnoses and interventions
acute pain, 1700
risk for disturbed sensory perception: visual, 1698–99
risk for injury, 1700
pathophysiology, 1697–98
refractive errors, 1696
trauma, 1694t, 1701–2. See also Eyes, trauma
ulcer, 1696–97
Corneal dystrophy, 1697
Corneal light (red) reflex, 1678t, 1680
Corneal reflex, 1520t, 1671
Corneal transplant:
graft harvest, 1697
indications, 342t
procedure, 1697–98, 1698f
success rate, 342t
Corneal ulcer, 1696–97
Cornstarch, 441t
Coronary angiography. See Cardiac catheterization
Coronary arteriography. See Cardiac catheterization
Coronary artery bypass grafting (CABG):
effectiveness, 977–78
nursing care
postoperative nursing diagnosis and interventions
acute pain, 981t
decreased cardiac output, 980t
disturbed thought processes, 982t
hypothermia, 980–81t
ineffective airway clearance/impaired gas exchange, 981t
risk for infection, 981t
preoperative, 980t

Nursing Care Plan
assessment, 983t
critical thinking in the nursing process, 983t
diagnoses, 983t
evaluation, 983t
expected outcomes, 983t
planning and implementation, 983t
off-pump, 978
procedure, 977f, 978–79
Coronary artery disease. See Coronary heart disease
Coronary circulation, 938, 938f
Coronary heart disease (CHD):
categories, 962
Chapter Highlights, 1019t
Framingham Heart Study, 962t
incidence and prevalence, 958
interdisciplinary care
complementary therapies, 968, 968t
diagnosis, 965–66
medications, 966–68, 967t
risk factor management
diabetes, 966
diet, 966, 966t
exercise, 966
hypertension, 966
smoking, 966
nursing care
assessment, 968
community-based care, 969
health promotion, 968
Medication Administration, 967t
nursing diagnoses and interventions
imbalanced nutrition: more than body requirements, 968–69
ineffective health maintenance, 969
pathophysiology
angina pectoris, 961t
atherosclerosis, 959, 960t
myocardial ischemia, 959, 961t, 962, 962t
racial/ethnic considerations, 958t
risk factors
diabetes mellitus, 587–88
modifiable
cigarette smoking, 964
diabetes mellitus, 963
diet, 964
emerging, 964
hyperlipidemia, 963, 963t
hypertension, 963
metabolic syndrome, 964, 964t
obesity, 964
overview, 963t
physical inactivity, 964
in women, 964
nonmodifiable, 962, 963t
rheumatoid arthritis, 1462, 1463
sudden cardiac death in, 1015
Coronavirus, 1276–77
Corpora cavernosa, 1744
Corpus callosum, 1505
Corpus luteum, 1753
Corpus spongiosum, 1744
Corrective lenses, 1697
Corticosteroids:
adverse/side effects, 344, 391, 1434, 1704
Medication Administration, 555t, 787–88t, 1328t, 1631t
site of action, 344f
in specific conditions
acute respiratory distress syndrome, 1367
acute respiratory failure, 1355
Addison's disease, 555t
asthma, 1326, 1328t

Corticosteroids—*continued*
  bacterial meningitis, 1566
  cancer, 391
  chronic obstructive pulmonary disease, 1334
  glomerular disorders, 890–91
  gout, 1445
  hypercalcemia, 232
  hypersensitivity responses, 338
  inflammation, 307, 441*t*
  inflammatory bowel disease, 786, 787–88*t*
  multiple sclerosis, 1627, 1631*t*
  myasthenia gravis, 1649
  organ transplantation, 344, 921
  pemphigus vulgaris, 460
  pruritus, 441*t*
  spinal cord injury, 1599
  systemic lupus erythematosus, 1473
  thrombocytopenia, 1141
  topical
    in pruritus, 440, 441*t*
    psoriasis, 444
    in stasis dermatitis, 1194
Cortisol, 524*t*, 549, 550*t*
Cortisol replacements, 555*t*
Cortisone, 555*t*
Cortisporin Otic. *See* Polymyxin B-neomycin-
      hydrocortisone
Corvert. *See* Ibutilide
Corynebacterium diphtheriae, 1241. *See also*
      Diphtheria
Coryza, 1229
Cosmetic surgery:
  frequency, 478*t*
  procedures
    blepharoplasty, 479
    rhinoplasty, 479
    rhytidectomy, 479
Cotton-wool spots, 1046
Coughing exercise, 72*t*
Coughing techniques, in respiratory disorders, 1341*t*
Cough-variant asthma, 1324
Coumadin. *See* Warfarin
Countercurrent exchange system, 833–34, 833*f*
Counterirritants, 1451
Coup-contrecoup head injury, 1554, 1554*f*
Cover–uncover test, 1678
Cowper's glands. *See* Bulbourethral glands
COWS (Clinical Opiate Withdrawal Scale), 117
COX-2 (cyclooxygenase-2) inhibitors, 178, 681,
      1451. *See also* Nonsteroidal anti-
      inflammatory drugs
Cozaar. *See* Losartan
CPAP. *See* Continuous positive airway pressure
CPB (cardiopulmonary bypass), 978, 979*f*
CPP (cerebral perfusion pressure), 1560*t*
CPR. *See* Cardiopulmonary resuscitation
CPS (central pain syndrome), 1582
Crackles, 1226*t*
"Cradle cap," 457
Cranberry juice, for urinary tract infection, 851
Cranial nerves:
  anatomy, 1509, 1510*f*
  assessment
    abnormal findings, 1223*t*, 1519–21*t*
    sample documentation, 1512
    technique/normal findings, 1223*t*, 1519–21*t*
  controlling eye muscles, 1671*f*
  disorders
    Bell's palsy. *See* Bell's palsy
    trigeminal neuralgia. *See* Trigeminal neuralgia
  functions, 1511*t*
Craniectomy, 1571
Craniocerebral trauma. *See* Traumatic brain injury
Craniopharyngioma, 1570*t*. *See also* Brain tumors

Cranioplasty, 1571
Craniotomy, 1571, 1571*f*
C-reactive protein (CRP):
  abnormal, possible causes, 386*t*
  in coronary heart disease, 965
  in inflammation, 306
  normal values, 386*t*
  in rheumatic fever, 1043
Creams, for skin disorders, 441*t*
Creatine kinase (CK):
  in acute coronary syndrome, 976
  in acute myocardial infarction, 986, 987*t*
  in musculoskeletal system assessment, 1388*t*
Creatine kinase-MB (CK-MB):
  in acute coronary syndrome, 976
  in acute myocardial infarction, 986, 987*t*
Creatine phosphokinase, 500
Creatinine, 834. *See also* Serum creatinine
Creatinine clearance:
  normal values, 890*t*
  in perioperative assessment, 61
  purpose and description, 836*t*
  related nursing care, 836*t*
  in specific conditions
    chronic renal failure, 918
    glomerular disorders, 890, 890*t*
Credé's method, 871
Cremasteric reflex, 1524*t*
Crepitation, 1392*t*
Crescendo–decrescendo pattern, 970
CREST syndrome, 1485
Creutzfeldt-Jakob disease:
  characteristics, 1658
  forms, 1658
  incidence, 1658
  interdisciplinary care, 1659
  manifestations, 1659
  nursing care, 1659
  physical assessment, 1659
Cricoid cartilage, 1211
Critical pathway, 15
Critical thinking:
  attitudes and mental habits for, 6
  definition, 6
  in nursing process, 6, 7*t*
  skills for, 6
Crixivan. *See* Indinavir
CRNA (certified registered nurse anesthetist), 65
Crohn's disease. *See also* Inflammatory bowel
      disease
  characteristics, 782*t*, 785
  complications, 786
  manifestations, 786
  pathophysiology, 785–86
  progression, 785*f*
Cromolyn sodium, 338, 1326, 1328*t*
Cross-tolerance, 103*t*
CRP. *See* C-reactive protein
CRRT (continuous renal replacement therapy),
      906, 907–8, 907*t*
Crushing, 256
Crust, skin, 431*t*, 433*t*
Cryoprecipitate, 263*t*
Cryosurgery, 453, 477
Cryptococcus, 354
Cryptorchidism, 1750*t*
Cryptosporidiosis, 778*t*, 779
Cryptosporidium, 354, 778*t*, 779
Crystalloid solutions, 277, 499
CT. *See* Computed tomography
cT$_n$I (cardiac-specific troponin I), 975–76,
      986, 987*t*
cT$_n$T (cardiac-specific troponin T), 975–76,
      986, 987*t*

Cultural background/practices. *See* Race/ethnicity;
      specific racial/ethnic groups
Culturally sensitive nursing care, 13*t*. *See also*
      Race/ethnicity; *specific racial/ethnic
      groups*
Cultures:
  blood. *See* Blood cultures
  in infection, 316
  skin, 428*t*
  urine. *See* Urine tests, culture
  vaginal, 1756*t*
Cuprimine. *See* Penicillamine
Curel, 441*t*
Curettage:
  for nonmelanoma skin cancer, 464
  postoperative care, 477
  procedure, 477
Curling's ulcers, 496, 677
Cushing's disease, 549
Cushing's response (triad), 1537
Cushing's syndrome:
  complications, 549
  definition, 548
  interdisciplinary care
    diagnostic tests, 524–25*t*, 549–50, 550*t*
    medications, 550
    surgery, 550, 550*t*
  management, 549, 549*t*
  manifestations, 548*f*
  nursing care
    assessment, 529–30*t*, 551
    of client having adrenalectomy, 550*t*
    community-based care, 552–53
    health promotion, 550
    nursing diagnoses and interventions
      disturbed body image, 552
      fluid volume excess, 551–52
      risk for infection, 552
      risk for injury, 552
    using NANDA, NIC, and NOC, 552, 553*t*
  Nursing Care Plan
    assessment, 551*t*
    critical thinking in the nursing process, 551*t*
    diagnoses, 551*t*
    evaluation, 551*t*
    expected outcomes, 551*t*
    planning and implementation, 551*t*
  pathophysiology, 548–49
Cushing's ulcers, 677
Cutaneous stimulation, 186
Cutaneous T-cell lymphoma, 1130*t*. *See also*
      Lymphomas
CVP. *See* Central venous pressure
Cyanide poisoning, 496
Cyanocobalamin. *See* Vitamin B$_{12}$
Cyanosis:
  assessment in light and dark skin, 426*t*
  in cardiogenic shock, 274
  causes, 426*t*, 1093*t*
  definition, 425, 1093*t*, 1266
Cyclobenzaprine hydrochloride, 1491, 1600*t*
Cyclooxygenase-2 (COX-2) inhibitors, 178, 681,
      1451. *See also* Nonsteroidal anti-
      inflammatory drugs
Cyclophosphamide:
  adverse/side effects, 392*t*
  Medication Administration, 345*t*, 1474*t*, 1631*t*
  nursing implications, 392*t*
  in specific conditions
    bone tumors, 1483*t*
    glomerular disorders, 891
    leukemia, 1123*t*
    multiple myeloma, 1137
    multiple sclerosis, 1627, 1631*t*

ovarian cancer, 1819
systemic lupus erythematosus, 1474t
target malignancies, 392t
Cyclosporine:
adverse/side effects, 344, 921
Medication Administration, 345t, 1474t
site of action, 344f
in specific conditions
inflammatory bowel disease, 786
organ transplantation, 344, 921
rheumatoid arthritis, 341
systemic lupus erythematosus, 1474t
Cycrimine, 1638t
Cyst:
definition, 1808
of female reproductive tissue
interdisciplinary care
diagnosis, 1809
medications, 1809
surgery, 1809
manifestations, 1809t
nursing care, 1809
pathophysiology, 1808
skin, 432t, 442
Cystectomy:
nursing care, 866t
nursing considerations, 864t
procedure, 864, 864t
Cystic fibrosis:
definition, 1340
genetic considerations, 152, 1220t, 1340t
incidence, 1340–41
interdisciplinary care
diagnosis, 1342
medications, 1342
surgery, 1342
treatments, 1342
manifestations, 1342
nursing care
community-based care, 1343
nursing diagnoses and interventions
anticipatory grieving, 1343
ineffective airway clearance, 1343
pathophysiology, 1341–42
Cystic medial necrosis, 1172, 1172t
Cystine stones, 856, 856t. See also Urinary
calculi
Cystitis. See also Urinary tract infection
bladder mucosa in, 847f
complications, 848
definition, 847
manifestations, 847–49, 848t
Cystocele, 1805, 1807t
Cystography, 837t
Cystometrogram (CMG):
purpose and description, 836t
related nursing care, 836t
in specific conditions
neurogenic bladder, 870
urinary incontinence, 874
urinary tract infection, 849
Cystoscopy:
purpose and description, 837t
related nursing care, 837t
in specific conditions
bladder cancer, 863
urinary calculi, 857
urinary tract infection, 849
Cytarabine, 1123t
Cytokines, 297, 299t
Cytomegalovirus (CMV):
cancers associated with, 375t
in HIV/AIDS, 353, 359t, 1718
Cytomel. See Liothyronine sodium

Cytosar. See Cytarabine
Cytotoxic agents, 1474t. See also
Chemotherapy
Cytotoxic cells, 297. See also T lymphocytes
Cytotoxic edema, 1537. See also Increased
intracranial pressure
Cytovene. See Ganciclovir
Cytoxan. See Cyclophosphamide

D

d4T. See Stavudine
Daclizumab, 344, 345–46t
Dalteparin, 1189t
Danazol, 1822
Dantrium. See Dantrolene
Dantrolene, 1631t
Daranide. See Dichlorphenamide
Darvocet-N. See Propoxyphene napsylate
Darvon. See Propoxyphene napsylate
DASH (Dietary Approaches to Stop Hypertension)
diet, 1159, 1160t
Daughter cell, 150
Daunorubicin, 1123t
Dawn phenomenon, 582
Daypro. See Oxaprozin
D&C (dilation and curettage), 1803, 1803t
DDAVP. See Desmopressin acetate
ddI. See Didanosine
D-dimer, 1349
De novo mutation, 155
Death and dying. See also End-of-life care; Loss
and grief
Chapter Highlights, 99t
cultural and spiritual practices, 88, 89t
definition, 85
development of concepts of, 87, 87t
family response, 94
Focus on Cultural Diversity, 89t
manifestations, 93, 94t
nurses' reaction to, 94, 94f
physiologic changes in dying client
altered levels of consciousness, 93
anorexia, nausea, and dehydration, 93
dyspnea, 92–93
hypotension, 93
Manifestations, 92
pain, 92
postmortem care, 94
support for client and family, 93
Death anxiety:
definition, 97
NANDA, NIC, and NOC Linkages, 97t
nursing interventions, 97
Debridement:
for burn injuries
definition, 504
enzymatic, 504
in healing process, 294
mechanical, 504
surgical, 502
for osteomyelitis, 1479, 1479t
Decadron. See Dexamethasone
Decadron Phosphate Respihaler. See
Dexamethasone sodium phosphate
Deceleration, in trauma, 256, 1596
Decerebrate posturing, 1525f, 1525t
Decompensation, 1025
Decongestants, 1230t
Decorticate posturing, 1525f, 1525t
Deep coma, 1529t. See also Altered level of
consciousness
Deep partial-thickness burn, 490, 490f. See also
Burns

Deep tendon reflexes (DTRs):
assessment, 1523f, 1523t
physiology, 1511
Deep venous thrombosis (DVT). See also
Pulmonary embolism; Venous thrombosis
complications, 1187
fracture and, 1406
incidence, 1186, 1347
locations, 1187f
manifestations, 1187, 1187t
Nursing Care Plan
assessment, 1191t
critical thinking in the nursing process, 1191t
diagnoses, 1191t
evaluation, 1191t
expected outcomes, 1191t
planning and implementation, 1191t
in ovarian cancer, 1818t
postoperative
assessment findings, 75
nursing care, 75
risk factors, 75
prevention, 1406
risk factors, 1186, 1186t, 1347, 1406, 1406t
treatment, 1406
Defecation, 743
Defeminization, 481
Deferasirox, 1116
Defibrillation, 1008, 1008f, 1008t
Deformation, 1596
Degenerative disease, 22t
Degenerative joint disease. See Osteoarthritis
Dehiscence, 78, 78f
Dehydration. See also Fluid volume deficit
definition, 203
in dying client, 93
surgical risk and nursing implications, 57t
Delavirdine, 358
Delayed ejaculation, 1771
Delayed union, 1407
Delegation, 14
Delirium tremens, 103t, 108
Delta cells, pancreas, 521, 564
Deltasone. See Prednisone
Demadex. See Torsemide
Demand pacing, 1010t. See also Pacemakers
Dementia:
in AIDS, 353
Alzheimer type. See Alzheimer's disease
causes, 1617, 1618t
definition, 1617
vs. delirium, 1617
family home care of older adult with
interventions, 43t
nursing diagnosis, 43t
outcome criteria, 43t
frontotemporal, 1618t
incidence, 1617
Lewy body, 1618t
pain assessment in, 175–76
in Parkinson's disease, 1636
vascular, 1618t
Demerol. See Meperidine HCl
Dendrite, 1504, 1504f
Dendritic cells, 289, 290
Dental health. See Oral health
Deoxyribonucleic acid. See DNA
Depade. See Naltrexone
Depakene. See Valproic acid
Depakote. See Valproic acid
Depen Titratable. See Penicillamine
Dependence, 103t, 179t. See also Substance abuse
Dependent rubor, 1177
Depolarization, 942, 942f

Diskectomy, 1608
Dislocation:
  causes, 1400–1401
  definition, 1400
  interdisciplinary care, 1401
  manifestations, 1401
  nursing care
    community-based care, 1401
    nursing diagnoses and interventions, 1401
  pathophysiology, 1401
Disopyramide, 1006t
Disorientation, 1529t
Dissecting aneurysm, 1170, 1592. See also Aortic dissection
Dissection, 1172. See also Aortic dissection
Disseminated intravascular coagulation (DIC):
  causes, 1146, 1146t
  definition, 1146
  interdisciplinary care
    diagnosis, 1148
    treatments, 1148
  manifestations, 1147, 1147t
  nursing care
    assessment, 1148
    community-based care, 1149
    nursing diagnoses and interventions
      fear, 1149
      impaired gas exchange, 1148–49
      ineffective tissue perfusion, 1148
      pain, 1149
  pathophysiology, 1146–47, 1147f
  in septic shock, 275
Distal dissection, 1172. See also Aortic dissection
Distraction, 186
Distributive shock, 274
Disulfiram:
  for alcohol abuse treatment, 112, 114t
  interaction with phenobarbital, 1551t
Dithranol. See Anthralin
Ditropan, Ditropan XL. See Oxybutynin
Diuretics:
  Medication Administration, 210t, 905t, 1033t, 1539t
  in specific conditions
    acute renal failure, 904, 905t
    chronic renal failure, 919
    fluid volume excess, 210, 210t
    heart failure, 1032, 1033t
    hyperkalemia, 225t
    hypertension, 1160, 1163
    increased intracranial pressure, 1538, 1539t
Diuril. See Chlorothiazide
Divalent, 196
Divergent thinking, 6
Diversity. See Race/ethnicity
Diverticular disease:
  characteristics, 814–15, 815f
  diverticulitis
    complications, 816
    definition, 815
    manifestations, 815–16
  diverticulosis, 815
  incidence, 815
  interdisciplinary care
    diagnosis, 816
    medications, 816
    nutrition, 816, 816t
    surgery, 816–17
  nursing care
    assessment, 817
    community-based care, 818
    health promotion, 817
    nursing diagnoses and interventions

  acute pain, 817
  anxiety, 817–18
  impaired tissue integrity: gastrointestinal, 817
  pathophysiology, 815
  risk factors, 815
Diverticulosis, 815. See also Diverticular disease
DKA. See Diabetic ketoacidosis
DMARDs (disease-modifying antirheumatic drugs), 341, 1464–66, 1465t
DNA, 149, 373t. See also Genetics
DNA-based tests, 157
DNR (do-not-resuscitate) order, 91
Dobutamine, 278t, 1034t
Dobutamine stress test, 944t. See also Stress/exercise tests
Dobutrex. See Dobutamine
Docusate:
  Medication Administration, 759t
  in specific conditions
    diverticulitis, 816
    hemorrhoids, 819
    intracranial aneurysm, 1593
    urine color changes caused by, 832t
Dofetilide, 1006t
Dolasetron, 672, 673t
Doll's eye movements, 1531, 1531f
Dolobid. See Diflunisal
Dolophine. See Methadone
Domestic violence. See Intimate partner violence
Donepezil, 189, 1621, 1621t
Dong quai, 1796
Donnagel-MB, 756t
Do-not-resuscitate (DNR) order, 91, 91t
Dopamine:
  functions, 1505
  Medication Administration, 278t, 1034t
  in specific conditions
    acute myocardial infarction, 989
    acute renal failure, 904
    heart failure, 1034t
    Parkinson's disease, 1635
    pulmonary edema, 1041
    shock, 278t
    substance abuse, 104, 104f
Dopamine agonists, 1638t
Dopamine antagonists, 672, 673t
Dopaminergics, 1637t
Dopar. See Levodopa
Doppler ultrasound, 1177, 1197
Dornase alfa, 1342
Dorsal recumbent position, 69f
Dorsiflexion, 1386t
Dorzolamide, 1709, 1710t
Dovonex. See Calcipotriene
Down syndrome. See Trisomy 21
Doxazosin, 1161t, 1779
Doxidan. See Docusate
Doxorubicin:
  adverse/side effects, 392t
  nursing implications, 392t
  in specific conditions
    bone tumors, 1483t
    leukemia, 1123t
  target malignancies, 392t
Doxy-Caps. See Doxycycline
Doxycin. See Doxycycline
Doxycycline:
  Medication Administration, 320t
  in specific conditions
    anthrax prophylaxis and treatment, 128t, 1294
    chlamydia, 1845, 1846
    Lyme disease, 1477
    pelvic inflammatory disease, 1851

  pneumonia, 1271t
  syphilis, 1849
Dramamine. See Dimenhydrinate
DRE. See Digital rectal examination
Dressings:
  biological and biosynthetic, 503–4
  for pressure ulcers, 474t
Dressler's syndrome, 986
DRGs (diagnosis-related groups), 38
Dronabinol, 672, 673t
Droperidol:
  Medication Administration, 673t
  preoperative use and nursing implications, 62t
  in specific conditions
    nausea and vomiting, 672, 673t
    vertigo, 1727
Droplet nuclei, 1280
Droplet precautions, 323t
Drowning, 1305–6, 1306f. See also Inhalation injury
Drug(s). See Medication(s)
Drug abuse, 179t. See also Substance abuse
Drug tolerance, 102, 103t, 179t
Drusen, 1714
"Dry drowning," 1306
Dry powder inhaler, 1324, 1325t
Dry skin, 441, 441t
DTRs. See Deep tendon reflexes
Dual diagnosis, 103, 103t
Dual disorder, 103
Dual energy x-ray absorptiometry (DEXA), 1387t, 1436
Dual-chamber pacing, 1009, 1010t. See also Pacemakers
DUB. See Dysfunctional uterine bleeding
Duchenne muscular dystrophy:
  genetic considerations, 1389t, 1458
  manifestations, 1459t
  progression, 1459t
Duct ectasia, 1821t, 1822
Duct of Wirsung, 726
Dulcolax. See Bisacodyl
Dullness, in lung percussion, 1224t
Dumping syndrome:
  after bariatric surgery, 638, 638t
  manifestations, 638, 690
  pathophysiology, 689–90, 690f
  treatment, 690–91
Duodenal string test, 779
Duodenal ulcers, 680. See also Peptic ulcer disease
Duodenum, 612, 742
DuoDerm. See Hydrocolloid dressing
Duplex Doppler ultrasound:
  in peripheral vascular disease, 1177
  in varicose veins, 1197
  in venous thrombosis, 1188
Durable power of attorney, 90. See also Advance directives
Duragesic. See Fentanyl
Dutasteride, 1779
DVT. See Deep venous thrombosis
Dwarfism, 530t
DynaCirc. See Isradipine
Dynapen. See Dicloxacillin
Dyrenium. See Triamterene
Dysarthria, 1518t, 1583
Dysfunctional uterine bleeding (DUB):
  definition, 1802
  interdisciplinary care
    diagnosis, 1803
    medications, 1803
    surgery
      dilation and curettage, 1803
      endometrial ablation, 1803
      hysterectomy, 1803–4

nursing care
  client having dilation and curettage, 1803t
  client having hysterectomy, 1804t
  community-based care, 1805
  nursing diagnoses and interventions
    anxiety, 1804–5
    sexual dysfunction, 1805
  pathophysiology, 1802
Dysmenorrhea:
  definition, 1800
  interdisciplinary care
    complementary and alternative therapies,
      1801–2
    diagnosis, 1801
    medications, 1801, 1802t
  manifestations, 1800, 1801t
  nursing care, 1802, 1802t
  pathophysiology, 1800
  primary, 1800
  secondary, 1800
Dyspareunia, 1758, 1795
Dysphagia, 668, 1520t
Dysphonia, 1518t
Dysplasia, 373
Dysplastic nevi, 466
Dyspnea:
  definition, 209, 1266
  in dying client, 92–93
  in fluid volume excess, 209
  paroxysmal nocturnal, 1027
Dysrhythmias. See Cardiac dysrhythmias
Dysuria, 839, 847

E

Ears. See also Hearing
  age-related changes, 1686t
  anatomy, physiology, and functions
    equilibrium, 1683
    external ear, 1680, 1682f
    inner ear, 1682
    middle ear, 1682–83, 1682f
    sound conduction, 1683
  assessment
    diagnostic tests, 1683–84, 1684t
    functional health pattern interview, 1685t
    genetic considerations, 1684, 1684t
    health assessment interview, 1684–85
    physical assessment
      external ear, 1688–89t, 1688f
      hearing, 1687–88t, 1687f, 1688f
      otoscope guidelines, 1686–87t, 1686f
    sample documentation, 1684t
  disorders
    acoustic neuroma, 1570t, 1727
    Chapter Highlights, 1734t
    Clinical Scenarios, 1738t
    foreign body, 1721
    hearing loss. See Hearing loss
    impacted cerumen, 1721
    inner ear. See Inner ear disorders
    mastoiditis. See Mastoiditis
    nursing care of the client having surgery
      for, 1725t
    otitis externa. See Otitis externa
    otosclerosis, 1725–26
Earthquake, 129t, 131
Eastern Cooperative Oncology Group, functional
      status scale, 401t
Eating disorders:
  anorexia nervosa, 650, 651t
  binge-eating disorder, 651, 651t
  bulimia nervosa, 650–51, 651t
  interdisciplinary care

diagnosis, 651–52
  treatment, 652
  nursing care, 652
EBCT (electron beam computed tomography), 965
Eccentric plaque formation, 959
Ecchymosis, 431t, 434f, 434t
Eccrine sweat glands, 424
ECF (extracellular fluid), 196–97, 196f, 197f
ECG. See Electrocardiogram
Echinacea:
  for benign prostatic hyperplasia, 1781
  for pneumonia, 1273
  for viral respiratory infections, 1231
Echocardiography:
  purpose and description, 943, 945t
  related nursing care, 945t
  in specific conditions
    acute myocardial infarction, 987
    angina, 971
    cardiomyopathy, 1067
    endocarditis, 1046
    heart failure, 1027
    pericarditis, 1051
    rheumatic heart disease, 1043t
    valvular heart disease, 1060
  types, 945t
Echolalia, 1620
Econazole, 450t
Ecotrin. See Aspirin
Ectopic beats, 996
Ectopic functioning, 380, 380t
Ectropion, 1701, 1701f
Eczema. See Atopic dermatitis
ED. See Erectile dysfunction
Edecrin. See Ethacrynic acid
Edema. See also Fluid volume excess
  in acute glomerulonephritis, 886
  assessment, 435f, 435t, 1097f, 1097t
  causes, 1093t
  cerebral, 1537. See also Increased intracranial
      pressure
  in cirrhosis, 715t
  definition, 209, 1093t
  grading, 1097f, 1097t
  in heart failure, 1027
  in metabolic acidosis, 245
  pulmonary. See Pulmonary edema
Edrophonium chloride, 1648, 1648t, 1649
Education level, health and, 19
Educator, nurse as, 13, 14f
EEG. See Electroencephalogram
E.E.S. See Erythromycin salts
Efavirenz, 358
Effector cells, 297. See also T lymphocytes
Efferent, 894
Effer-Syllium. See Psyllium hydrophilic mucilloid
Eflornithine, 778t
EGD. See Esophagogastroduodenoscopy
Egophony, 1226t
Ehlers-Danlos syndrome, 1172t
Ejaculatory dysfunction, 1771
Ejection fraction, 940, 1024
Elase. See Proteolytic enzymes
Elasticity, 1383
Elavil. See Amitriptyline
Elbows:
  epicondylitis, 1428
  fracture, 1413
  physical assessment, 1393t
Eldepryl. See Selegiline
Elder abuse, 256t
Elders. See Older adults
Elective lymph node dissection (ELND), 468
Elective procedure, 54t

Electrical bone stimulation, 1411–12, 1412f
Electrical burns, 488, 488t, 498. See also Burns
Electrocardiogram (ECG):
  interpretation, 949t
  intervals, 948f, 948t
  leads, 947f
  pacing artifacts, 1009, 1010f
  potassium levels and, 219, 219f
  in preoperative assessment, 60–61
  principles, 947–48t, 947f
  in specific conditions
    acute myocardial infarction, 987, 988f
    angina, 970, 971f
    cardiac dysrhythmias, 997–99t, 1004
    cardiomyopathy, 1067
    heart failure, 1027
    hypercalcemia, 232
    hypomagnesemia, 234
    metabolic acidosis, 245
    myocarditis, 1049
    pericarditis, 1051
    pulmonary embolism, 1349
    valvular heart disease, 1060
  waveforms, 947f, 947t
Electrodesiccation, 464
Electroencephalogram (EEG):
  in brain tumor diagnosis, 7, 1571
  health education for the client and family, 1515t
  nursing care, 1515t
  purpose and description, 1512, 1515t
Electrolarynx, 1256, 1258f, 1260t
Electrolytes. See also specific electrolytes
  in burns, 500
  composition of body fluid compartments, 197,
      197t
  definition, 196
  in fluid volume deficit, 205
  in fluid volume excess, 210
  functions, 196
  imbalances
    in acute renal failure, 904
    in altered level of consciousness, 1533
    calcium. See Hypercalcemia; Hypocalcemia
    in chronic renal failure, 918
    in cirrhosis, 716
    in glomerular disorders, 890, 890t
    in heart failure, 1027
    in inhalation injury, 1306–7
    magnesium. See Hypermagnesemia;
      Hypomagnesemia
    phosphate. See Hyperphosphatemia;
      Hypophosphatemia
    potassium. See Hyperkalemia; Hypokalemia
    sodium. See Hypernatremia; Hyponatremia
    surgical risk and nursing implications, 57t
  intravenous solutions, 207t
  normal values, 198t
  perioperative, significance and nursing
      implications, 60t
  in shock, 277
  units of measurement, 196
Electromyogram (EMG), 1388t, 1515t
Electron beam computed tomography (EBCT), 965
Electrophoresis, hemoglobin, 1110–11
Electrophysiology procedures, 1004–5
Electrosurgery, 477
Elimination disorders:
  bowel. See Bowel disorders
  urinary. See Urinary system, disorders
Elimination patterns:
  altered bowel elimination. See also Bowel
      disorders
    Build Clinical Competence, 824t
    Clinical Scenarios, 825t

Elimination patterns—*continued*
 altered urinary elimination. *See also* Urinary
  system
  Build Clinical Competence, 929*t*
  Clinical Scenarios, 930*t*
  NANDA nursing diagnoses, 739*t*
ELISA (enzyme-linked immunosorbent
  assay), 355
Ellis-van Creveld syndrome, 1389*t*
ELND (elective lymph node dissection), 468
Embolectomy, 1184
Embolic stroke, 1581. *See also* Stroke
Embolism:
 arterial. *See* Acute arterial occlusion
 definition, 1184
 fat, 1406
 pulmonary. *See* Pulmonary embolism
Embolization, uterine fibroid, 1810
Emergency:
 definition, 127
 vs. disaster, 127
 oncologic. *See* Oncologic emergencies
Emergency defibrillation, 1008, 1008*f*, 1008*t*
Emergency procedure, 54*t*
Emesis, 671. *See also* Nausea and vomiting
EMG (electromyogram), 1388*t*, 1515*t*
Emmetropia, 1696
Emollients, 441*t*
Emphysema, 1332, 1332*t*, 1360. *See also* Chronic
  obstructive pulmonary disease
Empyema:
 definition, 1269
 gallbladder, 698
 pleural, 1269, 1295
 treatment, 1296
E-Mycin. *See* Erythromycin
Enalapril, 1033*t*, 1161*t*
Enalaprilat, 1169*t*
Enbrel. *See* Etanercept
Encephalitis. *See also* Central nervous system
  infections
 arborvirus, 1565
 causes, 1565*t*
 viral, 1565. *See also* Rabies
Encephalopathy:
 hypertensive, 1158
 portal systemic, 704, 715, 715*t*
 spongiform. *See* Creutzfeldt-Jakob disease
Endarterectomy, 1178
Endocarditis:
 acute infective, 1046*t*
 complications, 1046
 definition, 1045
 incidence, 1045
 interdisciplinary care
  diagnosis, 1046
  medications, 1046–47
  prevention, 1046, 1047*t*
  surgery, 1047
 manifestations, 1045–46, 1046*t*
 nursing care
  assessment, 1047
  community-based care, 1048
  health promotion, 1047
  nursing diagnoses and interventions
   ineffective health maintenance, 1048
   risk for imbalanced body
    temperature, 1047
   risk for ineffective tissue perfusion,
    1047–48
 pathophysiology, 1045, 1045*f*, 1046*t*
 risk factors, 1045, 1046*t*
 subacute infective, 1046*t*
Endocardium, 937, 937*f*

Endocrine system:
 age-related changes
  in middle adults, 27*t*
  in older adults, 29*t*, 529*t*
 anatomy, physiology, and functions
  adrenal gland, 520–21, 520*f*
  gonads. *See* Ovaries; Testes
  overview, 518*f*, 519*t*
  pancreas, 521
  parathyroid glands, 520
  pituitary gland
   anatomy, 519*f*
   anterior, 519, 519*f*, 520
   posterior, 520
  thyroid gland, 520, 520*f*
 assessment
  diagnostic tests, 522, 523–25*t*, 526. *See also*
   specific tests
  genetic considerations, 527, 527*t*
  health assessment interview, 527
  physical assessment
   face, 529*t*
   hypocalcemic tetany, 531*t*
   motor function, 530*t*
   musculoskeletal function, 530*t*
   nails and hair, 529*t*
   overview, 527
   sample documentation, 527
   sensory function, 530*t*
   skin, 529*t*
   thyroid, 530*t*
 disorders
  adrenal glands
   Addison's disease (adrenocortical
    insufficiency). *See* Addison's disease
   Cushing's syndrome (hypercortisolism). *See*
    Cushing's syndrome
   pheochromocytoma, 557
  anterior pituitary gland
   acromegaly, 529*t*, 558, 558*f*
   gigantism, 558
   hyperfunction, 557
   hypofunction, 557
   interdisciplinary care, 558
   nursing care, 558
   pathophysiology, 557
  Clinical Scenarios, 601*t*
  pancreas. *See* Diabetes mellitus
  parathyroid glands
   hyperparathyroidism. *See*
    Hyperparathyroidism
   hypoparathyroidism. *See*
    Hypoparathyroidism
  posterior pituitary gland
   diabetes insipidus. *See* Diabetes insipidus
   syndrome of inappropriate antidiuretic
    hormone. *See* Syndrome of inappropriate
    diuretic hormone
  thyroid gland
   cancer, 546
   hyperthyroidism. *See* Hyperthyroidism
   hypothyroidism. *See* Hypothyroidism
End-of-life care. *See also* Death and dying; Loss
  and grief
 checklist for older adults, 95*t*
 comfort measures, 92*t*
 competencies, 89–90, 89*f*
 definition, 89
 health promotion, 95
 interdisciplinary care, 94–95
 legal and ethical issues
  advance directives. *See* Advance directives
  do-not-resuscitate orders, 91, 91*t*
  euthanasia, 91

 Nursing Research, 90*t*
 settings and services
  hospice. *See* Hospice
  palliative care, 92
  support for client and family, 93
  terminal weaning, mechanical ventilation, 1361
Endogenous, 304
Endogenous insulin, 566
Endoleak, 1173
Endolymphatic decompression, 1727
Endolymphatic hydrops. *See* Ménière's disease
Endometrial ablation, 1803
Endometrial biopsy, 1757*t*
Endometrial cancer:
 genetic considerations, 1755*t*, 1758
 incidence, 1816
 interdisciplinary care
  diagnosis, 1816
  medications, 1816
  radiation therapy, 1817
  surgery, 1816
 manifestations, 1816
 nursing care
  assessment, 1817
  community-based care, 1817
  health promotion, 1817
  nursing diagnoses and interventions
   acute pain, 1817
   disturbed body image, 1817
   ineffective sexuality pattern, 1817
 pathophysiology factors, 1816
 risk factors, 1816
 screening guidelines, 401*t*, 1817
 staging, 1816*t*
Endometrial cysts and polyps, 1808, 1809*t*
Endometriosis:
 definition, 1810
 interdisciplinary care
  diagnosis, 1810
  medications, 1811
  surgery, 1811
 manifestations, 1811*t*
 nursing care
  community-based care, 1812
  nursing diagnoses and interventions
   using NANDA, NIC, and NOC, 1812, 1812*t*
 Nursing Care Plan
  assessment, 1811*t*
  critical thinking in the nursing process, 1811*t*
  diagnoses, 1811*t*
  evaluation, 1811*t*
  expected outcomes, 1811*t*
  planning and implementation, 1811*t*
 pathophysiology, 1810
 risk factors, 1810
Endometritis, 1850
Endomyocardial biopsy, 1049
Endophytic, 1819
Endorphins, 172, 172*f*
Endoscopic retrograde cholangiopancreatography
  (ERCP), 616*t*, 727
Endoscopic sinus surgery, 1236–37
Endoscopic transduodenal sphincterotomy, 728
Endoscopy, 388*t*, 615*t*
Endothelins, 1158
Endotoxins, 312
Endotracheal tube:
 in acute respiratory failure, 1355–56, 1356*f*
 for airway management, 257, 257*f*
 suctioning procedure, 1363*t*
 vs. tracheostomy, 1356, 1357*t*
Endovascular stent grafts, 1173
End-stage renal disease (ESRD), 899. *See also*
  Chronic renal failure

Enemas, 760
Energy healing, for cancer, 399*t*
Enfuvirtide, 358
Engle, theory of loss and grief, 86, 86*t*
Enophthalmos, 1702
Enoxacin, 849
Enoxaparin, 1189*t*, 1585
Entacapone, 1638*t*, 1639
Entamoeba histolytica, 725, 778, 778*t*
Enteral nutrition:
  complications, 646
  in Crohn's disease, 788
  definition, 644
  feeding tube placement, 646*f*, 646*t*
  formulas, 646
  in malnutrition, 644–46
  Nursing Research
    aspiration prevention, 772*t*
    assessing gastric residual volume, 662*t*
    feeding tube placement methods, 647*t*
  tubes for, 645, 645*f*
Enteritis. *See* Gastroenteritis
Enterobiasis, 781*t*
Enterococci, vancomycin-resistant, 314
Entero-Test. *See* Duodenal string test
Entropion, 1694*f*, 1701
Entry inhibitors, 358
Enucleation, 1718
Environment, health and, 20, 37. *See also* Physical
    stressors
Enzymatic debridement, 504
Enzyme-linked immunosorbent assay (ELISA), 355
Enzymes, as tumor markers, 384, 384*t*
Eosinopenia, 307*t*
Eosinophilia, 307*t*, 779
Eosinophils:
  abnormal, possible causes, 307*t*, 387*t*
  characteristics, 288
  development, 289*f*, 1077*f*
  functions, 288, 288*t*, 1079
  location, 288*t*
  normal values, 307*t*, 387*t*, 1118*t*
Ependymoma, 1570*t*. *See also* Brain tumors
Ephedra, 1274, 1326
Epicardial pacemaker, 1009, 1009*f*. *See also*
    Pacemakers
Epicardium, 937, 937*f*
Epicondylitis, 1428. *See also* Repetitive use
    injury
Epidermis, 423, 423*t*, 424*f*. *See also* Skin
Epididymis:
  anatomy, physiology, and functions, 1745, 1745*t*
  physical assessment, 1750*t*
Epididymitis:
  definition, 1773
  interdisciplinary care, 1773
  nursing care, 1773
  pathophysiology, 1773
Epidural analgesia:
  benefits, 183
  nursing care, 184*t*
  procedure, 184*f*, 184*t*
Epidural anesthesia, 63
Epidural hematoma, 1557–58, 1557*f*, 1557*t*. *See*
    also Traumatic brain injury
Epiglottis, 1211
Epiglottitis, 1240–41
Epilepsy. *See also* Seizures
  genetic considerations, 1513*t*
  incidence and prevalence, 1547–48
  interdisciplinary care
    diagnosis, 1550
    medications, 1550–51, 1550*t*

surgery, 1551
  vagal nerve stimulation surgery, 1551
  nursing care
    assessment, 1552, 1553*t*
    of client having surgery for seizures, 1551*t*
    community-based care, 1553–54
    health promotion, 1551–52
    Medication Administration, 1550*t*
    nursing diagnoses and interventions
      anxiety, 1553
      risk for ineffective airway clearance,
        1552–53
    using NANDA, NIC, and NOC,
      1553, 1553*t*
  Nursing Care Plan
    assessment, 1552*t*
    critical thinking in the nursing process, 1552*t*
    diagnoses, 1552*t*
    evaluation, 1552*t*
    expected outcomes, 1552*t*
    planning and implementation, 1552*t*
  in older adults, 1548*t*
  pathophysiology, 1548
Epinephrine:
  in blood pressure regulation, 1155
  functions, 519*t*, 520
  Medication Administration, 1327*t*
  in specific conditions
    anaphylaxis, 337–38
    asthma, 1327*t*
    topical, for epistaxis, 1243
Epispadias, 872
Epistaxis:
  causes, 1243
  definition, 1243
  interdisciplinary care
    first aid measures, 1243
    medications, 1243
    nasal packing, 1244, 1244*f*
    surgery, 1244
  manifestations, 1243
  nursing care
    assessment, 1244
    of client with nasal packing, 1245*t*
    community-based care, 1245
    nursing diagnoses and interventions
      anxiety, 1245
      risk for aspiration, 1245
  pathophysiology, 1243
Epithalamus, 1506
Epitope, 290
Epivir. *See* Lamivudine
Epivir HBV. *See* Lamivudine
Epoprostenol, 1353
Eprosartan, 1161*t*
Epstein-Barr virus:
  cancers associated with, 375*t*
  in Hodgkin's disease, 1130
  in infectious mononucleosis, 1139
Eptifibatide, 976, 976*t*
Equal. *See* Aspartame
Equianalgesia:
  definition, 80, 179*t*
  drug chart with nursing considerations, 180*t*
Equilibrium, 1683
ERCP (endoscopic retrograde
    cholangiopancreatography), 616*t*, 727
Erectile dysfunction (ED):
  causes, 1768*t*, 1769
  in cirrhosis, 715*t*
  definition, 1768
  in diabetes mellitus, 595
  incidence, 1768–69

interdisciplinary care
  diagnosis, 1769
  mechanical devices, 1769
  medications, 1769
  surgery, 1769–70, 1770*f*
  nursing care
    community-based care, 1771
    nursing diagnoses and interventions
      sexual dysfunction, 1770
      situational low self-esteem, 1771
  pathophysiology, 1769
Erection, 1744
Ergonovine maleate, 971
Ergot alkaloid derivatives, 1545*t*
Ergotamine tartrate, 1544, 1545*t*
Erikson, psychosocial development theory, 25*t*
Erosion, skin, 433*t*
Erosive gastritis, 677. *See also* Stress ulcers
Ertapenem, 319*t*
ERV (expiratory reserve volume), 1214, 1214*t*
Erysipelas, 447
Erythema:
  assessment in light and dark skin, 426*t*
  causes, 426*t*
  definition, 425
  figurate, 431*t*
Erythema marginatum, 1043
Erythema migrans, 1477
Erythematous, 1229
Erythrocin. *See* Erythromycin salts
Erythrocyte sedimentation rate (ESR; sed rate):
  normal values, 1087*t*
  purpose and description, 1087*t*
  in specific conditions
    glomerular disorders, 889
    inflammation, 306
    lymphoma, 1131
    rheumatic fever, 1043
    rheumatic heart disease, 1043*t*
    systemic lupus erythematosus, 1473
Erythrocytes. *See* Red blood cells
Erythrocytosis. *See* Polycythemia
Erythromycin:
  Medication Administration, 320*t*
  in specific conditions
    endocarditis prophylaxis, 1047*t*
    Lyme disease, 1477
    pertussis, 1242
    pneumonia, 1271*t*
  topical
    for conjunctivitis, 1694
    for corneal infections, 1697
Erythromycin salts, 320*t*
Erythroplakia, 1253
Erythropoiesis, 1076, 1078, 1079*f*
Erythropoietin, 834, 1111
Escape rhythm, 1000
Eschar, 494
Escharotomy, 502, 502*f*, 502*t*
Escherichia coli:
  in hemorrhagic colitis, 774*t*, 775
  in liver abscess, 725
  in traveler's diarrhea, 774*t*, 775
  in urinary tract infections, 846
Esmolol:
  Medication Administration, 1006*t*
  in specific conditions
    acute myocardial infarction, 988
    aortic aneurysm, 1173
    cardiac dysrhythmias, 1006*t*
    hypertensive emergencies, 1169*t*
Esomeprazole, 665, 665*t*, 678
Esophageal acidity, 615*t*

Esophageal cancer:
  interdisciplinary care
    diagnosis, 669
    treatments, 669–70
  manifestations, 669, 669t
  nursing care
    assessment, 670
    community-based care, 670–71
    health promotion, 670
    nursing diagnoses and interventions
      anticipatory grieving, 670
      imbalanced nutrition: less than body
        requirements, 670
      risk for ineffective airway clearance, 670
  pathophysiology, 669
  risk factors, 669, 669t
Esophageal manometry, 615t, 665
Esophageal speech, 1256
Esophageal varices:
  in cirrhosis, 711
  pathophysiology, 704, 712–13t, 715t
  treatment, 718
Esophagectomy, 669–70
Esophagogastroduodenoscopy (EGD):
  purpose and description, 615t
  related nursing care, 615t
  in specific conditions
    esophageal cancer, 669
    gastritis, 678
    gastroesophageal reflux disease, 664
    peptic ulcer disease, 684
    upper gastrointestinal bleeding, 674, 675
Esophagojejunostomy, 689, 689f
Esophagus:
  anatomy, physiology, and functions, 610–11, 611f
  disorders
    cancer. See Esophageal cancer
    diagnostic tests, 615t
    gastroesophageal reflux disease. See
      Gastroesophageal reflux disease
    hiatal hernia. See Hiatal hernia
    impaired motility, 668, 668f
ESR. See Erythrocyte sedimentation rate
ESRD (end-stage renal disease), 899. See also
  Chronic renal failure
Essential tremor, 1513t
Estar. See Coal tar derivatives
Estradiol, 386t, 1753
Estrogen:
  functions, 1753
  osteoporosis and, 1434
  replacement therapy. See Hormone replacement
    therapy
  vaginal effects, 1752
ESWL. See Extracorporeal shock wave lithotripsy
Etanercept:
  in autoimmune disorders, 341
  in psoriasis, 444
  in rheumatoid arthritis, 1465
ETCO2. See Exhaled carbon dioxide
Ethacrynic acid:
  Medication Administration, 210t, 905t,
    1033t, 1539t
  in specific conditions
    acute renal failure, 905t
    fluid volume excess, 210t
    heart failure, 1033t
    increased intracranial pressure, 1538, 1539t
Ethambutol:
  dosage, 1288t
  Medication Administration, 1289t
  nursing implications, 1288t
  optic neuritis and, 1287, 1288t
  for tuberculosis, 1289t

Ether, abuse, 111
Ethics, 10. See also Nursing ethics
Ethinyl estradiol, 1802t
Ethmozine. See Moricizine
Ethnicity. See Race/ethnicity
Ethnopharmacology, 176
Ethosuximide, 1550t
Etidronate, 232
Etodolac, 178t, 1464t
Etoposide, 391, 393t, 1775
Euploidy, 150t
European Americans. See Caucasians/European
  Americans
Euthanasia, 91
Euthyroid. See Liotrix
Euthyroid, definition, 537
Evac-U-Gen. See Phenolphthalein
Evac-U-Lax. See Phenolphthalein
Evaluation, 7t, 10
Evening primrose, 1796
Eversion, 1386t
Evidence-based practice. See Nursing Research:
  Evidence-Based Practice
Evisceration, 78, 78f
Evista. See Raloxifene
Evoked potentials, 1515t
Evoked response, 1627
Exacerbation, 23
Excisional biopsy:
  breast, 1824, 1824f
  definition, 388t
  skin, 428t
Excitability, 995, 1383
Exelon. See Rivastigmine tartrate
Exenatide, 576
Exercise:
  in chronic obstructive pulmonary disease
    management, 1334–35, 1335t
  coronary heart disease risk reduction and,
    964, 966
  in diabetes management, 580–81
  in heart failure management, 1034
  in hypertension management, 1159–60
  in obesity treatment, 634, 634t, 635t
  osteoporosis risk and, 1434
  in rheumatoid arthritis treatment, 1466
Exercise ECG tests. See Stress/exercise tests
Exfoliative dermatitis, 457
Exhaled carbon dioxide (ETCO2):
  in acute respiratory failure, 1355
  in chronic obstructive pulmonary
    disease, 1334
  in pulmonary embolism, 1349
Exogenous, 304
Exogenous insulin, 566
Exophthalmos, 529t, 536, 536f
Exophytic, 1819
Exostoses, 1719
Exotoxins, 311
Expansion, infarct, 985
Expiration, 1215, 1215f
Expiratory reserve volume (ERV), 1214, 1214t
Expressive aphasia, 1583
Extended-spectrum beta-lactamase, 314
Extensibility, 1383
Extension, 1386t
Extension, infarct, 985
External auditory canal, 1680, 1682f, 1688
External AV shunt, 908
External fixation, 1410–11, 1411f, 1419t
External hemorrhoids, 818, 818f. See also
  Hemorrhoids
External rotation, 1386t
External sphenoethmoidectomy, 1237, 1237f

Extracapsular fracture, 1414, 1415f. See also Hip,
  fracture
Extracellular fluid (ECF), 196–97, 196f, 197f
Extracorporeal shock wave lithotripsy (ESWL):
  for gallstones, 700–701
  nursing care, 701, 859t
  for urinary calculi, 858, 858f
Extradural hematoma. See Epidural hematoma
Extranodal marginal zone lymphoma, 1130t. See
  also Lymphomas
Extubation, 1356
Exudate, 1295
Exudative macular degeneration, 1714
Eyelids:
  anatomy and functions, 1670, 1670f
  disorders
    interdisciplinary care, 1701
    nursing care, 1701
    pathophysiology and manifestations,
      1700–1701, 1701f
Eyes. See also Vision
  age-related changes, 1676t
  anatomy, physiology, and functions
    extraocular muscles, 1671f
    extraocular structures, 1670, 1670f
    intraocular structures
      aqueous fluid, 1671–72
      internal chamber, 1672
      iris, 1671
      overview, 1672f
      sclera and cornea, 1671
    refraction, 1673
    visual pathway, 1672–73, 1673f
  assessment
    diagnostic tests, 1674, 1675t
    genetic considerations, 1674, 1674t
    health assessment interview, 1674
    physical assessment
      external eyes, 1679–80t, 1679f
      eye movement, 1677–78t, 1677f
      internal eyes, 1680t, 1681t
      ophthalmoscope guidelines, 1681t
      pupils, 1678–79t
      vision, 1676–77t, 1677f
      visual fields, 1675–76t, 1676f, 1708f
  disorders
    age-related macular degeneration. See Age-
      related macular degeneration
    cataracts. See Cataracts
    Chapter Highlights, 1734t
    Clinical Scenarios, 1738t
    conjunctivitis. See Conjunctivitis
    corneal. See Corneal disorders
    diabetic retinopathy. See Diabetic retinopathy
    enucleation for, 1718
    eyelids
      interdisciplinary care, 1701
      nursing care, 1701
      pathophysiology and manifestations,
        1700–1701, 1701f
    glaucoma. See Glaucoma
    in HIV/AIDS, 1718
    incidence, 1692
    retinal detachment. See Retinal detachment
    retinitis pigmentosa, 1717–18
    uveitis. See Uveitis
  functional health pattern interview, 1675t
  prosthetic, removing and inserting, 1719t
  trauma
    blunt, 1702
    burns, 1702
    corneal abrasion, 1701–2
    in disasters, 129t, 131
    interdisciplinary care, 1702–3

nursing care
  community-based care, 1703
  health promotion, 1703
  nursing diagnoses and interventions, 1703
  pathophysiology and manifestations, 1701–2
  penetrating, 1702

F

F cells, pancreas, 521
Fab (antigen-binding fragment), 296, 297f
Face:
  assessment, 529t
  fracture, 1412
Facial nerve (cranial nerve VII):
  anatomy, 1510f
  assessment, 1520t
  functions, 1511t
Facial paralysis. See Bell's palsy
Facilitated diffusion, 200
Factor IX, 1144
Factor VIII, 1144
Factor XI deficiency. See also Hemophilia
  characteristics, 1143t
  pathophysiology, 1143
  treatment, 1143t
Fallopian tubes, 1751t, 1753, 1753f
Falls:
  hip fracture and, 1415. See also Hip, fracture
  prevention, 1418t, 1623t
False aneurysm, 1170
Famciclovir, 453, 1839
Familial adenomatous polyposis (FAP), 746t, 801
Familial Alzheimer's disease, 1618
Familial hypercholesterolemia, 950t
Family:
  of client with chronic illness, 33
  definition, 31
  developmental stages and tasks
    couple, 32
    family with adolescents and young adults, 33
    family with infants and preschoolers, 32
    family with middle adults, 33
    family with older adults, 33
    family with school-age children, 33
    overview, 31–32
  functions, 31
  in grieving process, 88
  risk factors for alterations in health, 32t
Famotidine:
  Medication Administration, 665t
  preoperative use and nursing implications, 62t
  in specific conditions
    burns, 502
    gastritis, 678
    gastroesophageal reflux disease, 502
Famvir. See Famciclovir
Fanconi anemia, 1109
FAP (familial adenomatous polyposis), 746t, 801
Far point of accommodation, 1673
Fascial excision, 502
Fasciculations, 1522t, 1645
Fasciectomy, 502
Fascioliasis, 781t
Fascioscapulohumeral muscular dystrophy, 1459t
FAST (focused assessment by sonography in trauma), 261
Fastin. See Phentermine
Fasting blood sugar, 386t, 526t. See also Blood glucose
Fast-tracking, 62
Fat embolism syndrome (FES), 1406
Fat necrosis, breast, 1821t
Fats, dietary:

in diabetes mellitus, 579
foods high in, 702t
recommended dietary guidelines, 606t
sources, 579, 608
types, 607–8
uses in body, 607f, 608
Fat-soluble vitamins, 608, 608t
F_c (crystallized fragment), 296, 296f
FCC (fibrocystic changes), 1820–21, 1821t, 1822f
Fecal impaction, 758
Fecal incontinence:
  causes, 763, 763t
  definition, 763
  interdisciplinary care, 764–65
  nursing care
    assessment, 765
    community-based care, 765–66
    health promotion, 765
    nursing diagnoses and interventions
      bowel incontinence, 765
      risk for impaired skin integrity, 765
    Nursing Research: self-care practices, 764t
  pathophysiology, 764
Fecalith, 766
Feces. See Stool
Feedback mechanisms, 521–22, 522f
Feeding tube. See Enteral nutrition
Feen-A-Mint. See Phenolphthalein
Feet:
  care
    in diabetes mellitus, 594t
    in peripheral vascular disease, 1178t
  deformities
    hallux valgus, 1492, 1492f
    hammertoe, 1492
    interdisciplinary care, 1493
    Morton's neuroma, 1492–93, 1493f
    nursing care
      community-based care, 1493
      nursing diagnoses and interventions, 1493
  in diabetes mellitus, complications, 590, 590f
  fracture, 1416
  physical assessment, 1394t
Feldene. See Piroxicam
Felodipine, 973–74t, 1162t
Female reproductive system:
  age-related changes, 27t, 29t, 1760t
  anatomy, physiology, and functions
    breasts, 1751, 1752f
    external genitalia, 1751–52, 1751t, 1752f
    internal organs, 1751t
    menstrual cycle, 1754–55, 1754f
    oogenesis and the ovarian cycle, 1754, 1754f
    sex hormones, 1753
  assessment
    diagnostic tests, 1755, 1756–58t
    functional health pattern interview, 1759–60t
    genetic considerations, 1755, 1755t
    health assessment interview, 1758
    physical assessment
      axillary lymph nodes, 1762f, 1762t
      breasts, 1761–62t, 1761f
      external genitalia, 1762–63t
      overview, 1760
    sample documentation, 1755
  disorders
    benign breast disorders
      fibrocystic changes, 1820–21, 1821t
      interdisciplinary care, 1821t, 1822
      intraductal, 1821–22, 1821t
      manifestations, 1820–22, 1821t
      nursing care, 1822
      pathophysiology, 1820–22
    breast cancer. See Breast cancer

cervical cancer. See Cervical cancer
Chapter Highlights, 1833t
Clinical Scenarios, 1855t
cysts or polyps
  interdisciplinary care, 1808–9
  manifestations, 1808
  nursing care, 1809
  pathophysiology, 1808
dysfunctional uterine bleeding. See Dysfunctional uterine bleeding
dysmenorrhea. See Dysmenorrhea
endometrial cancer. See Endometrial cancer
endometriosis. See Endometriosis
leiomyoma. See Leiomyoma
menopause-related. See Menopause
ovarian cancer. See Ovarian cancer
premenstrual syndrome. See Premenstrual syndrome
sexual dysfunction
  anorgasmia, 1795
  dyspareunia, 1795
  inhibited sexual desire, 1795
  nursing care, 1795
sexually transmitted infections. See Sexually transmitted infections
uterine displacement. See Uterine displacement
vaginal fistula, 1807–8
vulvar cancer. See Vulvar cancer
Femara, 1825
Femoral artery, 1097t, 1172
Femur:
  fracture of head or neck. See Hip, fracture
  fracture of shaft, 1414
Fenamates, 178t, 306
Fenofibrate, 967t
Fenoldopam, 1169t
Fenoprofen calcium, 178t, 179t, 1464t
Fentanyl, 62t, 190t
Ferric chloride, 465t
Ferrlecit. See Sodium ferric gluconate
Ferrous gluconate, 1112t
Ferrous sulfate, 716, 1112t
FES (fat embolism syndrome), 1406
FEV_1 (forced expiratory volume), 1214t
Fever blister. See Herpes simplex
Fexofenadine, 1230t
FFP (fresh frozen plasma), 263t
Fiber, dietary:
  in constipation, 760, 761
  for coronary heart disease risk reduction, 966
  in diabetes mellitus, 579
  in diverticular disease, 816, 817
  in irritable bowel syndrome, 763
  sources, 579, 816t
Fibercon. See Calcium polycarbophil
Fiberoptic bronchoscopy. See Bronchoscopy
Fibrates. See Fibric acid derivatives
Fibric acid derivatives, 967t, 968
Fibrin degradation products, 1148
Fibrin split products, 1148
Fibrin stabilizing factor, 1082t
Fibrinogen, 386t, 1082t
Fibrinolysis, 1081
Fibrinolytic therapy:
  nursing care
    during the infusion, 989t
    postinfusion, 989t
    preinfusion, 989t
  in specific conditions
    acute arterial occlusion, 1184
    acute myocardial infarction, 987–88
    pulmonary embolism, 1349
    thrombotic stroke, 1585
    venous thrombosis, 1188

Fibrinous exudate, 293
Fibroadenoma, 1821t
Fibrocystic changes (FCC), 1820–21, 1821t, 1822f
Fibroid tumor. See Leiomyoma
Fibromyalgia:
  incidence, 1486–87
  interdisciplinary care, 1487
  manifestations, 1487, 1487f
  nursing care, 1487
  pathophysiology, 1487
Fibrosarcoma, 1482t. See also Bone tumors
Fibula, fracture, 1416
Fifth vital sign, 170. See also Pain
Figurate erythema, 431t. See also Erythema
Filariasis, 1199
Filtration, 200, 200f
Finasteride, 1778
Fine-needle biopsy:
  breast, 1757t, 1824, 1824f
  definition, 388t
Fingers, 1393t
FIO₂ (oxygen concentration), 1360, 1360t
Fires, 487. See also Burns
First episode infection, 1839
First-degree AV block:
  causes, 1003
  ECG characteristics, 999t, 1003
  management, 999t
  pathophysiology, 1003
Fissures:
  anal, 820
  skin, 433t
Fistula:
  anorectal, 820–21
  in diverticular disease, 816
  vaginal, 1807–8
Fixed cells, 295
Flaccid neurogenic bladder, 870. See also
    Neurogenic bladder
Flaccidity:
  causes, 1522t
  definition, 1522t, 1584
  in stroke, 1584
Flagyl. See Metronidazole
Flail chest, 1303, 1303f, 1414. See also Thoracic
    trauma
Flap (closed) amputation, 1421, 1422t
Flash blindness, 131
Flashover effect, 488
Flat bones, 1380
Flat wart, 452, 1841. See also Genital warts
Flatus, 746
Flavoxate hydrochloride, 871, 871t
Flaxseed oil, 760
Flaxseeds, 761, 1796
Flecainide, 1006t
Fleet enema. See Phosphate enema
Fletcher's Castoria. See Senna
Flexall 454. See Counterirritants
Flexeril. See Cyclobenzaprine
Flexion, 1386t
Flolan. See Epoprostenol
Flomax. See Tamsulosin
Flovent. See Fluticasone propionate
Flow-cycled ventilators, 1358
Floxin. See Ofloxacin
Flu. See Influenza
Fluconazole:
  indications, 318, 321
  Medication Administration, 450t
  in specific conditions
    fungal meningitis, 1566
    thrush, 657t, 658
Flucytosine, 1566

Fludara. See Fludarabine
Fludarabine, 1123t
Fludrocortisone, 555t
Fluid challenge, 206
Fluid exudate, 292–93
Fluid replacement:
  in diarrhea, 755
  in increased intracranial pressure, 1539, 1539t
  Medication Administration, 1539t
Fluid restriction:
  in acute renal failure, 905
  in chronic renal failure, 919
  guidelines, 210t
Fluid resuscitation:
  for burns, 499
  definition, 499
  for diabetic ketoacidosis, 585–86
  for shock
    colloid solutions, 277–78
    crystalloid solutions, 277
Fluid volume deficit (FVD):
  causes, 203
  definition, 203
  interdisciplinary care
    assessment findings, 205t
    diagnosis, 205
    fluid challenge, 206
    fluid management
      intravenous therapy, 205–6
      oral rehydration, 205
    manifestations, 203, 204t, 205, 205t
    Multisystem Effects, 204t
  nursing care
    assessment, 207, 207t, 208t
    community-based care, 208–9
    health promotion, 206
    nursing diagnoses and interventions
      deficient fluid volume, 207–8
      ineffective tissue perfusion, 208
      risk for injury, 208
    of older adults, 203t
    using NANDA, NIC, and NOC, 208, 209t
  Nursing Research: weight vs. input-output
    records for assessment, 208t
  pathophysiology, 203
  third spacing, 203
Fluid volume excess:
  definition, 209
  interdisciplinary care
    assessment findings, 205t
    diagnosis, 210
    medications, 210, 210t
    treatment
      dietary management, 210–11
      fluid management, 210, 210t
    manifestations and complications, 205t, 209–10
  nursing care
    assessment, 211
    community-based care, 213
    health promotion, 211
    Medication Administration, 210t
    nursing diagnoses and interventions, 211
      excess fluid volume, 211–12
      risk for impaired gas exchange, 213
      risk for impaired skin integrity, 213
  Nursing Care Plan
    assessment, 212t
    critical thinking in the nursing process, 212t
    diagnoses, 212t
    evaluation, 212t
    expected outcomes, 212t
    planning and implementation, 212t
  pathophysiology, 209
Fluids. See Body fluids

Fluids and electrolytes:
  body fluid composition
    electrolytes, 196, 197, 197f. See also
        Electrolytes
    water, 195–96
  body fluid distribution, 196–97, 196f, 197f
  body fluid movement
    active transport, 200, 201f
    diffusion, 199–200, 200f
    filtration, 200, 200f
    osmosis
      definition, 198, 198f
      osmolarity and osmolality, 198
      osmotic pressure and tonicity, 198–99, 199f
  body fluid regulation
    antidiuretic hormone, 201–2, 202f
    atrial natriuretic peptide, 202
    kidneys, 201
    renin–angiotensin–aldosterone system, 201, 202f
    thirst, 200–201, 201f
  changes in older adults, 202
  Chapter Highlights, 252
  imbalances
    calcium. See Hypercalcemia; Hypocalcemia
    in chronic renal failure, 915–16
    fluid volume deficit. See Fluid volume
        deficit
    fluid volume excess. See Fluid volume
        excess
    magnesium. See Hypermagnesemia;
        Hypomagnesemia
    phosphate. See Hyperphosphatemia;
        Hypophosphatemia
    potassium. See Hyperkalemia; Hypokalemia
    sodium. See Hypernatremia; Hyponatremia
  normal gain and loss in an adult, 196t
Flumadine. See Rimantadine
Flunisolide, 1328t
Fluorescein angiogram, 1714
Fluorescein stain, 1694, 1697
Fluorescent treponemal antibody absorption (FTA-
    ABS), 1746t, 1756t, 1849
Fluoride therapy, 1436, 1437t
Fluoroquinolones:
  Medication Administration, 320t
  in specific conditions
    gonorrhea, 1846
    pneumonia, 1271, 1271t
5-Fluorouracil (5-FU):
  adverse/side effects, 392t
  nursing implications, 392t
  in specific conditions
    colorectal cancer, 805
    laryngeal cancer, 1254
    target malignancies, 392t
Fluoxetine:
  for eating disorders, 652
  for irritable bowel syndrome, 763
  for premenstrual syndrome, 1798
  for substance abuse/withdrawal treatment, 114t
Flurbiprofen, 178t, 1464t
Flutamide, 1787t
Fluticasone propionate, 1328t
Fluvastatin, 967t
Focal sclerosis, 888. See also Glomerular disorders
Focus on Cultural Diversity. See also
    Race/ethnicity
  breast cancer, 1822t
  cancer, 370t
  cirrhosis, 711t
  diabetes mellitus, 564t
  dying and death, 89t
  G6PD anemia, 1106t
  gallstones, 697

heart disease, 958t
heart failure, 1023t, 1035t
hemolytic anemias, 1106t
HIV/AIDS, 349t
hypertension, 1157t
inflammatory bowel disease, 782t
lactase deficiency, 798t
obesity, 631t
osteoarthritis, 1449t
osteoporosis, 1434t
prostate cancer, 1783t
sickle cell anemia, 1106t, 1107t
stroke, 1580t
substance use, 105t
testicular cancer, 1774t
thalassemia, 1106t
tuberculosis, 1281t
Focused assessment by sonography in trauma
    (FAST), 261
Folate. See Folic acid
Folic acid:
  for anemia in cirrhosis, 716
  deficiency
    causes, 1106, 1106t
    interdisciplinary care, 1110t, 1111t, 1112t
    manifestations, 1106
    neural tube defects and, 1106
    Nursing Care Plan
      assessment, 1113t
      critical thinking in the nursing process, 1113t
      diagnoses, 1113t
      expected outcomes, 1113t
      planning and implementation, 1113t
    pathophysiology, 1105–6
  functions, 609t
  recommended daily intake, 609t
  replacement therapy, 1112t
  sources, 609t, 1111t
  for substance abuse/withdrawal treatment, 114t
Folinic acid, 805
Follicle-stimulating hormone (FSH):
  functions, 520, 1753
  in ovarian cycle, 1754, 1754f
Follicular lymphoma, 1130t. See also Lymphomas
Follicular thyroid cancer, 546
Folliculitis, 446, 446f
Folvite. See Folic acid, replacement therapy
Food allergy:
  anaphylaxis caused by, 332, 332t
  testing, 337
Food Guide Pyramid, 21f
Food poisoning. See Gastroenteritis
Foot care. See Feet, care
Foradil. See Formoterol
Foraminotomy, 1610
Forced expiratory volume (FEV₁), 1214t
Forced vital capacity (FVC), 1214t
Foreign bodies:
  in ear, 1721
  retained after surgery, 59
Forequarter amputation, 1422t
Foreskin, 1749t, 1771
Formoterol, 1327t
Formulas, enteral feeding, 646t
Fornix, 1752
Fortaz. See Ceftazidime
Forteo. See Teriparatide
Forward effects, heart failure, 1026
Fosamax. See Alendronate
Foscarnet, 359t, 1718, 1839
Foscavir. See Foscarnet
Fosinopril, 1033t, 1161t
Fototar. See Coal tar derivatives
Fowler, spiritual development theory, 25t

Fractures:
  Case Study, 1499t
  classification, 1401–2, 1402f
  complications. See also Deep venous thrombosis
    compartment syndrome. See Compartment
      syndrome
    deep venous thrombosis, 1406, 1406t
    delayed union and nonunion, 1407
    fat embolism syndrome, 1406
    infection, 1406–7
    reflex sympathetic dystrophy, 1407
    Volkmann's contracture, 1406
  definition, 1401
  healing
    factors affecting, 1403t
    phases, 1402, 1404–5t
  interdisciplinary care
    diagnosis, 1407, 1407f
    emergency care, 1407
    medications, 1408
    pain management, 1408t
    treatments
      casts, 1409–10, 1410f, 1419t
      electrical bone stimulation, 1411–12, 1412f
      surgery, 1410–11, 1411f
      traction, 1408, 1409t, 1419t
  manifestations, 1402–3, 1403t
  nursing care
    assessment, 1417–18
    client in traction, 1409t
    client with a cast, 1410t
    client with internal fixation, 1412t
    clients with fracture of the humerus, 1413t
    community-based care, 1420–21
    health promotion, 1416–17
    nursing diagnoses and interventions
      acute pain, 1418
      impaired physical mobility, 1420
      risk for disturbed sensory perception:
        tactile, 1420
      risk for infection, 1419–20
      risk for peripheral neurovascular
        dysfunction, 1418–19, 1419f
    using NANDA, NIC, and NOC, 1420, 1420t
    Nursing Research: care of pin insertion sites, 1419t
    in osteoporosis, 1435
  pathophysiology, 1401
  of specific bones or areas
    clavicle, 1412–13
    elbow, 1413
    face, 1412
    femoral shaft, 1414
    hip. See Hip, fracture
    humerus
      characteristics, 1413
      nursing interventions, 1413t
    nose. See Nasal trauma
    pelvis, 1414
    radius and/or ulna, 1413
    rib, 1302–3, 1414. See also Thoracic trauma
    skull. See Skull fracture
    spine, 1412
    wrist or hand, 1413–14
Fragmin. See Dalteparin
Framingham Heart Study, 962t
Frank-Starling mechanism, 1024t, 1025
FRC (functional residual capacity), 1214t
Freestanding outpatient surgical facilities, 55
Fresh frozen plasma (FFP), 263t
Freud, theory of loss and grief, 85, 86t
Friction rub, 1226t
Friedreich's ataxia, 1513t
Frontal lobe, 1506f, 1506t
Frontotemporal dementia, 1618t

Frostbite, 476–77
Fructose, 579
FSH. See Follicle-stimulating hormone
FTA-ABS (fluorescent treponemal antibody
    absorption), 1746t, 1756t, 1849
5-FU. See 5-Fluorouracil
Fulguration:
  of bladder tumor, 864
  of colorectal tumors, 803
Full-thickness avulsion injuries, 259
Full-thickness burn, 490, 490f. See also Burns
Full-thickness graft, 478, 478f
Fulminant colitis, 784. See also Inflammatory
    bowel disease
Fulminant hepatitis, 706. See also Hepatitis
Fulvicin. See Griseofulvin
Functional colitis. See Irritable bowel syndrome
Functional disease, 22t
Functional health pattern interviews:
  ears, 1685t
  endocrine system, 528t
  eyes, 1675t
  female reproductive system, 1759–60t
  heart, 951–52t
  hematologic, peripheral vascular, and lymphatic
    systems, 1090t
  integumentary system, 429t
  intestinal tract, 747t
  male reproductive system, 1748t
  musculoskeletal system, 1390t
  neurologic system, 1517t
  nutritional status and gastrointestinal system, 618t
  respiratory system, 1221–22t
  urinary system, 840t
Functional health patterns:
  activity-exercise. See Activity-exercise
    patterns
  cognitive-perceptual. See Cognitive-perceptual
    patterns
  definitions, 9t
  elimination. See Elimination patterns
  nutritional-metabolic. See Nutritional-metabolic
    patterns
  sexuality-reproductive. See Sexuality-
    reproductive patterns
Functional residual capacity (FRC), 1214t
Functional urinary incontinence, 874t. See also
    Urinary incontinence
Fundoplication, 666
Fundoscopy, 1708
Fungi:
  characteristics, 311t
  lung infections
    aspergillosis, 1294
    blastomycosis, 1294
    coccidiomycosis, 1294
    geographic distribution, 1294
    histoplasmosis, 1294
    interdisciplinary care, 1294–95
    nursing care, 1295
    pathophysiology, 1294
  skin infections
    interdisciplinary care, 449–50, 450t
    nursing care, 450
    types
      candidiasis. See Candidiasis
      dermatophytoses, 448–49
Fungizone. See Amphotericin B
Furadantin. See Nitrofurantoin
Furazolidone, 778t, 780t
Furosemide:
  adverse/side effects, 1730
  Medication Administration, 210t, 717t, 905t,
    1033t, 1539t

Furosemide—*continued*
in specific conditions
acute renal failure, 904, 905*t*
ascites, 716, 717*t*
fluid volume excess, 210*t*
heart failure, 1033*t*
hyperkalemia, 225*t*
increased intracranial pressure, 1538, 1539*t*
pulmonary edema, 1041
Furoxone. *See* Furazolidone
Furstenberg diet, 1727
Furuncle, 446–47, 447*f*
Fusiform aneurysm, 1170, 1592
Fusiform excision, 477
Fuzeon. *See* Enfuvirtide
FVC (forced vital capacity), 1214*t*
FVD. *See* Fluid volume deficit

G

G6PD (glucose-6-phosphate dehydrogenase) anemia, 1106*t*, 1109
GABA (gamma aminobutyric acid), 1505
Gabapentin, 1550*t*, 1656
Gabitril. *See* Tiagabine
Gait, 1391*t*, 1522–23*t*
Galactorrhea, 1762*t*
Galantamine hydrobromide, 1621
Gallbladder:
anatomy, physiology, and functions, 611*f*, 613, 697
disorders
cancer, 703
diagnostic tests, 616*t*, 699
gallstones. *See* Gallstones
Gallstone ileus, 698
Gallstones:
complications, 698, 698*t*
ethnic considerations, 697
interdisciplinary care
diagnosis, 616*t*, 699, 699*t*
medications, 699
treatments
complementary therapies, 701
extracorporeal shock wave lithotripsy, 700–701
nutrition, 700
percutaneous cholecystostomy, 701
surgery, 699–700, 699*f*
manifestations, 698, 698*t*
nursing care
assessment, 701
community-based care, 703
health promotion, 701
nursing diagnoses and interventions
imbalanced nutrition: less than body requirements, 702–3
pain, 701–2, 702*t*
risk for infection, 703
Nursing Care Plan
assessment, 702*t*
critical thinking in the nursing process, 702*t*
diagnosis, 702*t*
evaluation, 702*t*
expected outcomes, 702*t*
planning and implementation, 702*t*
pathophysiology, 697–98
risk factors, 697*t*
GALT (gut-associated lymphoid tissue), 292
Gamma aminobutyric acid (GABA), 1505
Gamma benzene hexachloride, 451
Gamma glutamyltransferase (GGT), 386*t*
Gamma interferon, 299*t*. *See also* Interferon(s)
Gamma knife, 1572

Ganciclovir:
Medication Administration, 322*t*
in specific conditions
bone marrow transplant recipients, 344
cytomegalovirus infection, 359*t*, 1718
Gangrene, 588, 1093*t*
Gangrenous appendicitis, 766
Gantanol. *See* Sulfamethoxazole
Gantrisin. *See* Sulfisoxazole
Garamycin. *See* Gentamicin
Gardasil, 1815, 1841
Gardnerella vaginalis, 1842
Gardner-Wells tongs, 1601, 1601*f*
Garlic, 679, 1231
Gas gangrene, 267
Gastrectomy, 689, 689*f*
Gastric acid pump inhibitors. *See* Proton-pump inhibitors
Gastric analysis:
purpose and description, 615*t*
related nursing care, 615*t*
in specific conditions
gastritis, 678
Zollinger-Ellison syndrome, 684
Gastric bypass procedures, 636–37, 637*f*
Gastric cancer:
incidence, 688
interdisciplinary care
complications, 689–91
diagnosis, 689
gastrostomy, 691
gastrostomy/jejunostomy, 691*f*
surgery, 689, 690*f*
manifestations, 689
nursing care
assessment, 691
health promotion, 691
nursing diagnoses and interventions
anticipatory grieving, 693
community-based care, 694
imbalanced nutrition: less than body requirements, 691, 693
using NANDA, NIC, and NOC, 693, 693*t*
postoperative, 690*t*
preoperative, 690*t*
Nursing Care Plan
assessment, 692*t*
critical thinking in the nursing process, 693*t*
diagnoses, 692*t*
expected outcomes, 692*t*
planning and implementation, 692–93*t*
pathophysiology, 688, 689*f*
risk factors, 688
Gastric emptying studies, 616*t*
Gastric lavage:
for botulism, 777
closed-system irrigation, 676*f*, 676*t*
for esophageal varices, 718
for gastritis, 678–79
intermittent open system, 676
nursing responsibilities, 676*t*
for upper gastrointestinal bleeding, 675
Gastric mucosal barrier, 671
Gastric outlet obstruction, 681*t*, 684
Gastric residual volume, 662*t*. *See also* Enteral nutrition
Gastric ulcers, 680. *See also* Peptic ulcer disease
Gastritis:
definition, 677
interdisciplinary care
diagnosis, 678
medications, 665–66*t*, 678
treatments
complementary therapies, 679

gastric lavage, 678–79
nutrition, 678
manifestations, 677, 677*t*, 678
nursing care
assessment, 679
community-based care, 680
health promotion, 679
Medication Administration, 665–66*t*
nursing diagnoses and interventions
deficient fluid volume, 679
imbalanced nutrition: less than body requirements, 679–80
pathophysiology, 677–78
types, 677
Gastroduodenostomy (Billroth I), 689, 689*f*
Gastroenteritis:
complications, 774
definition, 773
interdisciplinary care
diagnosis, 776, 776*t*
dialysis, 777
gastric lavage, 777
medications, 776
nutrition and fluids, 776–77
plasmapheresis, 777
manifestations, 773, 773*t*
nursing care
assessment, 777
community-based care, 777
health promotion, 777
nursing diagnoses and interventions, 777
pathophysiology, 773
types
C. difficile colitis, 774*t*, 775
cholera, 774*t*, 775
hemorrhagic colitis, 774*t*, 775
salmonellosis, 774*t*, 775
shigellosis, 774*t*, 775
staphylococcal food poisoning, 774*t*, 775
traveler's diarrhea, 774–75, 774*t*
Gastroesophageal reflux, 663
Gastroesophageal reflux disease (GERD):
definition, 663
incidence, 663
interdisciplinary care
diagnosis, 664–65
medications, 665–66*t*
nutrition and lifestyle management, 666
surgery, 666
manifestations, 663–64, 664*t*
nursing care
assessment, 666
community-based care, 667
Medication Administration, 665–66*t*
nursing diagnoses and interventions, 667
using NANDA, NIC, and NOC, 667, 667*t*
pathophysiology, 663, 664*f*
Gastrografin. *See* Meglumine diatrizoate
Gastrointestinal bleeding:
causes, 674, 681. *See also* Esophageal varices; Gastritis; Peptic ulcer disease
complications, 674
interdisciplinary care
diagnosis, 674
treatments
endoscopy, 675
fluid and blood replacement, 674
gastric lavage. *See* Gastric lavage
nursing care
assessment, 675
community-based care, 677
health promotion, 675

nursing diagnoses and interventions
  decreased cardiac output, 675
  impaired tissue integrity: gastrointestinal, 675
pathophysiology, 674
Gastrointestinal system:
  age-related changes
    in middle adults, 27t
    in older adults, 29t, 619t, 746t
  anatomy, physiology, and functions
    esophagus, 610–11, 611f
    exocrine pancreas, 613
    gallbladder, 611f, 613
    large intestine, 742–43, 742f
    liver, 612–13, 613t
    mouth, 610, 611f
    overview, 605f
    pharynx, 611f
    rectum and anus, 743, 743f
    small intestine, 605f, 612, 742
    stomach, 611–12, 611f
  assessment
    diagnostic tests, 614, 615–17t. See also
      specific tests
    functional health pattern interview, 618t
    genetic considerations, 614, 614t
    health assessment interview, 614, 617–19
    physical assessment
      abdomen, 623–27t, 623f, 624f, 748–49t
      oral cavity, 622–23t
      overview, 619
  disorders
    anus and rectum
      anal fissure, 820
      anorectal abscess, 820
      anorectal fistula, 820–21
      hemorrhoids. See Hemorrhoids
      nursing care, 821
      pilonidal disease, 821
    Clinical Scenarios, 736t
    esophagus
      cancer. See Esophageal cancer
      diagnostic tests, 615t
      gastroesophageal reflux disease. See
        Gastroesophageal reflux disease
      hiatal hernia. See Hiatal hernia
      impaired motility, 668, 668f
    gallbladder
      cancer, 703
      diagnostic tests, 616t, 699
      gallstones. See Gallstones
    liver. See Liver, disorders
    mouth
      cancer. See Oral cancer
      stomatitis. See Stomatitis
    pancreas
      cancer. See Pancreatic cancer
      diagnostic tests, 526t, 616–17t, 728t
      endocrine function. See Diabetes mellitus
      pancreatitis. See Pancreatitis
    small and large intestine. See Bowel disorders
    stomach
      cancer. See Gastric cancer
      nausea and vomiting. See Nausea and
        vomiting
      peptic ulcer disease. See Peptic ulcer disease
    upper gastrointestinal bleeding. See
      Gastrointestinal bleeding
Gastrojejunostomy (Billroth II), 689, 689f
Gastroparesis, 589
Gastroscopy. See Esophagogastroduodenoscopy
Gastrostomy tube:
  characteristics, 691, 691f
  nursing care, 692t
Gate-control theory, of pain, 172, 172f

Gatifloxacin, 320t
Gaucher disease, 614t, 1089t
Gaviscon, 665, 666t
Gelusil, 666t
Gemfibrozil, 967t
Gender:
  cancer risk and, 370
  coronary heart disease risk and, 962–63
  health and, 20
General adaptation syndrome, 135t
General anesthesia, 61–63
Generalized seizures, 1549
Genes. See also Genetics
  alterations, 152
  characteristics, 151
  expression, 155
  function and distribution, 151
  mitochondrial, 151
  single nucleotide polymorphisms, 152
Genetic locus, 151
Genetics:
  cancer risk and, 370
  Chapter Highlights, 166t
  considerations in specific conditions
    Alzheimer's disease, 1513t
    amyotrophic lateral sclerosis, 1389t, 1513t
    ankylosing spondylitis, 1469
    asthma, 1220t
    atherosclerosis, 1089t
    cardiac disorders, 943, 950t
    chronic myeloid leukemia, 151, 1089t,
      1121, 1122f
    chronic obstructive pulmonary disease, 1331t
    chronic renal failure, 839t
    cystic fibrosis, 152, 1220t, 1340t
    diabetes mellitus, 527t, 565
    Duchenne muscular dystrophy, 1389t, 1458
    ear disorders, 1684t
    Ellis-van Creveld syndrome, 1389t
    endocrine system disorders, 527, 527t
    epilepsy, 1513t
    essential tremor, 1513t
    eye disorders, 1674t
    female reproductive system disorders, 1755t
    Friedreich's ataxia, 1513t
    Gaucher disease, 614t, 1089t
    hematologic, peripheral vascular, and
      lymphatic disorders, 1088, 1089t
    hemophilia, 1089t, 1143f, 1143t
    hirsutism, 427t
    hypertrophic cardiomyopathy, 950t
    integumentary system disorders, 427, 427t
    intestinal tract disorders, 745, 746t
    keloid, 427t
    lung cancer, 1220t
    lymphedema, 1199t
    lymphoma, 1129t
    male reproductive system disorders, 1747t
    Marfan syndrome, 950t, 1057t
    multiple sclerosis, 1389t, 1458
    musculoskeletal disorders, 1389t
    myotonic dystrophy, 155, 1389t
    narcolepsy, 1513t
    neurologic disorders, 1513t
    nutritional and gastrointestinal system
      disorders, 614, 614t
    obesity, 631
    Parkinson's disease, 1513t
    peripheral vascular disorders, 1088, 1089t
    polycystic kidney disease, 839t, 844, 884t
    porphyria, 1089t
    respiratory disorders, 1219, 1220t
    sickle cell anemia, 1089t, 1106, 1107f
    substance abuse, 104, 104t

    Tay-Sachs disease, 1513t
    thalassemias, 1089t
    thoracic aortic aneurysm, 1172t
    urinary system disorders, 839t
  health and, 19
  interdisciplinary care
    genetic testing
      diagnosing chromosomal alterations, 157
      diagnosing gene alterations, 157
      implications, 156
      indications, 156
      positive and negative outcomes, 156t
      quality and accuracy, 157–58
      types, 156–57
  nursing care
    assessment
      client intake and history, 159
      ethical implications, 164t
      genetic physical assessment, 160
      health promotion and health maintenance, 159
      pedigrees, 159–60, 160f, 161f, 162t, 163t
    evaluation, 165
    in genetic testing
      client education and rights, 158
      confidentiality and privacy issues, 158
      economic issues, 159
      psychosocial issues, 158–59
    nursing diagnoses and interventions
      client teaching, 163
      diagnoses to consider, 160–61
      genetic referrals and counseling, 161–62,
        163, 165t
      psychosocial care, 163–64
  in nursing practice
    "people first" approach, 149t
    scope and standards, 148–49, 149t
  principles
    cell division, 149–50
    chromosomes
      alterations in number, 150, 150t
      alterations in structure, 150–51
      structure, 149, 150f
    DNA, 149
    genes. See Genes
    inheritance. See Inheritance
Genital herpes:
  incidence, 1838
  interdisciplinary care
    diagnosis, 1839
    medications, 1839
    management, 1839t
    manifestations, 1839, 1839f
  nursing care
    community-based care, 1840
    nursing diagnoses and interventions
      acute pain, 1840
      sexual dysfunction, 1840
  pathophysiology, 1839
Genital warts:
  characteristics, 452
  incidence, 1840
  interdisciplinary care
    diagnosis, 1841
    medications, 1841, 1842t
    treatments, 1841
  manifestations, 1841, 1841f
  nursing care
    community-based care, 1842
    Medication Administration, 1842t
    nursing diagnoses and interventions
      anxiety, 1842
      deficient knowledge, 1841
      fear, 1842
  pathophysiology, 1840

Genitourinary system. *See* Female reproductive system; Male reproductive system; Urinary system
Genitourinary tuberculosis, 1283
Genotype, 151
Gentamicin:
  Medication Administration, 320*t*
  in specific conditions
    endocarditis, 1046
    eye trauma, 1703
    pelvic inflammatory disease, 1851
    peritonitis, 770
    skin infections, 441*t*
    urinary tract infection, 849
  topical
    for conjunctivitis, 1694
    for corneal infections, 1697
Gentran 40. *See* Dextran 40
Gentran 70. *See* Dextran 70
Gentran 75. *See* Dextran 75
Geocillin. *See* Carbenicillin
Geographic area, health and, 20
Geopen. *See* Carbenicillin
GERD. *See* Gastroesophageal reflux disease
Germ cell tumors, 1774
Germline mutations, 152
Gestational diabetes, 566*t*
GFR. *See* Glomerular filtration rate
GGT (gamma glutamyltransferase), 386*t*
GH. *See* Growth hormone
Giant cell tumor, 1482*t*
Giardia lamblia, 778, 779*t*
Giardiasis, 778, 778*t*
Gigantism, 523*t*, 558
Ginger:
  for diarrhea, 755
  for gastritis, 679
  for irritable bowel syndrome, 763
  for nausea and vomiting, 672, 709
  for premenstrual syndrome, 1800
Gingivitis, 623*t*
Ginkgo biloba, 1621
Ginseng, 1796
Glasgow Coma Scale, 1513*t*
Glatiramer acetate, 1627, 1631*t*
Glaucoma:
  angle-closure, 1684*t*, 1707–8, 1708*t*
  Case Study, 1739*t*
  definition, 1706
  genetic considerations, 1674*t*
  incidence, 1706
  interdisciplinary care
    diagnosis, 1708, 1708*f*, 1709*f*
    medications, 1709
    surgery, 1709
  manifestations, 1707, 1707*f*, 1708
  nursing care
    assessment, 1712
    community-based care, 1713
    health promotion, 1712
    nursing diagnoses and interventions
      anxiety, 1713
      disturbed sensory perception: visual, 1712
      risk for injury, 1712–13
    using NANDA, NIC, and NOC, 1713, 1713*t*
  Nursing Care Plan
    assessment, 1711*t*
    critical thinking in the nursing process, 1711*t*
    diagnoses, 1711*t*
    evaluation, 1711*t*
    expected outcomes, 1711*t*
    planning and implementation, 1711*t*
  open-angle, 1707, 1707*f*, 1708*t*

pathophysiology, 1706–7, 1707*f*
  risk factors, 1706
Gleevec. *See* Imatinib mesylate
Glimepiride, 578*t*
Glioblastoma, 1569, 1570*t*. *See also* Brain tumors
Glioma, 1570*t*
Gliosis, 1626, 1629*t*
Glipizide, 578*t*
Global aphasia, 1583
Glomerular capsule, 830, 885–86
Glomerular disorders:
  acute proliferative glomerulonephritis
    complications, 886–87
    manifestations, 886–87
    pathophysiology, 886, 886*f*, 887*t*
    prognosis, 887
  interdisciplinary care
    diagnosis, 889–90, 890*t*
    medications, 890–91
    treatments, 891, 891*t*
  nursing care
    assessment, 891
    health promotion, 891
    nursing diagnoses and interventions
      community-based care, 894
      excess fluid volume, 891–93
      fatigue, 893
      ineffective protection, 893
      ineffective role performance, 894
  Nursing Care Plan
    assessment, 892*t*
    critical thinking in the nursing process, 892*t*
    diagnoses, 892*t*
    evaluation, 892*t*
    expected outcomes, 892*t*
    planning and implementation, 892*t*
  pathophysiology, 885–86
  rapidly progressive glomerulonephritis, 887–88
Glomerular filtration rate (GFR):
  age-related changes, 883, 884*t*
  in chronic renal failure, 916*t*
  definition, 214, 831
  factors affecting, 831–33
  normal, 831, 831*f*
  in sodium balance regulation, 214
Glomerulonephritis, 886. *See also* Glomerular disorders
Glossitis:
  in anemia, 1106
  definition, 622*t*
  nursing interventions, 1114
  in nutritional deficiencies, 622*t*
Glossopharyngeal nerve (cranial nerve IX):
  anatomy, 1510*f*
  assessment, 1520*t*
  functions, 1511*t*
Glucagon:
  functions, 521, 564, 565*f*
  for severe hypoglycemia, 587
Glucocorticoids. *See also* Corticosteroids
  feedback mechanism, 519*t*
  functions, 519*t*, 521
  target organ and feedback mechanism, 519*t*
Gluconeogenesis, 272, 564
Glucophage. *See* Metformin
Glucose:
  blood. *See* Blood glucose
  in increased intracranial pressure, 1539*t*
  urine. *See* Urine tests, glucose
Glucose-6-phosphate dehydrogenase (G6PD) anemia, 1106*t*, 1109
Glucosuria, 566
Glucotrol. *See* Glipizide

Glucotrol XL. *See* Glipizide
Glulisine, 571*t*
Gluten:
  dietary sources, 796, 797*t*
  sensitivity to. *See* Sprue
Glyburide, 578*t*
Glycerol test, 1727
Glycogenolysis, 272, 564
Glycopyrrolate, 62*t*, 869
Glycosylated hemoglobin (Hb A$_1$C), 526*t*, 569
Glyset. *See* Miglitol
Goiter:
  definition, 536
  in hypothyroidism, 541
  physical assessment, 530*t*
  toxic multinodular, 536*f*
Gold salts, 1465, 1465*t*
Gold sodium thiomalate, 1465*t*
Goldenseal, 701, 1273, 1796
Golfer's elbow, 1428
Gonadotropin-releasing hormone agonists, 1798
Gonioplasty, 1709
Gonioscopy, 1708
Gonococcus, 1692
Gonorrhea:
  complications, 1846
  incidence, 1845
  interdisciplinary care
    diagnosis, 1746*t*, 1756*t*, 1846
    medications, 1846
  manifestations, 1845
  nursing care
    community-based care, 1846
    nursing diagnoses and interventions
      impaired social interaction, 1846
      noncompliance, 1846
  Nursing Care Plan
    assessment, 1847*t*
    critical thinking in the nursing process, 1847*t*
    diagnoses, 1847*t*
    evaluation, 1847*t*
    expected outcomes, 1847*t*
    planning and implementation, 1847*t*
  pathophysiology, 1845
  risk factors, 1845
Goodpasture's syndrome, 888. *See also* Glomerular disorders
Gout:
  complications, 1444
  definition, 1443
  incidence, 1444
  interdisciplinary care
    complementary therapies, 1445
    diagnosis, 1445
    medications
      acute attack, 1445
      Medication Administration, 1446*t*
      prophylactic therapy, 1445
    treatments
      nutrition, 1445, 1446
      rest, 1446
  manifestations
    acute gouty arthritis, 1444, 1444*t*
    hyperuricemia, 1444
    tophaceous (chronic) gout, 1444, 1444*t*
  nursing care
    community-based care, 1447
    Medication Administration, 1446*t*
    nursing diagnoses and interventions, 1447
  pathophysiology, 1444
  primary, 1443
  secondary, 1443
Gouty arthritis, 1433

Grafts, skin, 478, 478f
Graft-versus-host disease (GVHD):
  in bone marrow/stem cell transplantation, 343, 1124
    manifestations, 343, 1124
    pathophysiology, 343, 1124
Gram stain, urine, 849
Gram-negative bacteria, 311t
Gram-positive bacteria, 311t
Granisetron, 672, 673t
Granulocyte colony-stimulating factors, 1123
Granulocyte-macrophage colony-stimulating factors, 1123, 1139
Granulocytes, 288, 288t, 289f. See also White blood cells (WBCs)
Granuloma, 305
Granulopoiesis, 1138
Grape seed extract, 1326
Graphesthesia, 1522f, 1522t
Graves' disease. See also Hyperthyroidism
  manifestations, 534, 536, 536f
  Nursing Care Plan
    assessment, 540t
    critical thinking in the nursing process, 540t
    diagnoses, 540t
    evaluation, 540t
    expected outcomes, 540t
    planning and implementation, 540t
  pathophysiology, 534
Greater vestibular glands. See Bartholin's glands
Grief, 85. See also Loss and grief
Grieving:
  anticipatory, 86, 96
  definition, 85
Griseofulvin, 449, 450t
Group A beta-hemolytic streptococcus:
  in pharyngitis, 1238
  in rheumatic fever, 1042
  in skin infections, 447
Growth hormone (GH):
  diagnostic test, 523t
  feedback mechanism, 519t
  functions, 518, 519f, 519t
Guaifenesin, 1272
Guanfacine, 1162t
Guglielmi detachable coils, 1594
Guided imagery, 186
Guillain-Barré syndrome:
  characteristics, 1653
  incidence, 1653
  influenza vaccine and, 1234
  interdisciplinary care
    diagnosis, 1653
    medications, 1653–54
    nutrition and fluids, 1654
    physical and occupational therapy, 1654
    plasmapheresis, 1654
    surgery, 1654
  manifestations, 1653
  nursing care
    community-based care, 1655
    nursing diagnoses and interventions
      acute pain, 1654
      risk for impaired skin integrity, 1654–55
  pathophysiology, 1653
  stages, 1653t
Guillotine (open) amputation, 1421, 1422t
Gummas, 1848
Gums, 623t
Gut-associated lymphoid tissue (GALT), 292
GVHD. See Graft-versus-host disease
Gynecomastia:
  definition, 1749t
  nursing care, 1790

  pathophysiology, 1789–90
  physical assessment, 1749t
  in testicular cancer, 1774
  treatment, 1790
Gyrate atrophy, 1674t

H

H₂ receptor blockers. See Histamine₂ (H₂)-receptor blockers
Haemophilus influenzae, 1271t
Hageman factor, 1082t
Hair. See also Integumentary system
  age-related changes
    in middle adults, 27t
    in older adults, 29t
    in young adults, 26t
  anatomy, physiology, and functions, 425, 425f
  assessment, 435–36t
  disorders
    alopecia. See Alopecia
    hirsutism. See Hirsutism
    interdisciplinary care, 482
    nursing care, 482–83
    pathophysiology, 481–82, 482t
Haldol. See Haloperidol
Hallucinogens:
  abuse, 110–11
  overdose signs and treatment, 113t
  street names, 111t
  withdrawal signs and treatment, 113t
Hallux valgus, 1492, 1492f
Halo external fixation:
  characteristics, 1601, 1601f
  nursing care, 1602t
Haloperidol, 672, 673t, 1621
HALT acronym, relapse behaviors, 121t
Hammertoe, 1492
Hand:
  fracture, 1413–14
  physical assessment, 1393t
Handicap, 47
Haptoglobin, 386t
Hartmann procedure, 805
Hashimoto's thyroiditis, 543
Haversian system, 1380
Havighurst, developmental tasks, 25t
Hawthorn, 1036
Hazardous materials, 127
Hb A₁C (glycosylated hemoglobin), 526t, 569
hCG. See Human chorionic gonadotropin
Hct. See Hematocrit
HDL. See High-density lipoprotein
Head injury. See Traumatic brain injury
Headache:
  cluster, 1542t, 1543
  interdisciplinary care
    complementary and alternative therapies, 1544
    diagnosis, 1543–44
    medications, 1544, 1545–46t
  migraine, 1542–43, 1542t
  nursing care
    assessment, 1544
    community-based care, 1547
    health promotion, 1544, 1544t
    Medication Administration, 1545–46t
    nursing diagnoses and interventions, 1544, 1546
  Nursing Care Plan
    assessment, 1547t
    critical thinking in the nursing process, 1547t
    diagnoses, 1547t
    evaluation, 1547t
    expected outcomes, 1547t
    planning and implementation, 1547t

  pathophysiology, 1542
  tension, 1542t, 1543
Healing:
  burn wounds, 493. See also Burns
  impaired, 305, 306t
  nutrition and, 307–8
  phases, 294–95
  wound, 76–77, 76f, 77t
Health:
  Chapter Highlights, 33t
  community factors affecting
    community healthcare structure, 37
    economic resources, 37
    environment, 37
    social support systems, 37
  definition, 19
  factors affecting
    age, gender, and developmental level, 20
    cognitive abilities and educational level, 19
    genetic makeup, 19
    geographic area, 20
    lifestyle and environment, 20
    race, ethnicity, and cultural background, 20
    socioeconomic background, 20
  family-related risk factors for alterations in, 32t
  needs
    in middle adults. See Middle adults, health needs
    in older adults. See Older adults, health needs
    in young adults. See Young adults, health needs
  promotion and maintenance. See Health promotion and maintenance
  vs. wellness, 19
Health perception-health management pattern:
  Build Clinical Competence
    alterations in patterns of health, 143t
    dimensions of medical-surgical nursing, 49t
    pathophysiology and patterns of health, 416t
  NANDA nursing diagnoses, 2t
Health promotion and maintenance:
  healthy living
    dietary guidelines, 20t, 21f
    immunizations, 21t
    recommended practices, 20–21
  in middle adults, 28, 28t
  national goals and health indicators, 21, 22t
  in older adults, 30, 31t
  in young adults, 26, 27t
Healthcare professionals, core competencies, 5, 5t
Healthcare surrogate, 90. See also Advance directives
Healthcare-associated infections (HIAs). See Nosocomial infections
Health–illness continuum, 19, 19f. See also Disease; Health; Illness
Healthy People 2010, 22t
Hearing. See also Ears
  age-related changes
    in middle adults, 27t
    in older adults, 29t, 1686t
  physical assessment, 1687–88t, 1687f, 1688f
Hearing aids, 1730–31, 1731f
Hearing loss:
  conductive, 1729–30
  genetic considerations, 1684
  incidence, 1729
  interdisciplinary care
    amplification, 1730–31, 1731f
    diagnosis, 1730
    surgery, 1731–32, 1732f
  manifestations, 1729–30
  nursing care
    assessment, 1732
    community-based care, 1733–34

Hearing loss—*continued*
  health promotion, 1732
  nursing diagnoses and interventions
    disturbed sensory perception: auditory, 1732
    impaired verbal communication, 1732–33
    social isolation, 1733
    using NANDA, NIC, and NOC, 1733, 1733*t*
  pathophysiology, 1729–30
  presbycusis, 1730
  sensorineural, 1730
  special considerations in disasters, 140
Heart:
  anatomy, physiology, and functions
    action potential
      definition, 941–42, 942*f*
      depolarization, 942
      repolarization, 942–43
    cardiac cycle, 939–40, 939*f*
    cardiac output
      afterload, 940, 1023–24, 1024*t*
      clinical indicators, 940–41
      contractility, 940
      heart rate, 940
      normal ranges, 940
      overview, 1023
      preload, 940, 1023
    cardiac reserve, 1023
    chambers and valves, 937–38, 937*f*
    conduction system, 941, 941*f*, 995
    coronary circulation, 938–39, 939*f*, 959
    explanations for clients, 1024*t*
    layers of heart wall, 937, 937*f*
    location in thorax, 936*f*
    pericardium, 936–37, 937*f*
    pulmonary circulation, 938, 938*f*
    systemic circulation, 938, 938*f*
    valves, 1054
  assessing cardiac function
    age-related changes, 952*t*
    diagnostic tests, 943–46*t*
    electrocardiogram. *See* Electrocardiogram
    functional health pattern interview, 951–52*t*
    genetic considerations, 943, 950*t*
    health assessment interview, 943,
      949–50, 950*t*
    physical assessment
      apical impulse, 952–53*t*, 953*f*
      cardiac rate and rhythm, 953*t*
      heart sounds, 954–55*t*, 954*f*
      murmurs, 955*t*
      overview, 950, 952
    sample documentation, 943*t*
  disorders
    acute myocardial infarction. *See* Acute
      myocardial infarction
    angina pectoris. *See* Angina pectoris
    cardiomyopathy. *See* Cardiomyopathy
    Chapter Highlights, 1019*t*, 1068*t*
    coronary heart disease. *See* Coronary heart
      disease
    dysrhythmias. *See* Cardiac dysrhythmias
    endocarditis. *See* Endocarditis
    heart failure. *See* Heart failure
    myocarditis, 1049
    pericarditis. *See* Pericarditis
    rheumatic heart disease. *See* Rheumatic
      fever/heart disease
    sudden cardiac death. *See* Sudden cardiac
      death
Heart block, 996
Heart failure:
  Case Study, 1073*t*
  causes, 985, 1022, 1022*t*

classification
  acute vs. chronic, 1027
  left-side vs. right-sided, 1026–27, 1026*f*
  low-output vs. high-output, 1027
  systolic vs. diastolic, 1025–26
complications, 1027
definition, 1022
incidence and prevalence, 1022–23
interdisciplinary care
  cardiac transplantation. *See* Heart transplant
  cardiomyoplasty, 1036
  circulatory assistance, 1034–35
  complementary therapies, 1036
  diagnosis, 1027
  end-of-life care, 1036
  hemodynamic monitoring
    complications, 1029*t*
    intra-arterial pressure monitoring, 1029–30
    nursing care, 1031*t*
    principles, 1027, 1029, 1030*f*
    pulmonary artery pressure monitoring,
      1030–31
    venous pressure monitoring, 1030
  medications, 1031–32, 1033–34*t*, 1034
  nutrition and activity, 1034
  by stage, 1029*t*
  ventricular reduction surgery, 1036
manifestations, 1025–27, 1026*f*
Multisystem Effects, 1028*t*
nursing care
  assessment, 1036
  community-based care, 1039
  health promotion, 1036
  hemodynamic monitoring, 1031*t*
  home activity guidelines, 1040*t*
  Medication Administration, 1033–34*t*
  nursing diagnoses and interventions
    activity intolerance, 1038
    decreased cardiac output, 1037–38
    deficient knowledge: low-sodium diet,
      1038–39
    excess fluid volume, 1038
    of older adults, 1023*t*
    using NANDA, NIC, and NOC, 1039, 1039*t*
  Nursing Care Plan
    assessment, 1037*t*
    critical thinking in the nursing process, 1037*t*
    diagnoses, 1037*t*
    evaluation, 1037*t*
    expected outcomes, 1037*t*
    planning and implementation, 1037*t*
  pathophysiology, 1024–25, 1024*t*
  prognosis, 1023
  risk factors, 1023
  stages, 1029*t*
Heart rate, 940, 953*t*
Heart sounds:
  in aortic regurgitation, 1059
  in aortic stenosis, 1058
  assessment, 954–55*t*, 954*f*
  in dilated cardiomyopathy, 1065
  in heart failure, 1026
  in mitral regurgitation, 1056
  in mitral stenosis, 1055
  in valvular heart disease, 1055*t*
Heart transplant. *See also* Transplant procedures
  for cardiomyopathy, 1067
  complications, 1036
  for heart failure, 1035
  indications, 342*t*
  nursing care, 1035–36
  procedure, 1035, 1035*f*
  success rate, 342*t*, 1035

Heaves, 952
Heberden's nodes, 1393, 1450
Heel-to-shin test, 1523*f*, 1523*t*
Heimlich maneuver, 1249, 1249*f*
Helicobacter pylori:
  in chronic gastritis, 678
  diagnostic tests, 684*t*
  in gastric cancer, 688
  medications, 684
  in peptic ulcer disease, 680, 680*t*, 682–83*t*
Helminthic disorders:
  cestodes, 781*t*
  interdisciplinary care
    diagnosis, 779
    medications, 779–80
  nematodes, 781*t*
  nursing care, 780–81
  pathophysiology, 779
Helper T cells, 297, 298*f*. *See also* T lymphocytes
Hemangioblastoma, 1570*t*. *See also* Brain tumors
Hemangiomas, 430*t*, 443
Hematemesis, 674. *See also* Gastrointestinal
    bleeding
Hematochezia. *See also* Gastrointestinal bleeding
  in cirrhosis, 722
  definition, 674, 722
  in inflammatory bowel disease, 793
Hematocrit (Hct):
  abnormal, possible causes, 386*t*
  normal values, 386*t*, 1078*t*
  perioperative, significance and nursing
    implications, 60*t*
  in specific conditions
    fluid volume deficit, 205
    fluid volume excess, 210
    gastroenteritis and diarrhea, 776*t*
    leukemia, 1123*t*
    shock, 276
Hematologic system:
  age-related changes, 1091*t*
  anatomy, physiology, and functions
    blood cell formation from stem cells, 1077*f*
    blood composition, 1076
    hemostasis
      clot dissolution, 1081
      clot retraction, 1080
      coagulation factors, 1082*t*
      definition, 1079
      fibrin clot formation, 1080, 1081*f*
      platelet plug formation, 1080, 1080*f*
      vessel spasm, 1080
    platelets. *See* Platelets
    red blood cells. *See* Red blood cells
    white blood cells. *See* White blood cells
  assessment
    diagnostic tests, 1087, 1087*t*
    functional health pattern interview, 1090*t*
    genetic considerations, 1088
  disorders
    anemia. *See* Anemia
    Chapter Highlights, 1150*t*
    Clinical Scenarios, 1206*t*
    disseminated intravascular coagulation. *See*
      Disseminated intravascular coagulation
    hemophilia. *See* Hemophilia
    infectious mononucleosis, 1139
    multiple myeloma. *See* Multiple myeloma
    myelodysplastic syndrome. *See*
      Myelodysplastic syndrome
    neutropenia, 1139
    polycythemia. *See* Polycythemia
    thrombocytopenia. *See* Thrombocytopenia
Hematopoiesis, 1380

Hematopoietic growth factors, 396
Hematuria:
  definition, 839, 848
  in polycystic kidney disease, 885
  in urinary tract infection, 848
Hemianopia, 1582, 1582f
Hemilaryngectomy, 1255
Hemiparesis, 1584
Hemiplegia, 1584, 1584f
Hemodialysis:
  complications, 906–7
  definition, 609
  nursing care, 908t
  Nursing Research: promoting autonomy and
      acceptance, 926t
  principles, 609
  system components, 610f
Hemodynamic monitoring:
  complications, 1029t
  nursing care, 1031t
  principles, 1027, 1029, 1030f
  in specific conditions
    aortic aneurysm, 1173
    pericarditis, 1051
  types
    intra-arterial pressure monitoring, 1029–30
    pulmonary artery pressure monitoring,
        1030–31
    venous pressure monitoring, 1030
Hemodynamics, 1027
Hemoglobin (Hgb):
  abnormal, possible causes, 386t
  electrophoresis, 1110–11
  normal values, 386t, 1078t
  perioperative, significance and nursing
      implications, 60t
  in specific conditions
    fluid volume deficit, 205
    fluid volume excess, 210
    leukemia, 1123t
    shock, 276
  structure, 1076, 1078f
Hemoglobin-A, 60t
Hemolysis, 1078
Hemolytic anemias:
  causes, 1106, 1106t
  definition, 1106
  pathophysiology, 1106
  racial/ethnic considerations, 1106t
  sickle cell anemia. See Sickle cell anemia
Hemolytic jaundice, 704
Hemolytic reaction, 262
Hemolyze, 199
Hemophilia:
  definition, 1142
  genetic considerations, 1089t, 1143f, 1143t
  interdisciplinary care
    diagnosis, 1144
    medications, 1144
  manifestations, 1143–44
  nursing care
    assessment, 1144
    community-based care, 1146
    health promotion, 1144
    nursing diagnoses and interventions
      ineffective protection, 1145
      risk for ineffective health maintenance,
          1145–46
    using NANDA, NIC, and NOC, 1146, 1146t
  Nursing Care Plan
    assessment, 1145t
    critical thinking in the nursing process, 1145t
    diagnoses, 1145t

  evaluation, 1145t
  expected outcomes, 1145t
  planning and implementation, 1145t
  pathophysiology, 1142–43
  types
    factor XI deficiency (hemophilia C),
        1143, 1143t
    hemophilia A, 1089t, 1142–43, 1143f, 1143t
    hemophilia B, 1143, 1143f, 1143t
    von Willebrand's disease, 1143, 1143t
Hemoptysis, 1266
Hemorrhage:
  assessment in light and dark skin, 426t
  causes, 74
  definition, 74
  gastrointestinal. See Gastrointestinal bleeding
  in peptic ulcer disease, 681
  postoperative, 74–75
  in trauma, 258, 258f
Hemorrhagic exudate, 293
Hemorrhagic pleural effusion, 1295. See also
    Pleural effusion
Hemorrhagic stroke, 1581–82. See also Stroke
Hemorrhoidectomy, 819
Hemorrhoids:
  causes, 743
  characteristics, 818
  interdisciplinary care
    diagnosis, 819
    hemorrhoidectomy, 819
    medications, 819
    nutrition, 819
    sclerotherapy, 819
  locations, 818
  manifestations, 818–19
  nursing care, 819–20, 820t
  pathophysiology, 818–19
Hemostasis:
  clot dissolution, 1081
  clot retraction, 1080
  coagulation factors, 1082t
  definition, 1079
  disorders
    disseminated intravascular coagulation. See
        Disseminated intravascular coagulation
    hemophilia. See Hemophilia
    thrombocytopenia. See Thrombocytopenia
  fibrin clot formation, 1080, 1081f
  platelet plug formation, 1080, 1080f
  vessel spasm, 1080
Hemothorax:
  definition, 1295, 1302
  manifestations, 1302
  nursing care, 1302
  treatment, 1302
Hemotympanum, 1722
Heparin:
  low-molecular-weight. See Low-molecular-
      weight (LMW) heparins
  Medication Administration, 1189t
  in specific conditions
    acute myocardial infarction, 988
    disseminated intravascular coagulation, 1148
    ischemic stroke, 1585
    pulmonary embolism, 1349
    venous thrombosis, 1188
Heparin-induced thrombocytopenia (HIT),
    1140–41
Hepatic encephalopathy, 704, 715, 715t
Hepatic jaundice, 704
Hepatitis:
  definition, 705
  incidence, 705

  interdisciplinary care
    complementary therapies, 709
    diagnosis, 707
    medications, 708
    prevention
      postexposure prophylaxis, 302t, 707, 708t
      vaccines, 21t, 301t, 707, 708t
  manifestations, 705–6, 705t, 706t
  nursing care
    assessment, 709
    health promotion, 709
    nursing diagnoses and interventions
      community-based care, 710
      disturbed body image, 710
      fatigue, 709
      imbalanced nutrition: less than body
          requirements, 709–10
      risk for infection (transmission), 709
      using NANDA, NIC, and NOC, 710, 710t
  pathophysiology, 705–6
  types
    chronic, 706
    fulminant, 706
    hepatobiliary, 707
    toxic, 707
    viral, 705–6, 705t. See also Hepatitis A;
        Hepatitis B; Hepatitis C
Hepatitis A. See also Hepatitis
  characteristics, 705t, 706
  incidence, 705
  postexposure prophylaxis, 302t, 707, 708t
  vaccine, 707, 708t
Hepatitis B. See also Hepatitis
  cancers associated with, 375, 375t
  characteristics, 705t, 706
  incidence, 705
  interdisciplinary care
    medications, 708
  postexposure prophylaxis, 302t, 707, 708t
  vaccine
    characteristics, 707, 707t
    contraindications, 21t
    indications, 21t, 300, 301t, 707t
    nursing implications, 301t
Hepatitis C. See also Hepatitis
  characteristics, 705t, 706
  incidence, 705
  interdisciplinary care
    medications, 708
Hepatitis delta (D), 705t, 706
Hepatitis E, 705t, 706
Hepatobiliary hepatitis, 707. See also Hepatitis
Hepatocellular carcinoma, 723–24, 724t
Hepatorenal syndrome:
  cirrhosis and, 716
  definition, 704
  portal hypertension and, 704
Herbal supplements/therapy:
  for Alzheimer's disease, 1621
  for asthma, 1326
  for benign prostatic hyperplasia, 1781
  for cancer, 399t
  for chronic obstructive pulmonary disease, 1335
  for constipation, 760–61
  for coronary heart disease, 968
  for diarrhea, 755
  for gallstones, 701
  for gastritis, 679
  for heart failure, 1036
  for hepatitis, 709
  for inflammatory bowel disease, 792
  for irritable bowel syndrome, 763
  for menopausal symptoms, 1796

Hyperesthesias, 174
Hyperextension, 1596f, 1597
Hyperflexion, 1596f, 1597
Hyperglycemia, 565
Hyperkalemia:
  in acute renal failure, 904
  causes, 218t
  definition, 223
  ECG changes in, 219, 219f
  interdisciplinary care
    diagnosis, 224
    dialysis, 224
    medications, 224, 225t
  laboratory values, 218t, 224
  manifestations, 218t, 224
  nursing care
    assessment, 225
    community-based care, 227
    health promotion, 224–25
    Medication Administration, 225t
    nursing diagnoses and interventions
      risk for activity intolerance, 226
      risk for decreased cardiac output, 225–26
      risk for imbalanced fluid volume, 226–27
  Nursing Care Plan
    assessment, 226t
    critical thinking in the nursing process, 226t
    diagnoses, 226t
    evaluation, 226t
    expected outcomes, 226t
    planning and implementation, 226t
  pathophysiology, 223–24
Hyperkeratosis, 443
Hyperkinetic pulse, 1094t
Hyperlipidemia, 963, 963t, 1580
Hypermagnesemia:
  causes, 234t
  definition, 235
  interdisciplinary care, 235
  laboratory values, 234t
  manifestations, 234t, 235
  nursing care, 235–36
  pathophysiology, 235
Hypernatremia:
  causes, 214t
  definition, 213
  interdisciplinary care
    diagnosis, 216
    medications, 216
  laboratory values, 214t, 216
  manifestations, 214t, 216
  nursing care
    assessment, 217
    community-based care, 217
    health promotion, 217
    nursing diagnoses and interventions, 217
  pathophysiology, 216
Hyperopia, 1677t, 1696
Hyperosmolar hyperglycemic state (HHS):
  assessments, 584t
  laboratory findings, 584t, 585
  manifestations, 586
  pathophysiology, 586
  risk factors, 584t, 586, 586t
  treatment, 584t, 586
Hyperparathyroidism:
  definition, 547
  interdisciplinary care, 524t, 547
  manifestations, 547, 547t
  nursing care. See Hypercalcemia
  pathophysiology, 547
Hyperphosphatemia:
  causes, 236t, 237
  definition, 237

in hypocalcemia, 229
interdisciplinary care, 237–38
laboratory values, 236t
manifestations, 236t, 237
nursing care, 238
pathophysiology, 237
Hyperplasia, 373
Hyperresonance, in lung percussion, 1224t
Hypersensitivity:
  definition, 331
  interdisciplinary care
    diagnosis, 336–37, 337f
    goals, 336
    immediate care, 336
    medications, 337–38
    other therapies, 338
  nursing care
    assessment, 338
    community-based care, 339
    health promotion, 338
    nursing diagnoses and interventions
      decreased cardiac output, 339
      ineffective airway clearance, 338–39
      risk for injury, 339
  pathophysiology
    latex allergy, 335–36
    type I Ig-E mediated, 331–33, 332f
    type II cytotoxic, 333–34, 333f
    type III immune complex–mediated, 334–35
    type IV delayed, 335, 335f
  to transfusion, 262
Hypersensitivity pneumonitis, 1345–46
Hyperstat. See Diazoxide
Hypertension:
  Case Study, 1207t
  classification, 1156t
  complications, 1158
  coronary heart disease and, 963, 966
  definition, 1092t, 1154, 1156
  in diabetes mellitus, 588
  in end-stage renal disease, 916
  genetic considerations, 1156
  incidence, 1156
  interdisciplinary care
    algorithm, 1159f
    complementary therapies, 1163
    diagnosis, 1158
    goals, 1158
    lifestyle modifications
      alcohol and tobacco use, 1160
      diet, 1158, 1160t
      overview, 1159t
      physical activity, 1158–59
      stress reduction, 1160
    medications
      ACE inhibitors, 1161t, 1163
      alpha-blockers, 1161t, 1163
      ARBs, 1161t, 1163
      beta-blockers, 1161–62t, 1163
      calcium channel blockers, 1162t, 1163
      diuretics, 1160, 1163
      drug regimens, 1163
      sympatholytics, 1162t
      vasodilators, 1162t, 1163
  intracranial. See Increased intracranial pressure
  kidney disease and, 897
  manifestations, 1158
  nursing care
    assessment, 1164
    community-based care, 1166–67
    health promotion, 1163–64, 1164t
    Medication Administration, 1161–62t
    nursing diagnoses and interventions
      excess fluid volume, 1166

      imbalanced nutrition: more than body
        requirements, 1165–66
      ineffective health maintenance, 1164–65
      risk for noncompliance, 1165
    of older adults, 1157t
    using NANDA, NIC, and NOC, 1166, 1166t
  Nursing Care Plan
    assessment, 1168t
    critical thinking in the nursing process, 1168t
    diagnoses, 1168t
    evaluation, 1168t
    expected outcomes, 1168t
    planning and implementation, 1168t
  Nursing Research: relaxation training, 1164t
  in obesity, 632
  in older adults, 1157t
  pathophysiology, 1157–58
  racial/ethnic considerations, 1156, 1157t
  risk factors, 1156–57, 1156t
  secondary, 897, 1167
  stroke risk and, 1579
Hypertensive emergencies:
  complications, 894
  definition, 894, 1168
  manifestations, 1169, 1169t
  nursing care, 1170
  treatment, 1169–70, 1169t
Hypertensive encephalopathy, 1158
Hyperthermia, malignant, 61–62, 63t
Hyperthyroidism:
  definition, 534
  etiologies
    excess TSH stimulation, 536
    Graves' disease. See Graves' disease
    thyroid storm, 537
    thyroiditis, 536–37
    toxic multinodular goiter, 536, 536f
  interdisciplinary care
    diagnosis, 523–24t, 536t, 537
    medications, 537, 538t
    radioactive iodine therapy, 537
    surgery, 537–38
  Multisystem Effects, 535t
  nursing care
    assessment, 529–30t, 538
    of client having subtotal thyroidectomy, 539t
    community-based care, 541
    health promotion, 538
    Medication Administration, 538t
    nursing diagnoses and interventions
      disturbed body image, 541
      disturbed sensory perception: visual,
        539–40
      imbalanced nutrition: less than body
        requirements, 540–41
      risk for decreased cardiac output, 538–39
  pathophysiology, 534
Hypertonic dehydration, 216
Hypertonic dextrose, 225t
Hypertonic solutions, 198, 199f
Hypertrichosis. See Hirsutism
Hypertrophic cardiomyopathy. See also
    Cardiomyopathy
  genetic considerations, 950t
  management, 1065t
  manifestations, 1065t, 1066
  pathophysiology, 1065–66, 1065t
  prognosis, 1066
Hypertrophic obstructive cardiomyopathy, 1066
Hypertrophic scar, 493
Hypervolemia, 209. See also Fluid volume excess
Hyphema, 1702
Hypnotism, 185
Hypoalbuminemia, 704, 886

Hypocalcemia:
  causes, 228, 228*t*
  complications, 229
  definition, 227
  hypomagnesemia and, 229
  interdisciplinary care
    diagnosis, 229
    medications, 229, 230*t*, 548
    nutrition, 230, 230*t*
  laboratory values, 228*t*, 229
  manifestations, 228*t*, 229, 229*f*, 531*t*
  nursing care
    assessment, 230, 531*t*
    community-based care, 231
    health promotion, 230
    Medication Administration, 230*t*
    nursing diagnoses and interventions, 230–31
  pathophysiology, 228–29
  risk factors, 227–28
Hypocapnia, 239
Hypochromic RBCs, 1103
Hypoglossal nerve (cranial nerve XII):
  anatomy, 1510*f*
  assessment, 1521*t*
  functions, 1511*t*
Hypoglycemia:
  assessments, 584*t*
  definition, 586
  laboratory findings, 584*t*
  manifestations, 586–87, 587*t*
  medications causing, 586
  pathophysiology, 586–87
  risk factors, 584*t*
  treatment, 584*t*, 587
Hypoglycemia unawareness, 587
Hypokalemia:
  causes, 218*t*
  in diabetic ketoacidosis, 585
  ECG change in, 219, 219*f*
  interdisciplinary care
    diagnosis, 219, 221
    medications, 221, 221*t*
    nutrition, 221
  laboratory values, 218*t*, 219, 221
  manifestations, 218*t*, 219, 219*f*, 219*t*
  Multisystem Effects, 219*t*
  nursing care
    assessment, 221
    community-based care, 223
    health promotion, 221
    Medication Administration, 221*t*
    nursing diagnoses and interventions
      activity intolerance, 223
      acute pain, 223
      decreased cardiac output, 222
      risk for imbalanced fluid volume, 223
    using NANDA, NIC, and NOC, 223, 223*t*
  Nursing Care Plan
    assessment, 222*t*
    critical thinking in the nursing process, 222*t*
    diagnoses, 222*t*
    evaluation, 222*t*
    expected outcomes, 222*t*
    planning and implementation, 222*t*
  pathophysiology, 218–19
Hypokinetic pulse, 1094*t*
Hypomagnesemia:
  causes, 234*t*
  complications, 234
  definition, 233
  ECG changes in, 234
  hypocalcemia and, 229
  interdisciplinary care, 234, 235*t*
  laboratory values, 234*t*

manifestations, 234, 234*t*
  nursing care
    assessment, 235
    community-based care, 235
    health promotion, 235
    Medication Administration, 235*t*
    nursing diagnoses and interventions, 235
  pathophysiology, 233
  risk factors, 233
Hyponatremia:
  causes, 214*t*
  definition, 213, 214
  interdisciplinary care
    diagnosis, 215
    fluid and dietary management, 215
    medications, 215
  laboratory values, 214*t*, 215
  manifestations, 214–15, 214*t*
  nursing care
    assessment, 215
    community-based care, 216
    health promotion, 215
    nursing diagnoses and interventions
      risk for imbalanced fluid volume, 215
      risk for ineffective cerebral tissue
        perfusion, 216
  pathophysiology, 214
Hypoparathyroidism:
  definition, 548
  interdisciplinary care, 524*t*, 548
  manifestations, 548, 548*t*
  nursing care. *See* Hypocalcemia
  pathophysiology, 548
Hypophosphatemia:
  causes, 236–37, 236*t*, 1448, 1448*t*
  definition, 236
  interdisciplinary care, 237
  laboratory values, 236*t*
  manifestations, 236*t*, 237
  nursing care, 237
  osteomalacia and, 1448
  pathophysiology, 237
Hypophysis. *See* Pituitary gland
Hypoplasia, kidney, 883
Hypotension:
  in dying client, 93
  orthostatic. *See* Orthostatic hypotension
Hypothalamus, 270, 1506
Hypothermia, 58*t*, 59
Hypothyroidism:
  definition, 541
  etiologies
    Hashimoto's thyroiditis, 543
    iodine deficiency, 543
  interdisciplinary care
    diagnosis, 523–24*t*, 543, 543*t*
    medications, 543, 544*t*
    surgery, 543
  manifestations, 541
  medications causing, 541
  Multisystem Effects, 542*t*
  myxedema coma in, 543
  nursing care
    assessment, 529–30*t*, 543, 545*t*
    community-based care, 545
    health promotion, 543
    Medication Administration, 544*t*
    nursing diagnoses and interventions
      constipation, 544
      decreased cardiac output, 544
      risk for impaired skin integrity, 544–45
  Nursing Care Plan
    assessment, 546*t*
    critical thinking in the nursing process, 546*t*

diagnoses, 546*t*
    evaluation, 546*t*
    expected outcomes, 546*t*
    planning and implementation, 546*t*
  Nursing Research: thyroid hormone and calcium
    supplements, 545*t*
  pathophysiology, 541
Hypotonic dehydration, 215
Hypotonic solutions, 198, 199*f*
Hypovolemia, 203. *See also* Fluid volume deficit
Hypovolemic shock:
  assessment, 279
  in burns, 495
  definition, 273
  manifestations, 273, 274*t*
  in older adults, 273–74
  pathophysiology, 273
  stages, 273
Hypoxemia, 239, 1275
Hypoxis rooperi, 1781
Hysterectomy:
  in cervical cancer, 1813
  in endometrial cancer, 1816
  nursing care, 1804*t*
  in ovarian cancer, 1819
  procedure, 1803–4
Hysterosalpingogram, 1757*t*
Hytrin. *See* Terazosin

I

IABP (intra-aortic balloon pump), 990, 990*f*
Iatrogenic, 209
Iatrogenic disease, 22*t*
Iatrogenic pneumothorax, 1299. *See also*
  Pneumothorax
Ibandronate sodium, 1436
IBD. *See* Inflammatory bowel disease
IBS. *See* Irritable bowel syndrome
Ibuprofen:
  factors in selecting, 178*t*
  Medication Administration, 179*t*
  in specific conditions
    gout, 1445
    osteoarthritis, 1451
    rheumatoid arthritis, 1464*t*
Ibutilide, 1006*t*
ICF (intracellular fluid), 196, 196*f*, 197*f*
Ichthyol, 465*t*
Ichthyosis, 441
ICN (International Council of Nurses), Code of
  Ethics for Nurses, 10
ICSH (interstitial cell–stimulating hormone), 520
Icteric phase, hepatitis, 705, 706*t*
Icterus. *See* Jaundice
Icy Hot. *See* Counterirritants
I&D (incision and drainage), 304
Idamycin. *See* Idarubicin
Idarubicin, 1123*t*
Ideal body weight (IBW), 620*t*
IDET (intradiscal electrothermal therapy), 1610
Idiopathic aplastic anemia, 1109
Idiopathic disease, 22*t*
Idiopathic hypertrophic subaortic stenosis, 1066
Idiopathic thrombocytopenic purpura, 1140. *See
  also* Thrombocytopenia
Idoxuridine, 1694, 1697
Ifosfamide, 1483*t*
IgA (immunoglobulin A), 295*t*
IgD (immunoglobulin D), 295*t*
IgE (immunoglobulin E), 295*t*, 331–33, 332*f*
IGF-1 (insulin-like growth factor), 523*t*
IgG (immunoglobulin G), 295*t*
IgM (immunoglobulin M), 295*t*

Insensible water loss, 196
Inspiration, 1215, 1215f
Inspiratory capacity, 1214t
Inspiratory reserve volume (IRV), 1214, 1214t
Insulin:
    abnormal, possible causes, 386t
    administration
        continuous subcutaneous infusion, 572
        health education for client and family, 573t
        injection preparation, 574
        injection sites, 574–75, 575f, 575t
        intravenous, 586t
        lipodystrophy, 575
        mixing insulins, 575, 576t
        nursing responsibilities, 573t
        regimens, 575, 577t
        routes, 572
        sliding scale, 572–73, 574t
        syringe and needle selection, 573–74
    concentrations, 572
    functions, 521, 564, 565f
    for hyperkalemia, 224, 225t
    indications, 571
    laboratory tests, 380t
    Medication Administration, 573t, 586t
    normal values, 386t
    perioperative needs, 59t, 61, 572–73, 581–82
    preparations, 571–72, 571t
    sources, 571
Insulin glargine, 571t, 572
Insulin lispro, 571, 571t
Insulin pump, 570, 572
Insulin reaction, 586
Insulin resistance, 964, 1157, 1158
Insulin-like growth factor (IGF-1), 523t
Intal. See Cromolyn sodium
Integra, 503
Integrilin. See Eptifibatide
Integumentary system. See also Hair; Nails; Skin
    anatomy, physiology, and functions, 423t
    assessment
        abnormal findings, 431t
        diagnosis, 427, 428t
        functional health pattern interview, 429t
        genetic considerations, 427, 427t
        health assessment interview, 427, 429
        physical assessment, 429–30, 431t, 435–36t
        sample documentation, 427t
        technique/normal findings, 431t
Intercostal spaces, 1213, 1213f, 1223t
Interdisciplinary care, 54
Interferon(s). See also Alpha interferon; Beta interferon
    functions, 299t
    mechanism of action, 299t, 322t
    Medication Administration, 322t, 1631t
    production, 299t
    in specific conditions
        cancer, 396–97
        hepatitis, 708
        HIV/AIDS, 358
        leukemia, 1125
        multiple sclerosis, 1627, 1631t
Interferon beta-1a, 1631t
Interferon beta-1b, 1631t
Interleukin-1 (IL-1), 299t
Interleukin-2 (IL-2), 299t, 396–97
Interleukin-3 (IL-3), 299t
Interleukin-4 (IL-4), 299t
Interleukin-5 (IL-5), 299t
Intermittent claudication, 1172, 1176
Internal hemorrhoids, 818, 818f. See also Hemorrhoids
Internal rotation, 1386t

International Council of Nurses (ICN), Code of Ethics for Nurses, 10
International Normalized Ratio (INR), 1349
International Nursing Coalition for Mass Casualty Education (INCMCE), 126, 126t
International Prostate Symptom Score, 1778
International Society of Nurses in Genetics (ISONG), 148–49, 149t
Internet, for health information in older adults, 1458t
Interstitial cells. See Leydig's cells
Interstitial cell–stimulating hormone (ICSH), 520
Interstitial edematous pancreatitis, 726. See also Pancreatitis
Interstitial fluid, 196, 196f, 197f
Interstitial pneumonia, 1268t. See also Pneumonia
Intestinal decompression, 770, 771f, 813
Intestinal fluke, 780
Intestinal obstruction:
    interdisciplinary care
        diagnosis, 812–13
        gastrointestinal decompression, 813
        surgery, 813
    large-bowel
        complications, 812
        manifestations, 812
        pathophysiology, 812
    nursing care
        assessment, 813
        community-based care, 815
        health promotion, 813
        nursing diagnoses and interventions
            deficient fluid volume, 813–14
            ineffective breathing pattern, 814
            ineffective tissue perfusion:
                gastrointestinal, 814
            using NANDA, NIC, and NOC, 814
        in ovarian cancer, 1818t
    pathophysiology, 811
    small-bowel
        complications, 812
        manifestations, 812
        pathophysiology, 811–12
Intimate partner violence, 256t
Intra-aortic balloon pump (IABP), 990, 990f
Intra-arterial pressure monitoring, 1029–30
Intracapsular fractures, 1414, 1415f. See also Hip, fracture
Intracellular fluid (ICF), 196, 196f, 197f
Intracerebral hematoma, 1557t, 1558, 1558f. See also Traumatic brain injury
Intracoronary stents, 977
Intracranial aneurysm:
    complications
        hydrocephalus, 1593
        rebleeding, 1593
        vasospasm, 1593
    incidence and prevalence, 1592
    interdisciplinary care
        diagnosis, 1593
        medications, 1593
        treatments, 1593–94
    manifestations, 1592–93
    nursing care
        nursing diagnoses and interventions, 1594–95
    pathophysiology, 1592
Intracranial hypertension. See Increased intracranial pressure
Intracranial pressure:
    abnormal findings, 1560t. See also Increased intracranial pressure
    monitoring, 1540, 1540f, 1540t
    normal values, 1535, 1560t
Intradermal testing, 337, 337f

Intradiscal electrothermal therapy (IDET), 1610
Intraductal papilloma, 1821, 1821t
Intraductal papillomatosis, 1821
Intramural fibroid tumors, 1809, 1810f
Intraocular lens implant, 1705, 1705f
Intraoperative awareness, 67
Intraoperative period. See also Surgery
    definition, 54
    interdisciplinary care
        intraoperative awareness, 67
        malignant hyperthermia, 63t
        medications. See Anesthesia
        special considerations for older adults, 67, 70
        surgical environment
            surgical attire, 66–67, 66f
            surgical scrub, 66
            team members, 64–66, 66f
    nursing care, 73
Intraoperative radiotherapy, 1827
Intrarenal acute renal failure, 900t, 901–2. See also Acute renal failure
Intraspinal analgesia:
    nursing care, 184t
    procedure, 184f, 184t
Intravascular fluid. See Plasma
Intravenous administration:
    fluids
        in fluid volume deficit, 205–6
        in gastroenteritis, 777
        in hyponatremia, 215
        Medication Administration, 1539t
        types, 207t
    pain medication, 183, 183f
Intravenous pyelogram (IVP):
    client preparation, 836t
    health education, 836t
    purpose and description, 836t
    related nursing care, 836t
    in specific conditions
        acute renal failure, 904
        bladder cancer, 863
        polycystic kidney disease, 885
        urinary calculi, 857
        urinary incontinence, 874
        urinary tract infection, 849
Intraventricular conduction blocks, 1004
Intravesicular, 847
Intrinsic (intrarenal) acute renal failure, 900t, 901–2. See also Acute renal failure
Intrinsic factor, 611, 1105
Introitus, 1752
Intron A. See Interferon(s)
Intropin. See Dopamine
Inversion, 1386t
Invirase. See Saquinavir
Iodine:
    deficiency, 543
    Medication Administration, 538t
    radioactive. See Radioactive iodine therapy; Radioactive iodine uptake
    recommended daily intake, 610t
Iodoquinol:
    Medication Administration, 780t
    in specific conditions
        amebic liver abscess, 725
        protozoal bowel infections, 778t, 779, 780t
Ionamin. See Phentermine
Ionized calcium, 229
Ions, 196. See also Electrolytes
Ipratropium bromide, 1326, 1327–28t, 1334
Iranian culture, end-of-life practices, 89
Iraqi culture, death rituals, 88
Irbesartan, 1033t, 1161t
Iridectomy, 1709

Iridotomy, laser, 1709
Irinotecan (CPT-11), 805
Iris, 1671, 1672f, 1680
Iritis, 1703
Iron:
 deficiency. See Iron deficiency anemia
 diagnostic tests, 1110
 dietary sources, 1111t
 recommended daily intake, 610t
 replacement therapy, 1111, 1112t, 1114
Iron chelation therapy, 1116
Iron deficiency anemia. See also Anemia
 causes, 1105, 1105t
 interdisciplinary care
  diagnostic tests, 1110
  focus, 1110t
  medications, 1110, 1112t
  nutrition, 1111, 1111t
 manifestations, 642t, 1105
 pathophysiology, 1103, 1105, 1105f
Iron dextran injection, 1112t
Iron polysaccharide, 1112t
Iron sucrose, 1111, 1112t
Irregular bones, 1380
Irritable bowel syndrome (IBS):
 definition, 762
 interdisciplinary care
  complementary therapies, 763
  diagnosis, 762
  medications, 762–63
  nutrition, 763
 manifestations, 762, 762t
 nursing care
  assessment, 763
  community-based care, 763
  nursing diagnoses and interventions, 763
 pathophysiology, 762
Irritant laxatives, 759–60t
IRV (inspiratory reserve volume), 1214, 1214t
Ischemia, 969
Ischemic, 940
Ischemic stroke, 1581. See also Stroke
Islet cells:
 hormones secreted by, 564
 transplantation, 342t, 581
ISMO. See Isosorbide mononitrate
Isobutyl nitrite, 111
Isoetharine, 1327t
Isograft, 342
Isolation:
 in disasters, 134
 precautions, 321
ISONG (International Society of Nurses in
  Genetics), 148–49, 149t
Isoniazid:
 adverse/side effects, 1288t
 dosage, 1288t
 drug-induced lupus and, 1471
 Medication Administration, 1288t
 nursing implications, 1288t
 for tuberculosis, 1287, 1288t
Isoproterenol, 278t, 1327t
Isoptin. See Verapamil
Isordil. See Isosorbide dinitrate
Isosorbide dinitrate, 973t, 1032
Isosorbide mononitrate, 973t
Isotonic fluid volume deficit, 203. See also Fluid
  volume deficit
Isotonic solutions, 198, 199f
Isotretinoin, 458, 459t
Isradipine, 973–74t, 1162t
Israeli culture, death rituals, 88
Isuprel. See Isoproterenol
Itch–scratch–itch cycle, 440

ITP (immune thrombocytopenic purpura), 1140.
  See also Thrombocytopenia
Itraconazole, 1295
IVP. See Intravenous pyelogram

J

Jackknife position, 69f
Jacksonian march/seizure, 1549
Janeway lesions, 1046
Jannetta procedure, 1656
Jarisch-Herxheimer reaction, 1849
Jaundice:
 assessment in light and dark skin, 426t
 causes, 426t
 definition, 425t, 704
 pathophysiology, 704
 types, 704
Jejunostomy tube, nursing care, 692t
Jejunum, 612, 712
Jews, inflammatory bowel disease incidence, 782t
Joint(s):
 cartilaginous, 1383
 degenerative disease. See Osteoarthritis
 dislocation
  causes, 1400–1401
  definition, 1400
  interdisciplinary care, 1401
  manifestations, 1401
  nursing care
   community-based care, 1401
   nursing diagnoses and interventions, 1401
  pathophysiology, 1401
 fibrous, 1383
 functional classification, 1383t
 inflammatory disease. See Rheumatoid arthritis
 subluxation, 1401
 synovial, 1383, 1386, 1386f, 1386t
Joint arthroplasty, 1452. See also Total joint
  replacement
"Joint mice," 1450
Jugular venous pressure, 1095t
Junctional escape rhythm, 998t, 1001–2
Junctional tachycardia, 1002

K

K⁺. See Potassium
K + Care ET. See Potassium bicarbonate
Kaiser mouthwash, 409t
Kaletra. See Lopinavir; Ritonavir
Kanamycin, 320t
Kantrex. See Kanamycin
Kaolin, 465t
Kaolin and pectin, 756t
Kaon Elixir. See Potassium gluconate
Kaopectate, 756t
Kaposi's sarcoma (KS), 354, 354f, 359t, 1718
Karnofsky scale, functional status, 401t
Kaybovite. See Vitamin B₁₂, replacement therapy
Kayexalate. See Sodium polystyrene sulfonate
Keflex. See Cephalexin
Kegel exercises, 876, 877t, 1806
Kehr's sign, 617
Keloid:
 in burn injuries, 493
 characteristics, 433t, 442f
 definition, 442
 genetic considerations, 427t
 risk factors, 442
Kemadrin. See Procyclidine
Keratectomy, 1697
Keratin, 423
Keratitis, 1696, 1697
Keratoconjunctivitis, 1696

Keratoconus, 1697
Keratoplasty. See Corneal transplant
Keratoses, 430t, 443
Keratotic warts, 1841. See also Genital warts
Kerlone. See Betaxolol
Kernig's sign, 1524f, 1524t
Ketamine, 1772
Ketoconazole:
 Medication Administration, 450t
 in specific conditions
  Cushing's syndrome, 550
  hirsutism, 482
  thrush, 657t, 658
Ketonuria, 569
Ketoprofen, 178t, 1451, 1464t
Ketoprofen SR, 178t
Ketorolac tromethamine, 178t, 179t
Ketosis, 565
17-Ketosteroids, 525t
Kidney(s):
 age-related changes, 883, 884t
 anatomy and physiology, 800, 829–31, 830f,
  885–86
 biopsy, 838t
 in blood pressure regulation, 1085
 diagnostic tests, 836–38t
 disorders
  acute renal failure. See Acute renal failure
  calculi. See Urinary calculi
  Chapter Highlights, 927t
  congenital malformation, 883–84
  glomerular disorders. See Glomerular disorders
  incidence, 883
  polycystic kidney disease
   genetic considerations, 884, 884t
   interdisciplinary care, 885
   manifestations, 885
   nursing care, 885
   pathophysiology, 884, 885f
  tumors, 896. See also Renal cell carcinoma
  vascular
   hypertension, 894
   renal artery occlusion, 894–95
   renal artery stenosis, 895
   renal vein occlusion, 895
 functions
  in body fluid regulation, 201
  hormonal, 834
  maintenance of urine composition and volume,
   833–34, 833f
  in potassium balance, 217
  in sodium balance, 214
  urine formation
   glomerular filtration, 831–33, 831f
   tubular reabsorption, 831f, 833
   tubular secretion, 831f, 833
  waste clearance, 834
 physical assessment, 841t, 842–43t
 transplantation. See Kidney transplant
 trauma
  interdisciplinary care, 895–96
  manifestations, 895
  nursing care, 896
  pathophysiology, 895
Kidney, ureters, and bladder (KUB) x-ray, 857, 889
Kidney biopsy. See Renal biopsy
Kidney failure. See Acute renal failure; Chronic
  renal failure
Kidney transplant. See also Transplant procedures
 allocation of organs, 921t
 incidence, 920
 indications, 342t
 nursing care, 922t
 postoperative care, 921–23

Kidney transplant—*continued*
  procedure, 921, 921*f*
  results, 920
  source of organs, 920–21
  success rate, 342*t*
Kiesselbach's area, 1243
Killer T cells, 297, 298*f. See also* T lymphocytes
Kilocalorie (kcal), 613
Kimmelstiel-Wilson syndrome, 588
Kindling, 103, 103*t*
Kineret. *See* Anakinra
Kinesthesia, 1521*t*
Kinetic continuous rotation bed, 267, 267*f*
Kinins, 304*t*
Klean Prep. *See* Polyethylene glycol
K-Lease. *See* Potassium chloride
Klebsiella pneumoniae, 1271*t*
Klonopin. *See* Clonazepam
K-Lyte. *See* Potassium citrate
Knee:
  physical assessment, 1394*t*, 1395*f*, 1395*t*,
    1396*f*, 1396*t*
  replacement. *See* Total joint replacement
Kock pouch, 865*t*
Kock's ileostomy, 789, 789*f*
KOH (potassium hydroxide), 428*t*
Kohlberg, moral development theory, 25*t*
Korotkoff's sounds, 1092*t*
Korsakoff's psychosis, 103*t*, 108
KS (Kaposi's sarcoma), 354, 354*f*, 359*t*, 1718
Kübler-Ross, stages of loss and grief, 86–87, 86*t*
Kupffer cells, 289
Kussmaul's respirations, 244, 585*t*, 1051
Kwell. *See* Lindane
Kyphosis:
  definition, 1391*t*, 1487
  interdisciplinary care
    diagnosis, 1489
    treatments, 1489
  manifestations, 1488*f*, 1488*t*
  nursing care
    nursing diagnoses and interventions
      community-based care, 1490
      risk for injury, 1489
      risk for peripheral neurovascular
        dysfunction, 1489–90
  pathophysiology, 1488–89
Kytril. *See* Granisetron

L

Labetalol, 1161*t*, 1169*t*
Labia majora:
  anatomy, 1751, 1751*t*, 1752*f*
  physical assessment, 1762*t*
Labia minora:
  anatomy, 1751*t*, 1752, 1752*f*
  physical assessment, 1762*t*
Labile cells, 295
Labyrinth, 1683
Labyrinthectomy, 1727
Labyrinthitis, 1726. *See also* Inner ear disorders
Lacerations, 259, 259*f*
Lactase deficiency:
  ethnic considerations, 798*t*
  interdisciplinary care
    diagnosis, 799
    nursing care, 799
    nutrition, 799
  manifestations, 798
  pathophysiology, 798
Lactic dehydrogenase (LDH), 386*t*, 1775
Lactose breath test, 799
Lactose intolerance, 798. *See also* Lactase
  deficiency

Lactulose, 716, 717*t*, 759*t*
Laënnec's cirrhosis. *See* Alcoholic cirrhosis
Lamictal. *See* Lamotrigine
Laminectomy:
  nursing care, 1609–10*t*
  procedure, 1608
Lamivudine, 358, 708
Lamotrigine, 1550*t*
Laniazid. *See* Isoniazid
Lanoxin. *See* Digoxin
Lansoprazole, 62*t*, 665*t*, 678
Lantus. *See* Insulin glargine
Laparoscopic appendectomy, 767
Laparoscopic cholecystectomy:
  nursing care, 700*t*
  Nursing Research: postoperative pain
    management, 700*t*
  procedure, 699
Laparoscopic fundoplication, 666
Laparoscopy:
  definition, 388*t*
  in female reproductive system disorders
    nursing care, 1758*t*, 1801*t*
    purpose and description, 1758*t*, 1801, 1801*f*
Laparotomy:
  for appendectomy, 767
  for cholecystectomy, 699
  definition, 699
  for intestinal obstruction, 813
  for peritonitis, 770
Large intestine:
  anatomy, physiology, and functions, 742–43, 742*f*
  disorders. *See* Bowel disorders
  obstruction, 812. *See also* Intestinal obstruction
Large-bowel obstruction, 812. *See also* Intestinal
  obstruction
Larodopa. *See* Levodopa
Laryngeal cancer:
  interdisciplinary care
    chemotherapy, 1254
    diagnosis, 1254
    radiation therapy, 1254
    speech rehabilitation, 1255–56, 1255*f*, 1258*f*
    staging, 1254*t*
    surgery, 1254–55, 1255*f*
    treatments, 1254*t*
  manifestations, 1253, 1253*t*
  nursing care
    of client having total laryngectomy, 1256*t*
    community-based care, 1262–63
    health promotion, 1258
    nursing diagnoses and interventions
      anticipatory grieving, 1261
      imbalanced nutrition: less than body
        requirements, 1260–61
      impaired swallowing, 1260
      impaired verbal communication, 1259–60
      risk for impaired airway clearance, 1258
      using NANDA, NIC, and NOC, 1261, 1262*t*
    Nursing Research: use of speech-generating
      devices, 1260*t*
  pathophysiology, 1253, 1253*f*
  risk factors, 1253
Laryngectomy:
  nursing care
    postoperative, 1256*t*
    preoperative, 1256*t*
  Nursing Care Plan
    assessment, 1259*t*
    critical thinking in the nursing process, 1259*t*
    diagnoses, 1259*t*
    evaluation, 1259*t*
    expected outcomes, 1259*t*
    planning and implementation, 1259*t*

Nursing Research: use of speech-generating
      devices, 1260*t*
  partial, 1255
  procedure, 1255, 1255*f*
  total, 1255
Laryngitis, 1241
Laryngopharynx, 1211
Laryngospasm, 1249
Larynx:
  anatomy, physiology, and functions, 1211
  infections, 1240–41
  obstruction or trauma
    interdisciplinary care, 1249–50, 1249*f*
    manifestations, 1249
    nursing care, 1250
    pathophysiology, 1249
  tumors, 1252, 1253. *See also* Laryngeal cancer
Laser epithelial keratomileusis (LASEK), 1697
Laser eye surgery, 1697
Laser *in situ* keratomileusis (LASIK), 1697
Laser iridotomy, 1709
Laser lithotripsy, 858
Laser photocoagulation:
  of bladder tumors, 864
  of colorectal tumors, 803
  in diabetic retinopathy, 1716
  in peptic ulcer disease, 685
Laser surgery, 477–78, 1697
Laser thermokeratoplasty (LTK), 1697
Laser trabeculoplasty, 1709
Lasix. *See* Furosemide
Latanoprost, 1709, 1710*t*
Late phase response, in asthma, 1322
Latency, 1839
Latent syphilis, 1848
Lateral chest position, 69*f*
Lateral myocardial infarction, 984. *See also* Acute
  myocardial infarction
Lateral transtentorial herniation, 1538, 1538*f*
Latex allergy, 335–36, 456
Latin Americans, substance abuse in, 105*t*
Laudanum, 756*t*
Laxatives:
  bulk-forming, 759*t*
  in irritable bowel syndrome, 762
  irritant/stimulant, 759–60*t*
  lubricant, 760*t*
  magnesium-containing, 236*t*
  Medication Administration, 759–60*t*
  osmotic/saline, 759*t*
  wetting agents, 759*t*
LDH (lactic dehydrogenase), 386*t*, 1775
LDL. *See* Low-density lipoprotein
LE (lupus erythematosus) cell test, 341
Lead, pacemaker, 1010*t*. *See also* Pacemakers
Leader, nurse as, 14–15
LEEP (loop electrosurgical excision procedure),
  1757*t*, 1813
LEETZ (loop electrosurgical excision of
  transformation zone), 1757*t*
Leflunomide, 341, 1465
Left main coronary artery, 939*f*, 959
Left-sided heart failure, 1026, 1026*f. See also*
  Heart failure
Leg, ankle, and foot exercises, preoperative
  teaching, 73*t*
Legal issues:
  in end-of-life care, 12
  informed consent, 55, 56*f*
Legionnaire's disease, 1269, 1270*t*. *See also*
  Pneumonia
Leiomyoma:
  definition, 1809
  incidence, 1809

interdisciplinary care
  medications, 1810
  surgery, 1810
manifestations, 1809
pathophysiology, 1809
types, 1809, 1810f
Lens:
  age-related changes, 1676t
  anatomy, physiology, and functions, 1672, 1672f
  assessment, 1680
Lentigines, 430t
Lentigo maligna, 466–67
Lepirudin, 1141
Lescol. See Fluvastatin
Lesser vestibular glands. See Skene's glands
Leucovorin. See Folinic acid
Leukemia:
  classification, 1119, 1119t, 1121
  definition, 1118
  incidence, 1118
  interdisciplinary care
    biologic therapy, 1124–25
    bone marrow transplant, 1124, 1124f
    chemotherapy, 1123, 1123t
    complementary therapies, 1125
    diagnosis, 1122–23, 1123t
    stem cell transplant, 1124
  manifestations, 1119
  Multisystem Effects, 1120t
  nursing care
    anticipatory grief, 1128
    assessment, 1126
    community-based care
      encouraging self-care, 1129
      information about leukemia and
        treatment, 1129
      preventing infection and injury, 1129
      promoting nutrition, 1129
    health promotion, 1125–26
    imbalanced nutrition: less than body
      requirements, 1127
    impaired oral mucous membrane, 1127
    ineffective protection, 1127–28
    nursing diagnoses and interventions
      risk for infection, 1126–27
    using NANDA, NIC, and NOC, 1128, 1128t
  Nursing Care Plan
    assessment, 1125t
    critical thinking in the nursing process, 1125t
    diagnoses, 1125t
    evaluation, 1125t
    expected outcomes, 1125t
    planning and implementation, 1125t
  Nursing Research: care of physical problems
    during treatment, 1126t
  pathophysiology, 1119
  risk factors, 1118
  survival rates, 1119
  types
    acute lymphocytic. See Acute lymphocytic
      leukemia
    acute myeloid. See Acute myeloid leukemia
    chronic lymphocytic. See Chronic lymphocytic
      leukemia
    chronic myeloid. See Chronic myeloid
      leukemia
Leukeran. See Chlorambucil
Leukocyte esterase test, 849
Leukocytes. See White blood cells
Leukocytosis, 287, 307t, 1079
Leukopenia, 287, 307t, 1079, 1138
Leukoplakia, 623t, 1253
Leukotriene modifiers, 1326, 1328t
Leukotrienes, 292t, 304t

Leuprolide, 1787t, 1810
Levaquin. See Levofloxacin
Levatol. See Penbutolol
Level of consciousness, altered. See Altered level
  of consciousness
Levitra. See Vardenafil hydrochloride
Levobunolol, 1710t
Levodopa, 1637t, 1639
Levo-Dromoran. See Levorphanol
Levofloxacin, 320t
Levophed. See Norepinephrine
Levorphanol, 180t
Levothroid. See Levothyroxine sodium
Levothyroxine sodium, 544t
Levoxyl. See Levothyroxine sodium
Lewy body dementia, 1618t
Leydig's cells, 1744
LH. See Luteinizing hormone
Libido, 1768
Librium. See Chlordiazepoxide
Lichen planus, 460
Lichenification, 433t
Licorice root, 709, 1335
Lidocaine:
  adverse/side effects, 1006t
  for dysrhythmias, 1006t
  for long-term analgesia at home, 190t
  Medication Administration, 658t, 1006t
  viscous, for stomatitis, 657, 658t
Lifestyle:
  health and, 20
  modifications for hypertension, 1159–60,
    1159t, 1160t
Lifts, 952
Ligaments, 1380
Lightning injury, 488
Limb-girdle muscular dystrophy, 1459t
Limbic system, 1507
Lindane, 451
Lindemann, theory of loss and grief, 86, 86t
Linear fracture, skull, 1555, 1555t. See also Skull
  fracture
Linezolid, 320t
Linoleic acid, 608
Lioresal. See Baclofen
Liothyronine sodium, 544t
Liotrix, 544t
Lipancreatin. See Pancrelipase
Lipid profile:
  in coronary heart disease diagnosis, 965
  high-risk levels, 963t
  normal values, 944t, 963t, 965
  purpose and description, 944t
  related nursing care, 944t
Lipiduria, 888
Lipitor. See Atorvastatin
Lipoatrophy, 575
Lipodystrophy, 575
Lipoprotein (a), 965
Lipoproteins, 959. See also High-density
  lipoprotein; Lipid profile; Low-density
  lipoprotein
Liposuction, 479
Lisinopril, 1033t, 1161t
Lispro, 571, 571t
Lithiasis, 855
Lithotomy position, 69f
Lithotripsy. See also Extracorporeal shock wave
  lithotripsy
  nursing care, 859t
  procedure, 858
Liver:
  anatomy, physiology, and functions, 612–13,
    613t, 703–4

disorders
  abscess
    interdisciplinary care, 725
    manifestations, 725
    nursing care, 725
    pathophysiology, 725
  cancer
    causes, 724t
    incidence, 723–24
    interdisciplinary care, 724
    manifestations, 724, 724t
    nursing care, 724
    pathophysiology, 724
  cirrhosis. See Cirrhosis
  diagnostic tests
    laboratory, 716
    liver biopsy, 617t, 716
  hepatitis. See Hepatitis
  manifestations
    hepatocellular failure, 704
    jaundice, 704
    portal hypertension. See Portal hypertension
  surgical risk and nursing implications, 57t
  trauma
    interdisciplinary care, 725
    nursing care, 725
    pathophysiology, 725
  physical assessment, 625f, 625t, 627f, 627t
  transplantation. See Liver transplant
"Liver spots," 430t
Liver transplant. See also Transplant procedures
  contraindications, 719–20
  indications, 342t, 719
  nursing care, 720t
  success rate, 342t
Living will, 90. See also Advance directives
LMW (low-molecular-weight) heparins, 1188,
  1189t
Lobar pneumonia, 1268, 1268t, 1270t. See also
  Pneumonia
Lobectomy, 1312t
Local anesthetics:
  for long-term analgesia at home, 190t
  for pain management, 179
  for regional anesthesia, 63
  for skin disorders, 441t
Local nerve infiltration, 63
Locked-in syndrome, 1532. See also Altered level
  of consciousness
Lodine. See Etodolac
Lomotil. See Diphenoxylate
Long bones, 1380, 1393f
Long QT syndrome, 950t, 1002
Loniten. See Minoxidil
Loop diuretics:
  mechanism of action, 210
  Medication Administration, 210t, 905t, 1539t
  in specific conditions
    acute renal failure, 904, 905t
    fluid volume excess, 210t
    heart failure, 1032
    hyponatremia, 215
    increased intracranial pressure, 1538, 1539t
    pulmonary edema, 1041
Loop electrosurgical excision of transformation
  zone (LEETZ), 1757t
Loop electrosurgical excision procedure (LEEP),
  1757t, 1813
Loop ileostomy, 789
Loop of Henle, 830, 833–34, 833f
Loperamide hydrochloride, 756t, 762, 764
Lopid. See Gemfibrozil
Lopinavir, 358
Lopressor. See Metoprolol

Loratadine, 1230t
Lorazepam:
    preoperative use and nursing implications, 62t
    in specific conditions
        acute respiratory failure, 1355
        burns, 500
        nausea and vomiting, 672
        substance abuse/withdrawal treatment, 114t
        vertigo, 1727
Lordosis, 1391t
Losartan, 1033t, 1161t
Loss and grief. See also Death and dying; End-of-
        life care
    Chapter Highlights, 99t
    definitions, 85
    factors affecting response to
        age, 87, 87t
        cultural and spiritual practices, 88, 89t
        family, 88
        mourning rituals, 88
        social support, 87
    Meeting Individualized Needs, 98t
    nurses' response to clients', 88
    nursing care
        assessment
            physical, 95
            psychosocial, 96
            spiritual, 96
        community-based care, 97
        nursing diagnoses and interventions, 96
            anticipatory grieving, 96
            chronic sorrow, 96
            death anxiety, 96
        using NANDA, NIC, and NOC, 97, 97t
    Nursing Care Plan
        assessment, 98t
        critical thinking in the nursing process, 98t
        diagnoses, 98t
        evaluation, 98t
        expected outcomes, 98t
        planning and implementation, 98t
    teaching for clients experiencing, 98t
    theories of
        Bowlby: protest, despair, and detachment,
            85–86, 86t
        Caplan: stress and loss, 86, 86t
        Engel: acute grief, restitution, and long-term
            grief, 86, 86t
        Freud: psychoanalytic theory, 85
        Kübler-Ross: stages of coping with loss,
            86–87, 86t
        Lindemann: categories of symptoms, 86, 86t
    types, 85t
Lotensin. See Benazepril
Lotions, skin, 441t
Lotrol. See Diphenoxylate
Lou Gehrig's disease. See Amyotrophic lateral
        sclerosis
Lovastatin, 967t, 968
Lovenox. See Enoxaparin
Low back pain:
    causes, 1490t
    interdisciplinary care
        conservative treatment, 1491
        diagnosis, 1491
        medications, 1491
    manifestations, 1490, 1490t
    nursing care
        community-based care, 1492
        health promotion, 1491
        nursing diagnoses and interventions
            acute pain, 1491
            deficient knowledge, 1491–92
            risk for impaired adjustment, 1492

    pathophysiology, 1490
Low-density lipoprotein (LDL):
    functions, 959
    high-risk levels, 963, 963t
    normal values, 944t, 963t
Lower body obesity, 632. See also Obesity
Lower extremity:
    amputation sites, 1422f
    fracture, 1414, 1416
    physical assessment, 1096–97t, 1097f
Lower motor neurons, 1509
Lower respiratory disorders:
    Chapter Highlights, 1317–18t, 1372–73t
    hemothorax. See Hemothorax
    infections and inflammatory disorders
        acute bronchitis. See Acute bronchitis
        fungal infections
            aspergillosis, 1294
            blastomycosis, 1294
            coccidiomycosis, 1294
            geographic distribution, 1294
            histoplasmosis, 1294
            interdisciplinary care, 1294–95
            nursing care, 1295
            pathophysiology, 1294
        inhalation anthrax, 128t, 1293–94
        lung abscess. See Lung abscess
        in older adults, 315t
        pleural effusion. See Pleural effusion
        pleuritis, 1269, 1295
        pneumonia. See Pneumonia
        severe acute respiratory syndrome. See Severe
            acute respiratory syndrome
        tuberculosis. See Tuberculosis
    inhalation injury. See Inhalation injury
    interstitial pulmonary disorders
        occupational lung diseases. See Occupational
            lung diseases
        sarcoidosis, 1346–47
    lung cancer. See Lung cancer
    pneumothorax. See Pneumothorax
    pulmonary vascular disorders
        pulmonary embolism. See Pulmonary
            embolism
        pulmonary hypertension. See Pulmonary
            hypertension
    reactive airway disorders
        asthma. See Asthma
        atelectasis. See Atelectasis
        bronchiectasis. See Bronchiectasis
        chronic obstructive pulmonary disease. See
            Chronic obstructive pulmonary disease
        cystic fibrosis. See Cystic fibrosis
    respiratory failure
        acute respiratory distress syndrome. See Acute
            respiratory distress syndrome
        acute respiratory failure. See Acute respiratory
            failure
    surgical risk and nursing implications, 57t
    thoracic trauma. See Thoracic trauma
Low-molecular-weight (LMW) heparins, 1188,
        1189t
Low-output failure, 1027
Lozol. See Indapamide
LTK (laser thermokeratoplasty), 1697
Lubath, 441t
Lubricant laxative, 760t
Lubriderm, 441t
Lugol's solution. See Strong iodine solution
Lumbar puncture:
    client and family teaching, 1515t
    client preparation, 1515t
    in pneumonia, 1566
    purpose and description, 1515t

    related nursing care, 1515–16t
    in stroke, 1584
Lumbar spine:
    disk herniation, 1608. See also Herniated
        intervertebral disk
    physical assessment, 1392t, 1393f
Lumigan. See Bimatoprost
Lumpectomy, 1825, 1826f
Lund and Browder burn assessment method, 491, 492f
Lung:
    anatomy, physiology, and functions, 1211–12,
        1212f
    disorders. See Lower respiratory disorders
    physical assessment, 1224–26t, 1224f, 1225f
    transplantation. See Lung transplant
    trauma. See Thoracic trauma
Lung abscess:
    definition, 1280
    interdisciplinary care, 1280
    manifestations, 1280
    nursing care, 1280
    pathophysiology, 1280
    in pneumonia, 1269
Lung biopsy, 1219t, 1312
Lung cancer:
    Case Study, 418t
    complications, 1311
    course, 1311
    genetic considerations, 1220t
    incidence, 1308
    interdisciplinary care
        complementary therapies, 1313
        diagnosis, 1311–12
        medications, 1312
        radiation therapy, 1312–13
        staging, 1311, 1311t
        surgery, 1312, 1312t
    manifestations, 1309, 1311
    mortality rate, 1308
    Multisystem Effects, 1310t
    nursing care
        assessment, 1313–14
        of client having lung surgery, 1313t
        of client having radiation therapy, 1314t
        community-based care, 1316–17
        health promotion, 1313
        nursing diagnoses and interventions
            activity intolerance, 1315–16
            anticipatory grieving, 1316
            ineffective breathing pattern, 1314–15
            pain, 1316
        using NANDA, NIC, and NOC, 1316, 1317t
    Nursing Care Plan
        assessment, 1315t
        critical thinking in the nursing process, 1315t
        diagnoses, 1315t
        evaluation, 1315t
        expected outcomes, 1315t
        planning and implementation, 1315t
    pathophysiology, 1308–9
    risk factors, 1308
Lung compliance, 1216
Lung elasticity, 1216
Lung reduction surgery, 1335
Lung transplant:
    in chronic obstructive pulmonary disease, 1335
    in cystic fibrosis, 1342
    indications, 342t
    nursing considerations, 1336t
    success rate, 342t
Lupron. See Leuprolide
Lupus erythematosus (LE) cell test, 341
Lupus nephritis, 889. See also Glomerular
        disorders

Luteinizing hormone (LH):
functions, 520, 1753
in ovarian cycle, 1754, 1754f
Luteinizing hormone-releasing hormone
agonist, 1787t
Lyme disease:
cause, 1476
complications, 1477
incidence, 1476
interdisciplinary care, 1477
manifestations, 1477
nursing care, 1477
pathophysiology, 1476–77
Lymph, 1086, 1199
Lymph nodes:
assessment by palpation, 305f, 1098t, 1749t,
1762f, 1762t
biopsy, 1088t, 1131–32
functions, 291
locations, 291, 291f, 1086f
Lymphadenitis, 1098t
Lymphadenopathy:
causes, 1098t
definition, 1098t
in Hodgkin's lymphoma, 1130, 1131t
in non-Hodgkin's lymphoma, 1131, 1131f, 1131t
pathophysiology, 1199
treatment, 1199
Lymphangiography, 1088t, 1200
Lymphangitis, 1093t, 1199
Lymphatic system:
anatomy, physiology, and functions, 1085–86,
1086f. See also Lymph nodes
assessment
diagnostic tests, 1088, 1088t
functional health pattern interview, 1090t
genetic considerations, 1088
health assessment interview, 1089, 1091
physical assessment, 1091, 1098–99t, 1099f
disorders
lymphadenopathy. See Lymphadenopathy
lymphedema. See Lymphedema
Lymphedema:
after axillary node dissection, 1825
causes, 1093, 1199
definition, 1093, 1825
genetic considerations, 1199t
interdisciplinary care
diagnosis, 1200
treatments, 1200
manifestations, 1200
nursing care
community-based care, 1201
nursing diagnoses and interventions
disturbed body image, 1201
excess fluid volume, 1201
impaired tissue integrity, 1200–1201
in ovarian cancer, 1818t
pathophysiology, 1200
Lymphedema praecox, 1199t
Lymphedema tarda, 1199t
Lymphoblasts, 1122, 1123t
Lymphocytes:
abnormal, possible causes, 307t, 387t
development, 289f
differentiation, 290f, 1077f
functions, 289, 1079
in leukemia, 1123t
normal values, 307t, 387t, 1118t
types, 290, 290f. See also B lymphocytes;
Natural killer cells; T lymphocytes
Lymphocytic leukemia, 1119. See also Leukemia
Lymphocytopenia, 307t
Lymphocytosis, 307t

Lymphoid system, 291–92, 291f
Lymphomas:
in AIDS, 354, 359t, 1129
characteristics, 1129
definition, 1129
genetic considerations, 1129t
Hodgkin's disease. See Hodgkin's disease
incidence, 1129
interdisciplinary care
chemotherapy, 1132
complications of treatment, 1133
diagnosis, 1131–32
radiation therapy, 1132, 1132f
staging, 1132
stem cell transplant, 1132
manifestations, 1130–31, 1131t
non-Hodgkin's. See Non-Hodgkin's lymphoma
nursing care
assessment, 1133
community-based care, 1135–36
nursing diagnoses and interventions
disturbed body image, 1135
fatigue, 1133–34
nausea, 1134–35
risk for impaired skin integrity, 1133
sexual dysfunction, 1135
using NANDA, NIC, and NOC, 1135, 1136t
Nursing Care Plan
assessment, 1134t
critical thinking in the nursing process, 1134t
diagnoses, 1134t
evaluation, 1134t
expected outcomes, 1134t
planning and implementation, 1134t
Nursing Research: care of physical problems
during treatment, 1126t
pathophysiology, 1129–31
risk factors, 1129
Lymphoscintigraphy, 1200
Lynch syndrome, 801–2. See also Colorectal
cancer
D-Lysergic acid diethylamide (LSD), 111, 113t

M

M protein, 1136
Ma huang, 1274, 1326
Maalox, 665, 666t
MAC (midarm circumference), 621t, 622f, 622t
MAC (*Mycobacterium avium* complex), 353, 353f,
359t
Macrobid. See Nitrofurantoin
Macrodantin. See Nitrofurantoin
Macrodex. See Dextran 70
Macrolides, 320t, 1271, 1271t
Macrophages, 288, 288t, 289f
Macula, 1680, 1681t
Macular degeneration:
incidence, 1713–14
interdisciplinary care, 1714
manifestations, 1714, 1714f
nursing care, 1714
Nursing Research: effect on older adults, 1715t
pathophysiology, 1714
Macule, 432t
"Mad-cow disease," 1658
Mafenide acetate, 500, 501t
Magnesium (Mg^{2+}):
balance, 233
in body fluid compartments, 197t
foods high in, 234t
functions, 233
imbalances. See Hypermagnesemia;
Hypomagnesemia

medications containing, 236t
normal values, 198t
recommended daily intake, 610t
Magnesium citrate, 759t
Magnesium hydroxide, 759t
Magnesium salicylate, 178t
Magnesium silicate, 465t
Magnesium sulfate, 114t, 234, 235t
Magnetic resonance angiography (MRA):
brain and spinal cord, 1514t
in peripheral vascular disease, 1177
purpose and description, 1088t
related nursing care, 1088t
Magnetic resonance cholangiopancreatography
(MRCP), 616t
Magnetic resonance imaging (MRI):
abdominal, 744t, 1173
brain and spinal cord, 1514t
in cancer, 384
in deep venous thrombosis, 1188
heart, 944t
kidneys, 837t
lymphatic system, 1088t
musculoskeletal system, 1387t
pituitary gland, 523t
sinuses, 1236
stomach, 615t
thorax, 1218t
Magnetic resonance spectroscopy
(MRS), 1514t
Magnetoencephalogram (MEG), 1512, 1515t
Major burn injury, 491t. See also Burns
Major histocompatibility complex (MHC), 329
Major procedure, 54t
Malabsorption:
causes, 795, 795t
definition, 795
manifestations, 795–96, 796t
syndromes
lactase deficiency
ethnic considerations, 798t
interdisciplinary care, 798–99
manifestations, 798
nursing care, 799
short bowel syndrome
causes, 799
interdisciplinary care, 799
nursing care, 799–800
pathophysiology, 799
sprue. See Sprue
Malathion, 451
Maldigestion, 795, 795t
Male reproductive system:
age-related changes, 27t, 29t, 1749t
anatomy, physiology, and functions
breasts, 1744
overview, 1744f
penis, 1744
scrotum, 1744
sex hormones, 1745–46
testes, 1744
assessment
diagnostic tests, 1746–47, 1746t
functional health pattern interview, 1748t
genetic considerations, 1747, 1747t
health assessment interview, 1747
physical assessment
breasts and lymph nodes, 1749t
external genitalia, 1749–50t, 1749f, 1750f
overview, 1747–48
prostate, 1750t
disorders
benign prostatic hyperplasia. See Benign
prostatic hyperplasia

Male reproductive system—*continued*
  benign scrotal mass
    nursing care, 1773
    pathophysiology, 1772–73
  breast cancer, 1790. *See also* Breast cancer
  cancer of the penis
    incidence, 1772
    interdisciplinary care, 1772
    nursing care, 1772
    pathophysiology, 1772
  Chapter Highlights, 1790–91*t*
  Clinical Scenarios, 1855*t*
  ejaculatory dysfunction, 1771
  epididymitis, 1773
  erectile dysfunction. *See* Erectile dysfunction
  gynecomastia, 1749*t*, 1789–90
  orchitis, 1774
  phimosis, 1749*t*, 1771
  priapism, 1771–72, 1772*t*
  prostatitis. *See* Prostatitis
  sexually transmitted infections. *See* Sexually
    transmitted infections
  testicular cancer. *See* Testicular cancer
  testicular torsion, 1774
Malignant cells, 376–77, 377*t*. *See also*
    Cancer
Malignant disease, 22*t*. *See also* Cancer
Malignant hypertension. *See* Hypertensive
    emergencies
Malignant hyperthermia, 61–62, 63*t*
Malignant lymphoma. *See* Lymphomas
Malignant melanoma:
  classification
    acral lentiginous, 467
    lentigo maligna, 466–67
    nodular, 467
    superficial spreading, 466, 467*f*
  incidence, 465
  interdisciplinary care
    ABCD rule, 467
    diagnosis, 467
    identification, 467
    microstaging, 467, 468*f*
    treatments
      immunotherapy, 468
      new modalities, 468
      radiation therapy, 468
      surgery, 468
  nursing care
    assessment, 470, 470*t*. *See also* Skin,
      assessment
    community-based care, 471
    health promotion, 468–69
    nursing diagnoses and interventions
      anxiety, 471
      hopelessness, 470–71
      impaired skin integrity, 470
    using NANDA, NIC, and NOC, 471, 471*t*
  Nursing Care Plan
    assessment, 469*t*
    critical thinking in the nursing process, 469*t*
    diagnoses, 469*t*
    evaluation, 469*t*
    expected outcomes, 469*t*
    planning and implementation, 469*t*
  pathophysiology, 466
  precursor lesions
    congenital nevi, 466
    dysplastic nevi, 466
    lentigo maligna, 466
  risk factors, 466, 466*t*
Malignant pain, 174. *See also* Pain
Malleus, 1682, 1682*f*

Malnutrition:
  in cirrhosis, 715*t*
  conditions associated with, 641*t*
  definition, 641
  incidence and prevalence, 641
  interdisciplinary care
    diagnosis, 642, 644, 644*t*
    medications, 644, 645*t*
    nutrition
      enteral. *See* Enteral nutrition
      parenteral, 646, 647*f*, 648
  manifestations, 641, 642*t*
  Multisystem Effects, 643*t*
  nursing care
    assessment, 619*t*, 622–23*t*, 648
    community-based care, 650
    health promotion, 648
    Medication Administration, 645*t*
    nursing diagnoses and interventions
      imbalanced nutrition: less than body
        requirements, 648–49
      risk for deficient fluid volume, 649
      risk for impaired skin integrity, 650
      risk for infection, 649
    using NANDA, NIC, and NOC, 650, 650*t*
  Nursing Care Plan
    assessment, 649*t*
    critical thinking in the nursing process, 649*t*
    diagnoses, 649*t*
    evaluation, 649*t*
    expected outcomes, 649*t*
    planning and implementation, 649*t*
  in older adults, 641, 642*t*
  pathophysiology, 641
  risk factors, 641
  surgical risk and nursing implications, 57*t*
MALT (mucosa-associated lymphoid tissue), 292
Mammary duct ectasia, 1821*t*, 1822
Mammary glands, 1751*t*
Mammogram, 1755, 1756*t*, 1824*t*
Manager, nurse as, 14–15
Manganese, 610*t*
Manifestations, definition, 22
Manifestations of...:
  acute arterial occlusion, 1184*t*
  acute glomerulonephritis, 888*t*
  acute hepatitis, 706*t*
  acute myocardial infarction, 985*t*
  acute pyelonephritis, 848*t*
  Addison's disease, 554*t*
  Alzheimer's disease, 1620*t*
  amyotrophic lateral sclerosis, 1646*t*
  anaphylactic shock, 276*t*
  angina, 970*t*
  asthma, 1323*t*
  bacterial meningitis, 1564*t*
  Bell's palsy, 1658*t*
  bone tumors, 1483*t*
  brain tumors, 1569*t*
  breast cancer, 1823*t*
  cancer, 405*t*
  carbon monoxide poisoning, 496*t*
  cardiac tamponade, 1051*t*
  cardiogenic shock, 274*t*
  chronic venous insufficiency, 1194*t*
  cirrhosis, 715*t*
  compartment syndrome, 1403*t*
  concussion, 1558*t*
  Cushing's syndrome, 549*t*
  cystitis, 848*t*
  death, 94*t*
  deep venous thrombosis, 1187*t*
  diabetic ketoacidosis, 585*t*

  disseminated intravascular coagulation, 1147*t*
  dysmenorrhea, 1801*t*
  eating disorders, 651*t*
  endometriosis, 1811*t*
  esophageal cancer, 669*t*
  fracture, 1403*t*
  gastritis, 677*t*
  gastroenteritis, 773
  gastroesophageal reflux disease, 664*t*
  genital herpes, 1839*t*
  gout, 1444*t*
  herniated intervertebral disk, 1607*t*
  hiatal hernia, 668*t*
  HIV infection and AIDS, 351*t*
  Huntington's disease, 1643
  hydronephrosis, 857*t*
  hyperparathyroidism, 547*t*
  hypertensive emergencies, 1169*t*
  hypoglycemia, 587*t*
  hypovolemic shock, 274*t*
  impending death, 92*t*
  increased intracranial pressure, 1536*t*
  infective endocarditis, 1046*t*
  inflammation, 304*t*
  influenza, 1233*t*
  irritable bowel syndrome, 762*t*
  kyphosis, 1488*t*
  laryngeal cancer, 1253*t*
  liver cancer, 724*t*
  low back pain, 1490*t*
  metabolic acidosis, 244*t*
  metabolic alkalosis, 246*t*
  multiple sclerosis, 1627*t*
  musculoskeletal neoplasms, 1483*t*
  myasthenia gravis, 1648*t*
  nasal fracture, 1246*t*
  neurogenic shock, 276*t*
  nutrient deficiencies, 642*t*
  obstructive sleep apnea, 1251*t*
  oral cancer, 660*t*
  osteoarthritis, 1451*t*
  osteomalacia, 1448*t*
  osteomyelitis, 1479*t*
  Paget's disease, 1441*t*
  pancreatitis, 727*t*
  Parkinson's disease, 1636*t*
  perimenopausal period, 1796*t*
  peripheral vascular disease, 590*t*, 1177*t*
  peritonitis, 769*t*
  pertussis, 1242*t*
  pharyngitis, 1239*t*
  polycythemia, 1117*t*
  prostatitis and prostatodynia, 1777
  pulmonary edema, 1040*t*
  pulmonary embolism, 1348*t*
  pulmonary tuberculosis, 1283*t*
  renal tumors, 896
  retinal detachment, 1716*t*
  rheumatic fever, 1043*t*
  scoliosis, 1488*t*
  septic shock, 275*t*
  soft tissue sarcomas, 1483*t*
  spinal cord injury, 1598*t*
  spinal cord tumor, 1612*t*
  stroke, 1582*t*, 1583*t*
  syphilis, 1848*t*
  systemic lupus erythematosus, 1473*t*
  testicular cancer, 1775*t*
  tonsillitis, 1239*t*
  urinary calculi, 856*t*
  varicose veins, 1196*t*
  venous thrombosis, 1187*t*
Man-made disasters, 126–27. *See also* Disasters

Mannitol:
   Medication Administration, 905t, 1539t
   in specific conditions
      acute renal failure, 904, 905t
      increased intracranial pressure, 1538, 1539t
Manometer, 206t
Manometry, esophageal. See Esophageal
      manometry
Mantle cell lymphoma, 1130t. See also
      Lymphomas
Mantoux test, 1286, 1286f, 1286t
Manual traction, 1408
MAP. See Mean arterial pressure
Marfan syndrome:
   characteristics, 1389t
   genetic considerations, 950t, 1057t
   thoracic aortic aneurysm in, 1171, 1172t
Marginal blepharitis, 1700
Margination, 293, 293f
Marijuana, 107, 111t
Marinol. See Dronabinol
Marshall-Marchetti-Krantz procedure, 1806
Mass casualty incidents (MCIs). See also Disasters
   definition, 127
   educational competencies for registered nurses
      responding to, 126, 126t
Mass Trauma Data Instrument, 135, 136f
MAST (Michigan Alcohol Screening Test),
      116, 116f
Mast cell stabilizers, 1328t
Mastectomy:
   exercises following, 1832f
   nursing care, 1826t
   procedure, 1825, 1826f
   reconstruction following, 1828–29, 1828f, 1829f
Mastitis, 1821t
Mastoidectomy, 1724
Mastoiditis:
   characteristics, 1723
   complications, 1723–24
   incidence, 1723
   interdisciplinary care, 1724
   manifestations, 1724
   nursing care, 1724
   pathophysiology, 1723
Mavik. See Trandolapril
Maxair. See Pirbuterol
Maxalt. See Rizatriptan benzoate
Maxillofacial trauma, 257
Maxipime. See Cefepime
McBurney's point, 766, 766f
MCD (minimal change disease), 888. See also
      Glomerular disorders
McGill pain questionnaire, 187f
MCH (mean corpuscular hemoglobin), 1078t
MCHC (mean corpuscular hemoglobin
      concentration), 1078t
MCIs. See Mass casualty incidents
McMurray's test, 1395f, 1395t
MCV (mean corpuscular volume), 1078t
MD. See Muscular dystrophy
MDMA (Ecstasy), 111
MDR-TB (multidrug-resistant tuberculosis), 313
MDS. See Myelodysplastic syndrome
Meals-on-Wheels, 38
Mean arterial pressure (MAP):
   abnormal findings, 1560t
   definition, 269, 1030, 1085, 1154
   in heart failure, 1030
   in hypovolemic shock, 273f
   intra-arterial monitoring, 1030
   normal values, 1560t
   regulation, 1085

Mean corpuscular hemoglobin (MCH), 1078t
Mean corpuscular hemoglobin concentration
      (MCHC), 1078t
Mean corpuscular volume (MCV), 1078t
Measles, postexposure prophylaxis, 302t
Measles-mumps-rubella (MMR) vaccine:
   contraindications, 21t
   indications, 21t, 300, 300t
   nursing implications, 300t
Mebendazole, 779–80
Mechanical debridement, 504
Mechanical ventilation:
   complications
      barotrauma, 1360
      cardiovascular effects, 1360
      gastrointestinal effects, 1360
      nosocomial pneumonia, 1360
   indications, 1356
   modes of ventilators, 1358, 1359t
   Nursing Research: pain assessment in intubated
      clients, 1364t
   in specific conditions
      acute respiratory distress syndrome, 1367
      increased intracranial pressure, 1540
   terminal weaning, 1361
   types of ventilators, 1356–58, 1357f
   ventilator settings, 1358, 1360t
   weaning, 1360–61, 1360f
Mechlorethamine, 392t
Meclizine, 672, 673t, 1727
Meclofenamate, 178t, 1464t
Meclomen. See Meclofenamate
Mediastinoscopy, 1312t
Medicaid, 37
Medical-surgical nursing:
   Chapter Highlights, 16t
   definition, 5
   nurse's roles
      advocate, 14
      caregiver, 12–13, 12f, 13t
      educator, 13, 14f
      leader and manager
         in case management, 14
         delegation, 14
         evaluation of outcomes of nursing care, 15
         in primary nursing, 14
         in team nursing, 14
      researcher, 15
   practice. See Nursing practice
Medicare:
   coverage, 37
   home care reimbursement, 40, 40t
Medication(s). See also specific drugs
   administration. See Medication Administration
   affected by decreased glomerular filtration
      rate, 883
   causing alopecia, 482t
   causing constipation, 758t
   causing drug-induced lupus, 1471
   causing gout, 1443
   causing hearing loss, 1730
   causing hypoglycemia, 586
   causing hypothyroidism, 541
   causing platelet dysfunction, 1142t
   causing urinary retention, 869
   causing urine color changes, 832t
   surgical risk and nursing implications, 58t, 59
   topical. See Topical medications
   toxicity in older adults, 30
Medication Administration:
   acne medications, 459t
   adrenergic agonists (mydriatics), 1710t
   adrenergics, 278t, 1327t

alpha-adrenergic blockers, 1161t
angiotensin II receptor blockers (ARBs)
   for heart failure, 1033t
   for hypertension, 1161t
angiotensin-converting enzyme (ACE) inhibitors
   for heart failure, 1033t
   for hypertension, 1161t
antacids, 666t
antibiotics, 319–21t
anticholinergics
   for asthma, 1327–28t
   for neurogenic bladder, 871t
   for Parkinson's disease, 1638t
antidiarrheal preparations, 756t
antidysrhythmic drugs, 1006t
antiemetics, 673t
antiepileptic drugs, 1550t
antifungal agents, 450t
antihistamines
   for nausea and vomiting, 673t
   for upper respiratory infections, 1230t
antihypertensives, 1161–62t
antiprotozoal agents, 780t
antispasmodics, 1600t
antituberculosis drugs, 1288–89t
antiviral agents
   antiretroviral nucleoside analogs, 357t
   for oral herpes simplex, 658t
beta-blockers
   for angina, 973t
   for cardiac dysrhythmias, 1006t
   for hypertension, 1161–62t
   topical ophthalmic, 1710t
bisphosphonates, 1442t
blood transfusion, 264t
calcitonin, 1437t
calcium channel blockers
   for angina, 973–74t
   for cardiac dysrhythmias, 1006t
   for headache, 1545–46t
   for hypertension, 1162t
calcium supplements, 230t, 1437t
cannabinoids, 673t
carbonic anhydrase inhibitors, 1710t
cholesterol-lowering drugs, 967t
cholinergic drugs
   for Alzheimer's disease, 1621t
   to stimulate micturition, 871t
cholinesterase inhibitors, 1621t
corticosteroids
   for Addison's disease, 555t
   for asthma, 1328t
   for multiple sclerosis, 1631t
cortisol replacements, 555t
decongestants, 1230t
diuretics
   for acute renal failure, 905t
   for fluid volume excess, 210t
   for increased intracranial pressure, 1539t
dopamine agonists, 1638t
dopamine antagonists, 673t
dopaminergics, 1637t
ergot alkaloid derivatives, 1545t
ergotamine, 1546t
fluoride, 1437t
folic acid, 1112t
H₂-receptor blockers, 665t
hypertension, 1161–62t
immunomodulators, 1631t
immunosuppressive agents
   for multiple sclerosis, 1631t
   overview, 345–46t
insulin, 573t, 586t

Medication(s)—*continued*
intravenous fluids, 1539*t*
intravenous insulin, 586*t*
iron replacement, 1112*t*
laxatives and cathartics, 759–60*t*
leukotriene modifiers, 1328*t*
loop diuretics
for acute renal failure, 905*t*
for fluid volume excess, 210*t*
for increased intracranial pressure, 1539*t*
magnesium sulfate, 235*t*
mast cell stabilizers, 1328*t*
methylxanthines, 1327*t*
metoclopramide, 666*t*
monoamine oxidase inhibitors, 1638*t*
muscle relaxants, 1631*t*
narcotic analgesics (opiates/opioids), 182*t*
nonsteroidal anti-inflammatory drugs
for headache, 1546*t*
overview, 179*t*
oral hypoglycemic agents, 578*t*
osmotic diuretics
for acute renal failure, 905*t*
for increased intracranial pressure, 1539*t*
pancreatic enzyme replacement, 728*t*
prostaglandin analogs, 1710*t*
proton-pump inhibitors, 665*t*
serotonin receptor antagonists, 673*t*
serotonin selective agonists, 1545*t*
sodium channel blockers, 1006*t*
in specific conditions
acne, 459*t*
Addison's disease, 555*t*
Alzheimer's disease, 1621*t*
anemia, 1112*t*
angina, 973–74*t*
asthma, 1327–28*t*
burns, 501*t*
cardiac dysrhythmias, 1006*t*
cirrhosis, 717*t*
gastritis, 665–66*t*
gastroesophageal reflux disease, 665–66*t*
genital warts, 1842*t*
glaucoma, 1710*t*
gout, 1446*t*
headache, 1545–46*t*
heart failure, 1033*t*
hyperkalemia, 225*t*
hypersensitivity reactions, 673*t*
hypertension, 1161–62*t*
hyperthyroidism, 538*t*
hypokalemia, 221*t*
hypothyroidism, 544*t*
increased intracranial pressure, 1539*t*
inflammatory bowel disease, 787–88*t*
multiple sclerosis, 1631*t*
myasthenia gravis, 1649*t*
neurogenic bladder, 871*t*
obesity, 634*t*
oral herpes simplex, 658*t*
osteoporosis, 1437*t*
Paget's disease, 1442*t*
Parkinson's disease, 1637–38*t*
peptic ulcer disease, 665–66*t*
seizures, 1550*t*
shock, 278*t*
spastic bladder, 871*t*
spinal cord injury, 1600*t*
stomatitis, 658*t*
upper respiratory infections, 1230*t*
sucralfate, 666*t*
sympatholytics, 1162*t*
tamoxifen, 1825*t*
therapeutic baths, 441*t*

topical agents
antifungal, 658*t*
antimicrobial, 501*t*
local anesthetics, 658*t*
podophyllin, 1842*t*
trichloroacetic acid, 1842*t*
tricyclic antidepressants, 1545*t*
urinary anti-infectives and analgesics, 850*t*
vasodilators, 278*t*, 1162*t*
vitamin and mineral supplements, 645*t*
vitamin B_{12}, 1112*t*
Meditation, 186
Medrol. *See* Methylprednisolone
Medulla oblongata, 1505*f*, 1506
Medulloblastoma, 1570*t*. *See also* Brain tumors
Meeting Individualized Needs:
acute myocardial infarction in women and older
adults, 984*t*
amputation, home care, 1427*t*
assessing intimate partner violence, 256*t*
breast cancer in older women, 1823*t*
burns in older adults, 508*t*
client being discharged from acute care to home
care, 39*t*
client experiencing a loss, 98*t*
constipation in the older adult, 761*t*
dementing disorder in an older adult, family
home care, 43*t*
diet following bariatric surgery, 638*t*
epilepsy in older adults, 1548*t*
fall prevention in older adults, 1418*t*
foot care teaching, 594*t*
nutrition for older adults, 642*t*
prostate surgery discharge instructions, 1783*t*
ruptured intervertebral disk, client teaching, 1611*t*
safety interventions in Alzheimer's disease, 1623*t*
sexuality function in the aging woman, 1794*t*
sexually transmitted infections, health
promotion, 1838*t*
stroke risk factors in women, 1589*t*
substance abuse in older adults, 115*t*
trigeminal neuralgia, home care teaching, 1657*t*
Mefenamic acid, 178*t*
Mefoxin. *See* Cefoxitin
MEG (magnetoencephalogram), 1512, 1515*t*
Megestrol, 1787*t*
Meglitinides, 578*t*
Meglumine diatrizoate, 615*t*, 812–13
Meiosis, 150
Melanin, 423, 462
Melanoma. *See* Malignant melanoma
Melanosis coli, 758
Melena, 674, 750*t*. *See also* Gastrointestinal
bleeding
Mellaril. *See* Thioridazine
Melphalan, 1137
Memantine, 1621
Membranoproliferative glomerulonephritis, 888.
See also Glomerular disorders
Membranous glomerulonephropathy, 888. *See also*
Glomerular disorders
Mendelian inheritance. *See* Inheritance, Mendelian
patterns
Ménière's disease, 1726–27. *See also* Inner ear
disorders
Meninges, 1507, 1507*f*
Meningioma, 1570*t*. *See also* Brain tumors
Meningitis. *See also* Central nervous system
infections
bacterial
causes, 1564
complications, 1564*t*
manifestations, 1564, 1564*t*
definition, 1564

interdisciplinary care
diagnosis, 1566
medications, 1566
Nursing Care Plan
assessment, 1567*t*
critical thinking in the nursing process, 1567*t*
diagnoses, 1567*t*
evaluation, 1567*t*
planning and implementation, 1567*t*
pathophysiology, 1564
tuberculous, 1583
viral, 1564–65
Meningomyocele, 872
Menopause:
chemical, 1795
definition, 1795
hormone changes, 1753
interdisciplinary care
complementary and alternative therapies, 1796
diagnosis, 1796
medications, 1796
manifestations, 1796, 1796*t*
nursing care
assessment, 1797
health promotion, 1796–97
nursing diagnoses and interventions
deficient knowledge, 1797
disturbed body image, 1798
ineffective sexuality pattern, 1797
situational low self-esteem, 1797–98
physiology, 1795–96
premature, coronary heart disease risk
and, 964
sexuality function in, 1794*t*
surgical, 1795
uterine bleeding in. *See* Dysfunctional uterine
bleeding
Menorrhagia, 1802. *See also* Dysfunctional uterine
bleeding
Menstrual cycle, 1754–55, 1754*f*
Menstrual disorders:
dysfunctional uterine bleeding. *See*
Dysfunctional uterine bleeding
dysmenorrhea. *See* Dysmenorrhea
premenstrual syndrome. *See* Premenstrual
syndrome
Menstruation, 1753
Mental status assessment, 1518–19*t*
Mentax. *See* Butenafine
Meperidine HCl, 113*t*, 177, 180*t*
Meprobamate, 108
Mercaptopurine, 786
Meridia. *See* Sibutramine
Mcropenem, 319*t*
Mesalamine, 786, 787*t*, 788
Mestinon. *See* Pyridostigmine
Metabolic acidosis:
arterial blood gases in, 240*t*
causes, 242*t*
compensation, 243*t*
definition, 240, 241*f*
interdisciplinary care
diagnosis, 244
medications, 244
laboratory values, 242*t*
manifestations, 244, 244*t*
nursing care
assessment, 244–45
community-based care, 245
health promotion, 244
nursing diagnoses and interventions
decreased cardiac output, 245
risk for excess fluid volume, 245
risk for injury, 245

pathophysiology, 242–44
risk factors, 242
Metabolic alkalosis:
arterial blood gases in, 240t
causes, 242t
compensation, 243t
complications, 246
definition, 240, 241f
interdisciplinary care
diagnosis, 246
medications, 246
laboratory values, 242t, 245
manifestations, 246, 246t
nursing care
assessment, 246–47
community-based care, 247
health promotion, 246
nursing diagnoses and interventions
deficient fluid volume, 247
risk for impaired gas exchange, 247
pathophysiology, 246
risk factors, 246
Metabolic syndrome:
atherosclerosis risk and, 632
characteristics, 632, 964
coronary heart disease risk and, 632, 964
diabetes risk and, 567
Metabolism, 613
Metamucil. See Psyllium hydrophilic mucilloid
Metaplasia, 373
Metaprel. See Metaproterenol
Metaproterenol, 1327t
Metaraminol, 278t
Metastasis. See also Cancer
definition, 376
mechanisms, 378–79, 378f
sites, 378t
Metered-dose inhaler, 1324, 1325t
Metformin, 578t
Methadone:
characteristics and uses, 110
equianalgesic drug chart, 180t
nursing considerations, 180t
overdose signs and treatment, 113t
for substance abuse treatment, 114t
withdrawal signs and treatment, 113t
Methamphetamine, 109, 109f, 110. See also
Amphetamines
Methicillin, 319t
Methicillin-resistant S. aureus (MRSA), 313–14
Methimazole, 538t
Methocarbamol, 832t, 1491
Methotrexate:
adverse/side effects, 392t
Medication Administration, 345t
nursing implications, 392t
in specific conditions
autoimmune disorders, 341
bone tumors, 1483t
laryngeal cancer, 1254
rheumatoid arthritis, 1466
target malignancies, 392t
Methoxsalen, 445
Methyl methacrylate, 1452
Methylaminobenzine, 372t
Methylcellulose, 633, 759t
Methyldopa, 457, 1162t
Methylphenidate, 189
Methylprednisolone:
Medication Administration, 555t, 787–88t, 1631t
in specific conditions
Addison's disease, 555t
inflammatory bowel disease, 787–88t
multiple sclerosis, 1631t

nausea and vomiting, 672
organ transplantation, 344, 921
spinal cord injury, 1599
Methylxanthines, 1327t, 1355
Methysergide maleate, 1544, 1545t
Meticorten. See Prednisone
Metipranolol, 1710t
Metoclopramide:
Medication Administration, 666t, 673t
preoperative use and nursing implications, 62t
in specific conditions
gastroesophageal reflux disease, 665, 666t
nausea and vomiting, 672, 673t
Metolazone, 210t
Metoprolol:
Medication Administration, 973t, 1006t, 1161t
in specific conditions
acute myocardial infarction, 988
angina, 973t
aortic aneurysm, 1173
cardiac dysrhythmias, 1006t
hypertension, 1161t
Metronidazole:
Medication Administration, 321t, 780t
in specific conditions
amebic liver abscess, 725
diverticulitis, 816
peritonitis, 770
pneumonia, 1271t
protozoal bowel infections, 778t, 779, 780t
protozoal infections, 321
trichomoniasis, 1843
Metrorrhagia, 1802. See also Dysfunctional
uterine bleeding
Metzol. See Metronidazole
Mevacor. See Lovastatin
Mexate. See Methotrexate
Mexican Americans. See Hispanic Americans
Mexiletine, 1006t
Mexitil. See Mexiletine
Mezlin. See Mezlocillin
Mezlocillin, 319t
Mg²⁺. See Magnesium
MHC (major histocompatibility complex), 329
Miacalcin. See Calcitonin
Micardis. See Telmisartan
Michigan Alcohol Screening Test (MAST),
116, 116f
Miconazole, 450t
Microalbuminuria, 588
Microcytic RBCs, 1103
Microdiskectomy, 1610
Microglia, 289, 1628t
Micro-K 10. See Potassium chloride
Micronase. See Glyburide
Microstaging, malignant melanoma, 467, 468f
Microvilli, 612, 742
Micturition, 834–35, 869. See also Urinary
system
Midamor. See Amiloride HCl
Midarm circumference (MAC), 621t, 622f, 622t
Midarm muscle circumference (MMAC), 622t
Midazolam, 62t, 500, 1355
Midbrain, 1505f, 1506
Middle adults (ages 40 to 65):
family-related risk factors for alterations in
health, 32t, 33
health needs
assessment guidelines, 28
promoting healthy behaviors, 28, 28t
risks for alterations in health
cancer, 27
cardiovascular disease, 26–27
obesity, 26

physical and psychosocial stressors, 27
substance abuse, 27
physical changes, 27t
Miglitol, 578t
Migraine headache. See also Headache
characteristics, 1542t
classic, 1543
common, 1543
incidence, 1542
manifestations, 1542t
Nursing Care Plan
assessment, 1547t
critical thinking in the nursing process, 1547t
diagnoses, 1547t
evaluation, 1547t
expected outcomes, 1547t
planning and implementation, 1547t
risk factors, 1542t
triggers, 1543
Miliary pneumonia, 1268t. See also Pneumonia
Miliary tuberculosis, 1283
Milk of Magnesia. See Magnesium hydroxide
Milk thistle, 709
Milliequivalent, 196
Milrinone, 1034t
Milroy's disease, 1093t
Mind–body therapies:
for cancer, 399t
for hypertension, 1163, 1164t
for nausea, 672
Mineral oil, 441t, 760t
Mineralocorticoids, 519t
Minerals:
functions, 608
recommended daily intake, 610t
sources, 608
supplements, 645t
Minimal change disease (MCD), 888. See also
Glomerular disorders
Minimally invasive coronary artery surgery, 979
Minipress. See Prazosin
Minocin. See Minocycline HCl
Minocycline HCl, 320t
Minor burn injury, 491t. See also Burns
Minor procedure, 54t
Minor trauma, 256
Minoxidil, 482, 1162t
Mint oil aromatherapy, 679
Minute volume (MV), 1214t
Mirapex. See Pramipexole
Misoprostol, 685
Mithracin. See Plicamycin
Mithramycin, 232
Mitigation, disaster, 132–33
Mitochondria, 151
Mitochondrial DNA (mtDNA), 151
Mitosis, 149
Mitotane, 550
Mitotic inhibitors, 391. See also Chemotherapy
Mitral regurgitation. See also Valvular heart
disease
manifestations, 1056
murmur characteristics, 1055t
pathophysiology, 1056, 1056f
Mitral stenosis. See also Valvular heart disease
complications, 1055–56
manifestations, 1055
murmur characteristics, 1055t
pathophysiology, 1055, 1056f
Mitral valve, 937f, 938, 1054
Mitral valve prolapse. See also Valvular heart
disease
complications, 1057
manifestations, 1057

Mitral valve prolapse—*continued*
Nursing Care Plan
assessment, 1064*t*
critical thinking in the nursing process, 1064*t*
diagnoses, 1064*t*
evaluation, 1064*t*
expected outcomes, 1064*t*
planning and implementation, 1064*t*
pathophysiology, 1056–57, 1057*f*
in polycystic kidney disease, 884
Mittelschmerz, 1802
Mixed aphasia, 1583
Mixed incontinence, 873. *See also* Urinary incontinence
Mixed lymphocyte culture (MLC) assay tests, 343
MMAC (midarm muscle circumference), 622*t*
M-mode echocardiogram, 945*t*. *See also* Echocardiography
MMR vaccine. *See* Measles-mumps-rubella (MMR) vaccine
Mobitz type I AV block, 999*t*, 1003
Mobitz type II AV block, 999*t*, 1003
Modafinil, 189
Moderate burn injury, 491*t*. *See also* Burns
Modified radical mastectomy, 1825, 1826*f*. *See also* Mastectomy
MODS (multiple organ dysfunction syndrome), 259
Moexipril, 1033*t*, 1161*t*
Mohs surgery, 464
Moles. *See* Nevi
Molybdenum, 610*t*
Monistat. *See* Miconazole
Monoamine oxidase inhibitors (MAOIs), 58*t*, 1638*t*
Monoclonal antibodies. *See also specific drugs*
development, 317*t*, 344
Medication Administration, 345–46*t*
in organ transplantation, 344
site of action, 344*f*
Monocytes:
abnormal, possible causes, 307*t*, 387*t*
characteristics, 288–89
development, 289*f*
functions, 288–89, 288*t*, 1079
in leukemia, 1123*t*
location, 288*t*
normal values, 307*t*, 387*t*, 1118*t*
Monocytopenia, 307*t*
Monocytosis, 307*t*
Monogenic disorders, 152
Mono-Gesic. *See* Salsalate
Mononeuropathies, in diabetes mellitus, 589
Mononucleosis, infectious, 1139
Monopril. *See* Fosinopril
Monosomy, 150, 150*t*
Monro-Kellie hypothesis, 1535
Mons pubis, 1751, 1751*t*, 1752*f*
Mons veneris. *See* Mons pubis
Montelukast, 1328*t*
Mood disorders, in diabetes mellitus, 589
Moral development theory (Kohlberg), 25*t*
Morbid grief reaction, 86
Morbid obesity, 632
Moricizine, 1006*t*
Morphine sulfate:
in end-of-life care, 92*t*, 93*t*
equianalgesic drug chart, 180*t*
for long-term analgesia at home, 190*t*
Medication Administration, 182*t*
nursing considerations, 180*t*
overdose signs and treatment, 113*t*
preoperative use and nursing implications, 62*t*
in specific conditions

acute myocardial infarction, 987
burns, 500
pulmonary edema, 1040–41
street names, 111*t*
withdrawal signs and treatment, 113*t*
Morton's neuroma, 1492–93, 1493*f*
Mother cell, 150
Motofen. *See* Difenoxin
Motor function, assessment, 530*t*, 1522*t*
Motor speech area, 1506*t*
Motrin. *See* Ibuprofen
Mourning, 85, 88, 89*t*
Mouth:
anatomy, physiology, and functions, 610, 611*f*
disorders
cancer. *See* Oral cancer
stomatitis. *See* Stomatitis
physical assessment, 622–23*t*
Mouthwashes, for oropharyngeal pain control, 409*t*
6-MP. *See* Mercaptopurine
MRA. *See* Magnetic resonance angiography
MRCP (magnetic resonance cholangiopancreatography), 616*t*
MRI. *See* Magnetic resonance imaging
MRS (magnetic resonance spectroscopy), 1514*t*
MRSA (methicillin-resistant *S. aureus*), 313–14
MS. *See* Multiple sclerosis
mtDNA (mitochondrial DNA), 151
Mucomyst. *See* Acetylcysteine
Mucosa-associated lymphoid tissue (MALT), 292
Multidrug-resistant tuberculosis (MDR-TB), 313
Multifactorial conditions, 155–56
Multiple casualty incidents, 127
Multiple endocrine neoplasia, 527*t*
Multiple myeloma:
definition, 1136
incidence, 1136
interdisciplinary care
diagnosis and staging, 1137
treatment, 1137
manifestations, 1136
nursing care
assessment, 1137
community-based care, 1138
nursing diagnoses and interventions
chronic pain, 1137–38
impaired physical mobility, 1138
risk for injury, 1138
pathophysiology, 1136, 1137*f*
risk factors, 1136
Multiple organ dysfunction syndrome (MODS), 259
Multiple sclerosis (MS):
characteristics, 1626
classification, 1626
genetic considerations, 1513*t*
incidence and prevalence, 1626
interdisciplinary care
diagnosis, 1627
medications, 1627, 1631*t*
nutrition and fluids, 1632
rehabilitation, 1632
surgery, 1632
manifestations, 1626–27, 1627*t*
Multisystem Effects, 1630*t*
nursing care
assessment, 1632
community-based care, 1634–35
health promotion, 1632
Medication Administration, 1631*t*
nursing diagnoses and interventions
fatigue, 1632–33
self-care deficit, 1633–34
using NANDA, NIC, and NOC, 1634, 1634*t*

Nursing Care Plan
assessment, 1633*t*
critical thinking in the nursing process, 1633*t*
diagnoses, 1633*t*
evaluation, 1633*t*
expected outcomes, 1633*t*
planning and implementation, 1633*t*
Nursing Research: care of aging clients, 1634*t*
pathophysiology, 1626, 1628–29*t*
Multiple trauma, 256
Multisystem Effects:
anemia, 1104*t*
cirrhosis, 714*t*
diabetes mellitus, 583*t*
fluid volume deficit, 204*t*
heart failure, 1028*t*
hyperthyroidism, 535*t*
hypokalemia, 219*t*
hypothyroidism, 542*t*
inflammatory bowel disease, 783*t*
leukemia, 1120*t*
lung cancer, 1310*t*
malnutrition, 643*t*
multiple sclerosis, 1630*t*
premenstrual syndrome, 1799*t*
rheumatoid arthritis, 1462*t*
shock, 273*t*
systemic lupus erythematosus, 1472*t*
uremia (chronic renal failure), 917*t*
Mumps vaccine. *See* Measles-mumps-rubella vaccine
Murmurs. *See also* Valvular heart disease
in aortic regurgitation, 1055*t*, 1059
in aortic stenosis, 1055*t*, 1058
assessment, 955*t*
definition, 1054
in mitral regurgitation, 1055*t*, 1056
in mitral stenosis, 1055, 1055*t*
in mitral valve prolapse, 1057
in pulmonic regurgitation, 1059
in pulmonic stenosis, 1059
in tricuspid regurgitation, 1055*t*, 1059
in tricuspid stenosis, 1055*t*, 1059
Muromonab-CD3:
adverse/side effects, 921
Medication Administration, 345–46*t*
in organ transplantation, 344, 921
Murphy's sign, 627*f*, 627*t*
Muscle(s). *See also* Musculoskeletal system
anterior body, 1384*f*
contusion, strain, or sprain
interdisciplinary care, 1399–1400, 1400*t*
manifestations, 1399
nursing care, 1400
pathophysiology, 1399
function assessment. *See* Motor function
functional properties, 1383
posterior body, 1384*f*
range of motion assessment, 1391*f*, 1391*t*, 1392–94*t*, 1392*f*, 1393*f*
strength assessment, 1391*t*
structure, 1381
types, 1381, 1383*t*
Muscle relaxants, 1491, 1631*t*
Muscle wasting, in cirrhosis, 715*t*
Muscular dystrophy (MD):
definition, 1458
genetic considerations, 1389*t*, 1458
interdisciplinary care, 1458
manifestations, 1458
nursing care, 1459
pathophysiology, 1458
types, 1459*t*

Musculoskeletal system:
  age-related changes
    in middle adults, 27t
    in older adults, 29t, 1389t
    in young adults, 26t
  anatomy, physiology, and functions
    joints. See Joint(s)
    ligaments, 1386
    skeleton
      bones. See Bone(s)
      muscles. See Muscle(s)
      overview, 1380, 1381f
    tendons, 1386
  assessment
    abnormal findings, 530t
    diagnostic tests, 1386, 1387–88t, 1388
    functional health pattern interview, 1390t
    genetic considerations, 1388, 1389t
    health assessment interview, 1388–89
    physical assessment
      ballottement, 1395f, 1395t
      bulge sign, 1395f, 1395t
      gait and body posture, 1391t
      joints, 1392t
      McMurray's test, 1396f, 1396t
      muscle strength, 1391t
      overview, 1389–91
      Phalen's test, 1395f, 1395t
      range of motion, 1391f, 1391t, 1392–94t,
        1392f, 1393f
      Thomas test, 1396f, 1396t
    sample documentation, 1386
  autoimmune and inflammatory disorders
    ankylosing spondylitis. See Ankylosing
      spondylitis
    Lyme disease, 1476–77
    polymyositis, 1476
    rheumatoid arthritis. See Rheumatoid
      arthritis
  Chapter Highlights, 1429–30t, 1494t
  Clinical Scenarios, 1498t
  connective tissue disorders
    fibromyalgia. See Fibromyalgia
    scleroderma. See Scleroderma
    Sjögren's syndrome, 1486
  degenerative disorders
    muscular dystrophy. See Muscular dystrophy
    osteoarthritis. See Osteoarthritis
  infectious disorders
    osteomyelitis. See Osteomyelitis
    septic arthritis, 1481
  metabolic bone disorders
    gout. See Gout
    osteomalacia. See Osteomalacia
    osteoporosis. See Osteoporosis
    Paget's disease. See Paget's disease
  neoplastic disorders. See Bone tumors
  structural disorders
    foot deformities. See Feet, deformities
    kyphosis. See Kyphosis
    low back pain. See Low back pain
    scoliosis. See Scoliosis
  trauma
    amputation. See Amputation
    contusion, strain, or sprain
      interdisciplinary care, 1399–1400, 1400t
      manifestations, 1399
      nursing care, 1400
      pathophysiology, 1399
    dislocation
      causes, 1400–1401
      definition, 1400
      interdisciplinary care, 1401
      manifestations, 1401

    nursing care, 1401
    pathophysiology, 1401
  fractures. See Fractures
  repetitive use injury. See Repetitive use injury
Music therapy, 672
Musset's sign, 1059
Mustargen. See Mechlorethamine
Mutations, 152, 155
MV (minute volume), 1214t
Myambutol. See Ethambutol
Myasthenia gravis:
  characteristics, 1647
  complications, 1648, 1648t
  interdisciplinary care
    diagnosis, 1649
    medications, 1649, 1649t
    plasmapheresis, 1650, 1650t, 1651f
    surgery, 1649–50, 1650t
  manifestations, 1648, 1648f, 1648t
  nursing care
    client and family teaching, 1651t
    of client having a thymectomy, 1650t
    of client undergoing plasmapheresis, 1650t
    community-based care, 1651–52
    Medication Administration, 1649t
    nursing diagnoses and interventions
      impaired swallowing, 1651
      ineffective airway clearance, 1651
  Nursing Care Plan
    assessment, 1652t
    critical thinking in the nursing process, 1652t
    diagnoses, 1652t
    evaluation, 1652t
    expected outcomes, 1652t
    planning and implementation, 1652t
  pathophysiology, 1647–48, 1647f
Myasthenic crisis, 1648
Mycelex. See Clotrimazole
Mycobacterium avium complex (MAC), 353,
  353f, 359t
Mycobacterium tuberculosis, 1280. See also
  Tuberculosis
Mycophenolate mofetil, 344, 345t, 921
Mycoplasma, 311t
Mycoplasma pneumoniae, 1269, 1271t
Mycoses. See Skin infections/infestations, fungal
Mycosis fungoides, 1130t. See also Lymphomas
Mycostatin. See Nystatin
Mycotic aneurysm, 1592
Myelin sheath, 1504, 1504f
Myelodysplastic syndrome (MDS):
  interdisciplinary care
    diagnosis, 1115
    treatment, 1115–16
  manifestations, 1115
  nursing diagnoses and interventions
    activity intolerance, 1116
    community-based care, 1117
    risk for ineffective health maintenance, 1116
  pathophysiology, 1115
  risk factors, 1115
Myelogram, 1512, 1516t
Myeloid leukemia, 1119. See also Leukemia
Myidil. See Triprolidine
Mylanta, 665, 666t
Myleran. See Busulfan
Myocardial biopsy, 1067
Myocardial infarction. See Acute myocardial
  infarction
Myocardial ischemia:
  factors contributing to, 962t
  pathophysiology, 959, 962
  silent, 970
Myocardial perfusion imaging, 966

Myocardial remodeling, 984
Myocardial steal syndrome, 971
Myocarditis:
  definition, 1048
  interdisciplinary care, 1048
  manifestations, 1048
  nursing care, 1048
  pathophysiology, 1048
  risk factors, 1048
Myocardium, 937, 937f
Myochrysine. See Gold sodium thiomalate
Myofascial pain syndrome, 174
Myoglobin, 986
Myomectomy, 1810
Myopia, 1677t, 1696
Myotonia, 1794
Myotonic dystrophy:
  disease progression, 1459t
  genetic considerations, 155, 1389t
  interdisciplinary care, 1458
  manifestations, 1459t
  nursing care, 1459
Myringotomy, 1722, 1723
Mysoline. See Primidone
Mytelase. See Ambenonium
Myxedema, 541
Myxedema coma, 543t

N

Na⁺. See Sodium
Nabilone, 672, 673t
Nabumetone, 178t, 1464t
Nadolol:
  Medication Administration, 973t, 1161t, 1543t
  in specific conditions
    angina, 973t
    cirrhosis, 716
    headache, 1545t
    hypertension, 1161t
Naegleria, 1565t
Nafcillin, 319t, 1046, 1271t
NAHC. See National Association of Home Care
Nails. See also Integumentary system
  age-related changes, 29t
  anatomy, physiology, and functions, 425–26, 425f
  assessment, 436f, 436t, 529t
  candidiasis, 449t
  clubbing, 436f, 436t
  disorders
    interdisciplinary care, 483
    nursing care, 483
    pathophysiology, 483
  spoon-shaped, 436f, 436t
Nalbuphine HCl, 180t, 182t
Nalfon. See Fenoprofen calcium
Naltrexone, 112, 114t
Namenda. See Memantine
NANDA, NIC, and NOC Linkages:
  acute brain injury, 1562t
  acute myocardial infarction, 994t
  acute renal failure, 913t
  acute respiratory distress syndrome, 1371t
  acute respiratory failure, 1365t
  Alzheimer's disease, 1625t
  amputation, 1426t
  anemia, 1115t
  appendicitis, 769t
  brain tumor, 1575t
  breast cancer, 1831t
  cancer, 411t
  cervical cancer, 1815t
  chronic obstructive pulmonary disease, 1340t
  chronic pain, 190t

NANDA, NIC, and NOC Linkages—*continued*
cirrhosis, 723*t*
colorectal cancer, 809*t*
compound fracture, 1420*t*
Cushing's syndrome, 553*t*
death anxiety, 97*t*
deep venous thrombosis, 1193*t*
diabetes mellitus, 596*t*
diarrhea, 757*t*
endometriosis, 1812*t*
eye infection or inflammation, 1696*t*
fluid volume deficit, 209*t*
gastroesophageal reflux disease, 667*t*
glaucoma, 1713*t*
hearing loss, 1733*t*
heart failure, 1039*t*
hemophilia, 1146
hepatitis, 710*t*
herpes zoster, 455*t*
HIV infection, 365*t*
hypertension, 1166*t*
infections, 325*t*
inflammatory bowel disease, 795*t*
influenza, 1235*t*
inner ear disorders, 1728*t*
laryngeal cancer, 1262*t*
leukemia, 1128*t*
lung cancer, 1317*t*
lymphoma, 1136*t*
malignant melanoma, 471*t*
malnutrition, 650*t*
multiple sclerosis, 1634*t*
nasal trauma, 1248*t*
obesity, 640*t*
osteoarthritis, 1457*t*
osteoporosis, 1440*t*
pancreatitis, 731*t*
Parkinson's disease, 1642*t*
peptic ulcer disease, 688*t*
peripheral vascular disease, 1180*t*
peritonitis, 769*t*
pneumonia, 1276*t*
postoperative client, 80*t*
potassium imbalance, 223*t*
prostate cancer surgery, 1789*t*
pulmonary embolism, 1352*t*
respiratory acidosis, 250*t*
rheumatoid arthritis, 1469*t*
seizures, 1553*t*
shock, 283*t*
spinal cord injury, 1606*t*
stomatitis, 659*t*
stroke, 1592*t*
substance abuse problems, 120*t*, 121*t*
trauma, 268*t*
tuberculosis, 1293*t*
urinary incontinence, 879*t*
NANDA nursing diagnoses:
activity-exercise patterns, 933*t*
cognitive-perceptual patterns, 1501*t*
elimination patterns, 739*t*
health perception-health management patterns, 2*t*
nutritional-metabolic patterns, 420*t*
sexuality-reproductive patterns, 1501*t*
Naphthylalkanone, 178*t*
Naprosyn. *See* Naproxen
Naproxen:
factors in selecting, 178*t*
Medication Administration, 179*t*
in specific conditions
gout, 1445
osteoarthritis, 1451
rheumatoid arthritis, 1464*t*
venous thrombosis, 1188

Naproxen sodium, 178*t*
Naqua. *See* Trichlormethiazide
Narcolepsy, 1513*t*
Narcotic analgesics. *See also specific drugs*
abuse
by nurses, 121, 122*t*
prevalence, 110, 110*f*
in burns, 500
myths and misconceptions, 177
overdose signs and treatment, 113*t*
for pain management
in cancer, 399–400
effects, 182*t*
equianalgesic drug chart, 180*t*
health education for client and family, 182*t*
Medication Administration, 182*t*
myths, 179
nursing responsibilities, 182*t*
oral vs. parenteral dosage, 64*t*
postoperative, 64
preoperative use and nursing implications, 62*t*
in substance abuser, 181*t*
street names, 111*t*
withdrawal signs and treatment, 113*t*
Nasal continuous positive airway pressure, 1251, 1251*f*
Nasal endotracheal tube, 1357*t*. *See also* Endotracheal tube
Nasal packing:
nursing care, 1245*t*
procedure, 1244, 1244*f*
Nasal polyps:
definition, 1252
interdisciplinary care, 1252
manifestations, 1252
nursing care, 1252
pathophysiology, 1252
Nasal trauma:
complications, 1246
interdisciplinary care
diagnosis, 1246
surgery, 1246–47
treatments, 1246
manifestations, 1246, 1246*t*
nursing care
assessment, 1247
community-based care, 1248–49
health promotion, 1247
nursing diagnoses and interventions
ineffective airway clearance, 1247–48
risk for infection, 1248
using NANDA, NIC, and NOC, 1248, 1248*t*
Nursing Care Plan
assessment, 1247*t*
critical thinking in the nursing process, 1247*t*
diagnoses, 1247*t*
evaluation, 1247*t*
expected outcomes, 1247*t*
planning and implementation, 1247*t*
pathophysiology, 1246
NasalCrom. *See* Cromolyn sodium
Nasogastric tube, 719, 719*f*. *See also* Enteral nutrition
Nasopharynx, 1211
Nateglinide, 578*t*
National Academy of Sciences, core competencies for healthcare professionals, 5, 5*t*
National Association of Home Care (NAHC):
client's bill of rights, 41*t*
definition of home care, 38
Native Americans:
cancer incidence and mortality rates, 370*t*
cirrhosis incidence and mortality, 711
diabetes mellitus risk and incidence, 564*t*

end-of-life practices, 89
gallstone incidence, 697*t*
heart disease prevalence, 958*t*
lactate deficiency incidence, 798*t*
substance use, 105*t*
Native Hawaiians, substance use, 105*t*
Natriuretic hormone, 834
Natural disasters, 126. *See also* Disasters
Natural killer cells (NK cells, null cells):
development, 290, 290*f*
functions, 288*t*, 290
location, 288*t*
Naturetin. *See* Bendroflumethiazide
Nausea, 671. *See also* Nausea and vomiting
Nausea and vomiting:
in dying client, 93
interdisciplinary care
complementary and alternative therapies, 672
medications, 672, 673*t*
nursing care
community-based care, 674
Medication Administration, 673*t*
nursing diagnoses and interventions, 672
pathophysiology, 671
Near point of vision, 1673
Near-drowning, 1305–6, 1306*f*. *See also* Inhalation injury
Nebcin. *See* Tobramycin
Necrotizing pancreatitis, 726. *See also* Pancreatitis
Necrotizing ulcerative gingivitis, 657*t*. *See also* Stomatitis
Nedocromil, 1326, 1328*t*
Needle core biopsy, 388*t*
Needle thoracostomy, 258, 258*f*
Neglect syndrome, 1582
Neisseria gonorrhoeae, 1238, 1773. *See also* Gonorrhea
Nelfinavir, 358
Neo Tabs. *See* Neomycin sulfate
Neomycin sulfate, 716, 717*t*
Neoplasms:
benign, 376, 376*t*
classification, 382, 383*t*
malignant, 376, 376*t*. *See also* Cancer
Neoral. *See* Cyclosporine
Neostigmine, 870, 1649*t*
Neo-Synephrine. *See* Phenylephrine
Neotame, 579
Nephrectomy:
definition, 896
incisions for, 898*f*
in kidney trauma, 896
nursing care, 897
for renal tumors, 896–97
Nephrolithiasis, 855. *See also* Urinary calculi
Nephrolithotomy, 859
Nephrons, 830, 831*f*
Nephropathy, diabetic, 588–89, 889. *See also* Glomerular disorders
Nephrotic syndrome, 888. *See also* Glomerular disorders
Nephrox. *See* Aluminum hydroxide
Nerve blocks, 63, 183
Nervous system. *See* Neurologic system
Netilmicin, 320*t*
Netromycin. *See* Netilmicin
Neuralgias, 174
Neurectomy, 184, 185*f*, 1727
Neuro check, 1517*t*, 1518, 1518*t*
Neurofibrillary tangles, 1618, 1619*f*
Neurofibromatosis, 1684*t*
Neurogenic bladder:
flaccid, 870
interdisciplinary care

bladder retraining, 871
catheterization, 872
diagnosis, 870
medications, 870–71
nutrition, 871
surgery, 872
nursing care
assessment, 872
community-based care, 872
nursing diagnoses and interventions, 872
pathophysiology, 870
spastic, 870
Neurogenic shock:
assessment, 279
causes, 276
definition, 275
manifestations, 276, 276t
pathophysiology, 275
Neurologic system:
age-related changes, 1518t
anatomy, physiology, and functions
action potentials, 1504–5
blood–brain barrier, 1507
brain
brainstem, 1506, 1506t
cerebellum, 1505f, 1506t
cerebrum, 1505–6, 1505f, 1506f, 1506t
diencephalon, 1506, 1506t
ventricles, 1506
cerebral circulation, 1507, 1508f
cerebrospinal fluid
formation, 1506–7
functions, 1507
normal values, 1507t
nervous system, 1507
meninges, 1507, 1507f
neurons, 1504, 1504f
neurotransmitters, 1505
peripheral nervous system
autonomic nervous system, 1511. See also
Parasympathetic nervous system;
Sympathetic nervous system
cranial nerves, 1509, 1510f, 1511t
reflexes, 1510–11, 1511f
spinal nerves, 1508f, 1509, 1510f
reticular formation, 1507
spinal cord, 1508–9, 1508f, 1509f
assessment
diagnostic tests, 1512–13, 1514–16t
functional health pattern interview, 1517t
health assessment interview, 1513, 1516
physical assessment
abbreviated, 1518t
Brudzinski's sign, 1524f, 1524t
cerebellar function, 1522–23t
cranial nerves, 1519–21t
decerebrate posturing, 1525f, 1525t
decorticate posturing, 1525f, 1525t
Kernig's sign, 1524f, 1524t
mental status, 1518–19t
motor function, 1522t
overview, 1516, 1518
reflexes, 1523–24f, 1523–24t
sensory function, 1521–22t, 1522f
sample documentation, 1512
disorders
altered cerebral function
altered level of consciousness. See Altered
level of consciousness
brain tumors. See Brain tumors
epilepsy. See Epilepsy
headache. See Headache
increased intracranial pressure. See Increased
intracranial pressure

manifestations, 1528t
traumatic brain injury. See Traumatic brain
injury
cerebrovascular
arteriovenous malformation. See
Arteriovenous malformation
intracranial aneurysm. See Intracranial
aneurysm
stroke. See Stroke
Chapter Highlights, 1614t, 1663t
Clinical Scenarios, 1666t
degenerative
Alzheimer's disease. See Alzheimer's disease
amyotrophic lateral sclerosis. See
Amyotrophic lateral sclerosis
dementia. See Dementia
Huntington's disease. See Huntington's
disease
multiple sclerosis. See Multiple sclerosis
Parkinson's disease. See Parkinson's disease
infections. See Central nervous system
infections
peripheral nerves
Guillain-Barré syndrome. See Guillain-Barré
syndrome
myasthenia gravis. See Myasthenia gravis
spinal cord
herniated intervertebral disk. See Herniated
intervertebral disk
injury. See Spinal cord injury
tumor. See Spinal cord tumors
genetic considerations, 1513, 1513t
Neuromatrix theory, of pain, 172
Neuromuscular blockers, nondepolarizing,
1111, 1116t
Neurons, 1628t
Neurontin. See Gabapentin
Neuropathies, peripheral, 589
Neuro-specific enolase (NSE), 384t
Neurotransmitters:
functions, 1505
in pain impulse, 172f
in substance abuse, 104, 104f
types, 1505
Neutropenia:
causes, 307t, 1138
definition, 1138
interdisciplinary care, 1139
manifestations, 1138–38
nursing care, 1139
pathophysiology, 1138
Neutrophilia, 307t
Neutrophils:
abnormal, possible causes, 307t, 387t
development, 289f, 1077f
functions, 288, 288t, 1079
laboratory assessment, 316, 316t
in leukemia, 1123t
location, 288t
normal values, 307t, 387t, 1118t
Nevi:
characteristics, 442–43, 442f
congenital, 466
dysplastic, 466
Nevirapine, 358
Nevus flammeus, 443
New variant Creutzfeldt-Jakob disease, 1658
Newborn screening, 156
Nexium. See Esomeprazole
Niacin. See Nicotinic acid
Niaspan. See Nicotinic acid
Nicardipine:
Medication Administration, 973t, 1162t
in specific conditions

angina, 973–74t
hypertension, 1162t
hypertensive emergencies, 1169t
Nicobid. See Nicotinic acid
Nicolar. See Nicotinic acid
Nicotinamide. See Vitamin B_3
Nicotine, 106–7. See also Smoking
Nicotinic acid, 967t, 968
Nifedipine:
Medication Administration, 973–74t, 1545–46t
in specific conditions
angina, 973–74t
headache, 1545–46t
pulmonary hypertension, 1353
scleroderma, 1485
Night sweats, 1796, 1796t
Nikolsky's sign, 460
Nilstat. See Nystatin
Nimbex. See Cisatracurium
Nimodipine, 973–74t, 1593
Nimotop. See Nimodipine
Nipple, 1761–62t
Nipride. See Nitroprusside
Nisoldipine, 1162t
Nissen fundoplication, 666, 667f
Nitrates, 971, 973t, 1032
Nitric oxide, inhaled, 1367
Nitrite dipstick, 849
Nitrites, 113t
Nitro-Bid. See Nitroglycerin
Nitrodisc. See Nitroglycerin
Nitro-Dur. See Nitroglycerin
Nitrofurantoin, 832t, 850, 850t
Nitrogard. See Nitroglycerin
Nitroglycerin:
adverse/side effects, 987
Medication Administration, 278t, 973t
in specific conditions
acute myocardial infarction, 987
angina, 971, 973t
heart failure, 1032
hypertensive emergencies, 1169t
shock, 278t
Nitrol. See Nitroglycerin
Nitropaste. See Nitroglycerin
Nitroprusside:
Medication Administration, 278t
in specific conditions
aortic aneurysm, 1173
heart failure, 1032
hypertensive emergencies, 1169t
shock, 278t
Nitrous oxide, 111, 113t
NIX. See Permethrin
Nizatidine, 665, 665t, 678
Nizoral. See Ketoconazole
NK cells. See Natural killer cells
Nociception, age-related changes, 175
Nociceptors, 170, 171f
"No-code" order, 91, 91t
Nocturia:
definition, 839, 847, 1027
in heart failure, 1027
in urinary tract infection, 847
Nocturnal penile tumescence and rigidity
(NPTR), 1768
Nodes of Ranvier, 1504
Nodular melanoma, 467
Nodule/nodular lesions, 431t, 432t
Nolvadex. See Tamoxifen
Noncapture, pacemaker, 1011t
Nonconventional terrorist weapons, 127
Nondepolarizing neuromuscular blockers. See
Neuromuscular blockers

Nursing care—*continued*
  hypomagnesemia
    assessment, 235
    community-based care, 235
    health promotion, 235
    Medication Administration, 235*t*
    nursing diagnoses and interventions, 235
  hyponatremia
    assessment, 215
    community-based care, 216
    health promotion, 215
    nursing diagnoses and interventions, 215–16
  hypophosphatemia, 237
  metabolic acidosis
    assessment, 244–45
    community-based care, 245
    health promotion, 244
    nursing diagnoses and interventions, 245
  metabolic alkalosis
    assessment, 246–47
    community-based care, 247
    health promotion, 246
    nursing diagnoses and interventions, 247
  respiratory acidosis
    assessment, 249
    community-based care, 250
    health promotion, 249
    nursing diagnoses and interventions, 249–50
    using NANDA, NIC, and NOC, 250, 250*t*
  respiratory alkalosis
    assessment, diagnoses, and interventions, 251
    community-based care, 252
    health promotion, 251
gastrointestinal/nutritional disorders
  cirrhosis
    assessment, 720–21
    community-based care, 723
    health promotion, 720–21
    Medication Administration, 717*t*
    nursing diagnoses and interventions, 722–23
    using NANDA, NIC, and NOC, 723, 723*t*
  gallstones
    assessment, 701
    community-based care, 703
    health promotion, 701
    nursing diagnoses and interventions, 701–3
  hepatitis
    assessment, 709
    community-based care, 710
    health promotion, 709
    nursing diagnoses and interventions, 709–10
    using NANDA, NIC, and NOC, 710, 710*t*
  malnutrition
    assessment, 648
    community-based care, 650
    health promotion, 648
    Medication Administration, 645*t*
    nursing diagnoses and interventions, 648–50
    using NANDA, NIC, and NOC, 650, 650*t*
  obesity
    assessment, 638–39
    community-based care, 640–41
    health promotion, 638
    Medication Administration, 634*t*
    nursing diagnoses and interventions, 639–40
    using NANDA, NIC, and NOC, 640, 640*t*
  pancreatitis
    assessment, 729–30
    community-based care, 731
    health promotion, 729
    nursing diagnoses and interventions, 730–31
    using NANDA, NIC, and NOC, 731, 731*t*
genetic conditions. *See also* Genetics
  assessment, 159–60

evaluation, 165
nurse's role in genetic testing, 158–59
nursing diagnoses and interventions, 160–65
hematologic disorders
  anemias
    assessment, 1112–13
    community-based care, 1114–15
    health promotion, 1112
    Medication Administration, 1112*t*
    nursing diagnoses and interventions, 1113–14
    using NANDA, NIC, and NOC, 1114, 1115*t*
  disseminated intravascular coagulation
    assessment, 1148
    community-based care, 1149
    nursing diagnoses and interventions, 1148–49
  hemophilia
    assessment, 1144
    community-based care, 1146
    health promotion, 1144
    nursing diagnoses and interventions, 1144–46
    using NANDA, NIC, and NOC, 1146, 1146*t*
  leukemia
    assessment, 1126
    community-based care, 1129
    health promotion, 1125–26
    nursing diagnoses and interventions, 1126–28
    using NANDA, NIC, and NOC, 1128, 1128*t*
  lymphoma
    assessment, 1133
    community-based care, 1135–36
    nursing diagnoses and interventions, 1133–35
    using NANDA, NIC, and NOC, 1135, 1136*t*
  multiple myeloma
    assessment, 1137
    community-based care, 1138
    nursing diagnoses and interventions, 1137–38
  myelodysplastic syndrome
    community-based care, 1117
    nursing diagnoses and interventions, 1116
  neutropenia, 1139
  polycythemia, 1118
  thrombocytopenia
    assessment, 1141
    community-based care, 1142
    nursing diagnosis, 1141–42
HIV/AIDS
  assessment, 361–62
  community-based care, 365
  Medication Administration, 357*t*
  nursing diagnoses and interventions, 362–65
  prevention, 359–61, 361*t*
  using NANDA, NIC, and NOC, 365, 365*t*
hypersensitivity reaction
  assessment, 338
  community-based care, 339
  health promotion, 338
  nursing diagnoses and interventions, 338–39
immunization
  assessment, 302
  community-based care, 303
  health promotion, 301
  nursing diagnoses and interventions, 302
infections
  assessment, 322–23
  community-based care, 324–25
  health promotion, 322
  Medication Administration, 319–21*t*, 450*t*
  nursing diagnoses and interventions, 323–24
  using NANDA, NIC, and NOC, 324, 325*t*

inflammatory conditions
  assessment, 308
  community-based care, 309
  health promotion, 308
  nursing diagnoses and interventions, 308–9
integumentary disorders
  acne, 459, 459*t*
  bacterial skin infections, 447–48
  cutaneous and plastic surgery
    community-based care, 481
    nursing diagnoses and interventions, 479–81
  dermatitis, 457
  fungal skin infections, 450
  hair disorders, 482–83
  malignant melanoma
    assessment, 470, 470*t*
    community-based care, 471
    health promotion, 468–69
    nursing diagnoses and interventions, 470–71
    using NANDA, NIC, and NOC, 471, 471*t*
  nail disorders, 483
  parasitic infestations, 451
  pemphigus vulgaris, 460
  pressure ulcers
    community-based care, 476
    nursing diagnoses and interventions, 474–76, 475*t*
    in older adults, 474*t*
  psoriasis
    community-based care, 445–46
    nursing diagnoses and interventions, 445–46
  viral infections
    community-based care, 455
    nursing diagnoses and interventions, 453, 455
    using NANDA, NIC, and NOC, 455, 455*t*
kidney disorders
  acute renal failure
    assessment, 911
    community-based care, 913
    health promotion, 910–11
    Medication Administration, 905–6*t*
    nursing diagnoses and interventions, 911–13
    using NANDA, NIC, and NOC, 913, 913*t*
  chronic renal failure
    assessment, 923
    Case Study, 931*t*
    community-based care, 926
    health promotion, 923
    nursing diagnoses and interventions, 923–25
    in older adults, 914*t*
  glomerular disorders
    assessment, 891
    community-based care, 894
    health promotion, 891
    nursing diagnoses and interventions, 891–94
loss and grief. *See also* Death and dying
  assessment, 95–96
  community-based care, 98
  health promotion, 95
  nursing diagnoses and interventions, 96–97
  using NANDA, NIC, and NOC, 97, 97*t*
lymphedema
  community-based care, 1201
  nursing diagnoses and interventions, 1200–1201
male reproductive system disorders
  benign prostatic hyperplasia
    client having prostatectomy, 1780–81*t*
    community-based care, 1782
    discharge instructions after prostate surgery, 1783*t*
    nursing diagnoses and interventions, 1781–82
  benign scrotal mass, 1773
  cancer of the penis, 1772

epididymitis, 1773
erectile dysfunction
    community-based care, 1771
    nursing diagnoses and interventions, 1770–71
priapism, 1772
prostate cancer
    assessment, 1787
    client having prostatectomy, 1780–81t
    community-based care, 1789
    discharge instructions after prostate surgery, 1783t
    health promotion, 1786–87
    nursing diagnoses and interventions, 1787–89
    using NANDA, NIC, and NOC, 1789, 1789t
prostatitis, 1777
testicular cancer
    community-based care, 1776
    nursing diagnoses and interventions, 1776
musculoskeletal disorders
amputation
    assessment, 1424
    community-based care, 1426–27, 1427t
    health promotion, 1424
    nursing diagnoses and interventions, 1424–26
    using NANDA, NIC, and NOC, 1426, 1426t
ankylosing spondylitis, 1470
bone tumors
    community-based care, 1484
    nursing diagnoses and interventions, 1483–84
contusion, strain, or sprain, 1400
dislocations
    community-based care, 1401
    nursing diagnoses and interventions, 1401
fibromyalgia, 1487
foot deformities
    community-based care, 1493
    nursing diagnoses and interventions, 1493
fractures
    assessment, 1417–18
    Case Study, 1499t
    client in traction, 1409t
    client with a cast, 1410t
    client with internal fixation, 1412t
    clients with fracture of the humerus, 1413t
    community-based care, 1420–21
    health promotion, 1416–17
    nursing diagnoses and interventions, 1418–20
    using NANDA, NIC, and NOC, 1420, 1420t
gout
    community-based care, 1447
    Medication Administration, 1446t
    nursing diagnoses and interventions, 1447
Lyme disease, 1477
muscular dystrophy, 1459
osteoarthritis
    assessment, 1455
    client having total joint replacement, 1453–1545t
    community-based care, 1457
    health promotion, 1455
    nursing diagnoses and interventions, 1455, 1457
    using NANDA, NIC, and NOC, 1457, 1457t
osteomyelitis
    of client undergoing surgical debridement, 1479t
    community-based care, 1480–81
    nursing diagnoses and interventions, 1480
osteoporosis
    assessment, 1438–39

community-based care, 1400
health promotion, 1437–38
Medication Administration, 1437t
nursing diagnoses and interventions, 1439–40
using NANDA, NIC, and NOC, 1400, 1400t
Paget's disease
    community-based care, 1443
    Medication Administration, 1442t
    nursing diagnoses and interventions, 1443
polymyositis, 1476
reactive arthritis, 1470
repetitive use injury
    community-based care, 1429
    nursing diagnoses and interventions, 1428
rheumatoid arthritis
    assessment, 1468
    community-based care, 1469
    health promotion, 1466–68
    nursing diagnoses and interventions, 1468–69
    using NANDA, NIC, and NOC, 1469, 1469t
scleroderma
    community-based care, 1486
    nursing interventions, 1486
septic arthritis, 1481
spinal deformities
    community-based care, 1490
    nursing diagnoses and interventions, 1489–90
systemic lupus erythematosus
    community-based care, 1475
    Medication Administration, 1474t
    nursing diagnoses and interventions, 1474–75
neurologic system disorders
altered level of consciousness
    nursing diagnoses and interventions, 1534–35
    support of the family, 1533–34
Alzheimer's disease
    assessment, 1623
    communication techniques, 1624t
    community-based care, 1625–26
    health promotion, 1621, 1623
    Medication Administration, 1621t
    nursing diagnoses and interventions, 1623–25
    safety interventions, 1623t
    using NANDA, NIC, and NOC, 1625, 1625t
amyotrophic lateral sclerosis
    community-based care, 1647
    nursing diagnoses and interventions, 1646
arteriovenous malformation, 1595
Bell's palsy, 1656
botulism, 1662
brain tumor
    community-based care, 1575
    nursing diagnoses and interventions, 1572–75
    using NANDA, NIC, and NOC, 1575, 1575t
central nervous system infections
    assessment, 1567
    community-based care, 1569
    health promotion, 1567
    nursing diagnoses and interventions, 1567–68
    using NANDA, NIC, and NOC, 1568, 1568t
Creutzfeldt-Jakob disease, 1659
epilepsy
    assessment, 1552, 1553t
    client having surgery for seizures, 1551t
    community-based care, 1553–54
    health promotion, 1551–52

Medication Administration, 1550t
nursing diagnoses and interventions, 1552–53
using NANDA, NIC, and NOC, 1553, 1553t
Guillain-Barré syndrome
    community-based care, 1655
    nursing diagnoses and interventions, 1654–55
headache
    assessment, 1544
    community-based care, 1547
    health promotion, 1544, 1544t
    Medication Administration, 1545–46t
    nursing diagnoses and interventions, 1544, 1546
herniated intervertebral disk
    assessment, 1610
    of client having posterior laminectomy, 1609–10t
    client teaching, 1611t
    community-based care, 1611–12
    health promotion, 1610
    nursing diagnoses and interventions, 1610–11
Huntington's disease
    community-based care, 1645
    nursing diagnoses and interventions, 1644
increased intracranial pressure
    client and family education, 1541
    Medication Administration, 1539t
    nursing diagnoses and interventions, 1541–42
intracranial aneurysm
    nursing diagnoses and interventions, 1594–95
multiple sclerosis
    assessment, 1632
    community-based care, 1634–35
    health promotion, 1632
    Medication Administration, 1631t
    nursing diagnoses and interventions, 1632–34
    using NANDA, NIC, and NOC, 1634, 1634t
myasthenia gravis
    client and family teaching, 1651t
    of client having a thymectomy, 1650t
    of client undergoing plasmapheresis, 1650t
    community-based care, 1651–52
    Medication Administration, 1649t
    nursing diagnoses and interventions, 1651
Parkinson's disease
    assessment, 1639–40
    community-based care, 1642
    health promotion, 1639
    Medication Administration, 1637t
    nursing diagnoses and interventions, 1640–41
    using NANDA, NIC, and NOC, 1642, 1642t
postpoliomyelitis syndrome, 1660
rabies, 1660
spinal cord injury
    assessment, 1602
    of client with halo external fixation, 1602t
    community-based care, 1606–7
    health promotion, 1602
    Medication Administration, 1600t
    nursing diagnoses and interventions, 1602–6
    using NANDA, NIC, and NOC, 1606, 1606t
spinal cord tumor, 1613
stroke
    assessment, 1587
    Case Study, 1667t
    client having endarterectomy, 1586t
    community-based care, 1591–92

Nursing care—*continued*
 health promotion, 1587
 nursing diagnoses and interventions, 1587–91
 overview, 1586–87
 using NANDA, NIC, and NOC, 1591, 1591*t*
 tetanus, 1661
 traumatic brain injury
  assessment, 1560
  community-based care, 1562–63
  health promotion, 1560
  nursing diagnoses and interventions, 1560–62
  using NANDA, NIC, and NOC, 1562, 1562*t*
 trigeminal neuralgia
  of client undergoing percutaneous rhizotomy, 1656*t*
  community-based care, 1657
  nursing diagnoses and interventions, 1656–57
  teaching for home care, 1657*t*
pain
 assessment, 186–88
 community-based care, 190
 Medication Administration, 179*t*, 182*t*
 nursing diagnoses and interventions, 188–90
 using NANDA, NIC, and NOC, 190, 190*t*
peripheral vascular disorders
 acute arterial occlusion
  assessment, 1185
  community-based care, 1186
  nursing diagnoses and interventions, 1185–86
 aortic aneurysm
  assessment, 1173–74
  community-based care, 1175–76
  nursing diagnoses and interventions, 1174–75
  postoperative, 1174*t*
  preoperative, 1174*t*
 chronic venous insufficiency, 1195, 1196*t*
 hypertension
  assessment, 1164
  Case Study, 1207*t*
  community-based care, 1166–67
  health promotion, 1163–64, 1164*t*
  Medication Administration, 1161–62*t*
  nursing diagnoses and interventions, 1164–66
  in older adults, 1157*t*
  using NANDA, NIC, and NOC, 1166, 1166*t*
 peripheral vascular disease
  assessment, 1178
  community-based care, 1180
  health promotion, 1178
  nursing diagnoses and interventions, 1179–80
  in older adults, 1178*t*
  using NANDA, NIC, and NOC, 1180, 1180*t*
 Raynaud's disease/phenomenon, 1183
 thromboangiitis obliterans, 1182
 varicose veins
  assessment, 1197
  community-based care, 1199
  health promotion, 1197
  nursing diagnoses and interventions, 1197–99
 venous thrombosis
  assessment, 1190, 1191
  community-based care, 1193
  health promotion, 1190
  Medication Administration, 1189–90*t*
  nursing diagnoses and interventions, 1191–93
  using NANDA, NIC, and NOC, 1193, 1193*t*

respiratory disorders
 acute bronchitis, 1267
 acute respiratory distress syndrome
  community-based care, 1372
  nursing diagnoses and interventions, 1367, 1370–71
  using NANDA, NIC, and NOC, 1371, 1371*t*
 acute respiratory failure
  assessment, 1361
  community-based care, 1365
  endotracheal suctioning, 1363*t*
  health promotion, 1361
  nursing diagnoses and interventions, 1361–65
  using NANDA, NIC, and NOC, 1365, 1365*t*
 asthma
  assessment, 1326
  client teaching, 1325*t*
  community-based care, 1330
  health promotion, 1326
  Medication Administration, 1327–28*t*
  nursing diagnoses and interventions, 1329–30
 atelectasis, 1344
 bronchiectasis, 1344
 chronic obstructive pulmonary disease
  assessment, 1336
  Case Study, 1377*t*
  client teaching, 1341*t*
  community-based care, 1340
  health promotion, 1336
  nursing diagnoses and interventions, 1336–40
  using NANDA, NIC, and NOC, 1340, 1340*t*
 cystic fibrosis
  community-based care, 1343
  nursing diagnoses and interventions, 1343
 diphtheria, 1241–42
 epistaxis
  assessment, 1244
  of client with nasal packing, 1245*t*
  community-based care, 1245
  nursing diagnoses and interventions, 1244–45
 fungal lung infections, 1295
 influenza
  assessment, 1234
  community-based care, 1235
  health promotion, 1234
  nursing diagnoses and interventions, 1234–35
  using NANDA, NIC, and NOC, 1235, 1235*t*
 inhalation injury
  assessment, 1307
  community-based care, 1308
  health promotion, 1307
  nursing diagnoses and interventions, 1307–8
 laryngeal cancer
  assessment, 1258
  community-based care, 1261–62
  health promotion, 1258
  nursing diagnoses and interventions, 1258–61
  using NANDA, NIC, and NOC, 1261, 1262*t*
 laryngeal obstruction or trauma, 1250
 lung abscess, 1280
 lung cancer
  assessment, 1313–14
  Case Study, 418*t*
  of client having lung surgery, 1313*t*
  of client having radiation therapy, 1314*t*
  community-based care, 1316–17
  health promotion, 1313
  nursing diagnoses and interventions, 1314–16
  using NANDA, NIC, and NOC, 1316, 1317*t*

nasal polyps, 1252
nasal trauma
 assessment, 1247
 community-based care, 1248–49
 health promotion, 1247
 nursing diagnoses and interventions, 1247–48
 using NANDA, NIC, and NOC, 1248, 1248*t*
nursing care, 1302
obstructive sleep apnea, 1251–52
occupational lung diseases
 community-based care, 1346
 health promotion, 1346
 nursing diagnoses and interventions, 1346
pertussis, 1243
pharyngitis, 1239–40
pleural effusion, 1296, 1297*t*
pneumonia
 assessment, 1275
 community-based care, 1276
 health promotion, 1274
 nursing diagnoses and interventions, 1275–76
 of older adults, 1268*t*
 using NANDA, NIC, and NOC, 1276, 1276*t*
pneumothorax
 assessment, 1301
 client having chest tube insertion, 1300*t*
 community-based care, 1301–2
 health promotion, 1300–1301
 nursing diagnoses and interventions, 1301
pulmonary embolism
 assessment, 1350
 community-based care, 1351–52
 health promotion, 1349–50
 nursing diagnoses and interventions, 1350–51
 using NANDA, NIC, and NOC, 1351, 1352*t*
pulmonary hypertension, 1353
sarcoidosis, 1347
severe acute respiratory syndrome
 assessment, 1278
 community-based care, 1279–80
 health promotion, 1278
 nursing diagnoses and interventions, 1278–79
sinusitis
 assessment, 1237
 community-based care, 1238
 health promotion, 1237
 nursing diagnoses and interventions, 1237–38
thoracic trauma
 assessment, 1304
 community-based care, 1305
 health promotion, 1304
 nursing diagnoses and interventions, 1304–5
tonsillitis, 1239–40
tuberculosis
 assessment, 1290
 community-based care, 1293
 health promotion, 1289–90
 Medication Administration, 1288–89*t*
 nursing diagnoses and interventions, 1290–93
 of older adults, 1282*t*
 using NANDA, NIC, and NOC, 1293, 1293*t*
viral upper respiratory infections
 community-based care, 1231
 health promotion, 1231
 Medication Administration, 1230*t*
sexually transmitted infections
 chlamydia, 1845
 genital herpes

community-based care, 1840
  nursing diagnoses and interventions, 1840
genital warts
  community-based care, 1842
  Medication Administration, 1842*t*
  nursing diagnoses and interventions,
    1841–42
gonorrhea
  community-based care, 1846
  nursing diagnoses and interventions, 1846
pelvic inflammatory disease
  community-based care, 1852
  nursing diagnoses and interventions,
    1851–52
syphilis
  community-based care, 1849–50
  nursing diagnoses and interventions, 1849
vaginal infections
  community-based care, 1844
  nursing diagnoses and interventions,
    1844, 1844*t*
shock
  community-based care, 283*t*
  health promotion and assessment, 279–80
  Medication Administration, 278*t*
  nursing diagnoses and interventions, 280–83
  in older adults, 280*t*
  using NANDA, NIC, and NOC, 283, 283*t*
substance abuse
  assessment, 114–17
  community-based care, 120
  health promotion, 114
  nursing diagnoses and interventions, 117–20
  using NANDA, NIC, and NOC, 120,
    121, 122*t*
surgical client
  Clinical Scenarios, 144*t*
  community-based care, 80
  intraoperative nursing care, 73
  managing acute postoperative pain, 79–80
  postoperative complications, 74–79
  postoperative nursing care, 74
  preoperative client and family teaching, 71
  preoperative client preparation, 71–73
  preoperative nursing care, 71
  using NANDA, NIC, and NOC, 80, 80*t*
transplant procedures
  assessment, 346–47
  community-based care, 348
  health promotion, 349
  kidney transplant, 922*t*
  liver transplant, 922*t*
  Medication Administration, 345–46*t*
  nursing diagnoses and interventions, 347–48
trauma
  assessment, 265
  Case Study, 145*t*
  community-based care, 268
  health promotion, 265
  nursing diagnoses and interventions, 265–68
  using NANDA, NIC, and NOC, 268, 268*t*
upper gastrointestinal disorders
  esophageal cancer
    assessment, 670
    community-based care, 670–71
    health promotion, 670
    nursing diagnoses and interventions, 670
  gastric cancer
    assessment, 691
    community-based care, 694
    health promotion, 691
    nursing diagnoses and interventions,
      691, 693
    using NANDA, NIC, and NOC, 693, 693*t*

gastritis
  assessment, 679
  community-based care, 680
  health promotion, 679
  Medication Administration, 665–66*t*
  nursing diagnoses and interventions, 679–80
gastroesophageal reflux disease
  assessment, 666
  community-based care, 667
  Medication Administration, 665–66*t*
  nursing diagnoses and interventions, 667
  using NANDA, NIC, and NOC, 667, 667*t*
gastrointestinal bleeding
  assessment, 675
  community-based care, 677
  health promotion, 675
  nursing diagnoses and interventions, 675
nausea and vomiting
  community-based care, 674
  Medication Administration, 673*t*
  nursing diagnoses and interventions, 672
oral cancer
  assessment, 661
  community-based care, 663
  health promotion, 661
  nursing diagnoses and interventions, 661–63
peptic ulcer disease
  assessment, 685
  Case Study, 737*t*
  community-based care, 688
  health promotion, 685
  Medication Administration, 665–66*t*
  nursing diagnoses and interventions, 686–88
  using NANDA, NIC, and NOC, 688, 688*t*
stomatitis
  assessment, 658–59
  community-based care, 659–60
  health promotion, 658
  Medication Administration, 658*t*
  nursing diagnoses and interventions, 659
  using NANDA, NIC, and NOC, 659, 659*t*
urinary system disorders
  bladder cancer
    assessment, 865
    client undergoing cystectomy and urinary
      diversion, 866*t*
    community-based care, 868
    health promotion, 865
    nursing diagnoses and interventions, 865–68
  neurogenic bladder, 872
  urinary calculi
    assessment, 860
    community-based care, 862
    health promotion, 859
    nursing diagnoses and interventions, 860–61
  urinary incontinence
    assessment, 877
    client undergoing bladder neck suspension,
      876*t*
    community-based care, 879
    health promotion, 876
    nursing diagnoses and interventions, 877–79
    using NANDA, NIC, and NOC, 879, 879*t*
  urinary retention, 869–70
  urinary tract infection
    assessment, 852
    community-based care, 854–55
    health promotion, 851–52
    nursing diagnoses and interventions, 852–54
    in older adults, 315*t*, 873*t*
Nursing Care of the Client Having....:
  adrenalectomy, 550*t*
  aortic surgery, 1174*t*
  bladder neck suspension, 876*t*

  bowel surgery, 804*t*
  breast reconstruction, 1827*t*
  carotid endarterectomy, 1586*t*
  cast, 1410*t*
  chest tube insertion, 1300*t*
  colostomy, 806*t*
  coronary artery bypass graft, 980–82*t*
  cystectomy and urinary diversion, 866*t*
  dilation and curettage, 1803*t*
  ear surgery, 1725*t*
  eye surgery, 1699*t*
  fibrinolytic therapy, 989*t*
  gastric surgery, 690*t*
  gastrostomy or jejunostomy tube, 692*t*
  halo external fixation, 1602*t*
  hemodialysis, 908*t*
  hemodynamic monitoring, 1031*t*
  hysterectomy, 1804*t*
  ileostomy, 789–90*t*
  immunotherapy, 398*t*
  intraspinal analgesia, 184*t*
  kidney transplant, 922*t*
  laparoscopic cholecystectomy, 700*t*
  laparoscopy of female reproductive system, 1801*t*
  laryngectomy, 1256*t*
  lithotripsy, 859*t*
  liver transplantation, 720*t*
  lung surgery, 1313*t*
  mastectomy, 1826*t*
  nasal packing, 1245*t*
  nephrectomy, 897
  percutaneous coronary revascularization, 978*t*
  peritoneal dialysis, 910*t*
  permanent pacemaker implant, 1012*t*
  plasmapheresis, 1650*t*
  posterior laminectomy, 1609–10*t*
  prostatectomy, 1780–81*t*
  radiation therapy, 396*t*
  rhizotomy, 1656*t*
  subtotal thyroidectomy, 539*t*
  surgery for seizures, 1551*t*
  surgical debridement for osteomyelitis, 1479*t*
  thoracocentesis, 1297*t*
  thymectomy, 1650*t*
  total joint replacement, 1453–54*t*
  T-tube, 701*t*
  ureteral stent, 851*t*
  Whipple's procedure, 732*t*
Nursing Care of the Older Adult:
  age-related changes and effects on pain, 175*t*
  cancer, 371*t*
  cardiac dysrhythmias, 996*t*
  chronic venous insufficiency, 1196*t*
  end-of-life checklist, 95*t*
  fluid volume deficit, 203*t*
  heart failure, 1023*t*
  hypertension, 1157*t*
  hypothyroidism, 545*t*
  infections, 315*t*
  minimizing risk for urinary tract infection and
    urinary incontinence, 873*t*
  peripheral vascular disease, 1178*t*
  pneumonia, 1268*t*
  pressure ulcer prevention, 474*t*
  renal failure, 914*t*
  shock, 280*t*
  tuberculosis, 1282*t*
Nursing Care Plans:
  acute glomerulonephritis, 892*t*
  acute myocardial infarction, 991–92*t*
  acute renal failure, 912*t*
  acute respiratory distress syndrome, 1370*t*
  Addison's disease, 556*t*
  alcohol withdrawal, 119*t*

Nursing Care Plans—*continued*
Alzheimer's disease, 1622–23*t*
amputation, 1425*t*
appendicitis, 768*t*
bacterial meningitis, 1567*t*
bladder cancer, 867*t*
brain tumor, 1573*t*
breast cancer, 1828*t*
burns, 507*t*
cancer, 403–4*t*
cardiac dysrhythmia, 1013*t*
cervical cancer, 1814*t*
cholelithiasis, 702*t*
chronic obstructive pulmonary disease, 1338*t*
chronic pain, 191*t*
chronic renal failure, 924*t*
cirrhosis, alcoholic, 721*t*
client experiencing grief and loss, 98*t*
client having surgery, 80–81*t*
client with hand and foot injuries and suffering
    from trauma of natural disaster, 139*t*
client with multiple injuries, 266*t*
colorectal cancer, 807*t*
coronary artery bypass surgery, 983*t*
Cushing's syndrome, 551*t*
diabetes mellitus, 593*t*
endometriosis, 1811*t*
epilepsy, 1552*t*
fluid volume excess, 212*t*
folic acid deficiency anemia, 1113*t*
gastric cancer, 692–93*t*
glaucoma and cataracts, 1711*t*
gonorrhea, 1847*t*
heart failure, 1037*t*
hemophilia, 1145*t*
herpes zoster, 454*t*
hip fracture, 1417*t*
HIV infection, 363*t*
Hodgkin's disease, 1134*t*
hyperkalemia, 226*t*
hypertension, 1168*t*
hypokalemia, 222*t*
hypothyroidism, 546*t*
immunization, 303*t*
leukemia, 1125*t*
lung cancer, 1315*t*
malignant melanoma, 469*t*
malnutrition, 649*t*
migraine headache, 1547*t*
mitral valve prolapse, 1064*t*
multiple sclerosis, 1633*t*
myasthenia gravis, 1652*t*
nasal trauma, 1247*t*
obesity, 639*t*
oral cancer, 661*t*
osteoarthritis, 1456*t*
osteoporosis, 1438*t*
pancreatitis, acute, 729*t*
peptic ulcer disease, 686*t*
peripheral vascular disease, 1181*t*
peritonsillar abscess, 1240*t*
pneumonia, 1277*t*
prostate cancer, 1788*t*
respiratory acidosis, 249*t*
rheumatoid arthritis, 1467*t*
septic shock, 281*t*
spinal cord injury, 1603*t*
stroke, 1588*t*
subdural hematoma, 1561*t*
syphilis, 1850*t*
total joint replacement, 1456*t*
tuberculosis, 1291*t*
ulcerative colitis, 793*t*
urinary calculi, 861*t*
urinary incontinence, 878*t*
urinary tract infection, 853*t*
Nursing diagnosis. *See also* NANDA, NIC, and
    NOC Linkages; NANDA nursing
    diagnoses
critical thinking skills in, 7*t*
data analysis in, 8
functional health patterns and, 9*t*
overview, 8–9
reasoning in, 8
writing, 9
Nursing ethics:
codes
    American Nurses Association (ANA), 11, 11*t*
    International Council of Nurses (ICN), 10
dilemmas
    confidentiality, 12
    in end-of-life care, 12
    genetic information, 164*t*
    patients' rights, 12
Nursing Interventions Classification (NIC). *See*
    NANDA, NIC, and NOC Linkages
Nursing Outcomes Classification (NOC). *See*
    NANDA, NIC, and NOC Linkages
Nursing practice:
codes of ethics
    American Nurses Association (ANA), 11, 11*t*
    International Council of Nurses (ICN), 10
standards, 11, 11*t*
Nursing process:
benefits, 6–7
in clinical practice, 10
critical thinking skills in, 7*t*
definition, 6
steps, 7, 7*t*, 8*f*
Nursing research, 15
Nursing Research: Evidence-Based Practice:
acute myocardial infarction in women, 995*t*
antibiotic regimens, 310*t*
assisting older adults to communicate
    postoperative pain, 65*t*
breast cancer diagnosis and treatment in African
    American women, 1829*t*
burn injuries, prevention of pressure ulcers, 510*t*
chronic obstructive pulmonary disease
    management, 1335*t*
diabetes mellitus, individualized teaching about
    foot care, 591*t*
disaster preparedness training in nursing
    education, 138*t*
end-of-life care, 90*t*
enteral feeding in the critically ill client, 772*t*
family presence during resuscitation, 1066*t*
fecal incontinence, self-care practices, 764*t*
feeding tube placement methods, 647*t*
fluid volume imbalance assessment
    techniques, 208*t*
gastric residual volume assessment in enteral
    feeding, 662*t*
hemodialysis, 926*t*
HIV/AIDS, nurses' willingness to care for clients
    with, 360*t*
hormone replacement therapy, risks vs.
    benefits, 965*t*
hypertension, relaxation training in, 1164*t*
leukemia and lymphoma, care of physical
    problems during treatment, 1126*t*
male catheterization, 854*t*
multiple sclerosis in aging clients, 1634*t*
online health information use in older adults, 1458*t*
osteoporosis risk assessment, 1439*t*
pain assessment in intubated clients, 1364*t*
pain management, 189*t*
pain management after ambulatory surgery, 700*t*
pressure ulcer treatment and prevention, 475*t*
prostatectomy discharge teaching, 1785*t*
rheumatoid arthritis, use of Internet for client
    teaching, 1458*t*
skeletal pins, care of insertion sites, 1419*t*
smoking cessation for hospitalized patients, 106*t*
speech-generating devices after laryngectomy,
    1260*t*
stem cell transplant, fatigue and depression
    following, 1133*t*
stroke treatment, 1589*t*
thyroid hormone and calcium supplements, 545*t*
traumatic brain injury in young adults, caregiver
    burden, 1563*t*
tuberculosis screening in homeless persons, 1290*t*
urinary incontinence, stress vs urge, 876*t*
venous leg ulcers, rest periods for improved
    healing, 1196*t*
ventilator-associated pneumonia, prevention
    strategies, 280*t*
vision impairments in older adults, 1715*t*
Nutraderm, 441*t*
Nutrasweet. *See* Aspartame
Nutrients. *See also* Nutrition
carbohydrates
    recommended daily intake, 606
    sources, 606
    use by body, 606, 607*f*
deficiencies, 642*t*. *See also* Malabsorption;
    Malnutrition; *specific nutrients*
definition, 605, 631
dietary guidelines 2005, 605
fats
    sources, 579, 608
    types, 607–8
    use by body, 607*f*
proteins
    recommended daily intake, 606
    sources, 606
    uses in body, 606–7
Nutrition. *See also* Nutrients
assessment of status
    diagnostic tests, 642, 644, 644*t*
    functional health pattern interview, 618*t*
    in older adult, 642*t*
    physical assessment
        anthropometric assessment, 620–22*t*
        findings in malnutrition, 619*t*
        oral cavity, 622–23*t*
        overview, 619
        sample documentation, 613*t*
        by system, 402*t*
considerations in specific conditions
    acute renal failure, 906
    burns, 505
    chronic renal failure, 919
    diabetes mellitus
        alcohol, 579
        carbohydrates, 576–77
        diet plan for the older adult, 580
        fiber, 579
        goals, 576
        meal planning, 579–80
        protein, 577, 579
        sick-day management, 580
        sodium, 579
        sweeteners, 579
definition, 605
dietary guidelines, 20, 20*t*, 606*t*
disorders
    Clinical Scenarios, 737*t*
    eating disorders
        anorexia nervosa, 650, 651*t*
        binge-eating disorder, 651, 651*t*

bulimia nervosa, 650–51, 651t
  interdisciplinary care, 651–52
  nursing care, 652
malabsorption. See Malabsorption
malnutrition. See Malnutrition
obesity. See Obesity
Food Guide Pyramid, 21f
in healing process, 307–8
metabolic processes, 613, 631
postsurgical, 70
Nutritional supplements. See also Herbal
      supplements/therapy
  for cancer, 399t
  minerals, 645t
  vitamins
    in cirrhosis, 717
    Medication Administration, 645t
    in substance abuse/withdrawal treatment, 114t
Nutritional-metabolic patterns:
  altered endocrine function. See also Endocrine
      system
    Build Clinical Competence, 600t
    Clinical Scenarios, 601t
  altered integumentary structure and function. See
      also Hair; Integumentary system; Nails; Skin
    Build Clinical Competence, 513t
    Clinical Scenarios, 514t
  altered nutrition and gastrointestinal function.
      See also Nutrition
    Build Clinical Competence, 735t
    Clinical Scenarios, 736t
  NANDA nursing diagnoses, 420t
Nydrazid. See Isoniazid
Nystagmus:
  assessment, 1678
  definition, 1519t, 1678
  in labyrinthitis, 1726
Nystatin:
  Medication Administration, 450t, 658t
  for thrush, 359t, 657t, 658, 658t

O

OA. See Osteoarthritis
Oatmeal, in therapeutic baths, 441t
Obesity:
  cancer risk and, 372
  complications, 630t, 632
  coronary heart disease risk and, 964
  definition, 630, 964
  diabetes mellitus and, 567, 632
  ethnic considerations, 630t, 631t
  hypertension and, 1157
  incidence and prevalence, 630
  interdisciplinary care
    diagnosis, 632, 632t, 633t
    maintaining weight loss, 638
    medications, 633, 634t
    treatments
      behavior modification, 636, 637t
      dietary, 635, 635t, 636t
      exercise, 634, 634f, 635t
      surgical, 636–38, 637f, 638t
  in middle adults, 26
  nursing care
    assessment, 638–39
    community-based care, 640–41
    health promotion, 638
    Medication Administration, 634t
    nursing diagnoses and interventions
      activity intolerance, 640
      chronic low self-esteem, 640
      imbalanced nutrition: more than body
          requirements, 639–40

ineffective therapeutic regimen
    management, 640
  using NANDA, NIC, and NOC, 640, 640t
Nursing Care Plan
  assessment, 639t
  critical thinking in the nursing process, 639t
  diagnoses, 639t
  evaluation, 639t
  expected outcomes, 639t
  planning and implementation, 639t
osteoarthritis risk and, 1450
pathophysiology, 631–32
risk factors, 631
surgical risk and nursing implications, 57t
Obestin-30. See Phentermine
Objective data, 8
Oblique fracture, 1401, 1402f
Obstructive jaundice, 704
Obstructive shock, 274
Obstructive sleep apnea:
  complications, 1250–51, 1580
  incidence, 1250
  interdisciplinary care
    diagnosis, 1251
    surgery, 1251
    treatments, 1251, 1251f
  manifestations, 1250, 1251t
  nursing care, 1251–52
  pathophysiology, 1250
  risk factors, 1250
Obtundation, 1529t
ObyTrim. See Phentermine
Occipital lobe, 1506f, 1506t
Occult blood:
  definition, 744t
  stool
    in colorectal cancer diagnosis, 803
    definition, 674
    possible causes, 387t
    purpose and description, 744t
    related nursing care, 744t
Occupation, cancer risk and, 371, 372t
Occupational lung diseases:
  asbestosis, 1345
  causes, 1345t
  classification, 1344
  coal worker's pneumoconiosis, 1345
  hypersensitivity pneumonitis, 1345–46
  interdisciplinary care, 1346
  manifestations, 1345–46
  nursing care
    community-based care, 1346
    health promotion, 1346
    nursing diagnoses and interventions, 1346
  pathophysiology, 1345–46
  physiology review, 1344
  silicosis, 1345
Occupational therapy:
  in Guillain-Barré syndrome, 1654
  in Parkinson's disease, 1639
Octreotide:
  for cryptosporidiosis, 778t
  for Cushing's syndrome, 550
  for esophageal varices, 718
  for pancreatitis, 728
Oculocutaneous albinism, 427t
Oculomotor nerve (cranial nerve III):
  anatomy, 1510f
  assessment, 1519t
  functions, 1511t, 1671t
Ocupress. See Carteolol
Odynophagia, 1240
Off-pump coronary artery bypass (OPCAB), 978
Ofloxacin, 849, 1846

OGTT (oral glucose tolerance test), 526t, 569
Oil retention enema, 760
Oil slides, 428t
Ointments, for skin disorders, 441t
OKT3. See Muromonab-CD3
Older adults:
  chronic venous insufficiency, 1196t
Older adults (over age 65):
  abuse, 256t
  acute myocardial infarction, 984t
  age-related changes
    bowel elimination, 746t
    cardiac, 952t
    cardiovascular system, 29t
    ears, 1686t
    endocrine system, 529t, 545t
    eyes, 1676t
    female reproductive system, 1760t
    gastrointestinal system, 619t, 746t
    hematologic system, 1091t
    immune function, 330, 1091t
    kidneys, 883, 884t
    male reproductive system, 1749t
    musculoskeletal system, 1389t
    neurologic system, 1518t
    overview, 29t
    pancreas, 529t
    peripheral vascular system, 1091t
    respiratory system, 1214t, 1222t
    skin, 430t
    urinary system, 841t, 883, 884t
  age-related macular degeneration, 1715t
  breast cancer, 1823t
  burns, 508t
  cancer, 371t
  cardiac dysrhythmias, 996t
  constipation, 761t
  demographics, 28–29, 30f
  diabetes mellitus, 567–68, 568t, 580
  diversity, 28t
  end-of-life checklist, 95t. See also End-of-life
      care
  epilepsy, 1548t
  fall prevention, 1418t
  family-related risk factors for alterations in
      health, 32t, 33
  fecal incontinence self-care practices, 764t
  fire deaths, 487
  fluids and electrolytes
    changes with aging, 202
    fluid volume deficit, 203t, 207t
    hypocalcemia, 227–28
  health needs
    assessment guidelines, 30
    promoting health behaviors, 30, 31t
    risks for alterations in health
      injuries, 29–30
      pharmacologic effects, 30
      physical and psychosocial stressors, 30
  heart failure, 1023t
  hip fractures, 1415
  HIV/AIDS in, 349–50
  home care of dementing disorder, 43t
  hypertension, 1157t
  hypothyroidism, 545t
  infections, 314–15, 315t
  kidney function, 883, 884t
  malnutrition, 641, 642t
  medication toxicity, 30
  multiple sclerosis, 1634t
  nutritional needs, 642t
  online health information use, 1458t
  osteomyelitis, 1477
  pain management, 65t, 175, 175t

peripheral vascular disease, 1178*t*
pneumonia, 1268*t*
pressure ulcer, 474*t*, 475*t*
renal failure, 914*t*
sexuality function in women, 1794*t*
shock, 273–74, 280*t*
special considerations
  in disasters, 138
  in surgery
    intraoperative, 68, 70
    Nursing Research: assisting in
      communicating postoperative pain, 65*t*
    postoperative, 79, 80*t*
substance abuse, 115*t*
tuberculosis, 1282*t*
upper respiratory disorders, 315*t*
urinary incontinence, 873*t*
urinary tract infection, 315*t*, 847, 848, 873*t*
Olfactory nerve (cranial nerve I):
  anatomy, 1510*f*
  assessment, 1223*t*, 1519*t*
  function, 1511*t*
Oligodendrocytes, 1628*t*
Oligodendroglioma, 1570*t*. *See also* Brain tumors
Oligomenorrhea, 1802. *See also* Dysfunctional
  uterine bleeding
Oliguria, 839, 886
Olmesartan, 1161*t*
Olsalazine, 786, 787*t*
Omega-3 polyunsaturated fatty acids, 1326
Omeprazole:
  Medication Administration, 665*t*
  preoperative use and nursing implications, 62*t*
  in specific conditions
    gastritis, 678
    gastroesophageal reflux disease, 665
    pancreatitis, 728
    short bowel syndrome, 799
Ommaya reservoir, 1571, 1571*f*
Omnipen. *See* Ampicillin
Oncogenes, 374, 1121
Oncologic emergencies:
  hypercalcemia. *See* Hypercalcemia
  hyperuricemia, 410
  obstructive uropathy, 410
  pericardial effusions and neoplastic cardiac
    tamponade, 409
  sepsis and septic shock, 410
  spinal cord compression, 410
  superior vena cava syndrome, 409, 410*f*
  syndrome of inappropriate diuretic hormone, 410
  tumor lysis syndrome, 410–11
Oncology, 369
Oncology nurse, 369
Oncotic pressure. *See* Osmotic pressure
Oncovin. *See* Vincristine
Ondansetron, 672, 673*t*
Onycholysis, 483
Onychomycosis, 483
Oophorectomy, 1809, 1819
Oophoritis, 1850
OPCAB (off-pump coronary artery bypass), 978
Open (guillotine) amputation, 1421, 1422*t*. *See*
  also Amputation
Open commissurotomy, 1060
Open (compound) fracture, 1401, 1402*f*. *See also*
  Fractures
Open pneumothorax, 1299. *See also*
  Pneumothorax
Open reduction and internal fixation (ORIF):
  hip fracture, 1415, 1416*f*
  nursing interventions, 1412*t*
  procedure, 1411, 1411*f*
Open-angle glaucoma. *See* Glaucoma

Operating room technician (ORT), 66
Ophthalmoscope, guidelines for use, 1681*f*, 1681*t*
Opiates. *See* Narcotic analgesics
Opioids. *See* Narcotic analgesics
Opium, 756*t*
Opium derivatives, 756*t*
Opportunistic infections, in AIDS, 353–54, 359*t*
Opsonization, 293, 294*t*
Optic cup, 1706
Optic disc, 1680, 1681*f*, 1681*t*
Optic nerve (cranial nerve II):
  anatomy, 1510*f*, 1673*f*
  assessment, 1519*t*
  function, 1511*t*, 1672–73
OptiPranolol. *See* Metipranolol
Orabase, 657
Orajel, 658*t*
Oral cancer:
  incidence, 660
  interdisciplinary care, 660
  manifestations, 660, 660*t*
  nursing care
    assessment, 661
    community-based care, 663
    health promotion, 661
    nursing diagnoses and interventions
      disturbed body image, 663
      imbalanced nutrition: less than body
        requirements, 662
      impaired verbal communication, 662–63
      risk for ineffective airway clearance, 662
  Nursing Care Plan
    assessment, 661*t*
    critical thinking in the nursing process, 661*t*
    diagnoses, 661*t*
    evaluation, 661*t*
    expected outcomes, 661*t*
    planning and implementation, 661*t*
  pathophysiology, 660, 660*f*
  risk factors, 660
  staging, 660*t*
Oral contraceptives:
  coronary heart disease risk and, 964
  for dysfunctional uterine bleeding, 1803
  for dysmenorrhea, 1802*t*
  Medication Administration, 1802*t*
Oral endotracheal tube, 1357*t*. *See also*
  Endotracheal tube
Oral glucose tolerance test (OGTT), 526*t*, 569
Oral health:
  in diabetes mellitus, 592
  physical assessment, 622–23*t*
Oral hypoglycemic agents, 578*t*
Oral mucositis, 657*t*. *See also* Stomatitis
Oral rehydration:
  for diarrhea, 755
  for fluid volume deficit, 205
  for gastroenteritis, 776–77
Orasone. *See* Prednisone
Orbital blowout fracture, 1702
Orchiectomy:
  in advanced prostate cancer, 1787*t*
  in testicular cancer, 1775
  in testicular torsion, 1774
Orchitis, 1774
Oretic. *See* Hydrochlorothiazide
Organ donation:
  caring for donor, 265
  donor criteria, 342, 920
  process, 263–65
Organ transplantation. *See* Transplant procedures
Organic solvents, abuse by inhalation, 111
ORIF. *See* Open reduction and internal fixation
Orinase. *See* Tolbutamide

Orlistat, 633, 634*t*
Ornade. *See* Phenylpropanolamine
Ornish diet, 968*t*
Oropharynx, 1211
Orphenadrine citrate, 1600*t*
ORT (operating room technician), 66
Orthoclone. *See* Muromonab-CD3
Orthopnea, 209, 1026
Orthostatic hypotension:
  client teaching, 208
  definition, 1093*t*
  in fluid volume deficit, 205
Orthovisc. *See* Hyaluronan injections
Orudis. *See* Ketoprofen
Orudis KT. *See* Ketoprofen
Oruvail. *See* Ketoprofen SR
Oseltamivir, 1234
Osler's nodes, 1046
Osmolality:
  definition, 198
  serum. *See* Serum osmolality
  urine. *See* Urine, osmolality
Osmolarity, 198
Osmotic diuretics:
  Medication Administration, 905*t*, 1539*t*
  in specific conditions
    acute renal failure, 904, 905*t*
    increased intracranial pressure, 1538, 1539*t*
Osmotic laxatives, 759*t*
Osmotic pressure:
  in body fluid movement, 198
  definition, 198
  in glomerular filtration, 831, 996
Osseous metastases, 181
Ossicles, 1682, 1682*f*
Ossification, 1381
Osteitis deformans. *See* Paget's disease
Osteoarthritis (OA):
  complementary and alternative therapies, 1455
  complications, 1450–51
  definition, 1449
  hand, 1450, 1450*f*
  incidence, 1449
  interdisciplinary care
    conservative management, 1451–52
    diagnosis, 1451
    medications, 1451
    surgery
      arthroscopy, 1452
      joint arthroplasty. *See* Total joint replacement
      osteotomy, 1452
    viscosupplementation, 1452
  management, 1451*t*
  manifestations, 1450
  nursing care
    assessment, 1455
    community-based care, 1457
    health promotion, 1455
    nursing diagnoses and interventions, 1455,
      1457
    using NANDA, NIC, and NOC, 1457, 1457*t*
  Nursing Care Plan
    assessment, 1456*t*
    critical thinking in the nursing process, 1456*t*
    diagnoses, 1456*t*
    evaluation, 1456*t*
    expected outcomes, 1456*t*
    planning and implementation, 1456*t*
  pathophysiology, 1450
  racial/ethnic considerations, 1449*t*
  vs. rheumatoid arthritis, 1460*t*
  risk factors, 1450
Osteoblasts, 1380
Osteochondroma, 1482*t*

Osteoclasts, 1380
Osteocytes, 1380
Osteoid, 1482t
Osteolysis, 1482
Osteoma, 1482t
Osteomalacia:
  causes, 1447, 1448t
  in chronic renal failure, 918
  definition, 1447
  interdisciplinary care
    diagnosis, 1436t, 1448–49
    medications, 1449
  manifestations, 1448, 1448t
  nursing care, 1449
  vs. osteoporosis and Paget's disease, 1436t
  pathophysiology, 1436t, 1488
  risk factors, 1447–88
Osteomyelitis:
  from a contiguous infection, 1478
  definition, 1477
  hematogenous, 1478
  interdisciplinary care
    diagnosis, 1479
    medications, 1479
    surgery, 1479
  manifestations, 1479t
  nursing care
    of client undergoing surgical debridement
      health education for client and family, 1479t
      postoperative, 1479t
      preoperative, 1479t
    community-based care, 1480–81
    nursing diagnoses and interventions
      acute pain, 1480
      hyperthermia, 1480
      impaired physical mobility, 1480
      risk for infection, 1480
  in older adults, 1477
  pathophysiology, 1477–78, 1478f
  in vascular insufficiency, 1478
Osteophytes, 1450
Osteoporosis:
  in chronic renal failure, 918
  complications, 1435
  definition, 1433
  incidence, 1433
  interdisciplinary care
    diagnosis, 1436, 1436t
    medications, 1436, 1437t
    prevention, 1435
  manifestations, 1435, 1435f
  nursing care
    assessment, 1438–39
    community-based care, 1400
    health promotion
      exercise, 1438
      healthy behaviors, 1438
      nutrition, 1437–38
    Medication Administration, 1437t
    nursing diagnoses and interventions
      acute pain, 1440
      health-seeking behaviors, 1439
      imbalanced nutrition: less than body
        requirements, 1440
      risk for injury, 1439–40
    using NANDA, NIC, and NOC, 1400, 1400t
  Nursing Care Plan
    assessment, 1438t
    critical thinking in the nursing process, 1438t
    diagnoses, 1438t
    evaluation, 1438t
    expected outcomes, 1438t
    planning and implementation, 1438t
  Nursing Research: risk assessment, 1439t

vs. osteomalacia and Paget's disease, 1436t
  pathophysiology, 1434–35, 1436t
  racial/ethnic considerations, 1434, 1434t
  risk factors, 1433–34, 1433t, 1439t
Osteosarcoma, 1482t. See also Bone tumors
Osteotomy, 1452
Ostomy, 746. See also Colostomy; Ileostomy
Otitis externa:
  definition, 1718
  interdisciplinary care, 1719–20
  manifestations, 1719
  nursing care
    community-based care, 1720–21
    nursing diagnoses and interventions, 1720
    teaching to prevent, 1720t
  pathophysiology, 1719
  risk factors, 1719
Otitis media:
  acute, 1722
  chronic, 1724–25
  definition, 1721
  interdisciplinary care
    diagnosis, 1722
    medications, 1722
    surgery, 1723
  manifestations, 1722, 1722f
  nursing care
    assessment, 1723
    community-based care, 1723
    health promotion, 1723
    nursing diagnoses and interventions, 1723
  pathophysiology, 1721
  serous, 1721–22
Otorrhea, 1555
Otosclerosis, 1725–26
Otoscope, guidelines for use, 1686–87t, 1686f
Outcomes, 9
Outpatient surgery, 54–55
Output, pacemaker, 1010t. See also Pacemakers
Ovarian cancer:
  complications, 1818, 1818t
  genetic considerations, 1755t, 1758
  incidence, 1817
  interdisciplinary care
    diagnosis, 1818
    medications, 1818–19
    radiation therapy, 1819
    surgery, 1819
  manifestations, 1818
  nursing care, 1819
  pathophysiology, 1818
  risk factors, 1817
  staging, 1818, 1818t
Ovarian cycle, 1754, 1754f
Ovaries:
  anatomy, physiology, and functions, 1751t, 1753, 1753f
  cancer. See Ovarian cancer
  cysts, 1808, 1809t
  physical assessment, 1754–65t
Overdose:
  signs, 113t
  treatment, 112, 113t, 114t
Overflow urinary incontinence, 874t. See also
  Urinary incontinence
Oversensing, pacemaker, 1011t. See also
  Pacemakers
Overweight, 630. See also Obesity
Oviducts. See Fallopian tubes
Ovral. See Norgestrel/ethinyl estradiol
Oxacillin, 319t, 1046
Oxalate, 858, 858t
Oxaliplatin, 805
Oxaprozin, 178t, 1464t

Oxazepam, 114t, 716
Oxazolidinones, 320t
Oxicams, 178t, 306
Oxiconazole, 450t
Oximetry:
  pulse. See Pulse oximetry
  transcutaneous. See Pulse oximetry
Oxistat. See Oxiconazole
Oxybutynin, 871, 871t, 875
Oxycodone:
  abuse, 110, 110f
  equianalgesic drug chart, 180t
  for long-term analgesia at home, 190t
  nursing considerations, 180t
  preoperative use and nursing implications, 62t
OxyContin. See Oxycodone
Oxygen concentration (FIO$_2$), 1360, 1360t
Oxygen therapy:
  in acute respiratory failure, 1355
  in chronic obstructive pulmonary disease, 1335
  in pneumonia, 1272, 1272f, 1273f
Oxygen-hemoglobin dissociation curve, 1216, 1216f
Oxyhemoglobin, 1076, 1216
Oxymorphone HCl, 180t, 182t
Oxytetracycline, 320t
Oxytocin, 520

P

P wave, 948f, 948t
p24 assay, 355
PABA (p-aminobenzoic acid), 465t
Pacemakers:
  influence on ECG, 1009, 1010f
  client safety considerations, 1010t
  modes and functions, 1010t
  nursing care for implant procedure
    home care, 1012t
    postoperative, 1012t
    preoperative, 1012t
  problems and corrective strategies, 1011t
  types, 1008–9, 1009f
Pacific Islanders:
  substance use, 105t
  tuberculosis incidence, 1281t
Pacing spike, 1010t. See also Pacemakers
Packed red blood cells (RBCs), 263t
Paclitaxel, 391, 1819
PaCO$_2$:
  abnormal findings, 1560t
  definition, 239
  in gastroenteritis and diarrhea, 776t
  in metabolic acidosis, 242
  in metabolic alkalosis, 246
  normal values, 239, 240t, 1560t
  in respiratory acidosis, 242t, 247
  in respiratory alkalosis, 242t, 250
  significance, 240t
PACs. See Premature atrial contractions
Paget's disease:
  breast, 1823
  characteristics, 1441
  complications, 1441
  incidence, 1441
  interdisciplinary care
    diagnosis, 1436t, 1441–42
    medications, 1442, 1442t
    surgery, 1442
  manifestations, 1441, 1441t
  nursing care
    community-based care, 1443
    Medication Administration, 1442t
    nursing diagnoses and interventions

Paget's disease—*continued*
    chronic pain, 1443
    impaired physical mobility, 1443
    vs. osteoporosis and osteomalacia, 1436*t*
    pathophysiology, 1436*t*, 1441
Pagitane. *See* Cycrimine
Pain:
    acute
      definition, 173
      physical responses to, 173–74
      referred, 173, 173*f*
      somatic, 173
      visceral, 173
    breakthrough, 174
    cancer
      causes, 381
      management, 399–400
      types, 381
    central, 174
    Chapter Highlights, 192*t*
    chronic
      categories, 174
      conditions, 174
      definition, 174
    definition, 170
    factors affecting responses
      age, 175–76, 175*t*
      emotional status, 176
      knowledge, 177
      past experiences, 176
      sociocultural influences, 176
      source and meaning of pain, 176
    inhibitory mechanisms, 171–72
    interdisciplinary care
      complementary therapies
        acupuncture, 185
        biofeedback, 185
        cutaneous stimulation, 186
        distraction, 186
        hypnotism, 185
        relaxation, 185–86
      medications
        anticonvulsants, 179. *See also* Antiepileptic drugs
        antidepressants, 179. *See also* Antidepressants
        bisphosphonates, 181
        for cancer pain, 399–400
        dosing schedules, 181–82
        duration of action, 181
        local anesthetics, 179
        narcotic analgesics. *See* Narcotic analgesics
        nonnarcotic analgesics, 178
        nonsteroidal anti-inflammatory drugs, 178, 178*t*. *See also* Nonsteroidal anti-inflammatory drugs
        opiates/opioids. *See* Narcotic analgesics
        radiopharmaceuticals, 181
        routes of administration, 182–83, 183*f*
        WHO analgesic ladder, 177, 177*f*
      surgical procedures
        cordotomy, 184, 185*f*
        neurectomy, 184, 185*f*
        rhizotomy, 184, 185*f*
        sympathectomy, 184, 185*f*
        transcutaneous electrical nerve stimulation, 184–85, 185*f*
    myths and misconceptions, 177
    neurophysiology, 170, 170*t*, 171*f*
    nursing care
      acute postoperative pain, 79–80. *See also* Postoperative period, pain management
      assessment
        behavioral responses, 188
        client perceptions, 186–87

        McGill Pain Questionnaire, 187*f*
        pain scales, 187*f*
        physiologic responses, 188
        self-management, 188
      in client with a fracture, 1408*t*
      community-based care, 190, 190*t*
      in dying client, 92
      Medication Administration
        narcotic analgesics, 182*t*
        nonsteroidal anti-inflammatory drugs, 179*t*
      nursing diagnoses and interventions, 188–90
      using NANDA, NIC, and NOC, 190, 190*t*
      Nursing Care Plan
        assessment, 191*t*
        critical thinking in the nursing process, 191*t*
        diagnosis, 191*t*
        evaluation, 191*t*
        expected outcomes, 191*t*
        planning and implementation, 191*t*
      Nursing Research: observational studies of pain management, 189*t*
    pathway, 171, 171*f*
    phantom, 174
    postoperative. *See* Postoperative period, pain management
    psychogenic, 175
    theories, 172–73, 172*f*
Pain behaviors, 188
Pain scales, 186, 187*f*
Pain threshold, 175
Pain tolerance, 175
Palifermin, 658
Palliative care, 92
Palliative procedure, 54*t*
Pallidotomy, 1639
Pallor:
    assessment in light and dark skin, 426*t*
    causes, 426*t*, 1093*t*
    definition, 425*t*, 1093*t*
Pamidronate:
    Medication Administration, 1442*t*
    in specific conditions
      bony metastases, 181
      hypercalcemia, 232, 547
      Paget's disease, 1442, 1442*t*
p-aminobenzoic acid (PABA), 465*t*
Pancreas:
    age-related changes, 529*t*
    anatomy, 611*f*, 613
    cell types, 521
    disorders
      cancer. *See* Pancreatic cancer
      diagnostic tests, 526*t*, 616–17*t*, 728*t*
      endocrine function. *See* Diabetes mellitus
      pancreatitis. *See* Pancreatitis
    functions
      endocrine, 521, 564
      exocrine, 613, 725–26, 742
Pancreas transplant, 342*t*, 581. *See also* Transplant procedures
Pancreatic cancer:
    incidence, 731
    interdisciplinary care, 732–33
    manifestations, 731
    nursing care of client undergoing Whipple's procedure, 732*t*
    pathophysiology, 731
    risk factors, 731
Pancreatic polypeptide, 521
Pancreatitis:
    acute
      complications, 726–27
      manifestations, 726, 727*t*
      pathophysiology, 726

    chronic
      complications, 727
      manifestations, 727, 727*t*
      pathophysiology, 727
    definition, 726
    interdisciplinary care
      diagnosis, 616–17*t*, 727, 728*t*
      medications, 727–28, 728*t*
      treatments
        complementary therapies, 728
        nutrition, 728
        surgery, 728
    manifestations, 726, 727*t*
    nursing care
      assessment, 729–30
      community-based care, 731
      health promotion, 729
      Medication Administration, 728*t*
      nursing diagnoses and interventions
        imbalanced nutrition: less than body requirements, 730
        pain, 730
        risk for deficient fluid volume, 730–31
      using NANDA, NIC, and NOC, 731, 731*t*
    pathophysiology, 726–27
Pancreatoduodenectomy. *See* Whipple's procedure
Pancrelipase, 728*t*
Pancuronium bromide, 1356*t*
Pancytopenia, 1109
Pantoprazole, 502, 665, 665*t*
Pantothenic acid, 609*t*
PaO₂:
    abnormal findings, 1560*t*
    in acid–base imbalances, 242*t*
    definition, 239
    normal values, 239, 240*t*, 1560*t*
    significance, 240*t*
PAP (prostatic acid phosphatase), 384*t*
Papanicolaou smear (Pap test):
    classification systems, 1813*t*
    purpose and description, 1755, 1756*t*
    related nursing care, 1756*t*
Papaverine, 1769
Papillary thyroid carcinoma, 546
Papilledema, 1158
Papilloma:
    laryngeal, 1253
    urinary tract, 862, 862*f*
Papillomavirus. *See* Human papillomavirus
Papular warts, 1841. *See also* Genital warts
Papule, 432*t*
Paracentesis, 717, 719*t*
Paradoxic movement, 1303, 1303*f*
Paracsophageal hiatal hernia, 667, 668*f*
Paraflex. *See* Chlorzoxazone
Paraldehyde, 108
Paralytic ileus. *See also* Intestinal obstruction
    after abdominal surgery, 811
    in peritonitis, 770
    in spinal cord injury, 1599
Paraneoplastic syndromes:
    laboratory indicators, 380*t*
    in lung cancer, 1311
    pathophysiology, 380
    in renal cancer, 896
Paraphasia, 1620
Paraphimosis, 1771
Paraplatin. *See* Carboplatin
Paraplegia, 1584*f*, 1599
Parasites, 311*t*, 450–51
Parasympathetic nervous system:
    in blood pressure regulation, 1085
    effects of stimulation, 1512
    physiology, 1512

Parathyroid glands. *See also* Parathyroid hormone
  anatomy, physiology, and functions, 520
  disorders
    diagnostic tests, 524*t*
    hyperparathyroidism
      definition, 547
      interdisciplinary care, 547
      manifestations, 547, 547*t*
      nursing care. *See* Hypercalcemia
      pathophysiology, 547
    hypoparathyroidism
      definition, 548
      interdisciplinary care, 548
      manifestations, 548, 548*t*
      nursing care. *See* Hypocalcemia
      pathophysiology, 548
Parathyroid hormone (PTH):
  abnormal, possible causes, 387*t*
  in calcium balance, 227, 227*f*, 1381
  diagnostic test, 524*t*
  feedback mechanism, 519*t*
  functions, 520, 520*t*
  normal values, 387*t*, 524*t*
  in specific conditions
    cancer, 380
    hypercalcemia, 232
    osteomalacia, 1436*t*
    osteoporosis, 1436*t*
    Paget's disease, 1436*t*
    paraneoplastic syndromes, 380*t*
Paraurethral. *See* Skene's glands
Paregoric, 756*t*
Parenchyma, 294, 847
Parenteral nutrition. *See* Total parenteral nutrition
Paresthesian, 589, 1105
Parietal lobe, 1506*f*, 1506*t*
Parish nursing, 37
Parkinsonism, secondary, 1635
Parkinson's disease:
  characteristics, 1635
  complications, 1636*t*, 1637
  genetic considerations, 1513*t*
  incidence and prevalence, 1635
  interdisciplinary care
    deep brain stimulation, 1639
    diagnosis, 1637
    medications, 1637–38*t*
    rehabilitation, 1639
    surgery, 1639
  manifestations
    abnormal posture, 1636
    autonomic and neuroendocrine effects, 1636
    interrelated effects, 1636–37
    mood and cognition, 1636
    overview, 1636*t*
    rigidity and bradykinesia, 1635–36, 1636*f*
    sleep disturbances, 1636
    tremor, 1635
  nursing care
    assessment, 1639–40
    community-based care, 1642
    health promotion, 1639
    Medication Administration, 1637*t*
    nursing diagnoses and interventions
      disturbed sleep pattern, 1641
      imbalanced nutrition: less than body
        requirements, 1641
      impaired physical mobility, 1640–41
      impaired verbal communication, 1641
    using NANDA, NIC, and NOC, 1642, 1642*t*
  pathophysiology, 1635
  stages, 1635*t*
Parkland formula, 499
Parlodel. *See* Bromocriptine

Paromomycin, 778*t*, 780*t*
Paronychia, 483
Paroxetine, 1798
Paroxysmal, 1000
Paroxysmal nocturnal dyspnea (PND), 1027
Paroxysmal supraventricular tachycardia (PSVT),
  997*t*, 1001
Partial gastrectomy, 689, 689*f*
Partial laryngectomy, 1255
Partial parenteral nutrition, 648
Partial seizures, 1548–49
Partial thromboplastin time (PTT), 60*t*
Partial-thickness burn, 489*t*, 490, 490*f*. *See also*
  Burns
Partner abuse. *See* Intimate partner violence
Passive immunity, 299, 300*t*
Patch, skin, 432*t*
Patch test, 337, 428*t*
Patellar reflex, 1523*f*
Pathogens, 309, 310–12, 311*t*. *See also* Infections
Pathologic fracture, 1136, 1401
Pathophysiology Illustrated:
  acute glomerulonephritis, 887*t*
  acute renal failure, 901*t*
  acute respiratory distress syndrome, 1368–69*t*
  bone healing, 1404–5*t*
  cirrhosis and esophageal varices, 712–13*t*
  coronary heart disease, 960–61*t*
  multiple sclerosis, 1628–29*t*
  peptic ulcer disease, 682–83*t*
  sickle cell anemia, 1108*t*
  tuberculosis, 1284–85*t*
Patient-controlled analgesia, 183, 183*f*
Pavementing, 293, 293*f*
Pavulon. *See* Pancuronium bromide
PAWP (pulmonary artery wedge pressure),
  1031, 1032*f*
Paxil. *See* Paroxetine
PBSCT (peripheral blood stem cell
  transplantation), 398, 1132, 1333*t*. *See also*
  Stem cell transplant
PCOS (polycystic ovarian syndrome), 632,
  1808, 1809*t*
PCP. *See* Pneumocystis carinii pneumonia
PCP (phencyclidine), 110–11, 113*t*
PCR (percutaneous coronary revascularization),
  977, 977*f*, 978*t*
PCR (polymerase chain reaction), 1287
Peak expiratory flow rate (PEFR), 1324
Peau d'orange, 1761*t*, 1823
Pediculosis, 450–51
Pedigrees:
  challenges, 160
  characteristics, 159–60
  ethical implications, 164*t*
  facts and information included, 163*t*
  sample three-generation, 161*f*
  steps in drawing, 162*t*
  symbols used, 160*f*
Pedunculated polyps, 800, 800*f*. *See also* Polyps
PEEP (positive end-expiratory pressure),
  1358, 1359*t*
PEFR (peak expiratory flow rate), 1324
Pelvic exenteration, 1813
Pelvic floor muscle exercises, 876, 877*t*
Pelvic inflammatory disease (PID):
  in AIDS, 354
  Case Study, 51
  chlamydia and, 1845
  complications, 1851
  definition, 1850
  gonorrhea and, 1846
  incidence, 1851
  interdisciplinary care

    diagnosis, 1851
    medications, 1851
    surgery, 1851
  manifestations, 1851
  nursing care
    community-based care, 1852
    nursing diagnoses and interventions
      deficient knowledge, 1851–52
      risk for injury, 1851
  pathophysiology, 1851
Pelvis:
  bimanual examination, 1765*t*
  fracture, 1414
Pemphigus vulgaris:
  interdisciplinary care, 460
  manifestations, 460
  nursing care, 460
  pathophysiology, 460
Penbutolol, 1161*t*
Pendred syndrome, 527*t*
Penectomy, 1772
Penetrance, 155
Penetrating trauma, 256, 1702
Penetrex. *See* Enoxacin
Penicillamine, 1465*t*, 1466, 1485
Penicillin G:
  Medication Administration, 319*t*
  in specific conditions
    pneumonia, 1271*t*
    rheumatic fever, 1043
    syphilis, 1849
Penicillin V, 319*t*
Penicillin-resistant *Streptococcus pneumoniae*
  (PRSP), 314
Penicillins:
  Medication Administration, 319*t*
  in specific conditions
    endocarditis, 1046
    lung abscess, 1280
    tonsillitis, 1239
  topical
    in conjunctivitis, 1694
    in corneal infections, 1697
Penile implants, 1770, 1770*f*
Penis:
  age-related changes, 1749*t*, 1769
  anatomy, physiology, and functions, 1744, 1744*f*,
    1745*t*
  disorders
    cancer
      incidence, 1772
      interdisciplinary care, 1772
      nursing care, 1772
      pathophysiology, 1772
    phimosis, 1749*t*, 1771
    priapism, 1771–72, 1772*t*
    physical assessment, 1749–50*t*, 1749*f*, 1750*f*
Penred syndrome, 1684*t*
Pentamidine, 359*t*, 1271*t*
Pentazocine, 180*t*, 182*t*, 816
Pentoxifylline, 1177, 1182
Penumbra, 1580
Pepcid. *See* Famotidine
Peppermint tea, 792
Peptic ulcer disease (PUD):
  Case Study, 737*t*
  complications
    gastric outlet obstruction, 681*t*, 684
    hemorrhage, 681, 681*t*
    perforation, 681*t*, 684
  definition, 680
  incidence, 680
  interdisciplinary care
    diagnosis, 684

Platelet count—*continued*
  perioperative, significance and nursing
      implications, 60*t*
  in specific conditions
      disseminated intravascular coagulation, 1148
      leukemia, 1123*t*
Platelet transfusions, 1141
Platelets:
  disorders. *See* Thrombocytopenia
  formation, 1077*f*, 1140
  functions, 1079, 1080, 1080*f*, 1140
  medications affecting function, 1142*t*
  as volume resuscitation therapy, 263*t*
Platinol. *See* Cisplatin
Plavix. *See* Clopidogrel
Plendil. *See* Felodipine
Pletal. *See* Cilostazol
Plethora, 1117
Plethysmography, 1188
Pleura, 1213, 1295
Pleural cavity, 1295
Pleural effusion:
  causes, 1295
  definition, 1295
  interdisciplinary care
      thoracocentesis. *See* Thoracocentesis
      treatments, 1296
  manifestations, 1295–96
  nursing care, 1296, 1297*t*
  pathophysiology, 1295
Pleurisy. *See* Pleuritis
Pleuritic pain, 1269
Pleuritis:
  definition, 1295
  interdisciplinary care, 1295
  manifestations, 1295
  nursing care, 1295
  in pneumonia, 1269
Pleurodesis, 1296, 1299–1300
Plicamycin, 232
PMDD (premenstrual dysphoric disorder), 1798
PMNs (polymorphonuclear leukocytes). *See*
      Neutrophils
PMS. *See* Premenstrual syndrome
PND (paroxysmal nocturnal dyspnea), 1027
Pneumococcal vaccine:
  contraindications, 21*t*, 1274
  indications, 21*t*, 300, 301*t*, 1271
  nursing implications, 301*t*
Pneumocystis carinii pneumonia (PCP):
  in AIDS, 353, 359*t*, 1270
  manifestations, 353, 1270, 1270*t*
  pharmacologic treatment, 359*t*, 1271*t*
Pneumomediastinum, 1360
Pneumonectomy, 1312*t*
Pneumonia:
  acute bacterial
      complications, 1269
      manifestations, 1269, 1270*t*
      pathophysiology, 1268, 1269*f*
  aspiration, 1270
  classification, 1267
  community acquired, 1267*t*
  definition, 1267
  incidence, 1267
  interdisciplinary care
      complementary therapies, 1273–74
      diagnosis, 1270–71
      treatments
          chest physiotherapy, 1272–73,
              1273*f*, 1274*f*
          incentive spirometry, 1272
          oxygen therapy, 1272, 1272*f*, 1273*f*
  mortality from, 1267

  nosocomial, 313, 1267*t*. *See also* Ventilator-
      associated pneumonia
  nursing care
      assessment, 1275
      community-based care, 1276
      health promotion, 1274
      nursing diagnoses and interventions
          activity intolerance, 1275–76
          ineffective airway clearance, 1275
          ineffective breathing pattern, 1275
      of older adults, 1268*t*
      using NANDA, NIC, and NOC, 1276, 1276*t*
  Nursing Care Plan
      assessment, 1277*t*
      critical thinking in the nursing process, 1277*t*
      diagnoses, 1277*t*
      evaluation, 1277*t*
      expected outcomes, 1277*t*
      planning and implementation, 1277*t*
  in older adults, 1268*t*
  opportunistic, 1267*t*. *See also Pneumocystis
      carinii* pneumonia
  pathophysiology
      inflammatory response, 1267, 1267*f*
      organisms causing, 1267*t*
      pathogen entry routes, 1267
      patterns of lung involvement, 1268*t*
  physiology review, 1267
  postoperative
      assessment findings, 75
      nursing care, 76
  prevention. *See* Pneumococcal vaccine
  primary atypical, 1269, 1270*t*
  ventilator-associated. *See* Ventilator-associated
      pneumonia
  viral, 1269, 1270*t*
Pneumothorax:
  definition, 258, 1297
  interdisciplinary care
      diagnosis, 1299
      treatments
          surgery, 1300
  manifestations, 1298*t*
  in mechanical ventilation, 1360
  nursing care
      assessment, 1301
      of client having chest tube insertion, 1300*t*
      community-based care, 1301–2
      health promotion, 1300–1301
      nursing diagnoses and interventions
          impaired gas exchange, 1301
          risk for injury, 1301
  pathophysiology, 1297, 1298*t*, 1299
  spontaneous
      manifestations, 1297, 1298*t*
      pathophysiology, 1297, 1298*t*
  tension
      emergency treatment, 258, 258*f*
      manifestations, 258, 1298*t*, 1299
      pathophysiology, 258, 1298*t*, 1299
  traumatic
      causes, 1299
      manifestations, 1298*t*, 1299
      pathophysiology, 1298*t*
      types, 1299
"Pocket talker," 1731
Podofilox, 1841
Podofin. *See* Podophyllin
Podophyllin, 1841, 1842*t*
Podophyllum, 755
Poliomyelitis virus, 1659
Polycillin. *See* Ampicillin
Polycyclic hydrocarbons, 372*t*
Polycystic kidney disease:

  genetic considerations, 839*t*, 884, 884*t*
  interdisciplinary care, 885
  manifestations, 885
  nursing care, 885
  pathophysiology, 884, 885*f*
Polycystic ovarian syndrome (PCOS), 632, 1808,
      1809*t*
Polycythemia:
  definition, 1076, 1117
  interdisciplinary care
      diagnosis, 1117
      nursing care, 1118
      treatments, 1117–18
  manifestations, 1117
  pathophysiology, 1117
  primary, 1117
  in pulmonary hypertension, 1353
  relative, 1117
  secondary, 1117
Polycythemia vera, 1117
Polydipsia, 566
Polyethylene glycol, 759*t*
Polymerase chain reaction (PCR), 1287
Polymorphisms, 152
Polymorphonuclear leukocytes (PMNs). *See*
      Neutrophils
Polymyositis:
  definition, 1476
  interdisciplinary care, 1476
  manifestations, 1476
  nursing care, 1476
Polymyxin B-neomycin-hydrocortisone, 1719
Polyneuropathies, 589
Polypectomy, 1252
Polyphagia, 566
Polyploidy, 150*t*
Polyps:
  colon
      characteristics, 800, 800*f*
      definition, 800
      interdisciplinary care, 801
      laryngeal, 1253, 1253*f*
      manifestations, 801
      nursing care
          assessment, 801
          community-based care, 801
          health promotion, 801
          nursing diagnoses and interventions, 801
      pathophysiology, 800
  female reproductive tissue, 1808–9, 1809*t*
  laryngeal, 1252, 1253
  nasal. *See* Nasal polyps
Polysomnography, 1251
Polysporin, 441*t*
Polysubstance abuse, 103*t*, 115
Polytar. *See* Coal tar derivatives
Polythiazide, 210*t*
Polyuria:
  definition, 209, 566, 839
  in fluid volume excess, 209
  in type 1 diabetes mellitus, 566
Pons, 1505*f*, 1506
Ponstel. *See* Mefenamic acid
Popliteal artery, aneurysm, 1172, 1172*f*
Porphyria, 1089*t*
Port-access coronary artery bypass, 979
Portal hypertension, 704, 711
Portal systemic encephalopathy, 704, 715, 715*t*
Port-wine stain, 443
Positioning, surgical, 67, 69*f*
Positive end-expiratory pressure (PEEP), 1358,
      1359*t*
Positive pressure ventilators, 1357, 1357*f*. *See also*
      Mechanical ventilation

Positron emission tomography (PET):
  brain, 1512, 1514*t*, 1627
  heart, 945*t*
  in lymphoma, 1131
  thorax, 1218*t*
Postconcussion syndrome, 1558*t. See also*
    Traumatic brain injury
Posterior descending artery, 939*f*, 959
Posterior infarct, 984
Posterior laminectomy:
  nursing care, 1609–10*t*
  procedure, 1608
Posterior syndrome, 1597*t. See also* Spinal cord
    injury
Postherpetic neuralgia, 453
Posticteric/convalescent phase, hepatitis, 706, 706*t*
Postmenopausal women. *See also* Menopause;
    Older adults
  breast cancer in, 1823*t*
  coronary heart disease risk factors, 964
  hormone replacement therapy. *See* Hormone
    replacement therapy
Postoperative period. *See also* Surgery
  definition, 54
  interdisciplinary care, 70
  nursing care
    care after client is stable, 74
    immediate care, 74
    NANDA, NIC, and NOC Linkages, 80*t*
    postoperative complications
      cardiovascular, 74–75
      elimination-related, 78–79
      respiratory, 75–76
      special considerations for older adults, 79, 79*t*
      wound. *See* Wounds
  pain management. *See also* Pain
    interdisciplinary care, 64
    nursing care, 79–80
    Nursing Research
      assisting older adults to communicate
        postoperative pain, 65*t*
      pain management after ambulatory
        surgery, 700*t*
Postpoliomyelitis syndrome:
  characteristics, 1659
  interdisciplinary care, 1659
  manifestations, 1659
  nursing care, 1660
Postrenal acute renal failure, 900, 900*t. See also*
    Acute renal failure
Post-trauma syndrome, 268
Postural drainage, in chest physiotherapy,
    1273, 1274*f*
Postural hypotension. *See* Orthostatic hypotension
Postvoid residual urine, 836*t*, 870, 874
Potassium (K$^+$):
  in action potential, 1505
  balance, 217–18
  in body fluid compartments, 197*t*
  foods high in, 218*t*
  imbalances. *See* Hyperkalemia; Hypokalemia
  nurse, 217
  oral and parenteral administration, 221, 221*t*, 223
  recommended dietary guidelines, 606*t*
  serum levels
    abnormal, possible causes, 387*t*
    in gastroenteritis and diarrhea, 776*t*
    normal values, 198*t*, 387*t*
    perioperative, significance and nursing
      implications, 60*t*
Potassium acetate, 221*t*
Potassium bicarbonate, 221*t*
Potassium channel blockers, 1006, 1006*t*
Potassium chloride, 221*t*

Potassium citrate, 221*t*, 858
Potassium gluconate, 221*t*
Potassium hydroxide (KOH), 428*t*
Potassium iodide, 538*t*, 1272
Potassium permanganate, 441*t*, 449
Potassium phosphate, 232
Potassium-sparing diuretics, 210, 210*t*
Potassium-wasting diuretics, 225*t*
PPD (purified protein derivative), 1286, 1286*f*,
    1286*t*
PPE (personal protective equipment), 134–35, 134*t*
PQRST technique, pain assessment, 186
PR interval, 948*f*, 948*t*
Pramipexole, 1638*t*
Prandin. *See* Repaglinide
Pravachol. *See* Pravastatin
Pravastatin, 967*t*, 968
Prazosin, 1161*t*, 1485
Prealbumin, 642, 644*t*
Precose. *See* Acarbose
Precursor T-cell lymphoblastic
    leukemia/lymphoma, 1130*t. See also*
    Leukemia; Lymphomas
Prediabetes, 569
Predictive genetic testing, 157
Prednisolone, 555*t*, 787–88*t*
Prednisone:
  adverse/side effects, 393*t*
  as chemotherapy, 393*t*
  Medication Administration, 555*t*, 787–88*t*, 1631*t*
  nursing implications, 393*t*
  in specific conditions
    Addison's disease, 555*t*
    glomerular disorders, 890
    inflammatory bowel disease, 787–88*t*
    leukemia, 1123*t*
    multiple myeloma, 1137
    multiple sclerosis, 1631*t*
    organ transplantation, 344
Pregnancy:
  diabetes in, 566*t*
  hypertension in, 1167
  substance abuse in
    cocaine, 109
    marijuana, 107
    smoking, 107
Preicteric phase, hepatitis, 705, 706*t*
Preimplantation genetic diagnosis, 157
Preload, 940, 1023, 1024*t*
Premature atrial contractions (PACs):
  causes, 1000–1001
  ECG characteristics, 997*t*, 1001
  management, 997*t*
  manifestations, 1001
  pathophysiology, 1001
Premature ejaculation, 1771
Premature junctional contractions, 1002
Premature ventricular contractions (PVCs):
  after acute myocardial infarction, 985
  causes, 1002
  ECG characteristics, 998*t*
  in heart failure, 1034
  management, 998*t*
  patterns, 1002
  as warning signs, 1002
Premenstrual dysphoric disorder (PMDD), 1798
Premenstrual syndrome (PMS):
  definition, 1798
  incidence, 1798
  interdisciplinary care
    complementary and alternative therapies, 1800
    diagnosis, 1798
    medications, 1798, 1800
  manifestations, 1798

  Multisystem Effects, 1799*t*
  nursing care
    community-based care, 1800
    nursing diagnoses and interventions
      acute pain, 1800
      ineffective coping, 1800
  pathophysiology, 1798
Preoperative period. *See also* Surgery
  definition, 54
  interdisciplinary care
    client preparation
      positioning, 67, 69*f*
      shaving, 68*f*
      skin preparation, 67
    diagnosis, 60–61, 60*t*
    medications, 61, 62*t*
  nursing care
    client and family teaching
      coughing exercise, 72*t*
      diaphragmatic breathing exercise, 72*t*
      information needs, 71
      leg, ankle, and foot exercises, 73*t*
      turning in bed, 73*t*
    client preparation, 71–73
    nursing care, 71
    nursing diagnoses, 70*t*
Preparedness, disaster, 133. *See also* Disasters
Prerenal acute renal failure, 900, 900*t. See also*
    Acute renal failure
Presbycusis, 1730. *See also* Hearing loss
Presbyopia, 1677*t*
Pressure support ventilation, 1358, 1359*t*
Pressure trauma, in disasters, 129*t*
Pressure ulcer:
  definition, 472, 1093*t*
  incidence, 472
  interdisciplinary care
    diagnosis, 473
    medications, 473, 474*t*
    surgical treatment, 473
  nursing care
    community-based care, 476
    nursing diagnoses and interventions, 474–76,
      475*t*
    of older adults, 474*t*
  Nursing Research
    prevention in clients with major burn, 510*t*
    treatment and prevention in older adults, 475*t*
  pathophysiology, 472
  prevention, 474*t*, 475*t*
  risk factors, 472
  staging, 473*f*, 473*t*
Pressure-control ventilation, 1358
Pressure-cycled ventilators, 1358
Pretibial myxedema, 536
Prevacid. *See* Lansoprazole
Prevalence. *See* Omeprazole
Prilosec. *See* Omeprazole
Primacor. *See* Milrinone
Primary dysmenorrhea, 1800
Primary hypertension, 1155. *See also*
    Hypertension
Primary intention, wound healing by, 76, 76*f*
Primary lymphedema, 1199, 1199*t. See also*
    Lymphedema
Primary motor area, 1506*t*
Primary prevention, 24
Primary pulmonary hypertension, 1352
Primary syphilis, 1847–48, 1848*f*, 1848*t. See also*
    Syphilis
Primary tuberculosis, 1281. *See also* Tuberculosis
Primidone, 1550*t*
Prinivil. *See* Lisinopril

Race/ethnicity. *See also specific racial/ethnic groups*
considerations in specific disorders
breast cancer, 1822*t*
cancer, 370*t*
cirrhosis, 711*t*
diabetes mellitus, 564*t*
G6PD anemia, 1160*t*
gallstones, 697*t*
heart disease, 958*t*
heart failure, 1023*t*, 1035*t*
hemolytic anemias, 1106*t*
HIV/AIDS, 349*t*
hypertension, 1156, 1157*t*
inflammatory bowel disease, 782*t*
lactase deficiency, 798*t*
obesity, 630*t*, 631*t*
osteoarthritis, 1449*t*
osteoporosis, 1434, 1434*t*
prostate cancer, 1783*t*
sickle cell anemia, 1106–7, 1106*t*, 1107*t*
stroke, 1580*t*
substance abuse, 105, 105*f*, 105*t*
thalassemia, 1106*t*, 1199
tuberculosis, 1281*t*, 1291
death/dying experience and, 88, 89*t*
demographics of older adults, 28*t*
health and, 20
pain response and, 176
Radial pulse, 1096*t*
Radiation exposure:
burn injuries from, 488, 488*t*, 498. *See also* Burns
cancer risk and, 375–76
in nuclear detonation, 130*t*, 131
Radiation sickness, 131
Radiation therapy:
cancer sensitivity to, 396*t*
definition, 395
delivery methods, 395
nursing care
external radiation, 397*t*
internal radiation, 397*t*
lung cancer, 1314*t*
safety principles, 396*t*
in specific conditions
bladder cancer, 863
brain tumor, 1572
breast cancer, 1826–27
cervical cancer, 1813
colorectal cancer, 805
endometrial cancer, 1817
laryngeal cancer, 1254
leukemia, 1123–24
lung cancer, 1312–13
malignant melanoma, 468
nonmelanoma skin cancer, 464
ovarian cancer, 1819
spinal cord tumor, 1613
testicular cancer, 1775
Radical mastectomy, 1825. *See also* Mastectomy
Radical neck dissection, 660, 1255
Radical nephrectomy, 896. *See also* Nephrectomy
Radical orchiectomy. *See* Orchiectomy
Radical prostatectomy, 1785. *See also* Prostatectomy
Radioactive iodine therapy, 537
Radioactive iodine uptake (RIA), 524*t*, 537
Radioallergosorbent test (RAST), 336
Radiologic dispersion bomb, 128, 130*t*, 131
Radionuclide imaging:
in acute myocardial infarction, 987
in heart failure, 1027
liver and/or spleen, 1088*t*

Radionuclide stress tests, 944*t*, 970–71
Radiopharmaceuticals, 181
Radius, fracture, 1413
Radon, 1308
Raloxifene, 391, 1436, 1796
Ramipril, 1033*t*, 1161*t*
Range of motion (ROM), 1391, 1391*f*, 1392–94*t*, 1392*f*, 1393*f*
Ranitidine:
Medication Administration, 665*t*
preoperative use and nursing implications, 62*t*
in specific conditions
gastroesophageal reflux disease, 665
pancreatitis, 728
RAP (right atrial pressure), 1030
Rapamune. *See* Sirolimus
Rapid plasma reagin (RPR), 1746*t*, 1756*t*, 1849
Rapidly progressive glomerulonephritis, 887–88. *See also* Glomerular disorders
RAS (reticular activating system), 1529–30
RAST (radioallergosorbent test), 336
Raynaud's disease/phenomenon:
characteristics, 1182
interdisciplinary care, 1182–83
manifestations, 1182, 1183*f*
nursing care, 1183
pathophysiology, 1182
in scleroderma, 1485
vs. thromboangiitis obliterans, 1183*t*
Reactivation tuberculosis, 1281. *See also* Tuberculosis
Reactive airway disorders:
asthma. *See* Asthma
atelectasis. *See* Atelectasis
bronchiectasis. *See* Bronchiectasis
chronic obstructive pulmonary disease. *See* Chronic obstructive pulmonary disease
cystic fibrosis. *See* Cystic fibrosis
Reactive arthritis (ReA):
causes, 1470
interdisciplinary care, 1470
manifestations, 1470
nursing care, 1470
Reasoning, 6
Rebetol. *See* Ribavirin
Rebif. *See* Interferon(s)
Receptive aphasia, 1583
Reconstruction:
in disaster response, 133
in healing process, 294
Reconstructive procedure, 54*t*
Recovery, in disaster response, 133
Rectocele, 1805, 1807*t*
Rectovaginal fistula, 1808
Rectum:
anatomy and functions, 743, 743*f*
physical assessment, 750*f*, 750*t*
Recurrent infections, 1839
Red blood cells (RBCs):
abnormal
possible causes, 387*t*
types, 1103
anatomy, 1076, 1078*f*
destruction, 1078–79
disorders
anemia. *See* Anemia
myelodysplastic syndrome. *See* Myelodysplastic syndrome
polycythemia. *See* Polycythemia
formation, 1077*f*
functions, 1102
indices, 1078*t*
normal values, 387*t*, 890*t*, 1078*t*
packed, 263*t*. *See also* Blood transfusion

production and regulation, 1076, 1078, 1079*f*
in specific conditions
glomerular disorders, 890*t*
leukemia, 1123*t*
rheumatic heart disease, 1043*t*
tonicity and, 199*f*
in urine. *See* Urine, RBCs
Red (corneal light) reflex, 1678, 1680
Reducible hernia, 810. *See also* Hernia
Reed-Sternberg cells, 1130
Reentry phenomenon, 996
Refeeding syndrome, 236
Referral source, 39
Referred pain, 173, 173*f*
Reflection, 6
Reflex arc, 1511*f*
Reflex sympathetic dystrophy, 1407
Reflexes:
assessment, 1523–24*f*, 1523–24*t*
physiology, 1511, 1511*f*
Refludan. *See* Lepirudin
Reflux:
gastroesophageal. *See* Gastroesophageal reflux disease
urinary, 847, 847*f*
Refraction:
definition, 1673
errors of, 1696
testing, 1674*t*
Refractometry, 1674*t*
Refractoriness, 995
Regional anesthesia, 63
Regitine. *See* Phentolamine
Reglan. *See* Metoclopramide
Regonol. *See* Pyridostigmine
Regulator cells, 297. *See also* T lymphocytes
Regurgitation, 985, 1043, 1054. *See also* Valvular heart disease
Rehabilitation:
cancer, 412
cardiac, 990
in Parkinson's disease, 1639
Rehabilitation nursing, 47
Reiter's syndrome. *See* Reactive arthritis
Rejection, transplant, 342–43, 343*t*, 921–22. *See also* Transplant procedures
Relafen. *See* Nabumetone
Relaxation, 185–86
Relenza. *See* Zanamivir
Remicade. *See* Infliximab
Reminyl. *See* Galantamine hydrobromide
Remission, 23
Remodeling, in burn wound healing, 493
Remodulin. *See* Treprostinil
Renal arteriogram, 837*t*
Renal artery occlusion, 894–95
Renal artery stenosis, 895
Renal biopsy:
health education for the client and family, 838*t*
purpose and description, 838*t*
related nursing care, 838*t*
in specific conditions
chronic renal failure, 918
glomerular disorders, 889
renal failure, 904
Renal cell carcinoma:
incidence, 896
interdisciplinary care, 896–97
manifestations, 896, 896*t*
nursing care
community-based care, 899
nursing diagnoses and interventions
anticipatory grieving, 899
ineffective breathing pattern, 898

pain, 897–98
  risk for impaired urinary elimination, 898–99
pathophysiology, 896
staging, 896t
Renal colic, 856
Renal cortex, 830, 830f
Renal failure. *See also* Acute renal failure; Chronic renal failure
  definition, 899
  in diabetes mellitus, 588
  surgical risk and nursing implications, 57t
Renal medulla, 830, 830f
Renal osteodystrophy, 918
Renal pelvis, 830, 830f
Renal plasma clearance, 834
Renal replacement therapy:
  dialysis. *See* Dialysis
  kidney transplant. *See* Kidney transplant
Renal ultrasonography:
  purpose and description, 837t
  in specific conditions
    acute renal failure, 904
    chronic renal failure, 918
    polycystic kidney disease, 885
    renal mass, 896
Renal vein occlusion, 895
Renin, 201
Renin–angiotensin–aldosterone system:
  in blood pressure regulation, 1155
  in body fluid regulation, 201, 202f
  in heart failure, 1025
  in hypertension, 1157–58
  in shock, 270
  in sodium balance regulation, 214
RenoPro. *See* Abciximab
Repaglinide, 578t
Repetitive use injury:
  carpal tunnel syndrome, 1427–28
  interdisciplinary care
    conservative management, 1428
    diagnosis, 1428
    medications, 1428
    surgery, 1428
  nursing care
    community-based care, 1429
    nursing diagnoses and interventions
      acute pain, 1428
      impaired physical mobility, 1428
Repolarization, 942–43, 942f
Requip. *See* Ropinirole
Rescriptor. *See* Delavirdine
Researcher, nurse as, 15. *See also* Nursing research
Reserpine, 1162t
Residual urine test, 836t
Residual volume, 1214t
Residual volume (RV), 1214
Resistance, vascular, 1176
Resolution, in healing process, 294
Respiration. *See also* Respiratory system
  breathing techniques in respiratory disorders, 1341t
  factors affecting
    air pressures, 1214–15, 1215f
    airway resistance, lung compliance, and elasticity, 1216
    alveolar surface tension, 1216
    oxygen, carbon dioxide, and hydrogen ion concentrations, 1215–16
    respiratory volume and capacity, 1214, 1214t
  patterns in altered level of consciousness, 1530, 1530t
  phases, 1210
Respiratory acidosis:
  arterial blood gases in, 240t
  causes, 242t

compensation, 243t
definition, 240, 241f
interdisciplinary care
  diagnosis, 248
  medications, 248
  respiratory support, 248–49
laboratory values, 242t, 247
manifestations, 248, 248t
nursing care
  assessment, 249
  community-based care, 250
  health promotion, 249
  nursing diagnoses and interventions
    impaired gas exchange, 250
    ineffective airway clearance, 250
  using NANDA, NIC, and NOC, 250, 250t
Nursing Care Plan
  assessment, 249t
  critical thinking in the nursing process, 249t
  diagnoses, 249t
  evaluation, 249t
  expected outcomes, 249t
  planning and implementation, 249t
pathophysiology
  acute, 247–48
  chronic, 248
risk factors, 247
Respiratory alkalosis:
  arterial blood gases in, 240t
  causes, 242t
  compensation, 243t
  definition, 240, 241f
  interdisciplinary care
    diagnosis, 251
    medications, 251
    respiratory therapy, 251
  laboratory values, 242t, 250
  manifestations, 251, 251t
  nursing care
    assessment, diagnoses, and interventions, 251
    community-based care, 252
    health promotion, 251
  pathophysiology, 250–51
  risk factors, 250
Respiratory failure. *See* Acute respiratory distress syndrome; Acute respiratory failure
Respiratory rate:
  assessment, 1223t
Respiratory syncytial virus (RSV), 1231
Respiratory system:
  age-related changes
    in middle adults, 27t
    in older adults, 29t, 1214t, 1222t
    in young adults, 26t
  anatomy, physiology, and functions
    lower respiratory system
      airway response, 1322
      bronchi and alveoli, 1212f, 1213
      defense systems, 1267
      lungs, 1211–12, 1212f
      overview, 1212f
      pleura, 1213
      rib cage and intercostal muscles, 1213, 1213f
    upper respiratory system
      larynx, 1211
      nose, 1210–11
      overview, 1210f
      pharynx, 1211
      sinuses, 1211, 1211f
      trachea, 1211
  assessment
    diagnostic tests, 1217–19t, 1219, 1220t
    functional health pattern interview, 1221–22t
    genetic considerations, 1219

health assessment interview, 1220–21
physical assessment
  breath sounds, 1225–26t, 1225f
  nose, 1222–23t
  overview, 1222
  sinuses, 1223t
  thorax, 1223–25t, 1224–25f
sample documentation, 1217
blood gases
  carbon dioxide transport, 1216–17
  oxygen transport and unloading, 1216, 1216f
disorders
  Clinical Scenarios, 1376t
  genetic considerations, 1220t
  lower respiratory tract. *See* Lower respiratory disorders
  surgical risk and nursing implications, 57t
  upper respiratory tract. *See* Upper respiratory disorders
factors affecting ventilation and respiration
  air pressures, 1214–15, 1215f
  airway resistance, lung compliance, and elasticity, 1216
  alveolar surface tension, 1216
  oxygen, carbon dioxide, and hydrogen ion concentrations, 1215–16
  respiratory volume and capacity, 1214, 1214t
Respiratory tract infections. *See* Lower respiratory disorders; Upper respiratory disorders
Respite care, 38
Response, disaster, 133. *See also* Disasters
Rest pain, 1177
Restless leg syndrome, 916
Restrictive cardiomyopathy, 1066
Rete testis, 1745
Reteplase (rPA), 988
Reticular activating system (RAS), 1529–30
Reticular formation, 1507
Retina:
  age-related changes, 1676t
  anatomy, physiology, and functions, 1672, 1672f
  assessment, 1680, 1681t
  disorders
    diabetic retinopathy. *See* Diabetic retinopathy
    retinal detachment. *See* Retinal detachment
    retinitis pigmentosa, 1717–18
Retin-A. *See* Tretinoin
Retinal detachment:
  interdisciplinary care, 1716–17
  manifestations, 1716, 1716t
  nursing care
    community-based care, 1717
    nursing diagnoses and interventions
      anxiety, 1717
      ineffective tissue perfusion: retinal, 1717
  pathophysiology, 1716
Retinitis pigmentosa, 1717–18
Retinol. *See* Vitamin A
Retinoscopy:
  purpose and description, 1674t
  related nursing care, 1674t
Retraction, 952, 1386t
Retroflexion, uterus, 1805, 1806f
Retrograde amnesia, 1559
Retrograde conduction, 1001
Retrograde ejaculation, 1771
Retrograde pyelogram:
  purpose and description, 837t
  related nursing care, 837t
  in specific conditions
    acute renal failure, 904
Retropubic prostatectomy, 1781t, 1785
Retroversion, uterus, 1805, 1806f
Retrovir. *See* Zidovudine

Severe acute respiratory syndrome—*continued*
  medications, 1278
  treatments, 1278
  manifestations, 1278
  nursing care
    assessment, 1278
    community-based care, 1279–80
    health promotion, 1278
    nursing diagnoses and interventions
      impaired gas exchange, 1279
      risk for infection, 1279
  pathophysiology, 1276–77
Sex chromosomes, 149
Sex hormones:
  female, 1753. *See also* Estrogen
  male, 1745–46. *See also* Testosterone
Sex-determining region Y gene *(SRT)*, 1747t
Sexual activity:
  response cycle, 1794–95
  safer sex practices, 359, 361t
Sexual dysfunction:
  in cirrhosis, 715t
  in diabetes mellitus, 595
  in men
    ejaculatory dysfunction, 1771
    erectile dysfunction. *See* Erectile dysfunction
  in women
    anorgasmia, 1795
    dyspareunia, 1795
    inhibited sexual desire, 1795
    nursing care, 1795
Sexuality-reproductive patterns:
  altered reproductive function. *See also* Female
      reproductive system; Male reproductive
      system
    Build Clinical Competence, 1854t
    Clinical Scenarios, 1855t
  NANDA nursing diagnoses, 1501t
Sexually transmitted infections (STIs):
  Chapter Highlights, 1852t
  characteristics, 1837–38
  chlamydia. *See* Chlamydia
  definition, 1837
  genital herpes. *See* Genital herpes
  genital warts. *See* Genital warts
  gonorrhea. *See* Gonorrhea
  health promotion teaching, 1838t
  HIV/AIDS and, 1837
  incidence and prevalence, 1837
  pelvic inflammatory disease. *See* Pelvic
      inflammatory disease
  prevention and control, 1838
  resources, 1838t
  syphilis. *See* Syphilis
  vaginal infections. *See* Vaginal infections
  in young adults, 24
Shave skin biopsy, 428t
Shaving, preoperative, 67, 68f
Shearing, 256
Shigella, 774t, 775
Shigellosis, 774t, 775
Shingles. *See* Herpes zoster
Shock:
  assessment in light and dark skin, 426t
  cellular homeostasis and hemodynamics, 268–69
  Chapter Highlights, 283–84t
  definition, 268
  effect on body systems
    cardiovascular, 270, 272
    gastrointestinal and hepatic, 272
    Multisystem Effects, 273t
    neurologic, 272
    renal, 272

    respiratory, 272
    skin, temperature, and thirst, 272
  interdisciplinary care
    diagnosis, 276–77
    fluid replacement
      blood and blood products, 279
      colloid solutions, 277–78
      crystalloid solutions, 277
    medications, 277, 278t
    oxygen therapy, 277
  nursing care
    community-based care, 283
    health promotion and assessment, 279–80
    Medication Administration, 278t
    nursing diagnoses and interventions
      anxiety, 282–83
      decreased cardiac output, 280–82, 282f
      ineffective tissue perfusion, 282
    of older adults, 280t
    using NANDA, NIC, and NOC, 283, 283t
  Nursing Care Plan. *See* Septic shock, Nursing
      Care Plan
  pathophysiology, 269–70
  postoperative, 74
  stages, 269–70, 269t
  types
    anaphylactic, 276, 276t
    cardiogenic, 274, 274t
    distributive, 274
    hypovolemic, 273–74, 273f
    neurogenic, 275–76, 276t
    obstructive, 274
    septic, 275, 275t
Short bones, 1380
Short bowel syndrome:
  causes, 799
  interdisciplinary care
    diagnosis, 799
    medications, 799
    nursing care, 799–800
  pathophysiology, 799
Shoulder:
  physical assessment, 1394t
  replacement. *See* Total joint replacement
SIADH. *See* Syndrome of inappropriate
    antidiuretic hormone
Sibutramine, 633, 634t
Sick sinus syndrome, 1000
Sickle cell anemia:
  complications, 1107, 1109
  genetic considerations, 1089t, 1106, 1107f
  interdisciplinary care
    diagnostic tests, 1110
    focus, 1110t
    medications, 1111
  manifestations, 1107
  pathophysiology, 1107, 1108t
  physical assessment, 1107f
  racial/ethnic considerations, 1106–7, 1106t, 1107t
  stroke risk and, 1580
Sickle cell crisis, 1107
Sickle cell disease, 1107
Sickle cell test, 1110
Sickle cell trait, 1107
Sigmoid colon, 742f, 743
Sigmoid colostomy, 804
Sigmoidoscopy:
  in bowel disorders, 745t
  in cancer, 385
  in diarrhea, 755
  in gastroenteritis, 776
  in protozoal bowel infections, 779
Sildenafil citrate, 987, 1769

Silent myocardial ischemia, 970
Silicosis, 1345
Silvadene. *See* Silver sulfadiazine
Silver nitrate, 500, 501t, 1243
Silver sulfadiazine, 441t, 500, 501t
Silymarin, 709
Simple diffusion, 199–200
Simple (closed) fracture, 1401, 1402f. *See also*
    Fractures
Simple mastectomy, 1825
Simple obstruction, 811, 812f. *See also* Intestinal
    obstruction
Simple partial seizure, 1548–49
Simple Triage and Rapid Transport (START)
    System, 134t
Simulect. *See* Basiliximab
SIMV (synchronized intermittent mandatory
    ventilation), 1358, 1359t
Simvastatin, 98, 967t
Sinemet. *See* Carbidopa-levodopa
Single nucleotide polymorphisms (SNPs), 152
Single-chamber pacing, 1009, 1010t. *See also*
    Pacemakers
Single-gene disorders, 152
Single-photon emission computed tomography
    (SPECT), 1512, 1514t
Singulair. *See* Montelukast
Sinoatrial (SA) node, 941, 941f
Sinus arrhythmia:
  causes, 1000
  ECG characteristics, 997t
  management, 997t
Sinus bradycardia:
  causes, 1000
  ECG characteristics, 997t
  management, 997t
  manifestations, 1000
Sinus tachycardia:
  causes, 1000
  ECG characteristics, 997t
  management, 997t
  manifestations, 1000
  pathophysiology, 1000
Sinuses:
  anatomy, physiology, and functions, 1211,
      1211f, 1235
  infection. *See* Sinusitis
  physical assessment, 1223t
Sinusitis:
  complications, 1236, 1236t
  definition, 1235
  interdisciplinary care
    complementary therapies, 1237
    diagnosis, 1236
    medications, 1236
    surgery, 1236–37, 1237f
  manifestations, 1236
  nursing care
    assessment, 1237
    community-based care, 1238
    health promotion, 1237
    nursing diagnoses and interventions
      imbalanced nutrition: less than body
          requirements, 1237–38
      pain, 1237
  pathophysiology, 1235–36
  physiology review, 1235
Sirolimus, 345t
SIRS (systemic inflammatory response
    syndrome), 275
Sitz baths, 819, 821
Sjögren's syndrome:
  associated disorders, 1486

incidence, 1486
interdisciplinary care, 1486
nursing care, 1486
pathophysiology, 1486
Skeletal traction, 1408, 1409f
Skeletal tuberculosis, 1283
Skelid. See Tiludronate
Skene's glands:
  location and function, 1751t, 1752, 1752f
  physical assessment, 1763f, 1763t
Skin:
  age-related changes
    in middle adults, 27t
    in older adults, 29t, 430t
    in young adults, 26t
  anatomy, physiology, and functions
    anatomy, 424f
    dermis, 423–24
    epidermis, 423, 423t
    glands, 424–25
    skin color, 425
    superficial fascia, 424
  assessment
    abnormal findings, 431t, 435f, 435t, 529t, 1093t
    diagnosis, 427, 428t
    Genetic Considerations, 427, 427t
    health assessment interview, 427, 429
    sample documentation, 427t
    technique/normal findings, 431t, 435t, 529t
    variations in people with light and dark
      skin, 426t
  disorders
    benign lesions
      angiomas, 430t, 434t, 443
      cysts, 432t, 443
      keloid. See Keloid
      keratosis, 430t, 443
      nevi, 442–43, 442f
      in older adults, 430t
      primary, 432t
      secondary, 433t
      skin tags, 430t, 443
      terminology, 431t
      vascular, 434t
    Chapter Highlights, 483–84t
    Clinical Scenarios, 514t
    infections/infestations. See Skin
      infections/infestations
    inflammatory disorders
      acne. See Acne
      dermatitis. See Dermatitis
      lichen planus, 460
      malignant lesions
        actinic keratosis, 461, 461f
        malignant melanoma. See Malignant
          melanoma
        skin cancer. See Skin cancer
      medications for, 441t
      pemphigus vulgaris, 460
      pressure ulcer. See Pressure ulcer
      pruritus, 440, 441t
      psoriasis. See Psoriasis
      terminology, 431t
      toxic epidermal necrolysis, 460–61
      xerosis (dry skin), 441, 441t
    self-examination, 465t
    surgical procedures
      cutaneous
        chemical destruction, 478
        cryosurgery, 477
        curettage, 477
        electrosurgery, 477
        fusiform excision, 477

laser surgery, 477–78
sclerotherapy, 478
nursing care
  community-based care, 481
  nursing diagnoses and interventions, 479–81
plastic
  blepharoplasty, 479
  chemical peeling, 479
  dermabrasion, 479
  liposuction, 479
  rhinoplasty, 479
  rhytidectomy, 479
  skin grafts and flaps, 478–79, 478f
tenting, 435f, 435t
transplantation
  indications, 342t
  success rate, 342t
trauma
  burns. See Burns
  frostbite, 476–77
  injuries, 258–59, 259f
  pressure ulcer. See Pressure ulcer
turgor, 205, 435
Skin biopsy, 428t
Skin cancer:
  malignant melanoma. See Malignant
    melanoma
  nonmelanoma
    basal cell cancer, 462–63, 462t, 463f
    incidence, 461
    interdisciplinary care
      diagnosis, 463
      treatments, 463–64
    nursing care
      assessment, 470t
      community-based care, 465
      health promotion, 464, 464t, 465t
      risk factors, 461–62
      squamous cell cancer, 463, 463f
    prevention, 464t
Skin flap, 479
Skin grafts:
  in burns, 503, 503f
  types, 478, 478f
Skin infections/infestations:
  bacterial
    interdisciplinary care
      diagnosis, 447
      medications, 447
    nursing care
      community-based care, 448
      nursing diagnoses and interventions, 447–48
    pathophysiology, 446
    types
      carbuncles, 447
      cellulitis, 447, 447f
      erysipelas, 447
      folliculitis, 446, 446f
      furuncles, 446–47, 447f
  fungal
    interdisciplinary care, 449–50, 450t
    nursing care, 450
    types
      candidiasis. See Candidiasis
      dermatophytoses, 448–49
  parasitic
    interdisciplinary care
      diagnosis, 451
      medications, 451
    nursing care, 451
    types
      pediculosis, 450–51
      scabies, 451

viral
  interdisciplinary care
    diagnosis, 453
    medications, 453
  nursing care
    community-based care, 455
    nursing diagnoses and interventions,
      453, 455
    using NANDA, NIC, and NOC, 455, 455t
  types
    herpes simplex, 452, 452f
    herpes zoster. See Herpes zoster
    warts, 451–52
Skin tags, 430t, 443t
Skin tests:
  in hypersensitivity reactions, 337–38, 338f
  in immunity assessment, 300
  types and related nursing care, 428t
Skin traction, 1408, 1409f
Skull fracture. See also Traumatic brain injury
  definition, 1554
  interdisciplinary care, 1412, 1555
  nursing care, 1555–56
  pathophysiology, 1555
  types, 1555, 1555f
SLE. See Systemic lupus erythematosus
Sleep apnea:
  central, 1250
  definition, 1250
  obstructive. See Obstructive sleep apnea
  stroke risk and, 1580
Sleeve resection, lung, 1312t
Sliding hiatal hernia, 667, 668f
Slo-Phyllin. See Theophylline
"Slow codes," 91
Small intestine:
  anatomy, physiology, and functions, 605f, 612, 742
  disorders. See Bowel disorders
  obstruction. See Intestinal obstruction
Small-bowel obstruction. See Intestinal obstruction
Small-bowel series, 744t
Small-cell carcinoma, 1308, 1309t. See also Lung
  cancer
Smallpox, 128t
Smell, assessment, 1223t
Smoke inhalation/poisoning, 496, 1305. See also
  Inhalation injury
Smoking:
  cancer risk and, 371–72, 862, 1308, 1337t
  cessation
    in chronic obstructive pulmonary disease, 1334
    coronary heart disease risk reduction from, 966
    in hospital patients (Nursing Research), 106t
  chronic obstructive pulmonary disease and, 1331
  client teaching, 1337t
  coronary heart disease risk and, 964
  hypertension and, 1160
  nicotine characteristics, 106
  nursing diagnoses, 1337t
  nursing interventions, 1337t, 1340
  osteoporosis risk and, 1434
  rates in women, 106–7
  stroke risk and, 1580t
  surgical risk and nursing implications, 58t
  thromboangiitis obliterans and, 1180, 1182
Snellen chart, 1676–77, 1677f
Sniffing, 111
Snowstorm, 129t, 131
Soap-suds enema, 760
Social support systems, 37, 87
Socioeconomic factors:
  health and, 20, 37
  in heart disease, 958t

Sodium (Na$^+$):
  in action potential, 1505
  balance, 213–14
  in body fluid compartments, 197*t*
  foods high in, 211*t*
  in hypertension, 1157
  imbalances. *See* Hypernatremia; Hyponatremia
  intake in diabetes mellitus, 579
  intake in hypertension, 1157
  recommended dietary guidelines, 606*t*
  restriction
    in chronic renal failure, 919
    in cirrhosis, 717
    client teaching, 213*t*
    for fluid volume excess, 210–11
    in heart failure, 1034
    in hypertension, 1159
  serum levels
    abnormal, possible causes, 387*t*
    in gastroenteritis and diarrhea, 776*t*
    normal values, 198*t*, 387*t*
    perioperative, significance and nursing
      implications, 60*t*
Sodium bicarbonate:
  Medication Administration, 906*t*
  in specific conditions
    acute renal failure, 906*t*
    chronic renal failure, 919
    hyperkalemia, 225*t*
    metabolic acidosis, 244
    mouthwash, 658
    in therapeutic baths, 441*t*
Sodium channel blockers, 1005–6, 1006*t*
Sodium citrate, 62*t*
Sodium ferric gluconate, 1111, 1112*t*
Sodium fluoride. *See* Fluoride therapy
Sodium nitroprusside. *See* Nitroprusside
Sodium phosphate, 232
Sodium polystyrene sulfonate:
  Medication Administration, 225*t*, 906*t*
  in specific conditions
    acute renal failure, 904, 906*t*
    chronic renal failure, 919
    hyperkalemia, 224, 225*t*, 904
    tumor lysis syndrome, 411
Sodium salicylate, 178*t*
Sodium-potassium pump, 200, 201*f*
Soft tissue sarcomas, 1483*t*
Solganal. *See* Aurothioglucose
Solu-Medrol. *See* Methylprednisolone
Solutes, 198
Soma. *See* Carisoprodol
Somatic cells, 149
Somatic mutation, 152
Somatic neuropathies. *See* Peripheral neuropathies
Somatic pain, 173
Somatomedin C, 523*t*
Somatosensory evoked potential (SSEP), 1388*t*
Somatostatin, 521, 564, 718
Somatostatin analog. *See* Octreotide
Somogyi phenomenon, 582
Somophyllin. *See* Aminophylline
Sorbitol, 225*t*, 579, 759*t*
Sotalol, 1006*t*
Sound conduction, 1683
Spastic bowel. *See* Irritable bowel syndrome
Spastic hemiparesis, 1523*t*
Spastic neurogenic bladder, 870. *See also*
    Neurogenic bladder
Spasticity:
  causes, 1522*t*
  definition, 1522*t*, 1584
  in stroke, 1584

Specific gravity, urine. *See* Urine tests, specific
    gravity
Specific reactivity, 290
Specificity, test, 157–58
Spectazole. *See* Econazole
Speculum, vaginal, 1764*t*
Speech area, 1506*t*
Speech audiometry, 1730
Speech rehabilitation, 1255–56, 1255*f*
Speech-generating devices, 1258, 1258*f*, 1260*t*
Spermatocele, 1773, 1773*f*
Spermatogenesis, 1475
Spider angioma, 434*f*, 434*t*, 443, 624*t*
Spinal accessory nerve. *See* Accessory nerve
Spinal analgesia. *See* Epidural analgesia
Spinal anesthesia, 63
Spinal cord:
  anatomy, 1508–9, 1509*f*
  ascending tracts, 1508, 1509*f*
  compression, as oncologic emergency, 410
  descending tracts, 1508–9, 1509*f*
  disorders
    acute injury. *See* Spinal cord injury
    herniated intervertebral disk. *See* Herniated
      intervertebral disk
    tumor. *See* Spinal cord tumors
  upper and lower motor neurons, 1509
Spinal cord injury:
  complete, 1597
  complications
    autonomic dysreflexia, 1599
    by body system, 1598*t*
    paraplegia and quadriplegia, 1599
    upper and lower motor neuron deficits,
      1598–99
  incidence and prevalence, 1595
  incomplete, 1597, 1597*t*
  interdisciplinary care
    diagnosis, 1600
    emergency care, 1599, 1600*t*
    medications, 1600, 1600*t*
    treatments
      stabilization and immobilization,
        1600–1601, 1601*f*
      surgery, 1600
  manifestations, 1597–98, 1598*t*
  nursing care
    assessment, 1602
    of client with halo external fixation, 1602*t*
    community-based care, 1606–7
    health promotion, 1602
    Medication Administration, 1600*t*
    nursing diagnoses and interventions
      dysreflexia, 1604
      impaired gas exchange, 1602–3
      impaired physical mobility, 1602
      impaired urinary elimination and
        constipation, 1604–5, 1605*t*
      ineffective breathing patterns, 1604
      low self-esteem, 1606
      sexual dysfunction, 1605–6
    using NANDA, NIC, and NOC, 1606, 1606*t*
  Nursing Care Plan
    assessment, 1603*t*
    critical thinking in the nursing process, 1603*t*
    diagnoses, 1603*t*
    evaluation, 1603*t*
    expected outcomes, 1603*t*
    planning and implementation, 1603*t*
  pathophysiology
    anatomic considerations, 1596
    mechanisms, 1596–97, 1596*f*
    pathologic changes, 1596

  sites, 1597
  tissue repair, 1596
  risk factors, 1595
  self-catheterization procedure, 1605*t*
Spinal cord tumors:
  classification, 1612
  interdisciplinary care
    diagnosis, 1613
    medications, 1613
    radiation therapy, 1613
    surgery, 1613
  manifestations, 1612–13, 1612*t*
  nursing care, 1613
  pathophysiology, 1612
Spinal fusion, 1608
Spinal nerves, 1508*f*, 1509, 1510*f*
Spinal reflexes, 1511. *See also* Reflexes
Spinal shock, 1598, 1600*t*
Spine:
  fracture, 1412
  physical assessment, 1391*t*, 1392*t*, 1393*f*
Spinocerebellar ataxia, 1513*t*
Spiral fracture, 1401, 1402*f*
Spiramycin, 778*t*
Spiritual development, theories, 25*t*
Spiritual therapy, 399*t*
Spirituality:
  assessment in dying clients and their families,
    88, 96
  considerations in disasters, 140
Spiriva. *See* Tiotropium bromide
Spironolactone:
  Medication Administration, 210*t*, 717*t*, 1033*t*
  in specific conditions
    cirrhosis, 716, 717*t*
    heart failure, 1033*t*
Spleen:
  anatomy, 291, 291*f*
  enlargement. *See* Splenomegaly
  functions, 291, 1086
  physical assessment, 626*f*, 626*t*, 1098–99*t*, 1099*f*
Splenda. *See* Sucralose
Splenectomy, 1141
Splenomegaly, 711
Splinter hemorrhages, 1046
Split-thickness graft, 478, 478*f*
Spondylitis, tuberculous, 1283
Spongiform encephalopathy. *See* Creutzfeldt-
    Jakob disease
Spontaneous pneumothorax. *See also*
    Pneumothorax
  manifestations, 1297, 1298*t*
  pathophysiology, 1297, 1298*t*
Spoon-shaped nails, 436*f*, 436*t*, 1105
Sporadic Alzheimer's disease, 1618
Sportscreme. *See* Salicylates
Spousal abuse. *See* Intimate partner violence
Sprain:
  interdisciplinary care, 1399–1400, 1400*t*
  manifestations, 1399
  nursing care, 1400
  vs. strain, 1399
Sprue:
  celiac, 746*t*, 796, 1106
  definition, 796
  interdisciplinary care
    diagnosis, 797
    medications, 797
    nutrition, 797, 797*t*
  manifestations, 796
  nursing care
    assessment, 797
    community-based care, 798

nursing diagnoses and interventions
  diarrhea, 797–98
  imbalanced nutrition: less than body
    requirements, 798
  pathophysiology, 796
  tropical, 796
SPS Suspension. *See* Sodium polystyrene
    sulfonate
Sputum studies:
  procedure, 1220*t*
  purpose and description, 1217*t*, 1219
  related nursing care, 1217*t*
  in specific conditions
    lung cancer, 1311
    pneumonia, 1270
    severe acute respiratory syndrome, 1278
    tuberculosis, 1287
  types, 1217*t*
Squamous cell carcinoma:
  cervix. *See* Cervical cancer
  esophageal, 669. *See also* Esophageal cancer
  larynx. *See* Laryngeal cancer
  lung, 1309*t*. *See also* Lung cancer
  oral, 660. *See also* Oral cancer
  penis, 1772
  skin, 463, 463*f*. *See also* Skin cancer
SSEP (somatosensory evoked potential), 1388*t*
SSKI. *See* Potassium iodide
SSRIs (selective serotonin reuptake inhibitors),
    652, 763, 1798
St. John's wort, 709
ST segment, 948*f*, 948*t*
Stable angina, 969. *See also* Angina pectoris
Stable cells, 295
Stable fracture, 1402
Stadol. *See* Butorphanol
Staghorn stones, 856
Standard precautions, 321–22
Standards, 11, 11*t*
Stanford mouthwash, 409*t*
Stapedectomy, 1725
Stapedotomy, 1725
Stapes, 1682, 1682*f*
Staphcillin. *See* Methicillin
Staphylococcal food poisoning, 774*t*, 775
Staphylococcus aureus:
  antibiotic therapy, 1271*t*
  in endocarditis, 1045
  methicillin-resistant, 313–14
  in osteomyelitis, 1477, 1479
  in skin infections, 446–47
  vancomycin-resistant, 314
Staphylococcus saprophyticus, 846
Starling's law of the heart, 940
Starlix. *See* Nateglinide
START (Simple Triage and Rapid Transport)
    System, 134*t*
Starvation, 641. *See also* Malnutrition
Stasis ulcer, 1194, 1194*f. See also* Chronic venous
    insufficiency
Statins, 967*t*, 968
Status asthmaticus, 1323
Status epilepticus, 1549
Stavudine, 356
Steatorrhea:
  in cystic fibrosis, 1342
  definition, 727, 750*t*, 1342
  in pancreatitis, 727, 728
  in sprue, 797
  in Zollinger-Ellison syndrome, 684
Stein-Leventhal syndrome. *See* Polycystic ovarian
    syndrome
Stem cell transplant (SCT):

allogeneic, 1124
autologous peripheral blood
  advantages, 398
  Nursing Research: fatigue and depression
    following treatment, 1133*t*
  procedure, 1132
complications, 1124
in specific conditions
  leukemia, 1124
  lymphoma, 1132
  multiple myeloma, 1137
  myelodysplastic syndrome, 1116
Stenosis, 1043, 1054, 1054*f. See also* Valvular
    heart disease
Stents, intracoronary, 977
Steppage gait, 1523*t*
Stereotaxic thalamotomy, 1639
Stimate. *See* Desmopressin acetate
Stimulant laxatives, 759–60*t*
Stimulants. *See* Psychostimulants
STIs. *See* Sexually transmitted infections
Stokes-Adams attack, 1003
Stoma. *See also* Colostomy; Ileostomy
  characteristics, 789*f*
  definition, 789
  urinary. *See* Urinary diversion
Stomach:
  anatomy, physiology, and functions, 611–12,
    611*f*, 671
  disorders
    bleeding. *See* Gastrointestinal bleeding
    cancer. *See* Gastric cancer
    diagnostic tests, 615–16*t*
    nausea and vomiting. *See* Nausea and
      vomiting
    peptic ulcer disease. *See* Peptic ulcer disease
Stomafate suspension, 409*t*
Stomatitis:
  definition, 656
  interdisciplinary care
    medications, 657–58, 657*t*, 658*t*
    management, 657*t*
  manifestations, 656–87
  nursing care
    assessment, 658–59
    health promotion, 658
    Medication Administration, 658*t*
    nursing diagnoses and interventions
      community-based care, 659–60
      imbalanced nutrition: less than body
        requirements, 659
      impaired oral mucous membrane, 659
      using NANDA, NIC, and NOC, 659, 659*t*
  pathophysiology, 656
  risk factors, 656–57, 656*t*
Stool:
  assessment, 743, 750–51*t*
  characteristics, 750*t*
  tests
    culture, 744*t*
    occult blood, 744*t*
Strabismus, 1678*t*
Strain:
  interdisciplinary care, 1399–1400, 1400*t*
  manifestations, 1399
  nursing care, 1400
  vs. sprain, 1399
Strangulated hernia, 810. *See also* Hernia
Strangulated obstruction, 811. *See also* Intestinal
    obstruction
Stratum basale, 423, 424*f*
Stratum corneum, 423
Stratum granulosum, 423, 424*f*

Stratum lucidum, 424*f*
Stratum spinosum, 423, 424*f*
Streptococcus, group A. *See* Group A beta-
    hemolytic streptococcus
Streptococcus pneumoniae:
  antibiotic therapy, 1271*t*
  penicillin-resistant, 314
  in pneumonia, 1267, 1268, 1269*t. See also*
    Pneumonia
Streptokinase, 988, 1184, 1188
Streptomycin:
  adverse/side effects, 1287, 1288*t*
  dosage, 1288*t*
  Medication Administration, 320*t*, 1289*t*
  nursing implications, 1288*t*
  in tuberculosis, 1289*t*
Stress:
  cancer risk and, 370–71
  hypertension and, 1157
  reduction, 1160
  responses to, 135*t*, 370
Stress echocardiography, 945*t*
Stress fracture. *See* Pathologic fracture
Stress ulcers:
  in burn clients, 498
  in mechanical ventilation, 1360
  pathophysiology, 502
  prevention, 502
  in trauma clients, 272
Stress urinary incontinence, 874*t. See also* Urinary
    incontinence
Stress/exercise tests:
  nuclear dobutamine, 944*t*
  nuclear persantine (dipyridamole), 944*t*
  purpose and description, 943, 944*t*
  related nursing care, 944*t*
  in specific conditions
    angina, 970
    coronary heart disease, 965
    peripheral vascular disease, 1177
  thallium/technetium, 944*t*, 970–71
Stress-induced gastritis, 677. *See also* Gastritis;
    Stress ulcers
Striae, 624*t*, 748*t*
Stridor, 231
Stroke:
  Case Study, 1667*t*
  complications
    by body system, 1583*t*
    cognitive and behavioral changes, 1583
    communication disorders, 1583
    elimination disorders, 1584
    motor deficits, 1584, 1584*f*
    sensoriperceptual deficits, 1582–83, 1582*f*
  definition, 1579
  in diabetes mellitus, 588
  hemorrhagic, 1581–82
  incidence and prevalence, 1579
  interdisciplinary care
    diagnosis, 1584–85, 1585*t*
    goals, 1584
    medications
      acute stroke, 1585–86
      prevention, 1585
    rehabilitation, 1586
    surgery, 1586, 1586*f*, 1586*t*
  ischemic, 1581
  manifestations, 1582, 1582*t*, 1583*t*
  nursing care
    assessment, 1587
    of client having endarterectomy, 1586*t*
    community-based care, 1591–92
    health promotion, 1587

Stroke—*continued*
  nursing diagnoses and interventions
    impaired physical mobility, 1589–90, 1590*f*
    impaired swallowing, 1591
    impaired urinary elimination and risk for
      constipation, 1591
    impaired verbal communication, 1590–91
    ineffective tissue perfusion: cerebral,
      1587–89
    self-care deficit, 1590
  overview, 1586–87
  using NANDA, NIC, and NOC, 1591, 1591*t*
  Nursing Care Plan
    assessment, 1588*t*
    critical thinking in the nursing process, 1588*t*
    diagnoses, 1588*t*
    evaluation, 1588*t*
    expected outcomes, 1588*t*
    planning and implementation, 1588*t*
  Nursing Research: improving use of rapid
    treatment, 1589*t*
  pathophysiology, 1580
  racial/ethnic considerations, 1580*t*
  risk factors, 1579–80, 1580*t*, 1589*t*
Stroke volume (SV):
  definition, 269, 940, 1023
  in hypovolemic shock, 273*f*
  normal values, 940
Stroke-in-evolution, 1581
Strong iodine solution, 538*t*
Struvite stones, 856, 856*t*. *See also* Urinary calculi
Stuart factor, 1082*t*
Stunned, 984
Stupor, 1529*t*. *See also* Altered level of
  consciousness
Sty (hordeolum), 1700
Subacute infective endocarditis, 1045, 1046*t*. *See
  also* Endocarditis
Subarachnoid hemorrhage, 884, 1593. *See also*
  Intracranial aneurysm
Subcutaneous emphysema, 1360
Subdural hematoma. *See also* Traumatic brain
    injury
  causes, 1557*t*, 1558
  characteristics, 1557*f*, 1558
  manifestations, 1557*t*
  Nursing Care Plan
    assessment, 1561*t*
    critical thinking in the nursing process, 1561*t*
    diagnoses, 1561*t*
    evaluation, 1561*t*
    expected outcomes, 1561*t*
    planning and implementation, 1561*t*
Subendocardial infarction, 983. *See also* Acute
    myocardial infarction
Subjective data, 8
Sublimaze. *See* Fentanyl
Subluxation, 1401
Submucous fibroid tumors, 1809, 1810*f*
Subserous fibroid tumors, 1809, 1810*f*
Substance abuse:
  addictive substances
    alcohol. *See* Alcohol
    caffeine, 106
    central nervous system depressants, 108
    cocaine, 108–9
    hallucinogens, 110–11
    inhalants, 111
    marijuana, 107
    methamphetamine, 109–10, 109*f*
    nicotine, 106–7. *See also* Smoking
    opiates/opioids, 110, 110*f*. *See also* Narcotic
      analgesics

    psychostimulants, 108–10
    street names, 111
  cancer risk and, 372
  Chapter Highlights, 122–23*t*
  characteristics of abusers, 105
  definition, 102, 103*t*
  genetic considerations, 104*t*
  impaired nurses, 121, 122*t*
  interdisciplinary care
    diagnostic tests, 112
    overdose, 112, 113*t*, 114*t*
    withdrawal, 112, 113*t*
  in middle adults, 27
  nursing care
    assessment
      history of past substance abuse, 115
      medical and psychiatric history, 115
      open-ended questions for, 114–15, 115*t*
      psychosocial issues, 116
      relapse behaviors, 121*t*
      screening tools, 116–17, 116*f*
      withdrawal assessment tools, 117, 118*f*
    community-based care, 120–21
    health promotion, 114
    nursing diagnoses and interventions
      chronic low or situational low self-esteem,
        120
      deficient knowledge, 120
      disturbed sensory perceptions, 120
      disturbed thought processes, 120
      imbalanced nutrition: less than body
        requirements, 119
      ineffective coping, 117
      ineffective denial, 117
      risk for injury and risk for violence, 117
    settings, 114
    using NANDA, NIC, and NOC, 120, 120*t*, 121*t*
  in older adults, 115, 115*t*
  pain management considerations in, 181*t*
  pathophysiology, 102–3, 104, 104*f*
  in pregnancy. *See* Pregnancy, substance abuse in
  racial/ethnic considerations, 105*f*, 105*t*
  risk factors
    biologic, 104, 104*f*
    genetic, 104, 104*t*
    psychologic, 104
    sociocultural, 105, 105*t*
  stroke risk and, 1580
  vs. substance dependence, 102*t*
  terminology, 103*t*
  in young adults, 25
Substance dependence, 102, 102*t*, 103*t*
Substernal, 984
Sucking chest wound, 1299. *See also*
    Pneumothorax
Sucralfate, 665–66*t*, 678, 685
Sucralose, 579
Sudafed. *See* Pseudoephedrine
Sudden cardiac death (SCD):
  causes, 1015
  definition, 1015
  in hypertrophic cardiomyopathy, 1066
  interdisciplinary care
    advanced life support, 1016–17
    basic life support, 1016, 1016*f*, 1017*t*
    postresuscitation care, 1017
  manifestations, 1016
  nursing care, 1018
  Nursing Research: family presence during
    resuscitation, 1066*t*
  pathophysiology, 1016
  risk factors, 1015–16
Sular. *See* Nisoldipine

Sulfacetamide sodium, 1694, 1697
Sulfadiazine. *See* Silver sulfadiazine
Sulfamethizole, 321*t*
Sulfamethoxazole, 321*t*. *See also* Trimethoprim-
    sulfamethoxazole
Sulfamylon. *See* Mafenide acetate
Sulfasalazine:
  Medication Administration, 787*t*
  in specific conditions
    ankylosing spondylitis, 1470
    autoimmune disorders, 341
    inflammatory bowel disease, 786, 787*t*
    rheumatoid arthritis, 1465*t*, 1466
Sulfinpyrazone, 1446*t*, 1455
Sulfisoxazole, 321*t*, 832*t*
Sulfonamides, 321*t*, 832*t*
Sulfonylureas, 578*t*
Sulindac, 178*t*, 1445, 1464*t*
Sumatriptan, 1544, 1545*t*
Sun exposure:
  cancer risk and, 372*t*, 462
  minimizing, 464*t*
Sunburn, 493
Sundowning, 1620
Sunnette. *See* Acesulfame potassium
Sunscreens, 465*t*
Supartz. *See* Hyaluronan injections
Superficial burn, 489–90, 489*t*. *See also* Burns
Superficial partial-thickness burn, 490, 490*f*. *See
    also* Burns
Superficial venous thrombosis, 1187*t*, 1188. *See
    also* Venous thrombosis
Superior vena cava syndrome:
  in lung cancer, 1311
  nursing interventions, 409
  pathophysiology, 409, 410*f*
Supination, 1386*t*
Support garments, for burn wounds, 505, 505*f*
Suppressor T cells, 297, 298. *See also* T
    lymphocytes
Suprapubic prostatectomy, 1781*t*, 1785
Supraventricular aortic stenosis, 950*t*
Supraventricular dysrhythmias. *See also* Cardiac
    dysrhythmias
  causes, 1000–1001
  ECG characteristics, 997–98*t*
  management, 997–98*t*
  manifestations, 1000–1001
  pathophysiology, 1000–1001
Supraventricular rhythms, 996, 997*t*, 1000
Surface tension, alveolar, 1216
Surfactant, 1216, 1367
Surfak. *See* Docusate
Surge capacity, 133
Surgery:
  Chapter Highlights, 82*t*
  definition, 54
  interdisciplinary care
    client preparation
      positioning, 67, 69*f*
      shaving, 67, 68*f*
      skin preparation, 67
    diagnosis, 60–61
    intraoperative awareness, 67
    laboratory tests for perioperative
      assessment, 60*t*
    medications
      intraoperative, 61–64. *See also* Anesthesia
      postoperative, 64, 65. *See also* Postoperative
        period, pain management
      preoperative, 61, 62*t*
      sliding scale insulin, 572–73, 574*t*
    nutrition, 70

Practice Alerts, 64
special considerations in older adults, 68, 70
surgical environment
surgical attire, 66–67, 67f
surgical scrub, 67
team members, 64–66
legal requirements, 55
nursing care
Case Study, 145t
Clinical Scenarios, 144t
community-based care, 80
intraoperative phase, 73
laminectomy, 1609–10t
postoperative complications
cardiovascular, 74–75
elimination-related, 78–79
respiratory, 75–76
special considerations for older adults, 79, 79t
wound. See Wounds
postoperative phase
acute pain management, 79–80
care after client is stable, 74
immediate care, 74
preoperative phase
client and family teaching, 71, 72–73t
client preparation, 71–73
nursing care, 71
nursing diagnoses, 70t
for specific procedures
adrenalectomy, 550t
aortic aneurysm repair, 1174t
bladder neck suspension, 876t
bowel surgery, 804t
breast reconstruction, 1827t
carotid endarterectomy, 1586t
colostomy, 806t
coronary artery bypass graft, 980–82t
cystectomy and urinary diversion, 866t
dilation and curettage, 1803t
ear surgery, 1725t
eye surgery, 1699t
gastric surgery, 690t
gastrostomy or jejunostomy tube, 692t
halo external fixation, 1602t
hysterectomy, 1804t
ileostomy, 789–90t
kidney transplant, 922t
laparoscopic cholecystectomy, 700t
laryngectomy, 1256t
liver transplantation, 720t
lung surgery, 1313t
mastectomy, 1826t
nephrectomy, 897
percutaneous coronary revascularization, 978t
permanent pacemaker implant, 1012t
physiology review, 1783t
posterior laminectomy, 1609–10t
prostatectomy, 1780–81t
subtotal thyroidectomy, 539t
surgery for seizures, 1551t
surgical debridement for osteomyelitis, 1479t
thoracocentesis, 1297t
thymectomy, 1650t
total joint replacement, 1452–53
T-tube, 701t
ureteral stent, 851t
Whipple's procedure, 732t
using NANDA, NIC, and NOC, 80, 80t
Nursing Care Plan
assessment, 81t
case description, 80t
critical thinking in the nursing process, 81t
diagnoses, 81t
evaluation, 81t

expected outcomes, 81t
planning and implementation, 81t
phases, 54
procedures
cancer diagnosis, 388–89, 388t
cardiac
coronary artery bypass graft. See Coronary
artery bypass grafting
heart transplant. See Heart transplant
minimally invasive coronary artery surgery,
979
percutaneous coronary revascularization. See
Percutaneous coronary revascularization
transmyocardial laser revascularization, 979
valve replacement, 1060–61, 1061f, 1061t
valvuloplasty, 1060
cerebrovascular
carotid endarterectomy, 1586, 1586f
for intracranial aneurysm, 1594
classifications, 54t
cutaneous
chemical destruction, 478
cryosurgery, 477
curettage, 477
electrosurgery, 477
fusiform excision, 477
laser surgery, 477–78
sclerotherapy, 478
ear disorders
cochlear implant, 1731–32, 1732f
endolymphatic decompression, 1727
labyrinthectomy, 1727
mastoidectomy, 1724
myringotomy, 1722, 1723
tympanoplasty, 1724
vestibular neurectomy, 1727
endocrine
adrenalectomy, 550, 550t
thyroidectomy, 537–38, 539t
eye disorders
cataracts, 1705, 1705f
corneal transplant. See Corneal transplant
glaucoma, 1709
laser surgery, 1697
female reproductive system
breast reconstruction, 1825–26
colporrhaphy, 1806
conization, 1813, 1813f
dilation and curettage, 1803
hysterectomy, 1803–4, 1810
Marshall-Marchetti-Krantz procedure, 1806
mastectomy. See Mastectomy
myomectomy, 1810
pelvic exenteration, 1813
vulvectomy, 1819–20, 1820f
lower gastrointestinal
appendectomy, 766f, 767
bariatric, 636–38, 637f
cholecystectomy, 699, 700t
colectomy, 788, 788f
colostomy. See Colostomy
hemorrhoidectomy, 819
herniorrhaphy, 810
ileostomy, 789, 789f
Whipple's procedure, 732, 732f, 732t
male reproductive system disorders
prostatectomy, 1779, 1779f
musculoskeletal
fracture fixation, 1410–11, 1411f
total joint replacement, 1452–53
neurologic
brain tumor, 1571, 1571f
foraminotomy, 1610
intradiscal electrothermal therapy, 1610

laminectomy, 1608
microdiskectomy, 1610
pallidotomy, 1639
rhizotomy. See Rhizotomy
for seizure control, 1551
spinal fusion, 1608
stereotaxic thalamotomy, 1639
thymectomy, 1649–50
pain management
cordotomy, 184, 185f
neurectomy, 184, 185f
rhizotomy. See Rhizotomy
sympathectomy, 184, 185f
peripheral vascular
aortic aneurysm repair, 1173, 1174f, 1174t
varicose veins, 1197
venous thrombosis, 1190
plastic
blepharoplasty, 479
chemical peeling, 479
dermabrasion, 479
liposuction, 479
rhinoplasty, 479, 1246–47
rhytidectomy, 479
skin grafts and flaps, 478–79, 478f
respiratory
Caldwell-Luc procedure, 1237
endoscopic sinus surgery, 1236–37
external sphenoethmoidectomy, 1237, 1237f
laryngectomy, 1256t
in lung cancer, 1312, 1312t
transplant. See Transplant procedures
upper gastrointestinal
esophagectomy, 669–70
fundoplication, 666, 667f
gastrectomy, 689, 689f
urinary system
bladder neck suspension, 875, 876t
cystectomy, 864, 866t
kidney transplant. See Kidney transplant
nephrectomy, 896–97, 898f
urinary diversion, 864, 864f, 865t, 866t
risk factors, 55, 57–58t, 58–59
setting, 54–55
Surgical assistant, 65
Surgical debridement, 502
Surgical menopause, 1795
Surveillance, 127
Sustentacular cells, 1745
Sustiva. See Efavirenz
SV. See Stroke volume
SVR. See Systemic vascular resistance
Swan-Ganz catheter, 1030. See also Pulmonary
artery pressure monitoring
Swan-neck deformity, 1393, 1461, 1461f
Sweat analysis, in cystic fibrosis, 1342
Sweat glands, 424
Sweet & Low. See Saccharin
Sweeteners, 579
Swimmer's ear. See Otitis externa
Sycosis barbae, 446
Syme amputation, 1422t
Symmetrel. See Amantadine
Sympathectomy:
for pain management, 184
procedure, 185f
in thromboangiitis obliterans, 1182
Sympathetic nervous system:
in blood pressure regulation, 1085, 1155
effects of stimulation, 1512
in heart failure, 1024–25
physiology, 1511–12
Sympathetic tone, 269
Sympatholytics, 1162t

Tinidazole, 1843
Tinnitus, 1718, 1730. *See also* Hearing loss
Tinzaparin, 1189*t*
Tiotropium bromide, 1327–28*t*
TIPS (transjugular intrahepatic portosystemic
    shunt), 719, 719*f*
Tirofiban, 976, 976*t*
Tissue plasminogen activator (t-PA):
    for acute arterial occlusion, 1184
    for acute myocardial infarction, 988
    for thrombotic stroke, 1585
    for venous thrombosis, 1188
Tissue transplantation. *See* Transplant procedures
Titanium dioxide, 465*t*
Titrate, 183
TIVA (total intravenous anesthesia), 61
TLC (total lung capacity), 1214*t*
TMP-SMX. *See* Trimethoprim-sulfamethoxazole
TNF (tumor necrosis factor), 299*t*, 443
TNK (tenecteplase), 988
TNM staging:
    bladder cancer, 863*t*
    colorectal cancer, 803*t*
    laryngeal cancer, 1254*t*
    lung cancer, 1311*t*
    oral cancer, 660*t*
    overview, 383*t*
Tobacco use. *See* Smoking
Tobramycin, 320*t*
Tocainide, 1006*t*
Toes, 1394*t*
Tofranil. *See* Imipramine
Tolazamide, 578*t*
Tolbutamide, 578*t*
Tolcapone, 1638*t*, 1639
Tolectin. *See* Tolmetin
Tolerance:
    to drug or substance, 102, 103*t*, 179*t*
    to nitroglycerin, 971
    to pain, 175
Tolinase. *See* Tolazamide
Tolmetin, 178*t*, 1445, 1464*t*
Tolnaftate, 1720
Tolterodine, 871, 871*t*, 875
Tongue, assessment, 622*t*
Tongue turgor, 205
Tonic-clonic seizures, 1549, 1549*f*
Tonicity, 198, 199*f*
Tonocard. *See* Tocainide
Tonometry, 1674*t*, 1708, 1708*f*
Tonsillectomy, 1239
Tonsillitis:
    characteristics, 1238
    complications, 1239. *See also* Peritonsillar
        abscess
    interdisciplinary care, 1239
    manifestations, 1238, 1238*f*, 1239*t*
    nursing care, 1239–40
    pathophysiology, 1238
Topamax. *See* Topiramate
Tophi, 1443
Topical anesthetics, 657, 658*t*
Topical medications:
    antimicrobial
        for burns, 501*t*
        for conjunctivitis, 1694
        for corneal infections, 1697
        for eyelid infections, 1701
    beta-blockers, for glaucoma, 1709, 1710*t*
    guidelines for application, 444*t*
    for osteoarthritis, 1451
    for pruritus, 440, 441*t*
    for psoriasis, 444
    for stasis dermatitis, 1194

Topiramate, 1544
Toprol. *See* Metoprolol
Toradol. *See* Ketorolac tromethamine
Torecan. *See* Thiethylperazine
Toremifene, 1785, 1796
Tornado, 129*t*, 130
Tornalate. *See* Bitolterol
Torsades de pointes, 1002, 1003*f*
Torsemide, 210*t*, 905*t*
Torsion, testicular, 174
Total gastrectomy, 689, 689*f*
Total incontinence, 873. *See also* Urinary
    incontinence
Total intravenous anesthesia (TIVA), 61
Total joint replacement:
    cemented vs. uncemented, 1452
    definition, 1452
    elbow, 1453
    hip, 1452, 1452*f*
    knee, 1452–53, 1453*f*
    nursing care
        postoperative, 1454*t*
        preoperative, 1453–54*t*
    Nursing Care Plan
        assessment, 1456*t*
        critical thinking in the nursing process, 1456*t*
        diagnoses, 1456*t*
        evaluation, 1456*t*
        expected outcomes, 1456*t*
        planning and implementation, 1456*t*
    physical therapy and rehabilitation, 1455
    shoulder, 1453
Total laryngectomy, 1255. *See also* Laryngectomy
Total lung capacity (TLC), 1214*t*
Total parenteral nutrition (TPN):
    administration, 648
    catheter for, 647*f*
    complications, 648
    definition, 646
    indications, 648
    risks, 70
Total proctocolectomy with permanent
    ileostomy, 789
Toxic epidermal necrolysis (TEN):
    complications, 461
    interdisciplinary care, 461
    manifestations, 460
    pathophysiology, 460–61
Toxic hepatitis, 707. *See also* Hepatitis
Toxic megacolon, 785
Toxic multinodular goiter, 536, 536*f*
Toxic shock syndrome, 275
Toxoplasmosis, 354, 359*t*
TPN. *See* Total parenteral nutrition
Trabeculectomy, 1709
Trabeculoplasty, laser, 1709
Trachea:
    anatomy, physiology, and functions, 1211
    physical assessment, 1224*t*
Tracheoesophageal puncture, 1255–56
Tracheostomy:
    in acute respiratory failure, 1356
    vs. endotracheal intubation, 1356, 1357*t*
    nursing care, 1257*t*
Trachoma, 1693–94
Tracleer. *See* Bosentan
Tracrium. *See* Atracurium besylate
Traction:
    cervical, 1601, 1601*f*
    nursing interventions, 1409*t*
    types, 1408, 1409*f*
Tramadol, 62*t*, 178
Trandate. *See* Labetalol
Trandolapril, 1033*t*, 1161*t*

Transcellular fluid, 196*f*, 197
Transcranial Doppler study, 1515*t*
Transcutaneous electrical nerve stimulation
    (TENS), 184–85, 185*f*
Transcutaneous oximetry. *See* Pulse oximetry
TransCyte, 504
Transdermal administration, 182–83, 183*f*
Transderm-Nitro. *See* Nitroglycerin
Transesophageal echocardiography (TEE):
    in angina, 971
    in aortic aneurysm, 1173
    purpose and description, 943, 945*t*
Transfusion, 262. *See also* Blood transfusion
Transfusion reactions, 262
Transient ischemic attack (TIA), 1581. *See also*
    Stroke
Transjugular intrahepatic portosystemic shunt
    (TIPS), 719, 719*f*
Translocation, 151
Transmural infarction, 983
Transmyocardial laser revascularization, 979
Transparent dressing, 474*t*
Transplant procedures:
    indications, 342*t*
    interdisciplinary care
        diagnosis, 343
        medications, 343–44, 345–46*t*
    nursing care
        assessment, 346–47
        community-based care, 348
        health promotion, 346
        Medication Administration, 345–46*t*
        nursing diagnoses and interventions
            anxiety, 348
            ineffective protection, 347
            risk for impaired tissue integrity: allograft,
               347–48
    pathophysiology, 341–43
    rejection episodes, 342–43, 343*t*
    success rate, 342*t*
    types, 342*t*
        hair, 482
        heart. *See* Heart transplant
        kidney. *See* Kidney transplant
        liver. *See* Liver transplant
        lung. *See* Lung transplant
        pancreas. *See* Pancreas transplant
Transrectal ultrasonography, 1784
Transtentorial herniation, 1538, 1538*f*
Transthyretin. *See* Prealbumin
Transudate, 1295
Transurethral incision of the prostate (TUIP), 1779
Transurethral microwave thermotherapy, 1779
Transurethral needle ablation (TUNA), 1779
Transurethral resection:
    bladder tumor, 864*t*
    prostate (TURP)
        nursing care, 1780–81*t*
        procedure, 1779, 1779*f*
Transverse colon, 742*f*, 743
Transverse loop colostomy, 804
Trastuzumab, 1825
Trauma:
    Case Study, 145*t*
    Chapter Highlights, 283–84*t*
    components, 255–56
    definition, 255
    effects
        abdominal, 259
        airway obstruction
            assessment, 257
            in burn injuries, 258
            in cervical spine injury, 257
            in closed head injury, 257

in direct airway trauma, 257
    interventions, 257, 257f
    in maxillofacial trauma, 257
    on family, 260
    hemorrhage, 258, 258f
    integumentary, 258–59, 259f
    multiple organ dysfunction syndrome, 259
    musculoskeletal, 259. See also
        Musculoskeletal system, trauma
    neurological, 259. See also Traumatic brain
        injury
    tension pneumothorax, 258, 258f
interdisciplinary care
    emergency department care
        blood transfusions, 262, 263t
        brain death criteria, 265t
        diagnosis, 261
        emergency surgery, 263
        forensic considerations, 265
        medications, 261–62
        organ donation, 263–65
        volume resuscitation, 263t
    prehospital care
        critical interventions, 260–61, 260f
        injury identification, 260
        rapid transport, 261, 261f
        scoring systems, 260, 260t. See also Glasgow
            Coma Scale
    mechanisms, 255t
nursing care
    assessment, 265
    community-based care, 268
    health promotion, 265
    nursing diagnoses and interventions
        impaired physical mobility, 267, 267f
        ineffective airway clearance, 266
        post-trauma syndrome, 268
        risk for infection, 266–67
        spiritual distress, 267–68
    using NANDA, NIC, and NOC, 268, 268t
Nursing Care Plan
    assessment, 266t
    critical thinking in the nursing process, 266t
    diagnoses, 266t
    evaluation, 266t
    expected outcomes, 266t
    planning and implementation, 266t
Nursing Research: prevention of ventilator-
        associated pneumonia in clients with
        multiple trauma, 280t
types
    brain. See Traumatic brain injury
    chest. See Thoracic trauma
    classification, 256
    eye. See Eyes, trauma
    head. See Traumatic brain injury
    kidney, 895–96
    liver, 725
    nose. See Nasal trauma
    skin
        burns. See Burns
        frostbite, 476–77
        injuries, 258–59, 259f
        pressure ulcer. See Pressure ulcer
    spinal cord. See Spinal cord injury
Traumatic brain injury (TBI). See also Skull fracture
    airway obstruction in, 257
    caregiver considerations, 1563t
    causes, 1554
    classification, 1554
    definition, 1554
    diffuse
        classic cerebral concussion, 1559
        diffuse axonal injury, 1559

manifestations, 1558t
    mechanism, 1558
    mild concussion, 1559
    pathophysiology, 1558
focal
    contusion, 1557
    epidural hematoma, 1557–58, 1557f, 1557t
    intracerebral hematoma, 1557f, 1557t, 1558
    mechanisms, 1556
    pathophysiology, 1556
    subdural hematoma, 1557f, 1557t, 1558
interdisciplinary care
    acute injury, 1559, 1560t
    concussion, 1559
    diagnosis, 1559
    managing increased intracranial pressure, 1559
    surgery, 1560, 1560f
manifestations, 1557t, 1558t
mechanisms, 1554
nursing care
    assessment, 1560
    community-based care
        acute brain injury, 1563
        concussion, 1562
    health promotion, 1560
    nursing diagnoses and interventions
        decreased intracranial adaptive capacity,
            1560
        ineffective airway clearance, 1562
        ineffective breathing pattern, 1562
    using NANDA, NIC, and NOC, 1562, 1562t
Nursing Care Plan
    assessment, 1561t
    critical thinking in the nursing
        process, 1561t
    diagnoses, 1561t
    evaluation, 1561t
    expected outcomes, 1561t
    planning and implementation, 1561t
Nursing Research: considerations for caregivers
        of young adults, 1563t
    pathophysiology, 1556
    systemic effects, 1556, 1556t
Traumatic pneumothorax. See also
        Pneumothorax
    causes, 1299
    manifestations, 1298t, 1299
    pathophysiology, 1298t
    types, 1299
Travatan. See Travoprost
Travoprost, 1710t
Treadmill test, 944t. See also Stress/exercise tests
Tremors, 1522t, 1635
Trench mouth, 657t. See also Stomatitis
Trendelenburg test, 1197
Trental. See Pentoxifylline
Treponema pallidum, 1846, 1849. See also
        Syphilis
Treprostinil, 1353
Tretinoin, 458, 459t
Trexall. See Methotrexate
Triage, in disasters, 133–34, 134t
Triamcinolone acetate, 657–58, 658t
Triamcinolone acetonide, 1328t
Triaminic. See Phenylpropanolamine
Triamterene, 210t, 1033t
Triceps reflex, 1523f
Triceps skinfold thickness (TSF), 621t
Trichinosis, 779, 780, 781t
Trichlormethiazide, 210t
Trichloroacetic acid (TCA), 479, 1841, 1842t
Trichomonas vaginalis, 1843
Tricor. See Fenofibrate
Tricosal. See Choline magnesium trisalicylate

Tricuspid valve:
    anatomy, 937f, 938
    disorders, 1055t, 1059
    function, 1054
Tricyclic antidepressants:
    Medication Administration, 1545t
    in specific conditions
        fibromyalgia, 1487
        headache, 1545t
        irritable bowel syndrome, 763
        pain management, 179
Tridil. See Nitroglycerin
Trigeminal nerve (cranial nerve V):
    anatomy, 1510f
    assessment, 1520t
    functions, 1511t
    sensory and motor distribution, 1655, 1655f
Trigeminal neuralgia:
    characteristics, 1655
    interdisciplinary care
        medications, 1656
        surgery, 1656
    manifestations, 1656
    nursing care
        of client undergoing percutaneous
            rhizotomy, 1656t
        community-based care, 1657
        nursing diagnoses and interventions
            acute pain, 1656–57
            risk for altered nutrition: less than body
                requirements, 1657
        teaching for home care, 1657t
    pathophysiology, 1655
Trigger, 1358
Trigger zones, 1655
Triglycerides:
    formation, 631
    functions, 959
    serum levels. See Serum triglycerides
    uses in body, 608
Trihexyphenidyl, 1638t
Triiodothyronine (T₃):
    diagnostic tests, 523t, 536t, 537
    in hypothyroidism, 543t
    normal values, 523t, 536t
Tri-K. See Potassium acetate
Trilisate. See Choline magnesium trisalicylate
Trimethoprim, 850, 850t
Trimethoprim-sulfamethoxazole (TMP-SMZ):
    Medication Administration, 321t
    in organ transplantation, 343
    in specific conditions
        diverticulitis, 816
        epiglottitis, 1241
        gastroenteritis, 776
        otitis media, 1722
        P. carinii pneumonia, 359t
        pertussis, 1242
        pneumonia, 1271t
        urinary tract infection, 849, 850
Trimpex. See Trimethoprim
Triphenylethylene. See Tamoxifen
Triprolidine, 1230t
Trismus, 1611
Trisomy, 150t
Trisomy 21 (Down syndrome), 150
Trochlear nerve (cranial nerve IV):
    anatomy, 1510f
    assessment, 1519t
    function, 1511t, 1671t
Tropical sprue, 796. See also Sprue
Trousseau's sign, 229, 229f, 531t
True aneurysm, 1170
Trusopt. See Dorzolamide

Urinary tract infection (UTI)—*continued*
  manifestations, 847
  nosocomial, 313, 847, 848
  nursing care
    assessment, 852
    community-based care, 854–55
    health promotion, 851–52
    nursing diagnoses and interventions
      impaired urinary elimination, 852–54
      ineffective health maintenance, 854
      pain, 852
    of older adults, 315*t*, 873*t*
  Nursing Care Plan
    assessment, 853*t*
    critical thinking in the nursing process, 853*t*
    diagnoses, 853*t*
    evaluation, 853*t*
    expected outcomes, 853*t*
    planning and implementation, 853*t*
  obstruction as cause of, 850–51, 850*t*
  in older adults
    nursing care, 315*t*, 873*t*
    risk factors, 847
  pathophysiology, 847
  pyelonephritis, 848–49
  risk factors, 846, 846*t*
Urine:
  formation
    glomerular filtration, 831–33, 831*f*
    tubular reabsorption, 831*f*, 833
    tubular secretion, 831*f*, 833
  maintenance of normal composition and volume,
    833–34, 833*f*
Urine tests:
  24-hour
    in Cushing's syndrome, 549–50
    in hyponatremia, 215
  amylase, 728*t*
  for bacteria, 849
  in bladder cancer, 863
  creatinine
    in glomerular disorders, 890, 890*t*
  culture
    in chronic renal failure, 918
    in neurogenic bladder, 870
    purpose and description, 835*t*
    related nursing care, 835*t*
    in urinary tract infection, 849
  drug screen
    in substance abuse assessment, 112
    in trauma clients, 261
  glucose
    abnormal, possible causes, 832*t*
    in diabetes mellitus, 569
    normal values, 832*t*
  ketones
    abnormal, possible causes, 832*t*
    in diabetes mellitus, 569
    normal values, 832*t*
  osmolality
    abnormal, possible causes, 387*t*
    in fluid volume deficit, 205
    normal values, 387*t*
  protein
    abnormal, possible causes, 832*t*
    in diabetes mellitus, 569
    in glomerular disorders, 890*t*
    normal values, 832*t*, 890*t*
  RBCs
    abnormal, possible causes, 832*t*
    in glomerular disorders, 890*t*
    normal values, 832*t*, 890*t*
  specific gravity
    abnormal, possible causes, 832*t*

  in fluid volume deficit, 205
  in gastroenteritis and diarrhea, 776*t*
    normal values, 832*t*
  in urinary calculi, 857
  in urinary tract infection, 849
  WBCs, 832*t*
Urispas. *See* Flavoxate
Uroflowmetry, 836*t*, 874
Urokinase, 1184
Urolithiasis. *See* Urinary calculi
Uroxatral. *See* Alfuzosin
Ursodiol, 699
Urticaria, 333, 431*t*
Uterine cancer. *See* Endometrial cancer
Uterine displacement:
  classification, 1805, 1806*f*, 1807*f*
  interdisciplinary care
    diagnosis, 1806
    Kegel exercises, 1806
    pessary, 1806–7
    surgery, 1806
  manifestations, 1805, 1807*f*, 1807*t*
  nursing care
    community-based care, 1807
    nursing diagnoses and interventions
      anxiety, 1807
      stress incontinence, 1807
  pathophysiology, 1805
Uterine fibroid embolization, 1810
Uterine tubes. *See* Fallopian tubes
Uterus:
  anatomy, physiology, and functions, 1751*t*,
    1752–53, 1753*f*
  disorders
    displacement. *See* Uterine displacement
    dysfunctional uterine bleeding. *See*
      Dysfunctional uterine bleeding
    endometrial cancer. *See* Endometrial cancer
    endometriosis. *See* Endometriosis
    leiomyoma. *See* Leiomyoma
  physical assessment, 1764–65*t*
UTI. *See* Urinary tract infection
Uvea, 1672, 1672*f*
Uveitis:
  in ankylosing spondylitis, 1470
  manifestations, 1684*t*, 1704
  pathophysiology, 1703–4
  treatment, 1704
  in ulcerative colitis, 784
Uvulopalatopharyngoplasty (UPPP), 1251

V

V tach. *See* Ventricular tachycardia
Vaccines, 300. *See also* Immunizations; *specific
    vaccines*
Vacuum constriction device (VCD), 1769
Vacuum-assisted closure (VAC):
  for burns, 504, 504*f*
  for pressure ulcers, 474*t*
Vacuum-assisted mammotome, 1757*t*
VADs (ventricular assist devices), 990
Vagal nerve stimulation therapy, 1551
Vagina:
  anatomy and function, 1751*t*, 1752, 1753*f*
  cultures, 1756*t*
  infections. *See* Vaginal infections
  physical assessment, 1763–64*t*
Vaginal fistula:
  characteristics, 1807–8
  interdisciplinary care, 1808
  nursing care, 1808
Vaginal hysterectomy, 1804
Vaginal infections:

  bacterial vaginosis, 1842, 1843*t*
  candidiasis, 449*t*, 1842–43, 1842*t*, 1843*f*
  interdisciplinary care
    diagnosis, 1843
    medications, 1843
  manifestations, 1842–43, 1843*t*
  nursing care
    community-based care, 1844
    nursing diagnoses and interventions
      acute pain, 1844, 1844*t*
      deficient knowledge, 1844
  pathophysiology, 1842–43
  risk factors, 1842
  trichomoniasis, 1843, 1843*t*
Vaginismus, 1795
Vaginitis. *See* Vaginal infections
Vagus nerve (cranial nerve X):
  anatomy, 1510*f*
  assessment, 1520*t*
  functions, 1511*t*
Valacyclovir:
  Medication Administration, 658*t*
  in specific conditions
    genital herpes, 1839
    herpes zoster, 453
    oral herpes simplex, 658, 658*t*
Valium. *See* Diazepam
Valproic acid:
  interaction with phenobarbital, 1551*t*
  Medication Administration, 1550*t*
  for migraine prophylaxis, 1544
  for seizures, 1550*t*
Valsalva's maneuver, 743, 1013
Valsartan, 1033*t*, 1161*t*
Valtrex. *See* Valacyclovir
Valve replacement, 1060–61, 1061*f*, 1061*t*
Valves of Houston, 743
Valvular heart disease:
  aortic regurgitation, 1058–59, 1058*f*
  aortic stenosis, 1057–58, 1058*f*
  causes, 1053–54
  interdisciplinary care
    diagnosis, 1059–60
    medications, 1060
    percutaneous balloon valvuloplasty, 1060, 1060*f*
    surgery
      reconstructive, 1060
      valve replacement, 1060–61, 1061*f*, 1061*t*
  mitral regurgitation, 1056, 1056*f*
  mitral stenosis, 1055–56, 1056*f*
  mitral valve prolapse, 1056–57
  murmur characteristics, 1055*t*
  nursing care
    assessment, 1062
    community-based care, 1063
    health promotion, 1062
    nursing diagnoses and interventions
      activity intolerance, 1062
      decreased cardiac output, 1062
      ineffective protection, 1063
      risk for infection, 1062–63
  Nursing Care Plan
    assessment, 1064*t*
    critical thinking in the nursing process, 1064*t*
    diagnoses, 1064*t*
    evaluation, 1064*t*
    expected outcomes, 1064*t*
    planning and implementation, 1064*t*
  pathophysiology, 1054, 1054*f*
  pulmonic regurgitation, 1059
  pulmonic stenosis, 1059
  tricuspid regurgitation, 1059
  tricuspid stenosis, 1059
Valvuloplasty, 1060, 1060*f*

Vanceril. *See* Beclomethasone dipropionate
Vancocin. *See* Vancomycin
Vancomycin:
  adverse/side effects, 1730
  Medication Administration, 319*t*
  in specific conditions
    bacterial meningitis, 1566
    endocarditis prophylaxis, 1047*t*
    endocarditis treatment, 1046
    pneumonia, 1271*t*
Vancomycin-intermediate *S. aureus* (VISA), 314
Vancomycin-resistant *Enterococci* (VRE), 314
Vancomycin-resistant *S. aureus* (VRSA), 314
Vanillylmandelic acid, 557
VAP. *See* Ventilator-associated pneumonia
Vardenafil hydrochloride, 1769
Variable expression, 155
Variceal ligation, 718
Varicella, 302*t*. *See also* Herpes zoster
Varicella vaccine, 21*t*
Varicella-zoster immune globulin (VZIG), 302*t*
Varicocele, 1773, 1773*f*
Varicose veins:
  complications, 1196
  definition, 1093*t*, 1195
  incidence, 1195
  interdisciplinary care
    compression sclerotherapy, 1197
    diagnosis, 1197
    surgery, 1197
    treatments, 1197
  manifestations, 1196, 1196*t*
  nursing care
    assessment, 1197
    community-based care, 1198
    health promotion, 1197
    nursing diagnoses and interventions
      chronic pain, 1197–98
      ineffective tissue perfusion: peripheral, 1198
      risk for impaired skin integrity, 1198
      risk for peripheral neurovascular
        dysfunction, 1198–99
  pathophysiology, 1196
  physical assessment, 1096*t*
  risk factors, 1195
Vas deferens, 1745*t*
Vascor. *See* Bepridil
Vascular access devices:
  for chemotherapy, 394, 395*f*
  for dialysis, 908–9, 909*f*
Vascular dementia, 1618*t*
Vascular tunic. *See* Uvea
Vaseline, 441*t*
Vasoconstriction, 1176
Vasoconstrictors, 278*t*, 1243
Vasodilation, 1176
Vasodilators:
  avoidance in aortic aneurysm, 1173
  Medication Administration, 278*t*, 1162*t*
  in specific conditions
    heart failure, 1032
    hypertension, 1162*t*, 1163
    pulmonary edema, 1041
    pulmonary hypertension, 1353
    Raynaud's disease/phenomenon, 1182–83
    shock, 278*t*
Vasogenic edema, 1537. *See also* Increased
    intracranial pressure
Vasogenic shock, 274
Vasomotor rhinitis, 1229
Vasoocclusive crises, 1107
Vasopressin. *See* Antidiuretic hormone
Vasotec. *See* Enalapril
Vasotec IV. *See* Enalaprilat

VBG (vertical banded gastroplasty), 637, 637*f*
VCD (vacuum constriction device), 1769
Veins:
  anatomy, 1082, 1083*f*, 1085*f*
  assessment, 1094–95*t*
Vena caval filters, 1190, 1190*f*, 1349
Venereal Disease Research Laboratory (VDRL),
    1746*t*, 1756*t*, 1849
Venereal diseases. *See* Sexually transmitted
    infections
Venofer. *See* Iron sucrose
Venous lakes, 430*t*, 443
Venous pressure monitoring, 1030. *See also*
    Central venous pressure
Venous return, 1023
Venous star, 434*f*, 434*t*
Venous stasis, 426*t*, 1194. *See also* Chronic venous
    insufficiency
Venous thrombectomy, 1190
Venous thrombosis:
  complications, 1187
  definition, 1186
  interdisciplinary care
    diagnosis, 1188
    medications, 1188, 1189–90*t*
    prophylaxis, 1188
    surgery, 1190, 1190*f*
    treatments, 1190
  locations, 1187*f*
  manifestations, 1187, 1187*t*
  nursing care
    assessment, 1190, 1191
    community-based care, 1193
    health promotion, 1190
    Medication Administration, 1189–90*t*
    nursing diagnoses and interventions
      impaired physical mobility, 1192–93
      ineffective protection, 1192
      ineffective tissue perfusion:
        cardiopulmonary, 1193
      ineffective tissue perfusion:
        peripheral, 1192
      pain, 1191–92
      using NANDA, NIC, and NOC, 1193, 1193*t*
  Nursing Care Plan
    assessment, 1191*t*
    critical thinking in the nursing process, 1191*t*
    diagnoses, 1191*t*
    evaluation, 1191*t*
    expected outcomes, 1191*t*
    planning and implementation, 1191*t*
  pathophysiology, 1186–87
  risk factors, 1186, 1186*t*
Ventilation. *See* Respiration
Ventilation scan, 1349. *See also* Pulmonary
    ventilation/perfusion scan
Ventilation/perfusion scan (V/Q scan). *See*
    Pulmonary ventilation/perfusion scan
Ventilator-assisted breaths, 1358
Ventilator-associated pneumonia (VAP):
  Nursing Research: prevention strategies, 280*t*
  pathophysiology, 1360
Ventilator-controlled breaths, 1358
Ventolin. *See* Albuterol
Ventral hernia, 810. *See also* Hernia
Ventricles, 938
Ventricular aneurysm, 985
Ventricular assist devices (VADs), 990
Ventricular bigeminy, 1002
Ventricular dysrhythmias. *See also* Cardiac
    dysrhythmias
  causes, 1002–3
  ECG characteristics, 998–99*t*, 1002–3
  management, 998–99*t*

  manifestations, 1002–3
  pathophysiology, 996
Ventricular fibrillation:
  causes, 1002–3
  ECG characteristics, 999*t*
  management, 999*t*
  pathophysiology, 1002
Ventricular hypertrophy, 1024*t*, 1025
Ventricular remodeling, 1025
Ventricular tachycardia (VT, V tach):
  ECG characteristics, 998*t*
  management, 998*t*
  manifestations, 1002
  pathophysiology, 1002
Ventricular trigeminy, 1002
Venturi mask, 1272, 1273*f*
VePesid. *See* Etoposide
Verapamil:
  Medication Administration, 973*t*, 1006*t*, 1162*t*,
    1545–46*t*
  in specific conditions
    acute myocardial infarction, 988
    angina, 973–74*t*
    aortic aneurysm, 1173
    cardiac dysrhythmias, 1006*t*
    headache, 1545–46*t*
    hypertension, 1162*t*
    thromboangiitis obliterans, 1182
Verelan. *See* Verapamil
Vermox. *See* Mebendazole
Verruca plana, 452
Verruca vulgaris, 452, 452*f*
Verrucous, 1819
Versed. *See* Midazolam
Vertical banded gastroplasty (VBG), 637, 637*f*
Vertigo, 1722, 1726. *See also* Inner ear disorders
Very low calorie diets (VLCDs), 635
Very-low-density lipoproteins, 959
Vesicle/vesicular lesions, 431*t*, 432*t*
Vesicoureteral junction, 847, 847*f*
Vesicovaginal fistula, 1807
Vestibular neurectomy, 1727
Vestibule, 1683, 1751*t*, 1752, 1752*f*
Viagra. *See* Sildenafil citrate
Vibramycin. *See* Doxycycline
Vibration, in chest physiotherapy, 1273, 1273*f*
Vibrio cholerae, 774*t*, 775
Vicodin. *See* Hydrocodone
Vidarabine, 322*t*, 1566
Vidaza. *See* Azacitidine
Videx. *See* Didanosine
Vietnamese, end-of-life practices, 89
Villi, 612, 742
Villous adenomas, 800, 800*f*. *See also* Polyps
Vinblastine, 359*t*, 393*t*
Vinca alkaloids, 391, 393*t*
Vincristine:
  adverse/side effects, 393*t*
  nursing implications, 393*t*
  in specific conditions
    bone tumors, 1483*t*
    leukemia, 1123*t*
  target malignancies, 393*t*
Vinyl chloride polymers, 372*t*
Vioxx. *See* Rofecoxib
Vira-A. *See* Vidarabine
Viracept. *See* Nelfinavir
Viral encephalitis, 1565, 1565*t*
Viral meningitis, 1564–65. *See also* Central
    nervous system infections
Viral pneumonia, 1269, 1270*t*. *See also*
    Pneumonia
Viramune. *See* Nevirapine
Virazole. *See* Ribavirin

Virchow's triad, 1186
Virilization, 481
Virulence, 1267
Viruses:
cancer associated with, 374–75, 375t
characteristics, 311t
in hepatitis. See Hepatitis
herpes simplex. See Herpes simplex
herpes zoster. See Herpes zoster
HIV. See Human immunodeficiency virus (HIV)
infection
human papillomavirus. See Human
papillomavirus
influenza. See Influenza
in pneumonia, 1269, 1270t. See also Pneumonia
upper respiratory, 1229. See also Upper
respiratory disorders, viral infections
VISA (vancomycin-intermediate S. aureus), 314
Visceral neuropathies, 589
Visceral pain, 173
Viscosupplementation, 1452
Vision. See also Eyes
age-related changes
in middle adults, 27t
in older adults, 29t, 1676t
in young adults, 26t
impairments
incidence, 1692
nursing care, 1693t
Nursing Research: effect on older adults, 1715t
special considerations in disasters, 140
Visken. See Pindolol
Vistaril. See Hydroxyzine
Visual field testing:
in glaucoma diagnosis, 1708
procedure, 1675–76, 1676f, 1709f
Visual pathways:
age-related changes, 1676t
anatomy and physiology, 1672–73, 1673f
Vital capacity (VC), 1214, 1214t
Vitamin(s):
categories, 608
in healing process, 306t, 307
recommended daily intakes, 608t, 609t
supplements
in cirrhosis, 717
Medication Administration, 645t
in substance abuse/withdrawal treatment, 114t
Vitamin A (retinol):
deficiency, 642t
functions, 608t
in healing, 306t, 307
recommended daily intake, 608t
sources, 608t
Vitamin B complex, in healing, 306t, 307
Vitamin B₁ (thiamine):
deficiency, 642t
functions, 609t
recommended daily intake, 609t
sources, 609t
for substance abuse/withdrawal treatment, 114t
Vitamin B₂ (riboflavin):
deficiency, 642t
functions, 609t
recommended daily intake, 609t
sources, 609t
Vitamin B₃ (nicotinamide):
functions, 609t
recommended daily intake, 609t
sources, 609t
Vitamin B₆ (pyridoxine):
coronary heart disease risk and, 966
functions, 609t

recommended daily intake, 609t
sources, 609t, 966
Vitamin B₁₂ (cyanocobalamin):
deficiency
causes, 1105
interdisciplinary care
diagnostic tests, 1111
focus, 1110t
medications, 1111, 1112t
nutrition, 1111, 1111t
manifestations, 1105
pathophysiology, 1105
functions, 609t
recommended daily intake, 609t
replacement therapy, 1112t
sources, 609t, 1111t
Vitamin C (ascorbic acid):
coronary heart disease risk and, 966
deficiency, 642t
functions, 609t
in healing, 306t, 307
recommended daily intake, 609t
sources, 609t, 966
Vitamin D:
activation in kidney, 834
deficiency, 1447–48, 1448t
functions, 608t
limiting intake, in urinary calculi, 858
metabolism, 1448
recommended daily intake, 608t
sources, 608t, 1449
toxicity, 1449
Vitamin E:
functions, 608t
in gout treatment, 1445
recommended daily intake, 608t
sources, 608t
Vitamin K:
in cirrhosis, 415
functions, 608t
in healing, 307
recommended daily intake, 608t
sources, 608t
Vitiligo, 426t, 431t
Vitreous humor, 1672, 1672f
Vivox. See Doxycycline
VLCDs (very low calorie diets), 635
Voice sounds, assessment, 1226t
Voiding cystogram. See Cystometrogram
Voiding cystourethrography. See
Cystometrogram
Voiding diary, 875f
Volatile acids, 238
Volatile nitrites, 111, 113t
Volkmann's contracture, 1406, 1413
Voltaren. See Diclofenac sodium
Volume resuscitation therapies, 263t
Volume-cycled ventilators, 1358
Volutrauma, 1360
Vomiting, 671. See also Nausea and vomiting
Von Willebrand's disease, 1143, 1143t. See also
Hemophilia
VP-16. See Etoposide
V/Q scan. See Pulmonary ventilation/perfusion
scan
VRE (vancomycin-resistant Enterococci), 314
VRSA (vancomycin-resistant S. aureus), 314
VT. See Ventricular tachycardia
Vₜ (tidal volume), 1214, 1358, 1360t
Vulvar cancer:
incidence, 1819
interdisciplinary care, 1819–20
manifestations, 1819

nursing care
community-based care, 1820
nursing diagnoses and interventions, 1820
pathophysiology, 1819
Vulvar cysts, 1808, 1809t
Vulvectomy, 1819–20, 1820f
VZIG (varicella-zoster immune globulin), 302t

W

Waist circumference, 632
Waist-to-hip ratio, 622t, 631
Warfarin:
interaction with phenobarbital, 1551t
Medication Administration, 1189–90t
in specific conditions
ischemic stroke, 1585
pulmonary embolism, 1349
venous thrombosis, 1188
Warm phase, septic shock, 275, 275t
Warm zone, in disaster, 133t
Warts:
genital. See Genital warts
nongenital
interdisciplinary care, 453
manifestations, 452
pathophysiology, 451–52, 452f
Wasting syndrome, in AIDS, 353, 353f
Water. See also Body fluids
in body fluids, 195–96
function in body, 195
Water deprivation test, 216, 523t
Water-hammer pulse, 1059, 1094t
Water-soluble vitamins, 608, 609t
WBC count. See White blood cell (WBC) count
WBC differential. See White blood cell (WBC)
differential
WBCs. See White blood cells
Weaning, mechanical ventilation,
1360–61, 1361f
Weber test:
in hearing evaluation, 1730
in inner ear disorders, 1727
procedure, 1687f, 1687t
Wedge resection, lung, 1312t
Weepy lesions, 431t
Weight. See Body weight
Welchol. See Colesevelam
Wellferon. See Interferon(s)
Wellness, 19
Wernicke-Korsakoff syndrome, 108
Wernicke's aphasia, 1583
Wernicke's encephalopathy, 103t, 108
Westerhoff, spiritual development theory, 25t
Western blot testing, 355
Wetting agents, 759t
Wet-to-dry dressing, 474t
Wheal, 432t
Wheezes, 1226t
Whipple's procedure:
characteristics, 732, 732f
nursing care, 732t
Whisper test, 1688
Whispered pectoriloquy, 1226t
White blood cell (WBC) count:
abnormal, possible causes, 307t, 387t
normal values, 287, 387t, 1078t, 1118t
perioperative, significance and nursing
implications, 60t
in specific conditions
hypersensitivity reaction, 336
inflammation, 306
leukemia, 1123t

rheumatic heart disease, 1043*t*
shock, 277
White blood cell (WBC) differential:
abnormal, possible causes, 307*t*
normal values, 1118*t*
White blood cells (WBCs):
abnormal, possible causes, 387*t*
development and differentiation, 287, 298*f*,
1077*f*, 1079, 1118
disorders
leukemia. *See* Leukemia
neutropenia. *See* Neutropenia
functions, 290–91, 1118
in inflammatory response, 293, 293*f*
laboratory assessment. *See* White blood cell
(WBC) count
normal values, 387*t*
types
basophils. *See* Basophils
granulocytes, 288, 288*t*, 289*f*
lymphocytes. *See* Lymphocytes
monocytes, macrophages, and dendritic cells,
288–89, 288*t*, 289*f*. *See also* Monocytes
neutrophils. *See* Neutrophils
in urine. *See* Urine tests, WBCs
WHO. *See* World Health Organization
Whole blood, as volume resuscitation therapy, 263*t*
Whooping cough. *See* Pertussis
Wild-type gene, 152
Williams syndrome, 950*t*
Withdrawal:
assessment tools, 117, 118*f*
definition, 102
Nursing Care Plan
assessment of, 119*t*
critical thinking in the nursing process, 119*t*
diagnoses, 119*t*
evaluation, 119*t*
expected outcomes, 119*t*
planning and implementation, 119*t*
signs, 102, 113*t*
treatment, 112, 113*t*
Withdrawal symptoms, 102. *See also* Withdrawal
Withdrawal syndrome, 103*t*. *See also* Withdrawal
Wood's lamp, 428*t*
World Health Organization (WHO):
analgesic ladder, 177, 177*f*
definition of health, 19
Wounds:
burn. *See* Burns

complications
dehiscence, 78, 78*f*
evisceration, 78, 78*f*
infections, 77–78
nursing care, 77–78
drainage
devices, 77*f*
types, 77
healing, 76–77, 76*f*, 77*t*. *See also* Healing
Wrist:
fracture, 1413–14
physical assessment, 1393*t*, 1395*f*, 1395*t*

X

Xalatan. *See* Latanoprost
Xenical. *See* Orlistat
Xenograft, 342, 503
Xeroderma, 441
Xerophthalmia, 1486
Xerosis, 441, 441*t*
Xerostomia:
definition, 408, 1486
nursing interventions, 409
in Sjögren's syndrome, 1486
X-linked dominant inheritance, 155
X-linked recessive inheritance, 153–54, 153*f*, 154*t*
XomaZyme. *See* Immunotoxin
X-ray imaging:
in cancer, 384
in multiple myeloma, 1137
in musculoskeletal system assessment, 1387*t*
sinuses, 1236
skull and spine, 1514*t*
Xylitol, 570
Xylocaine, 441*t*. *See also* Lidocaine
Xyloxylin suspension, 409*t*

Y

Yodoxin. *See* Iodoquinol
Young adults (ages 18 to 40):
family-related risk factors for alterations in
health, 32*t*, 33
health needs
assessment guidelines, 26, 26*t*
promoting healthy behaviors, 26, 27*t*
risks for alterations in health
injuries, 24
physical and psychosocial stressors, 25–26

sexually transmitted infections, 24. *See also*
Sexually transmitted infections
substance abuse, 25. *See also* Substance
abuse
physical status and changes, 26*t*

Z

Zafirlukast, 1328*t*
Zanamivir, 1234
Zantac. *See* Ranitidine
Zarontin. *See* Ethosuximide
Zaroxolyn. *See* Metolazone
Zebeta. *See* Bisoprolol
Zelnorm. *See* Tegaserod mesylate
Zemuron. *See* Rocuronium
Zenapax. *See* Daclizumab
Zerit. *See* Stavudine
Zestril. *See* Lisinopril
Zetar. *See* Coal tar derivatives
Ziagen. *See* Abacavir
Zidovudine:
for cryptosporidiosis, 778*t*
in HIV infection, 356
Medication Administration, 322*t*, 357*t*
Zileuton, 1328*t*
Zinacef. *See* Cefuroxime
Zinc:
deficiency, 1223*t*
recommended daily intake, 610*t*
Zinc gluconate, 1231
Zinc oxide, 465*t*
Zithromax. *See* Azithromycin
Zocor. *See* Simvastatin
Zofran. *See* Ondansetron
Zoledronate (zoledronic acid), 181, 547
Zollinger-Ellison syndrome, 684
Zolmitriptan, 1544, 1545*t*
Zoloft. *See* Sertraline
Zometa. *See* Zoledronate
Zomig. *See* Zolmitriptan
Zostavax, 453
Zostrix. *See* Capsaicin
Zosyn. *See* Piperacillin-tazobactam
Zovirax. *See* Acyclovir
Zyflo. *See* Zileuton
Zyloprim. *See* Allopurinol
Zynol. *See* Sulfinpyrazone
Zyrtec. *See* Cetirizine

NURSING EXCELLENCE

Success in Skills, Review, & Test Preparation

Excellence in Nursing Skills

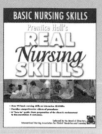
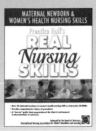

Prentice Hall's Real Nursing Skills on CD-ROMs

Prentice Hall Real Nursing Skills series offers you the complete foundation for competency in performing clinical skills. The CD-ROMs provide comprehensive procedures demonstrated in hundreds of videos, animations, illustrations, and photographs. These skills CD-ROMs are designed to help you visualize how to perform each skill and understand the concepts and rationales for each skill.

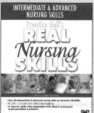
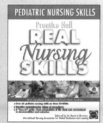

Basic Nursing Skills:
94 skills on 5 CD-ROMs. 2005, ISBN: 0-13-191526-6
Intermediate & Advanced Nursing Skills:
84 skills on 5 CD-ROMs. 2005, ISBN: 0-13-119344-9
Physical & Health Assessment Nursing Skills:
25 skills on 5 CD-ROMs. 2006, ISBN: 0-13-191525-8
Maternal-Newborn & Women's Health Nursing Skills:
24 skills on 2 CD-ROMs. 2005, ISBN: 0-13-191527-4
Pediatric Nursing Skills:
65 skills on 3 CD-ROMs. 2006, ISBN: 0-13-191524-X
Critical Care Nursing Skills:
35 skills on 2 CD-ROMs. 2005, ISBN: 0-13-119264-7

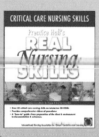
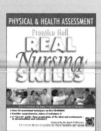

Excellence in NCLEX-RN® Review

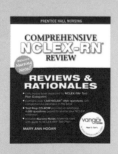

Prentice Hall's Comprehensive NCLEX-RN® Review is designed specifically to help you achieve nursing excellence by simplifying your review and making the most of your valuable study time. This review book is uniquely organized according to the April 2007 NCLEX-RN® Test Plan, providing you with both a comprehensive content review and practice questions in sections covering * Safe, Effective Care Environment * Health Promotion * Physiological Integrity, and * Psychosocial Integrity. Throughout this book, you will find:

- **Memory Aids** that help you remember key concepts.
- **NCLEX® Alerts** that identify critical concepts you are likely to see on the NCLEX-RN®.
- **Check Your NCLEX® IQ** boxes that help you to assess your readiness for the NCLEX-RN® on the topics covered in the chapter.
- **Practice Tests** at the end of the chapter that review the concepts from that chapter and provide comprehensive rationales and test-taking strategies to help you find the right answers.

2008, ISBN 0-13-119599-9

The **NCLEX-RN® Test Prep CD-ROM** that comes with your book simulates the test-taking environment by allowing you to practice questions on the computer. It contains all the questions in the book PLUS thousands of additional questions. You can choose to practice in Study, Quiz, or Exam modes, and you will receive detailed reports that will help you focus your preparation for NCLEX-RN®.

For additional information and resources

THE NEXT GENERATION
Success in Skills, Review, & Test Preparation

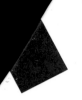

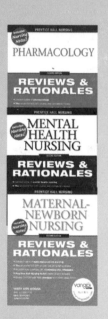
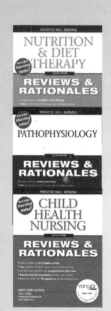
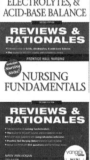
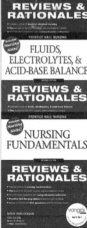
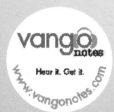